Medical-Surgical Care Planning

Fourth Edition

Medical-Surgical Care Planning

Fourth Edition

Nancy M. Holloway, RN, MSN

Critical Care Educator   Nancy Holloway & Associates   Orinda, California

LIPPINCOTT WILLIAMS & WILKINS
A **Wolters Kluwer** Company

Philadelphia • Baltimore • New York • London
Buenos Aires • Hong Kong • Sydney • Tokyo

STAFF

Publisher
Judith A. Schilling McCann, RN, MSN

Editorial Director
H. Nancy Holmes

Clinical Director
Joan M. Robinson, RN, MSN

Senior Art Director
Arlene Putterman

Senior Associate Editor
Jennifer P. Kowalak

Editors
Kate Jackson, Elizabeth Jacqueline Mills

Clinical Editor
Beverly Ann Tscheschlog, RN, BS (clinical project manager)

Copy Editors
Kimberly Bilotta (supervisor), Scotti Cohn, Tom DeZego,
Heather Ditch, Amy Furman, Dona Hightower Perkins,
Marcia Ryan, Dorothy P. Terry, Pamela Wingrod

Designers
Will Boehm (book design), Susan Sheridan (project manager)

Digital Composition Services
Diane Paluba (manager), Joyce Rossi Biletz (senior desktop
assistant)

Manufacturing
Patricia K. Dorshaw (senior manager), Beth Janae Orr (book
production coordinator)

Editorial Assistants
Megan Aldinger, Arlene Claffee, Linda Ruhf

Indexer
Barbara Hodgson

MSCP010703—020106

Library of Congress Cataloging-in-Publication Data
Medical surgical care planning / [edited by] Nancy M.
Holloway. — 4th ed.
    p.; cm.
    Includes bibliographical references and index.
    1. Nursing care plans. 2. Surgical nursing. 3. Nursing assessment.
    [DNLM: 1. Patient Care Planning. 2. Diagnosis-Related Groups.
    3. Nursing Diagnosis. WY 100 M4877 2003] I. Holloway, Nancy
    Meyer, 1947-
RT49.M45 2003
610.73—dc21
ISBN 1-58255-224-X (pbk. : alk. paper)   2003006907

Contents

vii *Contributors and consultants*

xi *Acknowledgments and dedication*

xiii *Preface*

Part 1
Introduction

2 Trends and issues in health care and nursing
9 Role of DRGs in delivering quality care
13 NANDA, NIC, and NOC
16 Care plans
19 Clinical pathways

Part 2
General care plans

24 Acute alcohol withdrawal
32 Acute pain
40 Anxiety
48 Cancer
63 Chronic pain
67 Compromised family coping
71 Confusion
78 Dying
92 Geriatric care
105 Grieving
111 Impaired physical mobility
124 Ineffective individual coping
129 Knowledge deficit
138 Nutritional deficit
146 Perioperative care

Part 3
Neurologic disorders

160 Alzheimer's disease
170 Craniotomy
181 Drug overdose
190 Increased intracranial pressure
205 Laminectomy
218 Multiple sclerosis
228 Seizures
236 Stroke

Part 4
Respiratory disorders

252 Acute respiratory distress syndrome
259 Asthma
267 Chronic obstructive pulmonary disease
281 Mechanical ventilation
297 Pneumonia
306 Pulmonary embolism
315 Thoracotomy

Part 5
Cardiovascular disorders

328 Abdominal aortic aneurysm repair
337 Acute myocardial infarction
355 Angina pectoris
366 Cardiac surgery
382 Cardiogenic shock
392 Carotid endarterectomy
404 Femoral popliteal bypass
411 Heart failure
424 Hypovolemic shock
432 Percutaneous transluminal coronary angioplasty
440 Permanent pacemaker insertion
449 Septic shock
459 Thrombophlebitis

Part 6
Gastrointestinal disorders

468 Colostomy
477 Duodenal ulcer, esophagitis, and gastroenteritis
487 Gastrointestinal hemorrhage
498 Inflammatory bowel disease
510 Parenteral nutrition

Part 7
Hepatobiliary and pancreatic disorders

524   Cholecystectomy
533   Liver failure
541   Pancreatitis

Part 8
Musculoskeletal and integumentary disorders

550   Amputation
559   Fractured femur
567   Major burns
582   Multiple trauma
594   Osteomyelitis
602   Skin grafts
612   Total joint replacement in a lower extremity

Part 9
Endocrine disorders

624   Diabetes mellitus
635   Diabetic ketoacidosis
645   Hyperosmolar hyperglycemic nonketotic syndrome
651   Hypoglycemia
656   Obesity

Part 10
Renal disorders

668   Acute renal failure
680   Chronic renal failure
697   Ileal conduit urinary diversion
707   Nephrectomy
713   Renal dialysis
724   Urolithiasis

Part 11
Hematologic and immunologic disorders

732   Acquired immunodeficiency syndrome
755   Anemia
764   Disseminated intravascular coagulation
771   Leukemia
789   Lymphoma

Part 12
Reproductive disorders

804   Hysterectomy
812   Mastectomy
826   Prostatectomy
838   Radioactive implant for cervical cancer

846   *Appendix A*
      Monitoring standards

848   *Appendix B*
      Acid-base imbalances

849   *Appendix C*
      Fluid and electrolyte imbalances

852   *Appendix D*
      Nursing diagnostic categories

854   *Appendix E*
      Critical care transfer criteria guidelines

855   *Appendix F*
      Quick-reference guide to laboratory test results

859   *Index*

Contributors and consultants

Deborah A. Andris, MSN, APNP
Nurse Practitioner, Minimally Invasive Gastrointestinal
  Surgery Division
Medical College of Wisconsin
Milwaukee

Marylou S. Anton, RN, BSN, OCN
Regional Manager, Cancer Services
North Broward Medical Center
Pompano Beach, Fla.

Melody C. Antoon, RN, MSN
Instructor
Lamar State College
Beaumont, Tex.

Diane S. Benson, RN, EdD(c)
Assistant Professor of Nursing
Humboldt State University
Arcata, Calif.

Cheryl Brady, RN, MSN
Adjunct Faculty
Youngstown (Ohio) State University

Marie O. Brewer, RN, LNC
Director of Performance Improvement
VNHS of Atlanta

Ruth Brewer, RN, PhD, CS
Professor of Nursing
McNeese State University
Lake Charles, La.

Barbara S. Broome, RN, PhD, CNS
Assistant Dean and Chair—Community/Mental Health
University of South Alabama College of Nursing
Mobile

Karen T. Bruchak, RN, MSN, MBA
Oncology Product Market Administrator
Siemens Health Services
Malvern, Pa.

Michelle M. Byrne, RN, MS, PhD, CNOR
Nursing Instructor and Independent Consultant
North Georgia College and State University
Dahlonega

Patricia C. Cloud, MSN, PhD
Independent Consultant
Orange, Tex.

Linda Carman Copel, RN, PhD, CS, DAPA
Associate Professor
Villanova (Pa.) University College of Nursing

Laurie Donaghy, RN
Charge Nurse, Emergency Department
Nazareth Hospital
Philadelphia

Eleanor Z. Franges, BSN, MSN, CNRN
Director, Neuroscience Services
Sacred Heart Hospital
Allentown, Pa.

Cynthia L. Frozena, RN, MSN
Medical Writer
Enzymatic Therapy
Green Bay, Wis.

Mary F. Gerard, RN, BSN, CCRN
Medical Information Specialist
Johnson & Johnson
Skillman, N.J.

Mary Hawkins, RDLD, CNSD
Nutrition Support Dietitian
Doctors Hospital
Columbus, Ohio

Connie S. Heflin, RN,MSN
Professor
Paducah (Ky.) Community College

Patricia F. Henry, RN, MS
Department Leader
Kaiser Permanente
Oakland, Calif.

Katherine Purgatorio Howard, RN, MS, BC
Instructor of Nursing
Charles E. Gregory School of Nursing
Raritan Bay Medical Center
Perth Amboy, N.J.

Lauren M. Isacson, RN, BSN, MPa., PHR
Manager, Human Resource Development
Meridian Health System
Neptune, N.J.

Patricia A. Lange-Otsuka, APRN, MSN, EdD, BC
Associate Professor of Nursing
Hawaii Pacific University
Kaneohe

Linda Laskowski-Jones, RN, MS, CCRN, CEN, CS
Director, Trauma, Emergency & Aeromedical Services
Christiana Care Health System—Christiana Hospital
Newark, Del.

Ellen P. Leber, RN, MSN, CCRN
Staff Nurse, CVICU
Doylestown (Pa.) Hospital

Virginia D. Lester, RN, MSN, CNS (inactive)
Assistant Professor in Nursing
Angelo State University
San Angelo, Tex.

Shirley L. Lewis, RN, MSN, CAN, OCN
Patient Care Director
Virginia Hospital Center
Arlington

Susan Luck, RN, BS, MA, CCN, HNC
Director of Nutrition Education—Special Immunology Services
Mercy Hospital
Coconut Grove, Fla.

Jeanne U. Magrath, RN, MSN
Cardiothoracic Clinical Nurse Specialist
Legal Nurse Consultant
Florissant, Mo.

Andrea Marino, RN, BSN, CCRN
Staff Nurse, Interventional Cardiology Unit
Doylestown (Pa.) Hospital

Dawna Martich, RN, BSN, MSN
Clinical Trainer
American Healthways
Pittsburgh

Kate McClure, RN, MS, CCRN
Case Manager/Project Manager
Kaiser Foundation Hospital
Oakland, Calif.

Marcella A. Mikalaitis, RN, MSN, CCRN
Staff Nurse, CVICU
Doylestown (Pa.) Hospital

Molly J. Moran, RN, MS, CS
Clinical Nurse Specialist
Arthur G. James Cancer Hospital and Richard J. Solove Research Institute
Columbus, Ohio

Sheryl Redlin-Frazier, RN, OCN
Clinical Research Specialist
Vanderbilt University Medical Center
Nashville, Tenn.

Terry Rodriguez, RN, BA, ET
Clinical Coordinator
Barry Gardiner, MD, Inc.
San Ramon, Calif.

Donna Scemons, RN, FNP, MSN, CNS, CWOCN
Healthcare Systems, Inc.
Panorama City, Calif.

Concha Carrillo Sitter, MS, APN, CGRN, FNP
Gastroenterology Nurse Practitioner
Sterling-Rock Falls Clinic
Sterling, Ill.

Cindy Wagner, RNC, MS, CNS
Gerontological Clinical Nurse Specialist
Doctors Hospital
Columbus, Ohio

Patricia Walters, RN, MSN, APN-C
Advanced Practice Nurse
Hackensack (N.J.) University Medical Center

Patricia Harvey Webb, RN,C, MS, EdD
Associate Professor
Samuel Merritt College
Oakland, Calif.

Karen Zulkowski, RN, DNS, CWS
Assistant Professor
Montana State University—Bozeman
Billings

The author wishes to thank those individuals who contributed to previous editions.

Sandra Allen, RN,C
Gerene S. Bauldoff, RN, MSN
Janice M. Beitz, RN, PhD, CETN, CNOR, CS
Nancy Newell Bell, RN, MN, MDiv, CCRN
Audrey J. Berman, RN, MSN, PhD, AOCN
Claudia J. Beverly, RN, PhD
Nancy E. Casali, RN, BSN
Karen L. Cooper, RN, MSN, CCRN, CNA
Dorothy B. Doughty, RN, MN, CETN

Phyllis R. Easterling, RN, EdD, FNP
Gayle Flo, RN, ARNP, MN, CCRN
Mary Kay Flynn, RN, DNSc, CCRN
Latrell P. Fowler, BSN, MN, PhD
Joanne Soldano Garcia, RN, MS, CCRN
Mel Herman, RN, BA, CCRN
Kathleen Hester, RN, BSN, CCRN
Margaret Hodge, RN, EdD
Beth Colvin Huff, RN, MSN, CS
Philip A. John, CCS
Donna M. Knisely, RN, MSN, CDE
Larry E. Lancaster, RN, MSN, EdD
Wendy M. Mancini, RN, MSN, CCRN, CNA, CNS
Cathy A. Machacyk, RN, BSN
Barbara Martin, RN, PhD
Scarlott K. Mueller, RN, MPH
Carolyn E. Munroe, RN,C, BS, ADN
Christine E. Ortiz, RN, MS, PhD(c)
Elizabeth Poulson, RN, MS, MA
Ellene Rifas, RN, EdD
Dennis G. Ross, RN, MAE, PhD
LuAnn E. Sanderson, RNP, MSN, CNS
Patricia C. Seifert, RN, MSN, CNOR, CRNFA
Debra Lynn Thelen, RN, MS, ACRN
M. Susan Theodoropoulos, RN,C, MSN
Charlene Thomas, RN, PhD
Nancy C. Thomas, RN, BSN, CCRN
Patricia Harvey Webb, RN,C, MS, EdD

Dedication

This book is dedicated to my family:
D. Michael Holloway, my husband; Jason Holloway, my son; and Willow Holloway, my daughter.
A friend told me, "A healthy relationship is one that brings out the best in you most of the time."
I am grateful beyond words to you for being there when I really needed you.

Acknowledgments

Publishing a book is never a sole creative endeavor. I extend a special thank you to our contributors and consultants, acknowledged by name in a separate section. My heartfelt thanks to Karen Bruchak for gallantly taking over the reins and helping to move this edition to publication. I also thank the talented publishing team at Lippincott Williams & Wilkins, especially Beverly Tscheschlog, the editor for which every author dreams. Bev, your vision and support through this difficult year brought this book to fruition, and I will be forever grateful.

Preface

Medical-Surgical Care Planning, Fourth Edition, is essential. Why? Because it integrates three major factors in nursing — care planning, nursing diagnoses, and diagnosis-related groups (DRGs) — and provides information nurses need to meet the 1992 Joint Commission on the Accreditation of Healthcare Organizations (JCAHO) Nursing Care Standards. Focusing on care of the adult medical-surgical patient, this book:
- distinguishes clearly between nursing's collaborative functions (those shared with medicine) and its independent functions (those unique to nursing)
- offers the bedside nurse, nursing student, and nursing educator comprehensive, realistic care plans to meet their educational needs.

WHY ARE CARE PLANS IMPORTANT?
Clinically, care plans offer a way to plan and communicate appropriate patient care. Legally, they offer a framework for establishing the standard of care for a given situation. Financially, they can validate the appropriateness of care and justify staffing levels and patient-care charges.

IF CARE PLANS ARE SO IMPORTANT, WHY DON'T MORE NURSES USE THEM?
Most nurses are first exposed to care plans as students. They soon learn that writing out individual plans can be frustrating and time consuming. After graduation, most nurses practice in a hectic, complex environment that allows little time for thoughtful care planning.

Even nurses who would like to use written care plans may be at a loss when trying to integrate nursing diagnoses into their planning. Overwhelmed, they may turn to previously published books for guidance, only to find the information too general or too theoretical, that common medical problems are renamed in nursing diagnosis terminology, or that nursing diagnoses aren't matched to medical disorders.

Yet *clinically relevant* care plans can help nurses answer many of the questions they ask daily:
- "What are the most important points to cover during a physical assessment when I haven't got time to check everything?"
- "Which laboratory tests and diagnostic procedures should I anticipate, and what do they typically show?"
- "What are this patient's nursing priorities?"
- "Which problems is this patient most likely to experience?"
- "Why are certain interventions important?"
- "Which complications can occur with this disorder?"
- "How long is this patient likely to be in the hospital?"
- "Realistically, how much patient teaching can I accomplish?"
- "From a nursing standpoint, how will I know when this patient is ready for discharge?"

THE SOLUTION: THIS BOOK
Medical-Surgical Care Planning, Fourth Edition, provides clinically relevant answers to common questions about patient care because it targets the needs of the "hands-on" nurse clinician through standardized care plans. Distinguishing features include:
- 15 general care plans covering conditions nurses encounter daily, such as impaired physical mobility and knowledge deficit
- 63 care plans, organized by body system, covering various medical-surgical conditions and procedures (including critical care disorders)
- 8 clinical pathways
- nursing diagnoses (using selected terminology from the North American Nursing Diagnosis Association) and collaborative problems (using familiar medical terminology such as shock) arranged in order of importance
- integration of nursing interventions classification (NIC) and nursing outcomes classification (NOC), following each nursing diagnosis in each care plan.

This approach will help you see the total picture of patient care; differentiate between collaborative and independent nursing responsibilities; apply the latest official nursing diagnoses; and avoid forcing all planning under nursing diagnoses, a process that only renames medical diagnoses and fosters confusion between nursing and medicine.

Each care plan presents the latest clinically relevant DRG information, including DRG numbers, principal diagnoses, and mean length of stay, to help you understand the reimbursement system responsible for today's cost-conscious health care environment and to help you anticipate the patient's recovery and plan patient teaching. Common historical and subjective findings are presented according to Gordon's functional health patterns, a widely accepted format that blends both traditional and contemporary methods of nursing assessment; objective findings are listed by body system. This assessment information will help you recognize pertinent signs and symptoms and understand how the nursing diagnoses and collaborative problems were identified.

The care plans build on a goal-directed, action-oriented approach to care planning that ranks problems and interventions in order of importance and identifies specific outcome criteria. This approach will help you determine the most important patient problems, decide what to do first, and recognize when a problem has been resolved.

JCAHO STANDARDS' IMPACT ON NURSING

The 1992 update represents the first major revision of the Nursing Care Standards since 1978. The JCAHO Nursing Standards Task Force, which included 23 representatives from various nursing services and educational programs, adopted the new standards after circulating two drafts and considering feedback from more than 50,000 nurses.

Where the former Nursing Services Standards focused on the process of care to determine if the nursing organization could provide quality care, the new Nursing Care Standards focus more on the patient and the outcomes of care to determine the quality of care provided. In addition, the new standards emphasize patient-family education and discharge planning. Consequently, nurses will play an even more important role in helping hospitals maintain accreditation. Such accountability is likely to *increase* interest in care planning.

The revised standards also place increased emphasis on documentation, requiring that nursing information involving assessment, nursing diagnoses or patient needs, interventions, and outcomes become a permanent part of the medical record. Care may be documented directly in the patient's record or indirectly through references to other documents. However, this documentation doesn't have to be the handwritten, complex, case-study approach to care planning that educators find helpful, or the routine, repetitive handwritten plan that many hospital nurses rightly dismiss as irrelevant and time consuming. Instead of being required to provide handwritten care plans for all patients, nursing departments now have more flexibility in documenting care. Nurses may now choose to document care planning through standards of care, clinical practice guidelines, critical paths, or preprinted care plans.

When individualized as recommended, the standardized plans in this book can help nurses meet all of the JCAHO's requirements. The care plans cover all the elements required for documentation of care planning and also include useful information about patient outcomes, patient-family education, and discharge planning.

STANDARDIZED VS. INDIVIDUALIZED PLANS

Major differences of opinion exist in nursing concerning standardized and individualized care plans. Opponents of standardization argue that it equals depersonalization. Advocates argue that standardization promotes efficiency, by limiting planning time without sacrificing quality, and fosters quality assurance. This disagreement can't be resolved easily; however, this book combines the advantages of standard care plans with unusual features that help minimize their disadvantages:

■ The care plans blend standardized and individualized aspects of care. Standardization works better in some areas of care planning than others: problems, priorities, and interventions can usually be standardized, but outcome criteria, timing of interventions, and discharge criteria require significant individualization. *Medical-Surgical Care Planning,* Fourth Edition, takes these factors into account and encourages flexibility in areas that vary significantly among patients.

■ Space is provided at the end of each problem for the nurse to add additional interventions and rationales specific to the individual patient's needs.

These unusual features challenge the nurse to think creatively. Because the resulting plan is pertinent and individualized, its clinical usefulness is ensured.

However, the most important point to remember in the debate over standardized versus individualized care plans is that a care plan doesn't cause depersonalized care; rather, the nurse's attitude is the culprit. The nurse who appreciates patients as individuals will use a standard plan as a starting point, staying attuned to the individual patient's responses while applying the art and science of nursing.

WHY NURSES WILL CONTINUE TO USE CARE PLANS

Care plans provide a valuable way to organize care, meet JCAHO's requirements for documentation, and prepare for site visits. In addition, many institutions have invested substantial time and money to develop systems of care planning appropriate for their patients. Before abandoning such systems, they would need to identify a better one and find the funds, time, and expertise to implement it — a difficult undertaking in this era of scarce resources. Finally, instructors in schools of nursing will continue to use care plans as a method for teaching patient care because of the plans' comprehensiveness.

Ultimately, any care plan is only as good as the nurse who provides the care. Conscientious nurses find care plans a resource for learning new information quickly, refreshing their knowledge, and focusing their energy on the most important problems their patients may encounter. The contributors to *Medical-Surgical Care Planning,* Fourth Edition, have based their plans on a blend of clinical expertise, nursing diagnosis, and care planning — always keeping in mind the nurse on the front line. This book will provide welcome help for nurses facing the daily challenge of providing quality patient care.

Nancy M. Holloway

Introduction

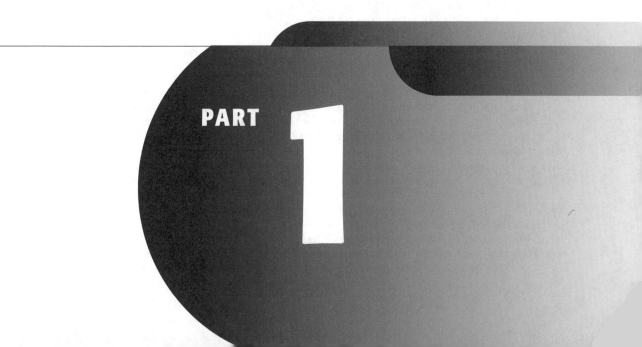

PART

1

Trends and issues in health care and nursing

Major developments in American society and the health care industry are producing revolutionary changes in health care delivery. The most significant of these include cultural diversity, the aging population (also known as the "graying of America"), chronic care, and restricted access to care. Other critical issues include the evolution of health care, its impact on the patient and on nursing, and opportunities for advanced practice.

Cultural diversity

The current health care arena reflects the increasing cultural diversity and awareness within America. Cultural awareness is defined as the deliberate, cognitive process by which health care providers become appreciative of and sensitive to the values, beliefs, life ways, practices, and problem solving strategies of clients' cultures.

There's no doubt that developing cultural competence can enhance our ability to provide care to people different from ourselves. Campinha-Bacote's model of cultural competence incudes personal awareness, knowledge, skill, encounters, and desire. Whereas cultural competence can't, in itself, be considered an outcome of nursing practice, its achievement can — and must — be an ongoing goal. Health care professionals must seek encounters and knowledge to challenge their sterotypic beliefs.

Cultural awareness also includes an examination of one's own biases. To understand cultural diversity, we must strive to acknowledge the prejudices we may already hold toward cultures different from our own.

The hospitals and health systems in which nurses typically work also constitute a culture — one into which nurses are socialized by both training and experience and one that has its own unique set of beliefs, values, and practices not understood by all patients.

Many of the values of the health care system have evolved from the socio-historic influences of wars, education, gender roles, and the availability of resources. Spector identified seven aspects of health care system culture, including beliefs, practices, likes and dislikes, customs, rituals, and recommendations.

BELIEFS
Beliefs are defined as ideas that a person accepts as true. As health care professionals, we know that a belief in standardization is the foundation of almost everything we do. Standardization is achieved through policies, procedures, critical pathways, forms, care plans, orders, flow sheets, and competency statements. However, the nurse must strike a careful balance between objectivity and standardization and creativity and individuality.

PRACTICES
The concepts of health maintenance and patient autonomy are embedded in nursing practices. Maintenance and preventive practices are key and include annual examinations and specific diagnostic procedures performed at certain ages. If diseases or conditions are identified, the goal is to cure the patient, thereby restoring his autonomy. Further, due to ever-changing reimbursement protocols and advances in medical care, current health care practices emphasize limited hospitalization, thereby allowing the patient to enter a post-acute care facility, or return home and resume his daily routine.

LIKES AND DISLIKES
In every human endeavor, elements exist that arouse either positive or negative feelings. To this end, health care practitioners certainly aren't immune to feelings of appreciation for some aspects of their profession and feelings of frustration for others. Promptness and compliance are valued by most health care practitioners. We want our patients to be prompt in arriving for appointments. Conversely, however, patients' appointments may be shorter than they expect, which may lead to frustration. So, although appointments run on a strict time schedule, it's up to the culturally competent nurse to be open-minded, respectful, and empathetic to the patient's own values, which may include asking a detailed set of questions during their visit, thus extending the appointment.

We want our patients to comply with taking medicine exactly as prescribed, seeking care when it's needed, and scheduling annual examinations, immunizations, and diagnostic tests. In this sense, most health care practitioners look to preventive measures to avert illnesses. Once again, however, the culturally competent nurse must accept that patients from different cultures have different views about when to seek professional help, treat oneself, or be treated by a family member or traditional healer.

CUSTOMS
In health care, customs can range from the basic to the complex. It's customary to wash your hands before (and

after) examinations and procedures—this common custom is consistently reinforced and for good reason.

An area where health care customs becomes more intricate, however, is when the health care professional, in order to complete forms and do work-ups, needs personal information, especially in sensitive areas involving intimate behavior and bodily functions. Patients from different cultures essentially know that they need care, but may have difficulty talking to strangers about personal matters. For example, in Asia, the Middle East, and to some extent, Latin America, one's dignity must be preserved at all costs. The culturally competent nurse must take care to spend extra time with her patient and should speak in soft, soothing tones to gain trust. By respecting and being sensitive to the customs of patients from other cultures, the nurse will simultaneously implement the customs of the health care culture.

RITUALS

Ritual is defined as a common and observable expression of culture. In our society the term ritual has developed connotations of primitive or "uncivilized" behavior—mention ritual and most people think of tribal rites of passage into adulthood or voodoo ceremonies. Western society, too, has its rituals. The health care industry, for example, has rituals that include the procedures performed prior to surgery and those common to physical examinations.

Many rituals are performed using instruments or artifacts. Cultural artifacts readily identifiable to most people include Christmas trees, Chanukah menorahs, and Buddhist prayer wheels. What most health care practitioners don't realize, however, is that their tools of the trade might also be considered artifacts to cultures unfamiliar with them. Otoscopes, penlights, tongue blades and blood pressure cuffs might be viewed as the artifacts of nurses.

RECOMMENDATIONS

As a health care provider who will interact with diverse clients and colleagues, it's important that you examine your personal and professional cultures. Ask yourself the following questions:
■ What's your ethnic heritage, religion, and community of origin?
■ What's your age-group, socio-economic background, and level of education?
■ What are your beliefs surrounding parenthood, family, and sexuality?
■ What characteristics do you like and dislike about your cultural group?

Nursing professionals care for many clients that abide by different religious, cultural, and gender beliefs and practices. Therefore, it's important to walk the fine line between learning about cultural variations, without stereotyping or generalizing. By doing this, the culturally

competent nurse will learn more about her own personal and professional culture. Lastly, knowledge about each culture can only enhance and add to the nurse's ability to communicate, learn, and change.

Population trends: The graying of America

By the year 2010, about 40 million Americans will be age 65 and older (13% of the population), with those age 85 and older constituting the fastest growing age-group. The percentage of elderly patients with disabilities is declining, partly due to the decline in diseases that cause disability in the elderly, such as stroke and heart disease. Despite this decline, however, the sheer number of people who are aging means that long-term disability will continue to be a major problem in the health care system. Older adults now account for 60% of adult ambulatory primary care visits, 80% of home care visits, 48% of hospital patients, and 85% of nursing home residents, according to the John A. Hartford Foundation Institute for Geriatric Nursing in New York University.

Only a small percentage of elderly citizens live in nursing homes; patients are usually discharged from acute care hospitals to their homes. Unfortunately, a consequence of shorter hospital stays is that nurses usually don't have enough time to educate caregivers. Additionally, a patient older than age 85 may have an elderly caregiver who also requires medical care or assistance with the activities of daily living.

Elderly patients require a range of services; the most important include home health care, homemaker or chore services, transportation, assistance with activities of daily living, nutrition services, and an emergency response system. Although integration of these services is important, in many cases it doesn't exist. Nurses could help bridge this gap.

Chronic care

The intersection of an aging population and a health care system focused on acute care creates another trend: the increasing importance of chronic care. This consists of medical care, rehabilitation, and assistance with activities of daily living.

Several factors affect the health status of older Americans. These patients commonly have multiple chronic disorders. According to the American Association of Retired Persons, the most common disorders in those older than age 50 are hypertension, arthritis, heart disease, hearing disorders, cataracts, sinusitis, orthopedic disorders, and diabetes—all chronic conditions that last for years. Although these patients may not necessarily be sicker with a given illness than they were a decade ago, they are more likely to have many concurrent or complex illnesses as they age. In addition, older people are at risk for receiving inadequate medical care because of poverty, forgetfulness, hearing or vision impairments, and transportation problems, among other factors. Finally, older people are at risk for experiencing unexpected adverse effects associated with complex drug regimens.

Access to care

According to the Census Bureau, about 39 million Americans are uninsured, making access to care a major issue in the current health care system. The nation's economic restructuring means that many higher-paying manufacturing jobs have been replaced by lower-paying service sector jobs that don't offer benefits. Of all uninsured children, most are from working families. During the coming years, the working poor will have less access to care, and the safety net will continue to deteriorate.

"The whole issue of the uninsured is the Achilles' heel of the reshaping of our health care system by market forces," says Kathryn Duke, a researcher from the University of California, San Francisco, Institute for Health Policy Studies. Compared to the insured, the uninsured are sick more often, less likely to seek care, more seriously ill, die sooner, and die more frequently from illness. Although some steps have been taken to achieve wider access to health care, the goals of universal coverage, a single-payer system, and a national health insurance plan remain unrealized.

Physicians, physician assistants, and nurse practitioners will increasingly control access to the health care system. However, their efforts to refer patients for specialized services will be hampered by spending caps and a limited number of specialists participating in insurance plans.

Evolution of health care

The evolution of health care continues to be characterized by reduced spending, increased governmental regulation, and changes in the site of health care delivery.

REDUCED REIMBURSEMENT

Enrollment in managed care plans continues to expand, especially among Medicaid recipients. Health care providers and plan administrators continually seek the most cost-effective ways to deliver care.

The health care system continues to reel from the reduced rate of Medicare and Medicaid spending. Most of the savings comes from reduced payments to providers, hospitals, and health maintenance organizations (HMOs).

GOVERNMENT REGULATION

Government regulation plays an increasing role in the health care field. State regulators are becoming more involved in policing managed care organizations (for ex-

ample, by citing hospitals for violating federal laws against patient dumping). Pressure from lawmakers and consumer groups continues to eliminate objectionable practices, such as excluding benefits for patients with preexisting conditions or canceling the policies of patients with catastrophic illnesses. Managed care organizations will likely respond to consumer backlash and temper their approaches primarily to avoid more restrictive legislation. Ongoing consolidation and mergers among health care facilities are forming large hospital chains that are monitored closely by the federal government for violations of antitrust laws. Vigorous federal prosecution of Medicare fraud will continue.

SITES OF CARE

Outpatient facilities and community programs — as opposed to inpatient acute care — have become popular sites of care. Many health care organizations have reduced the number of beds or closed units. Managed care is the major factor driving down hospital stays, with HMOs significantly limiting inpatient care. "Patients who used to be in the intensive care unit now are in medical-surgical units, while patients who were often hospitalized in a medical-surgical unit now are treated as outpatients," according to Kathy Reno, RN, executive vice president and chief operating officer of Clinical Services at Northwest Community Hospital in Arlington Heights, Ill.

Outpatient services are taking greater responsibility for complex care regimens previously managed by inpatient services. For example, AIDS patients today receive more of their care in ambulatory facilities. The trend toward same-day and outpatient surgery — driven by managed care, improved anesthesia, and advances in pain management — means that patients are commonly back home a few hours after a procedure or treatment.

Professionals caring for these patients need a different approach and greater range of skills than they did a few years ago. The demands of maintaining quality care within a shorter period of time present a daunting challenge for nurses. The nurse needs the ability to establish relationships quickly as well as excellent patient assessment skills. Managing these patients requires more critical thinking.

A patient's satisfaction with his care is directly related to his expectations of the experience. Preparation is one of the keys to achieving patient satisfaction. As one nurse notes, "Patients need to know that they're going to move through quickly. Patients think they're there for a day, but it's really a piece of a day; rarely is someone there 8 to 12 hours. That's information patients need to know up front — that they are being moved through not because we're rushing them but rather because criteria have been met and they're ready for discharge."

Consumers also are likely to see increased growth of long-term care facilities. "What we're seeing now is the diversification of long-term care," says David Kyllo, a spokesman for the American Health Care Association, which represents two-thirds of the nation's nursing homes. "Twenty-five years ago you had nursing homes doing the lighter care as well as the heavier care. Today, nursing homes have evolved to become the provider of more complex medical care. Lighter care has gone to assisted living or in-home care."

Nurses are likely to see an explosion of community-based programs, which are popular because most people want to live at home and because home care is cost-effective. Most nursing jobs will be in the community because of the increased need for health professionals in ambulatory care, home health, schools, and prisons. According to the American Medical Association, more than 80% of all health care takes place in the home. This shift in the site of health care requires a corresponding shift in the attitudes of health care professionals.

"Our hospital system in the past several decades has been built on an illness model: If you're sick, you go to the hospital," says Susan Odegaard Turner, a nurse who helped develop a guide for health care providers to assist nurses in making the transition to the new characteristics of health care. "Managed care is based on a wellness concept: You try to keep somebody out of the hospital and manage them in an off-site environment — an alternative site."

The shift of focus to ambulatory facilities is having a great impact on nurses, especially critical care nurses. Patients are either bypassing the intensive care unit or leaving it more quickly.

The addition of new care sites means today's nurses have a wider range of employment opportunities. Nurses may be hired to provide care in nontraditional settings, such as nurse advise lines or to work for case management firms, such as workers' compensation, disability, or health insurance carriers. Nurses may also seek employment as independent contractors or as nursing consultants for attorneys who handle cases concerning medical matters.

Impact on the patient

Reduced spending, increased governmental regulation, and shifts in the site of care significantly impact the patient. Health care providers need to focus more attention on patient satisfaction and patient education. The alternative health care trend is continuing as patients seek relief from stress and pain.

PATIENT SATISFACTION

Paul Schyve, a senior vice president of the Joint Commission on Accreditation of Health Care Organizations (JCAHO), says that "years ago, JCAHO based its assessments of the quality of care on standards like staffing and a facility's resources. Now JCAHO looks at other things, such as how healthy and satisfied patients are and how much their care costs." Patient satisfaction was evaluated in the American Hospital Association's "Eye on Patients," which surveyed 37,000 patients about the care they received in 1996 at 120 hospitals, clinics, or physicians' offices. Among the significant concerns patients mentioned were having little say in their treatment, receiving inadequate information, and experiencing posthospital "abandonment." As Sharon Ostwald, director of the Center on Aging at the University of Texas-Houston Health Science Center, comments, "The focus is on getting the patient out of the hospital, and we've sort of lost track of who is going to take care of them the day they walk out the door."

PATIENT EDUCATION

The past 15 years have brought three major changes in patient education: the increasing impact of technology, change in the site of health education, and the increasing sophistication of health care consumers.

The Internet has improved access to health information for millions and is bringing together people with similar health issues in forums and chat rooms. Hospital-associated learning centers are providing "one stop" education for patients and family. A growing number of hospitals now have sites on the World Wide Web, delivering health care information through cyberspace. The Internet isn't the only way technology is affecting the way care is delivered. Increasingly, phone-nursing experts are providing patients with information, advice, coaching, and referrals to specialists and, in some cases, providing care similar to case management.

State-of-the-art telemedicine systems (which use ordinary phone lines to transmit video, audio, and diagnostic information) allow nurses in an office to examine wound sites, evaluate heart or lung sounds, and check blood pressure, pulse, and temperature of a patient who's at home.

In many cases, the site of patient education has changed dramatically. Short stays and increased nursing responsibilities have virtually eliminated time for teaching and talking to patients in the hospital. Whereas most patient education previously occurred in the hospital, education now is occurring in health care providers' offices, patients' homes, and cyberspace.

Because of the shortened stays, most preoperative teaching has to be done on an outpatient basis. The teaching process now begins much earlier, in many cases in the physician's office. Many nurses use a combined approach of a preadmission phone call or visit, instruction before and after the procedure, and a follow-up call 24 hours after discharge.

Because of increased media coverage and public awareness, patients now are beginning to take more responsibility for their health care choices. Most consumers, however, don't have the knowledge or skills to evaluate available information about health care facilities, for example, report cards that contain complicated information.

ALTERNATIVE AND COMPLEMENTARY CARE

One intriguing development in health care is the widespread use of alternative and complementary approaches. Millions of patients are turning to herbalists, acupuncturists, homeopaths, chiropractors, and other health care practitioners. One reason for their popularity is their ability to offer chronically ill patients relief from stress or pain that traditional Western medicine hasn't treated successfully. In addition, the growing multiculturalism of American society introduces health care practices that are mainstream in their culture of origin such as the use of acupuncture in Chinese medicine.

Impact on nursing

Changes in the health care system offer nurses both challenges and opportunities. Challenges include the nursing shortage, changes in the nurse-patient relationship and in job expectations, and increased emphasis on collaboration and evidence-based practice. Nursing education and advanced practice nursing programs provide additional opportunities for nurses.

THE NURSING SHORTAGE

According to JCAHO, the nation's nursing shortage has had major consequences during the past 5 years. Inadequate nurse staffing has been a factor in 24% of the 1,609 cases involving death, injury, or permanent loss of function reported to JCAHO since 1997.

CHANGES IN THE NURSE-PATIENT RELATIONSHIP

"Nurses across the nation, in every setting and specialty, report that they're taking care of more patients, have been cross-trained to take on more nursing responsibilities, and have substantially less time to provide all aspects of nursing," according to an *AJN* survey. This reduction is probably due to a combination of factors, including cuts in the overall number of registered nurses, more patients assigned to each registered nurse, shorter lengths of stay, and increased complexity of patient care.

Nurses report having less time to teach patients, less continuity of care, an increase in unexpected readmissions (especially in emergency and psychiatric or mental health care), an increase in complications (especially in gerontology), and an increase in job-related injuries. The nurse's role has changed from providing direct care to managing nursing care and resources for a patient. Clinicians need to be more adept at managing care rather than simply delivering services.

CHANGES IN JOB EXPECTATIONS

Nurses increasingly are expected to provide more services with fewer resources, to carry heavier patient loads, and to work with more complex technology than in the past. In a recent national study of registered nurses by *Nurseweek* and the American Organization of Nurse Executives, nearly half the nurses said their jobs involved so many nonnursing tasks that they have little time left for nursing. Almost 90% said that the nursing shortage is a major problem that keeps them from spending time with patients. About two-thirds said the shortage affected the quality of nursing care, and 64% said it interferes with the ability to maintain patient safety. Because of extremely short stays, nurses must spend more time on discharge planning. In addition, they must be flexible and take on more supervisory responsibility. The increased responsibility for supervision is the result of two trends: the increased substitution of part-time or temporary registered nurses for full-time registered nurses, and the substitution of unlicensed assistive personnel (UAP) for registered nurses. Of *AJN* survey respondents, about 87% reported that the introduction of UAPs hasn't improved the quality of patient care. (See *Pros and cons of the nurse-patient relationship.*)

INCREASED EMPHASIS ON COLLABORATION

Working in collaboration with nurses and other professionals — rather than working in isolation or attempting to solve problems within a single discipline — is critical for success. Because nursing is so complex, and systems and technology change quickly, old ways have to be modified — but they need to be modified in collaboration with other professionals. Nurses must articulate their contributions and communicate across disciplines.

Collaboration between physicians and nurses is so important that it affects mortality. A recent study in the *New England Journal of Medicine,* "Nursing Staffing Levels and the Quality of Care in Hospitals," recapped a study released by the government showing that lower levels of hospital registered nurse staffing are associated with increased risk of potentially fatal patient complications.

The most recent and most famous study on the relationship between nurse staffing and quality of care in hospitals was led by Jack Needleman, PhD, of the Harvard School of Public Health and Peter Buerhaus, PhD, RN, FAAN, professor of nursing and senior associate dean for research at Vanderbilt University School of Nursing. The Needleman-Buerhaus study was released by the Department of Health and Human Services in the May 30, 2002 edition of the *New England Journal of Medicine.* This ambitious study analyzed outcomes for more than 6 million medical and surgical patients in 799 hospitals in 11 states across the country, using 1997 data. They focused on "outcomes potentially sensitive to nursing" because such outcomes can be prevented by good nursing care. These outcomes are pneumonia, shock, cardiac arrest, upper GI bleeding, blood poisoning, and blood clots. The authors found that patients in hospitals with lower registered nurse staffing were 3% to 9% more likely to develop these complications.

Pros and cons of the nurse-patient relationship

According to most nurses, the nurse-patient relationship continues to evolve under managed care. One readily apparent change is the more vigorous role a patient must play such as assuming responsibility for improving his condition by becoming an active partner in the collaborative efforts of the health care team.

Nurses, too, have witnessed changes in their roles. With family members commonly serving as the patients' primary caregivers, more and more nurses are seeing themselves as coordinators, coaches, patient advocates, and supervisors of others – including unlicensed assistive personnel – who provide some of the hands-on care that nurses once performed.

Nurses cite the following advantages and disadvantages of this relationship.

Pros	Cons
• Greater emphasis on assessment, planning, educating, and coordinating	• Less opportunity for direct, hands-on care
• Less task-based responsibility	• More emphasis on delegation and supervision
• Opportunities to be more directly available to patients such as by phone	• Less time for casual interaction with patients
• Greater patient knowledge of and active participation in their care	• Fewer immediate rewards

EVIDENCE-BASED PRACTICE

As a professional nurse, it's imperative that you provide the best possible care. But how do you know if what you're doing is the BEST for your patients? As a student, you acquire knowledge from textbooks and teachers. In the clinical setting, you gain knowledge and expertise from your personal experiences and patient preferences. Yet you must be conscious that basing your practice only on traditional practices or authority figures may lead to erroneous thinking. All nurses must be responsible for keeping their knowledge base accurate and updated.

Evidence-based practice is defined as the conscientious, explicit, and judicious use of the current best evidence when making decisions about the care of individual patients. In recent years, there has been an enormous increase in medical and nursing information. Using this knowledge to influence bedside practice so that nurses and physicians base their care on a sound rationale is at the forefront of evidence-based practice.

Evidence-based practice includes questioning why nurses are implementing some practices and not others. For example, nursing practice in wound care has changed dramatically in the past two decades. Twenty years ago, it was common practice to put sugar, Maalox, and heat lamps on open wounds; today, the scientifically based method to promote wound healing is to use colloidal dressings.

Nurses must ask difficult questions related to the risks and benefits associated with costly interventions or treatments. Do the nursing actions improve patient outcomes? Asking pertinent questions will help us determine the right course of action. Questions may include:
- Who determined the basis for this treatment?
- What's the rationale for making this decision?
- What are the clinical implications of this practice?

- Why is this being done, and why is it being done this way?
- Could it be done better, more efficiently, or more cost-effectively?
- Are these the highest achievable outcomes?

Ideally, nursing practice should be based on valid research, which nurses should be able to critique and integrate into their practice (the Internet is a valuable resource for performing literature searches). But, what if there's no formal nursing research on a topic? Identifying the need for research and asking "Why" are beginning steps toward promotion of evidence-based practice. Research may include qualitative studies, case studies, or an experimental design trial of a new technique or product. Remember that neither knowledge nor research is static. Research methodologies and statistical analysis procedures may be evolving as well. All types of research inquiries can be valuable in enhancing nursing's knowledge base.

All nurses should ask questions and be involved in finding answers. You'll increase your credibility with your patients, peers, and physicians when you integrate evidence-based protocols into your practice.

NURSING PRACTICE AND EDUCATION

Changes in health care practice result in tremendous opportunities for nursing education. For example, nurses in acute care need education about delegation and supervisory skills, stress management, and case management. Ambulatory care nurses need skills in assessment, prioritizing, and critical care. Professional organizations could play an important role in helping the nurse adapt to health care restructuring.

Nurses also need to develop familiarity with federal, state, and local laws governing health care delivery. This is especially important as facilities experiment with various staffing mixes, some of which may endanger patients, such as using more UAPs than registered nurses can safely supervise during a shift. Also, because some nurses have been terminated for whistle-blowing over patient endangerment and free-speech activities, there must be a drive for laws to protect whistle blowers.

The nursing profession must also develop continuing education programs to allow nurses to move from acute care to ambulatory care. Nurses need to become computer literate, too, particularly if they're involved in teaching. Computer-assisted instruction is used in 90% of programs surveyed by the American Association of Colleges of Nursing; however, computerization has barely begun in the care setting, where an estimated 90% of health care information is still paper-based.

OPPORTUNITIES FOR ADVANCED PRACTICE NURSING

The shifting trends of the health care system offer many opportunities for nursing. An increased number of advanced practice programs are preparing nurse practitioners for new roles and new settings. The greatest opportunities involve promoting health, preventing disease, and managing patients through the entire continuum of care. In the area of health promotion, programs aimed at reducing lifestyle risk factors — such as smoking cessation, exercise, nutrition, and family planning — will be areas of major growth. Other likely areas of growth include home health care, hospice nursing, and independent nurse clinics, particularly in rural and underserved areas. "Right now, people who have chronic problems have to integrate the care they receive from different providers themselves," points out Regina Herzlinger, Harvard Business School professor. Nurses could play a pivotal role in integrating patient care.

Conclusion

The coming years promise to be exciting for health care professionals. Major changes in American society and the health care arena will offer professionals extraordinary opportunities for professional growth. Nurses can greatly improve their chances of success by becoming aware of and preparing for these major changes.

References

Baldwin, D. "Community-Based Experiences and Cultural Competence," *Journal of Nursing Education* 38(5):195-96, May 1999.

Beyea, S. "Why Should Perioperative RN's Care About Evidence-based Practice?" *AORN Journal* 72(1):109-11, July 2000.

Byrne, M. "Uncovering Racial Bias in Nursing Fundamental Textbooks," *Nursing and Health Care Perspective* 22(6):299-303, 2001.

Byrne, M. Uncovering Racial Bias in Fundamental Nursing Textbooks: A Critical Hermeneutic Analysis of the Portrayal of African Americans. UMI Order # 9962688. Doctoral dissertation Georgia State University: Atlanta, Ga., 2000.

Campinha-Bacote, J. "A Model and Instrument for Addressing Cultural Competence in Health Care," *Journal of Nursing Education* 38(5):203-207, May 1999.

Clinical Evidence: *www.clinicalevidence.org.*

Coates, K. "Senior Class," *Nurseweek* 15:25-27, May 2002.

Craven, R., and Hirnle, C. *Fundamentals of Nursing.* Philadelphia: Lippincott Williams & Wilkins, 2000.

Domrose, C. "Changing Tides" *Nurseweek* 15:15-17, August 2002.

Domrose, C. "A Walk on the Wild Side," *Nurseweek* 14(17): 13-15, September 2001.

Dowdy, K.G. "The Culturally Sensitive Medical Interview," *Journal of the American Academy of Physician Assistants* 13(6):91-92, 98-99, 104, June 2000.

Duffy, M. "A Critique of Cultural Education in Nursing," *Journal of Advanced Nursing* 36(4):487-95, November 2001.

"Lack of Insurance Linked to Decline in Health," *Nurseweek* 15(11), June 3, 2002, reporting on National Academy of Sciences, Institute of Medicine: "Care Without Coverage: Too Little, Too Late," May 2002.

Lenburg, C., et al. *Promoting Cultural Competence in and through Nursing Education.* Washington DC: American Academy of Nursing, 1995.

"Nursing Shortage Contributes to Patient Injuries, Deaths," *Nurseweek* 15(15) August 2002, reporting on JCAHO report August 2002.

Spector, R. *Cultural Diversity in Health & Illness.* Upper Saddle River, N.J.: Prentice Hall Health, 2000.

U.S. Agency for Healthcare Research and Quality: evidence-based reports are at *www.ahcpr.gov/clinic/epgsix.htm*, and clinical practice guidelines are at *www.ahcpr.gov/clinic/edcix.htm.*

Role of DRGs in delivery quality

Medicare's prospective payment system (PPS) dramatically altered the U.S. health care system. Diagnosis-related groups (DRGs) provide the basis for payment to hospitals for the care of Medicare, Medicaid, and many commercially insured patients. The federal government adopted the DRG system to curb rising health care costs and to put a more measurable system of care versus cost in place. Faced with these restrictions and regulations affecting the delivery of health care, nurses are increasingly confronted with sicker patients and shorter allowable and paid hospital stays. Nurses play a key role in maintaining a hospital's financial viability in our competitive, market-driven health care environment. Documentation is crucial. Hospital executives closely evaluate case-mix because the nature and severity of overall patient illnesses plays heavily in budget projections. Nurses must continuously find ways to improve the quality of care and care outcomes while working within the ever-narrowing constraints of reimbursement.

Evolution of PPS

Charges for hospital care used to be based on a retrospective method of payment rather than the PPS used today. Hospital charges reflected what the market would bear and commonly were arbitrary, unrelated to the actual costs of delivering services. For the most part, nursing has been a nonbillable direct service that was bundled under room and board charges on the hospital bill. However, in recent years, third-party payers have demanded more explicit accounting for all services and appropriate charges for every area of health care delivery. In response, hospitals have begun to unbundle all units of service, including nursing.

As one of the nation's primary insurers, Medicare was the first to change its reimbursement method. PPS was an attempt to conserve the dwindling dollars in the Medicare trust fund set up in the 1960s to ensure health care access for America's elderly citizens.

Under Medicare's PPS, DRGs were developed to identify clinically homogeneous groups of diagnoses that use similar tests, treatments, and services and, therefore, could be reimbursed at similar rates. This federal system is now mandatory for Medicare recipients at all acute care hospitals. Besides standardizing payment, this classification system was designed to put acute hospitalized patients into groups that could be used to predict resource consumption.

At present, 511 DRGs are grouped into 25 Major Diagnostic Categories (MDC) plus one pre-MDC category that includes liver transplant, bone marrow transplant, and tracheostomy, for a total of 26. The predetermined rate of reimbursement for each DRG is based on such factors as principle diagnosis, patient age, comorbidities or complications, surgical intervention, and discharge type. Hospitals are reimbursed a flat rate based on the patient's combination of factors. Assuming patients with similar conditions and procedures will require similar care, each category of illness or treatment is assigned a DRG that's the main factor in determining reimbursement. Because DRG payments are standardized by diagnosis and treatment, hospitals can predict reimbursement prospectively, or before care is provided.

The DRG system is incongruous in many ways, the most important of which is that it doesn't consider the severity of the patient's illness. Thus, for two patients with the same illness (and therefore the same assigned DRG), a hospital would be reimbursed at the same rate even though one patient may be severely ill and need more services and a longer length of stay (LOS). DRGs are, in effect, an averaging system: A hospital loses money on cases in which the cost of care exceeds the amount paid for the assigned DRG, and it makes money on cases in which costs are less than the DRG payment. Many patients who would have been hospitalized in the past are now treated as outpatients and, conversely, only patients who meet strict criteria may be admitted to acute care facilities. Hospitals, therefore, typically have sicker patients to care for than in the past, and patient care must be managed as efficiently as possible for a hospital to remain financially viable.

How DRGs are assigned

After discharge, a patient is assigned a DRG based on the following factors:
- principal diagnosis — the diagnosis that necessitated admission to the hospital
- secondary diagnosis — all secondary conditions that exist at the time of admission or that develop during hospitalization and affect the treatment or LOS
- operative procedures — any surgical procedures performed for definitive treatment rather than for diagnostic or exploratory purposes
- age — for some conditions, a different reimbursement rate for patients younger than age 17 than for those age 17 and older
- discharge status — whether the patient was discharged home or transferred to another hospital

■ complications — any conditions arising during hospitalization that may prolong the LOS at least 1 day in approximately 75% of patients (such as diabetes)
■ comorbidity — a preexisting condition that will increase the LOS at least 1 day in about 75% of patients.

All these factors need to be considered and the presence or absence of each factor determined to identify the correct DRG.

How DRGs are used

Once the DRG has been determined, the administrator can identify further statistical measures affecting reimbursement, such as geometric mean LOS, relative weight, and outliers.

GEOMETRIC MEAN LOS

Each DRG has an assigned geometric mean LOS. The terms *geometric mean LOS* and *mean LOS* in this book refer to specific DRG statistical data for *groups* of patients. (The unqualified term *LOS* is a general abbreviation referring to an *individual* patient's LOS.) The geometric mean LOS is a statistical measure used in cost accounting solely to determine when a patient becomes a "day outlier." (See "Outliers" later in this entry.)

The geometric mean LOS is an average derived from data that indicated the mean LOS for patients with specific diagnoses or undergoing specific procedures at the time the DRG system was updated. This has four important implications:
■ The geometric mean LOS should be understood as an indicator of when most patients within each DRG *were* discharged during the period of data collection. It was never intended as a guide to determine when a specific patient *should* be discharged.
■ Current hospital stays are significantly shorter than the geometric LOS. This is due in part to other options, such as outpatient facilities and home health care for care delivery, which have become more available and desirable to the consumer. According to the Centers for Medicare and Medicaid Services (CMS) report for fiscal year 2000, the national average LOS by DRG for all categories and ages was 6.0 days.
■ The geometric mean LOS has nothing to do with the point after which a hospital loses money on a case. That point can be determined only after studying each case.
■ In most cases, a hospital begins losing money before the geometric mean LOS is reached because actual costs of caring for the patient usually exceed the reimbursement rate before this point. This is partly because hospital costs have continued to increase as the actual LOS has continued to decrease.

RELATIVE WEIGHT

Relative weight, a statistical term used in DRG reimbursement, determines the actual dollars a particular hospital is paid for a given DRG. Among other factors,

it's based on the categorization of the hospital as acute or chronic, teaching or nonteaching, and urban or rural. The weight assigned to each DRG is reevaluated and revised regularly. Because relative weights vary greatly from hospital to hospital and area to area and because of periodic revisions, they aren't specified in this book.

OUTLIERS

An outlier is a case that uses more than its assigned resources. There are two types of outliers — day and cost. Under the PPS, hospitals may receive additional payments to offset losses from high-cost cases if the costs surpass the DRG payment plus a threshold amount. The CMS is currently proposing to increase the threshold and estimates that as a result of the proposed higher threshold, total day outlier payments will equal 5.1% of total operating DRG payments. In most instances, day outliers are severely ill patients with multisystem failure. Preventing a patient from becoming a day outlier is rarely under the nurse's control.

An additional payment is made for atypical cases that generate extremely high costs (cost outliers) when compared to average cases in the same DRG. To qualify as a cost outlier in FY 2003, a hospital's charges for a case, adjusted to cost, must exceed the payment rate for the DRG by $33,560. The additional payment amount is equal to 80% of the difference between the hospital's entire cost for the stay and the threshold amount. Combined operating and capital costs for a case must exceed the combined threshold to qualify for an outlier payment.

Keys to success under DRGs

Several major factors affect a hospital's financial success under DRGs:
■ accurate coding of all medical record data upon the patient's discharge. A medical records professional must choose the diagnosis that was chiefly responsible for the admission and take into account all of the factors, such as complications and comorbidities, that will place the diagnosis in the highest-paying category. The coder depends on the documentation in the medical record when assigning the DRG.
■ effective and efficient management of the "products" of hospitals, such as hours of nursing care, laboratory tests, medications, supplies, and other services. The more efficiently care is delivered, the greater the hospital's profit.
■ an appropriate "case mix" (a hospital's mixture of patients, defined by the severity of illness and assigned DRGs). A hospital must maintain a mixture of patients with various DRGs to plan and manage resource allocation within defined reimbursement parameters.
■ using the appropriate site of care and LOS. Care will be reimbursed only if it's provided in the appropriate setting. For example, hospitals won't be reimbursed for care

that could have been appropriately provided in an outpatient setting. LOS also must be appropriate. Although patients can be discharged only when medically stable, the hospital must ensure that only necessary costs are incurred.

■ preventing complications. Because complications increase the likelihood that care costs will exceed reimbursement, their prevention is a key factor in maintaining fiscal control.

Nurse's role in a PPS

The overall impact of government regulations and third-party payers on the health care delivery system presents the nurse with challenges and opportunities. Nurses are instrumental in ensuring both the quality of care and the hospital's financial success under any PPS. They can take several steps, as outlined in this section, to exert a positive impact on a hospital's bottom line while maintaining the quality of patient care.

CARE PLANNING
The nurse must be able to prioritize and deliver care within the projected LOS, which means establishing and following an explicit care plan. Care planning is an essential means of determining goals and desired outcomes of care. Only through planning can care be managed effectively and efficiently. This book is designed to help the nurse provide quality care within the constraints of cost containment. Caring for a patient without a care plan is like starting an unfamiliar trip without a road map. You may eventually reach the desired destination, but most certainly it will involve many unnecessary detours and increased time, effort, and money. This book identifies the "destination" of care — the patient outcome criteria — as well as the most direct routes for getting there.

EARLY DISCHARGE PLANNING
The nurse must be involved in discharge planning from the moment of patient admission whenever possible. By beginning early, the nurse can help ensure that the patient is ready for discharge. For example, the nurse can emphasize patient and family education, maximize the patient's self-care abilities, and arrange for continued care, such as home care nursing or nursing home placement, when indicated.

PATIENT EDUCATION
Patient and family education is a key element in preventing readmissions. The patient's perception of quality care is also enhanced when the nurse promotes self-care and describes how to manage health problems after discharge.

DOCUMENTATION
Accurate documentation promotes communication among caregivers, maximizing the benefits of hospitalization while minimizing the LOS. Also, documentation is crucial to receiving appropriate reimbursement for services. Documenting complications and comorbidities is particularly important because they have even greater significance now than in the past.

QUALITY ASSURANCE
Quality assurance is a mandatory element that should include establishing specific nursing standards and monitoring adherence to those standards.

ECONOMICS OF HEALTH CARE
The nurse also needs to be aware of how the new economics of health care affect the professional status of nursing. This is a good time to advance the function and image of nurses as independent health care practitioners who can be judged not only on how they benefit patients, but also on how they contribute to a hospital's economic viability.

Retrospective review

In addition to DRGs, other changes in health care delivery continue to increase the pressure to provide care in the most efficient manner possible. Health maintenance organizations (HMOs) and other competitive medical plans, now a major source for health care reimbursement, have been particularly important.

The nurse should be aware of the complexity of reimbursement methods. Most third-party payers (not just Medicare) use a prospective payment mechanism to reimburse hospitals. For example, many HMOs currently pay hospitals on a negotiated rate not unlike DRGs. Also, all third-party payers are negotiating discounted rates for services provided in acute care facilities in return for guaranteeing that their subscribers will use specific facilities for their acute care needs. Such arrangements are important for hospitals because they ensure a constant source of admissions. With LOSs much shorter than they were before PPSs, hospitals must count on a stable census to ensure maximum efficiency and a constant cash flow.

For patients, incentives from PPSs to hospitals mean shorter stays and, possibly, fewer services. Because of perceptions of premature patient discharges and underuse of necessary services, state peer review organizations (PROs) were mandated to increase review of care provided in acute care facilities.

This mandate has led PROs to establish explicit review criteria for medical care. Within the DRG system, however, the Health Care Financing Administration and state PROs are developing and using generic and disease-specific criteria retrospectively to determine the appropriateness of admission and discharge and the quality of care. Such information could be useful to nurses in care planning. Although PROs are reviewing only Medicare cases now, in the near future all hospital admissions, outpatient procedures, home care services, and care in physicians' offices and long-term facilities will be reviewed in a similar manner.

Nursing challenge

Today, the nurse faces greater challenges than ever with sicker patients requiring more complex care during shorter hospital stays. This book features the expertise of colleagues who understand the complexities of those challenges and offer powerful help in meeting them.

References

Centers for Medicare and Medicaid Services; Inpatient Hospital Fiscal Year 2000; Published June 2001; Short Stay Inpatient by State and National Average LOS by DRG.

Centers for Medicare and Medicaid Services; Letter on Medicare Fiscal Year 2000 Hospital Inpatient Prospective Payment System Proposed Rule, Nancy-Ann Min DeParle; File Code HCFA (CMS)-1053-P.

Dray, P.B. "Déjà vu. When it Comes to Prospective Payment, Home Health Agencies Can Learn from the Experiences of Acute Care Hospitals with DRGs" *Health Management Technology* 23(10):44-46, 50, October 2002.

Hospital and Payor ICD-9-CM 1999. Salt Lake City, Utah: Medicode Publications.

Mazzocco, W. "Close-up on Reimbursement. Key Elements of Reimbursement Coding. A Guide for Nurse Practitioners," *Advance for Nurse Practitioners* 9(9):49-54, September 2001

Tarantino, D. "Making the Most of DRGs," *Physician Executive* 28(6):50-52, November-December 2002.

NANDA, NIC, and NOC

The languages

Three standardized nursing languages are recognized by the American Nurses Association. They are the diagnoses developed by the North American Nursing Diagnosis Association (NANDA), the interventions of the Nursing Interventions Classification (NIC), and the outcomes of the Nursing Outcomes Classification (NOC). A uniform nursing language serves several purposes, including the following:

- provides a language for nurses to communicate what they do among themselves, with other health care professionals, and the public
- allows the collection and analysis of information documenting nursing's contribution to patient care
- facilitates the evaluation and improvement of nursing care
- fosters the development of nursing knowledge
- allows for the development of electronic clinical information systems and the electronic patient record
- provides information for the formulation of organizational and public policy concerning health and nursing care
- facilitates teaching clinical decision making to nursing students.

Indeed, according to Marion Johnson, et al "the provision of links between these classifications is a major step forward in facilitating the use of these languages in practice, education, and research."

NANDA

Past diagnostic efforts have been hampered by the lack of a common language for labeling nursing problems. To overcome this barrier, the National Conference Group on the Classification of Nursing Diagnoses began identifying and classifying health problems that nurses treat. That organization, formed at the first National Conference on Classification of Nursing Diagnoses in 1973, became NANDA. Periodically, NANDA releases a list of diagnoses accepted for study and clinical testing. The current list appears in the appendix.

The American Nurses Association Social Policy Statement (1980) defines nursing as "the diagnosis and treatment of human responses to actual or potential health problems." The 1995 update, Nursing: A Social Policy Statement, further states that "Diagnoses facilitate communication among health care providers and the recipients of care and provide for initial direction in the choice of treatments and subsequent evaluation of the outcomes of care." NANDA defines nursing diagnosis as "a clinical judgment about individual, family, or community responses to actual and potential health problems or life processes. Nursing diagnoses provide the basis for selection of nursing interventions to achieve outcomes for which the nurse is accountable." Translated into nine languages, NANDA terminology is used in more than 20 countries

However, nurses have had difficulty with NANDA terminology. Many are frustrated by the categories' complexity, esoteric language, vagueness, wordiness, and differing levels of abstraction; some NANDA diagnostic labels aren't clinically useful. Because the clinical experts who wrote the care plans in this book found some NANDA diagnoses useful and others not, the editor made the following decisions:

- This book identifies nursing diagnoses using NANDA terminology whenever possible. If a diagnosis couldn't be found on the list to fit a patient problem that nurses treat independently, a new diagnosis was created.
- The official list is alphabetized by basic concept first, followed by modifiers, if any (for example, "airway clearance, ineffective"). In this book, diagnoses are modified to reflect usual conversational sequences.
- In an effort to avoid wordiness, one such example is that "Alteration in nutrition: Less than body requirements" has been replaced with "Nutritional deficit."

Two related issues have provoked substantial controversy within the nursing diagnosis community — the scope of nursing diagnosis and the possible renaming of medical diagnoses with nursing diagnostic language. This controversy stems, in part, from the continued difficulty nurses face in articulating the dimensions of their practice and, particularly, differentiating it from medical practice.

Many nurses believe that nursing diagnoses should describe only the independent domain of nursing, the area of clinical judgment in which the nurse functions in a self-directed way to prescribe definitive therapy for human responses to health problems, achieving outcomes for which the nurse is accountable. Others believe that nursing diagnoses should address all areas in which nurses make clinical judgments, including those in which they carry out medical treatments. This book uses nursing diagnoses for the independent domain of nursing only.

Renaming problems already defined by other disciplines simply perpetuates the confusion between nursing and medicine. In this book, such problems are clearly identified as *collaborative* problems requiring both medical and nursing interventions. They are named with familiar terminology, such as "cardiogenic shock" instead of "decreased cardiac output," "ischemia" instead of "impaired tissue perfusion," and "hypoxemia" instead of "impaired gas exchange."

In some cases, a nursing diagnosis fits a nonacute problem but not a related acute problem, such as "deficient fluid volume." In a nonacute fluid volume deficit, independent nursing interventions, such as providing preferred fluids and encouraging fluid intake, are paramount. In an acute fluid volume deficit, however, medical interventions, such as ordering the insertion of an I.V. catheter and prescribing specific I.V. solutions, are paramount. In this book, "deficient fluid volume" is used in the first situation and "hypovolemia" in the second for diagnostic clarity. The distinction between acute and nonacute may prove a fruitful path for exploration in further attempts to increase the clinical usefulness of nursing diagnoses.

Because some nursing schools and nursing services do use nursing diagnoses exclusively, this book provides a way to adapt its collaborative-problem format to exclusive use of NANDA diagnoses. Selected collaborative problems are starred, with the analogous nursing diagnosis specified at the bottom of the page.

NIC

In 1987, Joanne McCloskey and Gloria Bulecheck led a research team at the University of Iowa that used multiple research methods to develop the comprehensive NIC, a standardized classification of nursing interventions. An intervention is defined as "any treatment, based upon clinical judgment and knowledge, that a nurse performs to enhance patient/client outcomes." To use this classification, the nurse chooses the most appropriate activities for a specific individual or family from a list of about 10 to 30 activities for each intervention. The third edition of the regularly updated classification, published in 2000, describes 486 interventions divided into 30 classes. It also includes seven domains: (1) Physiological: Basic, (2) Physiological: Complex, (3) Behavioral, (4) Safety, (5) Family, (6) Health System, and (7) Community. The interventions are based on existing nursing practice. Original sources included textbooks, care planning guides, and nursing information systems. In addition to the clinical expertise of team members, more than 1,000 nurse specialists and approximately 50 professional associations provided input.

Individual nurses are expert in a limited number of interventions depending on their specialties. The NIC represents the expertise of *all* nurses in total and thus describes the domain of nursing. It's appropriate for use in all settings and by nurses in all specialties.

Current information about NIC can be found at the Center of Nursing Classification web page at *www. nursinguiowa.edu/cnc.*

NOC

Marion Johnson and Meridean Maas led a research team formed in 1991 at the University of Iowa for the purpose of developing a classification of nursing care patient outcomes. From this research grew a comprehensive, standardized classification of patient outcomes known as NOC, which allows a systematic evaluation of nursing interventions. This classification is now being used in several clinical sites to evaluate nursing practice. It's also being used as a tool to organize curricula and teach clinical evaluation to nursing students.

The effectiveness of nursing interventions is measured by patient outcomes, which gauge patients' responses, both physical and emotional, to the care they receive. Because patient outcomes are influenced not only by interventions but by additional variables, it's challenging for nurses to determine which outcomes are affected by nursing care.

To generate the outcomes, the NOC research team first evaluated 30 potential sources (current textbooks, care planning guides, and nursing information systems) to extract concrete outcome statements. Sources were evaluated and selected based upon the following criteria.
- They presented clear statements describing specific states or behaviors.
- They included a comprehensive list of outcome statements.
- They offered measurable outcome indicators.
- They offered outcome indicators specifically designed to evaluate nursing interventions.

The first edition of this book is cited as one of the 19 original outcome data sources accepted to sample for nursing-sensitive outcome statements.

In the NOC are individual, family, and community outcomes that can gauge progress or reveal lack of progress within an episode of care and in different care settings. They were devised to be useful in all nursing settings and specialties.

New outcomes are integrated into the continually revised classification and older outcomes are revised as research and user feedback dictate. The second edition contains 260 outcomes in 29 classes. They are grouped into seven domains: (1) Functional Health, (2) Physiologic Health, (3) Psychosocial Health, (4) Health Knowledge and Behavior, (5) Perceived Health, (6) Family Health, and (7) Community Health.

The NOC is also organized by 11 Functional Health Patterns developed by Marjorie Gordon. These are the same health patterns used to organize the Nursing History in the Focused Assessment Guidelines in this book.

The research methods used to develop the outcomes and the taxonomy are similar to those used in the development of NIC. About 1,200 expert nurses from 21 specialties were asked to evaluate indicators for determining outcomes and the degree to which they were influenced by nursing intervention. Nurses in nine clinical sites, including hospitals, home care, parish nursing, nursing centers, and long-term institutional care, are evaluating these outcomes.

Information about NOC can be found at the Center for Nursing Classification web page at *www.nursing.uiowa. edu/cnc.*

Conclusion

NANDA, NIC, and NOC, are included in the National Library of Medicine's *Metathesaurus for a Unified Medical Language System,* and the *Cumulative Index to Nursing Literature.* Collectively, they reflect the practice of nurses in all settings and specialties. They are in use, together or individually, in many clinical settings to document patient care and in many educational settings to educate nursing students. Cross-linking the classifications is a milestone in easing the use of the three languages in practice, education, and research.

References

Johnson., M., et al. *Nursing Diagnoses, Outcomes and Interventions: NANDA, NIC, and NOC Linkages.* St. Louis: Mosby–Year Book, Inc., 2001.

McCloskey, J., and Bulecheck, G., eds. *Nursing Interventions Classification (NIC),* 3rd ed. St. Louis: Mosby–Year Book, Inc., 2000.

North American Nursing Diagnosis Association. *Nursing Diagnoses: Definitions & Classification 2001-2002.* Philadelphia: NANDA, 2001.

Care plans

The past 15 years have introduced far-ranging changes in the health care delivery system. Factors affecting health care delivery include decreased financial resources for hospitals, an increasing number of elderly people, a shift from inpatient to outpatient care, and the AIDS crisis. As a result, health care has changed its focus from the process of delivering care to cost-effective patient outcomes. Interdisciplinary collaboration is critical to providing optimal care while conserving financial resources. Care plans are one way of providing cost-effective nursing care.

Using the plans

This book is intended as a guide to providing quality hands-on nursing care to patients. Consequently, these care plans are designed to give you the maximum amount of clinically relevant information within a minimal number of pages. Every care plan is divided into sections, each presenting a different type of information. Becoming familiar with the plans' basic format will enable you to use their practical information efficiently. Descriptions of each section follow, along with specific recommendations for using the care plans in practice.

DRG INFORMATION

Immediately after the title of each complete clinical plan, abbreviated *diagnosis-related group (DRG) information* appears:
- relevant DRG numbers
- mean length of stay (LOS) for the disorder.

Ideally, each care plan would include the average LOS for the disorder to guide patient and family teaching and provide a benchmark against which the nurse could assess the patient's progress toward discharge. Unfortunately, such information isn't available. However, this book provides the best substitute: the mean LOS. Use this information to anticipate when teaching and discharge planning should begin and when maximum hospital benefit usually has been reached. When the patient's needs permit, plan for a LOS shorter than the mean LOS. Remember that the mean LOS relates to discharge from the hospital, not transfer from one unit to another.

INTRODUCTION

In *Definition and time focus,* the disease, surgical procedure, or patient problem on which the plan focuses is briefly discussed within a specific time frame. Surgical care plans usually cover the immediate preoperative and postoperative phases of care. Medical care plans focus on the most acute phase of the illness, the period in which the patient is hospitalized in an acute care unit.

Etiology and precipitating factors lists factors that directly or indirectly contribute to the condition's development, grouped according to pathophysiologic mechanism when possible.

FOCUSED ASSESSMENT GUIDELINES

The assessment guidelines list specific findings common to most patients with the identified condition. These are intended to give you a vivid picture of the typical patient presentation.

The first assessment section, *Nursing history (functional health pattern findings),* presents subjective and historical data organized by Gordon's functional health patterns framework. (See *Functional health patterns.*) The health patterns represent 11 broad categories within the holistic wellness-illness system. Each of the health patterns provides useful parameters for assessing any patient. Because the emphasis of this section is on definitive or common findings, only those patterns with data relevant to the condition are included in the discussion of a specific disorder.

The second assessment section, *Physical findings,* presents typical objective findings for a patient with the identified condition. Physical findings are organized by body system, an approach familiar to most nurses.

Diagnostic studies, the next assessment section, provides information regarding laboratory and diagnostic tests usually performed for the diagnosis and treatment of the specified condition. Not all the tests listed may be performed on a particular patient; individual factors affect what's actually ordered. However, the astute nurse is aware of the significance of studies and tests pertaining to the patient's condition and, when indicated, collaborates with the physician to select such studies.

Finally, *Potential complications* lists the condition's most common complications. Because promoting wellness and preventing illness are a significant part of nursing practice, the nurse must be aware of potential complications to intervene appropriately on the patient's behalf.

NURSING DIAGNOSES AND COLLABORATIVE PROBLEMS

This section begins with a feature called *Clinical snapshot* that provides a sharp, concise picture of patient

Functional health patterns

The following health patterns represent broad categories within the wellness-illness continuum. These categories focus on a person's functional abilities.

1. Health perception–health management pattern
   - Perceived pattern of health and well-being
   - How health is managed
2. Nutritional-metabolic pattern
   - Food and fluid consumption relative to metabolic need
   - Pattern indicators of local nutrient supply
3. Elimination pattern
   - Patterns of excretory function
4. Activity-exercise pattern
   - Exercise, activity, leisure, and recreation
5. Sleep-rest pattern
   - Pattern of sleep, rest, and relaxation
6. Cognitive-perceptual pattern
   - Sensory-perceptual pattern
   - Cognitive pattern
7. Self-perception–self-concept pattern
   - Self-concept pattern
   - Perceptions of self
8. Role-relationship pattern
   - Role engagement – family, work, social
   - Relationships
9. Sexuality-reproductive pattern
   - Patterns of satisfaction
   - Dissatisfaction with sexuality pattern
   - Reproductive pattern
10. Coping–stress tolerance pattern
    - General coping pattern and effectiveness
    - Effectiveness of the pattern in terms of stress tolerance
11. Value-belief pattern
    - Values, beliefs (including spiritual), and goals

Adapted with permission from Gordon, M. *Nursing Diagnosis: Process and Application,* 3rd ed. St. Louis: Mosby–Year Book, Inc., 1994.

---

problems and the related outcomes criteria. In the left column are listed *Major nursing diagnoses and collaborative problems,* a brief itemization of key health problems that the nurse is likely to find in patients with the specific medical condition. Next, in the right column, is listed the corresponding *Key outcomes.* These outcomes, developed by clinical experts, provide specific guidelines for assessing the patient's readiness for discharge from the unit. They are particularly helpful when a rapid discharge or transfer decision must be made such as when the unit is full and a critically ill patient must be admitted from the emergency department. For critically ill patients, the criteria in this section supplement those in appendix E, Critical care transfer criteria guidelines. The criteria are intended to serve only as a guide; if a patient doesn't meet them, the health care team must make appropriate arrangements to fulfill any remaining needs.

Each clinical snapshot is followed by the main body of the care plan: the predictable patient health problems caused by the pathophysiology. Patients may have problems or be at risk for developing them. A problem is a condition with identifiable signs and symptoms that are present in all or most patients with the disorder. If the patient doesn't have signs and symptoms but is at risk for developing a disorder, the problem is labeled "Risk for."

Because nursing practice is based on both nursing and medical diagnoses, a patient problem is identified as either a *Nursing diagnosis* or a *Collaborative problem.*

Nursing diagnoses are those human responses the nurse identifies and treats independently. The nurse can prescribe nursing interventions that don't require other

professionals' approval and can assume accountability for the patient's response.

Collaborative problems are those that require the physician and nurse to work together to meet desired patient outcomes. Although the physician is accountable for definitive interventions, the nurse may initiate monitoring, implement medical orders, act under medically approved protocols, or institute measures to prevent complications.

In most plans, the most important patient problems are presented first. However, some surgical procedure plans present preoperative problems first in order to flow logically.

After problem identification, the *Nursing priority* indicates the focus for the nursing interventions that follow.

Each priority is followed by specific *Patient outcome criteria,* defined as ideal expected patient responses to the interventions, and are grouped according to ideal time periods for achievement. These criteria, based on the clinical expertise of the nurses who contributed to this book, focus on specific, measurable patient responses that can guide the nurse in evaluating care. However, these criteria are intended to serve only as a guide; individual variation is to be expected because outcomes depend on many factors.

Suggested NOC Outcomes lists NOC outcomes that relate to the patient outcome criteria. Suggested NIC Interventions includes selected interventions that relate to those discussed in the care plan's interventions.

Interventions and *Rationales* are presented in two columns. Interventions are based on clinical experience and nursing literature and thus represent a blend of practice and theory. The rationales are purposefully brief but incorporate relevant physiologic mechanisms whenever possible, along with other helpful data.

The most important interventions usually appear first. Key interventions are italicized. Interventions may be independent or collaborative in nature. The nurse may initiate independent functions according to the terms of professional licensure and the particular state's nurse practice act. Another health care provider, typically a physician, initiates collaborative functions. However, whether acting under direct or indirect supervision or according to protocol, the nurse must use sound nursing judgment when carrying out a collaborative function.

Nurses have long recognized that patients respond best to care that takes their personal characteristics and preferences into consideration. Consequently, space is provided at the end of each problem section for additional individualized interventions.

DISCHARGE PLANNING
The next section of the care plan includes three guides for planning discharge and documenting care: the *Discharge checklist*, *Teaching checklist*, and *Documentation checklist*.

The *Discharge checklist*, developed by clinical experts and a discharge planning expert, provides a brief summary of items that should be considered when planning for discharge.

The *Teaching checklist* ensures that the patient's and family's learning needs related to the condition have been considered. Ideally, teaching should begin on or before admission and continue throughout the patient's hospital stay and convalescence. Teaching interventions reflect only what may be reasonable to accomplish in a short period of time. Interventions related to teaching are interwoven throughout the plans or included in a special "Deficient knowledge" problem. (Refer to the "Knowledge deficit" care plan, page 129, for general teaching information.) The nurse can expect that various health care professionals, such as dietitians, physicians, clinical specialists, and social workers, will be responsible for different aspects of patient teaching, in addition to that which the nurse provides.

Finally, the *Documentation checklist* provides a summary of items that should appear in the patient record. Changes in health care payment systems and requirements of the Joint Commission on the Accreditation of Healthcare Organization make thorough documentation more essential than ever. Accurate documentation also helps protect the nurse in the event of case-related litigation. However, now, as always, the best way to avoid legal problems is to maintain high standards of care, impeccable professionalism, and warm, caring relationships with patients.

ASSOCIATED CARE PLANS AND REFERENCES
Finally, each care plan concludes with a list of *Associated care plans,* which refers you to related plans found elsewhere in this book, and *References,* which can help you seek further information.

Organization of the book
This book presents two types of plans: general care plans and care plans for specific disorders. The general plans provide detailed interventions for common patient problems, such as pain (acute or chronic), knowledge deficit, grieving, and dying. They're designed to be used with the diagnosis- or procedure-based comprehensive plans that constitute the main portion of the book. The plans for specific disorders contain the depth of detail appropriate for education and reference.

When using any of these care plans in clinical practice, you may benefit from closely reading the plan first. Thereafter, you can refer to the plan each shift, addressing problems and documenting interventions in the nurse's notes. Before the patient is discharged, you can review the appropriate sections and evaluate all teaching and documentation, using the checklists as guides.

Clinical pathways

The clinical pathway system is one approach to providing outcome-driven, interdisciplinary health care. The pathway documents the care plan and expected patient outcomes within a given time frame. Providers can track variances from the planned outcome and make needed adjustments to improve future outcomes.

First introduced as a case management tool in the mid-1980s, this system is known by a variety of names: critical paths, practice guidelines, clinical guidelines, clinical protocols or algorithms, and practice guidelines, among others. This book uses the term *clinical pathway* and presents pathways for selected disorders.

Benefits of clinical pathways

A clinical pathway tracks patient progress in a managed-care system and outlines the typical course of care for patients with similar, uncomplicated problems. It functions as a blueprint or map of the key events a patient might experience during care, organized according to time and tailored to a particular facility. This approach focuses on patient outcomes and includes only the most important steps in care. It serves as a clear, compact practice pattern, reminding clinicians of the most current guidelines for care. It promotes critical thinking, enhances collaboration among disciplines, provides optimal patient outcomes, and saves money.

Complement to care plans

The clinical pathway is a logical evolution of the nursing care plan because it integrates traditional care plans with a focus on outcomes and interdisciplinary collaboration. Clinical pathways may include nursing diagnoses, but many don't, so although collaborative nursing actions are included, independent nursing interventions may not be. In addition, by definition a clinical pathway for a clinical population doesn't reflect comorbidities (coexisting clinical problems). To reflect clinical problems not included in the pathway, the nurse can use a standard pathway plus individualized nursing diagnoses. A pathway can thus complement or replace the nursing care plan.

Best care, lowest cost

The goal of a clinical pathway system is to plan for the best care at the lowest cost by increasing collaboration and efficiency among clinicians and across disciplines,

promoting timely use of hospital resources, reducing system breakdowns, and focusing the health care team's attention on important aspects of care and the most current interventions likely to have a positive impact on patient outcomes. This system enhances collaboration by improving communication and helping team members understand the intricacies of patient care and the pattern of progress for specific groups of patients. This outcomes-driven system helps health care providers offer consistent patient care and collect data for continuous quality improvement. The pathway can also serve as a streamlined documentation tool.

Contents

The contents of clinical pathways are similar among institutions nationwide, but the organization of the contents may differ. Typically, the clinical pathway format consists of a time frame across the top of the page, with categories of data in a column along the left margin. The time frame may be measured in hours, days (the most common), weeks, or stages of care. The categories usually include assessments, tests, medications, other treatments, nutrition, activity, teaching, and discharge planning. The intersection of these two frames provides activities sequenced in the most logical order and interventions specific for each day.

The clinical pathway for a particular patient is kept in a convenient location for all health care team members to use. One of the benefits of the clinical pathway is that it can be used on every shift to plan and monitor care. Specifically, the pathway can answer ongoing questions the nurse or other clinician has, including:
- What should be happening this shift?
- What's really happening?
- What isn't being done and why?
- How should the problem be fixed?
- Who will do it and when?

For peak effectiveness, a clinical pathway is used as part of the overall system of patient care. This shift from activities to outcomes in providing care requires a long-term commitment to improve patient care. (See *Elements of clinical pathway–based patient care,* page 20.)

The clinical pathway can serve as a streamlined interdisciplinary documentation tool; activities can be checked off as they're performed. The pathway also serves as the basis for documentation by exception, a method that emphasizes abnormal findings, thereby eliminating repetitive narrative notes about normal find-

---

Elements of clinical pathway–based patient care

- Clinical pathways are designed by a multidisciplinary team of health care professionals representing all the disciplines involved in caring for the patient for whom the pathway is being designed.

- Clinical pathways are considered a description of the important interventions of care the health care team believes will achieve the optimal outcomes (maximum quality and minimum cost).

- Variances from the pathway are expected and considered desirable when warranted by the patient's clinical condition.

- Pathways are used by all clinicians to guide patient management decisions and are readily accessible to them throughout the episode of care.

- Pathways are integral to the process of patient care and add value to the patient care experience for caregivers and patients.

- Pathway variance data are correlated with patient outcome data and used to identify system breakdowns that require improvement to constantly improve patient care activities.

- Clinical pathways are regularly updated with the publication of new clinical practice guidelines, research studies, and other relevant practice parameters to ensure that they reflect the best available knowledge about caring for patients.

---

ings. Variances from the projected pathway can then be summarized for quality reviews.

Developing a pathway

The process of developing a clinical pathway begins with the formation of a health care team, made up of professionals from all disciplines involved in a particular area of care. The team identifies the types of patients who require significant resources. Usually, this population is characterized by high cost, high volume, or high risk. The team may also target such populations to decrease variability in physician practice. Note that the clinical pathway approach isn't used for patients with comorbidities, complex medical issues, or unpredictable outcomes.

Pathway-related software and other products are commercially available. The committee needs to decide whether the cost of research, development, and implementation of their own programs outweighs the purchase price and availability of packaged programs. If the team decides to proceed, it either creates pathways itself according to the following procedure or selects ready-made pathways based on a similar procedure.

Next, the team gathers information from such sources as professional literature, chart analysis, insurance reimbursement tables, and physician practice patterns.

Ideally, the team uses benchmarks, which have been identified as models of the most effective and efficient practices. Major types of benchmark data include community-based practice, research literature (especially useful because it summarizes a range of expert opinions), information from professional associations, and health care vendor studies. With these resources, team members identify desirable outcomes that represent realistic and measurable patient behaviors, and together the team determines the best way to manage that type of pa-

tient. After testing the pathway in a pilot program, the team revises it and then implements its system-wide.

Evaluating a pathway's effectiveness

Many factors are used to evaluate a pathway's effectiveness. An effective plan's organizational outcomes should include a decrease in length of stay (LOS) and patient charges. Postdischarge complications, as measured by LOS, emergency department visits, or hospital readmissions for the same disorder should decrease or at least remain the same. Finally, patient and clinician satisfaction should increase.

Patient teaching

Patient teaching is a crucial aspect of a clinical pathway. Ideally, the patient and family receive a simplified version of the pathway, which the nurse reviews with the patient daily. Standardized teaching protocols, described in the pathway, give the nurse detailed guides to teaching for both current and discharge needs. The nurse should review printed handouts with the patient and his family before discharge. Shorter LOSs make patient-teaching aids especially important because the patient may not be recovered enough at discharge to be ready for teaching. The nurse can review the handouts with family members, and the handouts can serve as a reference once the patient returns home.

Variances

A variance is a deviation from the clinical pathway that causes a delay in achieving an expected outcome. It's detected when the patient doesn't progress as expected or when an expected outcome isn't achieved. Because documenting and analyzing every single variance is time-consuming and isn't cost-effective, only significant variances — such as those that will prolong LOS, increase cost of care, or interfere with achieving expected outcomes — are tracked.

There are three different types of variance: patient, clinician, and system. A patient variance is a complication that affects care or discharge, such as a patient on a ventilator who develops pneumonia. A clinician variance is an intervention that isn't ordered (for example, a physician's failure to order oxygen therapy to be discontinued when it's no longer needed). A system variance is usually an interdepartmental problem that prolongs a stay such as the inability to schedule diagnostic testing on weekends.

It's important to detect, analyze, and correct variances, both for individual patients and for groups of patients. A three-step system is used to record and analyze variances. The bedside nurse first identifies and documents the variance, either on the clinical pathway or, more commonly, on a separate variance form. This allows for prompt intervention in the clinical setting. Next, the person in charge of the pathway system analyzes problems for groups of patients, providing management with data to eliminate system breakdowns. Finally, the interdisciplinary team that developed the pathway examines periodic reports and may revise the pathway if needed. Pathways are also updated regularly to incorporate developments in medical knowledge. In this way, the data serve as the basis for continual quality improvement. Variance analysis is the key for fine-tuning the pathway and the system.

Implementation

To date, nursing literature has focused on the benefits of using pathways and the steps taken to construct them. Relatively little information is available on critical items to include in the pathways and the process of defining outcomes, variance measures, or implementation difficulties.

Acceptance of the pathway system by the medical community is crucial. In addition to resistance by physicians, other potential causes of breakdown include lack of interdisciplinary acceptance, lack of leadership (especially failure to define clear goals), and unrealistic time frames for designing and implementing pathways.

Conclusion

Clinical pathways are evolving. Their widespread use in hospitals nationwide marks a growing awareness that health care delivery has changed dramatically in the last 15 years. Clinicians' acceptance of patient care systems based on clinical pathways highlights their growing

awareness that collaboration is the keystone of optimal patient care.

References

Ellershaw, J. "Clinical Pathways for Care of the Dying: An Innovation to Disseminate Clinical Excellence," *Journal of Palliative Medicine* 5(4):617-21, August 2002.

Pace K.B., et al. "Barriers to Successful Implementation of a Clinical Pathway for CHF," *Journal for Healthcare Quality* 24(5):32-38, September-October 2002.

General care plans

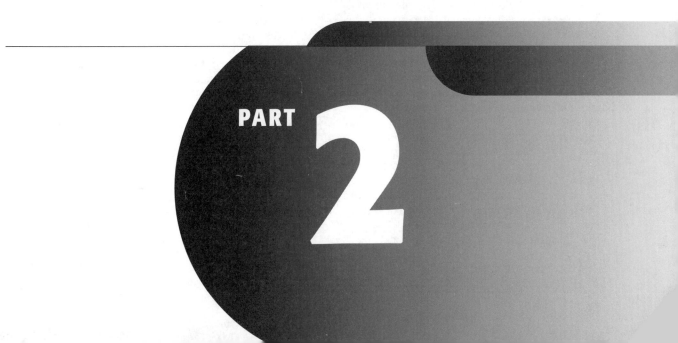

PART

2

Acute alcohol withdrawal

Introduction

DEFINITION AND TIME FOCUS

Acute alcohol withdrawal is a toxic, life-threatening result of alcohol abuse or alcoholism. The *Diagnostic and Statistical Manual of Mental Disorders*, Fourth Edition-Text Revision (*DSM-IV-TR*), lists two alcohol withdrawal syndromes: alcohol withdrawal and alcohol withdrawal delirium.

Alcohol withdrawal symptoms develop 6 to 8 hours after the last drink, peak after 24 hours, and rapidly subside in 48 hours. Early signs of alcohol withdrawal include an increase in vital signs (temperature, heart rate, respirations, and blood pressure), anxiety, tremulousness, anorexia, nausea and vomiting, diaphoresis, hyperreflexia, insomnia, and possible seizure activity.

Alcohol withdrawal can progress to alcohol withdrawal delirium, also known as delirium tremens. Alcohol withdrawal delirium develops approximately 48 to 72 hours after the last drink, peaks in 2 to 3 days, and subsides in 3 to 5 days.

The severity of symptoms experienced during the detoxification process depends on the length and extent of the drinking problem. Symptoms of alcohol withdrawal delirium include a continuation of many of the same symptoms seen in alcohol withdrawal, such as anxiety, diaphoresis, tachycardia, hypertension, and possible seizure activity. In addition, the patient experiences disorientation and severe perceptual disturbances such as visual, tactile, or auditory hallucinations. Paranoid delusions and agitated behavior are also common. Alcohol withdrawal delirium is a medical emergency, with a mortality of 5% to 10%, even if treated. Causes of death during alcohol withdrawal delirium may be cardiac or respiratory failure, peripheral vascular collapse, hyperthermia, dehydration, or liver disease.

Costs for treating acute alcohol withdrawal varies with the treatment setting. The current trend is to treat patients with mild to moderate withdrawal in outpatient ambulatory settings; whereas patients with more significant symptoms are treated in inpatient acute care settings, which are considered to be the safest for detoxification. The inpatient acute care settings generally use the pharmacologic approach to detoxification (medical detoxification), as opposed to nonpharmacologic treatment (nonmedical detoxification).

A holistic approach to nursing care, including attention to the body, mind, and spirit, is optimal for the patient experiencing alcohol withdrawal. The patient's dignity must be maintained while you care for physical and psychological disturbances in functional health patterns. This care plan focuses on the patient admitted to the acute care setting for the detoxification process, which includes alcohol withdrawal and possibly alcohol withdrawal delirium. The time frame is generally 3 to 5 days. (See *Clinical snapshot: Acute alcohol withdrawal,* page 26.)

ETIOLOGY AND PRECIPITATING FACTORS

Ethyl alcohol (ethanol) is absorbed directly into the bloodstream from the stomach and small intestine. Most of the alcohol (95%) is metabolized in the liver, with the remaining amount (5%) excreted through the lungs, kidneys, and skin. The liver enzyme dehydrogenase oxidizes alcohol to the acetaldehyde level, then to acetic acid. Finally, acetic acid is converted to carbon dioxide and water through the citric acid cycle.

Alcohol is a central nervous system (CNS) depressant, affecting all levels of the brain. Alcohol suppresses the inhibitory neurotransmitter gamma-aminobutyric acid (GABA). GABA exerts a "braking" effect on the CNS. Suppression of GABA results in a feeling of excitement or euphoria. With prolonged alcohol use, the cerebral cortex, cerebellum, and midbrain become depressed. This can lead to depression of the spinal reflexes, cardiac and respiratory systems, and temperature regulation, ultimately resulting in unconsciousness or death.

Physical dependence on alcohol (true addiction) occurs when the CNS requires alcohol for normal functioning. When the intake of alcohol is stopped, there is a rebound effect of excitability on the CNS. Symptoms of acute alcohol withdrawal are a direct result, depending on the severity of the alcohol problem and the physical condition of the patient. Less than 5% of these patients progress to alcohol withdrawal delirium. The presence of acute injury or other medical problems such as liver disease, pneumonia, gastrointestinal bleeding, hypoglycemia, or electrolyte imbalance may also precipitate alcohol withdrawal delirium.

Focused assessment guidelines

NURSING HISTORY
(FUNCTIONAL HEALTH PATTERN FINDINGS)
Nutritional-metabolic pattern

- Nausea
- Vomiting

- Diarrhea
- Diaphoresis
- Anorexia

Activity-exercise pattern
Alcohol withdrawal
- Tremors (the "shakes")
- Malaise or weakness

Alcohol withdrawal delirium
- Extreme psychomotor agitation

Sleep-rest pattern
- Restless sleep
- Nightmares

Cognitive-perceptual pattern
Alcohol withdrawal
- Transient visual or auditory hallucinations
- Complaints of strange skin sensations (tactile halluci-nations)
- Decreased attention span
- Illusions (especially at night)

Alcohol withdrawal delirium
- Delusions (especially paranoid type)
- Hallucinations (visual, tactile, or auditory)
- Illusions (especially at night)

Self-perception–self-concept pattern
Alcohol withdrawal
- Anxiety
- Nervousness
- Fear

Alcohol withdrawal delirium
- Heightened anxiety
- Fear
- Hopelessness

Coping–stress tolerance pattern
- Possible suicidal ideation

PHYSICAL FINDINGS
General appearance
- Malnourished appearance
- Weight loss

Integumentary
- Hyperhidrosis (profuse sweating)
- Bruises, abrasions, or other signs of trauma from falls
- Petechiae
- Telangiectasis (spider angiomas)

Eyes
- Red or bloodshot sclera
- Conjunctivitis
- Teariness

Nose and mouth
- Congested nose
- Reddened nose
- Rhinorrhea
- Oral mucosa red, irritated; tongue edematous and coated

Cardiovascular
- Hypertension

- Tachycardia (irregular)
- Hyperthermia (100° to 103° F [37.8° to 39.4° C])
- Possible arrhythmias

Respiratory
- Tachypnea (rapid, shallow, depressed)

Gastrointestinal
- Nausea
- Vomiting or dry heaves
- Diarrhea
- Epigastric tenderness
- Distended abdomen

Neurologic
- Disorientation to time, place, person, situation (alcohol withdrawal delirium)
- Irritability
- Seizures (absence or tonic-clonic)
- Hallucinations (visual, auditory, or tactile)
- Illusions (especially at night)
- Fatigue
- Impaired cognition
- Memory deficits
- Speech slurred or incoherent; distortions in volume and sound
- Decreased attention span
- Thought blocking

Musculoskeletal
- Coarse tremors (eyelids, tongue, or hands)
- Ataxia (unsteady gait)
- Weakness

DIAGNOSTIC STUDIES
Diagnostic studies are done to evaluate the severity of withdrawal and the extent of organ involvement.
Laboratory data
- Breathalyzer test — determines the blood alcohol level upon admission
- Toxicology screening (blood and urine) — identifies the types and levels of drugs present, including alcohol (polydrug use is common)
- Serum electrolyte tests — may indicate electrolyte alterations such as hypomagnesemia (resulting in seizures) or hypokalemia (resulting in arrhythmias)
- Serum glucose level — may indicate hypoglycemia, since alcohol disrupts gluconeogenesis and depletes liver glycogen stores (symptoms of hypoglycemia can be mistaken for intoxication)
- Complete blood count — may indicate anemia or infection, which can potentiate the state of withdrawal in developing delirium; the mean corpuscle value is elevated with alcohol abuse
- Liver function tests including gamma — glutamyltransferase, aspartate aminotransferase, alanine aminotransferase, alkaline phosphatase, and bilirubin-elevated levels of these liver enzymes help identify the degree of liver involvement

General care plans

- Serum folic acid (folate) level — may indicate a nutritional deficit, which is common in alcoholics
- HIV testing — indicates the presence of HIV, especially relevant if the patient is abusing intravenous drugs

Diagnostic procedures

- Electrocardiogram — an arrhythmia can result from stress of the withdrawal process, electrolyte imbalance, or cardiomyopathy
- Pulse oximetry — decreased blood oxygen saturation can lead to cerebral hypoxia, exacerbating the symptoms of withdrawal
- EEG — may indicate abnormal brain wave pattern
- Chest X-ray — may indicate an infectious process such as pneumonia, predisposing the patient to delirium
- Computerized tomography scan or magnetic resonance imaging — used to screen for head trauma

- Stool evaluation — to test for occult blood

POTENTIAL COMPLICATIONS

- Arrhythmia (related to electrolyte imbalance)
- Heart failure
- Seizures (absence and tonic-clonic)
- Hypoglycemia (related to liver involvement)
- Hepatic failure
- Cardiomyopathy
- Trauma (from falls)
- Immune system impairment
- Infections (such as pneumonia)
- Gastrointestinal bleeding
- Wernicke's encephalopathy
- Korsakoff's syndrome

CLINICAL SNAPSHOT

Acute alcohol withdrawal

Major nursing diagnoses	Key patient outcomes
Risk for injury	Remain free from injury.
Imbalanced nutrition: Less than body requirements	Eat a balanced diet with sufficient vitamins and nutrients for physiological needs.
Disturbed sensory perception (visual, auditory, or tactile)	Correctly interpret environmental stimuli.
Disturbed thought processes	Verbalize a feeling of safety.

Additional nursing diagnoses may include family processes, dysfunctional: alcoholism, hopelessness, ineffective individual coping (ineffective denial), risk for suicide, risk for trauma, and risk for violence (other-directed).

Nursing diagnosis

Risk for injury related to the abrupt withdrawal of alcohol

NURSING PRIORITIES

- Maintain patient's physical safety.
- Be alert for changes in status that may indicate development of complications.

PATIENT OUTCOME CRITERIA

Throughout the length of stay, the patient will:
- remain free from injury.
- maintain stable vital signs
- show no evidence of complications of withdrawal, such as seizures or infection.

INTERVENTIONS	RATIONALES
1. *Upon admission, make sure the patient can maintain an open airway.* *	1. The primary focus of care for the patient experiencing alcohol withdrawal or alcohol withdrawal delirium is on physical needs. Airway maintenance is essential to life.

---

*Italics indicate key interventions.

2. *Perform a baseline assessment of vital signs. Monitor vital signs every 15 minutes until stable, and then as ordered.*

2. Baseline assessment is essential to know what's normal for the patient and allow early detection of abnormalities. Frequent monitoring helps detect changes resulting from agitation, or other complications, such as hypertension, infection, circulatory collapse, or hyperthermia. Treatment may be based on changes in blood pressure readings.

3. *Complete a head-to-toe physical examination.* Complete the Clinical Institute Withdrawal Assessment-Alcohol, revised (CIWA-Ar), or other tool based on physical parameters of withdrawal (vital signs, diaphoresis, tremors, ataxia, GI disturbance, restlessness, anxiety, size and reactivity of pupils, and seizure activity).

3. The CIWA-Ar is a specific tool to quantify the severity of withdrawal. Evaluation of the physical parameters assists in assessing the degree of withdrawal and avoiding overmedication.

4. *When the patient is conscious, perform a mental status examination.* Assess level of orientation to person, place, time, and situation. Assess pattern of alcohol and other drug use. Determine amount and time of last drink. Determine if there are any complicating illnesses.

4. The mental status examination will determine orientation. Awareness of the pattern of alcohol and drug use allows prediction of problem areas. The presence of other physical illnesses may affect the severity of the withdrawal process.

5. Place patient in private room close to the nurse's station. Check on patient every 15 minutes. If needed, have a staff member assigned one-on-one with the patient.

5. The patient's condition may change rapidly. Increased monitoring will help decrease the risk of injury. The presence of another person has a calming effect.

6. Give sedating medication (for example, a benzodiazepine such as chlordiazepoxide [Librium]) on a decreasing dose schedule, as ordered. Check pulse, blood pressure, and presence of tremors before administering.

6. Sedating medication has a calming effect on the CNS. Such medication prevents or reduces agitation and exhaustion, and promotes sleep. Vital signs are checked before administration to avoid oversedation. Use of the CIWA-Ar can help reduce overmedication.

7. If blood pressure is dangerously high, give clonidine (Catapres) or other antihypertensive medication as ordered.

7. The blood pressure will rise because of CNS stimulation when alcohol (a CNS depressant) is no longer being ingested. In some patients, it may rise dangerously.

8. *Place patient on seizure precautions* according to your facility's policy. Give phenytoin (Dilantin) or other anticonvulsant medication, as ordered. Monitor magnesium level and administer magnesium sulfate, as ordered.

8. These interventions will prevent or control seizure activity. Low serum magnesium level potentiates seizure activity.

9. If possible, offer complementary therapies, such as warm herbal tea (chamomile) or therapeutic massage.

9. These therapies help promote rest and sleep without the use of medications.

10. *Use protective devices or restraints only when less restrictive measures have been tried,* in accordance with your facility's policy. Ensure that the restraints are applied properly, and check circulation and respirations on a regular schedule. Document the patient's response.

10. Restraints may be necessary to protect the patient from harming self or others. The least restrictive treatment that will protect the patient should be used. Restraints may increase agitation.

11. Additional individualized interventions: _____

11. Rationales: _____

General care plans

Nursing diagnosis
Imbalanced nutrition: Less than body requirements related to lack of food intake

NURSING PRIORITIES
- Ensure adequate intake of nutrients.
- Be alert for changes in nutritional status (body weight and fluid intake).

PATIENT OUTCOME CRITERIA
Through the length of stay, the patient will:
- maintain body weight and fluid hydration at acceptable levels
- eat a balanced diet with sufficient vitamins and nutrients for physiological needs
- maintain electrolyte balance within normal limits.

INTERVENTIONS

1. *Assess weight upon admission and daily* while hospitalized.

2. *Assess appetite and GI tolerance.* Inquire as to food preferences, considering patient's culture and background.

3. *Give the patient a high-protein diet*, as ordered.

4. *Encourage oral fluids if* the patient is dehydrated. Give water or fruit juice instead of caffeinated beverages or drinks high in sugar. Administer I.V. fluid replacement, as ordered. Maintain accurate intake and output. Document every 2 to 4 hours.

5. Give supplemental vitamin therapy as ordered. This will include multivitamins, folic acid, and thiamine (vitamin B_1). Give thiamine before glucose loading.

6. *Offer clear liquids or soft, bland, cold foods if the patient has gastric distress.* Give attapulgite (Kaopectate) or similar medications, as ordered, for diarrhea. Also give antacids or antiemetics as needed and ordered.

RATIONALES

1. Baseline assessment is essential to determine what is normal for the patient. Daily weight facilitates determination of fluctuations.

2. This information is part of baseline assessment. Considering the patient's preferences, culture and background offers a holistic approach to care.

3. A diet high in protein will help reverse the effects of malnutrition.

4. In mild withdrawal, only oral fluids are needed. In more severe withdrawal, fluid loss through diaphoresis, vomiting, diarrhea, or hyperthermia may necessitate I.V. fluid replacement. Fluid retention may occur as blood alcohol levels fall. Overhydrating the patient could result in heart failure. Caffeinated drinks or drinks high in sugar content can cause dehydration because of increased urination.

5. Alcohol interferes with absorption of vitamins, especially the B vitamins. Lack of thiamine can lead to Wernicke's encephalopathy. Thiamine is necessary for metabolism of glucose. If glucose is given without supplemental thiamine, severe and irreversible brain damage can result.

6. These types of foods are easier to digest and will decrease gastric distress. Antidiarrheal medication will help decrease gastric motility. Antacids decrease gastric acidity, and antiemetics help control nausea.

7. Observe for signs and symptoms of hypoglycemia. Administer parenteral dextrose, if ordered. Offer the patient orange juice, Gatorade, or other carbohydrate solutions if tremulous.

7. Alcohol depletes the liver's glycogen stores. Intake of carbohydrates will stabilize blood sugar and decrease tremulousness that accompanies hypoglycemia.

8. Give magnesium sulfate, as ordered.

8. Magnesium sulfate increases the effectiveness of thiamine, and helps raise the seizure threshold.

9. Additional individualized interventions: _____

9. Rationales: _____

> **Suggested NIC Interventions**
> *Fluid monitoring; Nutritional monitoring; Nutrition management; Weight gain assistance*

> **Suggested NOC Outcomes**
> *Nutritional status: Food and fluid intake; Nutritional status: Nutrient intake; Weight control*

General care plans

Nursing diagnosis

Disturbed sensory perception (visual, auditory, tactile) related to underlying pathophysiological changes in the nervous system

NURSING PRIORITIES
- Help patient to feel safe.
- Help patient reduce or eliminate misperceptions of environment.

PATIENT OUTCOME CRITERIA
Throughout the length of stay, the patient will:
- verbalize a feeling of safety
- correctly interpret environmental stimuli.

INTERVENTIONS

1. *Provide a calm, quiet environment.* Minimize staff and visitors in the patient's room.

2. Provide a staff person to stay with the patient, as needed. Document observation of the patient every 15 minutes.

3. *Don't argue with the patient about hallucinations or illusions.* Be respectful in your approach. Reorient the patient to reality as needed.

4. *Explain reasons for medications* and provide anticipatory guidance regarding procedures.

5. Administer benzodiazepines as prescribed, and evaluate the effectiveness of the medications.

6. *Keep room well lit*, especially at night. Keep closet and bathroom doors closed.

7. Additional individualized interventions: _____

RATIONALES

1. Decreasing CNS stimulation will decrease anxiety and possible agitation.

2. The presence of another person has a calming effect and helps maintain contact with reality.

3. The sensory perceptual alterations are real to the patient. Arguing about them displays a lack of respect for the patient.

4. This information may have a calming effect and will increase the patient's acceptance of treatment.

5. These medications help prevent agitation and possible seizure activity.

6. These activities help minimize hallucinations and nocturnal illusions.

7. Rationales:_____

Nursing diagnosis

Disturbed thought processes related to disruption in cognitive operations

NURSING PRIORITIES

- Reorient patient to reality.
- Effectively communicate with patient.

PATIENT OUTCOME CRITERIA

Throughout the length of stay, the patient will:
- verbalize a feeling of safety
- be able to express personal needs to the nurse
- verbalize a decrease in delusional thinking
- become grounded in reality.

INTERVENTIONS

1. *Perform a mental status examination* upon admission and every 8 hours, including assessment of suicidal ideation.

2. *Allow the patient to express fears regarding withdrawal.* Provide a nonjudgmental, caring approach. Reorient the patient to reality as needed.

3. *Don't argue with the patient about delusions.* Be respectful to the patient.

4. Additional individualized interventions: _____

RATIONALES

1. This examination will determine the type and the amount of delusional thinking. The patient may become suicidal due to cognitive distortions and a feeling of hopelessness.

2. Expressing feelings may lessen anxiety level, which in turn may decrease the intensity of the delusional material.

3. Delusions will lose their clarity as the patient improves.

4. Rationales: _____

Discharge planning

DISCHARGE CHECKLIST

Before discharge, the patient should show evidence of:
- ❏ stable vital signs
- ❏ stable weight
- ❏ accurate perception of reality, with absence of hallucinations, illusions, or delusions
- ❏ absence of physical complications associated with withdrawal
- ❏ ability to communicate needs to caregiver.

TEACHING CHECKLIST

Document evidence that the patient and family demonstrate an understanding of:
- ❏ physical and mental status at time of discharge

- ❐ the need to recognize postacute withdrawal symptoms
- ❐ the basics of disease concept of alcoholism and the addictive process
- ❐ the need to continue treatment in a rehabilitative program
- ❐ available support systems and community resources, such as Alcoholics Anonymous, Al-Anon, and certified addiction counselors.

DOCUMENTATION CHECKLIST

Using patient outcome criteria as a guide, document:
- ❐ mental status examinations upon admission, daily, and at discharge
- ❐ significant changes in clinical condition
- ❐ completion of laboratory tests and diagnostic studies
- ❐ vital signs and weight recorded upon admission, at regular intervals, and at discharge
- ❐ compete intake and output records
- ❐ results of daily physical assessment findings
- ❐ results of daily alcohol withdrawal scales
- ❐ patient and family teaching, including medication teaching
- ❐ discharge planning.

Associated care plans

- ▪ Anxiety
- ▪ Ineffective individual coping
- ▪ Nutritional deficit

References

"Acute Alcohol Withdrawal — Recognition and Treatment" [Online]. Available: *www.nursing.about.com/library/weekly/aa112101a.htm/* [2002, July 5].

Black, J.M., et al. *Medical-Surgical Nursing: Clinical Management for Positive Outcomes,* 6th ed. Philadelphia: W.B. Saunders Co., 2001.

Boyd, M.A. *Psychiatric Nursing: Contemporary Practice,* 2nd ed. Philadelphia: Lippincott Williams & Wilkins, 2002.

Carson, V.B. *Mental Health Nursing: The Nurse-Patient Journey,* 2nd ed. Philadelphia: W.B. Saunders Co., 2000.

Cox, H.C., et al. *Clinical Applications of Nursing Diagnosis: Adult, Child, Women's, Psychiatric, Geriatric, and Home Health Considerations,* 4th ed. Philadelphia: F.A. Davis Co., 2002.

Diagnostic and Statistical Manual of Mental Disorders — Text Revision, 4th ed. Washington, D.C.: American Psychiatric Association, 2000.

Fortinash, K.M., and Holoday-Worret, P.A. *Psychiatric Mental Health Nursing,* 2nd ed. St. Louis: Mosby–Year Book, Inc., 2000.

Frisch, N.C., and Frisch, L.E. *Psychiatric Mental Health Nursing: Understanding the Patient as well as the Condition,* 2nd ed. Albany, N.Y.: Delmar Pubs., 2002.

Ignatavicius, D.D., and Workman, M.L. *Medical-Surgical Nursing: Critical Thinking for Collaborative Care,* 4th ed. Philadelphia: W.B. Saunders Co., 2002.

Myrick, H., and Anton, R.F. Clinical Management of Alcohol Withdrawal: CNS Spectrums [Online]. Available: *www.medicalbroadcast.com/CMEReviews/pharmalcoholism/CNS200_Myrick.html/* [2002, July 11].

Smeltzer, S.C., and Bare, B.G. *Brunner and Suddarth's Textbook of Medical-Surgical Nursing,* 9th ed. Philadelphia: Lippincott Williams & Wilkins, 2000.

Stuart, G.W., and Laraia, M.T. *Principles and Practice of Psychiatric Nursing,* 7th ed. St. Louis: Mosby–Year Book, Inc., 2001.

Thompson, J.M., et al. *Mosby's Clinical Nursing,* 5th ed. St. Louis: Mosby–Year Book, Inc., 2002.

Varcarolis, E.M. *Foundations of Psychiatric Mental Health Nursing: A Clinical Approach,* 4th ed. Philadelphia: W.B. Saunders Co., 2002.

General care plans

Acute pain

Introduction

DEFINITION AND TIME FOCUS

Pain is an unpleasant sensory and emotional experience arising from actual or potential tissue damage. Pain is best prevented or relieved when the nurse continually anticipates it. Although individuals experience pain differently, pain's symbolic meaning as a danger and threat commonly heightens a patient's perceptions of it, leading to anxiety. Anxiety increases the perception of pain, thus creating a vicious cycle. Nursing interventions for pain management must address the emotional *and* physical component to pain. Sophisticated pain management demands patience, sensitivity, compassion, and a repertoire of pain-control techniques. Because of individual factors and the availability of the various pain-control techniques, the nurse must exercise keen judgment in selecting the best strategy for a particular patient at a particular time. This care plan focuses on the care of a patient with pain of sudden or slow onset, mild to severe, an anticipated or predictable end, and with a duration of fewer than 6 months. Acute pain subsides as healing takes place, making it self-limiting.

ETIOLOGY AND PRECIPITATING FACTORS

- Surgical or accidental trauma
- Inflammation
- Musculoskeletal disorders such as muscle spasm
- Visceral disorders such as myocardial infarction
- Vascular disorders such as sickle cell anemia
- Invasive diagnostic procedures
- Excessive pressure such as with immobility

Focused assessment guidelines

NURSING HISTORY
(FUNCTIONAL HEALTH PATTERN FINDINGS)

Health-perception–health-management pattern
- Acute physical discomfort, typically described as pain, pressure, tightness, soreness, or a crushing or burning sensation

Nutritional-metabolic pattern
- Anorexia, nausea, or vomiting

Activity-exercise pattern
- Intense fatigue and decreased ability to perform activities of daily living

Sleep-rest pattern
- Inability to rest or sleep

Cognitive-perceptual pattern
- Inability to concentrate

Self-perception–self-concept pattern
- Anxiety or depression

Role-relationship pattern
- Concern that others discount pain
- Decreased desire to interact with others

Coping–stress tolerance pattern
- Decreased ability to deal with frustration or other stress

Value-belief pattern
- Belief that suffering is punishment for wrongdoing or bad deeds
- Reluctance to take medication for pain relief because of religion, belief system, or fear of addiction

PHYSICAL FINDINGS

General appearance
- Tense, guarded posture
- Facial grimacing
- Crying
- Moaning

Musculoskeletal
- Muscle spasms
- Unnatural stillness
- Increased physical activity (uncommon)

Integumentary
- Diaphoresis
- Pallor

Neurologic
- Impaired concentration
- Irritability
- Restlessness

Cardiovascular
- Hypertension and tachycardia
- Hypotension and bradycardia (uncommon)

Respiratory
- Tachypnea
- Gasping

DIAGNOSTIC STUDIES

No specific studies indicate the presence or degree of pain. Various procedures may be indicated in the differential diagnosis of pain. For example, for chest pain, the patient may undergo a 12-lead electrocardiogram, chest X-ray, creatine kinase level measurements, and pulmonary ventilation scan to differentiate acute myocardial infarction from pulmonary embolism. See care plans on specific disorders for details.

POTENTIAL COMPLICATIONS
- Exhaustion
- Intractable pain

Nursing diagnosis
Acute pain related to tissue injury, ischemia, infarction, inflammation, edema, tension, or spasm

NURSING PRIORITY
Prevent or ameliorate pain.

PATIENT OUTCOME CRITERIA
Within 1 hour after the onset of pain, the patient will:
- rate pain as less than the goal level (typically less than 3 on a 0 to 10 pain rating scale)
- have a relaxed posture and facial expression
- have vital signs within normal limits.

INTERVENTIONS

1. *Monitor continually for possible indicators of pain,** including verbalization, grimacing, diaphoresis, tense posture, splinting, restlessness, irritability, emotional withdrawal, and changes in vital signs.

2. *Analyze and document pain characteristics* systematically. Use the PQRST mnemonic, for example:
P = precipitators
Q = quality
R = region and radiation
S = severity
T = time (frequency and duration).
   For severity, use a pain rating scale; the standard is the 0 to 10 Pain Intensity Scale with 0 indicating no pain and 10 indicating the worst possible pain.
– Ask the patient to rate his current level of pain as a baseline.
– Ask the patient to choose a goal pain level that allows him to eat, sleep, ambulate, and perform other required physical activities such as coughing after surgery.
– Assess pain frequency, at least with every vital sign check. Use ratings as indications of need for medication and treatment effectiveness.
– For information on assessing adults with language difficulty, see *Wong-Baker Faces Pain Rating Scale*, page 34.
– Promptly report any new or increased pain to the physician.

RATIONALES

1. The acutely ill patient may not be fully conscious because of the underlying disease or medications that blunt perception. As a result, verbal reports alone may not adequately indicate the presence and degree of pain. However, changes in vital signs don't need to be present for the nursing diagnosis of pain; physiological adaptation may return vital signs toward normal even in the presence of continued pain. Astute observation may provide ongoing protection against unreported or underreported pain.

2. Careful analysis of pain characteristics aids in the differential diagnosis of pain. Systematic analysis prevents hasty and possibly inaccurate conclusions about the quality or probable cause of pain. Standardized pain rating improves accuracy. Patient self-report is the most reliable indicator of the existence and intensity of pain in adults. New or increased pain requires prompt medical evaluation.

*Italics indicate key interventions.

General care plans

Wong-Baker Faces Pain Rating Scale

The Wong-Baker Faces Pain Rating Scale, used for pediatric patients ages 3 and older, can also be used for adult patients with language difficulties. Explain to the patient that each face shows either a person who feels happy because he has no pain or a person who feels sad because he has some or a lot of pain. Ask the patient to choose the face that best describes how he is feeling.

Face 0 is very happy because he doesn't hurt at all. Face 2 hurts just a little bit. Face 4 hurts a little more. Face 6 hurts even more. Face 8 hurts a whole lot. Face 10 hurts as much as you can imagine, although you don't have to be crying to feel this bad.

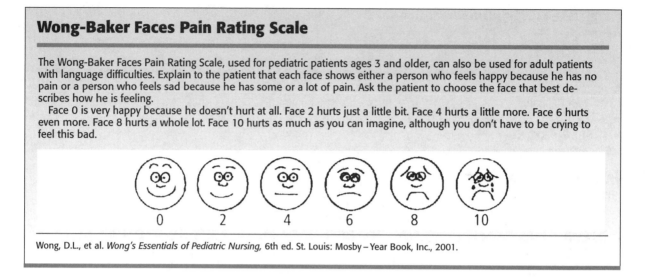

Wong, D.L., et al. *Wong's Essentials of Pediatric Nursing,* 6th ed. St. Louis: Mosby – Year Book, Inc., 2001.

3. Prepare the patient for brief, unavoidably painful experiences such as percutaneous skin puncture for arterial blood gas sampling. State clear expectations for behavior, such as "If it hurts, squeeze your wife's hand but hold your other arm still."

4. When preparing the patient for a painful experience, try to find out how much the patient wants to know. If possible, tailor the degree of detail to the patient's preference for information and the procedure's extensiveness.

5. During painful procedures, *provide ongoing support and positive reinforcement:*

– Use brief, simple directions, as needed. Use therapeutic touch, if accepted by the patient.

– When the experience is over, encourage the patient to express feelings, if desired. Convey acceptance for the way the patient handled pain, using praise generously when appropriate.

6. *Reduce factors that may increase pain,* such as anxiety that reports of pain won't be believed, a sense of isolation, and fatigue. Accept the patient's description of pain. Convey the sense that the patient isn't alone. Encourage the patient to rest sufficiently. Control environmental factors, such as noise, temperature, and lighting, when possible.

3. The psychological assault of unexpected pain can unnerve even the most stoic person and make coping with the pain needlessly stressful. Brief explanations decrease fear of the unknown and help the patient prepare for the experience. Positive suggestions provide an appropriate way to cope with the pain.

4. Patient teaching doesn't necessarily reduce anxiety; people vary in the degree of detail they find helpful. Some individuals seek information to reduce their anxiety, while others find detailed information increases their stress about impending situations. When possible, match teaching detail to the patient's preferred coping style.

5. Providing support and encouragement during the experience increases the patient's sense of security and control.
– Brief, simple directions are necessary because pain reduces comprehension and retention of information. Touch may convey comfort more profoundly than words.
– Discussing the pain experience afterward provides an opportunity for psychological integration and closure of the experience, which is necessary to "let go" of it. Conveying acceptance is particularly important for patients who scream or otherwise lose control because it reassures them and may relieve any residual feelings of shame.

6. Listening to the patient respectfully and implying an alliance against pain help reduce anxiety. Feeling well-rested increases tolerance of pain and the ability to cope with it. Environmental factors may exacerbate the pain. Constant, irritating noise, for example, may cause increased muscle tension and irritability.

7. For patients with ongoing pain, explicitly convey the goal of aggressive pain management. State the intent to prevent or "stay on top" of the pain. For acute pain that occurs most of the day, administer pain medication in "preventive" around-the-clock dosing. For acute pain, reevaluate dose and timing every 24 hours. Use a rating scale to compare the patient's current pain level to his chosen goal level as a measure of effectiveness. Once pain becomes intermittent, administer only as needed. Include low risk of addiction in teaching to encourage use of pain medication as needed.
– Use the pain rating scale to titrate dose and interval to keep rating as close to the patient goal as possible.
– Use regular pain assessment to ensure that pain is managed within "acceptable" levels, rather than allowed to become severe.

8. *Work with the patient to identify the most effective ways to control pain.* Explore various pain-control methods. Assess patient's usual pain relief measures at home. Use positive terms and the power of suggestion.

9. *Collaborate with the physician and clinical pharmacist as needed* to determine an effective analgesic regimen. Administer and document analgesics as ordered. Analgesics may include:
– nonnarcotic analgesics or nonsteroidal anti-inflammatory drugs (NSAIDs), such as aspirin, acetaminophen, ibuprofen, ketorolac, and other NSAIDs

– opioids (narcotics), such as codeine, morphine, and meperidine (Demerol). *Note:* Monitor for oversedation, hypotension, or respiratory depression. If they occur, limit the amount or interval before administering the next opioid dose. Obtain an order to discontinue meperidine within 48 hours.
– antiemetics, such as promethazine (Phenergan), metoclopramide (Reglan), or ondansetron (Zofran), to control nausea, a possible opioid adverse effect. Dose separately from opioids.

10. Use a combination of nonpharmacologic pain-control strategies:

7. Explicit goals imply that the situation is manageable, which is reassuring and reduces the fear of being overwhelmed by pain. Pain is more effectively controlled when a constant blood level is maintained. Less medication is needed to control pain when dosing is around-the-clock, rather than the peaks and valleys of dosing on an as-needed basis. In the presence of pain, risk of addiction is less than 1% if there's no previous history of addiction. It's improbable that addiction would occur with the short-term opioid use in acute pain.

8. Involving the patient in pain-control strategies promotes a sense of mastery that reduces fears of helplessness or loss of control. Using positive terms interrupts the cycle of negativity, in which pain worsens negativity and negativity worsens pain. Capitalizing on the power of suggestion creates an expectation that interventions will be successful. It may also help trigger release of endorphins, opiate-like analgesic substances that the body releases in response to certain stimuli.

9. Personalizing the analgesic regimen recognizes individual differences in pain perception and provides the most effective control for a particular patient.

– Nonnarcotic analgesics work peripherally, inhibiting formation of prostaglandins and bradykinins (inflammatory mediators that increase pain). These drugs are used alone for mild pain and in combination with opioids for moderate and severe pain. NSAIDs should be used as the basis for managing all types of pain. When used in combination with opioids, they may be dosed separately or in combination products. When using combination products, be aware of NSAID dose ceiling due to toxicity (bleeding or GI or hepatic damage).
– Opioids work by occupying central receptor sites, decreasing the perception of pain. They're used for moderate or severe pain, and they may cause sedation, respiratory depression, nausea, vomiting, or constipation.

– Controlling nausea improves tolerance of narcotic analgesics. Phenothiazines (such as Phenergan) have been found to be ineffective in potentiating analgesia and should be used only to control nausea. Meperidine has an active metabolite that's a central nervous system stimulant. It accumulates due to a half-life (15 to 20 hours) longer than the parent drug (3 to 6 hours).

10. Because various factors may cause or exacerbate pain, various techniques may bring relief. Trying a variety of pain-control measures allows for an individualized, multifaceted approach, which is more likely to be successful than a single strategy.

General care plans

– positioning (Cushion and elevate the painful area, if possible. Avoid pressure or tension. Encourage the patient to rest in a comfortable position, but also to change position every hour while awake. Explain the rationale for position changes, provide gentle reminders, and assist with movement, as necessary.)

– Cushioning increases comfort, while elevation reduces edema. Avoiding pressure or tension eliminates additional painful stimuli to an already sensitive area. Rest increases pain tolerance. Position changes improve perfusion, helping remove chemical mediators of inflammation and bringing oxygen and other nutrients to healing tissue. Position changes also help prevent complications of immobility. Because moving the painful area may temporarily increase pain, patient education, gentle but firm reminders, and active assistance may be necessary to ensure attention to this important need.

– cutaneous stimulation from massage or applications of heat, cold, or mentholated ointments

– Pain impulses are believed to be transmitted along peripheral nerve fibers to ascending spinal cord pathways to the brain. Sharp, acute pain is transmitted along small-diameter, type A fibers; whereas dull, chronic pain is transmitted along smaller type C fibers. Stimulation of large sensory (nonpain) fibers inhibits these ascending pain pathways (gate control). In addition, massage increases perfusion and lymphatic drainage and reduces muscle tension. Cold-induced vasoconstriction reduces edema. Cold can be used at any time and is especially helpful in the first 48 hours after injury. Heat increases circulation, mobility, and muscle relaxation, which is particularly helpful in decreasing painful reflex muscle spasms.

– contralateral stimulation, such as scratching or massage, when the injured area isn't directly accessible (for example, under a cast).

– Stimulation of the area opposite the painful one may provide relief, probably by gate control or triggering release of endorphins, opiate-like substances that relieve pain.

11. *Explore various behavioral pain-control strategies,* including:

11. Behavioral strategies divert attention from the pain, promote a sense of self-control, encourage muscle relaxation, and may stimulate endorphin release.

– distraction techniques, such as talking or listening to lively music

– Distraction is especially helpful for brief episodes of pain, but may increase pain perception and fatigue after the distracting stimulus is removed.

– relaxation techniques, such as rhythmic breathing, progressive muscle relaxation, listening to relaxation tapes or soothing music, or meditation

– These techniques reduce muscle tension, enhance rest, and promote a sense of well-being by stimulating the "relaxation response," which counteracts the physiologic arousal of the stress response.

– use of relaxation, breathing, and guided imagery during painful procedures.

– The image of flying and looking down on a peaceful setting is especially helpful to detach the patient from the painful experience.

12. *Minimize discomfort* from adverse effects of narcotic analgesics.

12. Narcotic analgesic use can result in constipation, nausea and vomiting, respiratory depression, urinary retention, stomatitis, and injury. (See *Preventing adverse effects of narcotic analgesics.*)

13. *Involve the family in pain-relief strategies.* Help them understand the patient's behavior in the context of the pain. Explain the rationale for pain-control techniques. Correct misconceptions, if present. When possible, have family members participate in providing pain relief such as massage. Explicitly acknowledge the difficulty in observing a loved one's pain, and provide emotional support.

13. Capitalizing on family bonds can provide a level of interpersonal comfort that exceeds what concerned, supportive staff can provide. Understanding pain behaviors may help the family be more patient, and correcting misconceptions (such as the danger of addiction) may relieve unwarranted anxiety. Acknowledgment of family members' emotional suffering conveys respect and concern for them, and nurturing family members increases their coping skills and ability to support the patient.

Preventing adverse effects of narcotic analgesics

Complication	Interventions	Rationales
Constipation	• Encourage bowel evacuation as soon as the urge to defecate occurs.	• Bowel evacuation can be delayed by voluntary inhibition of the urge to defecate, leading to constipation. Learning to defecate as soon as the urge occurs avoids this problem.
	• Encourage intake of at least eight 8-oz (240-ml) glasses of fluids daily and a high-fiber, well-balanced diet.	• Fluids promote optimal stool consistency; a diet high in fiber increases peristalsis.
	• Encourage moderate exercise, unless contraindicated, with emphasis on increasing abdominal muscle tone.	• Voluntary contraction of abdominal wall muscles helps expel feces.
	• Administer and document medications for increasing bowel elimination, as ordered.	• Stool softeners retard reabsorption of water and coat the intestinal lining. Laxatives stimulate peristalsis or add bulk.
	• Evaluate and document the frequency of elimination and consistency of stool.	• Monitoring elimination patterns determines the effectiveness of and need for continued use of laxatives.
Nausea and vomiting	• Instruct the patient that nausea may decrease after a few doses.	• Information helps reduce anxiety, which can increase nausea.
	• Eliminate noxious sights and smells from the environment.	• Noxious stimuli can stimulate the vomiting center.
	• Encourage the patient to move and change position slowly.	• Movement may stimulate the vomiting center in the medulla.
	• Encourage the patient to deep-breathe and swallow.	• Deep breathing and swallowing decrease the strength of the vomiting reflex.
	• Consult with the doctor about changing the narcotic analgesic.	• The patient may have less nausea and vomiting in response to another narcotic.
	• Administer and document an antiemetic, as ordered, using nursing judgment.	• Antiemetics decrease stimulation of the vomiting center and usually potentiate narcotic effects.
	• Evaluate and document the effects of antiemetics in relieving nausea and vomiting.	• Monitoring the response to medication determines its effectiveness and the need for continued antiemetics.
Stomatitis	• Encourage or provide mouth care at frequent intervals, after meals and as needed.	• Narcotic-induced mouth dryness may cause discomfort and contribute to mucous membrane breakdown (stomatitis). Cleanliness and moisture maintain the integrity of the mucous membrane.
	• Encourage the patient to breathe through the nose, if possible.	• Dryness of the oral mucous membrane may cause breakdown.
	• Encourage fluid intake of at least eight 8-oz (240-ml) glasses daily.	• Adequate hydration reduces discomfort and helps maintain the integrity of the oral mucous membrane.
	• Tell the patient not to use mouthwash or other products containing alcohol.	• Alcohol has a drying effect on the oral mucous membrane.
Injury	• Orient the patient to time and place, verbally and with touch, and explain the call system.	• Information provides support and relieves anxiety.
	• Instruct the patient to request assistance when getting out of bed.	• Assistance with ambulation will help prevent falls.
	• Secure the side rails and keep the bed at its lowest level.	• These measures prevent injuries and avert the possibility of the patient's falling out of bed.
	• Instruct the patient and family regarding the hazards of sedation when driving, smoking in bed, and so forth.	• Information about specific hazards helps prevent accidents and injury.

General care plans

14. If constant pain is present, collaborate with the patient, family, physician, and pharmacist to optimize pain relief through such measures as:

– continuous I.V. or subcutaneous infusion or patient-controlled analgesia devices that use bolus and continuous administration

– spinal (epidural or intrathecal) narcotic administration

– transcutaneous electrical nerve stimulation (TENS) or acupuncture

– hypnosis, guided imagery, and biofeedback.

15. Exert particular caution with spinal (epidural or intrathecal) narcotic administration. Follow agency protocol for monitoring adverse effects.

– Elevate head of bed at least 30 degrees at all times and monitor for respiratory depression.
– Double-check the dosage. Use infusion control pump with locking device.
– Reduce or discontinue the parenteral dosage, as ordered.

– Use preservative-free narcotics, such as morphine, meperidine, or fentanyl (Sublimaze).
– Maintain the catheter as prescribed by unit protocol.

16. *Evaluate and document the patient's response to pain-relief measures* hourly and as needed. Use the pain-rating scale to assess effectiveness. If the patient rates his pain higher than the goal he selected, medicate as needed. Be alert for "clock watching" for the next analgesic dose.

17. Additional individualized interventions: _____
_____

14. Persistent pain may demoralize the patient and make suffering seem unbearable. A collaborative approach using several options increases the likelihood of finding the optimal pain-control regimen for a given patient.
– Continuous infusions allow for more effective control by maintaining constant analgesic blood levels. Patient-controlled analgesia devices allow for immediate pain relief, increasing the patient's sense of control over pain and maintaining a constant blood level.
– These techniques deliver small doses of narcotics directly to endorphin receptor sites, allowing powerful pain control without the usual systemic effects of narcotics.
– TENS transmits an electrical stimulus to the painful area, and acupuncture uses needles to stimulate sensitive areas. These techniques are thought to stimulate endorphin and enkephalin release, thus providing analgesia, and block ascending pain transmission pathways.
– These techniques alter pain perception but require motivation and training, so they may not be appropriate for some patients.

15. Epidural and intrathecal narcotic techniques are used for long-term pain control in cancer and postoperative patients (such as after thoracotomy, orthopedic surgery, or abdominal surgery). They allow potent pain control with fewer adverse effects than systemic analgesics by delivering small doses of analgesic agents, such as morphine and local anesthetics, close to endogenous endorphin receptor sites.
– Head elevation prevents opioid traveling up the spinal cord to the respiratory control centers.
– Narcotic overdoses delivered by this route can be lethal.
–Central narcotic administration is so potent that continuation of normal parenteral dosage will result in narcotic overdose.
– The preservative in most commercial preparations causes meningeal irritation.
– Specific catheter care varies but includes maintenance of catheter patency and observation for catheter displacement.

16. Monitoring the effectiveness of pain relief determines the appropriateness of methods used. The main reason for "clock watching" behavior is inadequate pain relief.

17. Rationales:_____
_____

Suggested NIC Interventions
Medication management; Pain management; Patient-controlled analgesia (PCA) assistance; Analgesic administration; Conscious sedation

Suggested NOC Outcomes
Comfort levels; Pain control; Pain: Disruptive effects; Pain level

Discharge planning

DISCHARGE CHECKLIST
Before discharge, the patient should show evidence of:
- ❏ pain-relief measures effective in reducing pain to tolerable level
- ❏ stable vital signs.

TEACHING CHECKLIST
Document evidence that the patient and family demonstrate an understanding of:
- ❏ anticipated course of pain in relation to the medical condition
- ❏ all discharge medications' purposes, dosages, administration schedules, and adverse effects requiring medical attention (usual discharge medications are oral analgesics)
- ❏ nonpharmacologic relief strategies
- ❏ symptoms and severity of pain warranting medical care
- ❏ dates, times, and location of follow-up appointments
- ❏ how to contact the physician.

DOCUMENTATION CHECKLIST
Using outcome criteria as a guide, document:
- ❏ clinical status on admission
- ❏ significant changes in status
- ❏ pertinent laboratory and diagnostic test findings
- ❏ pain characteristics
- ❏ analgesic administration
- ❏ nonpharmacologic strategies
- ❏ behavioral strategies
- ❏ effectiveness of measures
- ❏ patient's and family's response to pain
- ❏ patient and family teaching
- ❏ discharge planning.

Associated care plans
- Anxiety
- Compromised family coping
- Confusion
- Impaired physical mobility
- Ineffective individual coping

References

American Pain Society. *Principles of Analgesic Use in the Treatment of Acute Pain and Cancer Pain,* 4th ed. Glenview, Ill.: The Society, 1999.

Mayer, D.M., et al. "Speaking the Language of Pain," *American Journal of Nursing* 101(20):44-49, February 2001.

McCafferty, M., and Pasero, C. *Pain: Clinical Manual,* 2nd ed. St. Louis: Mosby–Year Book, Inc., 1999.

Otis, J.A.D., and McGeenry, B. "Managing Pain in the Elderly," *Clinical Geriatrics* 9(5):82-88, May 2001.

Payne, R. "Limitations of NSAIDs for Pain Management: Toxicity or Lack of Efficacy?" *Journal of Pain* 1(3):14-18, Fall 2000

Peloso, P.M. "NSAIDs: A Faustian Bargain," *AJN* 100(6): 34-43, June 2000.

Puntillo, K.A., et al. "Patients Perceptions and Responses to Procedural Pain: Results from Thunder Project II," *American Journal of Critical Care* 10(4):238-51, July 2001.

The American Pain Society: *www.ampainsoc.org.*

The American Society of Pain Management Nurses: *www.aspmin.org.*

White, P.F. "Role of Non-pharmacologic Techniques in the Treatment of Pain and Emesis," *Current Reviews for Perianesthesia Nurses* 22(18):219-26, October 2000.

General care plans

Anxiety

Introduction
DEFINITION AND TIME FOCUS
When a person experiences anxiety, the internal message is that some part of life is out of balance. Indeed, anxiety may be a person's immediate response to an unsettling or threatening situation. According to NANDA, anxiety is "a vague unpleasant feeling of discomfort or dread accompanied by an autonomic response; the source is often nonspecific or unknown to the individual; a feeling of apprehension caused by anticipation of danger. It's an alerting signal that warns of impending danger and enables the individual to take measures to deal with threat."

Anxiety is commonly viewed along a continuum of mild (to moderate) to severe. With mild anxiety, the patient is coherent enough to vocalize and discuss what's distressing him. By relaying and working through his feelings, he can achieve change or a sense of accomplishment, thus promoting growth.

With severe anxiety, such as with receiving a life-threatening diagnosis, the patient may feel so overwhelmed or consumed that they perceive the situation to be paralyzing. Intense anxiety can manifest itself in a number of physical, emotional, relational, cognitive, and spiritual ways. For a medical-surgical patient, an intense level of anxiety may exacerbate the symptoms of an illness or cause an increase in physical or emotional pain.

Whenever a nurse identifies a patient who is experiencing anxiety, she must observe carefully for behaviors indicating withdrawal, avoidance, excessive irritability, or somatization and must initiate nursing interventions immediately. The nurse provides the opportunity for the patient to verbalize personal distress and the associated feelings and concerns connected with the distress. As a result, the patient can recognize the sources of anxiety and implement appropriate coping strategies. In addition, the nurse can utilize an important resource by incorporating family and support persons in the patient's ongoing care. Because patients manifest anxiety in a variety of different ways, the nurse must individualize care to address the specific needs of each patient. (See *Clinical snapshot: Anxiety,* page 42.)

This care plan addresses anxiety at any point during the health care experience, in any location.

ETIOLOGY AND PRECIPITATING FACTORS
- Hereditary predisposition
- Neurological or chemical abnormalities of the brain
- Fear of a known or unknown situation
- Unexpected news about one's health status
- Fear of death
- Conflict with another person
- Psychological trauma
- Inexperience or inadequate interpersonal skills
- Lack of or insufficient coping skills
- Cognitive distortions that induce stress
- Medication reaction or interaction
- Inappropriate use of drugs or alcohol
- Exposure to hazardous environmental conditions
- Medical conditions such as hypothyroidism, hyperthyroidism, hypoglycemia, hyperadrenocorticism, cardiac arrhythmia, heart failure, pulmonary emboli, pneumonia, chronic obstructive pulmonary disease, encephalitis, and neoplasms.

Focused assessment guidelines
NURSING HISTORY
(FUNCTIONAL HEALTH PATTERN FINDINGS)
A comprehensive assessment consists of both objective and subjective findings. The patient experiencing anxiety may manifest a variety of symptoms and behaviors. The patient tends to reveal individual difficulties and unhealthy coping methods during the nurse-patient interactions.

Health-perception–health-management pattern
- Difficulty understanding health problem and associated treatment
- Inability to remember or accurately verbalize health history or history of present illness
- Unrealistic expectations of treatment protocol
- Denial or uncertainty of role patient must play in effective management of illness

Nutritional-metabolic pattern
- Altered eating pattern due to level of stress
- Tendency to eat comfort foods since diagnosis was made
- Decreased fluid intake, placing patient at risk for dehydration

Elimination pattern
- Changes in elimination pattern due to level of distress
- GI irritability

Activity-exercise pattern
- Change in exercise habits because of health problem
- Increase in fatigue
- Verbalization of low energy level during the day; "I do what I need to do to get through the day"

- Difficulty sleeping due to worry and distressing dreams

Cognitive-perceptual pattern
- Ability to respond to history questions, but sometimes talking as if not thinking clearly
- Difficulty using coping methods that appeared to work in the past
- Verbalization about health using all-or-nothing thinking and worst-case situations
- Some difficulty concentrating
- Looking to family for interpretation of health care information and help with decision-making

Self-perception–self-concept pattern
- Concern expressed about health, surgery, or handling acute or chronic illness
- Verbalization of inability to care for self
- Change in usual hygiene or grooming habits

Role-relationship pattern
- Concern expressed about how illness, surgery, or both will interfere with family and job responsibilities
- Illness viewed as a burden to family, friends, and co-workers
- Concern voiced about who will do the things the patient normally takes care of at home or work while the patient is in the hospital

Sexuality-reproductive pattern
- Concern expressed about sexual functioning related to illness or surgery
- Concern communicated about ability to care for current or future children properly because of illness or surgery

Coping–stress tolerance pattern
- Tension demonstrated in body posture and positioning
- Anxious tone of voice during nurse-patient interaction
- Repeated questions asked due to difficulty processing the information supplied
- Demands made, some unrealistic, of family and staff
- Clumsy behavior exhibited because of excessive nervousness
- Unsettled behavior as noted by constant movement through fidgeting, pacing, or rearrangement of things
- Easily irritated or upset without much stimulation
- Wide range of emotions expressed, from nervous laughter to crying
- Negative thoughts and feelings communicated; difficulty verbalizing about things that are positive

Value-belief pattern
- No desire to have contact with clergy to obtain spiritual support

PHYSICAL FINDINGS
General appearance
- Lethargy
- Fatigue
- Difficulty sleeping or relaxing
- Nervous mannerisms

- Anxious facial expression
- Rapid speech
- Excessive perspiration

Integumentary
- Urticaria (hives)
- Skin irritations

Respiratory
- Hyperventilation
- Increased susceptibility to colds

Cardiovascular
- Hypertension
- Palpitations
- Coldness of extremities
- Cardiac arrhythmia

Neurologic
- Irritability
- Headaches
- Restlessness
- Tremors
- Depression or extreme negative thinking
- Tearfulness

Musculoskeletal
- Tense muscles
- Unsteady gait
- Lack of muscle strength

Gastrointestinal
- Change in appetite
- Change in weight
- Nausea
- Vomiting
- Diarrhea
- Bruxism (grinding teeth)

Genitourinary
- Frequent urination

Reproductive
- Lack of interest in sexual activity
- Impaired sexual functioning

POTENTIAL COMPLICATIONS
- Somatization
- Panic attacks
- Crises
- Depression

General care plans

Anxiety

Major nursing diagnoses	Key patient outcomes
Anxiety related to diagnostic information indicating a major change in health status	Discuss newly acquired information with the nurse, exhibiting comprehension of what it means.
Anxiety related to fear of the unknown and fear of dying	Address current fears and begin necessary anticipatory grieving.
Anxiety related to a knowledge deficit about coping with distress	Identify effects of increasing anxiety.
Anxiety related to alcohol use, illegal drug use, or reactions to medications	Verbalize if inappropriate use of drugs and alcohol is occurring.

Nursing diagnosis

Anxiety related to diagnostic information indicating a major change in health status

NURSING PRIORITIES
- Provide appropriate health information.
- Assist patient to apply information to current health situation.
- Promote patient recognition of methods to cope with health problems.

PATIENT OUTCOME CRITERIA
Within 1 week of receiving news about health situation, the patient will:
- discuss newly acquired information with the nurse, exhibiting comprehension of what it means
- verbalize an understanding about what treatment options are available and recommended
- decide on an appropriate treatment option or start the process to obtain a second opinion
- recognize the potential progression of the illness/injury/surgery process and the possible outcomes of treatment.

INTERVENTIONS	RATIONALES
1. *When the patient is ready, assist him to verbalize the concerns, issues, and feelings* associated with the change or alteration in health status.	**1.** Prior to addressing the patient's need for health information and treatment options, the nurse must allow the patient time to process this news. The patient needs to have the opportunity to integrate new information before the nurse can identify and address his teaching and learning needs.
2. Obtain written information, including diagrams of anatomy and appropriate pictures of procedures and treatments that the patient can review and have available for future reference. If this is suitable for the particular patient, supply appropriate web site information that has been reviewed by a health care professional.	**2.** Written materials allow the patient and family to have information for discussion and reference when questions arise. A packet of information may prevent confusion and misunderstanding of procedure or treatment details. When the patient is feeling anxious, it's common to forget or have difficulty recalling pertinent health care information.
3. *Discuss the advantages and disadvantages of a second health care opinion.*	**3.** A second health care opinion can promote peace of mind, decrease anxiety, detect possible errors in diagnosis, and perhaps open additional treatment options or alternative treatment modalities to the patient.

*Italics indicate key interventions.

4. When medically appropriate and logistically possible, ask if the patient would like to interact with a recovering person who has undergone and is recovering from a similar diagnosis, health condition, treatment procedure or protocol.

5. Additional individualized interventions: _____

4. The experience of interacting with a recovering person may alter positively the patient's perception of the medical or surgical experience about to be undertaken. It may also decrease anxiety and create a sense of empowerment for the patient.

5. Rationales: _____

> **Suggested NIC Interventions**
> Anxiety reduction; Anticipatory guidance; Coping enhancement

> **Suggested NOC Outcomes**
> Anxiety control; Coping

Nursing diagnosis
Anxiety related to fear of the unknown and fear of dying

NURSING PRIORITIES
- Minimize or prevent the escalation of the patient's anxiety.
- Provide a communication channel for the patient to release personal fears and frustrations.
- Help the patient to address current fears.
- Promote the overall well-being of the patient.

PATIENT OUTCOME CRITERIA
Within 1 week, the patient will:
- recognize the symptoms of anxiety resulting from identified fears
- verbalize a realistic view of health situation prior to the treatment procedures
- address current fears and begin necessary anticipatory grieving.

INTERVENTIONS	RATIONALES
1. *Monitor the patient for signs and symptoms of anxiety* while performing the nursing assessment.	**1.** Careful assessment of a patient experiencing anxiety enables the nurse to establish the priorities of care.
2. Focus discussion on types of stressors being experienced by the patient and what these stressors mean to the patient. Talk about the fears associated with the stressful feelings.	**2.** Focusing the discussion facilitates the patient's ability to gain an understanding of the verbalized fears and feelings rather than exacerbate them or create additional health problems. Talking about distress with a supportive person is one method to decrease anxiety level. The patient can clarify realistic and unrealistic perceptions and develop insight into appropriate ways of handling the distress.
3. *Discuss the patient's perceptions about death,* or misconceptions and fears related to dying.	**3.** Discussion of death and dying issues permits the patient to express self and explore concerns. Distressing feelings can emerge and be addressed with appropriate health care professionals. Patient energy can be refocused on coping methods rather than on unproductive behaviors.
4. *Address the issues of grief related* to change in or loss of functioning.	**4.** Both actual and anticipatory grieving are a normal part of handling loss. Once grief is acknowledged, the patient can attend to the grieving process and begin the journey toward grief resolution. Understanding that grief is a typical and universal response to what the patient is experiencing can be comforting.

5. Additional individualized interventions: _____ | **5.** Rationales: _____

Suggested NIC Interventions	**Suggested NOC Outcomes**
Anxiety reduction; Anticipatory guidance; Coping enhancement	Anxiety control; Coping

Nursing diagnosis

Anxiety related to a knowledge deficit about coping with distress

NURSING PRIORITIES
- Provide sufficient knowledge to promote effective coping.
- Assist patient to implement healthy coping strategies.

PATIENT OUTCOME CRITERIA
As individual readiness allows, the patient will:
- identify effects of increasing anxiety
- recognize sources of anxiety
- differentiate between healthy and unhealthy coping strategies
- learn and implement useful coping skills.

INTERVENTIONS	RATIONALES
1. *Provide the patient with information to assist in identifying the physical, emotional, and behavioral signs and symptoms of anxiety.*	**1.** Specific information on how anxiety manifests itself provides the patient with understanding and insight about what is being experienced.
2. *Assist patient to recognize sources of stress.*	**2.** Recognition of sources of stress assists the patient to acknowledge situations that promote stress. Anxiety escalation can be thwarted when early recognition of stress occurs. Knowledge about sources of stress provides the patient with opportunities to prevent self from becoming distressed or to institute early coping strategies.
3. *Explore the past and current coping mechanisms* used by the patient.	**3.** Building on current coping skills uses the patient's baseline and starts intervention from the place where the patient is comfortable. It further identifies unhealthy coping skills that need to be changed. The nurse can help the patient stop harmful behaviors and learn more useful coping skills.
4. Inform the patient about how to stop excessive worrying by limiting worry time to a specific interval of time at a particular hour of the day.	**4.** Worrying can become excessive and the patient may dwell on the negative to such a degree that unhealthy psychological and physiological changes can occur. The patient needs assistance to set limits on worrying, while still realizing that there are legitimate concerns about health that are natural to think about.
5. *Introduce the patient to new or more effective coping strategies.*	**5.** Learning effective coping strategies enables the patient to decrease anxiety and other negative thoughts and behaviors. This action allows the patient to take responsibility and participate in promoting and sustaining personal well-being.

6. Help the patient to identify appropriate resources and other sources of emotional and spiritual support.

6. Patients may need to be given information about available assistance and the potential ways to gain support. The nurse needs to facilitate the methods that the patient can use to acquire emotional and spiritual support.

7. Inform the patient of the adverse effects of using alcohol or nicotine as ways to cope with distress.

7. Use of alcohol or nicotine will initially have a depressant effect. However, the patient must use increasing amounts to achieve the same sedating effect, and increased use promotes addiction to the alcohol or nicotine and potential physiological complications.

8. Additional individualized interventions: _____

8. Rationales: _____

Suggested NIC Interventions
Anxiety reduction; Anticipatory guidance; Coping enhancement

Suggested NOC Outcomes
Anxiety control; Coping

Nursing diagnosis
Anxiety related to alcohol use, illegal drug use, or reactions to medications

NURSING PRIORITIES
- Assess for the abuse or misuse of alcohol, illegal drugs, and prescription medications.
- Monitor the actions and interactions of medications to prevent drug-induced anxiety.

PATIENT OUTCOME CRITERIA
As individual readiness allows, the patient will:
- verbalize if inappropriate use of drugs and alcohol is occurring
- recognize that a problem exists and take steps to resolve problematic drug and alcohol use.

INTERVENTIONS

1. *Assess for signs and symptoms of substance abuse* and determine if the patient uses denial as a coping strategy.

2. *Encourage the patient to talk about any drug and alcohol use,* especially if substance misuse or abuse is a means of coping with anxiety or other feelings of distress.

3. *Address the issue of self-medication* and how this practice can generate anxiety and be detrimental to the patient's overall well-being and current health problems.

RATIONALES

1. The use of denial under these circumstances may indicate that the patient has difficulty accepting responsibility for situations and taking accountability for personal feelings and actions.

2. Information about the patient's methods of coping, defense mechanisms, and high-risk behaviors can provide a background for understanding the patient's emotional state. Substance abuse or misuse problems need to be resolved prior to making decisions related to overall treatment.

3. Patients must realize that improper or inappropriate use of medications, illegal drugs, and alcohol can be physically and psychologically harmful. Anxiety is frequently an effect of drug use and a symptom associated with withdrawal from drugs and alcohol. Unexpected physical complications and dysfunctional behaviors, as well as interference with medical treatments and procedures, can occur with drug and alcohol use.

4. Ensure safety and provide support if the patient stops using any drug or alcohol. Perform appropriate treatment evaluations and make referrals as necessary. Be alert to anxiety as a symptom of withdrawal from substances.

5. Additional individualized interventions: _____

4. Evaluating and monitoring the patient enables the nurse to facilitate patient safety and develop a sound nurse-patient relationship. A strong sense of reliability and trustworthiness between the nurse and patient enables the patient to obtain maximum treatment benefits, preventing escalation of the current health condition or the development of additional health problems.

5. Rationales: _____

Suggested NIC Interventions
Anxiety reduction; Anticipatory guidance; Coping enhancement

Suggested NOC Outcomes
Anxiety control; Coping

Discharge planning
DISCHARGE CHECKLIST
Before discharge, the patient will:
- ❐ verbalize personal sources of stress
- ❐ describe the physical and behavioral symptoms of anxiety that were experienced
- ❐ state the difference between helpful and harmful methods of coping with stress
- ❐ begin to practice effective coping skills to eliminate or reduce anxiety
- ❐ acknowledge fears and concerns related to health status and fear of dying
- ❐ explain health information that focuses on current health condition, diagnosis, treatment, and related procedures
- ❐ verbalize the harmful effects of drugs and alcohol on the body and mind, especially the anxiety effect that accompanies drug and alcohol abuse
- ❐ verbalize a commitment to abstain from using drugs and alcohol as a coping mechanism to address stress.

TEACHING CHECKLIST
Document evidence that the patient and his family demonstrate an understanding of:
- ❐ physiological and psychological symptoms of anxiety
- ❐ sources of stress and anxiety
- ❐ effective coping skills
- ❐ differentiation between effective and ineffective coping skills
- ❐ preventing escalation of anxiety
- ❐ escalation of anxiety through the use of drugs and alcohol or as a result of abrupt withdrawal of the substance
- ❐ somatization as a result of increasing anxiety
- ❐ effective verbalization of feelings and personal concerns
- ❐ setting limits on excessive worrying

- ❐ information related to health condition, diagnosis, treatment, and procedures
- ❐ options, reasons for, and how to obtain a second opinion from another health care professional
- ❐ the grieving process and how grief is a necessary and normal part of potential loss or significant life change
- ❐ harmful effects of drug and alcohol use
- ❐ denial of stress and denial of the use of drugs or alcohol.

DOCUMENTATION CHECKLIST
Using outcome criteria as a guide, document:
- ❐ information provided on patient's health condition, diagnosis, illness progression, treatment options, second opinion option, and procedures
- ❐ written health information materials
- ❐ patient's verbalized understanding of health care information
- ❐ patient's stated feedback
- ❐ contact or visit from a person recovering from the same illness
- ❐ patient's baseline emotional status, including patient's fears and concerns
- ❐ manifested signs and symptoms of anxiety
- ❐ sources of anxiety
- ❐ patient's use of effective and ineffective coping methods
- ❐ patient's acknowledgment of actual or potential loss or lifestyle changes and anticipatory grieving
- ❐ patient's acknowledgment or denial of the inappropriate use of drugs and alcohol
- ❐ patient's knowledge of interaction of medications and illegal drugs or alcohol
- ❐ patient's plan to resolve drug and alcohol problem, if applicable.

Associated care plans

- Acute alcohol withdrawal
- Dying
- Grieving
- Ineffective individual coping
- Knowledge deficit
- Perioperative care

References

American Psychiatric Association. *Diagnostic and Statistical Manual of Mental Disorders,* 4th ed. Washington, D.C.: American Psychiatric Association, 2000.

Barlow, D.H. *Anxiety and its Disorders: The Nature and Treatment of Anxiety and Panic.* New York: Guilford Press, 2002.

Copel, L.C. *Nurse's Clinical Guide: Psychiatric and Mental Health Nursing,* 2nd ed. Springhouse, Pa.: Springhouse, 2000.

Frazier, S.K., et al. "Critical Care Nurses' Assessment of Patient's Anxiety: Reliance on Physiological and Behavioral Parameters," *American Journal of Critical Care* 11(1):57-64, January 2002.

Johnson, M., et al. *Nursing Diagnoses Outcomes, and Interventions: NANDA, NIC and NOC Linkages.* St. Louis: Mosby–Year Book, Inc., 2001.

Leahy, R.L., and Holland, S.J. *Treatment Plans and Interventions for Depression and Anxiety Disorders.* New York: Guilford Press, 2000.

LeDoux, J.E., and Gorman, J.M. "A Call to Action: Overcoming Anxiety Through Action," *American Journal of Psychiatry* 158(12):1953-55, December 2001.

Ninan, P.T. "Recent Perspectives on the Diagnosis and Treatment of Generalized Anxiety Disorder," *American Journal of Managed Care* 7(11 suppl.):S367-76, September 2001.

O'Brien, J.L., et al. "Comparison of Anxiety Assessments Between Clinicians and Patients with Acute Myocardial Infarction in Cardiac Critical Care Units," *American Journal of Critical Care* 10(2):97-103, March 2001.

Stuart, G.W., and Laraia, M.T. *Principles and Practice of Psychiatric Nursing.* St. Louis: Mosby–Year Book, Inc., 2001.

General care plans

Cancer

Introduction

DEFINITION AND TIME FOCUS

The term cancer refers to a group of more than 100 different diseases characterized by uncontrolled growth of abnormal cells. Each year, more than one million people in the United States are diagnosed with cancer. At current rates, it's estimated that one out of every two men and one out of every three women will develop cancer in their lifetime. While cancer can occur at any age, it remains a disease of later life, with more than 80% of all cancers diagnosed in people age 55 and older. The most common cancers in men are prostate, colon, and lung. Cancers of the breast, colon, and lung are the most common cancers in women.

Cancers are categorized according to their tissue of origin. Malignant neoplasms of epithelial origin are called carcinomas. If predominantly ductal or glandular, they are termed adenocarcinomas; if derived from a stratified squamous epithelium, squamous cell carcinomas. Sarcomas are malignant neoplasms of mesenchymal origin. Neoplasms of the hematopoietic system are categorized as leukemias or lymphomas with further differentiation by individual cell type and nature (acute versus chronic).

The stage of cancer defines the extent of tumor spread. After a thorough evaluation of multiple factors including tumor size, lymph node involvement, and metastatic spread, a numerical stage from I to IV is assigned. The lower the grade, the less extensive the disease and the greater likelihood of cure. (See *Clinical snapshot: Cancer*, page 50.)

ETIOLOGY AND PRECIPITATING FACTORS

While the exact cause of most cancers remains a mystery, risk factors can be grouped into several major categories:

- Behavioral and environmental — certain cancers are associated with smoking, alcohol consumption, obesity, high-fat diet, exposure to environmental and occupational carcinogens, chemicals, and radiation. It's estimated that 75% of all cancers diagnosed in the United States are caused by behavioral or environmental factors.
- Genetic disposition — certain genes have been isolated that are associated with a significantly greater risk of cancer. Typically, these cancers tend to develop at an earlier age and tend to be less responsive to conventional treatments.
- Health history — certain cancers are associated with prior viral infections, including Epstein-Barr virus and human papilloma virus.

Focused assessment guidelines

NURSING HISTORY (FUNCTIONAL HEALTH PATTERN FINDINGS)

Health-perception–health-management pattern
- Medical assistance sought either in response to a particular physical finding (lump in breast, persistent cough, visible blood in stools), abnormal examination result, or an overall sense that "something is wrong."

Nutrition-metabolic pattern
- Significant weight loss, anorexia, early satiety, changes in taste sensation, or reduced sensitivity to sweets

Elimination pattern
- Constipation along with abdominal discomfort or diarrhea

Activity-exercise pattern
- General fatigue and weakness

Sleep-rest pattern
- Sleep disturbed by cough, nausea, pain, or other symptom

Self-perception–self-concept pattern
- Inability to carry out routine activities that may cause questioning of self-worth and a feeling of powerlessness
- Fear related to diagnosis, physical disabilities, and possible death

Role-relationship pattern
- Inability to assume family tasks and occupational role
- Feelings of loss related to changing roles and possible death
- Loss of a significant relationship before diagnosis

Sexuality-reproductive pattern
- Inability to be sexually active without experiencing dyspnea

Coping–stress tolerance pattern
- Feelings of depression or despondency

Value-belief pattern
- Feeling of personal control over circumstances (common in the patient with an above-average chance for successful remission)
- Equating of cancer with death (common in the patient with a below-average chance for successful remission)

PHYSICAL FINDINGS

Physical findings will vary depending on type of cancer.

Cardiovascular
- Rapid pulse rate if anemia is present
- Possible arrhythmias

Pulmonary
- Cough (may be nocturnal)
- Rust-streaked or purulent sputum

- Crackles, wheezes, and friction rub in affected lung
- Hoarseness if vocal cords are involved
- Finger clubbing

Neurologic
- Headache, mental confusion, and unsteady gait if central nervous system (CNS) is involved
- Decreased mental alertness if anemia and hypoxemia are present

Gastrointestinal
- black tarry stools or visible blood from rectum
- abdominal tenderness, with or without swelling

Musculoskeletal
- Pathologic fractures with metastasis

DIAGNOSTIC STUDIES

- Carcinoembryonic antigen titer — high levels may be useful to monitor treatment responses; 50% of patients may have false-negative titers
- Arterial blood gas measurements — may reveal hypoxemia
- Hemoglobin values — may be low from anemia
- Hematocrit — may be low from anemia
- Platelet count — may be low from bone marrow suppression
- White blood cell (WBC) count — may be low from bone marrow suppression
- Sputum collection for cytology — may be useful to determine cell type (according to continuum of classes from normal to malignant)
- Serum albumin level — hypoalbuminemia may indicate malnutrition
- Serum creatinine level — indicates altered renal function related to chemotherapy
- 24-hour urine creatinine test — nutritional index that indicates changes in lean body weight when compared with individual's height; also indicates altered renal function related to chemotherapy
- Chest X-ray — may reveal tumor position; usually doesn't show early tumor involvement

- Computed tomography (CT) scan or magnetic resonance imaging (MRI) — outlines tumor's size, shape, and position
- Endoscopic examinations — useful in the visualization and biopsy of tumors. Depending on location of tumor, may include bronchoscopy, mediastinoscopy, colonoscopy, or upper endoscopy.
- Radioisotopic scans — performed to assess for metastasis
- Mammography — may reveal the presence of breast tumors or suspicious areas of abnormal tissue

POTENTIAL COMPLICATIONS
From cancer, depending on type
- Pleural effusion
- Pneumonitis
- Cardiac failure or arrhythmias
- Nerve involvement
- Cushing's syndrome
- Hypercalcemia
- Syndrome of inappropriate antidiuretic hormone secretion
- Peripheral neuritis
- CNS degeneration
- Dermatomyositis
- Superior vena cava syndrome
- Paralysis of diaphragm
- Pathologic fractures
- Disseminated intravascular coagulation

From chemotherapy
- Bone marrow suppression
- Immunosuppression
- Renal tubular necrosis
- Liver toxicity
- Cardiotoxicity
- Pulmonary toxicity
- Neurotoxicity
- Sterility (see *Chemotherapeutic agents,* page 51)

General care plans

Collaborative problem
Risk for hemorrhage related to depression of platelet production caused by chemotherapy

NURSING PRIORITY
Prevent or minimize hemorrhage.

PATIENT OUTCOME CRITERIA
Throughout chemotherapy, the patient will:
- exhibit vital signs within normal limits, typically: heart rate, 60 to 100 beats/minute; systolic blood pressure, 90 to 140 mm Hg; and diastolic blood pressure, 50 to 90 mm Hg
- have no evident bleeding
- follow safety measures to prevent bleeding.

Cancer

Major nursing diagnoses and collaborative problems	Key patient outcomes
CP: Risk for hemorrhage	Follow safety measures to prevent bleeding.
ND: Anxiety	Verbalize fears regarding diagnosis and treatment plan.
ND: Chronic pain	Express an increased sense of control over pain.
ND: Risk for infection	Display no signs of infection.
ND: Risk for peripheral neurovascular dysfunction	Have no complaints of paresthesia.
ND: Imbalanced nutrition: Less than body requirements	Control any nausea or vomiting with antiemetics.
ND: Risk for constipation	Maintain regular bowel elimination.
ND: Impaired urinary elimination	Maintain urine output.
ND: Activity intolerance	Perform ADLs with minimal assistance.
ND: Sleep deprivation	Report 8 to 10 hours of sleep during a 24-hour period.
ND: Risk for situational low self-esteem	Verbalize measures to improve self-esteem.
ND: Ineffective sexuality patterns	Discuss the desire for sexual expression and intimacy, if desired.

INTERVENTIONS

1. *Caution the patient to report any bleeding immediately,** including petechiae, ecchymoses, and oozing wounds.

2. *Initiate and monitor serum platelet counts* before, during, and after chemotherapy, as ordered.

3. *Caution the patient to use a soft or sponge toothbrush* for oral hygiene and to avoid spicy foods.

4. *Teach the patient to monitor urine and stools for signs of bleeding* and to report such signs at once.

5. *Instruct the patient to use an electric razor for shaving* or, if male, to grow a beard (unless alopecia is present).

6. Administer medications to suppress menses, as ordered. Make sure the patient doesn't use a vaginal douche.

7. *Instruct the patient to report any headaches, dizziness, or light-headedness immediately.*

RATIONALES

1. Hemorrhage may occur rapidly. The patient may be able to assume some responsibility for observing for signs of bleeding. Petechiae, ecchymoses, and oozing wounds indicate clotting problems.

2. Chemotherapeutic agents suppress bone marrow and affect platelet production. A patient with a platelet count below 20,000/mm³ is at high risk for spontaneous hemorrhage.

3. The oral mucosa may bleed if irritated from flossing or use of a hard toothbrush or a toothpick. Spicy foods also may irritate the oral mucosa.

4. Tea- or cola-colored urine or black, tarry, or blood-streaked stools indicate bleeding, which requires immediate attention.

5. An electric razor decreases the risk of lacerating the skin while shaving.

6. Prolonged menstrual bleeding may cause severe blood loss; douching may cause vaginal bleeding.

7. CNS bleeding may cause headaches, dizziness, or light-headedness. Dizziness and light-headedness also may indicate hypovolemia.

---

*Italics indicate key interventions.

Chemotherapeutic agents

Category	Mechanism of action	Cancers treated	Specific drugs	
Alkylating agents	Have ability to bind or crosslink with DNA, primarily interfering with DNA replication; most kill resting and dividing cells; cell cycle phase nonspecific	Chronic leukemias; Hodgkin's and non-Hodgkin's lymphomas; certain carcinomas of the breasts, lung, ovary, and prostate; multiple myeloma; testicular cancer, endometrial cancer; pancreatic and gastric cancer; sarcomas, malignant melanoma, neuroblastoma	Carboplatin Cisplatin Cyclophosphamide Thiotepa Ifosfamide Chlorambucil Dacarbazine Melphalan Mechlorethamine	Busulfan Temozolomide
Antimetabolites	Blocks or Interfere with DNA specific synthesis, halting normal development and reproduction; cell cycle S-phase specific	Acute and chronic leukemias; choriocarcinoma; certain cancers of the GI tract, breast, and ovaries; head and neck cancers; lymphomas, soft tissue sarcomas; osteosarcomas	5-Fluorouracil 6-Mercaptopurine Cytarabine Methotrexate Capecitabine Fludarabine Clardribine	Gemcitabine Floxuridine Thioguanine
Antitumor antibiotics	Reacts with or binds to DNA and prevents RNA synthesis; cell cycle phase nonspecific except Bleomycin-specific for G_2 and M phase	Widely used in the treatment of a variety of cancers, including breast, colon, rectal; Hodgkin's and non-Hodgkin's lymphoma; testicular; melanoma; sarcomas; ovarian; acute lymphocytic and non-lyphocytic leukemia	Daunorubicin & Daunorubicin Liposome Doxorubin & Doxorubicin Liposome Idarubicin Mitomycin-C Bleomycin	Epirubicin Mitoxantrone Dactinomycin Plicamycin Pentostatin Valrubicin
Plant (vinca) alkaloids	Blocks cell division during mitosis; cell cycle M-phase specific	Acute lymphoblastic leukemia, Hodgkin'sl ymphomas, neuroblastomas, Wilms' tumor; cancers of the breast, lung, and testes; brain tumors	Vinblastine Vincristine Etoposide Docetaxel Paclitaxel Vinorelbine	
Hormonal agonists/ antagonists	Interferes with protein synthesis and alters cell metabolism by changing the cell hormone environment	Widely used in the treatment of a variety of cancers, including breast, prostate, and endometrial	Diethylstilbesterol Estramustine Goserelin Tamoxifen Anastrozole (aromatase inhibitor)	Megestrol Leuprolide Exemestane Bicalutamide Letrozole
Nitrosureas	Function in a manner similar to alkylating agents interfering with DNA repair; cell cycle specific	Brain tumors, multiple myeloma, Hodgkin's disease, non-Hodgkin's lymphoma	Carmustine Lomustine	Pollifeprosan 20 with carmustine implant
Topoisomerase inhibitors	Inhibits topoisomerase I which leads to arrest of DNA replication and then, cell death	Colon, lung, cervical, gastric, ovarian, and pancreatic cancers; leukemia; lymphoma	Irinotecan Topotecan	
Immunomodulators	Exact mechanism by which it mediates antitumore activities unknown	Renal cell cancer, metastatic melanoma	Aldesleukin	
Biological response modifiers	Natural substances produced in small amounts by the body's immune system or manmade cellular products that target biologic functions	Hairy cell leukemia, malignant melanoma, Kaposi's sarcoma, renal cell carcinoma	Interferon alpha-2b Aldesleukin Rituximab	
Miscellaneous agents	Inhibits protein synthesis; cell-cycle specific	Acute lymphocytic leukemia	L-aspariginase Peg-L-aspariginase	
	Exact mechanism unknown	Hodgkin's disease	Procarbazine	
	Exact mechanism unknown	Acute promyelocytic leukemia	Tretinoin	
	Mechanism of action is at the G_2 phase of the cell cycle	Testicular and small cell lung cancers	Etoposide	
	Inhibits the proliferation of human tumor cells that overexpress HER2	Metastatic breast cancer with HER2 over-expression	Trastuzumab	
	Immediate inhibition of DNA synthesis	Melanoma; resistant chronic myelocytic leukemia; recurrent, metastatic or inoperable carcinoma of the ovary, concomitant with radiation therapy for primary squamous carcinomas of the head and neck, excluding lip	Hydroxyurea	
	Exact Mechanism unknown	Urinary bladder cancer	BCG live (intravesical)	

8. *Avoid intramuscular injections.* If they are unavoidable, apply pressure for at least 5 minutes after the injection. Don't take the patient's temperature rectally or allow the use of suppositories.

8. Decreased platelet counts prolong clotting time. Direct pressure for 5 minutes stops active bleeding in most patients. Objects inserted in the rectum may cause bleeding.

9. *Avoid administering aspirin and medications that contain aspirin.*

9. Aspirin decreases platelet aggregation and increases clotting time

10. *Apply ice packs to bleeding areas.*

10. Ice causes peripheral vasoconstriction, decreasing blood flow to the area and the risk of significant hemorrhage.

11. *Administer stool softeners, as ordered.*

11. Soft stools decrease the risk of tearing the rectal mucosa and help minimize straining on defecation, which increases intracranial pressure and may lead to intracranial bleeding.

12. Additional individualized interventions: _____

12. Rationales: _____

Nursing diagnosis
Anxiety related to diagnosis and treatment

NURSING PRIORITY
Support patient in coping strategies.

PATIENT OUTCOME CRITERIA
Throughout hospitalization, the patient will:
- exhibit signs and symptoms of diminished anxiety
- verbalize fears regarding the diagnosis and treatment plan.

INTERVENTIONS	RATIONALES
1. Consult the "Anxiety" care plan, page 40.	**1.** The "Anxiety" care plan details interventions useful to any patient in anxiety. This care plan contains interventions specific to cancer patients.
2. *Ascertain effectiveness of current coping skills.* Include patient in decisions, offering choices whenever possible .	**2.** Such collaboration promotes patient self-determination and diminishes feelings of powerlessness and hopelessness.
3. *Provide nonjudgmental atmosphere* and allow time for feelings and concerns to be expressed.	**3.** Cancer patients often are unable to express concerns and fears to family and significant others. By creating a supportive atmosphere, the nurse fosters the development of a therapeutic relationship.
4. *Provide uninterrupted periods.*	**4.** Such periods not only allow for necessary rest but also allow patient much needed time for personal reflection and planning.
5. *Offer supportive resources* in the community such as the American Cancer Society	**5.** Community-based resources offer support groups, information and other essential services necessary for long-term coping and success.
6. Additional individualized interventions: _____	**6.** Rationales: _____

> **Suggested NIC Interventions**
> *Anxiety reduction; Anticipatory guidance; Coping enhancement*

> **Suggested NOC Outcomes**
> *Anxiety control; Coping*

Nursing diagnosis
Chronic pain related to primary disease, metastasis, or chemotherapy

NURSING PRIORITY
Relieve pain and promote comfort.

PATIENT OUTCOME CRITERIA
Throughout chemotherapy, the patient will:
- request pain-relief medication before pain peaks
- rate pain at or less than individually-determined pain rating goal
- express an increased sense of control over pain
- demonstrate the correct procedure for administering pain medication.

INTERVENTIONS

1. *Instruct the patient to report pain or discomfort immediately.*

2. *Monitor the patient continually for signs or symptoms of pain or discomfort,* such as facial grimaces, splinting of the chest (painful area), diaphoresis, or restlessness.

3. *Involve the patient in pain-control strategies* by using imagery and relaxation techniques. See the "Chronic pain" care plan, page 63, for details.

4. *Administer pain medication, as needed,* according to a set schedule or medical protocol and nursing judgment. Teach the patient or a family member how to administer pain medication after discharge.

5. Additional individualized interventions: _____

RATIONALES

1. Early intervention provides more effective pain relief than measures employed after the pain has peaked.

2. The patient may not report pain or discomfort. Careful observation may allow detection of nonverbal indications that the patient is in pain.

3. Cognitive measures may decrease pain perception. The "Chronic pain" care plan contains general interventions for pain.

4. Pain medication ordered for a terminally ill patient may be given more frequently and in larger doses than routinely recommended (the patient receiving pain medication over a prolonged period may develop an increased tolerance). A set schedule may improve ongoing pain control because analgesics are more effective if given before pain becomes severe. Self-administration or administration of medication by a family member enables the patient to control pain at home.

5. Rationales: _____

> **Suggested NIC Interventions**
> *Pain management; Mood management; Patient contracting; Medication management; Behavior modification; Coping enhancement; Cognitive restructuring*

> **Suggested NOC Outcomes**
> *Comfort level; Depression control; Depression level; Pain control; Pain: Disruptive effects; Pain level; Pain: Psychological response*

Nursing diagnosis
Risk for infection related to immunosuppression from chemotherapy and malnutrition

NURSING PRIORITY
Prevent infection.

PATIENT OUTCOME CRITERIA
Within 1 day of admission, the patient will:
- isolate self from infected family members or friends.
  Throughout chemotherapy, the patient will:
- display no signs of infection and maintain normal temperature
- present no growth from cultures.

INTERVENTIONS	RATIONALES
1. Observe strict medical and surgical asepsis during wound care, venipuncture, and any invasive procedures.	**1.** The immunosuppressed patient easily contracts infections because of diminished host defenses. Maintaining strict medical and surgical asepsis decreases the risk of exposing the patient to pathogenic organisms.
2. Monitor and record temperature every 8 hours. Report even slight temperature elevations.	**2.** Elevated temperature is a sign of infection. The immunosuppressed patient may show slight or no temperature elevation even when extensive infection is present.
3. Instruct the patient to avoid crowds and persons with infections. Don't place the patient in reverse isolation unless laminar airflow or another method is available.	**3.** The risk of infection increases when a patient is exposed to individuals with contagious diseases. Reverse isolation is usually not effective unless laminar airflow is used because airborne organisms can still enter the patient's room.
4. Monitor WBC counts before, during, and after chemotherapy, as ordered.	**4.** Chemotherapy causes bone marrow depression, which may decrease the WBC count. Granulocyte counts below 1,000/µl increase the patient's risk of infection.
5. Initiate routine cultures of stool, urine, sputum, nasopharynx, oropharynx, and skin, as ordered.	**5.** Cultures provide information about bacterial colony growth that may produce infection. Early information about possible causes of infection guides the physician in prescribing appropriate antibiotic therapy.
6. Instruct the female patient to use sanitary napkins instead of tampons.	**6.** Tampons may traumatize the vaginal mucosa and provide a favorable environment for pathogen growth.
7. Avoid using indwelling urinary catheters.	**7.** Indwelling catheters may introduce pathogens into the bladder and increase the risk of urinary tract infections.
8. Additional individualized interventions: _____	**8.** Rationales: _____

Suggested NIC Interventions
Infection control; Protection

Suggested NOC Outcomes
Infection status

Nursing diagnosis
Risk for peripheral neurovascular dysfunction related to peripheral neuropathies caused by chemotherapy

NURSING PRIORITY
Prevent or minimize dysfunction caused by chemotherapy.

PATIENT OUTCOME CRITERIA
Throughout chemotherapy, the patient will:

- have no complaints of paresthesia
- have normal deep tendon reflexes.

INTERVENTIONS	**RATIONALES**
1. *Assess for, document, and report deficits in neurologic functioning,* including paresthesia and abnormal deep tendon reflexes.	**1.** Chemotherapeutic agents, such as vincristine (Oncovin), may cause peripheral neuropathies.
2. Discontinue or decrease the chemotherapy dosage, depending on the neuropathies' severity, as ordered.	**2.** Discontinuation or dosage reduction of medications such as vinca alkaloids may reverse adverse neurologic effects and will prevent further neuropathies.
3. *Explain that changes in sensation are related to chemotherapy,* and allow the patient to express fears related to this situation.	**3.** Fear may be reduced when the patient confronts the situation.
4. *Protect the area of decreased sensory perception from injury.* Use a bath thermometer; assess the skin every 8 hours for signs of trauma; apply dressings to injured areas; use a night-light; and avoid clutter in areas of activity to prevent abrasions, contusions, or falls.	**4.** Decreased perception at sensory nerve endings may reduce the patient's ability to judge temperature and pressure and may reduce pain sensation. Taking preventive measures reduces the potential for injury.
5. Additional individualized interventions: _____	**5.** Rationales: _____

> **Suggested NIC Interventions**
> *Peripheral sensation management*

> **Suggested NOC Outcomes**
> *Neurological status: Spinal sensory/motor function*

General care plans

Nursing diagnosis
Imbalanced nutrition: Less than body requirements related to cachexia associated with tumor growth, anorexia, changes in taste sensation, or stomatitis

NURSING PRIORITIES
- Minimize weight loss.
- Promote return to optimum achievable body weight.

PATIENT OUTCOME CRITERIA
Throughout chemotherapy, the patient will:
- plan meals appropriately, with or without family assistance
- control any nausea or vomiting with antiemetics
- exhibit pink oral mucosa, with no lesions.

INTERVENTIONS	**RATIONALES**
1. *Within 24 hours of admission, estimate the patient's required protein needs* based on ideal body weight and serum total protein level.	**1.** Caloric needs are altered by cancer-related cachexia. Serum total protein level reflects the status of visceral protein stores. Protein needs for a patient with cancer are calculated as 1 g/kg of ideal body weight (1 g of protein = 30 kcal).
2. *With the patient and dietitian, develop a diet plan based on calculated dietary needs* and the patient's food preferences.	**2.** Patient participation allows some feeling of control. Nutritional intake should increase if the patient's likes and dislikes are considered in planning meals.

3. Increase dietary protein levels by adding powdered milk to gravies, puddings, and milk products.

4. *Provide small frequent meals.*

5. *Document weight weekly.*

6. *Provide antiemetics, as ordered,* before administering chemotherapeutic agents. To reduce nausea, provide diversionary activities during chemotherapy and encourage the patient to lick salt or a lemon slice or sip sweetened ice water.

7. Daily assess the oral mucosa for stomatitis and document findings.

8. Provide a mild mouthwash with viscous lidocaine (Xylocaine) before meals.

9. After meals, clean the patient's mouth with $\frac{1}{4}$ tsp of sodium bicarbonate and $1\frac{1}{2}$ tsp salt mixed with 8 oz (240 ml) tap water. Follow with a 1:5 solution of hydrogen peroxide and water. Rinse with the sodium bicarbonate and salt solution. Don't use the hydrogen peroxide solution if bleeding occurs in the mouth, and don't use lemon-glycerin swabs.

10. Lubricate the patient's lips with petroleum jelly.

11. Assess oral mucosa daily for signs of lesions from opportunistic infections such as Candida.

12. Instruct the patient to swish and swallow with yogurt or buttermilk three times per day.

13. Administer oral nystatin (Mycostatin), as ordered.

14. Additional individualized interventions: _____

_____

3. Powdered milk increases protein content without increasing bulk.

4. Small, frequent meals increase total intake for the patient who experiences the early satiety common in cancer.

5. A weight record allows accurate assessment of changing nutritional needs. A patient with cancer commonly experiences significant weight loss.

6. The effects of chemotherapy on the CNS and gastric mucosa may induce vomiting. Granisetron (Kytril), ondansetron (Zofran), and prochlorperazine (Compazine) are effective antiemetics. Marijuana and tetrahydrocannabinol are being studied for control of nausea and vomiting. Nausea associated with chemotherapy may be psychogenic (it sometimes occurs before chemotherapy is administered); diversionary activities may distract the patient's attention and reduce nausea. The taste of lemon, salt, or sugar can relieve nausea in some patients.

7. Chemotherapeutic agents, such as methotrexate (Folex) and fluorouracil (Adrucil), affect cells that undergo rapid replication such as those in the GI system. Stomatitis interferes with the ability to eat.

8. The local anesthetic action of lidocaine decreases oral discomfort during meals.

9. Rinsing and cleaning with a sodium bicarbonate and salt solution followed by water and hydrogen peroxide reduces the bacterial count in the mouth and decreases the risk of infection. Using hydrogen peroxide in the presence of bleeding may disrupt clot formation. Lemon-glycerin swabs can dry the mouth, causing further discomfort.

10. Lubrication with petroleum jelly reduces lip drying and cracking.

11. Candida is an opportunistic organism that may cause infection in an immunosuppressed patient.

12. Yogurt and buttermilk restore to the GI tract the natural flora destroyed by chemotherapeutic agents. Growth of opportunistic organisms is decreased if normal flora is maintained.

13. Oral nystatin is effective against candidal infections.

14. Rationales:_____

_____

Suggested NIC Interventions
Nutritional monitoring; Nutrition management; Weight gain assistance

Suggested NOC Outcomes
Nutritional status; Nutritional status: Nutrient intake; Weight control

Nursing diagnosis

Risk for constipation related to chemotherapy

NURSING PRIORITY
Maintain normal bowel elimination.

PATIENT OUTCOME CRITERIA
Throughout chemotherapy, the patient will:
- maintain regular bowel elimination
- have soft stools.

INTERVENTIONS	RATIONALES
1. *Assess and document the patient's bowel elimination pattern* on admission. Reassess the patient's bowel elimination pattern before chemotherapy.	**1.** Chemotherapeutic agents may cause constipation or diarrhea. Information about the patient's previous bowel elimination pattern provides a baseline for evaluating bowel elimination during the hospital stay.
2. *Assess for signs of paralytic ileus* (such as diminished or absent bowel sounds and abdominal discomfort) every 8 hours. If present, report them to the physician immediately.	**2.** Paralytic ileus is a medical emergency that may be caused by chemotherapeutic agents.
3. *Prevent constipation by increasing dietary fiber, providing warm fluids, and promoting the optimal amount of exercise.* Don't check for fecal impaction if thrombocytopenia is present.	**3.** Bran, raw vegetables, fruits, and whole grain breads provide dietary fiber and promote bowel elimination. Liquids increase peristalsis. Exercise causes abdominal muscle contraction and promotes bowel elimination. Checking for fecal impaction may cause the thrombocytopenic patient to bleed.
4. *Administer stool softeners,* as ordered.	**4.** Stool softeners promote bowel elimination by increasing the water content of stools and easing their passage.
5. Additional individualized interventions:_____	**5.** Rationales:_____

> ### Suggested NIC Interventions
> *Bowel management; Constipation or impaction management; Fluid and electrolyte management*

> ### Suggested NOC Outcomes
> *Bowel elimination; Hydration; Symptom control*

Nursing diagnosis

Impaired urinary elimination related to possible development of renal toxicity or hemorrhagic cystitis from chemotherapy

NURSING PRIORITY
Maintain normal urinary elimination pattern.

PATIENT OUTCOME CRITERIA
Throughout chemotherapy, the patient will:
- maintain urine output within normal limits
- have amber-colored urine
- feel no pain on urination.

General care plans

INTERVENTIONS	RATIONALES
1. *Assess and document the patient's urinary elimination pattern* on admission.	**1.** Accurate assessment directs appropriate care planning.
2. *Force fluids and administer allopurinol (Lopurin)* before administering chemotherapeutic agents, as ordered.	**2.** Cyclophosphamide (Cytoxan) may cause hemorrhagic cystitis. Methotrexate may cause renal toxicity. Increasing fluid intake increases the glomerular filtration rate and reduces the risk of potentially toxic renal effects from chemotherapy. Allopurinol decreases uric acid calculi formation from chemotherapy by inhibiting uric acid synthesis.
3. *Alkalinize the patient's urine before and during chemotherapy* to prevent uric acid calculi formation.	**3.** Chemotherapy may cause uric acid calculi formation because acidic urine increases uric acid excretion. Fruits (such as oranges, tomatoes, and grapefruit), vegetables, and milk increase urine alkalinity and decrease uric acid calculi formation.
4. *Monitor serum creatinine and 24-hour urine creatinine,* as ordered, before chemotherapy.	**4.** Serum creatinine and 24-hour urine creatinine studies provide information about renal function. Normally functioning kidneys should clear creatinine.
5. Additional individualized interventions: _____	**5.** Rationales: _____

> **Suggested NIC Interventions**
> Urinary elimination management

> **Suggested NOC Outcomes**
> Urinary elimination

Nursing diagnosis

Activity intolerance related to weakness from cachexia, altered protein metabolism, muscle wasting, or hypoxia

NURSING PRIORITY

Optimize activity level without inducing exhaustion.

PATIENT OUTCOME CRITERIA

Within 1 week of admission, the patient will:
- manage activities with less exhaustion than on admission
- perform activities of daily living (ADLs) with minimal assistance.

INTERVENTIONS	RATIONALES
1. Immediately on admission, *determine what activities the patient can tolerate.*	**1.** Determining what activities the patient can tolerate guides activity recommendations.
2. *Instruct the patient to organize activities into manageable units.*	**2.** Activities performed without fatigue promote comfort.
3. *Teach proper body mechanics* to decrease the energy expenditure associated with ADLs: For example, explain the need to slide objects rather than carry them, work close to the body, sit when possible, use gravity, and avoid unnecessary bending or reaching.	**3.** The use of proper body mechanics reduces energy expenditure.
4. Additional individualized interventions: _____	**4.** Rationales: _____

> **Suggested NIC Interventions**
> Energy management

> **Suggested NOC Outcomes**
> Activity tolerance; Endurance; Energy conservation

Nursing diagnosis

Sleep deprivation related to anxiety, fear, pain, alterations in patterns of elimination or other sequelae of cancer

NURSING PRIORITY

Optimize sleep.

PATIENT OUTCOME CRITERION

Within 3 days of admission, the patient will report 8 to 10 hours of sleep within a 24-hour period, including 4 hours of uninterrupted sleep.

INTERVENTIONS	RATIONALES
1. *Assess and document sleep patterns on admission.* Discuss sleep patterns before the diagnosis was made.	1. Sleep goals should be based on the patient's perception of normal sleep patterns. Sleep deprivation, commonly caused by the psychological distress of the diagnosis and the physiologic sequelae of cancer, robs the patient of energy needed to cope with the illness.
2. *Provide quick, efficient monitoring and care* when needed.	2. Sleep disturbance is minimized if care is provided quickly and efficiently.
3. *Assist patient to control anxiety, fear, and pain.*	3. Anxiety, fear, and pain are notorious sleep disruptors.
4. Additional individualized interventions: _____	4. Rationales: _____

> **Suggested NIC Interventions**
> Energy management; Sleep enhancement

> **Suggested NOC Outcomes**
> Rest; Sleep; Symptom severity

Nursing diagnosis

Risk for situational low self-esteem related to weight loss, hair loss, role changes, and other sequelae of cancer

NURSING PRIORITY

Promote a positive self-concept.

PATIENT OUTCOME CRITERIA

Throughout chemotherapy, the patient will:
- wear well-fitting clothes
- express the desire to wear a wig, a hat, or scarf or verbalize acceptance of baldness
- verbalize measures to improve self-esteem
- initiate interaction with friends, family, and health care providers.

INTERVENTIONS	RATIONALES
1. *Approach the patient with an accepting attitude.*	1. An individual needs to experience acceptance from others to develop a positive self-concept.
2. *Assess and document the patient's self-concept and attitudes and responses to role changes.*	2. Accurate assessment of the patient's self-concept promotes appropriate care planning.

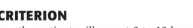

General care plans

3. *Encourage the patient and family to share feelings.*

4. *Discuss methods to accentuate the patient's positive features* through changes in hairstyle and clothing and minimize weight loss.

5. *Encourage frequent contact,* in person or by telephone, with loved ones.

6. *Discuss probable hair loss before chemotherapy starts* (keep in mind that hair loss may affect all parts of the body, not just the scalp). With the patient's permission, cut or shave hair before loss occurs. Natural hair may be used to fashion a wig, or the patient can be fitted for a wig before hair loss. The patient may want to wear a hat or scarf instead of a wig.

7. *Accept the patient's expression of acute distress or grief.* Remind the patient that hair loss isn't permanent and that hair grows back after chemotherapy ends. Be sure to mention that new hair may be different in color and texture.

8. Explain to the patient about scalp tourniquets and scalp hypothermia treatments that may diminish hair loss. Inform the patient that these procedures are time-consuming and may be unsuccessful.

9. Additional individualized interventions: _____
_____

3. Expression of feelings promotes honest, open relationships.

4. Clothing that fits well without accentuating weight loss improves general feelings of well-being. A well-groomed appearance improves self-concept.

5. Contact with others minimizes isolation and improves self-concept.

6. Knowledge about hair loss may decrease the anxiety associated with it. Hair loss is more manageable when hair is short. A wig, hat, or scarf helps minimize the impact of hair loss on body image and self-esteem.

7. For women in particular, hair loss may be very traumatic, as hair is a valued indicator of femininity in our culture. Hair regrowth usually begins within a few days to a few weeks after the end of chemotherapy.

8. Scalp tourniquets and scalp hypothermia treatments diminish the contact of chemotherapeutic agents with hair follicles and may decrease hair loss. The patient should be allowed to make an informed choice about whether to try them.

9. Rationales: _____
_____

Suggested NIC Interventions
Decision-making support; Grief work facilitation; Anticipatory guidance; Coping enhancement; Self-esteem enhancement

Suggested NOC Outcomes
Decision-making; Grief resolution; Psychosocial adjustment; Life change; Self-esteem

---

Nursing diagnosis
Ineffective sexuality patterns related to possible sterility, alterations in body image, and other sequelae of cancer

NURSING PRIORITIES
- Promote acceptance of optimal expressions of sexuality.
- Promote long-range plans for childbearing, if desired.

PATIENT OUTCOME CRITERIA
Throughout chemotherapy, the patient and spouse or partner will:
- discuss the desire for sexual expression and intimacy, if desired
- request time for privacy, if desired.

INTERVENTIONS

1. During initial assessment, *discuss any changes in patterns of sexual expression* that have resulted from the diagnosis and treatments.

2. *Help the patient and spouse or partner discuss their desires for sexual expression and intimacy.* Help them differentiate between the two needs and stress the importance of love and affection in maintaining a sense of closeness with each other.

3. *Discuss options for sexual expression within the patient's physical limitations.* For example, if intercourse is fatiguing or impossible for physical reasons and if the couple is receptive, suggest alternative forms of sexual and sensual expression that appeal to all senses, such as massage with scented oils, listening to music, sharing foods with various tastes and textures, and reading romantic literature.

4. *Encourage the use of supplemental oxygen during intercourse.*

5. *Provide privacy for the patient and spouse or partner to maintain intimacy* through such activities as private discussions and affectionate cuddling, if desired.

6. Explain that reduced sexual responsiveness may result from fatigue or chemotherapy.

7. *Explain that chemotherapy may cause sterility.* If appropriate, discuss sperm banking before chemotherapy. Inform the patient that childbearing plans should be postponed for at least 18 months after chemotherapy ends.

8. Additional individualized interventions: _____
_____

RATIONALES

1. Open discussion helps the patient to develop realistic goals and expectations related to sexual expression. Often the nurse is the only professional to raise this area of possible intense concern to the patient, family, or both.

2. Honest, caring communication between partners about their sexual needs promotes adjustment to cancer's impact on sexuality. Differentiating the desire for sexual activity from the desire for emotional closeness may allow the couple to focus on the strengths in their relationship, rather than on a loss of a specific sexual activity.

3. Sexual expression is closely tied to self-esteem, and the patient and spouse or partner may find that their self-esteem suffers when they can no longer participate in intercourse. Knowledge of alternative methods of sexual and sensual gratification can restore sexual intimacy and increase self-esteem when intercourse is no longer an option.

4. Exercise increases oxygen demands.

5. Intimacy is encouraged when individuals can share uninterrupted time.

6. Knowing the reasons for reduced sexual responsiveness decreases anxiety about sexuality.

7. Chemotherapy may affect gonadal function and diminish sperm and ovum production. Sperm may be saved in sperm banks for future fertilization. Drug-induced changes in sperm and ova should reverse by 18 months after the end of chemotherapy. Although the prognosis for these patients may be poor, discussion of future plans may help maintain hope.

8. Rationales: _____
_____

> *Suggested NIC Interventions*
> *Sexual counseling*

> *Suggested NOC Outcomes*
> *Sexual identity: Acceptance*

Discharge planning
DISCHARGE CHECKLIST
Before discharge, the patient shows evidence of:
- ❐ absence of fever and pulmonary or cardiovascular complications
- ❐ stable vital signs
- ❐ absence of infection
- ❐ nausea or vomiting and diarrhea controlled by oral medications
- ❐ adequate hydration
- ❐ normal renal function
- ❐ adequate nutritional and fluid intake
- ❐ ability to control pain using oral and subcutaneous medication

General care plans

❏ absence of bowel complications
❏ coughing controlled by medication
❏ minimal use of oxygen to assist breathing
❏ ability to demonstrate or explain proper oxygen administration technique, including how to acquire oxygen for home use
❏ ability to tolerate ADLs and ambulation with minimal difficulty
❏ adequate home support system or, if appropriate, referral to hospice, home care, or both
❏ knowledge of community support programs.

TEACHING CHECKLIST
Document evidence that the patient and family demonstrate an understanding of:
❏ diagnosis
❏ effects of chemotherapy
❏ prevention, detection, and management of bleeding
❏ use of supplemental oxygen
❏ smoking cessation
❏ breathing exercises
❏ purpose, dosage, administration schedule, and adverse effects requiring medical attention of all discharge medications; usual discharge medications include analgesics, antiemetics, and stool softeners or antidiarrheals, as appropriate
❏ pain-relief measures
❏ signs of and methods to prevent infection
❏ signs of neurologic changes
❏ dietary modifications
❏ measures to control nausea and vomiting
❏ measures to promote normal renal function
❏ measures to decrease dyspnea
❏ measures to minimize effects of changing body image
❏ plans for sexual expression
❏ date, time, and location of follow-up appointments
❏ how to contact the physician
❏ when and how to seek emergency medical care
❏ community resources.

DOCUMENTATION CHECKLIST
Using outcome criteria as a guide, document:
❏ clinical status on admission
❏ significant changes in status
❏ pertinent laboratory and diagnostic test findings
❏ response to chemotherapy
❏ episodes of dyspnea
❏ oxygen therapy
❏ bleeding episodes
❏ nutritional status
❏ bowel elimination
❏ urinary elimination
❏ activity tolerance
❏ sleep patterns

❏ patient and family teaching
❏ discharge planning.

Associated care plans
- Acute pain
- Anxiety
- Chronic pain
- Compromised family coping
- Dying
- Grieving
- Impaired physical mobility
- Ineffective individual coping
- Knowledge deficit

References
American Cancer Society (2002) Cancer Facts and Figures [Online]. Available: *www.cancer.org/eprise/main/doctroot/stt/stt_O.*

Karch, A. *2002 Lippincott's Nursing Drug Guide.* Philadelphia: Lippincott Williams & Wilkins, 2002.

Otto, S. *Oncology Nursing,* 4th ed. St. Louis: Mosby–Year Book, Inc., 2002.

Wilkes, G., et al. *2002 Oncology Nursing Drug Handbook.* Sudbury, Mass.: Jones and Barlett Publishers, 2002.

Chronic pain

Introduction

DEFINITION AND TIME FOCUS

Like acute pain, chronic pain represents physical and emotional suffering in response to a noxious stimulus. Unlike acute pain, chronic pain doesn't go away and usually isn't curable. Chronic pain is a constant daily companion. Because the body adapts to its continuous presence, vital signs are usually not elevated except when increased activity or breakthrough pain occurs. Through decreased endorphins, chronic pain lowers the pain threshold and decreases pain tolerance. Depression and chronic anxiety may occur as a result. Nursing care needs to include interventions for emotional as well as physical issues.

Chronic pain includes nonmalignant conditions, such as arthritis and neuropathies, where treatment is aimed at pain management over months and years and pain is usually stable. Chronic malignant pain is caused by cancer; the goal is control of pain until the disease is controlled or the end of life; 90% of malignant pain can be controlled by oral medications.

Many hospitalized patients have chronic pain, either malignant or non-malignant, and may also have acute pain related to the reason for hospitalization. Nursing management of chronic pain may be more challenging than that of acute pain, requiring compassionate understanding, a holistic view, and a multi-faceted approach toward pain management. This care plan focuses on the patient in chronic pain at any stage and in any location where care is provided.

ETIOLOGY AND PRECIPITATING FACTORS

- Joint inflammation, such as osteoarthritis and rheumatoid arthritis
- Musculoskeletal disorders such as muscle spasm accompanying other conditions
- Neuropathies secondary to such conditions as diabetes mellitus, acquired immunodeficiency syndrome, spinal nerve compression, or multiple sclerosis
- Cancer

Focused assessment guidelines

NURSING HISTORY (FUNCTIONAL HEALTH PATTERN FINDINGS)

Health-perception–health-management pattern

- Physical discomfort, usually described as pain, soreness, or a burning, tingling or cold sensation.

Nutritional-metabolic pattern

- Anorexia
- Constipation or diarrhea caused by autonomic neuropathy

Activity-exercise pattern

- Intense fatigue and decreased ability to perform activities of daily living (ADLs)

Sleep-rest pattern

- Inability to rest or sleep, leading to sleep deprivation

Cognitive-perceptual pattern

- Inability to concentrate on anything other than pain
- Preoccupation with pain

Self-perception–self-concept

- Depression from constant pain and changes in daily living

Role-relationship pattern

- Concern that others discount pain
- Decreased social interaction
- Alteration in family or intimate relationships

Coping–stress tolerance pattern

- Decreased ability to deal with any other stressors

Value-belief pattern

- Reluctance to take pain medication due to fear of addiction or belief system

PHYSICAL FINDINGS

General appearance

- Facial grimacing or mask-like face
- Tense, guarded posture
- Moaning or other utterances, especially with movement

Musculoskeletal

- Muscle spasms
- Joint deformity

Neurologic

- Decreased deep tendon reflexes (neuropathy)
- Decreased muscle tone or strength (neuropathy)
- Muscle tremors or weakness or paralysis
- Decreased sensation of extremities (numbness or paresthesia, neuropathy)
- Decreased bowel or bladder control (neuropathy)

DIAGNOSTIC STUDIES

No specific studies indicate the presence or degree of pain. Various studies may be used in differential diagnosis. X-rays may be used for musculoskeletal disorders or cancer. Computed tomography scans or magnetic resonance imaging may be used for cancer or neuropathies.

POTENTIAL COMPLICATIONS
- Paralysis (neuropathy or central nervous system [CNS] cancer)
- Incontinence (neuropathy or CNS cancer)
- Suicide

Nursing diagnosis
Chronic pain related to tissue injury, inflammation, nerve injury, or malignancy

NURSING PRIORITY
Control pain to enable optimal ability for ADLs.

PATIENT OUTCOME CRITERIA
The patient will:
- report that pain doesn't exceed the individually determined pain rating goal level
- maintain ability for self-care and ADLs.

INTERVENTIONS	RATIONALES
1. *Establish a baseline assessment of pain:* * location, characteristics and pain rating. (See the "Acute pain," care plan, page 32.) Have the patient choose a goal pain level. Monitor pain rating as the fifth vital sign. Report new or increased pain to the physician.	1. Baseline assessment provides a benchmark reference. The patient-selected goal is the pain level that allows him to eat, sleep, and perform activities of daily living. Standardized pain ratings are used as a baseline, to allow the nurse to determine changes in pain, and as an indicator of treatment effectiveness. New or increased pain may indicate a new disorder or extension of the disease process.
2. *State goal to aggressively manage or "stay on top" of the pain.* Give pain medication in "preventive" around-the-clock dosing. Use rating scale to compare current pain level to chosen goal level and titrate dose and interval to keep rating as close to the patient goal as possible.	2. Explicit goals imply that the pain is manageable, which is reassuring and reduces the anxiety and fear of chronic pain. Effective control of chronic pain requires the constant blood level achieved by around-the-clock dosing or long-acting preparations, or both.
3. *Work on a collaborative plan with the patient and family.* Use patient's usual pain relief measures if effective. Explore other pain-control measures and reaffirm goal to keep pain at acceptable level.	3. Involving the patient and family in pain-control plan fosters a feeling of control that reduces anxiety, helplessness and hopelessness.
4. *Encourage the patient to share feelings about chronic pain.* Use non-judgmental active listening. If possible, do the same with the family or significant other in an environment away from the patient.	4. People in chronic pain often have feelings of anxiety or depression which they hesitate to verbalize, especially around family or a significant other. Some patients feel relieved when they are able to share their feelings; others don't. Families share the same emotional burden of living with a person in chronic pain and may need to express their feelings in an accepting atmosphere away from their loved one.
5. *Collaborate with the physician to determine an effective analgesic regimen.* Administer and document analgesics as ordered; they may include:	5. Individualizing the analgesic regimen is essential for effective pain management since each person responds differently to various drugs.

---

*Italics indicate key interventions.

– nonnarcotic analgesics or nonsteroidal anti-inflammatory drugs (NSAIDs), such as acetaminophen, ibuprofen and other COX1 inhibitors, and celecoxib and other COX2 inhibitors.

– NSAIDs work peripherally, inhibiting formation of prostaglandins (inflammatory mediators that cause pain). NSAIDs are used as the basis for all analgesic regimens. They are used alone when possible for nonmalignant pain, especially inflammatory pain. When used in combination with opioids, they may be dosed separately or in combination products. When using combination products, be aware of NSAID dose ceilings due to toxicity (bleeding, GI or hepatic damage). COX2 inhibitors have a lower incidence of GI damage than COX1 inhibitors.

– opioids, such as morphine, fentanyl, methadone, and oxycodone.

– Opioids work by occupying central receptor sites, decreasing the perception of pain. They are used for chronic malignant pain and refractory nonmalignant pain. Side effects include sedation, respiratory depression, nausea, urinary retention, and constipation. With continued use, tolerance is developed to most side effects except constipation. Whenever possible, oral dosing is preferred.

– adjuvant agents, used for neuropathic and malignant pain

– Adjuvants aren't analgesics, but are other drugs effective with certain types of chronic pain. Neuropathic pain is caused by damage to nerves.

– tricyclic antidepressants, such as desipramine and amitriptyline, and selective serotonin reuptake inhibitors (SSRIs), such as sertraline and venlafaxine

– Tricyclic antidepressants and SSRIs increase the availability of serotonin, which inhibits the transmission of pain impulses at the level of the spinal cord.

– anticonvulsants, such as gabapentin, carbamazepine, and clonazepam
– skeletal muscle relaxants such as diazepam
– corticosteroids for refractory nonmalignant and malignant pain due to swelling and inflammation.

– Anticonvulsants inhibit nerve transmission in neuropathic and "phantom" pain.
– Muscle relaxants reduce muscle spasm.
– Steroids reduce swelling in joints and around nerves, reducing pressure.

6. *For chronic nonmalignant pain, use around-the-clock dosing of NSAIDs and adjuvant drugs as indicated.* Use long-acting drugs with individualized dosing to achieve pain management. For refractory pain, opioids may be ordered for both baseline and breakthrough pain management.

6. Most nonmalignant pain can be managed by a combination of nonopioid drugs and nondrug interventions. Long-acting drugs allow uninterrupted sleep. Refractory neuropathic pain may require opioids such as oxycodone with hydrocodone for breakthrough pain.

7. For chronic malignant pain, use all three drug groups. Don't use combination products. Reassure the patient that "addiction" isn't a consideration and that pain control is the goal. Once the opioid dose is determined, nonparenteral administration is used; usually, oral and transdermal opioids can control pain. Dosing includes baseline and rescue or breakthrough doses. Rescue doses are individualized; start with $1/10$ to $1/6$ of 24 hour oral dose. Dosing for elderly patients is lower initially and titrated for effect.

7. NSAIDs provide the foundation of cancer pain management. Morphine is the standard narcotic used because it comes in many different dosage forms, can be given by various routes, and there is no upper-end dose limit. Tolerance and physical dependence do develop; these don't indicate addiction (psychological dependence). Tolerance generally requires dosage increases; addiction is rare and physical dependence isn't an issue. Many health care professionals inappropriately undermedicate patients with cancer pain. Elderly patients may require lower doses due to diminished renal and hepatic function.

8. *Minimize discomfort from adverse effects of analgesics.* Tolerance is developed to most narcotic side effects except constipation. Monitor for respiratory depression with dosage increases. (See *Preventing adverse effects of narcotic analgesics,* page 37 in the "Acute pain" care plan.)

8. Constipation will occur with opioids and must be anticipated and prevented. A combination of diet, fluids, and stool softeners or laxatives must be individualized. Most adjuvant tricyclic antidepressants cause dry mouth and sedation; SSRIs may cause insomnia, dry mouth, diarrhea or sexual dysfunction.

General care plans

9. Use a combination of non-drug and behavioral pain-control strategies such as positioning, massage, cold or heat, relaxation, meditation, or guided imagery. (See the "Acute pain" care plan, page 32.)

10. *If pain can't be managed with the above measures, collaborate with the physician, patient, and family to optimize pain control through such measures as:*
– transcutaneous electrical nerve stimulation (TENS)

– acupuncture
– continuous subcutaneous opioid infusion (used for cancer pain)
– indwelling epidural with implanted pump (used for cancer pain)

11. Additional individualized interventions: _____

9. A variety of pain-control measures allows for an individualized, multifaceted approach, which is more likely to be successful than drug treatment alone.

10. In refractory pain, a collaborative approach using a variety of options increases chances of finding optimal pain management for an individual patient.
– TENS transmits an electrical stimulus, which uses a gate control mechanism to block ascending pain transmission.
– Acupuncture is thought to stimulate endorphin release.
– Continuous infusion maintains a constant blood level.

– Continuous spinal infusion concentrates drug with less systemic absorption.

11. Rationales: _____

Suggested NIC Interventions
Pain management; Mood management; Patient contracting; Medication management; Behavior modification; Coping enhancement; Cognitive restructuring

Suggested NOC Outcomes
Comfort level; Depression level; Depression control; Pain level; Pain control; Pain: Disruptive effects; Pain: Psychological response

---

Discharge planning
See the "Acute pain" care plan, page 32.

Associated care plans
- Acute pain
- Anxiety
- Cancer
- Dying

References
The American Chronic Pain Association: *www.theacpa.org.*
American Pain Society. *Principles of Analgesic Use in the Treatment of Acute Pain and Cancer Pain,* 4th ed. Glenview Ill: The Society, 1999.
American Pain Society: *www.ampainsoc.org.*
The American Society of Pain Management Nurses: *www.aspmn.org.*
Fillary, R. "Chronic Pain," *Vision* 6(11):15-19, November 2000.
Gloth, F.M. "Pain Management in Older Adults: Prevention and Treatment," *Journal of the American Geriatrics Society* 49(2):188-99, February 2001.
Guido, E.H. "Effects of Sympathetic Therapy on Chronic Pain in Peripheral Neuropathy Subjects," *American Journal of Pain Management* 12(1):31-34, January 2002.
Herndon, C.M., and Fike, D.S. "Continuous Subcutaneous Infusion Practices on U.S. Hospices," *Journal of Pain and Symptom Management* 22(6):1027-34, December 2001.
Heyckman-Stone, C., and Stone, C. "Pain Management Techniques Used by Patients with Multiple Sclerosis," *Journal of Pain* 2(4):205-208, August 2001.
Hunt, J. *Bedside Pain Manager.* Redway Calif.: Pain Management Resources, 2002.
McCaffery, M., and Pasero, C. *Pain: Clinical Manual,* 2nd ed. St. Louis: Mosby–Year Book, Inc., 1999.
Oliver, R.L., and Taylor, A. "Fatigue: The Art of Thorough Assessment in Chronic Pain Syndrome," *American Journal of Pain Management* 11(4):137-47, October 2001.
Panke, J.T. "Difficulties in Managing Pain at the End of Life," *American Journal of Nursing* 102(7):26-33, July 2002.

Compromised family coping

Introduction

DEFINITION AND TIME FOCUS

Compromised family coping occurs when "a usually supportive primary person (family member or close friend) is providing insufficient, ineffective, or compromised support, comfort, assistance, or encouragement" that the patient may need "to manage or master adaptive tasks related to his health challenge." This plan focuses on the family's ability to manage the stressors that affect them during the patient's hospital stay.

ETIOLOGY AND PRECIPITATING FACTORS

- Illness or injury of family member
- Disruption of usual family activities and routines
- Family disunity
- Loss of control by patient or family
- Role changes within the family
- Unfamiliar hospital environment
- Restricted visitation of loved ones
- Loss of income, cost of medical care
- Other situational crises occurring simultaneously

Focused assessment guidelines

NURSING HISTORY (FUNCTIONAL HEALTH PATTERN FINDINGS FOR FAMILY)

Nutritional-metabolic pattern
- Neglect of nutritional intake while family member is hospitalized

Sleep-rest pattern
- Inadequate sleep or rest while family member is hospitalized

Cognitive-perceptual pattern
- Inaccurate understanding of the patient's condition
- Failure to request clarification of information about the patient's situation
- Tendency to pay attention to only some aspects of the information given
- Lack of skills or education to understand complex medical information

Self-perception–self-concept pattern
- Inability to cope with current situation
- Anxiety, fear, or anger
- Unresolved guilt or hostility
- Unawareness of feelings or perceptions of other family members
- Discomfort with emotional reactions of other family members

Role-relationship pattern
- Lack of interaction among family members
- Difficulty communicating feelings and perceptions to other family members
- Difficulty reaching decisions
- Rigidly established roles within the family structure
- Inability to provide emotional support for each other
- Anger or disagreement over the care plan

Coping–stress tolerance pattern
- Use of inappropriate coping methods
- Use of non-growth-promoting methods (denial, depression, violence, or substance abuse) to handle past crises
- Failure to identify all coping strategies available within the family system
- Regression or increased dependence characterized by reliance on others to solve problems

Value-belief pattern
- Value conflicts among family members
- Unrealistic beliefs about health, disease, or roles and abilities of other family members

PHYSICAL FINDINGS
Not applicable

DIAGNOSTIC STUDIES
Not applicable

POTENTIAL COMPLICATIONS
- High anxiety levels among family members
- Transfer of anxiety from family to patient
- Unrealistic expectations of patient — for example, expecting full recovery of neurologic function in a brain-damaged person
- Unrealistic expectations of other family members — for example, expecting uncommunicative member to become emotionally supportive in crisis
- Inattention to family members' physical and psychosocial needs
- Inadequate preparation for the patient's discharge or death
- Disintegration of the family unit

Nursing diagnosis

Compromised family coping related to illness and hospitalization of family member

NURSING PRIORITY

Help the family identify, develop, and use healthy coping skills.

PATIENT OUTCOME CRITERIA

Within 2 days of the patient's admission, family members will:
- verbalize decrease in level of anxiety
- recognize their physical needs for food and rest.
  By the time of the patient's discharge, family members will:
- verbalize feelings appropriately to each other
- participate actively in caring for the ill family member
- use healthy coping mechanisms
- verbalize the need to adjust family roles
- demonstrate listening and supportive behaviors to each other
- identify resources within and outside the family
- develop a plan or strategy to provide necessary care and support for the ill family member after discharge.

INTERVENTIONS

1. *Assess and document the origins of the crisis and the family members' responses to it.* * Identify factors contributing to vulnerability in a crisis state. Observe nonverbal behaviors, such as eye contact and body posture.

2. *Demonstrate interest and concern for the patient's family members.* Acknowledge their feelings about the situation — for example, "This must be very difficult for you."

3. *Take measures to minimize the family members' level of anxiety:* Provide a quiet, private place for discussion; avoid elaborate information or unnecessary questions; and remain available to the family. Document the family's initial status and response to nursing interventions.

4. *Provide accurate, timely information about the patient's treatment and care.* Give explanations in lay terms, encourage questions, and introduce topics likely to be of interest. Reinforce information given by the physician. Document the information given to the family.

RATIONALES

1. Situational factors (such as illness or death), transitional states (developmental turning point or life-cycle phase), and sociocultural factors all can contribute to a crisis. Families in which several of these factors are present are at higher risk for crisis development. Nonverbal behaviors, such as clenched fists or lack of eye contact, provide valuable clues about the family's emotional state.

2. Approaching the family with a warm and respectful attitude lays the groundwork for developing a trusting relationship.

3. In states of heightened anxiety, the ability to think clearly, handle new information, and make appropriate decisions is impaired. Minimizing distractions reduces anxiety and helps family members regain control of their thinking processes.

4. Family members must be well informed to develop an accurate perception of the patient's illness or injury. Medical jargon may increase anxiety in some individuals. Clear, simple explanations will be understood best. Encouraging questions dispels possible discomfort over not knowing answers, while suggesting topics reduces possible discomfort over not knowing what to ask. Anxiety and misunderstanding can be minimized by giving explanations in lay terms and by reinforcing or clarifying information given by the physician. Family members who understand their own problems as well as the patient's can recognize their needs and identify appropriate solutions.

---

* Italics indicate key interventions.

5. *Clarify family members' perceptions of the information given to them.* Don't assume that what was stated was what the family heard and understood. Document the family's level of understanding.

6. *Reduce the stress associated with the hospital environment.* Individualize visitation privileges. Orient the family to hospital facilities. Arrange for a quiet place for the family to meet with the physician. Provide pillows and blankets for family members spending the night at the hospital.

7. *Assist family members in caring for their own physical and psychosocial needs.* Encourage them to find time for themselves every day. Encourage adequate rest periods. Reinforce the need for adequate dietary intake.

8. *Encourage family members to express their feelings* about the impact of the patient's illness. Ask open-ended questions. Listen carefully to each person. Support communication among family members. Observe how feelings are expressed and how family members behave. Document the family's response and behavior. Identify, when possible, the family member who is the primary health and illness resource for the family, and include that person in all teaching. Also, make sure that person has an adequate support system.

9. *Promote awareness of family strengths* by identifying areas in which the members work well together. Document identified family strengths and weaknesses. Direct nursing interventions toward encouraging family strengths — for example, support family efforts to learn care techniques or to bring in special items from home, as permitted.

10. *Facilitate family communication when dysfunctions are present.* Encourage verbalization and recognition of feelings. Provide referrals to other professionals (mental health liaison nurse, social worker, clinical specialist, clinical psychologist, or member of the clergy) when family problems lie outside the role of the staff nurse.

11. *Focus on immediate, concrete problems.*

5. Asking for feedback and clarification allows the nurse to determine the family members' actual level of understanding.

6. Manipulating the hospital environment decreases the family's physical distress in adjusting to the patient's hospitalization.

7. Development of problem-solving skills and effective coping strategies is impaired when family members are physically exhausted, malnourished, or stressed by unmet emotional or psychosocial needs.

8. Awareness of feelings and the ability to express them clearly and appropriately are important elements of healthy coping behaviors. Help-seeking behaviors are aided by intrafamily communication and realistic discussion of how the patient's illness may affect family functioning. By using open-ended questions, the nurse can guide the family's communication. Listening to the family and helping them clarify their feelings and perceptions will help the nurse identify areas where additional support is needed. Most families have one member who is the informed "health liaison person" who may act as caregiver, teacher, and interpreter. Acknowledgment of this role facilitates therapeutic intervention.

9. Acknowledging family strengths, such as closeness, open communication, or willingness to help each other, aids the family in identifying their resources for coping with the crisis.

10. The nurse's role is to listen, support, and clarify — not solve — the family's problems. The nurse helps the family to identify available resources and to make informed decisions about using them.

11. A primary nursing focus is to reduce the family members' anxiety so they can think constructively and make use of problem-solving skills. In many cases, anxiety can be decreased by attending to easily removable stressors; for example, refer an out-of-town family to the social services department to arrange for housing while the patient is hospitalized.

General care plans

12. Help the family develop a realistic appraisal of the situation and an action plan. Explore coping skills and support systems. Help them identify resources, such as friends or family members, self-help groups or home health care nurses. Ensure that the plan is appropriate to the family's functional level, dependence needs, and lifestyle.

12. In establishing a plan of action, family members need to match their own needs and the patient's with available resources. By providing such information, the nurse helps the family develop a plan to meet their needs.

13. Encourage independent decision making by family members.

13. Allowing family members to make decisions promotes their independence.

14. With the patient and family, follow up and evaluate the plan of action. Assist them to assume new roles

14. Evaluation of the plan of action with the patient and family reinforces successful strategies and may suggest additional or alternate interventions and provides positive feedback.

15. Avoid imposing personal values or codes of behavior on family members.

15. In order to intervene effectively with a family in crisis, the nurse must develop an awareness of personal value systems and beliefs related to cultural norms. This allows the nurse to view the family's problems without imposing personal values on the family system.

16. Additional individualized interventions: _____

16. Rationales:_____

Suggested NIC Interventions
Emotional support; Respite care; Caregiver support; Coping enhancement; Family involvement promotion; Family process maintenance

Suggested NOC Outcomes
Caregiver emotional health; Caregiver-patient relationship; Caregiver stressors; Family coping; Family normalization

---

Discharge planning

DISCHARGE CHECKLIST
Before discharge, the patient should show evidence of:
❐ identification of the impact of the patient's illness on family function
❐ plans for dealing with changes within the family
❐ identification of internal and external resources available to family members
❐ initial contact with selected external resources.

TEACHING CHECKLIST
Document evidence that the patient and family demonstrate an understanding of:
❐ extent and implication of the patient's illness and limitations
❐ changes in family roles and function such as new responsibilities each member must assume to facilitate care of the patient at home
❐ resources and referrals available to the family.

DOCUMENTATION CHECKLIST
Using outcome criteria as a guide, document:
❐ family's initial emotional status
❐ precipitating factors in crisis and the meaning of crisis to family members

❐ changes in emotional status related to nursing interventions
❐ treatment and care information given to family members
❐ family's level of understanding of information provided
❐ family members' ability to express feelings
❐ identified family strengths and weaknesses
❐ referrals to community resources.

Associated care plans
- Dying
- Grieving
- Ineffective individual coping
- Knowledge defect

References
Cox, H., et al. *Clinical Applications of Nursing Diagnosis: Adult, Child, Women's, Psychiatric, Geriatric, and Home Health Considerations*, 4th ed. Philadelphia: F.A. Davis Co., 2002.
Thompson, J.N., et al. *Mosby's Clinical Nursing*, 5th ed. St. Louis: Mosby–Year Book, Inc., 2002.

Confusion

Introduction

DEFINITION AND TIME FOCUS

Confusion may be classified as acute, chronic, or occurring simultaneously. Confusion isn't an actual disease entity, but rather a clinical state representing a symptom of neurologic instability that occurs when cognitive processes are disrupted. *Acute* confusion is defined as an abrupt onset of a cluster of global, transient changes and disturbances in attention, cognition, psychomotor activity, level of consciousness, and sleep/wake cycle. *Chronic* confusion is defined as an irreversible, long-standing and progressive deterioration of intellect and personality, characterized by decreased ability to interpret environmental stimuli and decreased capacity for intellectual thought processes, manifested by disturbances of memory, orientation, and behavior.

Acute confusion is commonly rapid in onset, occurring over several hours or days. It's fully developed within 3 days of onset. Chronic confusion may be long-term, continuing for several years.

Acute and chronic confusion can occur at any age across the life span, but they're most common in elderly people. Because the number of elderly people in the United States continues to grow rapidly, the nurse's ability to respond in an appropriate manner to this type of patient is of paramount importance.

Because hospitalized patients with acute confusion rerquire intensive nursing care, health care costs are enormous. These patients are commonly older than age 70 and three to five times more likely to have a longer recovery period than those patients who don't suffer from acute confusion. Patients with chronic confusion may be forced to live in long-term care facilities due to safety issues. The costs associated with long-term care in today's health care market may present a significant financial drain on the patient and the patient's family.

A holistic approach to nursing care, including body, mind, and spirit, is optimal for the confused patient. The patient's dignity must be maintained while you care for both physical and psychological disturbances in Functional Health Patterns. The confused patient can be found in any area of nursing practice, but especially in hospitals and extended care facilities. This care plan focuses on the patient displaying acute or chronic confusion, either in the acute care setting or in long-term care. (See *Clinical snapshot: Confusion,* page 73.)

ETIOLOGY AND PRECIPITATING FACTORS

Confusion is a sign of an underlying neurological disorder. Therefore, it's important to recognize confusion as soon as possible. Contributing factors to the development of confusion can be classified as physiological or psychosocial.

Physiological
- Fluid and electrolyte imbalances, related to hyponatremia
- Degenerative diseases such as dementia or Alzheimer's disease
- Metabolic disorders such as diabetes mellitus
- AIDS-related dementia
- Korsakoff's psychosis, related to organic changes in brain tissue from chronic alcoholism
- Mental illnesses, such as depression or schizophrenia, related to disturbances in thought processes
- Central nervous system infections (meningitis, encephalitis)

Brain tumors
- Seizures
- Head injury
- Vascular disorders, such as transient ischemic attacks or stroke
- Delay in metabolism and excretion of drugs
- Organ dysfunction caused by lack of oxygenation (renal, cerebral, gastrointestinal, or cardiopulmonary)
- Acute or chronic pain
- Shock
- Hypersensitivity to drugs
- Adverse effects of medications, particularly narcotic analgesics
- Carbon monoxide poisoning
- Electroshock therapy, postprocedure
- Length of surgery (exceeding 4 hours)
- Use of anesthetic agents
- Sleep deprivation
- Physical environment of critical care unit related to constant noise and light or lack of windows.
- Use of restraints

Psychosocial
- Anxiety
- Depression
- Use of alcohol or other drugs
- Recent relocation
- Lack of emotional or spiritual support systems

Focused assessment guidelines

NURSING HISTORY (FUNCTIONAL HEALTH PATTERN FINDINGS)

Activity-exercise pattern

Acute
- Restlessness, agitation
- Combative behavior
- Decrease in psychomotor activity (hypoactivity)

Chronic
- Wandering behavior

Sleep-rest pattern

Acute
- Disturbed sleep/wake cycle (circadian rhythm)
- Combines dreams with reality
- Stays awake at night and naps during day
- Vivid nightmares are common

Chronic
- Disturbed sleep/wake cycle

Cognitive-perceptual pattern

Acute
- Sudden onset of symptoms
- Hallucinations and illusions
- Problems worsen at night (sundowning syndrome)
- Short attention span
- Poor concentration
- Highly distractible
- Drowsiness

Chronic
- Disorientation to person, place, time, and situation
- Misinterpretation of stimuli
- Emotional lability
- Slurred speech or mumbling
- Inappropriate gestures
- Impaired memory
- Impaired ability to abstract or conceptualize
- Personality changes
- Progressive cognitive disturbance

Self-perception–self-concept pattern

Acute
- Anxiety over feeling "mixed up"
- Fear

Chronic
- Feelings of frustration due to inability to recognize or remember certain things
- Fear of "going crazy"

Role-relationship pattern

Acute
- Anger directed at health care workers for continued questioning about orientation status

Chronic
- Difficulty communicating with health care workers/family/significant others related to impaired cognition
- Impaired socialization

Coping–stress tolerance pattern

Acute
- Extreme agitation (attempts to climb out of bed)
- Displays combative behavior (hitting, kicking, biting)
- Responds to others in a loud voice, sometimes using profanity

Chronic
- Progressively decreased ability to tolerate any change in environment
- Depression
- Lowered stress threshold

PHYSICAL FINDINGS

General appearance

Acute or chronic
- Inappropriate dress
- Poor personal hygiene

Cardiovascular

Acute or chronic
- Potential tachycardia or hypertension

Gastrointestinal

Acute or chronic
- Potential constipation

Neurologic

Acute
- Disorientation to time, place, person, and situation
- Loss of short-term memory (loss of memory for recent events)

Chronic
- Difficulty finding the right word (aphasia)
- Difficulty recognizing well-known objects and people (agnosia)
- Inability to perform familiar activities (apraxia)
- Slowed speech

Integumentary

Acute or chronic
- Poor skin turgor
- Dry skin
- Bruising or other signs of trauma

Genitourinary

Acute or chronic
- Urinary retention

DIAGNOSTIC STUDIES

Diagnostic studies to determine the cause of acute or chronic confusion focus on the possible underlying etiologic factors.

Laboratory data

- Serum electrolyte tests — may indicate imbalances in electrolytes such as sodium; hyponatremia can cause a change in mental status
- Complete blood count with differential — may indicate anemia or infection (decreased oxygen transport to the brain or infection may cause acute confusion)
- Serum glucose level — may indicate hypoglycemia, which results in confusion if the brain isn't functioning properly

- Urinalysis with culture and sensitivity testing — may indicate an infectious process, which can result in confusion
- Renal function studies — may indicate a problem with the excretion of blood urea nitrogen and creatinine; elevated levels can cause confusion
- Thyroid function studies — may indicate hypothyroidism or hyperthyroidism, both of which can cause cognitive impairment
- Drug toxicity screening tests — may indicate toxicity from medications such as digoxin or antiseizure medications, as well as alcohol or other drug use
- Serum vitamin B_{12} and folic acid (folate) levels — may indicate pernicious anemia, degeneration in the spinal cord, or other neurological problems that cause confusion

Diagnostic procedures

- Electrocardiogram — may show an arrhythmia, resulting in heart failure, which can cause confusion
- Pulse oximetry — may reveal decreased blood oxygen saturation can lead to cerebral hypoxia, causing confusion
- EEG — may indicate abnormal brain wave pattern

- Computerized tomography scan — may indicate brain tumors, cerebral infarctions, or hydrocephalus
- Lumbar puncture — may indicate abnormality of the cerebrospinal fluid
- Chest X-ray — may indicate an infectious process such as pneumonia, leading to acute confusion

POTENTIAL COMPLICATIONS
Acute and chronic
- Arrhythmia (related to hypoxia or fluid and electrolyte imbalance)
- Dehydration (related to fluid loss and lack of replacement fluids)
- Urinary retention or constipation (patient doesn't remember to urinate or defecate)
- Self-injury (patient may injure self if sharp or breakable objects aren't secured; patient may become lost if wandering)
- Injury to others (patient may display combative or violent behavior)
- Inability to communicate (patient can't remember words or is slow to speak)

General care plans

CLINICAL SNAPSHOT

Confusion

Major nursing diagnoses	Key patient outcomes
Acute confusion related to physiological or psychological cause	Remain free from injury to self or others.
Chronic confusion related to physiological or psychological cause	Remain free from injury to self or others.

Nursing diagnosis
Acute confusion related to physiological or psychological cause

NURSING PRIORITIES
- Maintain patient safety.
- Be alert for changes in status that may indicate cerebral hypoxia or arrhythmia.
- Reorient patient to reality.
- Effectively communicate with patient.
- Assist with nightly sleep schedule.

PATIENT OUTCOME CRITERIA
Throughout the length of stay, the patient will:
- remain free from injury to self or others
- show no evidence of cerebral hypoxia or arrhythmia
- become reoriented to time, place, person, and situation
- communicate needs to health care professionals
- sleep continuously for 6 to 8 hours at night.

INTERVENTIONS

1. Upon admission, *perform a baseline assessment of vital signs and complete a head-to-toe physical examination.* * Focus on level of orientation and consciousness, skin turgor, lung sounds, and elimination pattern.

2. When possible, *perform a mental status examination* to confirm the nursing diagnosis. Complete one of the following: The Confusion Assessment Method; Confusion Rating Scale; NEECHAM Confusion Scale; Mini Mental State Exam.

3. *Maintain a safe environment by* placing patient in room close to nurse's station. Check patient frequently. Restrict patient's access to intravenous lines, oxygen tubing, and other equipment by concealing it (if appropriate) and offering an alternative object to hold (wash cloth or towel).

4. *Be alert for changes in vital signs, heart sounds, or complaints of chest pain,* especially during periods of agitation.

5. *Monitor for medication adverse effects.*

6. Initiate each interaction with patient by identifying yourself and the patient by name. Make direct eye contact. Use touch judiciously.

7. *During periods of aggression, focus on the underlying feelings* (usually anxiety or fear) and attempt to redirect the client.

8. *Use restraints only when less restrictive measures have been tried,* in accordance with your institution's policy.

9. *Monitor daily fluid intake.*

10. Give anticipatory guidelines for each procedure. Explain procedures in simple terms. Speak slowly, allowing patient time to process information.

11. *Provide visual cues for orientation,* such as a wall clock and calendar. Share the daily weather reports and news events, as appropriate.

12. Determine the patient's primary language and whether the patient is literate in this language or in English

13. If the patient is hallucinating or delusional, let the patient know that you aren't experiencing these states. Be calm and matter-of-fact. Speak in a low, calm voice, addressing the patient by name. Don't argue with the patient. Focus on the underlying feeling.

RATIONALES

1. Baseline assessment is essential to know what is normal for the patient. Look for problem areas.

2. The mental status exam and rating scale will help determine the severity of confusion, and whether it's acute. The exams mentioned have been validated clinically.

3. Patients with acute confusion have global, transient deficits that change rapidly. Increased surveillance can reduce the risk of injury.

4. These changes may indicate an arrhythmia.

5. Many medications can cause confusion, or exacerbate a confused state.

6. These actions assist with reality orientation and maintain the patient's dignity.

7. Focusing on the underlying feelings helps the patient feel understood. Redirecting the patient will lower the emotional tone of the aggression.

8. Restraints may be necessary to protect the patient from harming himself or others.

9. Dehydration may lead to electrolyte imbalance, which can worsen the state of confusion.

10. These actions will lessen anxiety about procedure. The ability to think abstractly is decreased with acute confusion.

11. These actions assist with reality orientation. They also promote the patient's self-esteem.

12. The patient may not understand English and may not be literate in the primary language or English as a second language.

13. These actions help the patient to feel safe and less anxious, while preserving the dignity of the patient.

---

*Italics indicate key interventions.

14. *Assess and document the patient's sleep/wake cycle.* Establish a sleep schedule with patient. If possible, implement bedtime routines used at home.

15. *Decrease lighting and noise level at night.* If possible, provide headphones with an audio cassette or compact disk player. Provide music therapy with soothing, instrumental music.

16. If possible, offer complementary therapies such as a warm herbal tea (chamomile) or therapeutic massage at bedtime.

17. Additional individualized interventions: _____
_____

14. This assessment will enable the nurse to know if sleep deprivation is a problem. The patient's normal sleep schedule should be continued for optimal rest.

15. Day/night cycles can be simulated by adjusting the lighting. Lowering the noise level promotes sleep. Music therapy decreases anxiety.

16. These therapies help promote rest and sleep without the use of medications. They also give the patient a feeling of being cared for.

17. Rationales:_____
_____

Suggested NIC Interventions
Delirium management; Delusion management; Reality orientation; Hallucination management; Cognitive stimulation; Cerebral perfusion promotion; Neurological monitoring; Environmental management: Safety; Fall prevention; Sleep enhancement

Suggested NOC Outcomes
Cognitive orientation; Distorted thought control; Information processing; Neurological status: Consciousness; Safety behavior: Personal; Sleep

General care plans

Nursing diagnosis
Chronic confusion related to physiological or psychological causes

NURSING PRIORITIES
- Maintain patient safety.
- Assist patient in achieving and maintaining optimal level of functioning.
- Reorient patient to reality.
- Be alert for changes in nutritional status (body weight and fluid intake).

PATIENT OUTCOME CRITERIA
Throughout the length of stay, the patient will:
- remain free from injury to self or others
- complete activities of daily living (ADLs) with maximum independence
- interacts with caregivers and others while maintaining emotional equilibrium
- maintain body weight and fluid intake at acceptable levels.

  The interventions and accompanying rationales listed under Acute confusion also apply to the patient with chronic confusion. Additional interventions for Chronic confusion are as follows:

INTERVENTIONS

1. *Assess the patient's ability to independently complete ADLs* (dressing, grooming, eating, mobility, toileting) and to maintain balance.

2. *Assess the patient's short-term memory* by determining if the patient can remember three objects after 5 minutes have passed. Assess long-term memory by the patient's ability to remember his birthplace, what happened yesterday, and other information.

RATIONALES

1. Baseline assessment is essential to know what deficits are present. The degree of imbalance is of paramount importance, because it determines the risk of fall.

2. Memory loss occurs with chronic confusion.

3. *Assess the patient's weight* upon admission and at regular intervals. Monitor fluid and food intake. Assess urine amount, odor, and color. Note characteristics of stool for signs of chronic constipation. Also assess skin turgor for signs of dehydration.

3. The confused patient may not eat. Failure to ear and wandering behavior can lead to weight loss. The patient may forget to drink fluids, or may be unable to tell you if he is thirsty. Fluid intake should be 1500 to 1800 ml per day. The patient may also not be able to communicate problems with elimination. Both dehydration and infection can compound confusion.

4. Encourage patient to wear assistive devices, such as hearing aids and glasses.

4. Use of assistive devices increases awareness of the environment, orientation, and comprehension. If sensory input isn't accurate, the patient may misinterpret the environment.

5. *Maintain a familiar environment* by providing personal items from home. Label the room with the patient's name and a picture of the patient. Provide the same room for the length of stay. Assign a primary nurse. Provide a structured daily routine, and post it where it can be seen.

5. This type of familiarity assists with orientation and promotes a feeling of safety and security.

6. If the patient displays wandering behavior, use a physical activity to redirect him. Approach the patient in an unhurried manner.

6. Physical activity helps decrease wandering behavior. Spending time with the patient in an activity helps increase self-esteem.

7. Talk with the patient about familiar topics. Encourage reminiscing about happy times.

7. Reminiscing helps give meaning to the patient's existence.

8. Ignore insults during periods of agitation. Focus on the underlying feeling. Set limits on physically abusive behavior.

8. Anger and fear are common emotions with chronic confusion. Focusing on the underlying feeling of the event can help to defuse aggressive behavior.

9. *Document episodes of agitation.* Note the specific behaviors and the context of the episodes.

9. Documentation will help identify "triggers" for agitation. Caregivers can then try to prevent these episodes from recurring.

10. *Decrease unnecessary environmental stimuli,* such as excessive noise from the television and multiple conversations.

10. Excessive noise may trigger an aggressive episode

11. *Provide quiet time* or a rest period each day.

11. Quiet time or a rest period helps decrease stress.

12. Encourage pet therapy (using the patient's own pet or one from an agency).

12. Pet therapy is a complementary therapy that has a calming influence on patients.

13. *Assess the family's response to the patient's condition.* Tell them how to respond during periods of agitation.

13. Teaching the family about the condition and how to respond will lessen caregiver role strain.

14. *Recommend frequent visitation from family and friends.* Encourage them to touch the patient.

14. Visits from family, friends, or both, along with touching, help to decrease sensory deprivation.

15. Additional individualized interventions _____

15. Rationales:_____

> ### *Suggested NIC Interventions*
> Cognitive stimulation; Dementia management; Mood management; Reality orientation; Anxiety reduction; Decision-making support; Family involvement promotion; Delusion management; Cognitive restructuring; Memory training; Cerebral perfusion promotion; Neurological monitoring

> ### *Suggested NOC Outcomes*
> Cognitive ability; Cognitive orientation; Concentration; Decision-making; Distorted thought control; Identity; Information processing; Memory; Neurological status: Consciousness

Discharge planning
DISCHARGE CHECKLIST
Before discharge, the patient with acute or chronic confusion shows evidence of:
- ❏ stable vital signs
- ❏ stable weight
- ❏ adequate fluid intake (1,500 to 1,800 ml daily)
- ❏ absence of cardiac complications
- ❏ ability to keep self safe (with assistance as needed)
- ❏ ability to communicate personal needs to caregiver
- ❏ sleeping continuously for at least 6 hours at night
- ❏ adequate social support to complete ADLs at an optimum level.

TEACHING CHECKLIST
Document evidence that the patient and family demonstrate an understanding of:
- ❏ the names of each medication (both generic and trade names), the reasons for taking them, and possible adverse effects
- ❏ the need for a written medication schedule, and how to devise a method for remembering to take each medication (medication dispensing box or a medication calendar
- ❏ the danger of taking herbal medications such as ginkgo biloba for memory enhancement without first checking with the advanced nurse practitioner or physician regarding possible interactions with other medications
- ❏ possible "triggers" for agitation
- ❏ how to respond to the patient during periods of agitation
- ❏ the level of care needed for the patient to complete ADLs
- ❏ modifications in home environment/home schedule necessary for patient safety
- ❏ available support systems and community resources, such as adult day care, home health care, homemaker services, transportation, Meals On Wheels, support groups, such as the Alzheimer's Association and the National Alliance for the Mentally Ill, and respite care.

DOCUMENTATION CHECKLIST
Using outcome criteria as a guide, document:
- ❏ level of confusion upon admission and at discharge
- ❏ significant changes in clinical condition
- ❏ completion of diagnostic studies and laboratory tests
- ❏ weight recorded upon admission, at regular intervals, and at discharge
- ❏ complete intake and output records
- ❏ results of daily physical assessment findings
- ❏ results of daily mental status examinations, including confusion scales
- ❏ sleep pattern
- ❏ periods of agitation, associated with aggravating factors
- ❏ patient and family teaching, including medication teaching
- ❏ discharge planning.

Associated care plans
- Alzheimer's disease
- Compromised family coping
- Geriatric care
- Ineffective individual coping
- Nutritional deficit

References
Cox, H., et al. *Clinical Applications of Nursing Diagnosis: Adult, Child, Women's, Psychiatric, Geriatric, and Home Health Considerations,* 4th ed. Philadelphia: F.A. Davis Co., 2002.

Harkreader, H. *Fundamentals of Nursing: Caring and Clinical Judgment.* Philadelphia: W.B. Saunders Co., 2000.

Ignatavicius, D.D., and Workman, M.L. *Medical-Surgical Nursing: Critical Thinking for Collaborative Care,* 4th ed. Philadelphia: W.B. Saunders Co., 2002.

Thompson, J.M., et al. *Mosby's Clinical Nursing,* 5th ed. St. Louis: Mosby–Year Book, Inc., 2002.

Urden, L.D., et al. *Thelan's Critical Care Nursing: Diagnosis and Management,* 4th ed. St. Louis: Mosby–Year Book, Inc., 2002

Working with Your Older Patient: A Clinician's Handbook [Online]. Available: *www.nia.nih.gov/health/pubs/clinicians-handbook/p8. htm* [2002, July 5].

Dying

Introduction

DEFINITION AND TIME FOCUS

Death, according to Dr. Elisabeth Kübler-Ross, is "the key to the door of life." Becoming aware of death's inevitability and contemplating our fears and feelings about it can lead to a heightened appreciation for life and a more courageous and thoughtful response to its challenges. Nurses are involved with death daily and thus have repeated opportunities to assist dying patients and their families.

More than any other professional, the nurse has close and continuing contact with patients, direct experience with those who die, and concern for meeting the emotional and physiologic needs of patients and their families. Death remains the "great unknown," but the patients and their loved ones have the right to continue sharing life until the end; the nurse can help. This care plan focuses on the needs of the dying patient and the bereaved family in the hospital setting. (See *Clinical snapshot: Dying*.)

ETIOLOGY AND PRECIPITATING FACTORS

Death may result from:
- disease (or, occasionally, complications of the treatment of disease)
- injury or accident
- debilitation
- suicide or homicide.

Focused assessment guidelines

NURSING HISTORY
(FUNCTIONAL HEALTH PATTERN FINDINGS)

Because etiologic factors vary so widely in dying persons, no typical findings exist. Thus, this section presents an assessment guide to help the nurse plan care for the patient who is admitted with a diagnosis suggesting impending death. However, no such guide is appropriate for all patients. The answers to the following questions may help the nurse intervene effectively on behalf of the dying and their families, but the nurse must use professional judgment in deciding what, when, and how much to ask a patient.

Health-perception–health-management pattern
- Is the patient aware of the prognosis? If so, for how long has he known? If not, whose decision was it not to tell him?
- If the patient isn't aware of the prognosis, what does he believe is the reason for hospitalization?

- What measures were taken to help support or improve the patient's physical or emotional condition before this hospitalization? Does the patient believe those measures have helped? If so, how?
- What are the patient's expectations about this hospital admission and the proposed treatment?

Nutritional-metabolic pattern
- Does the patient have any dietary preferences or intolerances?
- Has the patient been anorexic, vomiting, or dysphagic?

Elimination pattern
- What's the patient's present elimination status and pattern?
- Is the patient using any elimination aids?

Activity-exercise pattern
- What's the patient's current activity level and tolerance?

Sleep-rest pattern
- What are the patient's present sleeping habits?
- Does the patient feel rested? If not, why?

Cognitive-perceptual pattern
- Does the patient have pain? If so, how severe is it?
- Is the patient's pain controlled? If so, by what?

Self-perception–self-concept pattern
- Which events or achievements have brought the patient the most satisfaction?
- What does the patient most want to accomplish before dying?

Role-relationship pattern
- Who are the patient's significant others?
- Among these, does the patient have any long-standing or unresolved conflicts or other unfinished business?
- Has the patient been able to talk about dying and death with loved ones?
- How are loved ones handling the situation?

Coping–stress tolerance pattern
- If the patient is aware of the prognosis, how is he coping with it?
- What resources are available to help the patient cope?

Value-belief pattern
- What's the patient's religious or spiritual orientation?
- What does the patient believe about death?

PHYSICAL FINDINGS

Physical findings in dying patients vary widely, depending on the cause of impending death; see the plan related to the patient's specific disease or condition.

DIAGNOSTIC STUDIES

See the plan related to the patient's specific disease or condition.

CLINICAL SNAPSHOT ☀

Dying

Major nursing diagnoses	Key patient outcomes
Decisional conflict (end-of-life issues)	Participate in decisions related to the medical treatment plan.
Fear	Identify specific fears.
Powerlessness	Participate in decisions related to care.
Situational low self-esteem	Express acceptance of impending end-of-life, if queried.
Risk for spiritual distress	Maintain personally meaningful spiritual practices, if desired.
Acute pain	Describe pain level as being less than the goal level (typically 3 or below on a 0 to 10 pain rating scale).
Risk for deficient fluid volume	Experience minimum discomfort related to dehydration.
Interrupted family processes	(The family will) share concerns with the patient and each other.
Dysfunctional grieving	(The family will) make contact with support persons.

Nursing diagnosis

Decisional conflict (end-of-life issues) related to end-stage disease or condition

NURSING PRIORITY

Support the patient's rights to participate in health care decision making.

PATIENT OUTCOME CRITERIA

As appropriate, the patient will make the decisions to accept or refuse treatments to the maximum extent of his ability, consistent with what's medically, legally, and ethically sound.

INTERVENTIONS	RATIONALES
1. At the time of admission, *ask the patient if he has any type of advance directive** (living will and durable power of attorney for health care). If there's none, respect the competent patient's wishes. If there's no advance directive and the patient isn't competent or can't communicate his wishes, discuss treatment decisions with his next of kin.	**1.** End-of-life decisions are reached through an agreement among the physician, the competent patient, and the family. The patient has the right to decide that cardiopulmonary resuscitation, mechanical ventilators, or any other procedures be withheld. The patient also has the right to execute or revoke a formal advance directive or verbal declarations at any time. The patient may have appointed an agent (family or friend) to make these health care decisions if he can't do so himself.
2. *Request a copy of the advance directive for the medical record if* the patient has one.	**2.** The formal document is just one way for the patient to communicate his choices to the health care team and loved ones.

---

*Italics indicate key interventions.

3. *Offer to help the patient execute an advance directive* if he doesn't have one or can't locate a copy of the formal document. Seek the assistance of qualified staff members, such as a social worker, chaplain, or patient representative to give written information on advance directives to the patient and to help him write an advance directive. A patient's spouse or blood relative isn't allowed to legally serve as a witness. If the patient asks you to be a witness and you're uncomfortable with the request, seek the advice of an immediate supervisor. Notify the physician when a patient executes an advance directive.

3. Qualified personnel who understand and can explain the advance directive must give information to the patient and family and take time to allow the patient and family to ask questions so they fully understand their rights. Patients may wish to take time to talk about this decision with their families, physicians, or lawyers.

4. If the patient chooses to verbalize treatment choices, document in the medical record the substance of the conversation and notification of the patient's physician.

4. Although such verbalization doesn't constitute or take the place of a formal advance directive, it nevertheless provides an indication of the patient's wishes and warrants a conversation between patient and physician as soon as possible.

5. Discuss cultural issues, as appropriate, with the patient and family regarding end-of-life decision-making processes and death. Incorporate into the care plan any rituals important to the patient during the dying process and at the time of death.

5. Cultural beliefs and traditions should be upheld with the highest regard.

6. See "Risk for spiritual distress" page 84.

6. The information the plan contains is recognizing the significance of the spiritual dimension.

Suggested NIC Interventions
Anxiety reduction; Coping enhancement; Spiritual support

Suggested NOC Outcomes
Anxiety control; Fear control

Nursing diagnosis

Fear related to potential pain, loss, emotional upheaval, and the unknowns of dying

NURSING PRIORITY

Promote identification and confrontation of specific realistic fears.

PATIENT OUTCOME CRITERIA

At his own pace, the patient will:
- identify specific fears
- express feelings, as desired
- use appropriate resources.

INTERVENTIONS

1. Examine personal fears and feelings about death. Before becoming involved with the dying patient and his family, identify your previous experiences with death and be aware of personal emotions, religious, or spiritual beliefs and fears. If talking about death is too uncomfortable for you, refer the patient and family to another professional with the necessary skills.

RATIONALES

1. A caregiver's personal feelings about and experiences with death affect the ability to promote healthy emotional responses. While most health care providers feel some anxiety about discussing dying and death with their patients, nurses who have difficulty with issues of death are less able to empathize with the patient and family. Appropriate referrals allow the patient's emotional needs to be addressed.

2. *Assess the patient's coping style and previous experience with deaths of relatives or friends.* Observe the patient's behaviors, and confer with the family and other caregivers as needed.

2. Each person responds differently to the threat of death. When threatened, most people initially revert to familiar coping mechanisms, and caregivers must be aware of these when establishing therapeutic communication. Previous experiences with death shape behavioral responses and may contribute significantly to the patient's overall ability to cope.

3. Use role modeling to facilitate expression of feelings, as appropriate: "If I were facing what you face right now, I think I might feel scared (or 'angry' or 'depressed')."

3. The patient may need "permission" to discuss fears. Opening discussion by focusing on the caregiver's feelings allows the patient the option of responding with an expression of personal feelings (if ready) and reassures the patient that such feelings are normal and acceptable. For some patients, expression of fears reduces their impact.

4. *Support coping mechanisms. Avoid forcing the patient to confront emotional issues.*

4. Each patient moves through various stages, at various times, in coping with impending death. Forcing issues is counterproductive and may damage the therapeutic relationship. Showing respect for the individual promotes trust.

5. As indicated by the patient's responsiveness to role modeling, *help the patient identify and prioritize specific fears.* Acknowledge the unknowns.

5. Identifying specific fears helps reduce the sense of overwhelming threat. Pain, loss of control, and being a burden to others are common fears of dying patients; identifying fear-causing factors allows a patient to begin making specific plans to cope with them. Acknowledging unknowns reassures the patient that the caregiver recognizes the enormity of the questions faced.

6. *Identify the patient's support system and resource base.* Coordinate involvement of the patient, his family, and other members of the health care team in making plans to deal with anticipated problems and needs.

6. Coordination of resources and support for the patient is essential in reducing the sense of isolation, which contributes to fear. The nurse's "in-between" position can help facilitate teamwork.

7. As needed, *provide appropriate referrals,* such as to a psychiatric liaison nurse, social worker, hospice, chaplain, or support group related to the specific disorder.

7. The patient and family may not be aware of available resources. Even if referrals aren't used, knowledge of resource availability can be comforting.

8. Provide companionship when possible.

8. Simply sitting quietly beside the patient communicates concern and may decrease the sense of isolation the patient feels.

9. If the patient is confronting imminent unexpected death (for example, as a result of trauma), provide brief, clear explanations and offer to call a member of the clergy. Provide a support person for the family, and — if at all possible — allow a family member to see the patient before death.

9. Even in the emergency care setting, patients have the right to caring communication, which may help reduce fear. Survivors of near-death experiences report hearing conversation and being aware of activity around them even when they appeared unresponsive. Surviving spouses of victims of sudden death list their need to see their spouse during resuscitation or before death as the concern that produced the most anguish for them.

10. Additional individualized interventions: _____

10. Rationales: _____

Suggested NIC Interventions
Anxiety reduction; Coping enhancement; Security enhancement

Suggested NOC Outcomes
Anxiety control; Fear control

General care plans

Nursing diagnosis

Powerlessness related to the inevitability of death, lack of control over body functions, and dependence on others for care

NURSING PRIORITY

Increase the patient's sense of personal power while promoting acceptance of the condition.

PATIENT OUTCOME CRITERIA

According to individual readiness, the patient will:
- participate in decisions related to care
- verbalize inner strengths
- set realistic goals
- initiate activity to put his affairs in order.

INTERVENTIONS	RATIONALES
1. *Encourage personal decision making whenever possible.* Allow maximum flexibility for scheduling activities, treatments, or visitors. Include the dying patient in making care-related decisions, as appropriate.	**1.** Patients relinquish many freedoms, regardless of the reason for their hospitalization. Allowing as many choices as possible promotes a sense of control and increases their coping ability. "Taking over" by caregivers diminishes patient's self-esteem and should be avoided unless necessary.
2. *Recognize and support courageous attitudes.*	**2.** Regardless of external circumstances, individuals maintain the freedom to choose their attitudes and approaches to life and death. Acknowledgment of courageous attitudes reinforces feelings of self-worth.
3. Accept your personal powerlessness to alter the fact that the patient is dying.	**3.** Health care professionals are usually anguished when they can't save their patients. Realistic self-assessment is essential to prevent caregiver burnout and to maintain the potential for effective intervention in areas that can be altered.
4. *Help the patient identify inner strengths.* Ask him to recall past losses: How did he deal with them? What did he learn from them?	**4.** Recalling other losses may help the patient build on previously learned coping skills. Losses throughout life may have uniquely provided the individual with qualities that can be used in facing death.
5. *Encourage the patient to establish realistic goals for the remainder of life.*	**5.** Establishing goals provides a focus for energy and reduces helplessness. Realistic evaluation of capabilities helps acceptance.
6. *Help the patient, as needed, to put his affairs in order* — for example, planning the funeral and memorial, writing a will, settling economic affairs, and making arrangements for survivors.	**6.** Putting affairs in order increases the patient's sense of control and may help soften the anticipated effects of the death on loved ones. "Unfinished business" may interfere with the patient's ability to move through coping stages.
7. Additional individualized interventions: _____	**7.** Rationales: _____

General care plans

> ### *Suggested NIC Interventions*
> *Cognitive restructuring; Mood management; Self-esteem enhancement; Decision-making support; Family involvement promotion; Health education; Values clarification; Mutual goal setting; Self-responsibility; Facilitation; Financial resource assistance; Health system guidance*

> ### *Suggested NOC Outcomes*
> *Depression control; Family participation in professional care; Health beliefs: Perceived ability to perform; Health beliefs: Perceived control; Health beliefs: Perceived resources; Participation: Health care decisions*

Nursing diagnosis
Situational low self-esteem related to imminent threat of death

NURSING PRIORITY
Help the patient maintain and enrich personal sense of meaningfulness throughout the remainder of life.

PATIENT OUTCOME CRITERIA
At his own pace, the patient will:
- express acceptance of impending end-of-life, if queried
- maintain preferred coping behaviors
- recall and review life experiences
- participate in creative activity (as able)
- touch family members freely, if desired.

INTERVENTIONS

1. *Use active listening skills, paying special attention to nonverbal or symbolic communication.* Use reflective statements and open-ended observations to offer an opportunity for discussion of difficult issues.

2. *Accept and respect the patient's right to use denial or avoidance behavior.* Whatever the patient's response, try to communicate your understanding.

3. *Be honest with the patient when answering questions, but don't force discussion of issues the patient hasn't introduced* or to which he hasn't responded. Take care to maintain hope for meaningful experiences.

4. *Encourage reminiscence and review of life experiences.*

5. *Promote creative expression.* Encourage family and friends to provide materials the patient can use for drawing, painting, writing, or other creative pursuits, or obtain materials from the occupational therapy department.

RATIONALES

1. A patient facing death may use nonverbal or symbolic communication to describe experiences and to test another person's willingness to talk about them. Rushed or distracted behavior from caregivers may distance the dying patient and contribute to feelings of alienation. Active listening and sharing show concern and respect for the patient as an individual.

2. The patient may choose to use denial or avoidance to the end; if so, respect this choice. Denial correlates with longer survival, according to research.

3. Honesty, even when truths are painful, reflects respect for the patient as an individual. However, the patient has the right to choose which issues to discuss. Research suggests that hopelessness correlates with poorer prognosis.

4. Life experiences have helped to shape the patient's unique identity. Reminiscence helps the patient remain connected to important core experiences and provides the caregiver with additional information that may aid in understanding the patient's behavior and responding to family needs.

5. Creative activity gives voice to individual expression, helping the patient maintain a sense of uniqueness. Also, drawings, paintings, or other original work may provide clues to the patient's state of acceptance.

6. Explore the option of preparing audiotaped or video-taped messages or mementos for family and friends to share after the patient's death (or earlier, if the patient wishes).

6. The patient may feel more comfortable expressing feelings in this way. The process of recording helps achieve acceptance of impending death. Such mementos may offer the patient comfort in sensing that some aspect of individual identity will endure. These records may also be valued by families in preserving the memory of the loved one.

7. Use touch generously when providing care, unless it makes the patient uncomfortable. Encourage family affection, including holding, rocking, and even lying next to the patient.

7. Illness and hospitalization may reduce the frequency of physical contact with others, which normally helps provide body image self-definition. Encouraging family affection helps maintain physical contact. Also, touch provides comfort and communicates genuine caring more effectively than almost any other measure.

8. Additional individualized interventions: _____
_____

8. Rationales: _____
_____

Suggested NIC Interventions
Cognitive restructuring; Decision-making support; Family involvement promotion; Financial resource assistance

Suggested NOC Outcomes
Depression control; Family participation in professional care; Health beliefs: Perceived ability to perform; Perceived control; Perceived resources; Participation: Health care decisions

---

Nursing diagnosis
Risk for spiritual distress related to confrontation with the unknown

NURSING PRIORITY
Help the patient savor the remaining period of life and identify meaning in impending death.

PATIENT OUTCOME CRITERIA
Throughout the remainder of life, the patient will:
- maintain personally meaningful spiritual practices, if desired
- find pleasure in some activities.

INTERVENTIONS

1. *Support the patient's personal spiritual beliefs,* even if they seem unusual or unfamiliar.

RATIONALES

1. Spiritual beliefs provide comfort based on specific personal meaningfulness to the patient. Attempting to alter such beliefs or supplant them with others shows lack of respect for the patient's choices and may precipitate undue conflict and distress.

2. *Recognize that facing death and dealing with separation are developmental tasks for all humans.* Promote a focus on growth and learning, rather than on disease or injury.

2. Because our culture places such emphasis on youth, we lack the societal integration of death as part of life that many other cultures take for granted. To help a patient accept impending death, caregivers must acknowledge it as a stage of development and validate its importance. Non–disease-related interventions (discussed throughout this plan) help redirect coping efforts toward positive life closure.

3. *Acknowledge what dying patients have to teach others, and express this to the patient and family,* when appropriate.

4. *Provide privacy according to the patient's wishes.*

5. *Offer to call the spiritual advisor of the patient's choice* — for example, a member of the clergy, counselor, or friend. Obtain and provide religious texts and other inspirational readings if requested.

6. Explore the possibility of organ donation, if appropriate, with the patient and family. Be familiar with hospital and regional policies and procedures for arranging donation of organs. Consider the underlying disease before discussing donation of specific organs.

7. *Address the patient while providing care, even if the patient appears unresponsive or comatose.* Encourage family members to continue talking to the patient.

8. *Worry less about saying the "wrong thing" than about being afraid to communicate caring.* In this way, set an example that family members may follow.

9. *Maintain a positive attitude.* Promote activities that provide even a few moments of enjoyment. Avoid generalizations that attempt to explain the patient's suffering.

10. Additional individualized interventions:_____

_____

3. Nurses can learn much from dying patients that may help in caring for others. In this way, dying patients may touch the lives of others they will never meet. Recognition of the lessons a dying person may pass on to others can help the patient find meaning in death and a sense of connectedness with life.

4. The hospital environment may allow the patient little time to be alone. A patient struggling with spiritual issues may need uninterrupted time for prayer or meditation.

5. A spiritual advisor may provide guidance or perform rituals the patient views as essential. Religious readings may be satisfying to a patient with a traditional religious orientation, although others may find comfort in nonreligious literature that has special personal significance.

6. Patients and families can find meaning and consolation in knowing others may benefit from organ donation. Many programs now have broad interlinking systems for identification of donors and transplantation of donated organs. Underlying disease may make some organs unsatisfactory for donation, but others (such as skin) typically are usable and may not require immediate transplantation.

7. Survivors of near-death experiences and persons who recover from deep or prolonged coma have reported remembering conversation that took place around them while they were apparently unconscious.

8. Because of prolonged close contact with dying patients and interaction with their families, nurses are uniquely suited to help facilitate dialogue about dying between the patient and family. In many cases, patients and families are afraid to raise the subject directly, out of concern that they may cause emotional upset. The nurse may be able to act as a liaison to help communication, thereby reducing guilt and anxiety and further preparing the patient and family for separation.

9. The caregiver's positive attitude may help the patient maintain hope and find pleasure in living even while approaching death. Small pleasures may be extremely meaningful when the patient's world view is narrowed by illness. Generalizations or attempts to provide simplistic explanations (for example, "It may be a blessing") indicate shallow appreciation for the patient's situation and may be interpreted as dismissal of real concerns.

10. Rationales:_____

_____

General care plans

Suggested NIC Interventions
Dying care; Spiritual growth facilitation; Spiritual support; Hope instillation

Suggested NOC Outcomes
Dignified dying; Hope; Spiritual well-being

Nursing diagnosis

Acute pain related to injury; risk for chronic pain related to underlying disease

NURSING PRIORITY

Relieve pain, if present, while allowing the patient to remain as alert as possible.

PATIENT OUTCOME CRITERIA

Throughout the hospital stay, the patient will:
- participate in decisions regarding pain control (to the extent possible)
- describe his pain level as being less than the goal level (typically 3 or below on a 0 to 10 pain rating scale).

INTERVENTIONS	RATIONALES
1. See the "Acute pain" care plan, page 32 and the "Chronic pain" care plan, page 63.	**1.** These plans provide interventions useful for any patient in pain.
2. *Assess the patient's level of discomfort frequently.* Use pain scales as a concrete means for the patient to describe the pain. Compare his current level of pain with the goal level (typically 3 or lower on a 0 to 10 pain rating scale). Urge the patient to call for medication before the pain becomes severe.	**2.** A patient's level of discomfort has a significant impact on the emotional adjustment to limited life expectancy: Patients with poorly controlled pain tend to have more difficulty coping with other issues. Pain scales, used with other modes of subjective and objective assessment, can provide valuable confirmation or suggest the need to reevaluate assumptions about the patient's pain. Medication given early in the pain cycle is more effective.
3. *To the extent possible, include the patient in decisions regarding pain medications.*	**3.** Ability to control pain allows the patient to use limited energy for other, more rewarding, purposes.
4. *When possible, control pain with oral medication,* rather than with I.M. injections. If the patient is unable to tolerate oral medications, consider arranging for I.V. injections or infusions or subcutaneous injections or infusions. Investigate analgesic combinations, such as long- and short-acting medications or narcotics and nonsteroidal anti-inflammatory drugs (NSAIDs).	**4.** Repeated I.M. injections, particularly in the debilitated patient, traumatize skin and gradually become less effective as areas of scarring develop and inhibit absorption. Analgesic combinations may achieve better control over chronic and acute pain episodes. NSAIDs may be effective for bone pain. Around-the-clock medication administration may be required for effective pain control.
5. *Recognize that the usual safe dose levels may not apply to the terminally ill patient.* Consult the physician if the ordered dosage no longer seems effective.	**5.** A patient maintained on narcotic analgesics for an extended period may develop significant tolerance and require amounts of medication considerably larger than the usual dosage to achieve comparable effects.
6. *Assess for psychological factors that may exacerbate pain, and intervene to treat them.*	**6.** The patient's pain threshold may be lowered by boredom, anxiety, and loneliness.
7. *If abdominal distention causes pain, consider using return-flow enemas.* Ensure that routine stool softeners or laxatives have been prescribed, as indicated by the patient's condition.	**7.** Narcotic analgesics, lack of activity, and resultant slowing of peristalsis may cause painful abdominal distention and constipation. Gentle return-flow enemas may reduce discomfort. Medications can contribute further to constipation, and stool softeners or laxatives may be required regularly.
8. Additional individualized interventions: _____	**8.** Rationales: _____

Suggested NIC Interventions
For both: Medication management; Pain management; Patient-controlled analgesia (PCA) assistance; Analgesic administration; Conscious sedation
In addition, for chronic pain: Mood management; Patient contracting; Behavior modification; Coping enhancement; Cognitive restructuring

Suggested NOC Outcomes
For both: Comfort level; Pain control; Pain: Disruptive effects; Pain level
In addition, for chronic pain: Depression control; Depression level; Pain: Psychological response

Nursing diagnosis

Risk for deficient fluid volume related to anorexia and dehydration associated with imminent death

NURSING PRIORITY
Promote patient comfort during the dying process.

PATIENT OUTCOME CRITERION
During the final phase of the dying process, the patient will experience minimum discomfort related to dehydration.

INTERVENTIONS	RATIONALES
1. *Avoid vigorous fluid replacement for terminally ill patients.* Respect patient wishes regarding hydration and artificial feeding.	**1.** Dehydration is normal in terminal illnesses. I.V. hydration or artificial feeding may unnecessarily prolong discomfort. Patient wishes regarding hydration and artificial feeding must be honored.
2. *Offer frequent mouth care, ice chips, sips of water, or hard candy, as* indicated by the patient's condition.	**2.** These measures may help reduce discomfort related to mouth dryness and minimal oral intake.
3. *Provide meticulous skin care.* Use soap sparingly and lotion generously if dry skin is present. Turn the patient carefully to prevent shearing.	**3.** Dehydration and debilitation contribute to poor skin turgor and increased risk of skin breakdown. Soap dries skin, increasing irritation. Gentle massage with lotion and careful turning demonstrate care and help prevent complications.
4. Additional individualized interventions: _____	**4.** Rationales: _____

Suggested NIC Interventions
Acid-base management; Electrolyte management; Fluid and electrolyte management; Fluid monitoring; Hypovolemia management; Intravenous therapy (I.V.) therapy; Nutrition management; Nutritional monitoring

Suggested NOC Outcomes
Electrolyte and acid-base balance; Fluid balance; Nutritional status: Food and fluid intake

Nursing diagnosis

Interrupted family processes related to imminent death of a family member

NURSING PRIORITY
Promote family integrity by facilitating healthy coping, mutual support, and communication with the dying person.

PATIENT OUTCOME CRITERIA

Throughout the patient's hospital stay, the family will:
- participate in care
- share concerns with the patient and each other
- appear well rested most of the time.
  Throughout the hospital stay, the patient will:
- exhibit minimal anxiety over the family's well-being.

INTERVENTIONS	RATIONALES
1. See the "Compromised family coping" care plan, page 67.	**1.** The "Compromised family coping" care plan provides guidelines for helping families at risk for crisis.
2. *Assess the family's level of acceptance and coping by observing behaviors and interactions of individuals with the patient and by providing time for private discussions with family members,* as needed. Be alert to differences among individual family members and clues to the family's previous experiences with death, if any.	**2.** Effective intervention must be appropriately correlated with the stage of acceptance. Each member of the family may respond differently to the threat of loss. Previous family deaths may affect members' ability to cope in mutually supportive ways.
3. *Liberalize visiting policies,* as needed. Allow private time for the family to be with the patient. Encourage family members to participate in care, remaining alert for signs of possible anxiety or discomfort.	**3.** Family integrity is more likely to be maintained when members are able to continue their usual level of contact with one another. Helping with patient care reduces the family's sense of helplessness and provides special comfort to the patient. However, this shouldn't substitute for the nurse's cultivation of close involvement with the patient and family. The nurse must avoid giving the impression of dismissing or neglecting the patient.
4. *When possible, facilitate family dialogue,* remaining aware of established family roles and expectations. Offer to introduce topics, as appropriate; strive to promote face-to-face communication when possible.	**4.** Discussing issues surrounding death is difficult for most families and may be compounded by unresolved conflicts, guilt, or role demands. The nurse may be able to open up communication about sensitive issues. Family stability is related to long-standing patterns of behavior, so interventions that are at odds with these will be unsuccessful. Direct communication promotes maximum understanding and helps minimize guilt later over things left unsaid.
5. *Be aware of cultural attitudes* that may affect family response.	**5.** Every culture views death in a different way. Some observe specific rituals for the occasion; some emphasize withdrawal from others. Being aware of such differences helps the nurse plan interventions to support the family's cultural heritage.
6. *Help the family identify and mobilize external resources,* such as friends, clergy, and counselors, and financial resources. Provide referrals to a psychiatric clinician, social worker, or pastoral care, as needed.	**6.** A family coping with death, especially if the dying is prolonged, may require added support to deal with stresses. Other professionals may offer such assistance as spiritual or psychological counseling, temporary housing placement, and guidance in identifying programs to help with the financial burden of care.
7. *Encourage family members to maintain their physical and emotional strength.* Emphasize the importance of adequate rest, food, and exercise. Suggest that family members take turns at the bedside if they are reluctant to leave the patient unattended.	**7.** Maintenance of physical and emotional well-being is essential if family members are to continue providing support for the patient and each other. "Break times" help the family maintain contact with external resources and reduce the emotional strain of constant attendance to the dying person's needs.

8. Additional individualized interventions: _____

_____

8. Rationales: _____

_____

> **Suggested NIC Interventions**
> *Coping enhancement; Family support; Family integrity promotion; Family process maintenance; Normalization promotion*

> **Suggested NOC Outcomes**
> *Family coping; Family environment: Internal; Family functioning; Family normalization*

Nursing diagnosis

Dysfunctional grieving: Potential for growth related to ineffective management

NURSING PRIORITY
Facilitate the initiation of healthy grieving after death.

PATIENT OUTCOME CRITERIA
Before survivors leave the hospital, they will:
- view and touch the body, if desired
- express initial grief or disbelief
- make contact with support persons.

INTERVENTIONS

1. See the "Grieving" care plan, page 105.

2. If not already acquainted with the family, introduce yourself, identify your relationship as the patient's caregiver, and express sympathy.

3. *Allow family members to see and touch the body.* If death was sudden and unexpected, prepare them for the appearance of the body in advance, explaining that all measures were tried to restore life. *Ensure that the body is respectfully covered.* Don't remove all indications of emergency intervention before allowing the family into the room, but *leave side rails down and the patient's face and hands visible.*

4. Use direct, simple sentences, avoiding euphemisms, to describe the death. Provide comforting observations when possible such as, "He died quietly and appeared to have no pain" or "She told me last night about the good times you used to have, and she seemed very happy."

5. *Acknowledge the family's loss by gently reorienting them to the reality of death* with such statements as "It must be hard to accept that he's really dead." Avoid overly sentimental statements.

6. Avoid recommending or encouraging sedation of a family member unless severely dysfunctional behavior is present.

RATIONALES

1. The "Grieving" care plan contains general interventions helpful in caring for bereaved families.

2. If the family arrives after the patient has died, or if the family doesn't know caregivers from previous contact, such an introduction reassures them that the patient died with concerned caregivers at hand.

3. Seeing and touching the body of the loved one helps the family accept the reality of death. Advance preparation may help reduce distress. The face and hands invite touch if accessible; if not, the family may be reluctant to disturb coverings. Gross blood or other secretions should be removed before the family enters, but putting away all supplies and cleaning the room before the family sees the body may create doubts that "everything possible was done" for the patient.

4. Most family members are too anxious at this time to comprehend complex explanations. Euphemisms such as "passed on" may offend some family members and can interfere with reality orientation. Sharing selected, specific observations with family members may help minimize guilt and promote healthy grieving.

5. Shock and disbelief are normal initial responses to sudden death and, to a certain degree, even to expected death. Gentle reorientation aids in integrating death into reality. Overly sentimental utterances may be inappropriate to the family's actual relationship with the deceased.

6. Sedation may delay initiation of the normal grieving process.

General care plans

7. Offer to call a friend, member of the clergy, or counselor to help with immediate arrangements. If the family doesn't designate such a person, offer the services of the hospital chaplain, a liaison nurse, or another in-house professional skilled in dealing with grief.

8. *Prepare the family for the work of grieving.* Emphasize the normality of a wide range of emotional responses (such as anger, guilt, sadness, frustration, resentment, fear, and depression) and behaviors (such as crying, laughing, withdrawal, and confusion) in response to loss of a loved one. Provide information on bereavement counseling and support groups.

9. *Listen patiently to retellings of the story of the death,* especially if it was unexpected. Avoid statements that might be interpreted as judgmental.

10. *Reemphasize the need for health-promoting self-care behaviors during the grieving period.*

11. Ensure that significant others will be available to be with survivors after they leave the hospital.

12. If possible, provide a follow-up call to surviving family members 1 to 3 months after the death. Keeping a callback calendar on the unit can help in organizing this task.

13. Additional individualized interventions: _____
_____

7. During the initial stages of grieving, family members may exhibit indecision, disorganization, and disorientation. Providing an advocate may reduce the family's distress while they are making necessary arrangements, such as for disposition of the body.

8. Family members are sometimes unprepared for the various feelings experienced in the grieving process; some may feel they are "going crazy" when unexpected feelings occur. Understanding that such emotional disorganization is a normal and healthy response to loss can help the family deal with these feelings. Bereavement counseling and support groups can provide invaluable information and support.

9. Retelling of events by survivors is an essential part of reality acceptance and coping. Judgmental utterances may provoke severe guilt reactions in family members.

10. Grieving places additional stress on survivors, who are at increased risk for developing physical illness during mourning. Health-promoting behavior such as exercise can help release emotional energy and reduce the effects of stress.

11. Grieving is facilitated by sharing feelings with others. Few cases of loneliness are as profound as that of a bereaved person, newly alone.

12. Follow-up from caregivers to survivors is the final step in care of the dying patient and provides the family with added assurance that their loved one was special and received care accordingly. This call also provides an opportunity to identify dysfunctional grieving and make appropriate referrals, if needed.

13. Rationales:_____
_____

Suggested NIC Interventions
Caregiver support; Respite care; Family involvement promotion; Family support; Normalization promotion; Health education; Self-modification assistance; Decision-making support; Health system guidance

Suggested NOC Outcomes
Caregiver well-being; Family coping; Family normalization; Health promoting behavior; Health seeking behavior; Participation: Health care decisions

---

Discharge planning
DISCHARGE CHECKLIST
If the patient is discharged home before death occurs, the patient should have:
❏ referral to a hospice or to a home health care agency
❏ adequate support system for family members.

TEACHING CHECKLIST
If the patient is discharged home before death, document that the patient and family demonstrate an understanding of:
❏ support and resources available
❏ what to do when death is imminent
❏ what the family should do after death occurs
❏ what to expect in normal mourning and grieving.

DOCUMENTATION CHECKLIST

If the patient is discharged home before death, using outcome criteria as a guide, document:

❐ fears
❐ feelings expressed
❐ goals
❐ preferred coping behaviors
❐ spiritual or religious practices
❐ pain-control measures
❐ family members' behaviors
❐ patient and family teaching
❐ discharge planning.
   If death occurs in the hospital, document:
❐ time and circumstances of death
❐ request for autopsy
❐ request for organ and tissue donation
❐ disposition of body and effects
❐ family support measures implemented.

Associated care plans

- Acute pain
- Chronic pain
- Compromised family coping
- Grieving
- Ineffective individual coping

(See also the plan for the specific disease or disorder.)

References

Frankl, V.E. *Man's Search for Meaning.* New York: Pocket Books, 1997.

Hoff, L.A. *People in Crisis: Understanding and Helping,* 5th ed. San Francisco: Jossey-Bass, 2001.

Jung, C.G. *Modern Man in Search of a Soul.* New York: Harcourt, Brace, Jovanovich, 1996.

Kalish, R.A., ed. *The Final Transition.* Farmingdale, N.Y.: Baywood Publishing Co., 1985.

Kübler-Ross, E., ed. *Death: The Final Stage of Growth.* Englewood Cliffs, N.J.: Prentice-Hall, 1975.

Kübler-Ross, E. *Living with Death and Dying.* New York: Simon and Schuster, 1997.

Tatelbaum, J. *The Courage to Grieve: Creative Living, Recovery, and Growth through Grief.* New York: Harper & Row Publishers, 1984.

General care plans

Geriatric care

Introduction

DEFINITION AND TIME FOCUS
The geriatric patient is defined as a person age 75 or older who's admitted into an acute care hospital setting. This care plan focuses on care needs specific to aging and to the sudden impact of hospitalization. (See *Clinical snapshot: Geriatric care,* page 94.)

ETIOLOGY AND PRECIPITATING FACTORS
The geriatric patient is prone to health problems because of the following changes associated with aging:
- increased susceptibility to infection
- decreased muscle strength and generalized debility
- increased potential for chronic disease because of genetic flaws that appear with advancing age
- psychosocial isolation
- limited income and earning ability
- impaired compensatory mechanisms

Focused assessment guidelines

NURSING HISTORY (FUNCTIONAL HEALTH PATTERN FINDINGS)
Health-perception–health-management pattern
- Various presenting problems, depending on the underlying disease

Nutritional-metabolic pattern
- Decreased appetite resulting from trauma or disease and impact of hospitalization
- Preference for usual dietary pattern of frequent, small meals
- Appetite greatest during morning hours
- Chewing problems due to ill-fitting or lost dentures

Elimination pattern
- Constipation
- Regular use of laxatives or enemas
- Urinary incontinence or urine retention related to prostatic hyperplasia (males), relaxation of perineal support (females), immobility, or environmental changes

Activity-exercise pattern
- Stiffness resulting from bed rest and decreased activity
- Fear of falls because of general weakness

Sleep-rest pattern
- Shorter sleep cycles and early morning awakening

Cognitive-perceptual pattern
- Difficulty remembering or comprehending events that led to hospitalization
- Discomfort from forced confinement and limited physical activity
- Visual or sensory deficits

Self-perception–self-concept pattern
- Lack of self-confidence in maintaining independent activities
- Sense of despair because of inability to provide personal self-care (if ability is curtailed by disease or health problem)

Role-relationship pattern
- Social isolation
- Fear of uselessness and of becoming a family burden with increased care needs arising from health problem

Coping–stress tolerance pattern
- Anticipatory grief over loss of personal independence caused by chronic disease
- Dependence on others and loss of interest in living because of helplessness caused by illness

Value-belief pattern
- Mourning of loss of meaningful religious practices such as church attendance
- Anger at God, directed toward others or self, reflecting depression
- Inability to find meaning or purpose in existence
- Strong ethnic identity that may conflict with values of hospital and staff

PHYSICAL FINDINGS
General physiologic differences associated with aging are noted here. Specific physical findings related to particular disease or illness aren't discussed.

Gastrointestinal
- Decreased saliva and ptyalin secretion
- Decreased esophageal nerve function
- Decreased gastric and intestinal motility
- Decreased hydrochloric acid production
- Delayed gastric emptying
- Decreased fat and calcium absorption

Cardiovascular
- Increased systolic pressure
- Increased pulse rate
- Orthostatic hypotension
- Arterial insufficiency
- Narrowing of vessels
- Decreased blood flow to organs
- Increased systemic vascular resistance

Neurologic
- Decreased sense of smell, taste, vision, touch, and hearing
- Decreased deep tendon reflexes
- Reduced nerve conduction time

- Generally slower responses
- Reduced speed of fine motor movements
- Alteration in sleep patterns (3- to 4-hour sleep periods)

Integumentary
- Increased wrinkles
- Loss of skin turgor and elasticity
- Thinning skin (from reduced subcutaneous fat)
- Reduced sebaceous and sweat gland function
- Skin dryness
- Changes in nail thickness
- Brown or black wartlike areas of skin (seborrheic keratosis)
- Red-purple overgrowth of dilated blood vessels (cherry angioma)

Musculoskeletal
- Decreased bone mass, possible osteoporosis
- Decrease in height
- Flexed posture
- Calcified cartilage and ligaments
- Decreased muscle tone and strength
- Gait changes
- Decreased range of motion (may be due to osteoarthritis, rheumatoid arthritis, or gout)

Respiratory
- Decreased lung tissue compliance (elasticity)
- Calcification of vertebral cartilage, with reduced rib mobility and chest expansion
- Decreased vital capacity
- Decreased coughing efficiency

Genitourinary
- Enlarged prostate in male
- Decrease in number of renal nephrons
- Decrease in urine concentration ability
- Increased nocturia
- Reduced vaginal lubrication in female
- Stress incontinence in female due to decreased muscle tone, uterine prolapse, and decreased bladder capacity

Endocrine
- Thyroid — increased nodularity
- Parathyroid — decreased hormone release
- Pancreas — delayed insulin release from beta cells
- Adrenals — decreased aldosterone and ketosteroid levels

Eye
- Decreased light permeability of lens (cataracts) and cornea
- Decreased speed of adaptation to darkness
- Decreased accommodation
- Increased astigmatism
- Less efficient intraocular fluid absorption (can lead to glaucoma)
- White lipid deposit at edge of iris (arcus senilis)
- Drying of conjunctivae
- Increased nystagmus on lateral gaze

Ear
- Pure tone loss
- High-frequency loss
- Impacted cerumen
- Significant hearing loss in one-third of those older than age 65 and in one-half of those older than age 80

Nose
- Increase in coarse hairs

Mouth and throat
- Decreased saliva
- Increased dryness
- Loss of teeth
- Receding gums
- Atrophy of taste buds
- Slowed gag reflex

DIAGNOSTIC STUDIES
Tests ordered depend on the particular disease or on presenting pathophysiology or symptoms.

POTENTIAL COMPLICATIONS
- Mental confusion
- Contractures
- Fecal impaction
- Falls and fractures
- Urine retention and cystitis
- Pulmonary emboli
- Depression
- Hopelessness
- Loneliness
- Grief

General care plans

CLINICAL SNAPSHOT

Geriatric care

Major nursing diagnoses and collaborative problems	Key patient outcomes
ND: Disturbed thought processes: Slowed or diminished responsiveness	Adapt to hospital routine without agitation.
ND: Acute confusion	Maintain orientation at or above baseline.
ND: Risk for injury	Remain free from injury.
CP: Risk for renal impairment	Show no signs and symptoms of fluid overload.
ND: Imbalanced nutrition: Less than body requirements	Eat 50% or more of items on food tray, no unintentional weight loss.
ND: Impaired physical mobility	Show no new evidence of reddened skin areas.
ND: Disturbed sleep pattern	Report sleeping at least 5 to 6 hours at a time.
ND: Risk for situational low self-esteem	Initiate involvement with others.
ND: Social isolation	Maintain social contacts.
ND: Risk for spiritual distress	Verbalize or display satisfaction with provisions for spiritual needs.

Nursing diagnosis

Disturbed thought processes: Slowed or diminished responsiveness related to cerebral degeneration

NURSING PRIORITY
Allow ample time for all behaviors and responses.

PATIENT OUTCOME CRITERIA
Throughout the hospital stay, the patient will:
- perform self-care activities (to the degree possible) without evidence of feeling rushed
- adapt to hospital routine without agitation.

INTERVENTIONS

1. *Assess mental status:** Note orientation, remote and recent memory, ability to interpret and abstract, and general rapidity of response.

2. Depending on deficits identified, institute appropriate measures:

– Allow increased response time when speaking with an older person.
– Give information concisely and slowly.

– Allow ample time for activities of daily living and care-related procedures.

RATIONALES

1. The patient's mental status may be altered because of cerebral degeneration or other factors such as medications but must be assessed individually. Many elderly patients retain full alertness.

2. Compensation for any deficits can allow an older person to maintain dignity and active participation in daily activities.
– Thought processing may be slower in an older adult.

– Concise, slowed speech helps prevent information overload and decreases the risk of misunderstanding.
– Slower thinking may be accompanied by slower performance of tasks.

*Italics indicate key interventions.

– Avoid shouting at the patient or using baby talk when communicating.

– Slowed responses don't necessarily imply a hearing deficit. Shouting may increase the patient's anxiety, further impairing his performance of tasks. Use of baby talk is demeaning and may erode self-esteem already compromised by disability and dependence on others for care.

3. Once hospital activities are established, maintain a routine as much as possible.

3. Adaptation to change may be slower in an older patient. Routines provide security and reassurance. Major environmental alterations, particularly when accompanied by physiologic changes, may precipitate depression, confusion, or psychosis.

4. Additional individualized interventions: _____
_____

4. Rationales: _____
_____

Suggested NIC Interventions
Cognitive stimulation; Dementia management

Suggested NOC Outcomes
Cognitive ability; Concentration; Information processing

Nursing diagnosis
Acute confusion related to diminished perception of sensory data

NURSING PRIORITIES
- Promote increased clarity of sensory-perceptual stimuli.
- Decrease agitation related to confusion.

PATIENT OUTCOME CRITERIA
Throughout the hospital stay, the patient will:
- perform self-care activities (to the degree possible) without evidence of feeling rushed
- participate in prescribed therapy (such as physical therapy or occupational therapy)
- adapt to hospital routine without agitation.

INTERVENTIONS

1. When confusion is evident, attempt to identify the cause, such as a change in hearing, visual ability, or mental status (see previous diagnosis). Be aware of other factors that can cause confusion, such as metabolic alterations, hypoxemia, electrolyte imbalances, or medications. If possible, plan time to sit with the patient, engage in conversation, and provide reorientation to surroundings. If the patient is amenable, use touch often during communications.

2. Before speaking, alert the patient by touch; speak only when clearly in the patient's line of vision. Keep your face in the light.

3. Speak in a low tone. (If the patient's hearing is greatly impaired and no hearing aid is available, place a stethoscope into the patient's ears, then speak into the bell.) Provide a telephone amplifier.

4. Provide the patient's own glasses for reading, as needed.

RATIONALES

1. Confusion may be related to misunderstanding due to deafness or to disorientation due to visual impairment. Confusion may also be a symptom of more serious problems. Assuming that confusion is the normal mental state of a patient may allow problems that have physical or physiologic causes to go unrecognized. Touching and engaging in conversation can reduce the depersonalizing effects of hospitalization that may increase confusion.

2. If information isn't heard clearly, it may be misperceived and increase confusion. Older persons may compensate for hearing deficits by lipreading and must see your facial features to do so.

3. Loss of high-frequency hearing ability usually occurs first.

4. Distance accommodation decreases with aging.

5. Allow extra time for adjustment to changes in light levels. Turn on lights slowly if there are several in the room.

5. Light accommodation also decreases with aging.

6. Provide adequate illumination during the day and at night.

6. "Sundowning" is a condition in which the older patient tends to become confused at the end of the day, when fading light causes loss of visual cues. Commonly marked by wandering, it is reduced when the available lighting allows clear visualization of persons, objects, and surroundings.

7. Provide environmental cues to orient the patient — for example, a clock, a calendar, or pictures of loved ones.

7. Confusion and disorientation are reduced by the presence of familiar objects in the immediate environment.

8. Encourage the use of audiotaped or videotaped messages from family members if disorientation persists.

8. Taped messages provide the comfort of familiar voices (or voices and faces) when the family isn't able to visit and may decrease agitation and restlessness associated with disorientation.

9. Additional individualized interventions: _____

9. Rationales: _____

Suggested NIC Interventions
Cognitive stimulation; Dementia management; Mood management; Reality orientation; Anxiety reduction; Delusion management

Suggested NOC Outcomes
Cognitive ability; Cognitive orientation; Concentration; Distorted thought control; Information processing

Nursing diagnosis
Risk for injury due to a fall

NURSING PRIORITIES
- Prevent injury.
- Increase independent mobility.

PATIENT OUTCOME CRITERIA
Throughout hospital stay, the patient will:
- remain free from injury
- maintain or increase strength and range of motion
- maintain or increase independent mobility.

INTERVENTIONS

1. *Monitor blood pressure of patient in supine and sitting positions.* Teach the patient to rise slowly and sit at the edge of the bed for 3 to 5 minutes before standing.

2. *Observe the patient for impaired mobility:* gait, transfer, and balance. Request physical therapy (PT) and occupational therapy (OT) evaluation and treatment in hospital and PT/OT home safety evaluation upon discharge.

RATIONALES

1. Postural hypotension is a significant cause of falls and injury. Sitting at the edge of the bed prior to rising decreases the effect of postural hypotension.

2. Poor balance and gait impairment are frequent causes of falls. Five percent of falls result in fracture. PT/OT therapy can increase strength and independence and decrease the incidence of falls. Home safety evaluation can correct risk factors for falls and suggest the need for home safety equipment installation, such as grab bars anyd shower chairs.

3. *Use restraints judiciously and only with the permission of the patient or an individual who has his durable power of attorney for health care.* Monitor the use of benzodiazepines and sedative hypnotics (chemical restraints). Request a sitter for a patient at risk for falls as an alternative to employing restraints.

4. Additional individualized interventions:_____
_____

3. Restraints can contribute to falls, accidents, and circulatory injury, and can damage the patient's self-esteem. They should never be used as substitutes for adequate care or supervision. Use of physical or chemical restraints is carefully monitored by the Health Care Financing Association and other governing agencies.

4. Rationales:_____
_____

Suggested NIC Interventions
Surveillance: Safety; Fall prevention

Suggested NOC Outcomes
Safety status: Physical injury; Safety status: Falls occurrence

---

Collaborative problem

Risk for renal impairment related to physiologic degeneration of nephrons and glomeruli

NURSING PRIORITY

Compensate for decreased renal function.

PATIENT OUTCOME CRITERIA

Throughout the hospital stay, the patient will show:
- no medication-induced confusion or stupor
- no toxic adverse effects from medications
- no medication overdose from cumulative effect of reduced renal function
- no signs or symptoms of fluid overload.

INTERVENTIONS	RATIONALES
1. *Monitor the patient for toxic adverse effects.*	**1.** Altered and erratic renal function caused by aging may affect the drug excretion rate, causing toxicity at lower doses.
2. *Administer narcotics and sedatives judiciously.*	**2.** Normal doses of these drugs may create an overdose for the older person because of the cumulative effect of reduced renal excretion.
3. *Collaborate with the physician to adjust fluid intake.*	**3.** Impaired renal function may cause heart failure. In addition, the aging heart is less efficient, further contributing to the risk of heart failure.
4. *Monitor for signs of fluid overload,* such as neck vein distention, increased central venous pressure readings, crackles, dependent edema, increased pulse rate, and rapid weight gain.	**4.** Impaired renal function may cause fluid retention.
5. Additional individualized interventions:_____	**5.** Rationales:_____

Nursing diagnosis

Imbalanced nutrition: Less than body requirements related to taste bud atrophy, poor dentition, decreased saliva and ptyalin secretion, economic limitations, or poor dietary habits

NURSING PRIORITY

Promote optimal nutritional intake.

PATIENT OUTCOME CRITERIA
Within 1 day of admission, the patient will:
- verbalize dietary habits and preferences
- identify factors interfering with adequate nutritional intake
- eat 50% or more of items on food tray, if appropriate.
  By the time of discharge, the patient will:
- list dietary recommendations and specific foods to avoid or increase in diet, on request
- identify resources and referrals for assistance with meals, shopping, or financial needs (if appropriate)
- have no unintentional weight loss.

INTERVENTIONS	RATIONALES
1. *Assess the patient's dietary habits and history.* Request an evaluation by a dietitian if there has been: – recent unintentional weight loss – vomiting or diarrhea for 3 days – chewing or swallowing difficulty – tube feeding or total parenteral nutrition ordered – a wound – extended nothing-by-mouth status – surgery planned	1. Any of these factors place the patient at increased risk for infection, skin breakdown, and other complications. A high intake of saturated fats and salt may contribute to coronary artery disease and hypertension — two factors associated with mortality in elderly patients. Preferences must be considered, however, because an older patient may be reluctant to alter established dietary patterns.
2. With the patient and dietitian, plan to meet the patient's therapeutic dietary needs during hospitalization, providing foods according to the patient's usual pattern if the diet is nutritionally adequate. If the diet isn't adequate, teach the patient about dietary recommendations. Allow family members to bring food from home if appropriate.	2. Including the patient in diet planning promotes a sense of control and may improve compliance. Familiar foods are more likely to be eaten. Maintaining usual patterns whenever possible helps provide a sense of security — particularly important to the elderly person in an unfamiliar environment.
3. *Ensure that the diet plan is compatible with the patient's chewing capability.* Arrange for a dental consultation if poor dentition is a factor.	3. Chewing difficulty may compromise adequate nutritional intake.
4. Encourage liberal seasoning of food with herbs and spices, observing dietary limitations required for underlying conditions.	4. Because taste bud sensitivity diminishes with age, bland foods may be left uneaten.
5. Serve all meals when the patient is out of bed and seated in a chair, preferably in the company of others.	5. Eating meals in bed in a semi-Fowler's position can lead to aspiration. Socialization can help to increase the patient's dietary intake.
6. *Assess for environmental, physical, and emotional factors that may contribute to poor nutritional intake at home.* Examples include: – inadequate income – lack of transportation for shopping – lack of space or equipment for food preparation or storage – lack of energy for preparing food – loneliness and depression.	6. An elderly patient may be reluctant to verbalize reasons for poor nutrition unless questioned specifically about them.
7. Before discharge, make appropriate referrals to alleviate or eliminate any identified problems.	7. Careful predischarge assessment, problem solving, and referral are essential to prevent exacerbation of nutritional problems after discharge.
8. Additional individualized interventions:_____	8. Rationales:_____

> **Suggested NIC Interventions**
> *Fluid monitoring; Nutritional monitoring; Nutrition management; Eating disorders management; Weight gain assistance*

> **Suggested NOC Outcomes**
> *Nutritional status: Food and fluid intake; Weight control*

Nursing diagnosis

Impaired physical mobility related to general weakness, calcification around joints, arthritis, or debilitation from underlying disease

NURSING PRIORITY

Maintain healthy skin, optimal activity pattern, and bowel functions.

PATIENT OUTCOME CRITERIA

Throughout the hospital stay, the patient will:
- show no new evidence of reddened skin areas
- show no new dry skin areas
- show no pruritus
- show no new skin lesions or infections
- have no crackles, fever, or other evidence of pneumonia
- establish regular bowel elimination
- have stools that are normal in amount, color, and consistency.

INTERVENTIONS

1. *Provide appropriate skin care,* as follows:

– Omit soap during bathing.

– Apply oil to dry skin areas.

– Maintain the patient's usual bathing pattern — for example, every other day.
– Inspect the patient's skin twice daily for tissue breakdown.

2. *Promote appropriate activity,* as follows:

– Take the patient's history to identify activities of daily living (ADLs) and the need for special exercises. Encourage maintenance of the usual pattern of activity, keeping the patient out of bed most of the day.
– Institute active or passive exercise, or both, as soon as medical protocol permits.

– Maintain all parts of the patient's body in functional anatomic alignment.
– If the patient is on bed rest, turn him from back to side according to nursing protocol or at least every 2 hours during the day and every 4 hours at night.
– Encourage deep-breathing exercises hourly while the patient is awake. Each shift, assess the patient's breath sounds. Report decreased breath sounds, crackles, or other abnormal findings promptly.

RATIONALES

1. The stated measures will help ensure proper skin care.
– Soap is drying, and older persons have decreased function of sebaceous glands.
– Oil may prevent increasing dryness, which can lead to tissue breakdown.
– Increasing the frequency of baths may reduce normal skin flora and increase irritation and dryness.
– Pressure on bony prominences may produce pressure ulcers because older adults have less elastic body tissue and less fatty tissue.

2. Implementing the stated measures helps ensure adequate activity.
– Maintaining normal activity and exercise patterns is essential for optimal physiologic function. Special exercises may be required to maintain the tone of particular muscle groups.
– Exercise helps prevent thrombophlebitis, contractures, footdrop, and external rotation of the legs — complications associated with impaired mobility.
– Functional alignment prevents contractures and external rotation.
– Regular movement reduces the risk of hypostatic pneumonia and pressure ulcers.

– Decreased elasticity in lung tissue, commonly associated with aging, places these patients at increased risk for stasis of pulmonary secretions and resultant pulmonary infection. In this population, pneumonia is associated with higher mortality.

– Request an order for occupational therapy (OT) or physical therapy evaluation.

– OT can maximize independence in ADL function and the therapist can recommend valuable assistive devices. Physical therapists may recommend walkers or other safety devices to increase strength, mobility, safety, and independence.

3. *Promote normal bowel function.*

– Identify the patient's typical bowel care regimen. If the patient is dependent on enemas or laxatives, discuss more appropriate alternatives.
– Add bran, prune juice, or other acceptable roughage to meals, as the patient's medical condition allows.
– Ensure that the patient maintains adequate fluid intake.

– Administer and document the use of stool softeners or laxatives, as ordered.
– Provide assistance with the bedpan or commode, following the patient's schedule as closely as possible.

3. Implementing the stated measures helps ensure normal bowel function.
– Individualized care is essential for normal bowel function and a sense of emotional well-being.

– Decreased physical mobility contributes to constipation. Adding roughage to the diet stimulates peristalsis.
– Adequate fluid intake is essential to prevent drying of stool in the rectal vault, which can lead to fecal impaction.
– If the older patient is unable to assume a normal position on the toilet, he may need medicinal assistance.
– Maintaining routine timing facilitates bowel evacuation.

4. Additional individualized interventions: _____

4. Rationales: _____

Suggested NIC Interventions
Exercise therapy: Ambulation; Exercise promotion: Strength training; Exercise therapy: Joint mobility; Exercise therapy: Balance; Exercise therapy: Muscle control

Suggested NOC Outcomes
Ambulation: Walking; Joint movement: Active; Mobility level

Nursing diagnosis
Disturbed sleep pattern related to reduction in exercise, stress arising from concern with illness, anticipation of personal losses, unfamiliarity of surroundings, or discomfort associated with illness

NURSING PRIORITY
Minimize sleep disturbance during hospital stay.

PATIENT OUTCOME CRITERIA
Within 2 days of admission, the patient will:
■ appear rested
■ report sleeping at least 4 hours at a time.

INTERVENTIONS

1. *Provide frequent rest and sleep periods.*

2. Visit the patient frequently during the day and encourage participation in activities.

3. *Assess for and document factors that may cause sleep disruption.* Treat causes appropriately — for example, if pain causes wakefulness, administer analgesics before bedtime or provide other comfort measures. Group procedures to avoid interrupting sleep cycles.

RATIONALES

1. Older persons have less stage IV sleep and frequently awaken spontaneously. Shorter, more frequent sleep and rest periods are, in many cases, more appropriate than one long sleep period.

2. Boredom and inactivity contribute to sleep pattern disturbance.

3. Sleep deprivation may result in confusion, irritability, short-term memory loss, or other neuropsychiatric manifestations.

4. *Adapt the hospital environment to simulate the patient's home setting whenever possible.*

5. *Provide as quiet an environment as possible* (for example, turn off the radio or television if this reflects the usual home situation).

6. *"Shorten" the night by arranging activities around late bedtime and checking in early in the morning with food and conversation.*

7. Additional individualized interventions: _____

4. Moving the bed into a position similar to that at home or modifying other room details (such as the position of the radio or television) can produce a sense of security and familiarity and promote environmental comfort, inducing rest and sleep.

5. Similarity of environmental sounds to those at home enhances relaxation.

6. Because older people sleep for shorter periods, their night's sleep may be only 4 to 5 hours.

7. Rationales: _____

Suggested NIC Interventions
Energy management; Sleep enhancement; Coping enhancement

Suggested NOC Outcomes
Rest; Sleep; Well-being

Nursing diagnosis

Risk for situational low self-esteem related to dependent patient role, anxiety over loss of physical or mental competence, powerlessness to alter the aging process, or societal emphasis on youth

NURSING PRIORITY
Promote a positive self-image while providing opportunities to demonstrate competence.

PATIENT OUTCOME CRITERIA
Throughout the hospital stay, the patient will:
- participate in decision making
- participate in self-care to the extent possible
- set realistic goals and pursue them
- initiate involvement with others.

INTERVENTIONS

1. *Whenever possible, offer choices and include the patient in decision making related to care.*

2. *Involve the patient in self-care activities* as much as possible, paying special attention to grooming and hygiene needs.

3. *Affirm positive qualities* (for example, "You have a good sense of humor."). Help the patient identify and use coping behaviors they learned in dealing successfully with earlier situations.

4. *Move the conversation away from constant repetition of bodily problems.*

5. Review life activities that reflect accomplishments.

RATIONALES

1. Participating in decision making increases the patient's sense of personal competence and promotes independence.

2. "Taking over" by caregivers devalues the patient's abilities and may lead to dependence and depression. A neat personal appearance contributes to feelings of self-worth.

3. Hearing expressions of appreciation for positive attributes helps reinforce associated behaviors. Examining coping skills learned from previous experiences may help the patient build strengths in dealing with the current situation.

4. Repetition of negative thoughts only reinforces their impact.

5. Recognition of achievements bolsters a sense of societal usefulness.

6. *Allow time for verbalization of feelings,* such as sadness and powerlessness. Avoid overoptimistic responses.

6. Aging entails dealing with multiple losses, and feelings of sadness are a part of normal coping. Active listening and acceptance show respect for the patient as an individual and promote a sense of self-worth.

7. *Encourage realistic goal setting.*

7. Goal achievement fosters feelings of self-mastery.

8. Facilitate behavior that's considerate of others.

8. Focusing on others' needs reduces dependence and increases feelings of usefulness.

9. Provide diversionary activity appropriate to the patient's abilities, allowing opportunities for creative expression whenever possible. Refer the patient to the occupational therapist, as indicated.

9. Emotional well-being is enhanced by diversionary activities. Creative activities allow another avenue for expression of feelings and demonstration of unique abilities. The occupational therapist can help the patient select diversionary activities appropriate to functional capabilities.

10. Additional individualized interventions: _____

10. Rationales:_____

Suggested NIC Interventions
Decision-making support; Grief work facilitation; Anticipatory guidance; Coping enhancement; Self-esteem enhancement

Suggested NOC Outcomes
Decision making; Grief resolution; Psychosocial adjustment: Life change; Self-esteem

Nursing diagnosis

Social isolation related to decreased physical capacity, effects of illness, fear of burdening others, death or disability of peers, or sense of personal uselessness

NURSING PRIORITY
Promote social interaction and provide opportunities for positive feedback from others.

PATIENT OUTCOME CRITERIA
Within 3 days of admission, the patient will:
- maintain social contacts
- make no comments reflecting loneliness.
  Within 3 days of the patient's admission, family members will:
- approach nurses freely with care suggestions and questions.

INTERVENTIONS

1. *Consider ethnicity in initial and ongoing assessment* of adaptation to hospitalization.

2. *Assess the patient's social resources* and the willingness and ability of family, friends, and other caregivers to participate in care.

3. *Involve family members in the planning* — and, when possible, the provision of — care. Ask family members to identify specific needs or preferences the patient may have.

RATIONALES

1. Culturally sensitive care is essential to prevent social isolation.

2. Social isolation results from numerous factors. For example, the patient may hesitate to verbalize needs because of pride and independence; tactful intervention by the nurse may help link the patient with untapped social contacts.

3. Involvement of family members in care helps reduce isolation related to unfamiliar surroundings and prevents a sense of abandonment, which can occur in a hospitalized elderly patient. Participating in care for the hospitalized patient also allows family members to practice care techniques and ask questions in a "safe" setting. Family members are most attuned to the patient's special needs.

4. *Encourage generous use of touch and affectionate gestures in the provision of care, unless the patient appears uncomfortable with physical contact.*

5. Encourage family members to help the patient maintain previously established roles and functions in the family as much as possible.

6. Ensure telephone access. Discuss bedside telephone costs with the family or social worker, explaining the critical need for the patient to maintain communication with family and friends.

7. *Initiate a social services referral, as needed,* to arrange transportation for visitors, such as a senior citizens' or church group's van.

8. *Present socialization concerns and problems to other members of the hospital staff,* including the chaplain, dietitian, and housekeepers.

9. Additional individualized interventions: _____

_____

4. Older adults have diminished sensory capacities. Touch reduces "skin hunger" (the desire for human tactile contact) and communicates caring.

5. Maintaining roles—for example, as wise counselor or confidante—helps the older person maintain a sense of belonging and decreases feelings of uselessness.

6. For many elderly patients with impaired mobility, the telephone provides an essential link to the outside world. Also, elderly friends may be unable to visit, so the telephone may be their only means of offering support to the patient.

7. The patient and family may be unaware of available transportation resources.

8. Interaction with all members of the hospital staff may serve as a temporary replacement for the patient's normal social interactions.

9. Rationales: _____

_____

> **Suggested NIC Interventions**
> *Family integrity promotion; Socialization enhancement; Mood management; Family involvement promotion; Coping enhancement; Self-awareness enhancement*

> **Suggested NOC Outcomes**
> *Family environment: Internal; Loneliness; Mood equilibrium; Social involvement; Social support; Well-being*

Nursing diagnosis
Risk for spiritual distress related to inability to maintain usual religious and spiritual practices (if any) or loss of sense of life's meaning and purpose

NURSING PRIORITY
Provide for patient participation in meaningful religious and spiritual practices, if desired.

PATIENT OUTCOME CRITERIA
Throughout the hospital stay, the patient will:
- verbalize or display satisfaction with provisions for spiritual needs (if appropriate)
- express an ability to endure crisis (if appropriate).

INTERVENTIONS

1. *Identify the patient's normal preference and pattern for religious activities, if appropriate. Encourage participation in formal services if available. Arrange for visits by clergy as permitted,* or suggest that the family provide tapes of religious services. See the "Dying" care plan page 78.

2. If the patient wishes to read religious literature but can't do so, read it, get a volunteer to read it, or obtain it on a cassette tape.

RATIONALES

1. Maintaining the usual spiritual support increases the patient's coping ability. The "Dying" care plan contains other specific interventions for patients experiencing spiritual distress.

2. Maintaining continuity in religious experience provides special comfort.

3. *Provide privacy for personal prayer time,* when desired.

4. *Keep religious articles, such as rosary beads, conveniently available.*

5. Additional individualized interventions: _____
_____

3. If appropriate for the patient, encouraging expressions of trust and faith in God or a supreme being provides solace and a sense of providential care during crises.

4. Religious articles may provide reassurance and serve as a reminder of spiritual resources.

5. Rationales: _____
_____

> **Suggested NIC Interventions**
> *Hope instillation; Spiritual growth facilitation; Spiritual support*

> **Suggested NOC Outcomes**
> *Hope; Spiritual well-being*

Discharge planning
DISCHARGE CHECKLIST
Before discharge, the patient should show evidence of meeting discharge criteria for the specific disease or condition. The patient's medical record should show evidence of:
❒ appropriate referrals made for home care assistance as needed, or for care facility placement, if indicated
❒ understanding age-related needs, such as a hearing aid, eyeglasses, assistive devices, and home safety equipment
❒ appropriate referrals and special attention to age-related needs.

TEACHING CHECKLIST
Document evidence that the patient and family demonstrate an understanding of:
❒ the details specific to the patient's disease or condition
❒ the purpose, dosage, administration schedule, and adverse effects requiring medical attention of all discharge medications
❒ the care needs arising from illness
❒ dietary needs
❒ feeding assistance needs
❒ mental status changes: thought processing, insight, judgment, or confusion
❒ voiding needs
❒ mobility and transfer needs
❒ hygiene needs
❒ social and emotional needs to reduce loneliness and isolation
❒ the need for relationships with family and friends
❒ family and friends' access to a care facility, if placement has been planned
❒ the resources available for older persons
❒ how to contact the physician
❒ the use of durable medical equipment.

DOCUMENTATION CHECKLIST
Using outcome criteria as a guide, document:
❒ the clinical status on admission
❒ significant changes in status
❒ patient and family teaching
❒ discharge planning
❒ other data pertinent to the specific disease or condition.

Associated care plans
- Acute pain
- Alzheimer's disease
- Chronic pain
- Compromised family coping
- Dying
- Grieving
- Ineffective individual coping
- Knowledge deficit

(See also the plan for the patient's specific disease or condition.)

References
Tierney, L., et al., eds. *Current Medical Diagnosis and Therapy*, 41st ed. New York: Lange, 2002.

Grieving

Introduction

DEFINITION AND TIME FOCUS
Grief is the normal response to an actual or potential loss. It's a natural, necessary, and dynamic process. Anticipatory grieving occurs before an actual loss. Dysfunctional grieving is the ineffective, pathologic, delayed, or exaggerated response to an actual or potential loss. Theoretical phases of the grieving process have been outlined by various authors. As in all theoretical models, the phases overlap and may or may not be sequential; that is, the patient or family may move back and forth among these phases in a nonlinear fashion.

This care plan focuses on the patient and family members coping with impending or actual losses. (See *Clinical snapshot: Grieving*, page 106.)

ETIOLOGY AND PRECIPITATING FACTORS
■ Loss of body image or some aspect of the self (such as a social role or body part due to amputation, or scarring from burns or trauma)
■ Loss of a loved one or significant other through separation, divorce, death, or disappearance (presumed dead)
■ Loss of material objects (such as income, belongings, or companion pets)
■ Loss through a maturational or developmental process (such as aging or weaning an infant)
■ Loss of "ideal" or future expectations (such as through perinatal deaths, birth defects, chronic illness in children, or injuries or illness that alter lifestyle)

Focused assessment guidelines

NURSING HISTORY (FUNCTIONAL HEALTH PATTERN FINDINGS)
Health-perception–health-management pattern
■ Real or imagined loss
Nutritional-metabolic pattern
■ Nausea and vomiting, weight loss or gain, or anorexia
■ Increased food, drug, or alcohol intake as means of coping
Elimination pattern
■ GI upset, diarrhea, or constipation
Activity-exercise pattern
■ Shortness of breath
■ Exhaustion, weakness, inability to maintain organized activity patterns, or restlessness
Sleep-rest pattern
■ Insomnia caused by disruption of normal sleep pattern or frequent crying episodes

Cognitive-perceptual pattern
■ Guilt
■ Sorrow, emptiness, or "heaviness"
Self-perception–self-concept pattern
■ Powerlessness
■ Worthlessness
■ Decreased ability to fulfill personal life expectations
Role-relationship pattern
■ Episodes of withdrawal or social isolation (especially with dysfunctional grieving)
■ Support of family or lack thereof
Sexuality-reproductive pattern
■ Loss of sexual desire or hypersexuality
■ Menstrual irregularity in females
■ Abortions, miscarriages, or stillbirths
Coping–stress tolerance pattern
■ Difficulty expressing feelings about the loss
■ Rationalization or intellectualization of the loss to make it less painful, especially during the bargaining phase
■ Frequent crying episodes, usually associated with shock or with the denial or depression phases
■ Hostility during the anger phase in an attempt to resist the impact of the loss
■ Avoidance of any discussion of the loss (especially with dysfunctional grieving)
■ Previous experiences with depression
■ Repeated focus of events surrounding the loss
■ Preoccupation with lost object or image
■ Overwork until physical exhaustion
Value-belief pattern
■ Need for increased spiritual or pastoral support
■ Increased use of prayer or meditation
■ Doubts concerning religious beliefs
■ Specific cultural beliefs, rituals, or traditions related to death

PHYSICAL FINDINGS
Loss is a body stressor that can trigger physiologic as well as psychological stress and can decrease the immune system's resistance to infection and illness.
Cardiovascular
■ Palpitations
■ Hypertension
■ Arrhythmias
Pulmonary
■ Increased respirations
■ Deep sighing
Gastrointestinal
■ Vomiting

- Diarrhea or constipation

Neurologic
- Irritability
- Anxiety
- Agitation
- Paresthesia

Integumentary
- Diaphoresis
- Cold, clammy skin
- Flushed skin

Musculoskeletal
- Decreased muscle tone
- Weakness, fatigue, or both

Endocrine
- Change in menstrual patterns
- Changes in blood sugar levels

DIAGNOSTIC STUDIES

Physical debilitation and illness resulting from grieving may require studies but these will vary widely, depending on the signs and symptoms exhibited. For example, palpitations and pulse irregularities may indicate the need for an electrocardiogram to rule out significant cardiac problems.

Blood work can be used to eliminate other diseases or disorders, including problems with thyroid and pancreatic functioning or changes in serotonin levels.

POTENTIAL COMPLICATIONS

- Crisis state
- Major depression with suicidal or homicidal potential
- Physical deterioration
- Dysfunctional grieving

◀ CLINICAL SNAPSHOT ✳

Grieving

Major nursing diagnoses	Key patient or family outcomes
Anticipatory grieving	Communicate feelings, especially anger, guilt, or sorrow.
Dysfunctional grieving	Verify the absence of suicidal or homicidal thinking on request.

Nursing diagnosis

Anticipatory grieving related to impending or actual physical or functional loss

NURSING PRIORITY

Facilitate a healthy grieving process.

PATIENT OUTCOME CRITERIA

The patient or his family will, on request:
- identify the meaning of the loss
- communicate feelings, especially anger, guilt, or sorrow
- identify strategies to cope with the loss
- identify role and relationship changes
- identify and use spiritual support and resources
- perform self-care
- make decisions about care.

INTERVENTIONS

1. *Assess for and promote positive coping mechanisms** — for example, building and sharing close relationships, engaging in creative activities, exercising, and openly expressing feelings related to loss and readjustment. (See the "Dying" care plan, page 78.) Review your feelings and fears to minimize bias in care.

2. *Assess the relationship between the patient and his family for the type of support that might be available.*

RATIONALES

1. Coping with loss is a developmental task. Losses increase in occurrence and intensity throughout life. Adaptive coping methods are derived from previous losses. The "Dying" care plan contains general interventions helpful to those coping with loss. Caregivers' personal feelings can alter the patient's and family's grieving processes if caregivers lack empathy for the losses.

2. Sharing feelings with close friends and significant others helps the patient and family adjust to the loss.

---

*Italics indicate key interventions.

3. *Provide the patient and his family with accurate information before beginning any procedure or treatment that may affect appearance, physical or sexual functioning, or role performance.*

4. Assess and document the patient's and family's response to information about the disease, implications, and treatment. Include responses to experiences and numbers of past losses.

5. Discuss meaning of the loss with the patient or family, especially if no body is found; no funeral is scheduled (that is, MIAs, miscarriages); the loss is of social status; or the loss is one that may be disenfranchised by society (such as losses in homosexual relationships, in parent-child relationships caused by divorce, death from violence versus old age, or the loss of a long-time pet companion). Validate the patient's or family's need and right to mourn any loss they deem significant.

6. *Assess and discuss any cultural issues* that relate to the patient's or family's grief experience, and encourage rituals that are important to the patient and family.

7. Discuss changes in social roles or relationships that may result from the loss.

8. *Provide time to be with the patient and family.*

9. *Assess and document the patient's or family's current phase of grief.* Recognize that the bereaved may move back and forth among the stages of grief.

10. *Support and facilitate the expression of feelings associated with anger, guilt, sorrow, and sadness during any phase of grieving.* Listen nonjudgmentally. Recognize and accept any feelings of anger directed toward the health care team.

11. Encourage the release of emotion through crying. If the patient is receptive, hold the patient's hand and use touch liberally, if culturally appropriate.

12. *Provide spiritual support as needed* by the patient throughout grieving, or suggest appropriate resources.

13. Encourage participation in daily self-care activities.

14. *Provide positive reinforcement and realistic hope about the patient's progress.*

15. *Allow the patient to make decisions whenever possible.* Involve the family as directed by patient.

3. Accurate information prevents misconceptions and may decrease fears related to the loss.

4. Past experiences and values influence the current loss experience. Cumulative losses will result in different responses than will a single loss.

5. Establishing the significance of the loss enhances the person's ability to identify and release feelings related to the loss. The nurse's validation of the need and right to mourn regardless of lack of societal support shows respect for the dignity of the human spirit.

6. Cultural beliefs, rituals, or traditions may influence the response to the grief process.

7. Physical or functional loss may cause changes in social status associated with income, career, and relationships. Discussing these changes helps identify the impact of the loss and options for lifestyle adjustments.

8. The nurse's time spent with the patient and family can encourage the necessary review and processing of the loss. It may also decrease feelings of loneliness or social isolation and reassure the patient that caregivers perceive the loss as significant.

9. Identifying unresolved issues facilitates the grieving process. Often the family and patient are at different phases of grieving and should be treated accordingly.

10. Expressing feelings openly may enable the patient to move more easily through the phases of grieving. The nurse's nonjudgmental listening enables the patient to express feelings without fear of rejection.

11. The nurse's encouragement reassures the patient (and family, if indicated), that crying is a normal response to loss. Hand-holding and the use of touch provide reassurance and help the patient relax.

12. Spiritual support helps foster a sense of meaning, hope, love, and satisfaction with life.

13. Self-care promotes feelings of self-control and independence, increasing self-esteem.

14. Reinforcement and reassurance build self-confidence.

15. Decision making enables the person to maintain control.

General care plans

16. Assist activation of the patient's support system, such as significant others, agencies, and religious or professional staff.

16. The patient may need gentle guidance to identify resources. Appropriate referrals allow emotional needs to be met.

17. Seek support and discuss your own feelings about grieving. Encourage other staff members to do so too.

17. Support and encouragement allow staff to give themselves permission to grieve. Ignoring personal emotional needs will lead to "burnout."

18. Additional individualized interventions: _____

18. Rationales:_____

Suggested NIC Interventions
Anticipatory guidance; Coping enhancement; Grief work facilitation; Family support; Family integrity promotion

Suggested NOC Outcomes
Coping; Family coping; Family environment: Internal; Grief resolution; Psychosocial adjustment: Life change

---

Nursing diagnosis
Dysfunctional grieving related to unresolved feelings about physical or functional loss

NURSING PRIORITY
Identify dysfunctional grieving and make appropriate referrals.

PATIENT OUTCOME CRITERIA
At their own pace, the patient or his family will, on request:
- acknowledge the loss
- discuss the experience realistically
- report using healthy coping strategies
- understand and accept his (their) own and other's responses to the loss
- express and accept personal feelings
- identify resources within the family and community
- verify the absence of suicidal or homicidal thinking.

INTERVENTIONS

1. *Assess and document the patient's and his family's responses to the loss.* Identify feelings of unresolved guilt or anger. Recognize the patient or family's avoidance of discussing the loss. Be alert to possible use of alcohol or drugs as an escape.

2. *Assess and document the patient's daily activity level and ability to perform roles.*

3. *Assess the patient's physical well-being* and initiate a medical referral as indicated. Teach the importance of maintaining physical health.

4. *Monitor and document the administration of all medications* including tranquilizers, antidepressants, sedatives, narcotics, mood elevators, and herbal drugs.

RATIONALES

1. Accurate assessment allows the patient and family to understand the dynamics of the grieving process. Unresolved guilt and anger are common symptoms of pathologic grief and may result in major depression. Avoidance of discussion about the loss may indicate delayed grief. Drug or alcohol abuse contributes to a dysfunctional response to loss. Lack of family support can lead to dysfunctional grieving.

2. Withdrawal and social isolation commonly occur with chronic grieving.

3. Grieving requires emotional and physical energy. Prolonged grieving may result in physical illness and debilitation. Somatic symptoms may mask a depression resulting from delayed or unexpressed grief.

4. Tranquilizers and other medications may occasionally be helpful; however, overmedication may result in prolonging the grieving.

5. *Observe the patient for signs and symptoms of potential suicide* or homicide: increased agitation, insomnia, self-incrimination, and feelings of worthlessness, helplessness, and hopelessness.

6. Assess suicide risk by talking with the patient (see *Assessment of suicide potential,* page 110). Consult with the patient's physician regarding referral or intervention.

7. Involve other resource persons, such as social workers, chaplains, or psychiatrists, as indicated or requested by the patient and family.

8. Provide follow-up referral for the patient after discharge.

9. Additional individualized interventions: _____

5. Anxiety and depression may be exaggerated during chronic grieving states.

6. Frank discussion of suicide potential with the patient helps identify and define stressors and may relieve anxiety; it won't cause a suicide attempt. The greatest risk of suicide occurs as the patient is beginning to feel better and develops the energy needed to carry out a suicide plan.

7. Such referrals help identify financial, social, spiritual, and community resources. Psychiatric care identifies unhealthy responses and promotes healthy grieving.

8. Follow-up visits by nurses, chaplains, social workers, and other support persons should be based on patient need. During early grieving, weekly visits are likely to be helpful. Support groups may be helpful.

9. Rationales: _____

> **Suggested NIC Interventions**
> *Coping enhancement; Counseling; Grief work facilitation; Family integrity promotion; Family therapy*

> **Suggested NOC Outcomes**
> *Coping; Family coping; Grief resolution; Psychosocial adjustment: Life change*

Discharge planning
DISCHARGE CHECKLIST
Before discharge, the patient should show:
- ❏ acknowledgment of the loss and its meanings
- ❏ demonstration of positive coping behaviors
- ❏ identification of social and community support systems
- ❏ no display of suicidal or homicidal thinking.

TEACHING CHECKLIST
Document evidence that the patient and family demonstrate an understanding of:
- ❏ normal grief responses
- ❏ the phases of the grieving process
- ❏ information concerning role changes and physical and emotional losses
- ❏ the importance of maintaining physical health and well-being of the patient and family
- ❏ information about the patient's illness, medical treatment, and psychiatric treatment as needed
- ❏ the need to be understanding and accepting of those who are grieving and of social response to losses
- ❏ community resources including support groups and interagency referral.

DOCUMENTATION CHECKLIST
Using outcome criteria as a guide, document:
- ❏ past experiences and responses to losses
- ❏ current perception and meaning of losses
- ❏ changes in role relationships, body image, and self-esteem
- ❏ positive or maladaptive coping behaviors
- ❏ cultural influences
- ❏ support systems
- ❏ level of activity and participation in self-care
- ❏ medications including narcotics, herbs, tranquilizers, antidepressants, or sedatives
- ❏ signs and symptoms of suicidal or homicidal potential
- ❏ interdisciplinary referrals
- ❏ patient and family teaching
- ❏ discharge planning.

Associated care plans
- Compromised family coping
- Dying
- Ineffective individual coping

References
Boss, P. "Ambiguous Loss: Working with Families of the Missing," *Family Process* 41(1):14-18, Spring 2002.
"The Emotional Side of Amputee Care," *RN Magazine* 63(1):24-26, January 2000.
Foley, G. "Celebrating Legacies," *Cancer Practice* 8(6):263, November-December 2000.

General care plans

Assessment of suicide potential

The alert nurse is aware of suicide risk factors and specifically assesses patients at risk by asking direct questions.

Major risk factors	Questions	Additional risk factors
Intent Contrary to popular myth, asking patients directly about suicide doesn't cause attempts. Patients tend to answer truthfully and are typically relieved that someone has acknowledged their distress.	"Are you thinking about killing yourself?" or "Are you considering suicide?"	**Resources** Lack of social and personal resources to deal with external or internal crises, or a perception by the patient that such resources are unavailable, increases the likelihood of suicide.
Plan Patients who verbalize clearly defined, detailed plans for suicide are at greater risk than those who vaguely want to die.	"Do you have a plan to do it?"	**Recent loss or life changes** Loss or the threat of loss increases suicide risk. Even other kinds of change (a promotion, household move, or changes in roles or responsibilities) can increase stress and overwhelm the patient's coping abilities.
Lethality of method Highly lethal methods (such as firearms, hanging, or jumping from a height) greatly increase risk.	"How would you do it?"	**Physical illness** Physical illness may increase suicide risk, particularly if the illness involves major life changes or a threat to essential aspects of self-image.
Availability of means Patients who have the means readily available are at higher risk.	"Do you have a gun at home?"	**Alcohol or drug abuse** Substance abuse may increase impulsive behavior and contribute to depression, thus increasing suicide risk. Additionally, alcohol or drugs may increase risk by potentiating other drugs or decreasing a person's overall level of awareness, or give the energy needed to follow through on the plan for suicide.
Personal and family history Most people who succeed at suicide have made previous attempts. If previous attempts used highly lethal means or were unsuccessful only by accident (that is, if the plan didn't allow for rescue), risk is increased. Those who have lost loved ones to suicide are at greater risk.	"Have you tried to kill yourself before?" "How? What happened?" "Has anyone in your family committed suicide?"	**Sudden behavior change** Any abrupt change in behavior may signal suicidal intent. **Isolation** Physical or emotional isolation greatly increases suicide risk.
Goals If the patient is unable to envision or articulate future goals or plans, suicide potential is increased.	"Where do you see yourself next month? In 1 year? In 5 years?"	**Age, sex, marital status** Older males have a higher rate of successful suicide, possibly because they tend to choose more certain means. Risk of suicide may be increased for separated, widowed, or divorced persons. These parameters, however, are less reliable predictors than those above.

Fristad, M., et al. "The Role of Ritual in Children's Bereavement," *Omega: Journal of Death & Dying* 42(4):321-339, 2000-2001.

Furman, J. "Living with Dying," *Nursing* 31(4):36-42, April 2001.

Herkert, B. "Communicating Grief," *Omega: Journal of Death & Dying* 41(2):93-116, 2000.

Kempson, D. "Effects of Intentional Touch on Complicated Grief of Bereaved Mothers," *Omega: Journal of Death & Dying* 42(4):341-354, 2000-2001.

Lewes, L., et al. "Chronic Sorrow in Parents of Children with Newly Diagnosed Diabetes: A Review of Literature and Discussion of Implications for Nursing Practice," *Journal of Advanced Nursing* 32(1):41-49, July 2000.

Lipman, M. "The Dimensions of Grief," *Consumer Reports on Health* 13(7):11, July 2001.

"Long Grieving," *Harvard Mental Health Letter* 16(11):7, May 2000.

Meredith, R. "The Photography of Neonatal Bereavement at Wythenshawe Hospital," *Journal of Audiovisual Media in Medicine* 23(4), December 2000.

Papadatou, D. "A Proposed Model of Health Professionals' Grieving Process," *Omega: Journal of Death & Dying* 41(1):59-78, 2000.

Serb, C. "Click Here for Grieving and Coping," *H&HN: Hospital & Health Networks* 75(7):22, July 2001.

Stillion, J., et al. "Living and Dying in Different Worlds: Gender Differences in Violent Death and Grief," *Illness, Crisis & Loss* 9(3):247-260, July 2001.

Tully, J. "Good-bye, Old Friend," *AJN* 99(8):24-26, August 1999.

Wheeler, I. "Parental Bereavement: The Crisis of Meaning," *Death Studies* 25(1):51-67, January 2001.

Impaired physical mobility

Introduction

DEFINITION AND TIME FOCUS
Impaired physical mobility is a condition in which an individual has limited ability for independent physical movement. Acutely ill or injured patients are physically unable to engage in normal activities; physical recovery itself may demand activity limitations. Rest is essential for healing and should be encouraged; however, prolonged bed rest can result in well-documented physical and emotional disabilities that can add to the patient's problems. The effects of decreased mobility must be addressed early in the planning of care and reviewed frequently throughout the patient's hospital stay. This care plan focuses on the care of the patient whose condition causes impairment or requires restriction of physical mobility. (See *Clinical snapshot: Impaired physical mobility,* page 113.)

ETIOLOGY AND PRECIPITATING FACTORS
- Injury that prevents weight bearing (such as trauma)
- Illness that causes activity intolerance (such as cardiopulmonary disorders)
- Acute injury that causes paralysis or paresis (such as stroke or spinal cord injury)
- Chronic or acute disabling conditions (such as severe arthritis or Guillain-Barré syndrome)
- Sensory-perceptual alterations (as in stroke)
- Therapeutic restrictions
- Reluctance to attempt movement

Focused assessment guidelines

NURSING HISTORY (FUNCTIONAL HEALTH PATTERN FINDINGS)
This section presents a guide to assessing the patient with a mobility impairment.

Health-perception–health-management pattern
- Is the patient's mobility problem new, or does it reflect long-standing disability?
- What's the extent of the patient's activity limitation?
- Does the patient normally use any mobility aids at home (such as a walker, cane, or wheelchair)?
- Does the patient have a cast, splint, traction, or other immobilizing device?
- Does the patient have equipment that interferes with normal mobility, such as a ventilator or multiple I.V. lines?
- Does the patient have preexisting conditions that affect mobility, such as stroke or amputation, or a progressive debilitating disease, such as multiple sclerosis or acquired immunodeficiency syndrome?
- Does the patient have a history of blood disorders, integumentary problems, pulmonary disease, or cardiac disease?

Nutritional-metabolic pattern
- What's the patient's baseline nutritional status? (See the "Nutritional deficit" care plan, page 138.)
- Is the patient able or permitted to take oral nourishment?
- Is the patient receiving artificial nutrition, such as total parenteral nutrition or nasogastric or gastric tube feedings?

Elimination pattern
- When was the patient's last bowel movement?
- Does the patient normally use elimination aids, such as laxatives or enemas?
- Does the patient have a preexisting condition requiring a bowel regimen that includes removal of impacted feces?
- Does the patient have a history of calculi, renal disease, or recurrent urinary tract infections?
- If the patient has an indwelling urinary catheter, when was it placed?

Activity-exercise pattern
- Is the patient able to perform any self-care activity?
- What was the patient's baseline activity tolerance before hospitalization?
- Are all joints capable of full range of motion?

Cognitive-perceptual pattern
- Is the patient conscious and alert?
- Does the patient have any sensory deficits (such as blindness, deafness, or hemiparesis)?

Self-perception–self-concept pattern
- What's the patient's attitude toward resuming physical activity?

Role-relationship pattern
- Does the patient's occupation require full mobility?
- Does the patient have a supportive social network?
- Are family members involved in care of the patient at home?

Sexuality-reproductive pattern
- Does the patient's mobility impairment have the potential to affect sexual function?

Coping–stress tolerance pattern
- Has the patient used physical activity as a primary coping behavior or stress-relieving measure?

PHYSICAL FINDINGS

This section focuses on some of the major physiologic effects of immobility on body systems.

Cardiovascular

- Orthostatic hypotension (related to reduced autonomic neurovascular reflex response)
- Reduced stroke volume
- Gradually increasing tachycardia (related to deconditioning effects)
- Decreased oxygen uptake
- Venous pooling (related to lack of muscle activity)
- Plasma volume loss
- Blood volume loss
- Reduced cardiac reserve

Respiratory

- Restricted diaphragmatic and costal excursion
- Reduced ciliary activity
- Reduced vital capacity
- Reduced gas exchange (related to gravitational effects)
- Reduced production of surfactant

Gastrointestinal

- Decreased peristalsis
- Increased sphincter tone
- Abdominal distention
- Anorexia

Neurologic

- Decreased sensorium
- Paralysis or paresis related to stroke or spinal cord injury

Integumentary

- Reduced skin turgor
- Impaired wound healing
- Dependent edema

Musculoskeletal

- Reduced muscle mass
- Decreased strength and endurance
- Bone demineralization (at increased rate)
- Fibrosis or ankylosis
- Calcium deposition in soft tissue

Renal

- Hypercalciuria and precipitation of calcium salts (related to bone demineralization)
- Increased renal blood flow
- Initial diuresis (related to decreased antidiuretic hormone [ADH] release)
- Bladder distention
- Urinary stasis

Metabolic

- Increased rate of catabolism
- Decreased basal metabolic rate
- Increased excretion of electrolytes

DIAGNOSTIC STUDIES

Because no diagnostic studies specifically apply to all patients with impaired mobility, only the usual laboratory test findings related to the physiologic changes described in the preceding section are presented here. Laboratory tests may include:

- serum protein level — usually decreased from accelerated catabolism
- serum and urine calcium and phosphate levels — increased from bone demineralization
- arterial blood gas (ABG) measurements — may show reduced partial pressure of arterial oxygen (Pao_2) and increased partial pressure of arterial carbon dioxide, indicating hypoventilation and impaired gas exchange
- blood urea nitrogen level — may be elevated from catabolic activity
- urine pH — may be elevated from decreased levels of acid end products released by muscle activity
- hematocrit — may be increased from plasma and blood volume losses and diuresis.

POTENTIAL COMPLICATIONS

- Thromboembolic phenomena
- Atelectasis
- Pneumonia
- Infections
- Skin breakdown, potential pressure-ulcer formation
- Constipation
- Contractures
- Osteoporosis
- Muscle wasting
- Urinary calculi
- Difficulty coping

CLINICAL SNAPSHOT

Impaired physical mobility

Major nursing diagnoses and collaborative problems	Key patient outcomes
ND: Ineffective airway clearance	Maintain a clear airway.
CP: Risk for pulmonary embolism	Display no signs of pulmonary embolism.
ND: Risk for impaired skin integrity	Maintain clear, intact skin.
ND: Ineffective tissue perfusion (renal)	Maintain urine output of at least 60 ml/hour.
ND: Risk for constipation	Maintain normal bowel elimination.
ND: Risk for disuse syndrome	Perform exercises as taught, if condition permits.
ND: Situational low self-esteem	Express feelings related to losses, if desired.

General care plans

Nursing diagnosis

Ineffective airway clearance related to reduced diaphragmatic and costal excursion, stasis of secretions, decreased ciliary activity, weakness, and underlying disease process

NURSING PRIORITIES
- Maintain a clear airway.
- Prevent pulmonary complications.

PATIENT OUTCOME CRITERIA
Throughout the hospital stay, the patient will:
- maintain a clear airway
- change position (or be turned) at least every 2 hours
- perform pulmonary hygiene measures at least every 2 hours while awake, as the patient's condition permits
- exhibit no evidence of pneumonia, atelectasis, or pulmonary embolus.

INTERVENTIONS

1. *Assess pulmonary capabilities at least every 2 hours** while the patient is awake, as appropriate. Evaluate the patient's level of alertness, ability to cough and deep breathe, respiratory rate and effort, and breath sounds.

2. *Evaluate the patient for risk factors that affect pulmonary status, such as obesity, lung disease, incisions, abdominal distention,* neuromuscular dysfunction, chest wall pathology, and medications that depress respirations.

3. *Monitor vital signs, fluid intake and output, hemodynamic pressures, and electrocardiogram* findings according to appendix A, Monitoring standards, or unit protocol. Report changes or abnormal findings promptly.

RATIONALES

1. Initial and ongoing assessments provide direction for planning care. The factors listed are crucial determinants of the patient's ability to counteract the effects of bed rest on pulmonary function.

2. The risk factors listed are associated with increased incidence of serious pulmonary complications.

3. Bed rest has significant effects on cardiovascular function, including a reduction in stroke volume (which may induce tachycardia), redistribution of blood flow (which may contribute to orthostatic hypotension), and decreased cardiovascular reserve (resulting in reduced exercise tolerance and general deconditioning). Careful monitoring of cardiovascular parameters aids in early detection of preventable complications.

*Italics indicate key interventions.

4. *Obtain and monitor ABG measurements,* as ordered. Monitor vital capacity and other pulmonary function studies, as ordered, and report any abnormal findings promptly.

5. *Initiate measures to promote effective breathing:*

– Place the patient in Fowler's or semi-Fowler's position, as condition permits, and change his position at least every 2 hours while he's awake.

– Encourage deep breathing at least every 2 hours while he's awake, and help the patient use an incentive spirometer, as ordered. Check with the physician about including orders for coughing with deep breathing.

– Teach the patient to splint incisions, if applicable, and provide assistance, if necessary.
– Reduce abdominal distention, when possible, through the use of gastric suction, return-flow enema, or other measures, as ordered.

6. *Initiate measures to promote airway clearance:*

– Provide humidification of inspired air.

– Encourage an adequate fluid intake, typically eight to twelve 8-oz (237-ml) glasses a day as the patient's condition allows.
– Suction, as needed, providing supplemental oxygen before and after the procedure.

– Perform chest physiotherapy every 4 hours while the patient is awake (or more frequently, as indicated).

7. *Monitor the patient for pulmonary complications associated with bed rest,* as follows:
– pneumonia — crackles, rhonchi, chest pain, fever, productive cough, tachypnea, tachycardia, whispered pectoriloquy, infected sputum specimen and increased white blood cells (WBCs), or consolidation or effusion on chest X-ray

4. ABG measurements provide direct evaluation of ventilatory status. Pulmonary function studies aid further classification and evaluation of the effects of bed rest on the lungs (bed rest is associated with decreased ventilatory capacity).

5. Maintaining an effective breathing pattern reduces the risk of developing pulmonary complications.
– Patients on bed rest commonly assume a slumped position, decreasing the adequacy of chest expansion. Frequent repositioning helps facilitate drainage of secretions by gravity.
– Deep breathing and incentive spirometry may increase inspiratory reserve volume, promote maximum alveolar inflation, and improve ventilation-perfusion ratios. Deep breathing may actually reverse microatelectasis related to hypoventilation. The incentive spirometer also provides a goal for the patient. The effectiveness of coughing as an airway clearance measure is controversial because its direct effects on small airways haven't been shown, and coughing may increase intrathoracic pressure and lead to alveolar microatelectasis. Some clinicians believe coughing may result in a "milking" effect from smaller to larger airways. If coughing is used, it should always be followed by several deep breaths to help reinflate alveoli.
– Splinting may decrease the fear of pain and promote deeper breathing and fuller chest wall expansion.
– Abdominal distention exerts upward pressure on the diaphragm, reducing chest excursion.

6. Pulmonary hygiene measures help reduce the risk of developing pulmonary complications.
– Humidification may help decrease the viscosity of secretions and helps minimize upper airway irritation if constant supplemental oxygen is required.
– Rehydration of dehydrated patients can promote increased mucociliary clearance.

– Suctioning may be necessary for airway clearance, especially in persons with weak or absent cough or artificial airways. Supplemental oxygen is essential because suctioning can cause significant reduction in Pao_2.
– Chest physiotherapy may help prevent pooling of secretions and loosen mucus plugs. When used in combination with postural drainage, it can help bring secretions into larger airways for easier expectoration.

7. Pulmonary insult complicates treatment and increases mortality risk in the acutely ill patient.
– Prompt detection and treatment of pulmonary infections is essential because their presence exacerbates ventilatory compromise. Purulent sputum is more tenacious because it contains viscous leukocyte deoxyribonucleic acid. In addition, proteolytic enzymes released from destroyed leukocytes can increase inflammation, resulting in bronchoconstriction.

– atelectasis — bronchial or decreased breath sounds, dull percussion note over affected side, tachypnea, tachycardia, restlessness, tracheal shift toward affected side on chest X-ray, or cyanosis (in advanced macroatelectasis)

– pulmonary embolism — see "Risk for pulmonary embolism" below.

8. Additional individualized interventions: _____

– Bed rest aids the development of atelectasis because of reduced chest expansion, ventilatory capacity, and secretion clearance. Microatelectasis is common and may appear on chest X-ray. When atelectasis occurs, ventilatory capacity is reduced because inspired air can't reach the affected areas.
– Pulmonary embolus is the most immediately life-threatening complication associated with bed rest.

8. Rationales: _____

> ### Suggested NIC Interventions
> *Airway management; Airway suctioning; Aspiration precautions; Positioning; Cough enhancement; Acid-base monitoring; Oxygen therapy; Respiratory monitoring; Ventilation assistance*

> ### Suggested NOC Outcomes
> *Aspiration control; Respiratory status: Airway patency; Respiratory status: Gas exchange; Respiratory status: Ventilation*

Collaborative problem

Risk for pulmonary embolism related to venous pooling, loss of vasomotor tone, lack of skeletal muscle contraction, and increased blood viscosity

NURSING PRIORITY
Prevent or promptly detect and treat thromboembolic complications.

PATIENT OUTCOME CRITERIA
Throughout the hospital stay, the patient will:
- perform leg exercises at least every 2 hours during waking hours as instructed or receive passive range-of-motion exercises
- increase activity to maximum level permitted
- display no signs of pulmonary embolus or thrombophlebitis.

INTERVENTIONS	RATIONALES
1. *Evaluate the patient for factors that increase the risk of thromboembolism,* including: – previous history of deep vein thrombosis – abdominal, pelvic, or orthopedic surgery – trauma – history of varicosities, cancer, smoking, stroke, or bleeding disorders – use of oral contraceptives or other medications that affect clotting – dehydration – obesity – hypertension, diabetes mellitus, or renal disease – paralysis – decreased alertness – age (older than age 40).	1. Any factor that contributes to venous stasis, hypercoagulability, trauma, or degeneration of blood vessels increases the risk of thromboembolism. Because bed rest can cause thromboembolism, noting any additional contributing factors will help to identify the highest-risk patients and plan their care.
2. *Initiate measures to promote venous return and decrease venous pooling:*	2. Venous stasis is associated with increased incidence of thromboembolic complications.

General care plans

– Teach the patient to perform leg exercises every 1 to 2 hours while awake, such as flexion and extension of the feet and quadriceps setting. Elevate the patient's legs 15 degrees.

– Don't jackknife the bed (raising both the head and feet simultaneously). Instruct the patient to avoid crossing his legs or placing pillows directly under the popliteal area.

– Apply graded antiembolism stockings, taking care to remove them at least three times daily for 30 to 60 minutes, or according to unit protocol. Discuss use of pneumatic devices, such as special boots, with the physician.

– Increase the patient's activity to permit ambulation as soon as his condition allows. Use caution when first getting the patient out of bed.

3. *For high-risk patients, administer prophylactic anticoagulants, if ordered* (typically low-dose heparin or warfarin [Coumadin]). Monitor clotting studies (prothrombin time [PT], international normalized ratio [INR], or partial thromboplastin time [PTT]) daily for these patients, as ordered. Question anticoagulant orders for trauma patients and others with possible cardiovascular instability or bleeding problems. Monitor patients receiving anticoagulant therapy for signs and symptoms of occult bleeding such as a positive test for hemoglobin in stool or urine.

4. *Monitor the patient for evidence of thromboembolic complications,* including:

– pulmonary embolism — tachypnea, sudden dyspnea, pleuritic chest pain, restlessness, feelings of impending doom, diaphoresis, hypotension, pallor, or cyanosis. If these signs and symptoms occur, elevate the head of the bed, administer oxygen, obtain a specimen for an ABG study, and notify the physician immediately.

– thrombophlebitis — erythema, edema, tenderness, venous patterning or engorgement, positive Homans' sign, cording, or calf pain. Avoid deep palpation of the affected area. If swelling is suspected, initiate daily measurements of leg circumference at a designated point (make an indelible mark on the patient for subsequent measurement). If these signs and symptoms occur, notify the physician immediately and elevate the affected extremity.

5. Additional individualized interventions: _____
_____

– Leg exercises cause muscle contraction, promoting venous return toward the heart. Leg elevation promotes gravity drainage from peripheral vessels.

– These measures may cause venous compression or occlusion, increasing the risk of complications.

– Antiembolism stockings "squeeze" superficial vessels and may promote venous return. Removal of the stockings permits skin examination and allows drying of accumulated moisture. Pneumatic devices may also promote venous return; their use is particularly desirable if heparin is contraindicated.

– Weight bearing increases muscle contraction and decreases bone demineralization associated with immobility. Clots from immobility are most likely to embolize when the patient first resumes activity.

3. Heparin inactivates fibrin, thus preventing fibrin clot formation and reducing the risk of enlargement of existing clots. Warfarin interferes with vitamin K production, thus decreasing production of clotting factors. Monitoring PT, INR, or PTT permits dosage adjustment as needed. Anticoagulants may induce bleeding in susceptible patients.

4. Early detection and treatment of thromboembolic phenomena may minimize their effects.

– Pulmonary embolism is the blockage of a pulmonary artery by a thrombus. As a result, alveoli are ventilated but not perfused, resulting in increased alveolar dead space in the affected lung tissue. A large embolus may significantly increase pulmonary vascular resistance, which may lead to right-sided heart failure. Pulmonary infarction may also occur if the embolus is large. ABG findings guide intervention.

– Thrombophlebitis may occur in superficial or deep veins; the leg veins are usually affected. Superficial thrombophlebitis, although not dangerous, can cause significant discomfort; deep vein thrombophlebitis, however, may lead to life-threatening movement of clots to the lung. Initial erythema, swelling, and tenderness are related to inflammatory changes, while later signs (such as cording and a positive Homans' sign) represent actual thrombus formation. Deep palpation may cause dislodgment of clots. Measuring leg circumference provides an objective evaluation of swelling. Elevating the affected extremity helps minimize venous stasis.

5. Rationales: _____
_____

Nursing diagnosis

Risk for impaired skin integrity related to impeded capillary flow, possible altered sensation, or venous stasis

NURSING PRIORITY
Prevent skin breakdown.

PATIENT OUTCOME CRITERIA
Throughout the hospital stay, the patient will:
- maintain clear, intact skin
- exhibit no evidence of skin breakdown
- maintain adequate nutritional intake.

INTERVENTIONS

1. On the patient's admission to the unit, and at least daily thereafter, *inspect the skin carefully, evaluating color, texture, turgor, dryness, sensation, and capillary refill.*

2. *Evaluate for factors that increase the risk of skin breakdown,* such as nutritional deficit, obesity, diabetes mellitus (or other conditions affecting vascular status), incontinence, decreased sensation, infection, excessive moisture, old age, decreased alertness, and paralysis.

3. *Initiate measures to prevent skin breakdown,* including:
– turning and repositioning every 1 to 2 hours, massaging areas of pressure and bony prominences

– careful turning technique

– judicious use of lotion, avoidance of harsh soaps, and careful cleaning, especially for the incontinent patient, followed by gentle but thorough drying

– use of convoluted foam mattress, flotation pad or water bed, sheepskins, air mattress, air-fluidized bed system (Clinitron therapy bed), low-air-loss bed, or kinetic (RotoRest) bed, as available and indicated
– adequate nutrition.

4. *Monitor for evidence of impending skin breakdown:* edema, blanching, coldness, tenderness, redness, or blistering. Brief reactive hyperemia of the skin is normal following relief from pressure. If reactive hyperemia doesn't resolve after 15 minutes, institute additional protective measures for the affected area.

RATIONALES

1. Initial and ongoing assessment is the first step in providing individualized care. Abnormal findings may provide clues to problems and can be used to guide care planning.

2. Bed rest alone places any patient at increased risk for skin problems because pressure areas may develop rapidly if motion is restricted or impossible. The patient with one or more of the conditions listed should be considered at extremely high risk. Early evaluation of such factors allows for preventive measures.

3. Preventing skin breakdown is much easier than treating a problem after it develops.
– Repositioning allows redistribution of pressure. Massage stimulates circulation and promotes comfort; bony prominences are the most common sites of skin breakdown.
– Rapid or overly vigorous turning may cause delicate skin to shear.
– Dry skin is more prone to cracking and peeling, but excessive moisture provides a medium for bacterial growth and may lead to maceration. Soaps may be irritating. Urine and feces, if left in contact with skin, may cause chemical irritation and contribute to rapid breakdown of tissue.
– Special bedding or beds may help improve patient comfort, distribute pressure more evenly, and reduce the deleterious effects of impaired mobility. Special beds don't eliminate the need to turn and reposition the patient.
– Immobility contributes to increased catabolism and tissue breakdown; also, using stored fats as an energy source may reduce adipose tissue that provides cushioning. Protein is essential for maintaining and rebuilding tissue.

4. Early detection of impending problems permits treatment before skin breakdown occurs. The signs and symptoms listed result when pressure and immobility diminish perfusion. Pressure ulcers can result from as little as 1 hour of pressure and immobility, if the pressure is great enough to impede capillary flow. Additionally, subcutaneous tissue and muscle have usually suffered ischemia before the ulcer becomes apparent on the skin surface, so early detection and treatment are vital.

5. *If a pressure ulcer develops, institute a therapeutic regimen immediately,* according to the physician's orders or unit protocol.

6. Additional individualized interventions: _____

_____

5. Treatment of pressure ulcers varies among practitioners and institutions. Prompt treatment is essential to avert development of additional complications, such as osteomyelitis.

6. Rationales: _____

_____

Suggested NIC Interventions
Pressure management; Pressure ulcer care; Skin surveillance; Incision site care; Wound care

Suggested NOC Outcomes
Tissue integrity: Skin and mucous membranes; Wound healing: Primary intention; Wound healing: Secondary intention

---

Nursing diagnosis

Ineffective tissue perfusion (renal) related to diuresis, stasis of urine, positioning, or bone demineralization

NURSING PRIORITIES
- Promote normal urine elimination.
- Prevent urinary system complications.

PATIENT OUTCOME CRITERIA
Throughout the hospital stay, the patient will:
- maintain urine output of at least 60 ml/hour
- maintain fluid intake of at least eight 8-oz (237-ml) glasses daily, unless contraindicated
- exhibit no signs of urinary tract infection or calculi.

INTERVENTIONS	RATIONALES
1. *Assess the patient's normal urine elimination pattern,* if possible, by noting the following: – frequency, time, and amount of voidings – any change in the usual pattern – continence – special measures used to initiate or control voiding; note color, odor, and appearance (including inspection for increased sedimentation).	**1.** Assessment of the patient's normal elimination status is the first step in planning individualized care.
2. *Evaluate factors that may increase the risk of urinary complications,* such as: – dehydration – incontinence – indwelling catheters – narcotics, sedatives, diuretics, or other medications that affect renal function or alertness – diabetes – neurogenic bladder dysfunction – pregnancy – immunosuppression – shock – altered acid-base or electrolyte status.	**2.** Immobility has several effects on urinary elimination. Bed rest increases the solute load of the kidneys because tissue breakdown and bone demineralization both occur at an increased rate. The increased thoracic blood volume associated with the supine position triggers decreased ADH release, resulting in diuresis. The supine position also contributes to urinary stasis, because downward urine flow is normally enhanced by gravity. Additionally, complete bladder emptying may be harder to achieve in the supine position. Any additional factors, such as those listed, contribute further to the risk of complications and must be considered in care planning.
3. *Initiate measures to promote normal urine elimination:*	**3.** Measures to promote normal elimination may help reduce the risk of developing urinary system complications.

– Have a female patient sit on a bedside commode and allow a male patient to stand to urinate, condition permitting.

– Encourage adequate fluid intake (eight to twelve 8-oz [237-ml] glasses daily), unless contraindicated.

– Promote as much activity as the patient's condition permits — turning, sitting, leg dangling, standing, walking, or range-of-motion exercises.
– Provide privacy during attempts to void.

– Use measures to promote full emptying of the bladder, as needed, such as running water nearby, pouring warm water over the perineum, and applying manual pressure over the bladder.
– Use urinary catheterization only as needed to prevent distention and stasis. Exercise strict aseptic technique during insertion and care of catheters.

4. *Measure urine output hourly and report values less than 60 ml/hour for 2 hours. Assess for bladder distention at least every 8 hours. Measure urine pH every 8 hours and report levels greater than 6. Monitor routine urine cultures, as ordered.*

5. *Monitor for indications of urinary tract complications, as follows:*
– infection — burning, frequency, and urgency (if voiding voluntarily); cloudy, foul-smelling urine; hematuria; fever; low back pain; or increased WBC count

– calculi — severe flank pain, lower abdominal pain, hematuria, nausea, or altered urine stream (if a calculus lodges in the bladder neck or urethra).

6. If indications of urinary complications are detected, notify the physician promptly and collaborate in treatment.

7. Additional individualized interventions: _____
_____

– The upright position facilitates improved urine flow from the ureters and bladder and usually is more comfortable for the patient. In addition, studies report no significant differences in oxygen consumption and cardiovascular response between in-bed and out-of-bed toileting. Weight-bearing exercise of any kind, including the effort to sit or stand, may also help reduce deleterious orthostasis and bone demineralization.
– Calcium precipitation and resultant calculi formation are less likely to occur in dilute urine. Also, an adequate quantity of dilute urine increases frequency of urination, reducing the likelihood of infection from stasis.
– Position changes promote urine drainage, minimize stasis, and reduce protein breakdown associated with immobilization.
– The sphincter relaxation necessary for voiding may be difficult to achieve unless privacy is ensured.
– Bladder distention may cause back pressure and eventual nephron damage. Incomplete bladder emptying is also associated with increased risk of infection.

– Urinary catheterization is associated with a high incidence of nosocomial infections. Placement of a catheter in the normally sterile urinary tract exposes the patient to pathogens that may cause infection.

4. Urine output of less than 60 ml/hour may indicate impending renal failure or other complications. Bladder distention and resultant urinary stasis may occur even in a catheterized patient if the tube becomes obstructed by sediment, blood clots, or calculi. Alkaline urine contributes to the formation of calcium calculi. Routine urine cultures allow early detection of infection.

5. Urinary tract complications usually result from several interrelated factors.
– Urinary tract infection may be related to stasis, dehydration, bladder distention, or any factor that damages the protective mucosal lining of the bladder, such as calculi or catheterization.
– Calcium excretion is increased in a patient on prolonged bed rest because of increased bone breakdown. Most calculi are composed of calcium salts. Such factors as stasis, infection, and decreased urine volume contribute to calculi formation. Also, because of low levels of muscle contraction, a smaller-than-normal quantity of acid end products is excreted, and the urine becomes increasingly alkaline, a condition that favors calculi formation.

6. Treatment of urinary pathology in acutely ill patients must be carefully coordinated with treatment of the patient's primary condition to avoid further complications.

7. Rationales: _____
_____

Nursing diagnosis

Risk for constipation related to weakness of abdominal muscles, loss of defecation reflex, slowed peristalsis, altered nutritional intake, or psychological inhibition

NURSING PRIORITY

Promote normal bowel elimination.

PATIENT OUTCOME CRITERIA

Throughout the hospital stay, the patient will:
- maintain normal bowel elimination
- perform abdominal exercises as taught, if the condition permits
- exhibit no signs of constipation.

INTERVENTIONS

1. *Assess the patient's normal bowel elimination pattern,* if possible, noting the frequency, times, color, and consistency of stools; any change in the usual pattern; continence; use of laxatives or enemas; date and time of last bowel movement; and bowel sounds. Monitor bowel status daily.

2. *Evaluate the patient for factors that may increase the risk of constipation,* including dehydration; narcotics, iron intake, anticholinergics, or other medications affecting peristaltic function; paralysis; age (because of reduced colon tone); cachexia; emphysema (because of reduced ability to increase intra-abdominal pressure); abdominal surgery; abdominal tumors; pregnancy; ascites; hemorrhoids; nothing-by-mouth status; and trauma.

3. *Initiate measures to promote normal bowel elimination:*
– Allow the use of a bedside commode or toilet, if the patient's condition permits. Encourage the patient to attempt defecation at usual times or when the urge arises.
– Encourage the patient to contract abdominal muscles while exhaling during defecation attempts. Instruct the patient to avoid Valsalva's maneuver.

– As the patient's condition permits, teach exercises to maintain or strengthen abdominal muscles, such as contracting and relaxing abdominal muscles several times per hour and performing leg lifts.
– Encourage adequate fluid intake, unless contraindicated.
– Encourage the use of natural laxatives and high-fiber foods, as permitted and tolerated.

RATIONALES

1. Assessment of the patient's normal elimination status is the first step in planning individualized care. Daily monitoring helps in the early identification of potential problems.

2. Because normal bowel motility depends in part on abdominal muscle contraction and physical activity, immobility predisposes the patient to constipation. Any additional factors, such as those listed, contribute further to the risk of complications and must be considered in care planning.

3. Maintaining normal bowel elimination reduces the risk of the development of bowel complications.
– The normal defecation position facilitates evacuation. If defecation is suppressed despite impulses from rectal distention, colon motility eventually may be inhibited.
– Contraction of abdominal muscles increases intra-abdominal pressure and aids in evacuation. Valsalva's maneuver causes a vagal response and, in susceptible patients, may result in bradycardia, heart block, or other cardiovascular complications.
– Bed rest results in generalized muscle atrophy. Weakness of the abdominal muscles may render the patient unable to assist with evacuation.

– Inadequate fluid intake may cause dry, hard stools that are more difficult to expel.
– Whole-grain cereals, fruits and vegetables, and prune juice help promote natural elimination.

– Provide privacy and comfort measures during toileting, such as ensuring warmth and providing air freshener.

4. *Assess for indications of constipation,* such as absence of bowel movements; hard, dry, small stools; sensation of rectal fullness; abdominal distention or mass; headache; decreased appetite; hard stool felt in rectal vault on digital examination; or ribbonlike diarrhea.

5. *As necessary, collaborate with the physician to select appropriate elimination aids,* such as laxatives, suppositories, enemas, or stool softeners.

6. Additional individualized interventions: _____
_____

– Bowel activity may be inhibited if the patient is anxious, embarrassed, or uncomfortable.

4. In the absence of normal bowel elimination, water continues to be reabsorbed from the stool that remains in the bowel, and the stool becomes harder, dryer, and more compacted. As softer stool collects behind it, increasing peristaltic pressure may result in a forceful expulsion of diarrhea past the hard stool mass.

5. Laxatives, suppositories, and enemas may be necessary occasionally, but their frequent use may disrupt normal bowel functioning. Stool softeners may help in the natural expulsion of stool and aren't habit-forming.

6. Rationales: _____
_____

> **Suggested NIC Interventions**
> *Bowel management; Constipation/impaction management; Fluid and electrolyte management*

> **Suggested NOC Outcomes**
> *Bowel elimination; Hydration; Symptom control*

Nursing diagnosis
Risk for disuse syndrome: Muscle atrophy and joint contractures related to disuse, nonfunctional positioning, and reduced muscle tone

NURSING PRIORITY
Maintain maximum functional integrity of bone and muscle.

PATIENT OUTCOME CRITERIA
Throughout the hospital stay, the patient will:
- perform exercises as taught, if the condition permits
- maintain functional alignment of all joints.

INTERVENTIONS

1. *Evaluate the patient for factors that increase the risk of significant muscle, bone, and joint complications,* including preexisting conditions that reduce mobility (such as arthritis, paralysis, paresis, or debilitation), decreased level of alertness, spinal injury or surgery, major burns, and trauma.

2. *Initiate measures to preserve motor functions and strength.*

RATIONALES

1. Normal bone and muscle functions depend on activity, which maintains and increases muscle strength, maintains balanced muscle tone, and promotes normal bone formation. When a muscle is immobilized, 10% to 15% of its strength may be lost in as little as 1 week, and it may atrophy to half its size within 1 month. Disuse atrophy leads to shortening of muscle fibers and reduces joint motion. Immobilization decreases osteoblastic deposition of bone matrix, but normal osteoclastic destruction continues, depleting calcium and other minerals essential for bone stability. The other factors listed may add to the risk of significant bone- and muscle-related complications.

2. Maintaining healthy bone and muscle function is easier than restoring function after disability.

– weight bearing, as the patient's condition permits, even if he is only standing at the bedside or on a tilt table several times daily

– Weight-bearing exercise stimulates osteoblastic activity by providing normal stress to bones. Lack of weight bearing is the primary contributor to osteoporosis, a condition in which the bones are so weakened that the patient is prone to fractures.

– active exercise, as the patient's condition permits, including hourly ankle rotation and flexion and extension of the feet and quadriceps during waking hours
– complete range of motion (ROM) to all joints at least four times daily, as the condition permits

– Active exercises promote maximum muscle contraction and help maintain strength and endurance.

– Putting the joint through its full ROM stretches the surrounding muscle fibers and maintains the coordinated function of joint structures.

– careful positioning to maintain functional alignment, using such devices as trochanter rolls, hand rolls, splints, footboards, and padding between thighs (if hip adduction is a problem); alternating flexion and extension of extremities when turning; and repositioning at least every 2 hours.

– If functional alignment isn't maintained, serious joint contractures may result, requiring surgical intervention or prolonged corrective physical therapy.

3. Additional individualized interventions: _____

3. Rationales: _____

Suggested NIC Interventions
Activity therapy; Exercise therapy: Joint mobility; Exercise therapy: Muscle control

Suggested NOC Outcomes
Endurance; Immobility consequences: Physiological; mobility level

---

Nursing diagnosis
Situational low self-esteem related to dependent patient role

NURSING PRIORITY
Promote positive self-image.

PATIENT OUTCOME CRITERIA
Throughout the hospital stay, the patient will:
- express feelings related to losses
- participate in decision making related to care
- exercise healthy coping behaviors.

INTERVENTIONS

1. Assess the effects of reduced mobility on the patient's self-concept. Encourage expression of feelings and identification of primary losses.

2. Encourage the patient's participation in self-care and decision making, as the condition permits.

3. Anticipate such behaviors as regression, withdrawal, aggression, apathy, and crying. Try to help the patient interpret these normal responses to loss.

RATIONALES

1. Identifying what the loss of normal mobility means to the individual is the first step in care planning. A patient's reaction to immobility can vary enormously, depending on baseline activity level and the importance of physical functioning to identity.

2. Participating in self-care, even in small ways, preserves a patient's sense of identity and integrity.

3. Immobility may cause disorganization of the psyche as the individual attempts to cope with the profound loss of usual roles, stimulation, and independence. Helping the patient to understand the normalcy of his reactions may reduce psychic disequilibrium and facilitate healthy coping strategies.

4. See the "Confusion" care plan, page 71.

4. Immobility results in significant reduction in normal sensory stimulation. This can contribute to decreased motivation, reduced ability to learn and solve problems, sleep disturbances, and other problems that may compound the patient's distress. The "Confusion" care plan contains detailed information on preventing, detecting, and treating this problem.

5. See the "Ineffective individual coping" care plan, page 124.

5. The "Ineffective individual coping" care plan contains further interventions that may be helpful in caring for the patient with low self-esteem.

6. Additional individualized interventions: _____

6. Rationales: _____

Suggested NIC Interventions
Cognitive restructuring; Decision-making support; Family involvement promotion; Financial resource assistance

Suggested NOC Outcomes
Depression control; Family participation in professional care; Health beliefs; Health beliefs: Perceived ability to perform; Health beliefs: Perceived control; Health beliefs: Perceived resources; Participation: Health care decisions

Discharge planning
DISCHARGE CHECKLIST
Before discharge, the patient should show no evidence of life-threatening or disabling complications of immobility.

TEACHING CHECKLIST
Document evidence that the patient and family demonstrate an understanding of:
- ❏ activity recommendations, restrictions, and limitations
- ❏ measures to avert orthostatic hypotension and activity intolerance
- ❏ indicators of clinically significant activity intolerance
- ❏ signs of complications related to impaired mobility
- ❏ use of mobility aids.

DOCUMENTATION CHECKLIST
Using outcome criteria as a guide, document:
- ❏ clinical status on admission
- ❏ significant changes in status
- ❏ pertinent laboratory and diagnostic test findings
- ❏ protective measures initiated
- ❏ response to resumption of activity
- ❏ complications of immobility, if any
- ❏ patient and family teaching
- ❏ discharge planning.

Associated care plans
- Confusion
- Geriatric care
- Ineffective individual coping
- Nutritional deficit

References
Daley, J., et al. "Use of Standardized Nursing Diagnoses and Interventions in Long-Term Care," *Journal of Gerontological Nursing* 21(8):29-36, August 1995.

Kozier, B., et al. *Fundamentals of Nursing: Concepts, Process and Practice.* Menlo Park, Calif.: Addison-Wesley-Longman Publishing Co., 1995.

Oullet, L., and Rush, K. "A Study of Nurses' Perception of Client Mobility," *Western Journal of Nursing Research* 18(5):565-79, October 1996.

Roberts, B., et al. "The Congruence of Nursing Diagnoses and Supporting Clinical Evidence," *Nursing Diagnosis* 7(3):108-15, July-September 1996.

Ineffective individual coping

Introduction

DEFINITION AND TIME FOCUS

NANDA defines ineffective individual coping as an "inability to form a valid appraisal of the stressors, inadequate choices of practical responses, and/or inability to use available resources (NANDA 2001-2002)."

ETIOLOGY AND PRECIPITATING FACTORS

- Stimuli likely to cause ineffective coping in illness
–Pain and incapacitation
–Lack of sleep
–Stressful hospital environment and treatment procedures
–Loss of control over what's happening to self
–Loss of hope
–Lack of meaningful contact with loved ones
–Uncertain future
- Conditions necessary for a stimulus to cause ineffective coping
–Perception of a harmful stimulus or cues that a harmful stimulus is imminent
–Perception that the harmful stimulus threatens the individual's goals or values
–Perception that the patient's resources aren't equal to coping with the threat

Focused assessment guidelines

NURSING HISTORY
(FUNCTIONAL HEALTH PATTERN FINDINGS)

Health-perception–health-management pattern
- Perception of illness and hospitalization as a loss of control that threatens fulfillment of usual roles or threatens life itself
- Drastically reduced ability to solve problems effectively
–Selecting course of action without weighing alternatives
–Feeling overwhelmed by alternatives and being unable to select a course of action
- Failure to follow plan of treatment

Nutritional-metabolic pattern
- Anorexia, nausea, or vomiting
- Weight loss from anorexia
- Frequent overeating to deal with stress

Elimination pattern
- Diarrhea or constipation from dietary changes or stress

Activity-exercise pattern
- Occasional hyperactivity and inability to rest
- Occasional withdrawal, listlessness, or fatigue

Sleep-rest pattern
- Sleep disturbance
–More than usual amount of sleep
–Difficulty falling asleep
–Early awakening followed by inability to return to sleep (early morning insomnia)
–Frequent night-time awakening

Cognitive-perceptual pattern
- Diminished ability to view the world objectively
- Decreased ability to take in information
- Lack of information necessary to make decisions
- Suspicion surrounding intentions of caregivers

Self-perception–self-concept pattern
- Feeling that the threat is greater than available internal resources to combat it
- Inability to control events affecting the situation

Role-relationship pattern
- Decreased ability to communicate needs
- Feelings of isolation and inability to respond to caring from others
- Occasional inability to control impulsive behavior, possibly leading to hostility, aggression, or suicidal behavior

Sexuality-reproductive pattern
- Loss of libido, impotence, or orgasmic dysfunction

Coping–stress tolerance pattern
- Physiologic responses related to sympathetic nervous system stimulation such as tachycardia
- Increased number of infections related to alteration in the immune system
- Denial of symptoms and delay in seeking treatment
- Various negative coping behaviors, depending on individual and environmental factors
–Anger and hostility
–Anxiety and hyperactivity
–Depression and withdrawal
–Suicidal ideation
- Behavior that alienates caregivers and removes a source of support
- History of ineffective coping mechanisms, such as drug or alcohol abuse, nicotine addiction, or overeating

Value-belief pattern
- Loss of faith related to feelings of hopelessness and abandonment

PHYSICAL FINDINGS
General appearance
- Anxious facial expression
- Flat affect
- Poor eye contact
- Slumped posture

Cardiovascular
- Elevated blood pressure
- Increased heart rate
- Increased ventricular arrhythmias (occasionally)

Pulmonary
- Increased rate and depth of respirations

Gastrointestinal
- Vomiting
- Diarrhea
- GI bleeding (if stress ulcer develops)

Neurologic
- Dilated pupils, as sympathetic nervous system response (occasionally)
- Restlessness
- Lethargy

Integumentary
- Diaphoresis (occasionally)

Musculoskeletal
- Increased muscle tension and pain

DIAGNOSTIC STUDIES
In the clinical setting, laboratory tests aren't normally done to identify ineffective coping. Remember, however, that physiologic responses to stress can mimic disease.
- Arterial blood gas measurements may reveal respiratory alkalosis from an increased rate and depth of respiration (hyperventilation).
- White blood cell count may be increased.
- Mental status examination
–Appearance may yield clues about self-perception (patients coping ineffectively may not care about their appearance).
–Behavior (body movements, tone of voice) is an indicator of the person's self-expression ability, an important coping skill; behavior may vary, depending on the patient's expressive style. The relationship of the patient with caregivers is also important to assess: Is the patient controlling, passive, aggressive, suspicious, or uncooperative?
–Impaired cognitive function (orientation, memory, and judgment) may be demonstrated by the inability to solve problems.
–Feelings shown indicate which emotions the patient expresses and their appropriateness to the situation; a wide variety of feelings are possible, ranging from anxiety to anger to depression and typically including isolation and hopelessness
–Perceptions indicate the patient's view of the situation; perceptions of a threat are based on previous experience, values, and beliefs along with perception of inadequate resources in relation to the magnitude of the threat. Which coping mechanisms were used in the past? Which were useful? Which are potentially harmful — for example, smoking, alcohol use, or drug use?
- Suicide assessment — a patient who feels hopeless and helpless needs to be asked about presence of suicidal thoughts; this question doesn't cause a patient to think about suicide but instead provides an opportunity to talk about these disturbing feelings. Factors associated with high risk include:
–high level of anxiety or panic
–severe depression
–minimal ability to perform activities of daily living
–few or no sources of support or significant others
–continued abuse of alcohol or drugs, or both
–negative view of previous psychiatric help (if applicable)
–one or more previous suicide attempts
–marked hostility
–frequent or constant thoughts of suicide
–suicide plan that's specific in method and timing
–possession of means to carry out the plan, such as physical capacity and weapon. (See also *Assessment of suicide potential,* page 110, in the "Grieving" care plan.)

POTENTIAL COMPLICATIONS
- Physiologic
–Increased risk of falls and accidents
–Ventricular arrhythmias
–Increased susceptibility to infections
- Psychological
–Suicide or homicide
–Major depression
–Reactive psychosis
–Disintegration of family unit

General care plans

Nursing diagnosis

Ineffective coping related to stress of illness and hospitalization

NURSING PRIORITIES

- Establish rapport and trust.
- Accurately identify threat and coping resources.
- Intervene to optimize coping skills.
- Evaluate the effectiveness of interventions.

PATIENT OUTCOME CRITERIA

Within 2 days of the identification of ineffective coping, the patient will:

- describe his emotional state to the nurse
- express an accurate understanding of the current situation and plan of treatment
- state that any pain is within tolerable limits
- participate in developing a plan of care
- use support offered by caregivers.

INTERVENTIONS

1. *Form a positive relationship with the patient.* *
– Convey a sense of caring and concern for what happens to the patient.
– Use appropriate eye contact.
– Convey feelings of comfort and relaxation by approaching the patient calmly, including the patient in all bedside conversations, and speaking in a well-modulated tone.
– Identify personal reactions to the patient's coping style that could interfere with formation of a helping relationship. Avoid judging the patient's behavior.

2. *Rule out organic causes for such behavioral changes as decreased alertness, impaired memory, confusion, restlessness, or depression.*

3. *Provide factual information about the illness and plan of treatment.* Reinforce information the patient has received from the physician. Be prepared to repeat information in clear, concise language.

4. *With the patient, identify the source of the threat.*

RATIONALES

1. Patients report that feelings of not being cared for interfere with their recovery and contribute to feelings of hopelessness. An ineffective relationship with caregivers drains energy that could be better used for healing. Conversely, patients who feel positive about their nurses say this gives them an energy that helps with healing, decreases isolation, and increases coping ability. People express anxiety, pain, and needs for privacy and intimacy in various ways, depending on their cultural and personal biases. The patient's behavior is an individual pattern used to decrease anxiety. For example, if the patient who feels comfortable expressing pain openly is cared for by a nurse who believes that pain should be tolerated in silence, an ineffective nurse-patient relationship may result. Recognizing one's own cultural and personal biases is the first step in avoiding prejudicial responses to the patient's behavior.

2. Behavioral changes that appear to be signs of ineffective coping may actually represent such physiologic problems as hypoxia, electrolyte imbalance, or drug toxicity. Assuming that all behavioral responses are related to psychological mechanisms may delay needed medical treatment.

3. For problem solving to begin, the patient needs accurate information. Patients who are coping ineffectively have a decreased ability to hear and assimilate information.

4. Whether a stimulus is felt as threatening depends on values, beliefs, and the perception of available resources. The patient may not perceive an obvious, identifiable threat (such as a diagnosis of cancer) as the primary threat. Conversely, what seems routine to the nurse may be frightening to the patient.

*Italics indicate key interventions.

5. *Help the patient be specific about what seems threatening.*

5. Patients may have misconceptions about what's happening to them. If they can specify their fears, the nurse can plan specific actions such as providing information that helps the patient see the situation realistically. Verbalizing feelings of fear can help to reduce them.

6. *With the patient, identify modifiable components of the threat.*

6. In many cases, people coping ineffectively are unable to separate their situation into manageable parts; instead, they view the problem as overwhelming and unmanageable. If they can view the problem in its component parts, their anxiety may be reduced and effective coping behaviors become more possible.

7. *Help the patient identify personal strengths and external resources, such as family, friends, and economic means.*

7. People in crisis may not identify their strengths. They will need assistance in assessing resources and identifying ways to activate them.

8. *Identify external resources and make appropriate referrals — for example, for social services, spiritual counseling, or psychiatric interventions.*

8. Expansion of the patient's base of support helps decrease the perceived magnitude of the specific threat.

9. *Keep pain at a tolerable level.*

9. Pain is a common source of fear. Uncontrolled pain increases anxiety and decreases the energy available for coping.

10. *Ensure adequate nutrition and sleep.*

10. Inadequate diet and lack of sleep are stressors themselves and, as such, decrease the amount of energy available for coping and adaptation.

11. *Control environmental stimuli that drain adaptive energy* needed to maintain psychological equilibrium: Provide privacy for all invasive procedures and for nursing and self-care activities; eliminate conversation around the bedside that doesn't include the patient; and decrease environmental noise.

11. Every stimulus in the environment is a potential threat. Stimuli not normally viewed as threatening may, in combination, create more stress and decrease coping ability.

12. *Offer alternative strategies to counteract the effects of the threat — for example, guided imagery, relaxation techniques, or back rubs.*

12. The relaxation response is the physiologic opposite of anxiety. Relaxation techniques may help the patient cope with stress and regain control.

13. *Give choices related to the patient's care and situation* whenever possible.

13. Maintaining some ability to control one's life helps to combat feelings of helplessness.

14. *Provide opportunities for loved ones to interact with the patient in meaningful ways.*

14. A positive response from loved ones encourages a more positive response to treatment and decreases the sense of isolation.

15. *Assess responses to nursing interventions,* and collaborate with the physician to determine if pharmacologic intervention would be helpful.

15. Antianxiety medications may be helpful in decreasing potentially harmful physiologic and psychological effects of anxiety. Antidepressants may be useful in patients with signs of depression.

16. Additional individualized interventions: _____
_____

16. Rationales:_____
_____

General care plans

Suggested NIC Interventions

Anger control assistance; Environmental management: Violence prevention; Impulse control training; Coping enhancement; Decision-making support; Learning facilitation; Learning readiness enhancement; Role enhancement; Family involvement promotion; Support group; Support system enhancement

Suggested NOC Outcomes

Aggression control; Decision making; Impulse control; Information processing; Role performance; Social support

Discharge planning

DISCHARGE CHECKLIST
Before discharge, the patient should show evidence of:
❒ recognition of personal ineffective coping behaviors
❒ perception of increased ability to cope with the situation
❒ ability to name resources appropriate to the situation
❒ increased ability to manage the current situation by defining the problem and reasonable solutions.

TEACHING CHECKLIST
Document evidence that the patient and family demonstrate an understanding of:
❒ personal ineffective coping behaviors
❒ diagnosis, plan of treatment, and prognosis
❒ expected physiologic responses during recovery
❒ community resources appropriate to perceived problems
❒ appropriate alternative coping strategies
❒ how to contact the physician.

DOCUMENTATION CHECKLIST
Using outcome criteria as a guide, document:
❒ coping status on admission
❒ significant changes in appearance, affect, behavior, perception, and cognitive function
❒ psychological responses to hospitalization and interventions
❒ significant physiologic stress responses
❒ sleep patterns
❒ nutritional intake
❒ pain control
❒ response to caregivers
❒ response to interventions designed to increase coping skills
❒ suicide risk
❒ referrals made
❒ patient and family teaching
❒ discharge planning.

Associated care plans

- Acute pain
- Chronic pain
- Compromised family coping
- Dying
- Grieving
- Knowledge deficit

References

Jordan, K. (ed.) Emergency Nursing Core Curriculum. *Emergency Nurses Association.* Philadelphia: W.B. Saunders Co., 2000.

Lee, A., and Craft-Rosenberg, M. "Ineffective Family Participation in Professional Care: A Concept Analysis of a Proposed Nursing Diagnosis," *Nursing Diagnosis* 13(1):5-14, January-March 2002.

Lynn-McHale, D.J., and Carlson, K.K. American Association of Critical Care Nurses *AACN Procedure Manual for Critical Care*, 4th ed. Philadelphia: W.B. Saunders Co., 2001.

Shoemaker, W.C., et al. *Textbook of Critical Care*, 4th ed. Philadelphia: W.B. Saunders Co., 2002.

Thompson, J.M., et al. *Mosby's Clinical Nursing*, 5th ed. St Louis: Mosby–Year Book, Inc., 2002.

Knowledge deficit

Introduction

DEFINITION AND TIME FOCUS

A knowledge deficit is an absence or deficiency of cognitive information related to a specific topic. This teaching plan focuses on the acutely ill patient and his family. Even in today's hectic health care environment, you can capitalize on unexpected teaching opportunities to meet immediate learning needs as well as to identify long-range learning needs. The latter are usually addressed after the patient has been discharged or transferred to an environment more conducive to learning.

Through expert teaching, the nurse can provide a context for the patient and family to understand the rationale for therapeutic interventions. Teaching is most effective when it pervades all phases of patient care.

Because of the importance of knowledge deficit as a patient problem and the number of possible interventions, problems in this plan are subdivided by cause. (See *Clinical snapshot*: *Knowledge deficit*, page 130.)

ETIOLOGY AND PRECIPITATING FACTORS

- Unfamiliar diagnostic procedure
- New diagnosis
- Alteration in existing health problem
- Unfamiliar or altered treatment plan
- Complex treatment regimen
- Denial
- Anxiety

Focused assessment guidelines

NURSING HISTORY (FUNCTIONAL HEALTH PATTERN FINDINGS)

Because each patient's knowledge deficit will be individual, this section presents a guide for assessment of teaching and learning factors.

Health-perception–health-management pattern

- Did the patient delay seeking medical attention?
- Does the patient lack knowledge about the disorder?
- Does the patient express lack of confidence in managing the condition?
- Does the patient express misconceptions about health status?
- Has the patient failed to comply with recommended health practices?
- Does the patient fail to carry out self-care, even though physically able?

Nutritional-metabolic pattern

- Does the patient express concerns about the effects of the disorder on nutrition and eating habits?
- Has the patient had difficulty staying on a prescribed dietary regimen?

Activity-exercise pattern

- Does the patient express concerns about life-changing physical limitations because of the disorder?

Cognitive-perceptual pattern

- Does the patient express concerns about specific details of a diagnostic or therapeutic procedure?
- Does the patient have sensory deficits, such as visual or hearing impairments?
- Does the patient lack psychomotor skills needed to maintain a home treatment regimen?
- Has the patient experienced confusion or changes in thought processes from the disorder?
- Has the patient shown signs of misinterpreting information such as by asking inappropriate questions?

Self-perception–self-concept pattern

- Does the patient express concerns about an inability to maintain the treatment regimen?
- Does the patient report anxiety about changes in body image from the disorder?

Role-relationship pattern

- Does the patient want a family member present or available during procedures?
- Does the patient express concerns about job, income, family responsibilities, or the family's response to lifestyle changes because of the disorder?

Sexuality-reproductive pattern

- Does the patient report concern about the disorder's impact on sexual activity?
- Does the patient express concern about the impact of changes in sexual activity on a spouse or partner?

Coping–stress tolerance pattern

- Does the patient display an unusual amount of anxiety?
- Does the patient display denial of the disorder?
- Does the patient report depression because of lifestyle changes caused by the disorder?
- Does the patient express concerns about coping behaviors and motivation?

PHYSICAL FINDINGS

Not applicable

DIAGNOSTIC STUDIES
Not applicable

POTENTIAL COMPLICATION
■ Exacerbation of disorder

CLINICAL SNAPSHOT ☀

Knowledge deficit

Major nursing diagnoses	Key patient outcomes
Deficient knowledge related to lack of readiness to learn	Display motivation to learn.
Deficient knowledge related to teaching program inappropriate for current needs	Identify high-priority learning needs.
Deficient knowledge related to inadequate or ineffective implementation of teaching plan	Have teaching accomplished during stay documented in chart. Indicate interest in learning during care activities.
Deficient knowledge related to lack of needed modification in teaching	Express satisfaction with teaching plan.

Nursing diagnosis
Deficient knowledge related to lack of readiness to learn

NURSING PRIORITY
Determine readiness to learn.

PATIENT OUTCOME CRITERIA
Before initiation of teaching, the patient will:
■ be physiologically stable
■ discuss current knowledge of the disorder when asked
■ identify primary perceived learning needs
■ display motivation to learn such as by asking appropriate questions.

INTERVENTIONS	RATIONALES
1. *Assess the impact of the patient's disorder on lifestyle.* *	1. The degree of impact determines the extent of teaching necessary. Areas of impact provide foci around which learning experiences should be structured.
2. *Determine the patient's stage of adaptation to the disorder:* shock and disbelief, developing awareness, or resolution and reorganization. Consider psychological issues when planning teaching objectives and content during each phase.	2. Different psychological work occurs in each of these phases. Attempting to provide teaching inappropriate for a particular phase results in increased learner anxiety or irritation and inability to absorb information.
3. *Assess the patient's physical readiness to learn:* Is the patient physiologically stable, rested, and pain-free? If not, defer teaching.	3. Teaching is most effective when the patient is ready to learn. Readiness to learn depends on physical as well as psychological factors. Determining readiness to learn requires weighing the interaction of numerous variables. Learning requires energy that won't be available if the patient is unstable, tired, or in pain. Because of shortened hospital stays, few patients reach physical or emotional readiness to learn extensive amounts of information before discharge.

*Italics indicate key interventions.

4. *Determine the patient's motivation to learn.* For example, has the patient asked appropriate questions about status or care? Is the patient preoccupied, distracted, or emotionally labile?

4. Motivation is the crucial variable in learning and may be absent initially because of anxiety or preoccupation with personal needs. Prolonged absence of interest in learning about the condition may be a clue to an underlying emotional disorder requiring treatment before the patient can assume independent self-care. Motivation may be developed through teaching by linking relevant information to the patient's particular concerns.

5. *Determine the general pattern of health maintenance;* for example, has the patient sought regular medical checkups, followed previous health recommendations, eaten a balanced diet, and exercised regularly?

5. The general pattern can provide clues to overall acceptance of responsibility for self-care and receptivity to teaching.

6. *Assess the patient's current knowledge of the disorder* and its implications, the likelihood of complications, and the likelihood of cure or disease control. Specifically ask about the physician's explanations, the patient's past experiences, and information received from family, friends, and the media.

6. Adults learn best when teaching builds on previous knowledge or experience. Assessing recall of the physician's explanations as well as the patient's past experiences and exposure to health information provides an opportunity for evaluating attitudes and the accuracy and completeness of knowledge.

7. *Ask how much the patient wants to know,* if possible. Consider the patient's preference for information in planning teaching. When possible, appropriately match preference and teaching to respect individual differences and support the patient's preferred learning style.

7. Research suggests that the common assumption that teaching reduces anxiety or otherwise helps the patient isn't always true; people vary in the degree of detail they find helpful. Those who cope with a threatening experience by avoiding it generally want to know relatively little about impending experiences, whereas those who cope by learning as much as possible about the threatening experience want to know a great deal. Providing the first type of patient with detailed information increases anxiety, whereas withholding it from the second type of patient increases stress. When possible, appropriately matching preference and teaching style and supporting the patient's preferred learning style shows respect for individual differences.

8. *Determine learning needs.* Consider needs expressed by the patient and family; predictable disorder-related concerns and responses; and activities necessary to monitor health status, prevent disease, implement prescribed therapy, and prevent complications or recurrence.

8. Learning needs determine appropriate content. Learning occurs most rapidly when it's relevant to current needs and past experiences. Responding to expressed needs displays sensitivity to the patient's and family's concerns. Identifying predictable concerns and responses and necessary self-care activities helps the nurse fulfill learning needs of which the patient and family may be unaware.

9. *Estimate learning capacity.* Assess the patient's age; language skills; ability to read, write, and reason; and educational, religious, and cultural background.

9. Sociocultural factors affect the speed and degree of learning. Awareness of the patient's age, background, and general capacity for logical thought and self-expression helps the nurse present material at an appropriate learning level.

10. Additional individualized interventions:_____

10. Rationales:_____

> **Suggested NIC Interventions**
> *Teaching: Prescribed diet; Teaching: Disease process; Teaching: Prescribed activity/exercise; Teaching: Procedure/treatment; Teaching: Prescribed medication; Teaching: Psychomotor skill; Teaching: Preoperative; Health education; Health system guidance; Infection protection; Risk identification; Preparatory sensory information*

> **Suggested NOC Outcomes**
> *Knowledge: Diet; Knowledge: Disease process; Knowledge: Energy conservation; Knowledge: Health behaviors; Knowledge: Health resources; Knowledge: Illness care; Knowledge: Infection control; Knowledge: Medication; Knowledge: Prescribed activity; Knowledge: Treatment procedures; Knowledge: Treatment regimen*

Nursing diagnosis

Deficient knowledge related to teaching program inappropriate for current needs

NURSING PRIORITY

Plan an individualized teaching strategy.

PATIENT OUTCOME CRITERIA

Before discharge, the patient will:
- identify high-priority learning needs
- have learning needs documented in chart.

INTERVENTIONS

1. *Determine realistic goals for learning while the patient is in the health care setting.* Work with the patient and family to ensure that goals are mutually acceptable.

2. *Determine what to teach by assessing what's essential from the patient's viewpoint.* Set priorities for content by dividing it into "need to know now" and "need to know later" categories.

3. *Provide a logical sequence to the information presented.* In general, teach the acutely ill patient only:
– information about expressed concerns

– high-priority information-specific teaching without which the patient's condition may be seriously jeopardized.

4. *Select appropriate teaching methods,* such as individual bedside instruction, discussions, and demonstrations.

RATIONALES

1. Goals determine content. Goal-directed learning is more efficient than fragmented, unfocused learning. Active participation in goal setting increases the likelihood that the patient and family will understand goals and support them.

2. Because the patient's attention span may be limited and the health care setting stay may be short, set priorities for content. Content largely determines the appropriate teaching method.

3. Proper sequencing allows the patient to build on current knowledge and experience.
– Learning is strongest when it fulfills perceived needs. Dealing with initial concerns displays sensitivity to the patient, helps establish rapport and trust, and frees the patient's energy to focus on further learning. In general, only crucial questions are answered for the acutely ill patient; the remainder is deferred.
– Presenting essential information early in the teaching period helps ensure that all the critical information will have been covered by the time of discharge.

4. Although various teaching methods exist (see *Teaching strategies*), individual instruction, discussion, and demonstration are most appropriate in the hospital because of constraints imposed by the patient's condition and the environment.

Teaching strategies

Method	Characteristics	Appropriate uses	Disadvantages
Individual bedside instruction	• One-on-one interaction between teacher and patient • Immediate feedback • Informal	• Acute phase • Sensitive topics • "Private" patient • Emotionally labile patient • Patient with language difficulties • Patient with limited education	• Time consuming
Group session	• Small or large number of patients • Informal • Interchange of ideas	• General content • Patients at similar readiness levels	• Lack of individualization
Lecture	• Highly structured • Efficient	• Large amount of factual content • Rehabilitation program	• Lack of opportunity for teacher-patient interaction • Possible failure to engage the patient's interest (Disadvantages may be overcome by alternating lectures with interactive learning opportunities, such as question-and-answer periods or skill demonstrations.)
Discussion	• Interchange of ideas • More informal than lecture • More opportunity to adapt content and evaluate patient comprehension	• Acute phase • Sensitive topics • When attitudinal change is desired • Highly verbal patient	• Time consuming • Possibly uncomfortable for some patients because of cultural norms that discourage expression
Demonstration and return demonstration	• Observation and supervised practice • Immediate feedback	• Teaching psychomotor skills	• Requires actual equipment

5. *Be creative in choosing appropriate teaching materials,* such as booklets, instruction sheets, films, videotapes, models or dolls, slides, and audiotapes. Consider the educational level, advantages and availability of various teaching materials, patient's preferred learning style, and the learning environment.

5. The more senses involved in learning, the more likely the patient will retain the information. Printed materials offer consistency, reinforce orally presented information, and provide a source to which the patient can refer as needed. Models (for example, of the heart or a pacemaker) help the patient visualize how something works. Dolls may be useful adjuncts for teaching. Slides, audiotapes, films, and videotapes can vividly present an experience — for example, by showing a diagnostic procedure from the patient's viewpoint. These audiovisuals may not be suitable, however, unless the patient is stable enough to focus attention on them and the learning environment is conducive to using them. If used, they should be supplemented by a one-on-one follow-up discussion.

6. *Determine how best to teach the content to an individual patient* at a particular time. Consider the advantages and disadvantages of various teaching methods, the appropriateness and availability of educational materials, and the patient's personality.

6. In many cases, combinations of teaching methods and educational materials can achieve a desired goal. Selecting the combination most appropriate to this patient enlivens the learning experience.

7. *Decide who should teach what:* Consider the primary nurse, a nurse with special related expertise, and other health care professionals. Mention the availability of visitors from community or self-help groups when the patient is more stable physiologically.

7. Depending on the content and patient preferences, different teachers may be necessary or appropriate to reinforce learning. Support groups may provide especially relevant information based on personal experience with the patient's disorder. In many cases, their credibility makes them invaluable in helping the patient accept the need for long-term education and rehabilitation. Their visits may need to be deferred until after the patient has stabilized and can benefit from their insights and competencies. Knowing that others have coped productively with similar experiences may provide the patient with hope that facilitates the necessary learning.

8. *Decide when to teach.*

8. Choosing appropriate times to teach capitalizes on learning readiness. Appropriate sequencing builds on previously presented material and enhances integration of learning.

9. *Plan evaluation strategies based on goals and objectives,* such as observing, questioning, and having the patient demonstrate new skills.

9. Evaluation commonly is interwoven with the presentation. Clear evaluation plans help ensure measurable goals and increase the likelihood that the nurse will recognize spontaneous opportunities for evaluation and respond appropriately to them.

10. *Communicate the teaching strategy to other professionals* involved in the patient's care.

10. Communication enhances consistency of information provided by caregivers, permits appropriate reinforcement, and minimizes unnecessary repetition.

11. *Identify and document long-range learning needs.* If the patient is transferred to another unit, communicate learning needs to colleagues on the receiving unit and arrange for continuation of the teaching plan.

11. The patient's condition, extensiveness of learning needs, and the busy unit atmosphere may complicate the patient's learning before transfer. Documentation and communication of long-range learning needs allow personalization of ongoing educational efforts.

12. Additional individualized interventions: _____

12. Rationales:_____

Suggested NIC Interventions
Teaching: Prescribed diet; Teaching: Disease process; Teaching: Prescribed activity/exercise; Teaching: Procedure/treatment; Teaching: Prescribed medication; Teaching: Psychomotor skill; Teaching: Preoperative; Health education; Health system guidance; Infection protection; Risk identification; Preparatory sensory information

Suggested NOC Outcomes
Knowledge: Diet; Knowledge: Disease process; Knowledge: Energy conservation; Knowledge: Health behaviors; Knowledge: Health resources; Knowledge: Illness care; Knowledge: Infection control; Knowledge: Medication; Knowledge: Prescribed activity; Knowledge: Treatment procedures; Knowledge: Treatment regimen

Nursing diagnosis
Deficient knowledge related to inadequate or ineffective implementation of the teaching plan

NURSING PRIORITY
Implement an individualized teaching plan that maximizes learning, retention, and compliance.

PATIENT OUTCOME CRITERION
At his own pace, the patient will indicate interest in learning during care activities.

INTERVENTIONS

1. *Incorporate teaching into other nursing activities.* Be alert for unexpected teaching opportunities; for example, use symptomatic episodes (such as an insulin reaction in a newly diagnosed diabetic) to help the patient and family learn to identify symptoms.

2. *Present yourself as enthusiastic, knowledgeable, and approachable.*

3. *Present manageable amounts of information at any one time.*

4. *Provide simple explanations, using easy-to-understand terminology.*

5. *Use review and repetition judiciously, considering individual factors.*

6. *Before planned teaching, assess for physiologic needs* (such as thirst or an urge to void) *and intense emotions.* Meet any physiologic needs first, and encourage the patient to express any strong emotions.

7. *Provide opportunities for immediate application of learning.* For example, after you have taught pulse taking, have the patient count your radial pulse while you take your carotid pulse for comparison.

8. *Ask for feedback:* Were the words understandable? Was the presentation too fast, too slow, too detailed, or too scant? Adjust terminology, pace, and amount of information accordingly.

9. *Be alert for signs of pain, fatigue, confusion, or boredom,* such as grimacing, fidgeting, yawning, agitation, or lack of eye contact.

10. *Promote a positive outlook;* solicit feelings and convey confidence in the patient's ability to learn.

11. *Encourage active participation.* Use interactive teaching methods.

12. *Document teaching sessions.* Communicate progress to appropriate caregivers.

RATIONALES

1. The hectic pace of most units allows little time for extended teaching sessions. Incorporating teaching into other activities increases the likelihood that it will be accomplished and contributes to an atmosphere of naturalness and informality. Activity-related teaching (for example, teaching stoma care whenever the stoma is visible) also reinforces learning. The immediacy of a symptomatic episode makes it a powerful teaching tool for establishing the importance of the patient's and family's active involvement in learning.

2. Enthusiasm is contagious. Presenting yourself as knowledgeable increases credibility, and maintaining approachability allows the patient to feel comfortable capitalizing on your expertise.

3. Too much information at one time causes confusion. The patient may lose sight of key points.

4. Medical and nursing jargon distances the patient and family members. Intricate explanations may confuse or overwhelm them.

5. Physiologic changes, pain medications, anxiety, the unit environment, and the patient's age may contribute to a short attention span and poor retention. (Elderly persons commonly have difficulty remembering details.)

6. Unmet physiologic needs and strong emotions interfere with the ability to concentrate on learning.

7. Immediate application improves retention.

8. The patient may be reluctant to reveal lack of understanding. Soliciting feedback demonstrates respect for the learner and permits adjustments before the patient becomes lost, overwhelmed, or bored.

9. These nonverbal signs may provide clues to the need for modification or conclusion of the teaching session.

10. The patient may initially feel overwhelmed and insecure about learning because of the magnitude, urgency, or unfamiliarity of necessary adaptations to illness.

11. Adults learn best when they are actively involved. Active participation also facilitates changes needed to allow recovery from or adaptation to the patient's disorder.

12. Documentation provides a teaching record for legal purposes and enhances continuity of teaching among caregivers.

General care plans

13. Additional individualized interventions: _____ | **13.** Rationales: _____

> **Suggested NIC Interventions**
> *Teaching: Prescribed diet; Teaching: Disease process; Teaching: Prescribed activity/exercise; Teaching: Procedure/treatment; Teaching: Prescribed medication; Teaching: Psychomotor skill; Teaching: Preoperative; Health education; Health system guidance; Infection protection; Risk identification; Preparatory sensory information*

> **Suggested NOC Outcomes**
> *Knowledge: Diet; Knowledge: Disease process; Knowledge: Energy conservation; Knowledge: Health behaviors; Knowledge: Health resources; Knowledge: Illness care; Knowledge: Infection control; Knowledge: Medication; Knowledge: Prescribed activity; Knowledge: Treatment procedures; Knowledge: Treatment regimen*

Nursing diagnosis
Deficient knowledge related to lack of needed modification in teaching

NURSING PRIORITIES
- Evaluate learning.
- Modify teaching when appropriate.

PATIENT OUTCOME CRITERIA
According to individual readiness, the patient will:
- demonstrate learning
- display minimal anxiety about self-care
- express satisfaction with teaching plan
- display realistic appraisal of continuing learning needs
- identify appropriate learning resources.

INTERVENTIONS	**RATIONALES**
1. *During and after teaching, determine what learning has occurred.* For example, observe the patient, ask questions, or have the patient demonstrate a new skill.	**1.** Determining learning accomplishment permits resolution of some learning needs and provides guidance for meeting others.
2. With the patient, *compare learning to date against previously identified goals.*	**2.** Comparison indicates whether goals have been achieved or whether their appropriateness should be reevaluated.
3. *Modify the teaching plan as indicated* by unmet goals or new learning needs.	**3.** Frequent evaluation and modification of the teaching plan ensures that the teaching is tailored to individual learning capabilities and ongoing learning needs.
4. Refer the patient and family to health care and community agencies, as appropriate, before discharge.	**4.** Needs not met by the time of discharge require follow-up.
5. Additional individualized interventions: _____	**5.** Rationales: _____

> **Suggested NIC Interventions**
> *Teaching: Prescribed diet; Teaching: Disease process; Teaching: Prescribed activity/exercise; Teaching: Procedure/treatment; Teaching: Prescribed medication; Teaching: Psychomotor skill; Teaching: Preoperative; Health education; Health system guidance; Infection protection; Risk identification; Preparatory sensory information*

> **Suggested NOC Outcomes**
> *Knowledge: Diet; Knowledge: Disease process; Knowledge: Energy conservation; Knowledge: Health behaviors; Knowledge: Health resources; Knowledge: Illness care; Knowledge: Infection control; Knowledge: Medication; Knowledge: Prescribed activity; Knowledge: Treatment procedures; Knowledge: Treatment regimen*

Discharge planning

DISCHARGE CHECKLIST
Before discharge, the patient should show evidence of:
- ❏ being able to identify learning needs
- ❏ the teaching accomplished during the stay.

TEACHING CHECKLIST
Document evidence that the patient and family demonstrate an understanding of:
- ❏ key pathophysiologic aspects of the disorder
- ❏ signs and symptoms requiring medical attention
- ❏ dietary modifications, if appropriate
- ❏ medications
- ❏ other therapies
- ❏ community resources for adjustment to lifestyle changes.

DOCUMENTATION CHECKLIST
Using outcome criteria as a guide, document:
- ❏ assessment of readiness for learning
- ❏ identification of factors that may inhibit learning
- ❏ identification of learning goals
- ❏ response of the patient and family to the teaching plan
- ❏ problems encountered in teaching
- ❏ evaluation of learning.

Associated care plans

- Acute pain
- Anxiety
- Chronic pain
- Compromised family coping
- Confusion
- Ineffective individual coping

(See also the plan for the specific disorder.)

References

Gordon, M. *Manual of Nursing Diagnosis, 1997-1998.* St. Louis: Mosby–Year Book, Inc., 1997.

Gordon, M. *Nursing Diagnosis: Process and Application,* 3rd ed. St. Louis: Mosby–Year Book, Inc., 1994.

Nutritional deficit

Introduction
DEFINITION AND TIME FOCUS
A nutritional deficit exists when a patient doesn't ingest or absorb the nutrients necessary to meet metabolic needs. Adequate nutrition is vitally important to patients recovering from critical illness. Besides glucose needs for cellular metabolism and energy production, there are many other nutritional needs. For example, calories, protein, and potassium are necessary to rebuild injured tissue; proteins, fatty acids, and phosphate are necessary to fight infection; and trace elements are necessary for optimal functioning of enzyme systems. This care plan focuses on the acutely ill patient whose survival and recovery may be threatened by inadequate nutrition. Because it's so wordy, this book uses "Nutritional deficit." (See *Clinical snapshot: Nutritional deficit*, page 140.)

ETIOLOGY AND PRECIPITATING FACTORS
- Contraindications to eating, as with peptic ulcer or pancreatitis
- Decreased appetite
- Nothing by mouth for more than 4 days
- Inability to chew, as with jaw wiring or poor dentition
- Impaired swallowing, as with stroke, coma, or obstruction
- Preexisting malnutrition, as with cancer or anorexia nervosa
- Decreased GI motility, as with paralytic ileus
- Failure to absorb nutrients, as with malabsorption syndrome, ulcerative colitis, or acquired immunodeficiency syndrome
- Hypermetabolic state, as with burns or trauma
- Protein loss from wounds (pressure ulcers, surgical wounds)
- Insufficient finances or transportation to obtain food
- Depression, dementia, delirium

Focused assessment guidelines
NURSING HISTORY (FUNCTIONAL HEALTH PATTERN FINDINGS)
Health-perception–health-management pattern
- History of chronic GI disorder
- Preexisting debility
Nutritional-metabolic pattern
- Anorexia, indigestion, nausea, or vomiting
- Difficulty or pain on swallowing
- Refusal to eat

Activity-exercise pattern
- Weakness or lack of energy
Cognitive-perceptual pattern
- Abdominal pain
Coping–stress tolerance pattern
- Depression

PHYSICAL FINDINGS
General appearance
- Emaciation (if preexisting malnutrition exists)
- Weakness
- Recent unintentional weight loss
Gastrointestinal
- Weak mastication or swallowing muscles
- Inflamed oral cavity or tongue
- Vomiting
- Absent bowel sounds
- Diarrhea
- Hepatomegaly
Neurologic
- Lethargy
- Decreased level of consciousness (LOC)
- Paresthesia
- Confusion
- Disorientation
Integumentary
- Subcutaneous fat loss
- Dry, scaly skin
- Poor skin turgor
- Sparse, lackluster, or easily plucked hair
- Dry, cracked lips; red cracks at corners of mouth
- Thin, brittle nails
Musculoskeletal
- Weakness
- Body weight at least 20% below ideal weight for height and frame
- Poor muscle tone
- Muscle wasting

DIAGNOSTIC STUDIES
See *Diagnostic studies in nutritional deficit.*

POTENTIAL COMPLICATIONS
- Reduced immunocompetence
- Electrolyte imbalances
- Poor wound healing

Diagnostic studies in nutritional deficit

Various diagnostic studies may be performed in the care of a patient with a nutritional deficit. These studies can be used to assess weight loss, muscle protein stores, or visceral protein stores; estimate body fat reserves; or obtain additional information on the patient's nutritional status.

To assess weight loss and significance
Use the following calculations along with midarm muscle circumference and skin-fold measurements.

Calculating usual body weight
To calculate the patient's usual body weight percentage, use this formula:
current weight ÷ usual body weight ÷ 100
Malnutrition is rated as mild (85%), moderate (75% to 84%), or severe (less than 74%).

Calculating weight loss
To calculate the patient's weight loss as a percentage, use this formula:
([usual weight–current weight] ÷ usual weight) × 100
Weight loss is considered severe if the percentage is more than 5% over 1 month, more than 7.5% over 3 months, or more than 10% over 6 months.

Calculating body mass index (BMI)
To calculate the patient's BMI, use this formula:
BMI = weight in kilograms ÷ height in square meters
The normal range is 20 to 25 kg/m².

To assess muscle protein stores
Height-weight ratio
About 85% or less of the expected value indicates significant protein-calorie malnutrition. (Height and weight are the most significant factors in determining malnutrition.) In the Harris-Benedict equation, the patient's height-weight ratio predicts calorie expenditure. The height-weight ratio is compared with the patient's historical height-weight ratio to determine the severity of malnutrition and the preferred method of feeding the patient.

Midarm circumference (MAC) and midarm muscle circumference (MAMC)
These tests estimate fat and skeletal muscle mass. Measurements are compared to a standard table: 35% to 40% of normal indicates mild depletion of muscle and fat; 25% to 34%, moderate depletion; and less than 25%, severe depletion. MAMC is calculated using MAC and skin-fold measurements and evaluated in comparison with standard tables.

24-hour urine urea nitrogen excretion
This test indicates the severity of protein catabolism. The normal range is 4 to 10 g/day; greater than 10 g/day in a patient with major injuries or sepsis indicates hypermetabolism and a need for increased calories or nitrogen for tissue repair. In a patient who is stable, has no injuries, and is gaining weight, a 24-hour urine urea greater than 10 g/day can indicate overfeeding. (To ensure a positive nitrogen balance in the catabolic patient, approximately 4 to 6 g of nitrogen is given in excess of the amount excreted in the urine.)

Creatinine height index
This shows the relationship between creatinine level and the patient's height and indirectly measures depletion of muscle mass. A range of 60% to 80% of normal represents moderate protein depletion; less than 60% indicates severe depletion. (Creatinine excretion varies directly according to loss of skeletal muscle mass; creatinine height index is obtained by comparing creatinine and height-weight ratio with charts listing normal creatinine excretion for height and weight. Increased creatinine excretion indicates skeletal muscle breakdown.)

Nitrogen balance
The value is obtained by comparing urine urea nitrogen excretion with nitrogen intake (calculated from protein intake). In malnutrition, negative nitrogen balance reveals a catabolic state. A positive nitrogen balance of 2 to 3 g is ideal; in severe illness, zero nitrogen balance may be the realistic maximum attainable.

To assess visceral protein stores
These include plasma proteins, hemoglobin, clotting factors, hormones, antibodies, and enzymes.

Total lymphocyte count (TLC)
This study helps evaluate immunocompetence; a value of 1,200 to 2,000/mm³ indicates mild lymphocyte depletion; 800 to 1,199/mm³, moderate depletion; and less than 800/mm³, severe depletion. (Severe depletion indicates inadequate antibody production and an impaired ability to fight infection. Nutritional repletion is indicated to improve the body's defense mechanisms. TLC is not an accurate indicator of nutritional status in patients on immunosuppressive therapy.)

Albumin
A serum level of less than 3 g/dl correlates with increased severity of illness. A value of 2.8 to 3.5 g/dl indicates mild visceral protein depletion; 2.1 to 2.7 g/dl, moderate depletion; and less than 2.1 g/dl, severe depletion. Because the albumin level falls slowly, it isn't a reliable early indicator of malnutrition. Prealbumin (PAB) is more responsive than albumin to changes in nutrition because of its short half-life (2 days) and small body pool. It increases 1 mg/dl/day with nutritional support. Levels can be affected by stress, liver and renal dysfunction, or acute inflammation. A PAB level below 8 mg/dl indicates severe malnutrition; levels of 10 to 16 mg/dl indicate moderate malnutrition.

Transferrin
This study measures the level of a protein synthesized in the liver. A serum level of 150 to 200 mg/dl indicates mild visceral protein depletion; 100 to 149 mg/dl, moderate depletion; and less than 100 mg/dl, severe depletion. Serum concentration levels fall rapidly with starvation and stress over approximately 8 days. Serial serum transferrin levels indicate response to nutritional therapy.

(continued)

Diagnostic studies in nutritional deficit *(continued)*

Skin-test antigens

This study evaluates cell-mediated immunity, which can decrease with severe malnutrition. This may be assessed using skin-test antigens, such as mumps, *Candida*, streptokinase, or streptodornase. If a negative reaction occurs, malnutrition may be the cause, and the body lacks defense mechanisms to fight infection. A positive reaction is induration exceeding 5 mm, in response to at least two antigens, within 24 to 48 hours.

To estimate body fat reserves
Skin-fold measurements (such as triceps skin fold)

These measurements help estimate the patient's body fat reserves. Measurements are compared with a standard table of values: 35% to 40% of normal indicates mild fat depletion; 25% to 34%, moderate depletion; and less than 25%, severe depletion. The measurements are difficult to evaluate if the patient has edema or can't sit. Serial measurements made by the same observer are more accurate.

Other studies
Total iron-binding capacity (TIBC)

This measures the ability of iron to bind with transferrin transported in the blood. Followed serially, TIBC indicates if nutritional support is correcting the patient's nutritional state.

Serum electrolyte levels

Levels are obtained to serve as baseline values and to guide replacement therapy; in patients with malnutrition, they typically reveal hyponatremia, hypokalemia, hypomagnesemia, and hypophosphatemia.

Serum cholesterol

Levels below 150 mg/dl can indicate malnutrition. Evaluate with other tests.

CLINICAL SNAPSHOT ✳

Nutritional deficit

Major nursing diagnoses	Key patient outcomes
Imbalanced nutrition: Less than body requirements related to difficulty chewing or swallowing, sore throat after endotracheal intubation, or dry mouth	Swallow without choking.
Imbalanced nutrition: Less than body requirements related to anorexia	Eat and retain at least three-quarters of prescribed diet, if able.
Imbalanced nutrition: Less than body requirements related to inability to digest nutrients or hypermetabolic state	Tolerate enteral or parenteral feedings, if any, without adverse effect.

Nursing diagnosis

Imbalanced nutrition: Less than body requirements related to difficulty chewing or swallowing, sore throat after endotracheal extubation, or dry mouth

NURSING PRIORITY
Compensate for eating difficulties.

PATIENT OUTCOME CRITERIA
At his own pace, the patient will:
- eat the prescribed diet without difficulty
- swallow without choking.

INTERVENTIONS

1. *Assess and document causes of nutritional deficit.** Initiate referrals as appropriate — for example, to a dentist or speech pathologist.

2. *Assess the patient's LOC and ability to chew and swallow, and check for gag reflex.* Observe for coughing or moist voice after eating.

3. In collaboration with the dietitian or nutritional support nurse and as ordered, provide a diet appropriate to the patient's abilities — for example, liquids, soft foods, or food requiring little cutting.

4. If the patient has a sore mouth or throat, obtain an order for viscous lidocaine (Xylocaine). If the patient has been extubated recently, explain that the sore throat usually resolves spontaneously within a few days.

5. *Place the patient sitting upright for meals,* with his head flexed forward about 45 degrees, unless contraindicated.

6. *Have suction equipment available nearby but out of the patient's sight.* Suction food, fluids, and accumulated saliva, as needed.

7. Provide assistance, as needed. If the patient has had a stroke, place food in the unaffected side of the mouth.

8. *Document feeding technique and food intake.*

9. Additional individualized interventions: _____
_____

RATIONALES

1. Some eating difficulties call for diagnosis or interventions beyond the scope of nursing. For example, a dentist may be able to diagnose jaw pain or a speech pathologist may be able to teach swallowing technique.

2. Alertness, ability to chew and swallow, and a gag reflex determine if the patient can safely ingest nutrients orally.

3. An appropriate diet minimizes patient frustration when eating.

4. Use of viscous lidocaine, a topical anesthetic, reduces discomfort. Knowing that the sore throat, common after extubation, will probably disappear after extubation may increase the patient's tolerance of the discomfort.

5. This position maintains esophageal patency, facilitates swallowing, and minimizes the risk of aspiration.

6. If the patient has sudden difficulty swallowing, prompt suctioning prevents aspiration. Keeping the equipment out of sight creates a more pleasant eating environment.

7. Providing assistance increases food intake. Placing the food in the unaffected side facilitates use of the tongue to move food toward the back of the mouth.

8. Documenting the technique provides for continuity of care; records are necessary to monitor the adequacy of food intake.

9. Rationales: _____
_____

> ### Suggested NIC Interventions
> *Diet staging; Eating disorders management; Nutrition management; Weight gain assistance; Fluid monitoring; Nutritional monitoring*

> ### Suggested NOC Outcomes
> *Nutritional status: Food and fluid intake; Nutritional status: Nutrient intake; Weight control*

Nursing diagnosis
Imbalanced nutrition: Less than body requirements related to anorexia

NURSING PRIORITY
Promote appetite.

PATIENT OUTCOME CRITERION
At his own pace, the patient will eat and retain at least three-quarters of the prescribed diet.

---

*Italics indicate key interventions.

INTERVENTIONS

1. *Assess possible causes of anorexia,* such as nausea and vomiting, unpleasant sights and odors, depression, and medications. Determine food preferences.

2. *Provide a pleasant eating environment.* For example, place an emesis basin nearby but out of direct sight (if someone will be staying at the bedside); remove tissues containing sputum.

3. Before meals, promote rest; administer analgesics or antiemetics, as needed and ordered; avoid painful procedures; and provide oral hygiene.

4. *Emphasize the importance of eating.* Use positive terms when presenting food; for example, "Here's a milkshake to help you regain your strength," rather than "Do you think you'll be able to keep this down?"

5. *Provide social interaction* during meals, preferably with family and friends.

6. *Offer small, frequent feedings* of highly nutritious foods, including the patient's preferences whenever possible.

7. *Limit fluid intake at mealtimes.*

8. *If the patient begins to feel nauseated, encourage slow, deep breathing.* If vomiting occurs, document the amount and type of emesis. Provide oral hygiene afterward.

9. *Praise the patient for signs of increased appetite.*

10. Additional individualized interventions:_____
_____

RATIONALES

1. Accurate identification of the cause of the anorexia facilitates selection of appropriate interventions.

2. Removal of noxious sights and smells may decrease anorexia, nausea, and vomiting.

3. Adequate rest conserves the energy necessary to eat. Analgesics, antiemetics, and avoidance of painful procedures remove the influences of pain, nausea, and emotional stress. Oral hygiene removes unpleasant tastes.

4. Emphasizing the importance of eating encourages the patient to eat despite anorexia. Positive terms capitalize on the power of suggestion to influence the subconscious mind.

5. Social interaction increases food intake by providing a pleasant distraction from anorexia. Involving family and friends strengthens interpersonal bonds.

6. Small meals promote prompt gastric emptying, lessening anorexia, and nausea. When food intake is low, every mouthful must count toward meeting nutrient needs.

7. Large amounts of fluid distend the stomach, causing early satiety and promoting nausea.

8. Deep breathing helps to diminish the vomiting reflex. Documentation of emesis is necessary to maintain accurate intake and output records and to evaluate the adequacy of oral nutrition. Oral hygiene removes unpleasant tastes.

9. Praise acknowledges the patient's efforts to overcome anorexia and reinforces desired behavior.

10. Rationales:_____
_____

Suggested NIC Interventions
Diet staging; Eating disorders management; Nutrition management; Weight gain assistance; Fluid monitoring; Nutritional monitoring

Suggested NOC Outcomes
Nutritional status: Food and fluid intake; Nutritional status: Nutrient intake; Weight control

---

Nursing diagnosis

Imbalanced nutrition: Less than body requirements related to inability to digest nutrients or hypermetabolic state

NURSING PRIORITY

Provide nutrients in a form that can be assimilated.

PATIENT OUTCOME CRITERIA

Within 7 days of admission, the patient will:
- tolerate enteral or parenteral feedings (if ordered) without adverse effects
- gain up to 2½ lb (1 kg) per week.

INTERVENTIONS	RATIONALES
1. *Stay alert for increased nutrient needs,* such as from trauma, burns, infection, surgical wounds, and fever. Also observe the patient for indicators (such as diarrhea) of possible inability to absorb nutrients.	**1.** Early recognition of the patient's decreased absorptive ability or increased needs helps provide adequate nutrition before debilitation occurs.
2. Collaborate with the dietitian, nutritional support service, and physician to obtain a comprehensive nutritional assessment.	**2.** A comprehensive assessment includes anthropometric and laboratory measurements performed by colleagues with special nutritional expertise. These measurements document the type and degree of nutritional deficit and provide guidelines for selecting appropriate nutritional interventions.
3. *Assess and document bowel sounds and abdominal distention every 4 hours.*	**3.** Bowel sounds indicate whether the patient can tolerate enteral feedings or whether parenteral feedings are necessary. Abdominal distention suggests paralytic ileus.
4. Collaborate with nutritional experts to establish nutrient requirements, depending on whether the following exist: – starvation – hypermetabolism.	**4.** Nutrient requirements vary depending on whether the patient is merely nutritionally depleted or is experiencing a hypermetabolic state. – Early starvation is characterized by various compensatory mechanisms, including glycogenolysis, lipolysis, proteolysis, and gluconeogenesis. Rapid catabolism produces rapid weight loss, osmotic diuresis, and urinary nitrogen loss. After approximately 10 days, the metabolic rate slows and weight loss continues at a slower rate while the body uses fat as its primary energy source. After several months, exhaustion of fat stores causes the body to use visceral protein for energy. – The release of catecholamines, glucocorticoids, mineralocorticoids, and cytokines in response to stress cause the traumatized or infected patient to develop greater glucose mobilization than the starved patient. Rapid weight loss and osmotic diuresis are delayed for approximately 24 to 48 hours after trauma.
5. *Provide the appropriate nutritional replacement, as ordered.* Options include the following: – enteral feeding (via nasogastric, gastrostomy, or jejunostomy tubes), such as: – meal replacements – nutrient supplements – defined-formula diets – parenteral nutrition (PN) – peripheral parenteral nutrition (PPN)	**5.** Nutritional replacement methods depend on the patient's needs. – Enteral feeding is preferred for the patient with a functioning GI tract. – Meal replacements are nutritionally complete but require digestive and absorptive abilities. – Supplements, although nutritionally incomplete, can replace one or more specific nutrients. – Defined-formula diets are nutritionally complete and require little digestion. – PN is appropriate for patients who can't meet nutritional needs through GI absorption. It's administered peripherally or centrally. – PPN may be prescribed if caloric needs are relatively low, relatively short-term GI dysfunction is anticipated, and peripheral veins are adequate.

General care plans

– central venous nutrition or total nutrient admixture.

– Central venous nutrition is appropriate for patients with relatively high calorie needs because these solutions have greater calorie and protein content than peripheral venous solutions.

6. Perform these interventions if the patient is receiving tube feedings:
– Check tube placement before each feeding.

6. Nursing measures for tube feedings are designed to facilitate absorption and prevent complications.
– Checking tube placement confirms that the tube is in the stomach or jejunum, as appropriate. Checking a nasogastric tube ensures that it hasn't migrated upward into the trachea.

– Monitor bowel sounds, bowel movements, residual stomach content amounts, abdominal girth, intake and output, and weight.

– Monitoring promotes early identification of complications, such as ileus or obstruction.

– Keep the head of the bed elevated during, and for 1 hour after, feedings.

– Elevation prevents reflux into the esophagus.

– Begin with small amounts (25 to 50 ml/hour) of full strength isotonic solution; dilute hypertonic (greater than 300 mOsm/kg) solutions. Increase the amount and concentration as tolerated (usually 25 ml every 12 hours). Don't increase the concentration and rate at the same time.

– Large amounts of concentrated solution may provoke osmotic diarrhea. Gradual increases allow time for the GI system to adapt to the increased volume and solute load.

– Use a bolus, intermittent, or continuous method as ordered.

– The method of delivery can depend on the patient's disease and ability to tolerate feedings. Intermittent or continuous methods are less likely to cause adverse GI effects such as nausea or diarrhea.

7. If the patient is receiving PN, ensure delivery of the solutions and monitor for complications. Refer to the "Parenteral nutrition" care plan, page 510, for details.

7. PN is a complex therapy with numerous nursing considerations.

8. Additional individualized interventions: _____

8. Rationales: _____

> ### Suggested NIC Interventions
> *Diet staging; Eating disorders management; Nutrition management; Weight gain assistance; Fluid monitoring; Nutritional monitoring*

> ### Suggested NOC Outcomes
> *Nutritional status: Food and fluid intake; Nutritional status: Nutrient intake; Weight control*

Discharge planning
DISCHARGE CHECKLIST
Before discharge, the patient should show evidence of:
❐ assessment of nutritional status
❐ implementation of appropriate nutritional support.

TEACHING CHECKLIST
Document evidence that the patient and family demonstrate an understanding of:
❐ importance of nutrition to recovery
❐ rationale for selection of a specific nutritional support method.

DOCUMENTATION CHECKLIST
Using outcome criteria as a guide, document:
❐ clinical status on admission
❐ significant changes in status

❐ pertinent diagnostic test findings
❐ specific nutritional support method
❐ patient tolerance of method
❐ complications, if any
❐ daily nutritional intake
❐ medications administered, if any
❐ attitude toward eating
❐ patient and family teaching
❐ discharge planning.

Associated care plans
■ Parenteral nutrition
(See also the plan for the specific disorder.)

References

American Society for Parenteral and Enteral Nutrition (A.S.P.E.N.) Board of Directors and Clinical Guidelines Task Force: Guidelines for Use of Parenteral and Enteral Nutrition in Adult and Pediatric Patients. *Journal of Parenteral and Enteral Nutrition* 26 (suppl):15A-1365A, 2002.

Case, K., et al., "Nutrition Support in the Critically Ill Patient," *Critical Care Nursing* 22(4):75-79, January 2000.

Finch, C. "How to Provide Nutrition Support," *Nutrition* 16(4)1555-557, July, 2000.

Hamilton, S. "Detecting Dehydration and Malnutrition in the Elderly," *Nursing* 31(12):56-57, March 2002.

Hess, C. *Clinical Guide: Wound Care,* 3rd ed. Springhouse, Pa. Springhouse Corp., 2000.

Jacelon, C. "Rehabilitation and Iatrogenic Complications of Critical Care," *Critical Care Nursing Clinics of North America* 13(3):365-70, May 2001.

Mahan, L., and Escott-Stump, S., eds. *Krause's Food, Nutrition and Diet Therapy,* 10th ed., Philadelphia: W.B. Saunders Co., 2000.

Mahesh, C., et al., "Extended Indications for Enteral Nutrition Support," *Nutrition* 16(6):129-132, August 2000.

Minei, J. "Metabolism and Nutrition in Surgical Patients," *Selected Readings in General Surgery* 28(5):2-34. September 2001.

Omran, M.L., and Morley, J.E. "Assessment of Protein Energy Malnutrition in Older Persons. Part I: History, Examination, Body Composition and Screening Tools," *Nutrition* 16(1): 50-63, January 2000.

Omran, M.L., and Morley, J.E. "Assessment of Protein Energy Malnutrition in Older Persons Part II: Laboratory Evaluation," *Nutrition* 16(2):131-140, February 2000.

Rakel, R, ed. *Saunders Manual of Medical Practice,* 2nd ed. Philadelphia: W.B. Saunders Co., 2000.

Scolapio, J., et al. "Enteral versus Parenteral Nutrition: The Patient's Preference," *Journal of Parenteral and Enteral Nutrition* 26(4):248-250, March 2002.

Wilmore, D. "Metabolic Response to Severe Surgical Illness: Overview," *World Journal of Surgery* 24(6):705-11, April 2000.

Wilmore, D. "Nutrition and Metabolic Support in 21st Century," *Journal of Parenteral and Enteral Nutrition* 24(2):1-3, January 2000.

General care plans

Perioperative care

Introduction

DEFINITION AND TIME FOCUS

Surgery is an important medical therapy used for diagnostic, curative, restorative, palliative, or cosmetic reasons. This care plan focuses on care of perioperative patients. (See *Clinical snapshot: Perioperative care.*)

ETIOLOGY AND PRECIPITATING FACTORS

Precipitating factors aren't applicable in this general care plan.

Focused assessment guidelines

Nursing history and physical findings aren't applicable in this general care plan.

DIAGNOSTIC STUDIES

- Urinalysis
- Complete blood count (CBC)
- Prothrombin time and partial thromboplastin time
- Electrolyte panel
- Blood urea nitrogen and creatinine levels
- Blood typing and cross-matching
- Chest X-ray
- 12-lead electrocardiogram (ECG)
- Pregnancy test screen
- Special studies depending on the disorder

POTENTIAL COMPLICATIONS

- Shock
- Atelectasis
- Pulmonary embolism
- Thrombophlebitis
- Wound infection, dehiscence, and evisceration
- Paralytic ileus
- Acute renal failure
- Urine retention
- Aspiration
- Malignant hyperthermia
- Hypothermia
- Latex allergy

Nursing diagnosis

Deficient knowledge (perioperative routines) related to lack of familiarity with hospital procedures

NURSING PRIORITY

Prepare the patient for perioperative routines.

PATIENT OUTCOME CRITERIA

Before surgery, the patient will:
- verbalize understanding of perioperative routines
- demonstrate ability to cough, deep-breathe, use the incentive spirometer, and perform leg exercises.

INTERVENTIONS	RATIONALES
1. See the "Knowledge deficit," care plan, page 129.	1. Generalized interventions regarding patient teaching are included in the "Knowledge deficit" care plan.
2. *Instruct the patient in the various aspects of perioperative routines,* * such as time of surgery, food or fluid restrictions, type of anesthesia, insertion of I.V. and intra-arterial lines, personnel, the environments of the operating and recovery rooms and surgical intensive care unit, type of wound and dressing, tubes, drains, and postoperative respiratory care. Include demonstrations and return demonstrations of coughing, deep breathing, spirometry, splinting the incision, and leg exercises.	2. Patients will be more likely to remember and comply with perioperative procedures if they understand the rationale for them, have been instructed before surgery, and have practiced activities where appropriate.

*Italics indicate key interventions.

CLINICAL SNAPSHOT ✳

Perioperative care

Major nursing diagnoses and collaborative problems	Key patient outcomes
ND: Deficient knowledge (perioperative routines)	Demonstrate ability to cough, deep-breathe, use incentive spirometer, and perform leg exercises.
CP: Risk for postoperative shock	Have a pulse rate of 60 to 100 beats/minute, a systolic blood pressure of 90 to 140 mm Hg, and a diastolic blood pressure of 50 to 90 mm Hg.
ND: Acute pain	Rate pain as less than the chosen goal level (typically less than 3 on a 0 to 10 pain rating scale).
ND: Impaired gas exchange	Manifest clear breath sounds in all lobes.
CP: Risk for postoperative thromboembolic phenomena	Show no signs of thromboembolic phenomena.
ND: Risk for injury	Ambulate without injury.
ND: Risk for infection	Perform wound care.
ND: Urinary retention	Show no signs of urine retention.
CP: Risk for postoperative paralytic ileus, abdominal pain, or constipation	Have normal bowel sounds.
ND: Risk for imbalanced body temperature	Show no signs of malignant hyperthermia or hypothermia.
CP: Risk for nausea or vomiting	Be free from nausea or vomiting.

3. Additional individualized interventions: _____

_____

3. Rationales: _____

_____

Suggested NIC Interventions
Teaching: Preoperative

Suggested NOC Outcomes
Knowledge: Diet; Knowledge: Energy conservation; Knowledge: Illness care; Knowledge: Infection control; Knowledge: Medication; Knowledge: Prescribed activity/exercise; Knowledge: Treatment procedure; Knowledge: Treatment regimen

General care plans

Collaborative problem
Risk for postoperative shock related to hemorrhage, hypovolemia, or ineffective tissue perfusion

NURSING PRIORITY
Detect shock.

PATIENT OUTCOME CRITERIA
Within 12 hours after surgery, the patient will:
- have a pulse rate of 60 to 100 beats/minute, a systolic blood pressure of 90 to 140 mm Hg, and a diastolic blood pressure of 50 to 90 mm Hg
- display minimal bloody drainage on dressing and in wound drains
- maintain a urine output greater than 60 ml/hour.
  Within 2 days after surgery, the patient will:
- display balanced fluid intake and output.

INTERVENTIONS

1. *Monitor and document vital signs on admission to the post-anesthesia care unit (PACU) and every 4 hours.* If vital signs have changed significantly from recovery room findings, monitor and document every 15 to 30 minutes until stable. Report abnormalities. Estimate intraoperative blood loss from the surgical record and laboratory blood studies.

2. *Assess the surgical dressing on admission to the unit, every hour for 4 hours, then every 4 hours.* Mark any drainage, and note on the dressing the date and time it occurred. Document and report excessive drainage.

3. *Assess the amount and character of drainage from wound-drainage tubes when assessing the surgical dressing.* Report bright red bloody drainage.

4. *Reinforce the surgical dressing as needed.* Don't change the original surgical dressing unless specifically ordered to do so.

5. *Assess the surgical area for swelling or hematoma.* Remember to examine multiple port sites if it was a laparoscopic procedure. Document and report abnormalities.

6. *Monitor for changes in mental status and level of consciousness (LOC).* Be alert for restlessness and a sense of impending doom. Document and report such signs.

7. *Assess and maintain I.V. line patency.* Maintain I.V. fluids at the ordered rate.

8. *Monitor urine output every hour for 4 hours, then every 4 hours, during the immediate postoperative period.* Report urine output of less than 60 ml/hour and, in such cases, measure urine specific gravity. Administer I.V. fluids and diuretics as ordered, to maintain urine output at greater than 60 ml/hour and specific gravity at 1.010 to 1.025.

9. *Monitor hemoglobin level and hematocrit, as ordered.* Determine availability of blood and blood products.

10. *Monitor fluid intake and output every 8 hours* with an accumulated total every 24 hours for at least 3 to 4 days after surgery.

RATIONALES

1. Hypotension and tachycardia may indicate hemorrhage. Estimated blood loss guides fluid and blood replacement.

2. Hemorrhage typically occurs within the first several hours after surgery. Frequent assessments allow for its prompt detection. Marking the extent of drainage permits objective serial measurements.

3. Bright red blood from drainage tubes may indicate arterial hemorrhage.

4. Changing the surgical dressing may disrupt the wound edge, cause bleeding, and introduce bacteria.

5. Swelling or hematoma may indicate internal bleeding.

6. Changes in mental status or LOC may reflect cerebral hypoxia, indicating decreased cerebral perfusion from hemorrhage or hypovolemia.

7. A patent I.V. line is essential to fluid replacement. Fluids will be ordered according to the surgeon's preference. At times, fluid replacement is the only treatment necessary for hypovolemic shock.

8. Urine output decreases if the patient is bleeding or is hypovolemic. The kidneys retain fluid to maintain intravascular pressure. Urine specific gravity will reveal urine concentration as the body attempts to conserve fluid. Additionally, blood flow to the kidneys is reduced if the patient is in shock, thereby decreasing the glomerular filtration rate and urine output. I.V. fluids and diuretics help maintain the glomerular filtration rate to prevent acute tubular necrosis.

9. Hemoglobin level and hematocrit don't drop immediately with excessive blood loss because plasma is lost along with red blood cells. If bleeding persists, the blood remaining in the vessels will become more dilute as kidneys conserve water and as fluid shifts from interstitial to intravascular spaces; then hemoglobin level and hematocrit will drop. Rapid administration of blood and blood products may be necessary; confirming their availability avoids delays in initiating therapy.

10. For the first 48 hours after surgery, intake may exceed output because of fluid loss (from hemorrhage, vomiting, or diaphoresis) and increased secretion of antidiuretic hormone and aldosterone.

11. Additional individualized interventions: _____

11. Rationales: _____

Nursing diagnosis

Acute pain related to surgical tissue trauma, positioning, and reflex muscle spasm

NURSING PRIORITY

Relieve pain.

PATIENT OUTCOME CRITERION

Within 1 hour of reporting pain, the patient will rate pain as less than the chosen goal level (typically less than 3 on a 0 to 10 pain rating scale).

INTERVENTIONS	RATIONALES
1. See the "Acute pain" care plan, page 32.	**1.** The "Acute pain" care plan contains detailed information on pain assessment and management.
2. Additional individualized interventions: _____	**2.** Rationales: _____

> ### *Suggested NIC Interventions*
> *Medication management; Pain management; Analgesic administration; Patient-controlled analgesia (PCA) assistance; Conscious sedation*

> ### *Suggested NOC Outcomes*
> *Comfort level; Pain control; Pain: Disruptive effects; Pain level*

Nursing diagnosis

Impaired gas exchange, ciliary depression from anesthesia and positioning

NURSING PRIORITY

Promote normal gas exchange.

PATIENT OUTCOME CRITERIA

Throughout the postoperative period, the patient will:
- display a respiratory rate of 12 to 20 breaths/minute
- have nonlabored, deep respirations
- manifest clear breath sounds in all lobes.

INTERVENTIONS	RATIONALES
1. *Maintain a patent airway.* Suction as needed.	**1.** Airway patency is critical to normal gas exchange.
2. *Assess vital signs according to unit protocol for the first day after surgery, then every 4 hours.* Note the characteristics of respirations. Monitor the amount and characteristics of sputum. Document and report abnormalities.	**2.** Elevated temperature may indicate atelectasis, which can lead to pneumonia. Respirations may be shallow after anesthesia.
3. *Auscultate for breath sounds every 4 hours on the first postoperative day, then once per shift.* Document and report abnormalities.	**3.** Breath sounds may be diminished postoperatively because air exchange is decreased in atelectatic areas.
4. *Instruct and coach the patient in diaphragmatic breathing and chest splinting.*	**4.** Diaphragmatic breathing increases lung expansion by allowing the diaphragm to descend fully. Chest splinting reduces pain and facilitates breathing.

5. *Assist the patient in using the incentive spirometer—* 10 breaths every hour during the day, every 2 hours at night. In the first 24 hours, coach the patient on its use; then, once the patient is alert, encourage independent use and assess its effectiveness.

5. Use of the incentive spirometer promotes sustained maximal inspiration, which inflates alveoli as fully as possible.

6. *Help the patient turn at least every 2 hours* unless contraindicated.

6. Position changes provide for better ventilation of all lobes of the lungs and promote drainage of secretions.

7. Help the patient progressively increase ambulation.

7. Ambulation promotes adequate ventilation by increasing the respiratory rate.

8. *Encourage adequate fluid intake.*

8. Respiratory secretions will be thinner and more easily expectorated if the patient is well hydrated.

9. Additional individualized interventions: _____

9. Rationales: _____

> ### Suggested NIC Interventions
> *Airway management; Vital signs monitoring; Respiratory monitoring; Ventilation assistance*

> ### Suggested NOC Outcomes
> *Respiratory status: Airway patency; Respiratory status: Ventilation; Vital signs status*

Collaborative problem
Risk for postoperative thromboembolic phenomena related to immobility, dehydration, and possible fat particle escape or aggregation

NURSING PRIORITY
Prevent thromboembolism.

PATIENT OUTCOME CRITERIA
- Throughout the postoperative period, the patient will show no signs of thromboembolic phenomena.
- By the time of discharge, the patient will be able to identify an appropriate postdischarge activity schedule.

INTERVENTIONS

1. *Instruct and coach the patient to do leg exercises* hourly while awake: foot flexion and extension, ankle rotation, knee flexion and extension, and quadriceps setting.

2. *Assess the patient twice daily for signs of thromboembolic phenomena.* If any of these signs or symptoms is present, alert the physician promptly:

– thrombophlebitis (redness, swelling, increased warmth along the vein, possibly a positive Homans' sign, and pain)
– pulmonary thromboembolism (sharp, stabbing chest pain, worsening on deep inspiration or coughing; hemoptysis; pleural friction rub; and tachypnea)
– fat embolism (dyspnea, restlessness, and petechiae)

RATIONALES

1. Leg exercises promote blood flow in the legs. Muscle contractions compress the veins and help prevent venous stasis, a major cause of clot formation.

2. Systematic observations aid in prompt detection of thromboembolic phenomena. Prompt treatment reduces the risk of clot extension, pulmonary infarction, or pulmonary arrest.
– Vessel wall inflammation and clot formation produce signs and symptoms of thrombophlebitis.

– Pulmonary thromboembolism occurs when a clot detaches from a vessel and lodges in the lungs.

– Fat embolism is a risk after orthopedic trauma or surgery (such as femoral fractures or sternum-splitting incisions). It may result from the escape of fat particles from bone marrow or from an aggregation of fat particles in the bloodstream.

– peripheral vascular thromboembolism (pallor, weak pulse, loss of sensation).

– Blood clots and sclerotic plaques can detach and lodge in the peripheral vascular bed.

3. Administer heparin as ordered; monitor and report increased bleeding.

3. Heparin is an anticoagulant that can prevent thrombus formation.

4. *Encourage early ambulation after surgery.*

4. Ambulation promotes blood flow in the legs.

5. Avoid using the Gatch bed or placing pillows under the patient's knees.

5. Pressure on the popliteal blood vessels can slow blood circulation to and from the legs. Appropriate positioning also decreases venous stasis.

6. *Encourage adequate fluid intake* (in the initial postoperative period, I.V. fluids will be administered).

6. Inadequate fluid intake causes dehydration, which leads to increased blood viscosity — another major contributor to clot formation.

7. Apply antiembolism stockings, if ordered. Remove them twice daily for 1 hour.

7. Antiembolism stockings compress the leg veins and prevent venous stasis. Stockings should be removed periodically to allow for thrombophlebitis assessment and skin inspection.

8. Apply and monitor lower extremity pneumatic compression devices as ordered by physician.

8. Intermittent pneumatic compression devices are effective in preventing deep vein thrombus.

9. Before discharge, teach the patient and family about guidelines for resuming normal activity.

9. Patients and families probably will have specific questions or concerns about the type and progression of allowable activity after discharge. Providing guidelines promotes the resumption of activity at an appropriate pace, which in turn lessens immobility-related complications and promotes a sense of well-being.

10. Additional individualized interventions:_____
_____

10. Rationales:_____
_____

General care plans

Nursing diagnosis
Risk for injury related to possible changes in LOC or mental status secondary to anesthesia, analgesia, and surgical positioning

NURSING PRIORITY
Prevent injury.

PATIENT OUTCOME CRITERIA
Within 24 hours after surgery, the patient will:
- be free from injury
- seek appropriate assistance with activity from the nurse.

INTERVENTIONS

1. Assess the patient's LOC, orientation, and ability to follow directions every 30 to 60 minutes in the first 8 to 10 hours postoperatively. Compare to preoperative LOC and mental status.

2. Assess skin condition, range of motion (ROM), and neurovascular status within the first 4 to 8 hours of postoperative period. Notify the surgery and/or anesthesia personnel about any abnormalities.

RATIONALES

1. A greater risk of injury exists if the patient is drowsy or disoriented. Frequent observation allows prompt detection of injury risk factors, if present. Preoperative status provides a baseline for comparison.

2. Alterations in skin condition, ROM, or neuropathies that appear with the immediate postoperative period, often are attributed to intraoperative causes.

3. *Position the drowsy patient in a side-lying position;* have suction equipment available.

3. In a side-lying position, the patient has less risk of aspirating secretions or vomitus. Suction equipment at the bedside facilitates prompt airway clearance of secretions or vomitus.

4. *Keep side rails up in the initial postoperative period,* until the patient is awake and alert.

4. Side rails help prevent falls.

5. Keep the call cord within the patient's reach.

5. If the call cord is within reach, the patient is more likely to ask the nurse for assistance.

6. Keep the bed in the low position.

6. The low bed position is safer for the patient.

7. *Monitor postural vital signs and assist the patient with initial postoperative activity.* Observe for a pulse rate increase of more than 20 beats/minute, a systolic blood pressure decrease of more than 10 mm Hg, a decreased LOC, diaphoresis, and cyanosis. If present, discontinue activity and alert the physician.

7. When first ambulating, the patient may feel dizzy or have an unsteady gait from orthostatic hypotension. This occurs because immobility compromises the ability of peripheral vessels to constrict when the patient assumes an upright position. Orthostatic hypotension can also occur if the patient is hypovolemic, producing the more alarming signs listed and requiring medical evaluation and I.V. fluid replacement.

8. Additional individualized interventions: _____
_____

8. Rationales: _____
_____

Suggested NIC Interventions
Fall prevention; Surveillance: Safety

Suggested NOC Outcomes
Safety status; Falls occurrence; Safety status: Physical injury

---

Nursing diagnosis
Risk for infection related to surgical wound

NURSING PRIORITY
Promote wound healing.

PATIENT OUTCOME CRITERIA
Within 3 days after surgery, the patient will:
- be afebrile
- show healing wound with no signs of infection.
  Within 7 days after surgery, the patient will:
- have a clean, dry, and well-approximated surgical wound.

INTERVENTIONS

1. *Identify risk factors for surgical wound infection:*

– obesity

– smoking history

– extremes of age

– immunosuppression
– poor nutritional status
– diabetes mellitus.

RATIONALES

1. Knowledge of risk factors enables the nurse to individualize patient care.
– Adipose tissue is poorly vascularized, retarding healing.
– The poor tissue perfusion resulting from smoking is one cause of dehiscence.
– The very young and the very old have less physiologic reserve.
– A compromised host is at greater risk for infection.
– A catabolic state retards wound repair.
– Impaired glucose metabolism delays healing.

2. *Assess the surgical wound and other invasive sites once per shift for:*
– evidence of normal healing, such as approximation of wound margins and absence of purulent or foul-smelling drainage

– signs of dehiscence, such as poorly approximated wound edges and serous drainage from a previously nondraining wound (If dehiscence occurs, notify the physician immediately.)
– signs of evisceration, such as disruption of the surgical wound with protrusion of the viscera. (If evisceration occurs, cover the viscerated organs with sterile saline-soaked gauze and notify the physician immediately.)

3. Determine wound classification:

– I. clean — minimal endogenous contamination present (such as with breast biopsy)

– II. clean-contaminated — possible endogenous bacterial contamination present (such as with appendectomy)

– III. contaminated — contamination present (such as with trauma)
– IV. dirty — infected tissue present (such as with abscess).

4. *Monitor temperature every 4 hours.* Document and report elevations.

5. *Maintain a clean, dry incision.* Teach patient and family to perform wound care as ordered.

6. *Use aseptic technique* or no-touch clean technique *when performing wound care.* Instruct the patient and family in hand-washing technique; aseptic or clean technique; and wound care, including dressing change and application, irrigations and cleaning procedures, proper disposal of soiled dressings, and bathing by shower (not tub) until the wound is healed.

7. *Instruct the patient and family in signs and symptoms of infection:* elevated temperature, abdominal pain, and purulent or foul-smelling wound drainage.

8. *Encourage adequate nutritional intake* every shift. Document intake every shift.

9. Additional individualized interventions: _____
_____

2. Regular assessment promotes early detection of sub-optimal healing.
– The normally healing wound is well approximated and without evidence of infection. (The surgical wound, however, may be reddened in the first 3 postoperative days — the normal inflammatory response.)
– Wound dehiscence most commonly occurs 3 to 11 days after surgery.

– Eviscerated organs must be kept sterile, moist, and surgical intervention must be prompt because blood supply to tissues is compromised when organs herniate.

3. Wound classification is a predictor of surgical wound infection.
– I. In this wound class, the respiratory, alimentary, or genitourinary tract isn't entered during surgery so the likelihood of contamination is minimal.
– II. In this wound class, the respiratory, alimentary, or genitourinary tract is entered under controlled conditions, but infection isn't noted and the risk of postoperative infection is increased only slightly.
– III. In this wound class, gross GI spillage or traumatic wounds place the patient at higher risk for infection.
– IV. In this wound class, retained devitalized tissue or existing infection pose the greatest risk of infection.

4. A low-grade temperature present in the first 3 postoperative days is associated with the normal inflammatory response. Fever that persists may signify infection.

5. A clean, dry incision is at less risk for infection. Moisture can harbor microorganisms.

6. Aseptic and clean techniques prevent cross-contamination and transmission of bacterial infections to the surgical wound.

7. Educating the patient and family promotes their sense of control and minimizes anxiety and fear during preparation for discharge.

8. Sufficient intake of protein, calories, vitamins, and minerals is essential to promote tissue healing.

9. Rationales: _____
_____

> **Suggested NIC Interventions**
> *Incision site care; Wound care; Infection control; Infection protection; Circulatory care: Arterial insufficiency*

> **Suggested NOC Outcomes**
> *Infection status; Wound healing: Primary intention; Wound healing: Secondary intention*

General care plans

Nursing diagnosis

Urinary retention related to neuroendocrine response to stress, anesthesia, and recumbent position

NURSING PRIORITY
Prevent urine retention.

PATIENT OUTCOME CRITERION
Within 1 day after surgery, the patient will void at least 200 ml of clear urine at a time.

INTERVENTIONS	RATIONALES
1. *Assess for signs of urine retention.* Include subjective complaints of urgency as well as objective signs, such as bladder distention, urine overflow, and marked discrepancy between the fluid intake amount and the time of the last voiding.	1. The distended bladder can be palpated above the level of the symphysis pubis. Overflow incontinence occurs when intravesical pressure exceeds the restraining ability of the sphincter and enough urine flows out to decrease the intravesical pressure to a level at which the sphincter can control urine flow. A difference of several hundred milliliters between fluid intake and output, with the passage of several hours since the last voiding, implies retention.
2. *Initiate interventions to promote voiding* as soon as the patient begins to sense bladder pressure.	2. Prompt treatment of potential voiding problems may reduce anxiety, which can further impair the ability to void.
3. *Provide noninvasive measures to promote voiding* such as normal position for voiding, ambulation to the bathroom if possible, running water, relaxation, a warm bedpan if needed, pouring warm water over the perineum, or privacy.	3. These measures are designed to promote relaxation of the urinary sphincter and facilitate voiding. Successful use of noninvasive measures prevents unnecessary catheterization and related psychological strain and urethral trauma.
4. Provide a supportive atmosphere: Use conscious positive suggestion; reassure the patient that voiding usually occurs eventually; don't threaten catheterization.	4. Conscious positive suggestion and reassurance promote relaxation and set up expectations for spontaneous voiding.
5. *If the patient complains of bladder discomfort or hasn't voided within 8 hours after surgery, obtain an order for straight catheterization.*	5. Straight catheterization poses less risk of infection than indwelling catheterization; an indwelling catheter can provide a pathway for bacteria to ascend into the bladder.
6. If the patient requires catheterization, drain the bladder of no more than 1,000 ml at a time. If urine output reaches 1,000 ml, clamp the catheter, wait 1 hour, then drain the rest of the urine from the bladder.	6. Draining more than 1,000 ml from the bladder releases pressure on the pelvic vessels. The sudden release of pressure allows subsequent pooling of blood in these vessels. Rapid withdrawal of this blood from the central circulating volume may cause shock.
7. *After catheterization, assess for dysuria, hematuria, pyuria, burning, and frequency and urgency of urination as well as for suprapubic discomfort.* Assess and document the amount, appearance, odor, and clarity of urine. Report any signs of urinary infection.	7. Urine retention (stasis) and the introduction of a urethral catheter increase the risk for lower urinary tract infection.
8. Additional individualized interventions: _____	8. Rationales: _____

> **Suggested NIC Interventions**
> *Urinary catheterization: Intermittent; Urinary elimination management; Urinary retention care*

> **Suggested NOC Outcomes**
> *Urinary continence; Urinary elimination*

Collaborative problem

Risk for postoperative paralytic ileus, abdominal pain, or constipation related to immobility, surgical manipulation, anesthesia, and narcotic analgesia

NURSING PRIORITIES
- Detect paralytic ileus.
- Prevent constipation.

PATIENT OUTCOME CRITERIA
Within 2 days after surgery, the patient will:
- have normal bowel sounds.
  Within 4 days after surgery, the patient will:
- have soft, formed bowel movements
- not strain while defecating.
  Within 7 days after surgery, the patient will:
- establish a regular bowel elimination pattern.

INTERVENTIONS

1. *Assess the abdomen twice daily for bowel sounds and distention.* Assess for the presence of flatus or stool. Question the patient about abdominal fullness.

2. If paralytic ileus occurs, implement measures, as ordered, such as instructing the patient not to eat or drink anything, connecting a nasogastric (NG) tube to low intermittent suction, using a rectal tube to expel flatus, and administering I.V. fluids.

3. *Implement comfort measures if paralytic ileus occurs:* Provide frequent mouth care and position and tape the NG tube carefully.

4. Provide a diet appropriate to peristaltic activity. Make sure peristalsis has returned before progressing from nothing-by-mouth status to liberal fluid and solid food intake.

5. *Encourage fluid intake of at least eight 8-oz (237-ml) glasses per day unless* contraindicated (such as by heart failure). Provide fluids that the patient prefers.

6. *Encourage frequent position changes and ambulation.*

7. Provide privacy for the patient during defecation. Assist with ambulation to the bathroom, if necessary.

8. Consult with the physician concerning use of laxatives, suppositories, or enemas.

RATIONALES

1. Bowel sounds will be hypoactive initially but should return to normal within the first 2 days after surgery. The presence of flatus or stool signals the return of peristalsis. Abdominal distention and absence of bowel sounds, flatus, and stool may indicate paralytic ileus.

2. These measures help prevent abdominal distention while promoting return of peristalsis. I.V. fluids maintain fluid and electrolyte balance while the patient has no oral intake.

3. Maintaining patient comfort is important for the prevention of further anxiety.

4. If peristalsis hasn't returned, feeding the patient will cause distention.

5. Sufficient fluid intake is required for proper stool consistency. Providing preferred fluids promotes hydration.

6. Activity promotes peristalsis.

7. Providing privacy eliminates possible embarrassment.

8. A laxative, suppository, or enema may be needed to promote bowel evacuation. These supplements should be used judiciously to avoid bowel dependence or possible damage to healing tissues.

9. Additional individualized interventions: _____

9. Rationales: _____

Nursing diagnosis
Risk for imbalanced body temperature

NURSING PRIORITY
Maintain patient's core body temperature within normal range.

PATIENT OUTCOME CRITERIA
- Body temperature will continuously remain within expected range (98.6° F to 100.4° F [37° C to 38° C]).
- Throughout the postoperative period, the patient won't show any evidence of malignant hyperthermia.

INTERVENTIONS	RATIONALES
1. *Assess the patient's temperature immediately upon his arrival at the PACU, and every thirty minutes if* he's hypothermic. If he's normothermic, assess his temperature every two to four hours.	**1.** Anesthetic agents impair the body's ability to control and conserve heat by inhibiting vasoconstriction. Patients at risk include those with: – extremes of age – long intraoperative time – peripheral vascular disease.
2. *Assess the patient for evidence of malignant hyperthermia.* Assess for a familial pattern in the preoperative phase of care to prevent its onset. Postoperatively, notify anesthesia personnel STAT if the patient exhibits: – ventricular arrhythmias – tachypnea – hot, diaphoretic, mottled skin – elevated temperature – excessive muscle rigidity – oliguria or anuria.	**2.** Malignant hypothermia is an inherited skeletal muscle disorder causing a hypermetabolic state induced by anesthetic agents. It is imperative to alert anesthesia personnel if it's suspected during the perioperative phase of care.
3. If the patient is hypothermic (displaying shivering or piloerection, complaining of being cold and having a body temperature of less than 97°F [36°C]), initiate active warming measures: – apply forced air warming – apply passive insulation (warm blankets, socks, and head covering) – increase ambient room temperature – warm I.V. fluids, if possible.	**3.** Hypothermia can contribute to cardiac events, delayed wound healing, blood coagulopathies, and altered drug metabolism.
4. Additional individualized interventions: _____	**4.** Rationales: _____

Suggested NIC Interventions
Temperature regulation; Vital signs monitoring; Fever treatment; Fluid management; Postanesthesia care

Suggested NOC Outcomes
Thermoregulation

Collaborative problem

Risk for nausea or vomiting related to GI distention, rapid position changes, or cortical stimulation of the vomiting center or chemoreceptor trigger zone

NURSING PRIORITY
Prevent or relieve nausea or vomiting.

PATIENT OUTCOME CRITERIA
Within 1 hour of onset of nausea or vomiting, the patient will:
- verbalize relief of nausea
- be free from vomiting.

INTERVENTIONS	RATIONALES
1. *Prevent GI overdistention: Maintain patency of the nasogastric tube;* change the patient's diet only as tolerated.	1. Overdistention of the GI tract, particularly the duodenum, triggers the vomiting reflex.
2. Limit unpleasant sights, smells, and psychic stimuli, such as intense anxiety and pain.	2. These factors stimulate the chemoreceptor trigger zone in the medulla, which causes vomiting.
3. *Caution the patient to change position slowly.*	3. Rapid position changes also stimulate the trigger zone.
4. As soon as possible, advance the patient from narcotics to other analgesics (as ordered), and then to nonpharmacologic pain-control measures.	4. Medications, especially narcotics, may excite the chemoreceptor trigger zone.
5. Administer antiemetics, as ordered.	5. Agents that depress the vomiting center or trigger zone responsiveness may be necessary when the measures described above are inappropriate or ineffective.
6. Additional individualized interventions: _____	6. Rationales: _____

Discharge planning
DISCHARGE CHECKLIST
Before discharge, the patient should show evidence of:
- ❏ return to preoperative LOC
- ❏ normothermia
- ❏ absence of pulmonary and cardiovascular complications
- ❏ stable vital signs
- ❏ healing wound with no signs of infection
- ❏ hemoglobin level and white blood cell count within normal ranges
- ❏ I.V. lines discontinued for at least 24 hours
- ❏ ability to tolerate oral food intake
- ❏ ability to perform wound care independently
- ❏ ability to void and have bowel movements as before surgery
- ❏ ability to ambulate and perform activities of daily living as before surgery
- ❏ knowledge of activity restrictions
- ❏ ability to control pain using oral medications
- ❏ adequate home support, or referral to home care or nursing home if indicated by lack of home support system or by inability to perform self-care.

TEACHING CHECKLIST
Document evidence that the patient and family demonstrate an understanding of:
- ❏ a plan for resumption of normal activity
- ❏ wound care
- ❏ signs and symptoms of wound infection or other surgical complications
- ❏ all discharge medications' purpose, dosage, administration, and adverse effects requiring medical attention (postoperative patients may be discharged with oral analgesics)
- ❏ when and how to contact the health care provider
- ❏ the date, time, and location of follow-up appointment with the surgeon
- ❏ community resources appropriate for postoperative rehabilitation performed such as a home health nurse.

DOCUMENTATION CHECKLIST

Using outcome criteria as a guide, document:

❑ clinical status on admission
❑ allergies
❑ familial history of malignant hypothermia
❑ significant changes in preoperative status (level of consciousness, emotional status, baseline physical data)
❑ preoperative teaching and its effectiveness
❑ preoperative checklist (includes documentation regarding preoperative consent, urinalysis, CBC, 12-lead ECG, chest X-ray, preoperative medication administration, surgical skin preparation, voiding on call from the operating room, and removal of nail polish, jewelry, prostheses, dentures, glasses, and hearing aids)
❑ clinical status on admission from the recovery room
❑ amount and character of wound drainage (on dressing and through drains)
❑ skin condition
❑ vital signs
❑ patency of tubes (I.V., nasogastric, indwelling urinary catheter, drains)
❑ pulmonary hygiene measures
❑ pain-relief measures
❑ activity tolerance
❑ nutritional intake
❑ elimination status (urinary and bowel)
❑ pertinent laboratory test findings
❑ patient and family teaching
❑ discharge planning.

Associated care plans

▪ Acute pain
▪ Anxiety
▪ Chronic pain
▪ Confusion
▪ Grieving
▪ Impaired physical mobility
▪ Ineffective individual coping
▪ Knowledge deficit

References

Association of Operating Room Nurses. Perioperative Nursing Data Set. Denver: AORN Publications Department, 2002.

Jeran, L. "Patient Temperature: An Introduction to the Clinical Guideline for the Prevention of Unplanned Perioperative Hypothermia," *Journal of Perianesthesia Nursing* 16(5):303-314, October 2001.

Neurologic
disorders

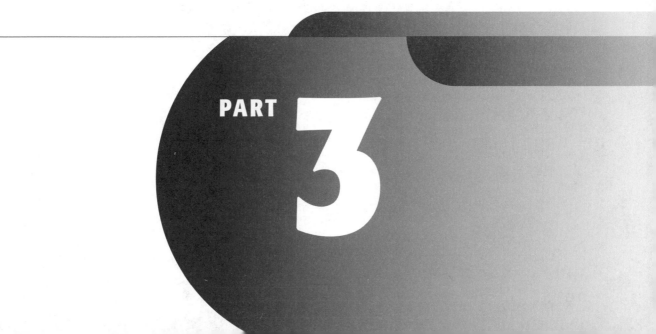

PART

3

Alzheimer's disease

DRG INFORMATION
DRG 012   Degenerative Nervous System Disorders.
          Mean LOS = 8.1 days
Additional DRG information: Patients are rarely admitted with only Alzheimer's disease (AD); usually, another disorder, such as pneumonia or dehydration, is the primary diagnosis.

Introduction
DEFINITION AND TIME FOCUS
Dementia is a syndrome exhibited by the development of multiple cognitive deficits. The most commonly identified problem is a memory deficit, but the syndrome can include aphasia, agnosia, difficulty with reason and judgment, and inappropriate behavior and social responses.

The most commonly identified dementia is AD, which affects as many as 4 million people in the United States, although there may be many reasons other than AD for cognitive decline. (See *Types of dementia,* page 162.) AD is a chronic, irreversible neuronal degeneration of the central nervous system, leading to severe disorders of cognition in the absence of other neurologic manifestations. Senile plaques (conglomerations of protein) and neurofibrillary tangles (twisted nerve fibers) characterize the insidious, relentless progression of structural brain atrophy.

Although the care plan may be the same regardless of the reason, making the differential diagnosis regarding the dementia's underlying cause is key to the treatment and outcomes. (See *Clinical snapshot: Alzheimer's disease,* page 162.)This care plan focuses on the AD patient admitted at any stage of the disease.

ETIOLOGY AND PRECIPITATING FACTORS
Although the etiology is obscure, ongoing research suggests the following possible causes of AD:
- neurochemical deficiency of the neurotransmitters acetylcholine and somatostatin (important for cognition and memory)
- neurometabolic disorder that diminishes cellular protein synthesis
- genetic and environmental factors, with autosomal-dominant transmission in certain families
- aluminum deposits in senile plaques and neurofibrillary tangles in the hippocampus of the brain, a cortical area necessary for memory
- slow viruses (those that invade the host but remain dormant for years before symptoms develop) whose effects sometimes resemble those of AD

- immune system dysfunctions.

Focused assessment guidelines
NURSING HISTORY
(FUNCTIONAL HEALTH PATTERN FINDINGS)
Health-perception–health-management pattern
- Belief that memory loss results from normal aging
- Use of learned social skills and fabrication to disguise confusion and disorientation
- Family reports of patient's mental decline

Nutritional-metabolic pattern
- Anorexia (patient forgets to eat or doesn't recognize hunger signs)
- Weight loss
- Fatigue and malaise
- Dysphagia (in later stages)

Elimination pattern
- Constipation related to forgetfulness, disorientation, and inadequate fluid intake.
- Urinary and fecal incontinence in later stages

Activity-exercise pattern
- Limitation of activity to familiar environments as confusion and disorientation increase
- Growing inability to perform activities of daily living as patient loses ability to perform actions sequentially
- Deterioration in personal hygiene and appearance
- Incompetence in performing complex tasks, such as shopping, telephoning, and banking
- Personal safety jeopardized through wandering behavior or loss of locomotion

Sleep-rest pattern
- Nocturnal restlessness with insomnia
- Altered sleep-wake cycle
- Growing difficulty in awakening as the disease progresses

Cognitive-perceptual pattern
- Progressively impaired judgment
- Progressively impaired ability to orient self in the environment
- Loss of immediate, recent, and remote memory, including episodic (events) and semantic (knowledge) memory
- Incongruent, inconsistent, often depressed affect
- Progressively reduced conceptualization, attention, arousal, concentration, and abstract thinking
- Progressively impaired expressive language and increased receptive aphasia
- Repetitive actions or perseveration

Self-perception–self-concept pattern
- Attempt to sustain an internal center of control, dignity, and self-esteem

Role-relationship pattern
- Altered family dynamics resulting from role reversals and increased patient dysfunction
- Increased social withdrawal (isolationism)

Sexuality-reproductive pattern
- Rejection of intimate contact

Coping–stress tolerance pattern
- Defense mechanisms, such as rationalization, denial, and projection
- Apathy, depression, and helplessness
- Primary emotional lability, characterized by irritability, anger, fear, and agitation
- Symptoms of ego disintegration, including hallucinations, illusions, and suicidal ideation

Value-belief pattern
- Altered value system resulting from defective mental faculties

PHYSICAL FINDINGS
Neurologic
- Confusion
- Disorientation
- Memory loss
- Language disintegration
- Irritability
- Cognitive dysfunction
- Labile affect
- Clinical depression

Integumentary
- Poor skin turgor or other signs of dehydration

Musculoskeletal
- Decreased activity tolerance
- Lack of coordination
- Immobility
- Limited range of motion

Genitourinary
- Urine retention
- Urinary incontinence

Gastrointestinal
- Fecal incontinence

DIAGNOSTIC STUDIES
Diagnostic tests are performed to rule out other diseases and allow the clinical diagnosis of AD, although postmortem brain biopsy is the only definitive diagnostic test.
- Hematologic measurements of neurotransmitters and neurotransmitter metabolites — low levels indicate a biochemical deficiency as the cause
- Complete blood count, Venereal Disease Research Laboratory test, blood chemistries, endocrine studies —

performed for differential diagnosis of reversible cognitive impairment
- Vitamin B_{12} levels — low levels indicate a nutritional deficit
- Computed tomography scan — may indicate cortical atrophy and widening of the ventricles
- Lumbar puncture for cerebrospinal fluid examination — commonly shows abnormal protein levels
- Positron emission tomography — may reflect diminished brain metabolism
- Skull X-rays — may reflect cerebral atrophy
- EEG — may show decreased electrical activity contributing to dysfunction
- Magnetic resonance imaging — performed to rule out reversible cognitive impairment
- Language ability tests — performed for differential diagnosis
- Vision and hearing tests — establish sensory deficits (as opposed to cognitive impairment) as the cause of selected symptoms
- 12-lead electrocardiography — may indicate coronary insufficiency contributing to symptoms

POTENTIAL COMPLICATIONS
- Total loss of mental faculties
- Pneumonia
- Injury

Neurologic disorders

Types of dementia

- *Normal cognitive aging* — Research has demonstrated that the cognitive decline commonly thought to be part of the normal aging process may actually reflect mild dementia. Primary and recognition memory along with tasks involving well-learned knowledge decline little with age. The ability to learn new information does decline slightly but not as significantly as was previously thought. In the absence of disease, the cognitive changes associated with a truly healthy aging individual are minimal.
- *Mild cognitive impairment* — Mild cognitive impairment is a dementia characterized by objective memory complaints in the absence of comorbid disease states. It may also include cognitive dysfunction related to adverse drug reactions and sleep disorders.
- *Lewy body dementia* — This is thought to be the second most common cause of dementia after AD. Diagnosis of Lewy body dementia is based upon the presence of dementia and at least one of the following: visual hallucina-

tions, parkinsonism, and fluctuation of cognitive status. In general, patients with this type of dementia have increased extrapyramidal symptoms with better memory performance than patients with AD.
- *Vascular dementia (multi-infarct dementia)* — Thought to be the result of small-vessel disease, cerebral white matter changes are thought to play a significant role in the development of dementia related to vascular compromise. Controlling modifiable risk factors for cerebrovascular disease, most notably hypertension, reduces the risk of developing this type of dementia.
- *Frontotemporal dementia* — Usually the result of an underlying disease process like Pick's disease or Creutzfeldt-Jakob disease, this form of dementia presents with a disturbance in behavior or language. The symptoms are disinhibition, impulsivity, and impaired judgment, which are more pronounced than with AD. This form of dementia also has an earlier onset than AD.

CLINICAL SNAPSHOT ✳

Alzheimer's disease

Major nursing diagnoses	Key patient outcomes
Chronic confusion	Perform self-care as much as possible.
Imbalanced nutrition: Less than body requirements	Gain a predetermined number of pounds or maintain a stable weight.
Risk for injury	Avoid injury.
Constipation	Regularly eliminate soft, formed stools.
Caregiver role strain	(The family is expected to) arrange a plan for care and mutual support.

Nursing diagnosis

Chronic confusion related to degenerative loss of cerebral tissue

NURSING PRIORITIES
- Provide a safe, structured environment.
- Promote an optimum level of functioning.
- Establish effective communication patterns.

PATIENT OUTCOME CRITERIA
Within 1 day of admission and then continuously, the patient will:
- remain free from injury
- perform self-care as much as possible
- communicate needs as clearly as possible
- wear some means of identification.

INTERVENTIONS

1. *Assess the patient's level of cognitive functioning** using a functional rating scale for symptoms of dementia or a mini-mental status exam (see *Assessing Alzheimer's disease,* page 164). Prepare the patient for psychological testing.

2. *Assign the patient to a room close to the nursing station* for frequent observation.

3. *Minimize hazards in the environment.*

4. *Maintain consistency in nursing routines.*

5. *Promote self-care* within the scope of the patient's abilities; assist when necessary. Identify specific needs in the care plan.

6. Establish and maintain a therapeutic relationship by communicating with the patient in a calm, reassuring, affirming, and nonthreatening manner.

7. *Give simple, specific directions for accomplishing tasks;* use eye contact and unobtrusive guidance.

8. *Orient the patient to reality* frequently and repetitively.

9. Administer and document medications as ordered.

10. *Use aids* to improve language skills, and use verbal repetition and pictures to improve recall.

11. *Minimize communication barriers.* Be aware that anxiety, cultural influences, spiritual beliefs, and language difficulties may contribute to paranoia and withdrawal.

12. *Encourage social interaction* by including the patient in unit activities when possible, allowing maximum flexibility in visiting hours, and providing occupational therapy referrals.

RATIONALES

1. Information obtained from the patient and his family provides a guide for planning care. Psychological testing will provide information necessary to structure a therapeutic regimen.

2. The patient may wander or require frequent attention.

3. The confusion and faulty judgment that result from AD make the patient more prone to injury.

4. Taking such measures as assigning the same nurse, serving meals on time, and scheduling rest periods provides the patient with structure in an unfamiliar environment.

5. Allowing the patient to provide self-care preserves self-esteem. As the disease progresses, complete physical care — bathing, dressing, and toileting — becomes necessary. Identifying needs in the care plan promotes appropriate care.

6. Trust must be established to achieve any goal because of the patient's suspicions and increasing paranoia.

7. The effects of memory loss and a reduced attention span can be minimized with clear directions and appropriate guidance.

8. Although repetitive reorientation may not reduce disorientation, it may reduce the patient's anxiety.

9. Donepezil (Aricept) or rivastigmine (Exelon) for improving memory and bethanechol (Urecholine) for increasing neurotransmission may be used. Antianxiety drugs may be helpful. Other drugs may include ergoloid mesylates (Hydergine) or lecithin for cognition and memory; doxepin (Sinequan), nortriptyline (Pamelor), or amitriptyline (Elavil) as antidepressants; and temazepam (Restoril) or a similar drug for sleep maintenance. Vitamin E and ginkgo biloba, thought to enhance memory function early on, can be used as adjunct therapy.

10. Both methods may assist the patient with word recall.

11. Knowing and understanding the patient's cultural background and beliefs can further open communication.

12. Continued social interaction reinforces reality and contributes to a sense of self-worth and identity.

Neurologic disorders

---

*Italics indicate key interventions.

Assessing Alzheimer's disease

Understanding how Alzheimer's disease progresses helps the nurse plan appropriate care and maximize the patient's functional ability. This chart summarizes the stages of disease progression.

Stage	Duration	Signs and symptoms	Nursing considerations
Early	2 to 4 years	• "Fishing" for words • Forgetfulness progressing to inability to recall details of recent events • Irritability or apathy • Occasional episodes of getting lost • Periods of disorientation • Significantly impaired reasoning ability and judgment	• The patient can typically manage most daily activities and doesn't require institutionalization. • The patient senses a decrease in mental faculties and may use denial to cope with this. Don't force the patient to "face the facts."
Middle	2 to 12 years	• Reduced vision, hearing, and pain sensation • Hyperorality (chewing or tasting anything within reach) • Inability to recognize familiar things (may not recognize own mirror reflection) • Increased aphasia (language defect) • Increased appetite without weight gain • Perseveration (repeating the same word or action over and over) • Seizures • Social inappropriateness, such as poor table manners, personal hygiene, and grooming • Has difficulty following simple instructions • Wanders particularly at night • Loses important papers • Neglects personal hygiene • Forgets to pay bills	• Assist the patient with hygiene and grooming to preserve self-esteem and dignity. • Avoid using puns or jokes because these will confuse the patient • Call the patient by name, rather than "Honey," "Grandma," or another belittling term. • If the patient has trouble walking, accompany him on walks several times per day to prevent muscle contractures and other complications of immobility. • Maintain a consistent, calm environment to orient the patient. • Make sure that the patient wanders only in safe areas. • Monitor the items the patient places in his mouth. • Maintain the patient on a toileting schedule to minimize incontinence. • Stay with the patient during meals to observe for swallowing problems and assist with table manners.
Late	1 year	• Apraxia (inability to perform purposeful movements, even on command) • Bladder and bowel incontinence • Decreased appetite • Disappearance of perseveration and hyperorality • Generalized tonic-clonic seizures • Muteness • Unresponsiveness to verbal and physical stimuli	• Maintain a consistent routine. • Monitor the patient's skin for breakdown and pressure ulcers. • Monitor all body systems carefully for physiologic deterioration. • Perform passive range-of-motion exercises at least four times per day to prevent contractures if the patient is bedridden.

13. *Prevent excessive stimulation and promote a regular sleep-wake pattern.*

13. Moderate stimulation helps orient the patient, but excessive stimulation and sleep deprivation contribute to confusion.

14. Be attentive. Keep your verbal and nonverbal responses to the patient consistent.

14. Nurse-patient dialogue must reflect trust and understanding. Consistent verbal and nonverbal responses reduce cognitive dissonance.

15. When talking with the patient, *encourage reminiscences.*

15. Remembering past events helps the patient maintain self-identity. Distant memory may remain even when recent memory is impaired.

16. Additional individualized interventions: _____
_____

16. Rationales:_____
_____

Suggested NIC Interventions
Cognitive stimulation; Dementia management; Mood management; Reality orientation; Anxiety reduction; Decision-making support; Family involvement promotion; Delusion management; Cognitive restructuring; Memory training; Cerebral perfusion promotion; Neurologic monitoring

Suggested NOC Outcomes
Cognitive ability; Cognitive orientation; Concentration; Decision making; Distorted thought control; Identity; Information processing; Memory; Neurologic status: Consciousness

Nursing diagnosis

Imbalanced nutrition: Less than body requirements related to memory loss, difficulty swallowing, and inadequate food intake

NURSING PRIORITY

Stabilize and improve nutritional status.

PATIENT OUTCOME CRITERION

By discharge, the patient will gain a predetermined number of pounds or maintain a stable weight.

INTERVENTIONS

1. *Assess present nutritional status:* Weigh the patient and record customary dietary intake on admission. See the "Nutritional deficit" care plan, page 138, and the "Parenteral nutrition" care plan, page 510, for more information on nutritional assessment.

2. *Offer a balanced diet* consisting of small meals at regular intervals and nutritious snacks between meals. Provide finger foods when possible.

3. Prepare the tray in advance — cut the meat, provide a spoon, open containers, and so forth — with appropriate portions of food arranged so that the patient may eat unassisted.

4. Provide time and privacy for meals.

5. *Monitor and record daily weight and intake,* including the amount and type of food. Adjust the dietary plan accordingly.

6. Provide dietary information to the home caregiver.

7. Additional individualized interventions:_____
_____

RATIONALES

1. Assessing the patient's nutritional status provides necessary information for determining actual deficits; an appropriate dietary regimen may then begin.

2. Regularly scheduled meals help maintain a structured environment. Small quantities may appeal to the patient and provide a sense of achievement when all the food is consumed. Finger foods are easier to handle than food that must be eaten with a utensil.

3. The patient may develop coordination difficulties, which impairs his ability to use utensils. Preparing food servings in advance decreases the patient's frustration and prevents humiliation of being unable to provide self-care.

4. The patient who has difficulty chewing or swallowing will need more time to eat. Lack of coordination may result in socially unacceptable eating habits.

5. Evaluating weight and intake provides guidelines for modifying the dietary plan.

6. The patient will probably continue to need assistance in menu selection, cooking, and eating after discharge. The person shopping, cooking, and offering meals to the patient may need instruction in the patient's specific dietary needs.

7. Rationales: _____
_____

Neurologic disorders

<table>
<tr><td>

Suggested NIC Interventions
Diet staging; Nutrition management; Weight gain assistance; Fluid monitoring; Nutritional monitoring

</td><td>

Suggested NOC Outcomes
Nutritional status; Nutritional status: Nutrient intake; Nutritional status: Food and fluid intake; Weight control

</td></tr>
</table>

Nursing diagnosis

Risk for injury related to wandering behavior, aphasia, agnosia, or hyperorality

NURSING PRIORITY

Prevent injury while maximizing independence.

PATIENT OUTCOME CRITERIA

Throughout the hospital stay, the patient will:
- remain on the unit
- be appropriately dressed for the temperature
- walk about only when attended
- perform daily exercise to the best of his ability
- avoid injury.
    By the time of the patient's discharge, the family will:
- list five safety measures for the home environment.

INTERVENTIONS	RATIONALES
1. Consider alarms or other audible signal.	**1.** Wandering and restlessness characterize the later stages of AD. If unattended, the patient may become lost, even in familiar surroundings.
2. *Prepare an identity card, a bracelet, or a name tag for the patient.* Include his name, address, phone number, medical problem, and other pertinent information.	**2.** Should the patient wander, identification information can help in the patient's prompt return.
3. *Ensure that the patient is dressed appropriately* for the temperature. Provide shoes that fit well.	**3.** The patient may not make appropriate choices about dress and may have a reduced ability to identify or verbalize discomfort. Loose shoes may be lost or contribute to injuries from falls.
4. *Avoid using restraints.*	**4.** Restraints increase the patient's agitation and paranoia and may contribute to injury.
5. *Recommend specific safety measures to the family* to prepare for home care, including: – safely storing knives, medications, matches, firearms, and cleaning solutions and other toxic household chemicals – using night-lights – storing small objects safely – securing door locks – making sure objects remain in the same place – explaining the patient's condition to neighbors.	**5.** An unprepared home environment may contribute to injuries. – The patient may not recognize familiar objects (agnosia) and thus may inadvertently injure himself or others. – Night-lights may decrease the risk of falling and help reorient the patient to the environment. – AD patients may be prone to hyperorality (chewing or tasting anything within reach) and may put small objects in their mouths, swallowing or choking on them. – Door locks may help prevent wandering. – Consistency may help reorient the patient to the environment. – If neighbors are aware of the patient's illness, they can alert the family if they see the patient wandering or engaging in unsafe behaviors.

6. Encourage a regular exercise program as tolerated.

6. Regular exercise decreases restlessness and agitation, promotes muscle tone, and contributes to a sense of well-being. Overactivity, however, may contribute to fatigue and confusion.

7. *Watch for nonverbal cues to injury,* such as grimacing, rubbing, panting, or protecting an injured area, and note repetitive use of words or seemingly inappropriate statements. Alert the family to cues observed.

7. The patient may be unable to identify or express discomfort but may reveal illness or injury through nonverbal cues. Because aphasia may make expressions of discomfort convoluted, such words as *cold* or *hurt,* especially if repeated, may warrant investigation.

8. Additional individualized interventions: _____
_____

8. Rationales: _____
_____

Suggested NIC Interventions	*Suggested NOC Outcomes*
Surveillance: Safety	Safety status: Physical injury

Nursing diagnosis

Constipation related to memory loss about toileting behavior, inadequate diet, or inadequate fluid intake

NURSING PRIORITY

Establish an effective elimination pattern.

PATIENT OUTCOME CRITERIA

Within 2 days of admission, the patient will:
- demonstrate knowledge of bathroom location
- regularly eliminate soft, formed stools.

INTERVENTIONS

1. *Identify the bathroom clearly*—symbols or color codes may be helpful.

2. *Prompt the patient at regular intervals to use the toilet.* With an incontinent patient, use standard precautions.

3. *Encourage a therapeutic diet* with ample fluid and fiber intake during waking hours.

4. *Observe the patient for nonverbal clues* that signal the need for elimination.

5. *Administer and document use of elimination aids* (stool softener, laxative, or cathartic) as ordered.

6. *Monitor and document the frequency of elimination.*

7. Additional individualized interventions: _____
_____

RATIONALES

1. A patient with AD may develop constipation because he forgets the location of the bathroom.

2. When memory fails, the patient may neglect toileting. Reminders, with assistance at regular intervals, promote a regular elimination pattern and help prevent accidents.

3. Proper diet promotes effective elimination. Ample fluids and fiber help prevent constipation.

4. The patient may become restless, pick at clothing, or clutch the genitals but may be unable to verbalize the need to eliminate.

5. Such aids may help promote regular elimination.

6. Noting the frequency of elimination helps identify a regular bowel pattern and minimizes problems.

7. Rationales: _____
_____

Neurologic disorders

<table>
<tr><td>

Suggested NIC Interventions
Bowel management; Fluid and electrolyte management; Constipation and impaction management

</td><td>

Suggested NOC Outcomes
Bowel elimination; Hydration; Symptom control

</td></tr>
</table>

Nursing diagnosis

Caregiver role strain related to the patient with AD who requires constant attention because of progressive mental deterioration

NURSING PRIORITY

Aid in developing necessary role transitions while maintaining family integrity.

PATIENT OUTCOME CRITERIA

Throughout the hospital stay, the family will:
- be involved in teaching and providing care.
  By the time of the patient's discharge, the family will:
- arrange a plan for care and mutual support
- identify community support resources.

INTERVENTIONS

1. *Involve the family in all teaching.* Use teaching as an opportunity to assess family roles, resources, and coping behaviors. See the "Compromised family coping" care plan, page 67.

2. *Offer support, understanding, and reassurance to the family.* Support efforts to provide care for the patient in the home setting. Provide examples of caregiving schedules. Encourage family members to give each other breaks and "holidays." Encourage the use of adult day-care programs.

3. *Involve a social worker or discharge planner* in decisions regarding home care or nursing home placement. If appropriate, encourage family members to express their feelings about the decision to place the patient in a nursing home.

4. Provide information about community resources, such as home care, financial and legal assistance, and an Alzheimer's support group. Encourage use of all available resources.

5. Additional individualized interventions: _____
_____

RATIONALES

1. Because AD patients require long-term care, the family must be taught how to cope effectively with this chronic, progressive disease. If the patient develops a childlike dependence after holding a strong provider role, others must assume new roles to maintain family stability. Assessment of family status provides a baseline for determining the best approach and needed interventions. The "Compromised family coping" care plan contains additional information.

2. In many cases, caring for the AD patient is a frustrating and thankless task, involving endless repetition and, commonly, emotional confrontations that may leave family members drained. However, maintaining a stable home environment with familiar caregivers helps give the patient a sense of worth, reduces isolation, and may minimize disorientation. Frequent breaks from caregiving help increase family cohesiveness and prevent burnout.

3. Patient needs may become unmanageable at home. The social worker or discharge planner may offer special expertise in answering questions about long-term care. Family members may feel guilt, relief, anguish, or other conflicting emotions and will need support if this decision becomes necessary.

4. Community support may help lessen the family's burden and promote healthy adaptations to change. The AD patient is likely to appear in the emergency department when the family becomes overwhelmed. A social service referral may decrease such inappropriate use of resources and help avert family crises.

5. Rationales: _____
_____

Discharge planning
DISCHARGE CHECKLIST
Before discharge, the patient shows evidence of:
- ❏ vital signs that are stable and within normal limits for this patient
- ❏ adequate nutritional intake
- ❏ regular bowel and bladder elimination
- ❏ adequate home support system or referral to home care or a nursing home if indicated.

See also the discharge checklist for the primary diagnosis if other than AD.

TEACHING CHECKLIST
Document evidence that the family demonstrates an understanding of:
- ❏ the diagnosis and disease process — for example, through literature from the Alzheimer's Association (919 North Michigan Avenue, Suite 1100, Chicago, IL 60611)
- ❏ plans for adequate supervision and behavior management
- ❏ recommended steps for minimizing environmental hazards
- ❏ instructions for promoting self-care independence
- ❏ recommended procedures for reorienting the patient to the home environment
- ❏ the need for an identification bracelet or other medical alert device
- ❏ the purpose, dosage, administration schedule, and adverse effects of prescribed medications
- ❏ techniques for continued improvement of language skills
- ❏ recommendations for meeting nutrition and elimination needs
- ❏ available community resources
- ❏ the need for restoring family equilibrium as roles change and patient dependence increases
- ❏ the probability of total patient regression
- ❏ how to contact the physician.

DOCUMENTATION CHECKLIST
Using outcome criteria as a guide, document:
- ❏ the patient's clinical status on admission, including level of cognitive function
- ❏ a planned approach to maintain patient safety, security, and orientation
- ❏ laboratory data and diagnostic findings
- ❏ any change in the patient's behavioral response
- ❏ the patient's level of communication and social interaction

- ❏ the patient's dietary intake and elimination patterns
- ❏ patient and family teaching
- ❏ discharge planning.

Associated care plans
- ▪ Compromised family coping
- ▪ Geriatric care
- ▪ Grieving
- ▪ Ineffective individual coping
- ▪ Knowledge deficit

References
Agency for Healthcare Policy and Research Clinical Practice Guidelines. *Early Recognition and Treatment of Alzheimer's Disease.* AHCPR Publication No. 96-0704.

Alzheimer's Disease Association Web site: *www.alz.org.*

Diseases, 3rd edition. Springhouse, Pa.: Springhouse Corp., 2001.

Kukull, W.A., and Ganguli, M. "Epidemiology of Dementia: Concepts and Overview," *Neurologic Clinics* 18(4):923-50, November 2000.

Patient Teaching Reference Manual. Springhouse, Pa.: Springhouse Corp., 2002.

Neurologic disorders

Craniotomy

DRG INFORMATION

DRG 001   Craniotomy. Except for trauma. Age 17+.
              Mean LOS = 9 days
DRG 002   Craniotomy for Trauma. Age 17+.
              Mean LOS = 10 days
DRG 003   Craniotomy. Ages 0 to 17.
              Mean LOS = Not available

Introduction

DEFINITION AND TIME FOCUS

Craniotomy, the most common neurosurgical procedure, is the surgical opening of the skull to provide access to the brain. It's performed to treat intracranial disease — for example, to remove tissue for biopsy or to remove a mass lesion (a substance that occupies the cranial cavity, compromising either the space or the integrity of the brain). The surgery involves making a series of small holes, called burr holes, in the cranium with a special drill, then cutting between the holes to allow removal of a flap of bone and scalp. At the end of the surgery, the flap is replaced and the muscle and scalp are realigned and sutured.

Although the surgical approach depends on the lesion's location, surgery is performed in two general areas. In the supratentorial craniotomy, the cranium is incised above the tentorium (the fold of dura mater that separates the cerebral cortex from the cerebellum and brain stem). This approach is used for lesions in the frontal, parietal, temporal, and occipital lobes of the cerebral hemispheres. The infratentorial approach, by which the cranium is incised below the tentorium, is used for lesions in the brain stem (midbrain, pons, and medulla) and cerebellum.

A craniotomy may be an emergency procedure for cerebral decompression or removal of a rapidly expanding lesion, such as a hematoma or intracranial abscess; an elective procedure to resect or remove a slow-growing, space-occupying lesion such as a benign tumor; or to clip or remove an aneurysm or arteriovenous malformation. This care plan focuses on the immediate preoperative and postoperative care (in the intensive care unit) of a patient undergoing an elective craniotomy. (See *Clinical Snapshot: Craniotomy,* page 172.)

ETIOLOGY AND PRECIPITATING FACTORS

- Tumor, abscess, aneurysm, chronic hematoma, cyst, or arteriovenous malformation
- Condition requiring repair of a cerebral injury

Focused assessment guidelines

NURSING HISTORY (FUNCTIONAL HEALTH PATTERN FINDINGS)

Health-perception–health-management pattern
- History of headache that's worse on arising in the morning and is aggravated by movement or straining at stool
- Personality changes
- Mental changes or mood swings
- Age (adults are at increased risk)
- Family or personal history of diabetes mellitus, intolerance to previous operative procedures, history of adrenocorticosteroid use, or signs and symptoms of endocrine dysfunction

Nutritional-metabolic pattern
- Vomiting

Activity-exercise pattern
- Recent hospitalization or bed rest
- Restricted physical activity because of motor or sensory deficits

Cognitive-perceptual pattern
- Changes in vision, hearing, touch, taste, or smell, depending on lesion's location and duration
- Language and memory problems (with chronic lesion)

Self-perception–self-concept pattern
- Negative self-image because of body disfigurement (if patient is undergoing radiation or chemotherapy for chronic lesion)
- Anger, embarrassment, or denial

Role-relationship pattern
- Altered role as spouse and breadwinner (depending on lesion's duration)

Sexuality-reproductive pattern
- Impaired sexual functioning (depending on lesion's location)

Coping–stress tolerance pattern
- Ineffective coping patterns
- Anticipatory grieving

Value-belief pattern
- Fear of the unknown and death brought on by the possible need for surgery, resulting in a delay in seeking medical attention
- Frustration with health care system if vague symptoms delayed diagnosis

PHYSICAL FINDINGS

Signs and symptoms depend on the lesion's site. The following are general findings that point to cerebral dysfunction.

Neurologic
- Decreased level of consciousness (LOC)
- Mental changes, such as impaired memory, lack of initiative, or mood changes
- Visual deficits, such as decreased visual acuity, blurred vision, diplopia, or changes in extraocular eye movements
- Sensory deficits
- Motor deficits
- Seizures
- Papilledema
- Cranial nerve dysfunction

Gastrointestinal
- Vomiting

DIAGNOSTIC STUDIES
- Complete blood count — decreased hemoglobin level may indicate anemia or blood dyscrasia as well as the need for blood transfusion before surgery to ensure adequate transport for oxygen in the blood; increased white blood cell (WBC) count may signal infection or an abscess, a contraindication for surgery (unless the abscess is in the brain)
- Blood urea nitrogen (BUN) level, serum creatinine — used to monitor renal function; increased values may indicate an impaired ability to cope with the sodium and water retention that results from the body's stress reaction to surgery
- Electrolyte analyses — used to monitor fluid status and detect hypokalemia and hyperkalemia; the patient may develop diabetes insipidus (DI) or syndrome of inappropriate antidiuretic hormone (SIADH)
- Fasting blood glucose levels — used to detect diabetes mellitus, which would need to be controlled before and after surgery
- Typing and crossmatching — used to determine patient blood type and have blood products readily available in case the patient requires blood replacement from surgical loss
- Computed tomography (CT) scan — used to diagnose cerebral lesions, such as hematomas, tumors, cysts, hydrocephalus, cerebral atrophy, cerebral infarction, and cerebral edema; serial scanning may be done before and after surgery
- Cerebral angiography — used to diagnose cerebrovascular aneurysms, cerebral thrombosis, hematomas, tumors with increased vascularization, vascular plaques or spasm, arteriovenous malformations, cerebral fistulas, or cerebral edema
- Radionuclide imaging (brain scan) — used to diagnose intracranial masses, such as malignant or benign tumors, abscesses, cerebral infarctions, intracranial hemorrhage, arteriovenous malformations, or aneurysms; has been largely replaced by CT scans

- Magnetic resonance imaging — used to assess brain edema, hemorrhage, infarction, blood vessels, and tumors and to measure fluid flow
- Chest X-ray — can rule out congestion, pneumonia, atelectasis, or other pulmonary diseases that would compromise respiration
- Electrocardiography — can detect cardiac abnormalities such as arrhythmias that would be aggravated by the stress of a prolonged surgical procedure and drug therapy

POTENTIAL COMPLICATIONS
- Increased intracranial pressure (ICP)
- Cerebral edema
- Shock (hemorrhagic or hypovolemic or from intracranial bleeding)
- Hematoma (subdural or epidural)
- Atelectasis
- Pneumonia
- Seizures
- Neurogenic pulmonary edema
- DI
- SIADH
- Meningitis
- Wound infection
- Neurologic deficits, such as decreased LOC, motor weakness, or paralysis
- Loss of corneal, pharyngeal, or palatal reflexes
- Arrhythmias
- Thrombophlebitis
- Hyperthermia
- Postoperative hydrocephalus
- GI ulceration and bleeding
- Cranial nerve III damage (eye drop) and visual disturbances
- Personality changes
- Cerebrospinal fluid (CSF) leakage
- Injury from falls
- Loss of airway
- Fluid and electrolyte imbalances

CLINICAL SNAPSHOT ✳

Craniotomy

Major nursing diagnoses and collaborative problems	Key patient outcomes
ND: Deficient knowledge (impending craniotomy)	Verbalize understanding of upcoming surgery and its potential effects and complications.
CP: Risk for cerebral ischemia	Demonstrate improved neurologic status.
ND: Risk for infection	Have no signs or symptoms of wound or systemic infection or meningitis.
CP: Risk for respiratory failure	Have a normal respiratory rate and pattern.
ND: Risk for injury	Remain free from injury.
ND: Risk for imbalanced fluid volume	Have electrolyte levels, BUN level, hematocrit, serum osmolality, and urine output within normal limits.
ND: Risk for deficient fluid volume	Maintain urine output within normal limits.
ND: Disturbed body image	Verbalize feelings of self-worth.
ND: Deficient knowledge (follow-up care)	Verbalize questions about follow-up care.

Nursing diagnosis

Deficient knowledge (impending craniotomy) related to lack of exposure to information

NURSING PRIORITY
Prepare the patient and his family for the craniotomy.

PATIENT OUTCOME CRITERIA
Before surgery, the patient and his family will:
- verbalize understanding of the upcoming surgery and its potential effects and complications
- describe their anxieties and how they're coping with them.

INTERVENTIONS

1. *Implement the measures in the "Knowledge deficit" care plan,** page 129, as appropriate.

2. *Assess what the patient and his family know* about the impending craniotomy and what they want to know. Consider the patient's educational level, LOC, mental changes, and memory loss. As appropriate, ask the patient or his family what they have learned from the physician, other family members, or someone who has had a craniotomy.

3. *Describe the preoperative procedure,* including neurologic assessment, weight measurement, the need for taking nothing by mouth after midnight, hair washing, and the possibility that long hair will be braided.

RATIONALES

1. The "Knowledge deficit" care plan contains detailed general information about teaching. This plan covers only specific information about craniotomy.

2. LOC, mental changes, and memory loss affect the patient's knowledge base. Although the physician should have informed the patient and his family about the procedure and potential complications, anxiety, memory loss, or limited comprehension may interfere with understanding and retention. Also, the patient and his family may have limited or confusing information. Assessing the knowledge base allows the nurse to reinforce appropriate information, correct misconceptions, and fill in gaps.

3. Knowing what to expect usually decreases anxiety.

*Italics indicate key interventions.

4. *Explain that the patient's hair is cut and the scalp shaved in the operating room.* Explain the rationale and allow time for the patient to express any feelings. If the operating room personnel are willing to save the patient's hair, ask whether the patient wants it saved. Explain that, if desired, all hair can be shaved to promote uniform regrowth. If possible, have the family present during this explanation.

4. Hair is an important component of body image and self-concept. Having the hair cut may be extremely distressing to the patient. Knowing why it must be removed and that it may be saved may alleviate some of the distress and sense of loss. Allowing time for the patient to express feelings conveys sensitivity and validates the patient's emotions. Having the family present may provide the support necessary to help them cope with this situation and prepare them for how the patient will look after surgery.

5. *Discuss what the intensive care unit will be like and what the effects of the craniotomy will be during the immediate postoperative period.* Mention that headaches and altered consciousness may occur as well as postoperative eye or facial swelling and periorbital ecchymosis. Describe intravascular lines, intracranial catheters, and other invasive lines that may be present postoperatively.

5. Knowing in advance what the unit will be like may increase the patient's sense of security when he awakens after surgery. Knowing that headaches and altered consciousness are common after the operation may help decrease anxiety.

6. *Encourage the patient and his family to express fears and concerns about the impending surgery.*

6. Fear of death, anxiety over other possible outcomes, and anticipatory grieving for the possible loss of body function interfere with learning. Providing an environment in which the patient is comfortable discussing these feelings may improve learning and reduce preoperative and postoperative anxiety.

7. Additional individualized interventions: _____

7. Rationales: _____

> **Suggested NIC Interventions**
> *Teaching: Procedure/treatment*

> **Suggested NOC Outcomes**
> *Knowledge: Treatment regimen*

Collaborative problem
Risk for cerebral ischemia related to increased ICP

NURSING PRIORITIES
- Decrease ICP.
- Minimize fluctuations in cerebral perfusion pressure.

PATIENT OUTCOME CRITERIA
Within 72 hours after surgery, the patient will:
- have an ICP of 0 to 15 mm Hg and a cerebral perfusion pressure greater than 60 mm Hg
- have a mean arterial pressure greater than 60 mm Hg
- display no clinical signs of increased ICP or herniation.
  Within 1 week after surgery, the patient will:
- demonstrate improved neurologic status.

INTERVENTIONS

1. *Implement the measures in "Risk for cerebral ischemia," page 192, in the "Increased intracranial pressure" care plan.*

RATIONALES

1. Several factors can raise ICP to dangerous levels after a craniotomy, including surgical trauma, cerebral edema, blood pressure fluctuations, and nursing activities. The care plan for "Increased intracranial pressure" covers this problem in detail.

2. Additional individualized interventions: _____

_____

2. Rationales: _____

_____

Nursing diagnosis

Risk for infection related to surgery, invasive techniques, continuous intracranial monitoring, ventricular drains, or CSF leakage

NURSING PRIORITY

Prevent or promptly detect signs of infection.

PATIENT OUTCOME CRITERIA

By 72 hours after surgery, the patient will:
- have a normal temperature and WBC count
- have no positive cultures.
  By the time of discharge, the patient will:
- have no signs or symptoms of wound or systemic infection or meningitis.

INTERVENTIONS	RATIONALES
1. *Implement the measures in "Risk for infection,"* page 196, *in the "Increased intracranial pressure" care plan.*	**1.** The "Increased intracranial pressure" plan provides general measures for prevention, assessment, and treatment of infection. This plan discusses additional care specific to the craniotomy patient.
2. *Administer antibiotics as ordered,* usually immediately before surgery begins.	**2.** Wound infection occurs in 0.7% to 5.7% of neurosurgical patients. Prophylactic antibiotic administration helps prevent infection by establishing the optimal tissue concentration of antibiotic before possible contamination. Antibiotic administration may also be repeated during a lengthy procedure. Antibiotics may be discontinued at the completion of surgery.
3. *Assess for respiratory infection:* – Auscultate the lungs every 2 hours and as necessary for adventitious sounds. – Assess sputum for color, consistency, amount, and odor; culture if necessary. – Observe for temperature elevation and WBC elevation.	**3.** The overall pulmonary infection rate in the neurosurgery patient is 13% to 16%. Impaired mobility, characteristic of the surgical and postoperative periods, compromises the respiratory system by slowing the movement of secretions; this promotes atelectasis and produces generalized hypoxia. Dehydration makes the sputum thicker, increasing the risk of consolidation and pneumonia. Adventitious breath sounds, purulent or foul-smelling sputum, fever, and WBC elevation strongly suggest the development of pulmonary infection.
4. *Observe the surgical wound daily for signs and symptoms of infection,* such as redness, edema, suture stretch, pigskin appearance of the epidermis, tenderness, or drainage. Also observe for systemic signs of infection, including fever, malaise, leukocytosis, or tachycardia.	**4.** Scalp margin necrosis, wound dehiscence, CSF leakage, the presence of a drain and monitoring device, possible scratching and manipulation by the patient, and environmental factors increase the risk of wound infection in the postcraniotomy patient. A stitch abscess may appear before a major wound infection develops. A true wound infection rarely occurs before the 2nd day after surgery and usually occurs within the first 2 weeks.

5. *Monitor the patient for signs and symptoms of meningitis,* such as temperature elevation, chills, lethargy, severe headache, nausea and vomiting, nuchal rigidity, positive Kernig's and Brudzinski's signs, photophobia, irritability, decreased LOC, or generalized seizures. Assist with CT scan and lumbar puncture if necessary.

5. Patients at risk for developing acute inflammation of the meninges of the brain or spinal cord include those with cranial or spinal wound infections, CSF fistulae following operative procedures on the dura mater, and subarachnoid bolts or ventricular drains. All of these are possible risk factors for the postcraniotomy patient. Abnormal lumbar puncture findings typically confirm the diagnosis. These findings include a positive culture, an elevated opening pressure of 200 to 700 mm H_2O, WBC count increased from 10 to 1,000 cells/μl, an increased protein count, decreased glucose and chloride levels and, in purulent bacterial meningitis, a tan or milky appearance of the fluid. A CT scan may be performed before the lumbar puncture to determine the risk of brain herniation from the sudden removal of CSF from the spinal canal.

6. Additional individualized interventions: _____

6. Rationales: _____

> **Suggested NIC Interventions**
> *Infection control; Infection protection; Incision site care; Wound care*

> **Suggested NOC Outcomes**
> *Infection status; Wound healing: Primary intention*

Collaborative problem
Risk for respiratory failure related to decreased LOC, neurologic deficits, effects of anesthesia, immobility, altered respiratory patterns, and tenacious secretions associated with fluid loss and decreased fluid intake

NURSING PRIORITY
Maintain effective gas exchange.

PATIENT OUTCOME CRITERIA
Within 24 hours after surgery, the patient will:
- have an airway free from secretions
- have arterial blood gas (ABG) levels within desired limits.
  By the time of discharge, the patient will:
- have a normal respiratory rate and pattern
- have normal ABG levels
- have a clear chest X-ray.

INTERVENTIONS

1. *Implement the measures discussed in "Risk for respiratory failure," page 199, in the "Increased intracranial pressure" care plan.*

2. Additional individualized interventions: _____

RATIONALES

1. The neurosurgical patient requires meticulous respiratory assessment, support of oxygenation and ventilation, and pulmonary hygiene.

2. Rationales: _____

Neurologic disorders

Nursing diagnosis

Risk for injury related to decreased LOC, effect of anesthetics, seizures, or drug therapy

NURSING PRIORITY
Prevent injury.

PATIENT OUTCOME CRITERION
Throughout the hospital stay, the patient will remain free from injury.

INTERVENTIONS	RATIONALES
1. *Implement the measures discussed in "Risk for injury," page 203, in the "Increased intracranial pressure" care plan.*	**1.** Although the risk factors for injury for the neurosurgical patient differ somewhat from those for the patient with increased ICP, the measures used to prevent them are the same.
2. Additional individualized interventions: _____ _____	**2.** Rationales: _____

> **Suggested NIC Interventions**
> *Surveillance: Safety*

> **Suggested NOC Outcomes**
> *Safety status: Physical injury*

Nursing diagnosis

Risk for imbalanced fluid volume related to physiologic stress response to surgery, steroid therapy, or SIADH

NURSING PRIORITY
Maintain fluid volume within prescribed limits.

PATIENT OUTCOME CRITERIA
By the time of discharge, the patient will:
- display electrolyte levels, BUN level, hematocrit, and serum osmolality within normal limits
- have a urine output within normal limits
- manifest hemodynamic values within normal limits.

INTERVENTIONS	RATIONALES
1. *Implement the measures discussed in "Excess fluid volume," page 201, in the "Increased intracranial pressure" care plan.*	**1.** The "Increased intracranial pressure" care plan discusses the potential for excess fluid volume in detail.
2. Additional individualized interventions: _____	**2.** Rationales: _____

> **Suggested NIC Interventions**
> *Fluid management; Fluid monitoring; Fluid and electrolyte management; Hypervolemia management*

> **Suggested NOC Outcomes**
> *Electrolyte and acid-base balance; Fluid balance; Hydration*

Nursing diagnosis

Risk for deficient fluid volume related to diuretic therapy, fluid restriction, DI, hyperthermia, or GI suction

NURSING PRIORITY
Maintain fluid volume within prescribed limits.

PATIENT OUTCOME CRITERIA
By the time of discharge, the patient will:
- maintain a urine output within normal limits
- have electrolyte levels, hematocrit, BUN level, and serum osmolality within normal limits
- maintain hemodynamic values within normal limits.

INTERVENTIONS	RATIONALES
1. *Implement the measures discussed in "Risk for deficient fluid volume," page 200, in the "Increased intracranial pressure" care plan.*	1. DI most commonly occurs after neurosurgery. The "Increased intracranial pressure" care plan discusses this problem in detail.
2. Additional individualized interventions: _____	2. Rationales: _____

> **Suggested NIC Interventions**
> *Acid-base management; Electrolyte management; Fluid and electrolyte management; Hypovolemia management; Intravenous (I.V.) therapy*

> **Suggested NOC Outcomes**
> *Electrolyte and acid-base balance; Fluid balance; Hydration*

Nursing diagnosis

Disturbed body image related to hair loss, possible disruption in sensory or motor function, or possible alteration in personality and thought processes

NURSING PRIORITIES
- Promote a healthy body image.
- Minimize damage to self-concept.

PATIENT OUTCOME CRITERIA
Within 5 to 7 days after surgery, the patient will:
- verbalize feelings of self-worth
- participate in self-care
- demonstrate an interest in personal appearance
- demonstrate an interest in occupational therapy, activities of daily living (ADLs), and a potential rehabilitation program.

INTERVENTIONS	RATIONALES
1. *Encourage the patient to express feelings, beliefs, and concerns* about changes resulting from the diagnosis and craniotomy. Offer emotional support as appropriate, based on knowledge of the diagnosis and the success of surgery.	1. The patient may have fears or misconceptions that can be clarified. Some residual effects of surgery are temporary. Recovery may be slow (months or years).

Neurologic disorders

2. *Implement measures to minimize the patient's reaction to loss of hair and to the misshapen skull, if a bone flap was removed.*
– Provide a surgical cap or scarf to wear; encourage usual grooming, makeup habits, and wearing a wig; reinforce that hair will regrow.

– Use therapeutic touch and visit frequently.

3. *Provide appropriate stimuli:*
– Place the patient in a room with a window if possible.
– Provide a clock and calendar.
– Provide objects of interest to the patient such as photographs of loved ones.
– Play the radio, tapes, or television, if the patient wishes.
– Talk with the patient.
– Encourage the family to interact with the patient.

4. *Implement the measures in the "Impaired physical mobility" care plan,* page 111, as appropriate. Encourage participation in self-care, occupational therapy, ADLs, and ambulation, as permitted.

5. Additional individualized interventions: _____
_____

2. Specific interventions to minimize the body image changes may make the patient feel less self-conscious.

– These measures to improve appearance and help the patient become aware of the temporary nature of body image alterations may encourage greater acceptance of the changes.
– Therapeutic touch and frequent visits convey acceptance, which may facilitate the patient's self-acceptance.

3. These measures provide stimulation and reality orientation. Talking with the patient and encouraging family interaction are particularly important because they reinforce a sense of human connection in the unfamiliar hospital environment.

4. The measures in the "Impaired physical mobility" care plan prevent deformities and other complications resulting from the enforced immobility associated with major surgery. Maintaining motor function, muscle strength, and joint mobility are particularly important in preserving the patient's ability to benefit from later rehabilitation programs. Participation in activities fosters the patient's belief that independence can be reestablished.

5. Rationales: _____
_____

> **Suggested NIC Interventions**
> *Body image enhancement; Grief work facilitation; Anticipatory guidance; Coping enhancement; Self-esteem enhancement*

> **Suggested NOC Outcomes**
> *Body image; Grief resolution; Self-esteem*

Nursing diagnosis
Deficient knowledge (follow-up care) related to lack of exposure to information

NURSING PRIORITY
Provide early teaching regarding rehabilitation and follow-up care.

PATIENT OUTCOME CRITERIA
By the time of discharge, the patient and his family will:
■ verbalize questions about follow-up care
■ express satisfaction with the staff's willingness to answer questions
■ begin identifying long-range learning needs.

Neurologic disorders

INTERVENTIONS	RATIONALES
1. *Implement measures in the "Knowledge deficit" care plan, page 129, as appropriate.* Wait to start formal teaching until the patient's condition stabilizes.	1. In the first days after surgery, the craniotomy patient is usually too ill for a structured teaching program, and the attention of the patient and his family is directed toward more immediate needs. Formal teaching works best after the patient's condition has stabilized and the patient has been transferred to a better environment for learning.
2. *Provide informal teaching as appropriate.* Encourage questions, provide brief explanations about the current situation, and clarify misconceptions.	2. Capitalizing on informal opportunities conveys a willingness to meet the learning needs of the patient and his family.
3. *Instruct the patient to avoid activities producing sudden changes in ICP,* such as bending, lifting, straining, and the Valsalva maneuver.	3. The Valsalva maneuver commonly occurs with position changes in bed and straining with a closed epiglottis. Teach the patient to continue to breathe deeply through the mouth when changing position in bed. Use stool softeners and other therapies to prevent constipation and straining at stool which can result in significant increases in blood pressure and ICP.
4. *Provide information about seizure precautions and what to do if a seizure occurs.* See the "Seizures" care plan, page 228.	4. Seizures can occur postoperatively up to a year. The patient and his family should know how to recognize seizure activity, safety precautions, and actions to take if a seizure occurs.
5. *Identify and document long-range teaching needs* as the patient or his family raises questions or demonstrates a specific need. Upon the patient's discharge, communicate these needs to the receiving staff.	5. Planning for discharge teaching is most effective based on the specific needs of the patient and his family. Documentation and colleague-to-colleague communication enhance continuity of care.
6. Provide information to the patient and his family about community agencies and support groups, such as head injury support groups, vocational rehabilitation, and the American Cancer Society.	6. These organizations provide many forms of support for patients and their families. In many cases, their credibility allows them to provide invaluable practical information on long-range education and rehabilitation. Knowing that others have coped with similar experiences may provide a sense of rapport and trust that encourages the learning necessary to adjust successfully to cranial surgery and possible residual deficits.
7. Additional individualized interventions: _____	7. Rationales: _____

> **Suggested NIC Interventions**
> *Teaching: Procedure/treatment*

> **Suggested NOC Outcomes**
> *Knowledge: Treatment regimen*

Discharge planning
DISCHARGE CHECKLIST
Before discharge, the patient shows evidence of:
- ❏ stable vital signs
- ❏ stable neurologic function
- ❏ ICP within normal limits
- ❏ healing incision
- ❏ headache controlled by oral analgesics
- ❏ absence of pulmonary, cardiovascular, or GI complications
- ❏ normal fluid and electrolyte balance
- ❏ absence of infection
- ❏ absence of fever.

TEACHING CHECKLIST
Document evidence that the patient and his family demonstrate an understanding of:

❑ the diagnosis and extent of surgery
❑ wound care
❑ the extent of neurologic deficits if present
❑ the extent and demands of the rehabilitation process
❑ the need for continued family support
❑ date, time, and location of follow-up care
❑ purpose, dosages, and potential adverse effects of discharge medications.

DOCUMENTATION CHECKLIST

Using outcome criteria as a guide, document:
❑ the patient's clinical status on admission
❑ significant changes in status
❑ pertinent laboratory and diagnostic test findings
❑ fluid intake and output
❑ neurologic status
❑ neurologic deficits if present
❑ GI bleeding if any
❑ wound condition
❑ seizures if any
❑ rehabilitation program needs
❑ patient and family teaching
❑ discharge planning.

Associated care plans

■ Acute pain
■ Compromised family coping
■ Impaired physical mobility
■ Increased intracranial pressure
■ Ineffective individual coping
■ Knowledge deficit
■ Nutritional deficit
■ Perioperative care
■ Seizures

References

Biller, J. (ed). *Practical Neurology*, 2nd ed. Philadelphia: Lippincott Williams & Wilkins, 2002.

Black, J.M., et al. *Medical-Surgical Nursing Clinical Management for Positive Outcomes*, 6th ed. Philadelphia: W.B. Saunders Co., 2001.

Hickey, J.V. *The Clinical Practice of Neurological and Neurosurgical Nursing*, 5th ed. Philadelphia: Lippincott Williams & Wilkins, 2002.

Ignatavicius, D.D., and Workman, M.L. *Medical-Surgical Nursing. Critical Thinking for Collaborative Care.* Philadelphia: W.B. Saunders Co., 2002.

Lewis, S.M., et al. *Medical-Surgical Nursing Assessment and Management of Clinical Problems,* 5th ed. St. Louis: Mosby–Year Book, Inc., 2000.

Urden L.D., et al. *Thelan's Critical Care Nursing Diagnosis and Management,* 4th ed. St. Louis: Mosby–Year Book, Inc., 2002.

Urden L.D., and Stacey, K.M. *Priorities in Critical Care Nursing,* 3rd ed. St. Louis: Mosby–Year Book, Inc., 2002.

Drug overdose

DRG INFORMATION

DRG 449   Poisoning and Toxic Effects of Drugs with Complication or Comorbidity (CC). Age 17+.
Mean LOS = Not available

DRG 450   Poisoning and Toxic Effects of Drugs without CC. Age 17+.
Mean LOS = 3.8 days

DRG 451   Poisoning and Toxic Effects of Drugs. Ages 0 to 17.
Mean LOS = 2.1 days

Introduction

DEFINITION AND TIME FOCUS

The patient admitted after a drug overdose is a challenge. He may be comatose, withdrawn, agitated, somnolent, or otherwise unable to provide clear historical data. The type of drug involved may be unknown, or evidence may suggest that the patient took more than one drug. If illegal substances are involved, family members may be reluctant to provide a full history because they fear possible criminal prosecution, even if they're assured of medical confidentiality.

Even when the patient or his family clearly identifies a specific drug that was taken, the nurse must consider the potential interaction of the drug with other medications and the possibility that the patient took more than one drug. For the purposes of this care plan, overdose is defined as an intentional act by which the patient ingests, injects, sniffs, inhales, or otherwise self-administers a dose that proves to be toxic.

Using this definition, the plan omits discussion of overdoses from accidental poisoning, toxic reactions to prescribed medications taken at recommended dosages, and industrial or agricultural exposure to toxic substances. This care plan focuses on the patient who's admitted to a hospital for treatment of an intentional overdose, commonly associated with a suicide gesture or attempt. (See *Clinical Snapshot: Drug overdose,* page 184.)

ETIOLOGY AND PRECIPITATING FACTORS

For each patient, different factors may cause the overdose event, but usually one or more of the following are involved:
- Drug or alcohol abuse or addiction
- Unhealthy coping patterns
- Unusually stressful life event or circumstances
- Despair, depression, anger, or the desire for revenge

Focused assessment guidelines

NURSING HISTORY (FUNCTIONAL HEALTH PATTERN FINDINGS)

Health-perception–health-management pattern
- History of short- or long-term drug or alcohol abuse or addiction
- Intent to commit suicide
- Previous suicide attempt

Sleep-rest pattern
- History of insomnia or early morning awakening (associated with depression)

Cognitive-perceptual pattern
- Poor concentration or memory impairment
- Difficulty making decisions

Self-perception–self-concept pattern
- Helpless or hopeless self-perception (common)
- Self-deprecating statements

Role-relationship pattern
- Lack of significant other
- Recent conflict or breakup with significant other
- Recent or chronic job difficulties
- Recent death of a loved one

Coping–stress tolerance pattern
- Habitual use of unhealthy coping behavior such as drug abuse

Value-belief pattern
- Surprise or disbelief about the seriousness of overdose

PHYSICAL FINDINGS

Because physical findings vary widely with the drug taken, this section is omitted. See *Nurse's guide to common drug overdoses,* pages 182 and 183, or consult pharmacologic references for findings associated with specific drug overdoses.

DIAGNOSTIC STUDIES

Appropriate laboratory tests vary widely, depending on the drug taken. The following are commonly performed for toxicity screening and evaluation.
- Serum electrolyte levels — may be abnormal; several drugs commonly seen in overdose cases, including salicylates and alcohol, may cause electrolyte abnormalities
- Arterial blood gas (ABG) values — essential for monitoring the adequacy of respiratory efforts; salicylates and other drugs cause acid-base abnormalities
- Liver enzyme levels — may reveal liver damage; many medications can cause liver damage at toxic levels, most notably acetaminophen and alcohol

(Text continues on page 184.)

Nurse's guide to common drug overdoses

Drug	Therapeutic effects	Signs and symptoms of overdose	Treatment	Complications
Acetaminophen	Reduces fever and raises pain threshold; exact mechanisms unclear; metabolized in liver	• Anorexia • Nausea and vomiting • Diaphoresis • Right upper quadrant abdominal pain • Hypotension • Altered level of consciousness (LOC)	• Drug level measured every 4 hours to guide treatment • Emesis or lavage • Cathartics • Acetylcysteine (Mucomyst) given orally, if more than 7.5 g ingested within 24 hours and serum level in toxic range 4 hours after ingestion	• Hepatic failure • Coagulation defects • Renal failure • Hepatic encephalopathy • Shock
Alcohol (ethanol)	Central nervous system (CNS) depression, peripheral vasodilation	• Ataxia • Reduced comprehension • Vomiting • Respiratory depression • Hypotension • Seizures • Flushing • Coma	• Emesis or lavage, if ingested within 4 hours • I.V. fluids • Ventilatory support, especially in multiple-drug overdose • Observation for withdrawal, including anxiety, tremors, diaphoresis, tachycardia, and hypertension (usually occurs 24 to 48 hours after last alcohol intake) • Sedation (if withdrawal symptoms are noted)	• Respiratory depression • Aspiration • Hepatic failure • GI tract bleeding • With chronic abuse: –Esophageal varices –Portal hypertension –Hepatic encephalopathy • Additive effects if taken with another CNS depressant
Barbiturates	CNS depression	• Cardiopulmonary depression • Hypotension • Tachycardia • Sluggish pupil response • Nystagmus • Bullae • Hypothermia • Confusion • Ataxia • Coma	• Ventilatory support • Emesis or lavage (if ingested) • Activated charcoal • Cathartics • I.V. fluids • Observation for withdrawal, including tremors, vomiting, weakness, and hallucinations • Dialysis possible for large doses	• Arrhythmias • Respiratory arrest • Shock • Seizures • Pulmonary edema • Coma
Benzodiazepines	CNS depression	• Lethargy • Hypotension • Tachycardia • Respiratory depression • Confusion • Ataxia • Coma	• Ventilatory support • Emesis or lavage (if ingested) • Activated charcoal • Cathartics • Flumazenil (Romazicon) given I.V. in repeated doses • I.V. fluids *Note:* Hemodialysis and forced diuresis *aren't* effective	• Taken alone, usually not fatal but when taken with other CNS depressants, additive effects can lead to respiratory depression, coma, and death

Nurse's guide to common drug overdoses *(continued)*

Drug	Therapeutic effects	Signs and symptoms of overdose	Treatment	Complications
Cocaine	CNS stimulation, local anesthesia	• Hyperexcitability • Anxiety • Hypertension or hypotension • Fever • Tachypnea • Tachycardia • Confusion • Hallucinations • Dilated pupils • Diaphoresis • Seizures, coma	• Sedatives • Anticonvulsants • Cardiac monitoring • Emesis or lavage (if ingested) • Activated charcoal (if ingested) • Cathartic (if ingested) • Fever control measures	• Myocardial infarction • Cerebral hemorrhage • Respiratory arrest • Status epilepticus • Cardiomyopathy • Rhabdomyolysis (rare)
Opiates	CNS depression, analgesia, peripheral vasodilation	• Respiratory depression • Constricted pupils • Reduced LOC • Hypothermia • Hypotension • Bradycardia	• Ventilatory support • Naloxone (Narcan) I.V. in repeated doses • Close monitoring, because respiratory depression may recur • Cardiac monitoring • Emesis or lavage (if ingested)	• Respiratory arrest • Shock • Arrhythmias • Coma
Salicylates	Analgesia	• Nausea and vomiting • Hyperthermia • Electrolyte imbalances • Acid-base imbalances (usually respiratory alkalosis and metabolic acidosis) • Hyperglycemia (in children, hypoglycemia) • Hyperpnea • Hyperventilation • Oliguria • Tinnitus • Confusion • Seizures • Petechiae	• Ventilatory support • Cardiac monitoring • I.V. fluids • Cooling measures • Correction of electrolyte and acid-base abnormalities • Emesis or lavage • Activated charcoal • Cathartics • Alkalinization of urine with sodium bicarbonate and potassium chloride (a urine pH between 7.5 and 8.5 promotes increased renal excretion)	• Respiratory failure • Arrhythmias or other life-threatening conditions caused by electrolyte or acid-base abnormalities • Renal tubular necrosis • GI bleeding • Hepatotoxicity • Pulmonary edema • Shock • Interference with normal clotting • Increased gastric motility
Tricyclic antidepressants	Relieves symptoms of depression in patients with mood disorders	• Lethargy • Dry mouth • Dilated pupils • Confusion • Tremors • Urine retention • Tachycardia • Hypotension • Respiratory depression • Cardiac conduction delay • Hypothermia • Seizures • Coma	• Ventilatory support • Cardiac monitoring • Emesis or lavage • Activated charcoal • Cathartics • I.V. fluids • Sodium physostigmine • Cardiac pacing (if complete heart block) • Anticonvulsants • Alkalinization with sodium bicarbonate • Temperature regulation measures *Note:* Dialysis *not* effective	• Arrhythmias • Myocardial depression • Complete heart block • Heart failure • Shock • Paralytic ileus • Central and peripheral anticholinergic effects, myocardial depression

Neurologic disorders

- Blood alcohol level — an important screening test in any overdose because alcohol potentiates many drug effects, thus increasing central nervous system (CNS) depression
- Toxicology screening assay — checks for various substances, depending on the laboratory, but usually includes barbiturates, narcotics, amphetamines, salicylates, and acetaminophen
- Serum salicylate level — may reveal toxicity; time-elapsed nomograms are obtained in cases of acute overdose to assess toxicity levels; because salicylates have a prolonged half-life, the sample should be obtained at least 6 hours after drug ingestion; a level greater than 150 mg/ml is considered toxic
- Urine narcotic level — determines the presence and concentration of narcotics; most narcotics are excreted in urine within 48 hours of administration; toxic levels vary depending on the narcotic

- Serum barbiturate level — determines the concentration of barbiturates in the blood; salicylates may interfere with the test and alcohol ingestion may increase barbiturate levels; toxic levels vary depending on the barbiturate taken
- Serum antidepressant level — identifies and determines the concentration of antidepressant in the blood; toxic levels vary, depending on the antidepressant; for most tricyclic antidepressants, the toxic level is greater than 1,000 ng/ml
- Abdominal X-rays — can reveal a mass of pills in the stomach
- Gastroscopy — may be performed to remove substances if X-rays reveal a coalesced mass of material that can't be removed by lavage

POTENTIAL COMPLICATIONS

See *Nurse's guide to common drug overdoses*, pages 182 and 183.

CLINICAL SNAPSHOT

Drug overdose

Major nursing diagnoses and collaborative problems	Key patient outcomes
ND: Ineffective airway clearance	Maintain a clear airway.
CP: Risk for multiple organ dysfunction syndrome	Maintain vital organ function.
ND: Hopelessness	Participate as much as possible in self-care and care planning.

Nursing diagnosis

Ineffective airway clearance related to reduced alertness, decreased or absent gag reflex, obstruction by tongue, vomiting, or lavage procedures

NURSING PRIORITY

Maintain a clear airway.

PATIENT OUTCOME CRITERIA

Throughout the hospital stay, the patient will:
- maintain a clear airway
- maintain a spontaneous respiratory rate of 12 to 24 breaths/minute or be placed on mechanical ventilation.

INTERVENTIONS	RATIONALES
1. *Assess the patient's airway status continually** by noting the adequacy of spontaneous respiratory efforts, chest excursion, breath sounds, gag reflex, skin color, and level of consciousness (LOC).	**1.** Initial and ongoing airway evaluation is essential in the patient who has taken a drug overdose because many medications cause CNS depression. If several medications were taken, their combined effects may further reduce the patient's ability to clear the airway.

---

*Italics indicate key interventions.

2. *Place the patient in a side-lying position.* Ensure that suction equipment is ready at the bedside.

3. *If lavage is initiated, ensure airway protection by placing the patient in a head-down position;* if the patient is sedated, assist with placement of a cuffed endotracheal tube.

4. If the patient's gag reflex is reduced or absent or if respirations are less than 12 or more than 24 per minute, shallow, or labored, anticipate and assist with endotracheal intubation and mechanical ventilation. See the "Mechanical ventilation" care plan, page 281, for details.

5. *Monitor ABG levels, as ordered.* See appendix B, Acid-base imbalances.

6. Additional individualized interventions: _____

_____

2. The side-lying position makes drainage from the mouth easier and reduces the probability of aspiration. Suctioning may be needed if the patient vomits.

3. Aspiration of gastric contents may lead to aspiration pneumonitis, a complication associated with increased morbidity and mortality.

4. Toxic CNS effects may interfere with vital functions. Unless promptly corrected, respiratory impairment results in permanent damage to the brain and other organs.

5. Changes in ABG levels may provide early warning of impaired ventilatory status before clinical evidence is apparent. Also, toxic levels of many medications cause acid-base abnormalities; ABG studies serve as a guide for intervention.

6. Rationales: _____

_____

> **Suggested NIC Interventions**
> *Airway management; Airway suctioning; Acid-base monitoring; Aspiration precautions; Positioning; Respiratory monitoring; Ventilation assistance*

> **Suggested NOC Outcomes**
> *Aspiration control; Respiratory status: Airway patency; Respiratory status: Gas exchange; Respiratory status: Ventilation*

Collaborative problem
Risk for multiple organ dysfunction syndrome related to systemic toxic drug effects

NURSING PRIORITIES
- Support and monitor vital organ functions.
- Identify and counteract drug effects.

PATIENT OUTCOME CRITERIA
- Within 1 hour of admission to the hospital, the patient will receive initial treatment for a specific drug overdose.
- Throughout the hospital stay, the patient will maintain vital organ functions.

INTERVENTIONS

1. *Collect as much information as possible about the overdose* by questioning the patient, family, friends, and other caregivers. If possible, determine:
– what was taken
– how much was taken
– when the drug was taken
– how it was taken (for example, ingested or injected)
– whether there was also alcohol use
– if the patient has underlying health problems
– what other medications were taken
– what has been done for the patient so far.

RATIONALES

1. A thorough history may be difficult to obtain, but it provides vital clues for effective intervention and ongoing monitoring.

Neurologic disorders

2. *Monitor vital signs, hemodynamic pressures, and electrocardiogram findings* according to appendix A, Monitoring standards, or unit protocol.

3. Collaborate with the physician and regional poison control center personnel in selecting and initiating measures to reverse or eliminate the drugs from the body (some measures may have been implemented in the emergency department). Initiate one or more of the following as appropriate:
– induced vomiting with ipecac syrup, 30 ml orally with 10 to 12 oz (295 to 355 ml) of fluids. Observe for onset of vomiting within 15 to 30 minutes. If no vomiting occurs, the dose may be repeated once. If the patient still doesn't vomit, consult the physician and prepare for gastric lavage. Never administer ipecac if the patient has an absent gag reflex, signs of decreasing alertness, a history of seizures, or ingested corrosives. Consult with the poison control center before administering ipecac to a patient who has ingested a hydrocarbon or has taken an overdose of an antiemetic drug.

– gastric lavage, using a large-bore Ewald tube and normal saline solution or other ordered irrigant. Lavage with 100- to 200-ml fluid boluses and avoid overdistending the stomach. Lavage until return is clear, unless otherwise ordered, usually 1,000 to 1,500 ml total. Monitor inflow and outflow volumes and report discrepancies. Save aspirated fluid for analysis as needed. Monitor serum electrolyte levels in conjunction with large-volume or prolonged lavage.

– dilution, usually with milk or water, unless the patient is obtunded.

– gut lavage, using a peristaltic pump to deliver warmed electrolyte solution to the stomach.
– activated charcoal, usually 25 to 50 g in a slurry, administered orally or via gastric tube after emesis or lavage is completed. Don't give charcoal at the same time as ipecac syrup.

– cathartics as ordered, usually mixed with charcoal; cathartics ordered include magnesium sulfate and magnesium citrate.
– specific antidotes or antagonists used as ordered.

2. At toxic levels, many drugs can interfere with the vasomotor center's control of cardiac function and blood vessel constriction. Baseline and ongoing assessment of these parameters provides early warning of cardiovascular dysfunction.

3. Since the institution of regional poison control centers, with their hot line consultative services, mortality from poisonings has fallen significantly. The poison control center provides expert advice on treating all types of drug overdoses.

–Ipecac syrup is thought to act centrally and locally on the GI tract to stimulate vomiting. Fluids are given with ipecac because without adequate gastric volume, esophageal injury may occur from forceful retching. Doses greater than 60 ml may have cardiotoxic effects. Ipecac administration is contraindicated if the patient's condition may result in aspiration. Also, vomiting of corrosives may cause or increase damage to esophageal and oropharyngeal mucosae. The treatment of hydrocarbon ingestion depends on the specific substance. Ipecac may not be effective if the patient has taken an overdose of antiemetic medication such as a phenothiazine.
– Gastric lavage is used when vomiting is contraindicated (for example, if the patient has a reduced or absent gag reflex). It effectively removes ingested substances from the stomach but is thought to be somewhat less effective than induced emesis. The choice of fluid is controversial and may depend on the drug ingested. Fluid boluses larger than 200 ml are thought to wash the toxin into the small bowel. A discrepancy between the amounts of instilled irrigant and returned fluid may indicate a need to reposition the patient to promote drainage or may indicate fluid reabsorption and the risk of fluid overload. The aspirate may be examined for diagnostic clues. Electrolyte imbalances and their cardiovascular sequelae may result from prolonged or large-volume lavage.
– Dilution is used primarily to treat ingestion of corrosives or other substances that preclude emesis. Distending the abdomen with fluid if the patient isn't conscious may increase the risk of aspiration.
– Gut lavage is a relatively new therapy that may be used to aid clearance of certain herbicides from the bowel.
– Activated charcoal is an inert substance that absorbs toxins. It shouldn't be given at the same time as ipecac syrup because it will inactivate the ipecac and prevent emesis. Opinions vary on whether the charcoal should be removed after a given time or allowed to pass through the intestines.
– Saline cathartics stimulate peristaltic activity by drawing fluid into the bowel through osmosis, thus hastening drug excretion and reducing absorption from the gut.
– A few drugs, notably narcotics and acetaminophen, are effectively treated with antidote-antagonist substances; however, because the patient may have taken more than one drug, close monitoring is still necessary.

– other measures, as recommended by the physician or poison control center, may include forced diuresis, peritoneal dialysis, hemodialysis, exchange transfusions, or gastroscopy.

– Forced diuresis may be used if the drug involved is excreted primarily through the urinary tract. Dialysis may help remove certain substances, but its effectiveness depends on the drug's pharmacologic properties and its distribution within body tissues. Exchange transfusions may be used for certain drugs if the dosage is massive and recent enough that tissue absorption hasn't taken place. Gastroscopy may be performed if abdominal X-rays reveal a coalesced mass of pills in the stomach.

4. *Perform careful serial evaluations of LOC, mental status, and gag and corneal reflex status every 1 to 2 hours* during the first 24 hours or until the patient's condition stabilizes.

4. Decreasing alertness and diminished or absent protective reflexes indicate CNS impairment and the likely need for airway management or ventilatory support. Serial evaluations allow early detection of subtle changes.

5. *Monitor fluid intake and output* and promptly report a dropping urine output (less than 60 ml/hour) to the physician.

5. Because many medications are detoxified or excreted through the renal system, the possibility of renal failure from toxic effects must always be considered. Also, a dropping urine output is a clue to the early development of shock, another potential complication of drug toxicity.

6. *Assess and monitor initial or serial laboratory test findings,* as ordered, for overdose substances.

6. Specific initial and serial urine or serum studies provide information about the amount of drug taken and the rate of absorption, guiding treatment.

7. Additional individualized interventions: _____
_____

7. Rationales: _____
_____

Nursing diagnosis
Hopelessness related to low self-esteem, emotional disorganization, or a sense of having inadequate resources to cope with life

NURSING PRIORITIES
- Promote a sense of hope.
- Foster self-esteem.

PATIENT OUTCOME CRITERIA
Before discharge from the unit, the patient will:
- discuss reasons for the overdose and identify precipitating factors
- participate as fully as possible in self-care and care planning
- begin to display healthy coping behaviors
- make contact with follow-up care providers.

INTERVENTIONS

1. Examine your attitudes toward suicide and drug abuse. *Maintain a concerned but nonjudgmental attitude* when providing care, avoiding all punishing behavior. If your feelings about suicide or drug abuse interfere with patient care, transfer the patient's care to another nurse, seek peer support, or consult with a psychiatric liaison nurse.

RATIONALES

1. Many health professionals have difficulty caring for a suicidal or self-abusive patient. Frustration and anger are common when the patient seems to be undermining the efforts of health care providers. Punishing attitudes, however, tend to further decrease the patient's fragile self-esteem and reduce coping ability. The patient may interpret such behavior as "just one more sign I'm no good for anything," adding to self-directed anger and hopelessness. Peer or psychiatric liaison support can help professionals address and resolve issues raised by an abusive or noncompliant patient.

2. *Foster communication.*

– Use touch as appropriate.

– Use active listening skills.

– Note and acknowledge nonverbal cues (body posture and gestures, facial expression, tone of voice, and silences).
– Make eye contact.

3. *Encourage the patient to participate in care-related decisions* as soon as possible.

4. *Arrange a referral to psychiatric resources* (such as a psychiatric nurse specialist, psychiatrist, or other mental health professional). Place the patient on suicide precautions if appropriate.

5. See the "Ineffective individual coping" care plan, page 124, and the "Dying" care plan, page 78.

6. *Ensure appropriate follow-up care arrangements* before discharge from the unit, including continuation of suicide precautions, if appropriate.

7. Additional individualized interventions: _____
_____

2. Usually, the patient who has taken an overdose perceives a lack of personal resources or can't communicate feelings because of emotional disorganization. Opening communication is the first step in identifying more positive responses to the problems that may have led to the overdose.
– Touch can convey profound messages of acceptance and caring and, for some patients, may be less threatening than verbal interaction as a way to initiate the therapeutic relationship.
– Active listening involves an attentive attitude, feedback, and rephrasing or reflection to help the patient clarify feelings and ideas. This reaffirms a sense of self-worth and the importance of feelings.
– Acknowledging nonverbal communication may help verify expressed feelings or open discussion of unexpressed feelings.
– Making eye contact in a nonthreatening manner expresses interest and the intent to communicate.

3. Considering the patient's stated wishes may, in many cases, be secondary to saving the patient's life. However, as the patient's condition stabilizes, a return to participation in self-care helps bolster self-respect and reduces feelings of powerlessness.

4. Any patient admitted with an intentional overdose warrants psychiatric evaluation and counseling as part of the plan of treatment. Careful evaluation of suicide potential is essential. If suicidal ideation is present, suicide precautions are warranted.

5. The "Ineffective individual coping" care plan contains interventions for patients struggling with emotional adjustments. The "Dying" care plan addresses issues that may relate to the care of the patient who has attempted suicide.

6. The patient who has been severely depressed may try suicide again when physical energy has been restored and personal appearance seems improved. Careful follow-up, both on the unit to which the patient is transferred and after discharge from the hospital, is vital in helping the patient make the transition to everyday life.

7. Rationales: _____
_____

Suggested NIC Interventions
Decision-making support; Mood management; Resiliency promotion; Hope instillation

Suggested NOC Outcomes
Decision making; Depression control; Depression level; Hope; Mood equilibrium; Quality of life

Discharge planning
DISCHARGE CHECKLIST
Before discharge, the patient shows evidence of:
❒ spontaneous respirations and airway clearance
❒ stable vital signs for at least 12 hours
❒ completion of specific measures to remove or reverse drugs consumed
❒ drug levels (if applicable) declining since admission
❒ urine output greater than 60 ml/hour
❒ ABG values within normal limits
❒ initial psychiatric evaluation and follow-up arrangements made
❒ implementation of suicide precautions if appropriate.

TEACHING CHECKLIST
Document evidence that the patient and his family demonstrate an understanding of:
❒ toxic effects of drugs and possible later complications
❒ the treatment measures undertaken
❒ the signs and symptoms of potential complications
❒ healthy coping behaviors
❒ resources available for help.

DOCUMENTATION CHECKLIST
Using outcome criteria as a guide, document:
❒ clinical status on admission
❒ significant changes in status
❒ pertinent laboratory and diagnostic test findings
❒ effectiveness of measures to promote elimination of drug or reversal of drug effects
❒ mental health measures
❒ suicide precautions if used
❒ follow-up plans
❒ patient and family teaching
❒ discharge planning.

Associated care plans
■ Acute renal failure
■ Confusion
■ Dying
■ Grieving
■ Impaired physical mobility
■ Ineffective individual coping
■ Mechanical ventilation

References
Jordan, K. (ed). *Emergency Nursing Care Curriculum.* Emergency Nurses Association. Philadelphia: W.B. Saunders Co., 2000.

Lynn-McHale, D.J., and Carlson, K.K. American Association of Critical Care Nurses *AACN Procedure Manual of Critical Care,* 4th ed. Philadelphia: W.B. Saunders Co., 2001.

Phipps, W.J., et al. *Medical-Surgical Nursing, Health and Illness Perspectives,* 7th ed. St. Louis: Mosby–Year Book, Inc., 2003.

Shoemaker, W.C. et al. *Textbook of Critical Care,* 4th ed. Philadelphia: W.B. Saunders Co., 2002.

Thompson, J.M., et al. *Mosby's Clinical Nursing,* 5th ed. St. Louis: Mosby–Year Book, Inc., 2002.

Neurologic disorders

Increased intracranial pressure

DRG INFORMATION

Increased intracranial pressure (ICP) is a sign of an underlying problem and not a condition in and of itself in terms of coding guidelines. The DRG assigned for increased ICP depends entirely on the underlying cause that requires hospitalization, such as hemorrhage, hematoma, head trauma, abscess, or radiation. The length of stay depends solely on the principal diagnosis.

Introduction

DEFINITION AND TIME FOCUS

Increased ICP occurs when the components of the intracranial cavity — brain tissue, cerebral blood volume, and cerebrospinal fluid (CSF) — exceed the cavity's compensatory capacity. The volume of these three components usually remains relatively constant, with a normal ICP of 0 to 15 mm Hg.

Autoregulatory mechanisms in the brain compensate for volume changes of the contents, so an increase in one component is counteracted by a decrease in another. These mechanisms include displacement of CSF from the cranial cavity to the subarachnoid space surrounding the spinal cord (the primary compensatory mechanism), increased CSF reabsorption, and the reduction of cerebral blood volume by compression of the venous system, displacing venous blood from the intracranial cavity into the systemic circulation. Displacement of brain tissue without concurrent decompensation is extremely limited and occurs primarily with a slowly expanding mass, such as a tumor or chronic subdural hematoma.

When these autoregulatory mechanisms can no longer compensate for changes in the components of the intracranial cavity, increased ICP results. When ICP is sufficiently elevated to reduce cerebral perfusion pressure, irreversible brain damage may occur. This care plan focuses on the critically ill patient with acutely increased ICP. (See *Clinical snapshot: Increased intracranial pressure*, page 192.)

ETIOLOGY AND PRECIPITATING FACTORS

- Increased brain volume (caused by intracranial hemorrhage or hematoma, cerebral edema caused by surgical or head trauma, rapidly growing tumors, abscess, metabolic coma, radiation, chemotherapeutic agents, infarction, and anoxic events)
- Increased cerebral blood volume (from loss of autoregulation; hyperthermia; vasodilation caused by hypoxemia, hypercapnia, anesthetic agents, or narcotics;

venous outflow obstruction caused by compression of the internal jugular veins or intrathoracic or intra-abdominal pressure; fluctuations above a mean arterial pressure [MAP] of 160 mm Hg or below 60 mm Hg)
- Obstruction of CSF outflow (because of hematomas in the posterior fossa; brain shift and herniation; or impaired reabsorption from the subarachnoid space caused by inflammation of the meninges either by subarachnoid hemorrhage or infection, or obstruction of arachnoid villi by blood cells or bacteria)

Focused assessment guidelines

NURSING HISTORY (FUNCTIONAL HEALTH PATTERN FINDINGS)

Health-perception–health-management pattern

- Sudden change in level of consciousness (LOC), ranging from flattening of affect to coma; possible loss of consciousness for less than 24 hours
- History of head trauma resulting from a motor vehicle accident, fall, assault, gunshot or stab wound, or recreational accident; males between ages 15 and 24 are at an increased risk because of this group's higher incidence of head injury from motor vehicle accidents
- History of infection, particularly in middle ear, mastoid cells, or paranasal sinuses
- History of receiving anesthetics, narcotics, radiation, or chemotherapeutic drugs
- History of hypoxia from hypoventilation, apnea, chest trauma, pneumonia, or ventilation-perfusion abnormalities

Nutritional-metabolic pattern

- Vomiting (uncommon); if present, it isn't preceded by nausea

Cognitive-perceptual pattern

- Headache (uncommon); if present, it's worse on arising in the morning; straining or movement may increase the pain.

Self-perception–self-concept pattern

- Anxiety or apprehension if the patient is alert enough to understand that something abnormal is happening

PHYSICAL FINDINGS

Many of the classic signs and symptoms of increased ICP now are considered indicators of brain shift and brain stem dysfunction. Clinical signs and symptoms alone aren't reliable in determining if ICP is elevated, in detecting early increased ICP, or in determining the severity of increased ICP. Frequent neurologic assessment and ICP monitoring are the most reliable methods for detecting early deterioration.

Neurologic
Early findings
- Decreasing LOC (most sensitive indicator of increased ICP), indicated by such signs as confusion, restlessness, or lethargy
- Pupillary abnormalities, with the pupil dilating gradually and becoming slightly ovoid and sluggish in the eye ipsilateral to the cause of the increased ICP
- Visual deficits, such as decreased visual acuity, blurred vision, diplopia, and changes in extraocular eye movements
- Motor weakness (monoparesis or hemiparesis) contralateral to the cause of increased ICP

Later findings
- Coma
- Pupillary abnormalities, including dilated and nonreactive (fixed) ipsilateral pupil; with herniation, pupils become bilaterally fixed and dilated
- Loss of deep tendon reflexes
- Hemiplegia and abnormal posturing (sometimes termed *decorticate* or *decerebrate posturing*), which may be unilateral or bilateral; as death approaches, the patient becomes bilaterally flaccid
- Positive Babinski's sign
- Hyperthermia from hypothalamic injury
- Loss of brain stem reflexes, including corneal, oculocephalic (doll's eyes), and oculovestibular reflexes (the oculovestibular reflex isn't as readily compromised as the oculocephalic and is a more sensitive indicator of any remaining brain stem function); gag, cough, and swallowing reflexes also are lost
- Papilledema (rarely); more common with chronically increased ICP

Cardiovascular
Later findings
- Cushing's reflex (compensatory mechanism to provide adequate cerebral perfusion pressure [CPP]) — rising systolic blood pressure, widening pulse pressure, and bradycardia; Cushing's triad (hypertension, bradycardia, and bradypnea)

Pulmonary
- Irregular respirations, commonly in patterns that relate to the level of brain dysfunction; Cheyne-Stokes respirations, central neurogenic hyperventilation, and ataxia are common in later stage of increased ICP; may be difficult to assess with the mechanically ventilated patient

Gastrointestinal
- Vomiting (uncommon); if present, not preceded by nausea

DIAGNOSTIC STUDIES
Although no laboratory test for diagnosing increased ICP exists, tests may include the following:

- Arterial blood gas (ABG) measurements — used to monitor the patient's acid-base balance and to detect hypoxemia and hypercapnia, which increase ICP
- Complete blood count — may reveal elevated white blood cell (WBC) count, which may signify the beginning of an infection or abscess
- Electrolyte panel — used to monitor the patient's fluid status and potassium and sodium levels; sodium is retained during stressful events and potassium is lost; sodium and potassium levels also are altered in diabetes insipidus (DI) and syndrome of inappropriate antidiuretic hormone secretion (SIADH), two abnormalities that may occur with increased ICP
- Serum creatinine, blood urea nitrogen (BUN) levels — used to monitor renal function, particularly if osmotic diuretics are administered
- Blood glucose test — used to monitor for hyperglycemia if dexamethasone (Decadron) therapy is used
- Serum osmolality — used to monitor for hyperosmolality when mannitol therapy is used and aids in establishing a diagnosis of DI or SIADH
- Urine specific gravity — may indicate DI if low or SIADH if high
- Urine glucose and acetone levels — may reveal glucose in the urine, which may be an adverse reaction to dexamethasone therapy
- Computed tomography (CT) scan — can differentiate among many conditions that cause increased ICP; clearly outlines ventricles and shows size and position in relation to midline structures; useful in diagnosing cerebral edema, hematomas caused by intracranial bleeding, abscesses, cerebral infarctions, and tumors; serial scanning useful in a deteriorating patient or one who doesn't improve as rapidly as expected; may show intracranial hematomas in a patient whose initial CT scan was normal
- Skull X-rays — useful in detecting linear and depressed skull fractures (high incidence of developing masses and intracranial hemorrhage occurs with linear fractures); may demonstrate intracranial shifts; should be considered when the patient has an altered LOC any time after injury, focal neurologic signs, or CSF discharge from the nose or ears
- Cerebral echoencephalography — may be used if a CT scan isn't available; useful in detecting shifts of normally midline structures but isn't reliable in detecting generalized cerebral edema that doesn't produce a midline shift
- Cerebral angiography — may be used if a CT scan isn't available; can reveal space-occupying lesions, such as subdural or epidural hematoma, and cerebral edema; an invasive study, therefore, the CT scan preferred
- Cerebral blood flow studies — determine whether blood flow is within normal limits, increased, or decreased
- Magnetic resonance imaging — gives clearer images of soft tissues than a CT scan and can detect brain edema,

hemorrhage, infarction, and blood vessel disruptions more clearly; has limited usefulness at this time, for a patient with increased ICP because it can't be used on a patient whose care requires use of such metal devices as electrocardiogram (ECG) electrodes, or a patient who's on mechanical ventilation

■ ICP monitoring — may reveal values of 15 to 40 mm Hg, indicating moderately elevated ICP, or 40 mm Hg or greater, indicating severely elevated ICP

■ EEG monitoring — useful in identifying changes in electrical activity that could indicate cerebral ischemia or subclinical seizures and in assessing responses to treatment

■ ECG — useful in assessing changes, such as the development of tall T waves in early increased ICP that become progressively flatter or inverted with an ICP greater than 45 mm Hg; ST-segment changes occur with transient changes in ICP and return to normal with the return of ICP to previous levels; low levels of increased ICP produce abnormally shortened QT intervals; prolonged QT intervals occur with ICP greater than 65 mm Hg

POTENTIAL COMPLICATIONS

■ Brain herniation
■ Permanent neurologic deficits
■ Seizures
■ Pneumonia
■ Atelectasis
■ GI ulceration and hemorrhage
■ Infection
■ DI
■ SIADH
■ Neurogenic pulmonary edema

CLINICAL SNAPSHOT ✳

Increased intracranial pressure

Major nursing diagnoses and collaborative problems	Key patient outcomes
CP: Risk for cerebral ischemia	Demonstrate improved neurologic function.
ND: Risk for infection	Display no indications of infection.
CP: Risk for increased cerebral metabolism	Maintain a normal temperature.
CP: Risk for respiratory failure	Have a normal respiratory rate and pattern.
ND: Risk for deficient fluid volume	Maintain a urine output within normal limits.
ND: Excess fluid volume	Maintain a urine output within normal limits.
ND: Risk for injury	Remain free from additional injury.

Collaborative problem

Risk for cerebral ischemia related to fluctuations in arterial blood pressure, ICP, stressful events, nursing activities, hypoxemia, or hypercapnia

NURSING PRIORITY

Minimize fluctuations in cerebral perfusion pressure.

PATIENT OUTCOME CRITERIA

Within 72 hours of admission, the patient will:
■ have an ICP of 0 to 15 mm Hg and a CPP greater than 60 mm Hg
■ have an MAP greater than 60 mm Hg
■ display no clinical signs of increased ICP and herniation.
Within 1 week of admission, the patient will:
■ demonstrate improved neurologic status.

INTERVENTIONS

1. *Assess the patient's LOC, behavior, motor and sensory function, pupillary reactions (size, position, and reactivity), and respiratory patterns** every hour and as necessary. Notify physician of changes.

2. *Monitor ICP* (if an ICP monitoring device is in place) *and MAP continually* and compare readings with a desirable level. Correlate with clinical assessments and CPP. Document every hour or as changes occur. Calculate CPP as changes occur (see appendix A, Monitoring standards). Report ICP greater than 15 mm Hg or MAP less than 60 mm Hg, or as ordered.

3. *Monitor cerebral blood flow continuously* via Transcutaneous Doppler (TCD) as ordered.

4. *Maintain MAP at a level that will result in a CPP of 60 mm Hg or more.*

– Administer blood products, colloids, or albumin to increase blood pressure as ordered. Assess intake and output closely to prevent fluid overload. Monitor ICP, MAP, and CPP closely for efficacy of therapy.
– If pharmacologic support of blood pressure is needed, administer dopamine hydrochloride (Intropin) or other vasopressors as ordered.

– If systemic hypertension is present, titrate fluid restriction, vasodilator administration, sedative or analgesic agents, or other therapies according to CPP, as ordered.

RATIONALES

1. Changes in any of these parameters may indicate a deterioration in the patient's neurologic condition. The LOC is the most sensitive and reliable indicator of increasing ICP. A change in respiratory patterns, also a sensitive indicator of increased ICP, is an early indicator of hypoxemia or hypercapnia, which also lead to increased ICP.

2. ICP indicates how well the intracranial cavity's three components are balanced. CPP is the blood pressure gradient across the brain and is calculated as the difference between the incoming MAP and the opposing mean ICP (CPP = MAP−ICP). Alterations in either MAP or intracranial volume affect CPP and the integrity of brain tissue. A CPP of at least 60 mm Hg must be maintained to provide a minimally adequate blood supply to the brain. A CPP of 30 mm Hg or less results in cell death.

3. TCD is a noninvasive method of indirectly monitoring cerebral blood flow at the bedside. Correlation of TCD and ICP values allows for assessment of the individual patient's response to nursing interventions and treatments.

4. Blood pressure must be carefully controlled to ensure adequate CPP. Between a MAP of 60 and 160 mm Hg, the brain automatically regulates blood vessel diameter to maintain constant cerebral blood flow (CBF) and thus CPP. If the autoregulatory mechanism is lost, CBF and cerebral blood volume passively depend on the blood pressure and CPP so that hypotensive episodes provoke ischemia, whereas hypertensive bursts push fluid into the brain.
– Increased systemic blood pressure can be achieved via vascular expansion, resulting in an increased MAP and CPP.

– An increase in systemic hypotension worsens cerebral ischemia and necrosis. If autoregulation is intact, use of vasopressors with a resultant increase in blood pressure can cause vasoconstriction and reduced CBF and CPP.
– Administration of a sedative or analgesic agent may control increased blood pressure due to noxious stimuli or pain. Treating hypertension may be difficult because blood pressure may be elevated as a compensatory mechanism for ischemia. Antihypertensive agents like nitroprusside and nitroglycerine are cerebral vasodilators and should be avoided or used with caution. Using beta-adrenergic blockers concomitantly may help reduce the cerebral vasodilatory effect common to some degree in all antihypertensives. CPP is considered the best guide for gauging the effects of therapies to control systemic hypertension in a patient with increased ICP.

---

*Italics indicate key interventions.

5. *Monitor ABG levels as ordered.* Maintain ABG levels within prescribed parameters, typically partial pressure of arterial oxygen (Pao_2) greater than 80 mm Hg and partial pressure of arterial carbon dioxide ($Paco_2$) at 35 ($+/-2$) mm Hg, or as ordered. Monitor arterial oxygen saturation (Sao_2) continuously via pulse oximetry. Keep Sao_2 at 96% or greater, or as ordered.

6. *Use an ICP monitoring device to observe ICP levels,* particularly during activities known to cause sustained increases in ICP, such as suctioning, moving the patient, emotional upsets, noxious stimuli, arousal from sleep, coughing, sneezing, or Valsalva's maneuver.

7. *Instruct the alert patient to avoid the following activities that increase ICP: straining at stool, holding breath while moving or turning in bed, coughing, nose blowing, and extreme hip flexion (90 degrees or more).*

8. *Instruct the alert patient to avoid pushing his feet against a footboard or his arms against the bed.*

9. Administer pharmacologic agents as ordered for shivering and abnormal posturing, typically chlorpromazine (Thorazine) for shivering and propofol (Diprivan) or neuromuscular blocking agents (atracurium or vecuronium) for severe abnormal posturing. Document administration and effects.

10. *Structure the environment to reduce unpleasant stimuli:*
– Avoid unnecessary or unintended emotionally stimulating conversation (for example, about prognosis or condition).
– Provide a quiet room.
– Avoid jarring the patient's bed.
– Provide soft stimuli, such as a soft voice, soft music, and a gentle touch when necessary.
– Increase sedation before necessary interventions that are known to increase ICP.
– Space painful nursing or medical procedures.
– Use lidocaine (Xylocaine) to decrease effect of coughing and suctioning.
– Encourage the presence of calming visitors.
– When necessary to awaken the patient, use gentle touch and a soft voice.
– Avoid unnecessary disturbances.
– Restrict disturbing visitors as needed.

11. *Assess the patient's level of comfort* and administer ordered medications as needed, documenting administration and effectiveness:
– analgesics when permitted for headache and pain
– antiemetics for nausea and vomiting
– stool softeners for constipation.

5. Hypoxemia (Pao_2 less than 60 mm Hg) and hypercapnia ($Paco_2$ greater than 45 mm Hg) have a potent vasodilatory effect on cerebral vessels and increase CBF and ICP. Keeping the patient well-oxygenated and on the lower limits of eucapnia helps limit CBF and therefore helps control ICP.

6. Clinical symptoms of increased ICP aren't always present, even when a substantial increase in pressure occurs. By maintaining an awareness of activities that produce spikes in ICP and by monitoring ICP levels, you can modify or terminate these activities as ICP increases.

7. These activities increase intrathoracic and intra-abdominal pressure, which are transmitted to the jugular veins, impeding cerebral venous return and increasing ICP.

8. These activities produce isometric muscle contractions, which increase muscle tension without lengthening the muscle. These contractions elevate systemic blood pressure and result in increased ICP.

9. Shivering commonly occurs in response to hypothermia, which may be used to control ICP increase due to increased temperature. Shivering is a form of isometric contraction and thus can increase ICP. Abnormal posturing also produces muscle contractions, which elevate ICP.

10. Unpleasant or noxious stimuli can increase ICP. They also increase systemic blood pressure, which may increase ICP in the patient with poor or absent autoregulation. Calming visitors who provide soothing touch may decrease ICP.

11. Pain, nausea, vomiting, and constipation are noxious stimuli that increase ICP. Vomiting also increases intra-abdominal and intrathoracic pressure, impeding venous return from the brain.

12. *Use restraints only when absolutely necessary* and as ordered.

12. Restraints may cause the patient to struggle. The stimulation and the resulting increased activity (producing increased heart rate and increased blood flow to the brain) elevate ICP.

13. *Space activities when possible,* especially routine care activities, such as turning, baths, mouth care, and bed changes. Don't provide care for routine reasons only. Use pressure-relieving mattresses. If activity results in a sharp rise in ICP with concomitant decrease in CPP, stop the activity until ICP returns to baseline.

13. Closely spaced activities can have a cumulative effect, causing a greater and more prolonged elevation of increased ICP than a single activity.

14. *Maintain venous drainage from the brain* by proper alignment and positioning; logroll when turning to maintain alignment. Assess the optimal position for each patient and maintain that position during the critical stage. Avoid extreme flexion of the arms and hips.

14. Because the cerebral venous system has no valves, jugular vein compression causes increased pressure throughout the system, impeding drainage from the brain and increasing ICP. Placing the patient flat or in the Trendelenburg position prevents venous drainage as well; the Trendelenburg position increases blood flow to the brain. Extreme flexion of the arms and hips increases intra-abdominal and intrathoracic pressure, decreasing cerebral venous drainage and increasing ICP.

15. *Maintain appropriate head of bed position.* Assess the patient's response to various position changes. Maintain CPP of 60 mm Hg or more and ICP at 20 mm Hg or less, or as ordered. If ICP monitoring isn't in use, keep head of bed elevated 15 to 30 degrees or as ordered.

15. Although elevating the head of the bed improves venous drainage, thus decreasing ICP, it may also decrease CPP. The degree of head elevation should be based on assessment of the individual patient's ICP, MAP, and CPP. Assessing the patient's clinical response to various positions will also help determine changes in CPP and ICP, particularly if the patient isn't being monitored with an ICP catheter. Medications, such as Dopamine, may be used to increase CPP by increasing MAP, thus allowing for increased elevation of the head of bed.

16. Implement therapeutic measures, as ordered:

– corticosteroids, usually dexamethasone (Decadron) or methylprednisolone (Solu-Medrol)

16. Interventions help maintain ICP at a level consistent with optimal CPP.
– Although the value of corticosteroids in reducing ICP is controversial, clinicians usually consider these drugs effective in reducing cerebral edema in some clinical problems such as tumors. They're still used by many clinicians for treatment of severe head injury, although research doesn't support their use. Their exact mechanism of action is unknown.

– diuretics, commonly mannitol (Osmitrol) and furosemide (Lasix) (see "Excess fluid volume" page 201); maintain serum osmolality of 300 to 320 mOsm/kg to prevent renal failure

– Diuretics limit cerebral intracellular and extracellular swelling and CSF volume.

– CSF drainage via an intraventricular drain

– Draining CSF helps control erratic ICP increases and is most helpful when decreased CSF absorption is causing increased ICP.

Neurologic disorders

– drugs to control metabolic demand: benzodiazepines (sedatives, hypnotics, or antianxiety medications), such as midazolam (Versed) and lorazepam (Ativan); opioid narcotics, such as fentanyl and morphine; anesthetics propofol; and neuromuscular blocking agents such as Vecuronium and atracurium (Adjust level of administration to the individual patient's response to keep ICP stable and CPP optimal. Monitor closely and provide care related to ICP monitoring and mechanical ventilation. Use propofol or neuromuscular blocking agents only with adequate analgesia, and use neuromuscular blocking agents with sedation.)

– barbiturate coma, typically with pentobarbital (Nembutal) or thiopental (Pentothal), for severe, persistent, refractory increased ICP in adults

– hypothermia using hypothermia blankets. Place hypothermia blanket over and under the patient. Avoid shivering as this increases ICP and oxygen demand. Assess for changes in skin condition and pneumonia (see the "Pneumonia" care plan, page 297 and the "Impaired physical mobility" care plan, page 111), neutropenia and infection, arrhythmias at body temperature less than 82.4° F (28° C), renal dysfunction, and clotting abnormalities.
– hyperventilation: if using hyperventilation with $Paco_2$ less than 30 mm Hg, monitor CPP and ICP closely to identify cerebral ischemia; avoid $Paco_2$ less than 25 mm Hg; evaluate oxygen delivery at the cellular level via jugular bulb or cerebral tissue oxygen monitoring

17. When noninvasive therapeutic interventions don't control ICP, prepare the patient and his family for surgical intervention (see the "Craniotomy" care plan, page 170).

18. Additional individualized interventions: _____
_____

– These drugs, individually or in combination, are used to control increased cerebral metabolic demand and ICP. The preferred therapeutic regimen begins with antianxiety, sedation, analgesic medications. Propofol and neuromuscular blockers are added if ICP isn't controlled. Assessment of the neurologic system is limited by sedation so the patient should have ICP monitoring in place. The patient needs to be mechanically ventilated and extensively monitored because these drugs induce respiratory depression, paralysis, or anesthetic effects. Propofol or neuromuscular blockers should never be used without adequate analgesia because neither affect the pain threshold. In addition, neuromuscular blockers should be used in conjunction with sedation because they cause skeletal muscle paralysis but don't affect anxiety or agitation.
– Barbiturate coma therapy is a controversial treatment that rapidly induces cerebral vasoconstriction and decreases cerebral metabolism and blood flow, thus lowering ICP, preserving ischemic cells, and preventing irreversible damage. Because barbiturate coma requires complete life support and extensive nursing supervision, it's used to manage uncontrolled intracranial hypertension unresponsive to conventional treatment. This therapy is used primarily in patients with head injuries, cerebral hemorrhage, encephalitis, and Reye's syndrome.
– Rapid induction of hypothermia may be used for increased ICP refractory to barbiturate coma, particularly in severe head injury. Cerebral metabolic rate increases 5% to 7% for each degree increase in temperature, which increases cerebral oxygen demand and blood volume and thus ICP. Reducing the temperature to 92.3° to 94.1° F 33.5° to 34.5° C may reduce the risk of hypoxemia and ischemia.

– Prophylactic hyperventilation may be used when sustained ICP doesn't respond to standard treatment. Once a standard therapy, hyperventilation is now believed to produce ischemia by causing cerebral vasoconstriction with a resulting decrease in ICP but also a decrease in cerebral blood volume and CPP.

17. Surgical intervention may be necessary to control a cause such as intracranial hematoma or to gain time to prevent herniation while slower therapies reduce swelling — for instance, removing a bone flap to allow brain expansion.

18. Rationales: _____
_____

Nursing diagnosis
Risk for infection related to invasive techniques, immunosuppression, or surgical or other trauma

NURSING PRIORITIES
- Prevent infection.
- Monitor for signs and symptoms of infection.

PATIENT OUTCOME CRITERIA

Within 48 to 72 hours of admission, the patient will:
- have a normal body temperature
- have a WBC count within normal limits.
  By the time of discharge, the patient will:
- display no indicators of infection.

INTERVENTIONS	RATIONALES
1. *Maintain strict sterile technique* as appropriate for catheterization, endotracheal (ET) tube care, and closed intracranial drainage system care. Wash hands before contact with patient and wear gloves. As appropriate, maintain standard precautions.	1. Sepsis is the primary concern with any invasive equipment or procedure. Using the appropriate technique will help prevent infection.
2. *Change dressings as ordered,* using sterile technique. Change the dressing at the intracranial monitoring device site every 24 to 48 hours or as ordered. Apply antibiotic ointment around the insertion site only if ordered.	2. Preventing infection and sepsis is crucial, particularly at sites with direct access to the brain. Cerebral infection increases the cerebral metabolic rate and CBF, thus increasing ICP. Practices regarding use of antibiotic ointment around the insertion site vary.
3. *Maintain ICP monitoring devices as closed systems.* Don't flush the system routinely. Instill antibiotic solutions via the ICP monitoring line every 24 to 48 hours, followed by normal saline solution, only if ordered.	3. Maintaining a closed system may be critical in preventing infections in the CSF. Flushing an ICP monitoring line isn't a routine procedure and isn't considered a safe practice by many clinicians, so it should be performed only on specific orders. Prophylactic instillation of antibiotics may help control infection but is highly controversial.
4. *Assess periodically for signs and symptoms of infection:* – redness, tenderness, or warmth around insertion sites or wounds (check daily) – cloudy or foul-smelling drainage (check daily) – fever (check every 4 hours) – elevated WBC count (monitor as ordered) – positive urine, sputum, blood, or wound cultures (monitor as ordered) – infiltrates on chest X-ray (monitor as ordered).	4. Early detection of infection allows for prompt and appropriate intervention. An elevated WBC count may confirm an infection; however, the value may be elevated if the patient is on steroids.
5. *Administer antibiotics as ordered,* typically if the patient has an ICP monitoring device or ventricular drainage system or if signs and symptoms of infection are present. Document your actions and monitor for effectiveness and adverse reactions.	5. Broad-spectrum antibiotics may be ordered prophylactically for direct access to the brain. After infection has been documented, choice of antibiotic depends on culture results.
6. Administer antipyretic drugs and use hypothermia blankets and tepid sponge baths, as ordered, for increased temperature. Monitor for shivering.	6. An increase in temperature can increase ICP (see "Risk for cerebral ischemia," page 192). Vigorous sponge baths can also increase ICP and should only be used after an assessment of the patient's ICP levels. Rapid cooling may also cause shivering which can increase ICP and should be treated with appropriate medications.
7. Additional individualized interventions: _____	7. Rationales: _____

Neurologic disorders

Collaborative problem

Risk for increased cerebral metabolism related to temperature elevations caused by infection and hypothalamic injury

NURSING PRIORITY

Maintain normal body temperature.

PATIENT OUTCOME CRITERION

By the time of discharge, the patient will maintain a temperature within normal limits without the aid of a hypothermia blanket.

INTERVENTIONS	RATIONALES
1. Monitor and document temperature every 4 hours and as needed. Maintain temperature of 100.4° F (38° C) or less.	**1.** In the later stages of increased ICP, pressure on the hypothalamus may cause hypothalamic injury, disrupt normal thermoregulatory mechanisms, and cause extremely elevated temperatures. Because an elevated temperature increases systemic and CBF as well as oxygen demand and consumption, and contributes to increased ICP, it should be controlled as soon as possible.
2. *Administer antipyretics as ordered,* typically acetaminophen (Tylenol). Administer tepid sponge baths as ordered.	**2.** With infection, the temperature rises because interleukin-1 (IL-1) may act as a pyrogen. Both IL-1 and the fever it triggers activate the body's defense mechanisms. These measures, along with antibiotic administration discussed earlier, may be sufficient to control an elevated temperature caused by infection.
3. *Apply a hypothermia blanket as ordered* for an elevated temperature that doesn't respond to more conservative measures.	**3.** Temperature elevation from hypothalamic injury and loss of autoregulatory control usually requires more aggressive intervention to return the temperature to normal levels.
4. *Take appropriate precautions when using the hypothermia blanket:* – Cover the hypothermia blanket with a sheet or bath blanket. – Check the patient's rectal temperature every 15 minutes or use a rectal probe for continuous monitoring. – Turn the blanket off when the rectal temperature slightly exceeds desired temperature, according to unit protocol. – Control shivering by administering medication as ordered, usually chlorpromazine.	**4.** Hypothermia has numerous physiologic effects that may result in injury. – Direct contact between the patient's skin and the hypothermia blanket can cause skin damage similar to frostbite. – The degree of hypothermia must be controlled carefully to prevent adverse reactions. A rectal thermometer or probe more accurately measures body temperature. – The patient's temperature will continue to drop and will return to normal gradually because the solution inside the blanket remains cold. – Shivering is a form of isometric contraction that results in increased ICP.
5. Remove excessive bed clothes, use rotating fans, and allow for adequate ventilation in the patient's room.	**5.** Inadequate ventilation and excessive bed clothes increase the time needed to reduce the patient's temperature to normal.
6. Additional individualized interventions:_____	**6.** Rationales: _____

Collaborative problem

Risk for respiratory failure related to increased ICP, cerebral dysfunction, obstructed airway, absence of spontaneous respirations and gag or cough reflexes, aspiration, atelectasis, ventilation-perfusion abnormalities, altered LOC, or neurogenic pulmonary edema

NURSING PRIORITY
Maintain effective gas exchange.

PATIENT OUTCOME CRITERIA
Within 24 hours of admission, the patient will:
- have an airway free from secretions
- have ABG levels within desired limits
- have clear breath sounds in all lobes.
  By the time of discharge, the patient will:
- have a normal respiratory rate and pattern
- have normal ABG levels
- have a clear chest X-ray.

INTERVENTIONS

1. *Assess and document the respiratory rate, depth, and pattern every 15 to 60 minutes.* Notify the physician of a rate less than 14 breathes/minute or greater than 24 breaths/minute, shallow respirations, or changes in the respiratory pattern. Assist with intubation if the patient can't maintain an adequate airway, respiratory depth, and respiratory pattern.

2. *Auscultate for breath sounds every 2 hours and as needed to determine adequacy of aeration and the presence of adventitious sounds.* Observe for anxiety, restlessness, dyspnea, and tachycardia. Assess for cyanosis around the mouth, in nail beds, and in earlobes.

3. *Assess the color, amount, and consistency of respiratory secretions.* Culture as needed.

4. *Monitor ABG levels as ordered.* Maintain ABG levels within prescribed parameters, as described in "Risk for cerebral ischemia," page 192. Obtain chest X-rays as ordered. Correlate the findings with clinical observations.

5. *Position the patient with the head of the bed elevated to the prescribed height and the patient's hips at the break in the bed.*

6. *Turn the patient every 2 hours if ICP levels allow.* Administer increased sedation before turning.

RATIONALES

1. Respiratory status is the result of a complex interplay of factors, including airway patency and medullary and pontine control mechanisms. The respiratory rate is a sensitive indicator of airway patency and increasing ICP; the respiratory pattern may correlate with the level of brain stem dysfunction. If the patient can't maintain adequate gas exchange, intubation and mechanical ventilation may be necessary to avert cardiopulmonary arrest.

2. Adventitious sounds may signal the need for intervention such as suctioning. Restlessness and tachycardia are key findings in early hypoxemia. Cyanosis, a late finding, indicates inadequate gas exchange.

3. Secretions may indicate infection or the need for hydration to help clear secretions.

4. Objective documentation of pulmonary status is an important adjunct to clinical observations.

5. Proper positioning allows for complete lung expansion.

6. Dependent lung lobes can't fully expand, thus compromising gas exchange. Turning allows for full expansion of all lobes and aids in preventing atelectasis and pneumonia, which interfere with gas exchange. However, turning may increase ICP levels, so the benefits of turning must outweigh the risks. Administering increased sedation before turning may decrease the risk of increased ICP.

Neurologic disorders

7. *Suction as needed,* preoxygenating with 100% oxygen before and after suctioning and limiting suctioning to no more than 10 seconds for each catheter pass and no more than two passes in a suctioning episode. Administer lidocaine through an ET tube or I.V. line as ordered. Monitor for seizures, depressed respirations, or cardiac arrhythmias. If you give it I.V., administer it 2 minutes before suctioning; if you give it endotracheally, administer it 5 minutes before suctioning.

8. Implement care related to mechanical ventilation, if used. See the "Mechanical ventilation" care plan, page 281.

9. Additional individualized interventions: _____
_____

7. A decision to suction should always be based on adventitious breath sounds or presence of sputum in the ET tube. Suctioning-induced hypoxemia contributes to increased ICP and compromised CPP. Suctioning can raise ICP up to 100 mm Hg. Used topically, lidocaine limits elevation of ICP in response to suctioning. When given as an I.V. bolus, lidocaine can sustain this effect over time. Lidocaine overdoses may cause seizures, respiratory arrest, or cardiac arrest.

8. Carbon dioxide and oxygen levels are more precisely controlled when the patient is intubated and ventilated mechanically. The "Mechanical ventilation" care plan contains detailed information about this intervention.

9. Rationales: _____
_____

Nursing diagnosis

Risk for deficient fluid volume related to diuretic therapy, fluid restriction, DI, hyperthermia, or GI suction

NURSING PRIORITY
Maintain fluid volume within prescribed limits.

PATIENT OUTCOME CRITERIA
By the time of discharge, the patient will:
- maintain a urine output within normal limits
- maintain electrolyte and BUN levels, hematocrit, and serum osmolality within normal limits
- maintain hemodynamic values within normal limits.

INTERVENTIONS

1. See appendix C, Fluid and electrolyte imbalances.

2. *Monitor and correlate fluid intake and output,* both hourly and cumulatively. Measure and document urine specific gravity every 1 to 4 hours. Report the following:

– urine output greater than 200 ml/hour for 2 hours, with specific gravity 1.001 to 1.005

RATIONALES

1. The Fluid and electrolyte imbalances appendix contains general information; this plan focuses on fluid and electrolyte problems specific to increased ICP.

2. Diuretic therapy, hyperthermia, restricted fluid intake, and DI may produce an overwhelming fluid deficit. Hourly and cumulative measurements allow prompt detection of any deficit. Fluid restriction is used less commonly now because it can adversely affect CBF and CPP.
– Urine output greater than 200 ml/hour usually indicates DI. In a patient with increased ICP, DI results from failure of the pituitary gland to secrete ADH because of damage to the hypothalamus, the supraopticohypophysial tract, or the posterior lobe of the pituitary gland. Such damage occurs most commonly after neurosurgery, but it can also occur secondary to vascular lesions or severe head injury. Because ADH is absent, the renal tubules fail to conserve water, resulting in the excretion of large volumes of dilute urine. The low specific gravity reflects the dilute urine. Urine output of this magnitude can rapidly create a fluid volume deficit.

– urine output less than 30 ml/hour for 2 hours, with specific gravity greater than 1.025.

– A urine output less than 30 ml/hour for 2 hours with a high specific gravity indicates that a fluid volume deficit exists.

3. *Monitor laboratory values,* as ordered. Report the following:
– urine osmolality, less than 200 mOsm/kg
– serum osmolality, greater than 300 mOsm/kg
– serum sodium, greater than 145 mEq/L
– BUN levels and hematocrit elevated.

3. Laboratory values provide objective evidence of an imbalance. The low urine osmolality reflects diuresis; the elevated serum osmolality and serum sodium levels and hematocrit reflect hemoconcentration.

4. *Monitor the ECG and hemodynamic pressures continually.* Promptly report:
– the appearance of U waves, prolonged QT interval, depressed ST segment, and low T waves

– arrhythmias, particularly bradycardia and atrial arrhythmias, first-degree and second-degree heart block, and premature ventricular contractions (PVCs)
– low hemodynamic pressure and cardiac output.

4. Continual monitoring provides early warning of potentially fatal conditions.
– ECG signs reflect the decreased responsiveness of cardiac cells to stimuli — the result of hypokalemia secondary to renal potassium washout.
– Bradycardia, heart block, atrial arrhythmias, and PVCs reflect hypokalemia. Prompt treatment is necessary to prevent hypokalemic arrest.
– Low pressure reflects hypovolemia and decreased cardiac output indicates insufficient preload.

5. *Administer replacement therapy as ordered,* usually isotonic solution with potassium chloride added if serum potassium is low. Monitor the I.V. flow rate closely. Anticipate increased fluid requirements if hyperthermia or infection is present.

5. Isotonic solution is the replacement fluid of choice for lost body fluids. Blood products, colloids, or albumin may be used to increase the MAP and thus CPP. Close monitoring is needed to prevent fluid volume overload. Solutions with potassium should be carefully monitored because potassium irritates the vein and rapid potassium infusion can cause hyperkalemia, possibly leading to complete heart block, ventricular fibrillation, or ventricular standstill. Hyperthermia and infection accelerate fluid loss by increasing metabolic rate and increasing skin and respiratory fluid excretion.

6. *Administer exogenous antidiuretic hormone* (ADH), such as vasopressin (Pitressin) or desmopressin (DDAVP). Monitor intake and output, urine and serum osmolality, specific gravity, and electrolytes. Weigh daily and assess for edema.

6. DI occurs when circulating ADH is diminished or absent, resulting in massive free-water loss. A short-acting drug such as vasopressin or a long-acting drug such as desmopressin controls water loss.

7. Additional individualized interventions: _____

7. Rationales: _____

Suggested NIC Interventions
Acid-base management; Fluid and electrolyte management; Fluid monitoring; Hypovolemia management; Intravenous (I.V.) therapy

Suggested NOC Outcomes
Electrolyte and acid-base balance; Fluid balance; Hydration

Nursing diagnosis
Excess fluid volume related to stress, steroid therapy, or SIADH

NURSING PRIORITY
Maintain fluid volume within prescribed limits.

PATIENT OUTCOME CRITERIA

By the time of discharge, the patient will:

- display serum osmolality, electrolyte and BUN levels, and hematocrit within normal limits
- have a urine output within normal limits
- maintain hemodynamic values within normal limits.

INTERVENTIONS	RATIONALES
1. See appendix C, Fluid and electrolyte imbalances.	**1.** The Fluid and electrolyte imbalances appendix contains general information on fluid and electrolyte problems. This plan focuses on problems specific to increased ICP.
2. *Monitor and correlate fluid intake and output hourly.* Report a urine output less than 30 ml/hour for 2 hours with a specific gravity greater than 1.025. Insert an indwelling urinary catheter if necessary and as ordered.	**2.** Carefully monitoring fluid intake and urine output helps detect potential problems that increase ICP. Decreased urine output may reflect a fluid volume deficit or SIADH; high specific gravity reflects increased water reabsorption. SIADH is characterized by abnormally high levels or continuous secretion of ADH, resulting in water being continuously reabsorbed from the renal tubules. Increased ADH secretion is caused by several factors related to increased ICP, including hyperthermia, hypotension, trauma, stress response, and administration of drugs, such as chlorpromazine, barbiturates, and acetaminophen. Sodium and water retention also are caused by corticosteroids and the stress response. Awareness of water retention may prevent further complications such as pulmonary edema.
3. *Monitor urine and serum osmolality, serum electrolyte studies, hematocrit, and BUN levels* daily or as ordered. Report the following: – urine osmolality (usually high) – serum osmolality (usually less than 280 mOsm/kg) – serum sodium (usually less than 126 mEq/L) – BUN levels and hematocrit (usually low)	**3.** High urine osmolality reflects water retention. Low serum osmolality, serum sodium, hematocrit, and BUN levels reflect hemodilution.
4. *Monitor the ECG and hemodynamic pressures continually.* Report promptly: – the appearance of U waves, prolonged QT interval, depressed ST segment, or low T waves – arrhythmias, particularly bradycardia and atrial arrhythmias, first-degree and second-degree heart block, and PVCs – elevated hemodynamic pressures and decreased cardiac output.	**4.** Constant monitoring provides early warning of impending problems. – These ECG findings reflect dilutional hypokalemia. – These rhythms are commonly caused by hypokalemia. – Elevated hemodynamic pressures indicate fluid overload, and decreased cardiac output results when the heart can't handle the excessive preload.
5. Institute the following therapies, as ordered. Carefully monitor intake and output with: – fluid restriction – diuretics, generally mannitol and furosemide.	**5.** An increase in cerebral blood volume increases ICP, requiring therapy. – Fluid restriction helps decrease extracellular fluid. – Mannitol is an osmotic diuretic that moves water from the brain and CSF into plasma by an osmotic gradient, thus decreasing ICP. Furosemide, a loop diuretic, inhibits distal tubular reabsorption, promoting diuresis. Furosemide also appears to dehydrate injured cerebral tissue selectively, thus reducing cerebral edema and ICP.

– potassium (if furosemide has been given).

– When furosemide is used, potassium is excreted along with fluid, so it may need replacement.

6. Additional individualized interventions: _____

6. Rationales: _____

> **Suggested NIC Interventions**
> *Fluid monitoring; Fluid and electrolyte management; Hypervolemia management*

> **Suggested NOC Outcomes**
> *Electrolyte and acid-base balance; Fluid balance; Hydration*

Nursing diagnosis

Risk for injury related to decreased LOC, seizures, and drug therapy

NURSING PRIORITY
Maintain patient safety.

PATIENT OUTCOME CRITERION
Throughout the hospital stay, the patient will remain free from new injury.

INTERVENTIONS	RATIONALES
1. *Observe the patient closely at all times.* Keep side rails up except during direct nursing care.	**1.** Decreased LOC is one of the earliest indications of increased ICP. The patient may not be aware of surroundings and possible dangers.
2. *Assess for seizures.* Implement seizure precautions, such as making sure that the bed has padded side rails and that airway and suction equipment is at the bedside. Assess oxygenation status during the seizure using oximetry. Administer and document antiseizure medication as ordered, typically phenytoin (Dilantin) or Phenobarbital (Luminal).	**2.** Seizures may be caused by the altered neuronal function associated with increased ICP. If the patient has a seizure, padded side rails lessen the potential for such physical injuries as cuts, abrasions, and fractures. A patient may need help maintaining a patent airway or may need suctioning after a seizure. If an oral ET tube is in place for airway management, a bile block may need to be inserted to prevent closure of the ET tube during the seizure, with resulting hypoxemia.
3. *Assess for gastric bleeding.* Administer medications as ordered, usually an antacid, such as aluminum and magnesium hydroxide (Maalox), and such histamine-2 (H_2) blockers as cimetidine (Tagamet), ranitidine (Zantac), or famotidine (Pepcid).	**3.** Gastric irritation and GI bleeding are major adverse reactions to corticosteroid therapy. Also, gastric bleeding occurs with increased ICP, although the exact mechanism is unknown. Increased ICP hypothetically stimulates the vagal nuclei directly, resulting in hypersecretion of gastric acid and hyperacidity. A patient with increased ICP is usually placed on prophylactic antacid and H_2-blocker therapy to decrease the risk of bleeding.
4. *Assess for an absent corneal reflex and apply artificial tears and eye patches,* as needed.	**4.** During the later stages of increased ICP, brain stem dysfunction results in the loss of the corneal reflex. Artificial tears lubricate the eyes, and the tears and patches prevent injury to the cornea.
5. Additional individualized interventions:_____	**5.** Rationales: _____

Suggested NIC Interventions	**Suggested NOC Outcomes**
Surveillance: Safety	Safety status: Physical injury

Discharge planning

DISCHARGE CHECKLIST

Before discharge, the patient shows evidence of:
- ❏ stable ICP within normal limits
- ❏ stable vital signs
- ❏ absence of cardiopulmonary complications
- ❏ absence of GI bleeding
- ❏ normal fluid and electrolyte balance
- ❏ ABG levels within normal limits
- ❏ stable temperature
- ❏ stable neurologic function
- ❏ removal of ICP monitoring line.

TEACHING CHECKLIST

Document evidence that the patient and his family demonstrate an understanding of:
- ❏ the causes of increased ICP
- ❏ the extent of neurologic deficits if present
- ❏ the need for continued family support
- ❏ the requirements for rehabilitation program if known
- ❏ the date, time, and location of follow-up appointments
- ❏ the purpose, dosage, and potential adverse effects of discharge medications.

DOCUMENTATION CHECKLIST

Using outcome criteria as a guide, document:
- ❏ clinical status on admission
- ❏ significant changes in status
- ❏ pertinent laboratory and diagnostic test findings
- ❏ fluid intake and output
- ❏ neurologic status
- ❏ neurologic deficits if present
- ❏ GI bleeding if any
- ❏ seizures if any
- ❏ patient and family teaching
- ❏ discharge planning.

Associated care plans

- Acute pain
- Anxiety
- Compromised family coping
- Impaired physical mobility
- Ineffective individual coping
- Knowledge deficit
- Mechanical ventilation
- Nutritional deficit
- Pneumonia
- Seizures

References

Deglin, J.H., and Vallerand, A.H. *Davis's Drug Guide for Nurses,* 8th ed. Philadelphia: F.A. Davis Co., 2003.

Hickey, J.V. *The Clinical Practice of Neurological and Neurosurgical Nursing,* 5th ed. Philadelphia: Lippincott Williams & Wilkins, 2002.

Iacono, L.A. "Exploring the Guidelines for the Management of Severe Head Injury," *The Journal of Neuroscience Nursing* 32(1):54-60, February 2000.

Ignatavicius, D.D., and Workman, M.L. *Medical-Surgical Nursing. Critical Thinking for Collaborative Care.* Philadelphia: W.B. Saunders Co., 2002.

Littlejohns, L.R., and Bader, M.K. "Guidelines for the Management of Severe Head Injury: Clinical Applications and Changes in Practice," *Critical Care Nurse* 21(6):48-65, December 2001.

March, K. "Intracranial Pressure Monitoring and Assessing Intracranial Compliance in Brain Injury," *Critical Care Nursing Clinics of North America* 12(4):429-36, December 2000.

Urden, L.D., et al. *Thelan's Critical Care Nursing Diagnosis and Management,* 4th ed. St. Louis: Mosby–Year Book, Inc., 2002.

Urden, L.D., and Stacy, K.M. *Priorities in Critical Care Nursing.* 3rd ed. St. Louis: Mosby–Year Book, Inc., 2002.

Laminectomy

DRG INFORMATION

DRG 499   Back and Neck Procedures except Spinal Fusion with Complication or Comorbidity (CC).
Mean LOS = 4.7 days

DRG 500   Back and Neck Procedures except Spinal Fusion without CC.
Mean Los – 2.6 days

Introduction

DEFINITION AND TIME FOCUS

Laminectomy is a major spinal surgery in which one or more vertebral laminae are removed to expose the spinal cord and nearby structures. Most commonly, it's performed to allow the removal of part or all of a disk (nucleus pulposus) that has herniated and is pressing on a spinal nerve root and to remove bony fragments or disk material from the spinal cord. Almost all herniated disks occur in the lumbar spine, 90% to 95% occurring at the level of L4 or L5 to S1. Cerebral herniation usually occurs between C5 and C6.

A laminectomy also may be performed to relieve spinal cord compression from a fracture, dislocation, hematoma, or abscess and to allow for spinal nerve surgery or the removal of a spinal cord tumor or vascular malformation. Less commonly, it may be performed to treat intractable pain by sectioning posterior nerve roots or interrupting spinothalamic tracts.

Lumbar laminectomy is more common than cervical laminectomy. A posterior surgical approach is used most commonly for lumbar laminectomy and an anterior approach for cervical laminectomy.

If the spine is unstable or repeated laminectomies are performed, the spine may be fused to stabilize the affected area, and may require hardware (rods, plates) to achieve vertebral stability. Typically, iliac crest bone fragments or bone chips from a donor bone are grafted between the vertebrae. Recovery takes longer with fusion because the bone graft heals slowly.

This care plan focuses primarily on the patient undergoing lumbar laminectomy for lumbar disk herniation that hasn't responded to conservative medical management. Exceptions or differences between spinal fusion and cervical laminectomy are noted. (See *Clinical snapshot: Laminectomy,* page 206.)

ETIOLOGY AND PRECIPITATING FACTORS

For a herniated disk, causes include:
- disk degeneration

- trauma — for example, an accident, strain, or repeated minor stresses
- osteoarthritis
- poor body mechanics that cause low back strain
- congenital predisposition.

Focused assessment guidelines

NURSING HISTORY (FUNCTIONAL HEALTH PATTERN FINDINGS)

Health-perception–health-management pattern
- Pain in lumbosacral area accompanied by varying degrees of sensory and motor deficit
- Pain and spasms in cervical area, arm, and neck.
- Dull pain in the buttocks followed by unilateral or bilateral leg pain that may extend to the foot, depending on the level of disk herniation
- Severe burning or stabbing pain, possibly
- Numbness and tingling in the toes and feet
- Pain that usually increases with activities that cause increased intraspinal pressure (such as sitting, sneezing, coughing, straining, and lifting)
- Natural deformity of the lumbar spine
- Obesity
- History of chronic low back pain
- History of employment involving straining, lifting, or twisting
- Gender and age (male patients between ages 20 and 45 are at increased risk)

Nutritional-metabolic pattern
- Dietary history consistent with obesity (high-calorie, high-fat intake)

Activity-exercise pattern
- Altered mobility because of asymmetrical gait
- Lack of physical activity because of pain

Sleep-rest pattern
- Sleep disturbances related to chronic low back pain, aggravated by sleeping on the stomach

Role-relationship pattern
- Greatest concern about the ability to return to work, especially if work involves lifting

PHYSICAL FINDINGS

General appearance
- Anxious or pained facial expression

Cardiovascular
- Radiating pain elicited by jugular vein compression with patient in a standing position (Naffziger's test)

Gastrointestinal

- Constipation (related to inactivity or pressure on spinal nerve roots)

Genitourinary

- Urine retention (related to pressure on spinal nerve roots)

Neurologic

- Increased pain in affected leg with straight leg raising (positive Lasègue's sign)
- Sensory and motor deficit in affected leg and foot
- Paresthesia or numbness in involved limb
- Pain with extension of knee when both hip and knee are at 90-degree flexion (positive Kernig's sign)
- Pain with deep palpation over the affected area
- Decreased or absent Achilles tendon and patellar reflexes
- Deformity of lumbar spine
- Cervical — arm and leg pain, pain around back of shoulder blades, numbness or weakness in arm; rarely, difficulty with hand dexterity or walking

Musculoskeletal

- Muscle spasms (also with cervical disk problems)
- Stabbing, continuous pain in muscle closest to affected disk
- Muscle weakness or atrophy in the affected leg and foot
- Asymmetrical gait
- Decreased ability to bend forward
- Restricted lateral movement
- Leaning away from affected side during standing or ambulation
- Absence of normal lumbar lordosis and presence of lumbar scoliosis with reflex muscle spasms
- Tense posture

DIAGNOSTIC STUDIES

- Cerebrospinal fluid (CSF) — protein level may be elevated 70 to 100 mg/dl
- Hemoglobin level and hematocrit — performed as a prerequisite for surgery and as a baseline for comparison with postoperative values to detect bleeding
- Computed tomography (CT) scan — may show disk protrusion or prolapse
- Spine X-ray — may show narrowed vertebral interspaces at the level of disk degeneration, with flattening of the lumbar curve
- Magnetic resonance imaging (MRI) — may reveal herniated disk, disk pressure on the spinal cord or nerve root
- Myelogram — may confirm a herniated disk and show the precise level of herniation
- Electromyogram — may indicate neural and muscle damage as well as the level and site of injury

POTENTIAL COMPLICATIONS

- Unrelieved acute pain
- Muscle weakness and atrophy
- Paralysis
- Altered bowel or bladder function
- Chronic pain
- Impaired mobility

CLINICAL SNAPSHOT ✳

Laminectomy

Major nursing diagnoses and collaborative problems	Key patient outcomes
ND: Deficient knowledge (impending surgery)	Verbalize understanding of preoperative instructions.
CP: Risk for sensory and motor deficits	Have circulatory, motor, and sensory function improve or return to prehospitalization level.
CP: Risk for cerebrospinal fistula	Have no CSF drainage from the incision.
ND: Acute pain	Describe pain as within tolerable limits (typically less than 3 on a 0 to 10 pain rating scale).
CP: Risk for paralytic ileus	Have normal bowel sounds.
ND: Risk for deficient fluid volume	Have stable vital signs, typically: heart rate, 60 to 100 beats/minute; systolic blood pressure, 90 to 140 mm Hg; and diastolic blood pressure, 50 to 90 mm Hg.
ND: Ineffective tissue perfusion (renal)	Show balanced fluid intake and output.
ND: Deficient knowledge (home care)	Verbalize understanding of recommended follow-up home care.

Nursing diagnosis

Deficient knowledge (impending surgery) related to lack of exposure to information

NURSING PRIORITY

Prepare the patient to cope with the surgical experience.

PATIENT OUTCOME CRITERIA

By the day of surgery, the patient will:
- verbalize understanding of preoperative instruction
- correctly demonstrate logrolling, leg exercises, use of an incentive spirometer, and coughing and deep breathing.

INTERVENTIONS

1. *Provide specific preoperative teaching** for the patient who will have spinal surgery. Also provide general preoperative teaching (see the "Perioperative care" care plan, page 146 for details).
–Give instructions and fit the patient for a brace if required postoperatively.
–For spinal fusion, explain the type of graft to be used, the donor site, and the amount of expected postoperative pain.

2. *Explain what will happen postoperatively,* including:
– frequent taking of vital signs and neurovascular observations of the extremities, and inspection of the operative site and donor site, if present
– turning by logrolling during the first 48 hours
– positioning with pillows under the thigh of each leg when the patient is in a supine position, between legs in side-lying position, to maintain proper body alignment
– keeping the head of the bed flat
– coughing and deep breathing with the back firmly against the mattress or with a pillow held against the chest for splinting purposes
– using a urinal or bedpan while the patient lies flat in bed
– wearing antiembolism stockings or sequential compression devices and performing ankle and foot exercises
– beginning progressive activity 24 to 48 hours after surgery, depending on the physician's preference
– avoiding flexing, hyperextending, turning, or twisting the lumbar spine
– using the correct method for moving from the lying to the standing position (for example, maintaining spinal alignment, keeping the back straight, and using arm and leg muscles to change position)
– sitting in a straight-backed chair with feet on the floor
– exercising as ordered to strengthen arm, leg, and abdominal muscles
– with spinal fusion, being on bed rest for the first 24 hours and logrolling every two hours

RATIONALES

1. The patient having a spinal surgery usually has undergone a long period or intermittent periods of conservative treatment. The surgery is preceded by chronic pain, a decrease in physical activity, and possible absence from work. The patient may view the surgery with relief but also with anxiety about the possible results. Information about the specific procedure will help to allay anxieties about having spinal surgery. The "Perioperative care" care plan provides detailed information on general preoperative teaching.

2. The patient's understanding of the postoperative routine helps avoid complications, such as increased pressure on the operative site or twisting of the spinal column. Correct body alignment should be maintained in all positions to prevent trauma to the surgical site and to decrease discomfort. Other potential complications, such as pneumonia or atelectasis and thromboembolism, also may be prevented by proper postoperative care.

Neurologic disorders

---

*Italics indicate key interventions.

– with cervical laminectomy or fusion, having the head of the bed elevated 30 to 45 degrees or as ordered; using a small towel or pillow under the head to maintain spinal alignment
– if the patient is wearing a brace or collar, having no position restrictions
– having a nurse assess the patient's airway functioning and swallowing frequently.

3. *Demonstrate logrolling, leg exercises, incentive spirometry, coughing and deep breathing, and have the patient practice these techniques before surgery.*

3. Practicing these techniques before surgery will help the patient perform them more effectively postoperatively, helping to prevent circulatory and respiratory complications.

4. *Explain the sources of postoperative pain.* Tell the patient that preoperative numbness or pain in the affected leg will remain for some time after the surgery because of nerve irritation and edema. Also explain that muscle spasms may occur.

4. This knowledge helps allay the patient's anxiety that the surgery might not be successful when numbness or tingling occurs or when weakness makes moving the extremities difficult. Muscle spasms that typically occur on the 3rd or 4th postoperative day are accompanied by severe pain.

5. *Provide information about comfort measures,* including:
– the importance of communication with the staff about the patient's pain (characteristics and tolerance) and anxiety
– the availability of analgesics

– giving injections in the least painful area

– positioning.

5. The patient should know that measures are available to promote postoperative comfort.
– Pain tolerance is individual, and the patient who's anxious about the potential for injury from movement may feel more discomfort.
– Medicating as needed and encouraging the patient to request medication before pain becomes severe can help maintain comfort.
– I.M. injections given in the unaffected buttock, or in the deltoid muscle if both buttocks are affected, cause the least pain.
– Proper body alignment increases patient comfort.

6. Additional individualized interventions: _____

6. Rationales: _____

Suggested NIC Interventions
Teaching: Procedure/treatment

Suggested NOC Outcomes
Knowledge: Treatment regimen

Collaborative problem

Risk for sensory and motor deficits related to the surgical procedure, edema, or hematoma at the operative site

NURSING PRIORITY
Prevent or minimize neurovascular impairment.

PATIENT OUTCOME CRITERIA
Within 48 hours after surgery, the patient will:
■ have normal circulatory, motor, and sensory function in the lower extremities (the same as before hospitalization or improved)
■ have no signs or symptoms of hematoma
■ maintain correct body alignment.

INTERVENTIONS

1. *Document the neurovascular status of the extremities every 2 hours or as needed* for 24 to 48 hours: skin color and temperature, sensation and motion, edema, peripheral pulses, capillary refill time, ability to flex and extend the foot and toes, muscle strength, numbness or tingling in the extremities, and tone and strength in the quadriceps. Compare bilateral findings. Report new tingling, paresthesia, or muscle weakness.

2. *Assess pain* in the neck or upper extremities for cervical laminectomy or lower extremities for lumbar surgeries. Determine exact location and whether the pain is diminishing or worsening.

3. *Assess for hematoma formation at the surgical site,* looking for such indications as severe incision pain unrelieved by analgesics and decreased motor function and sensation in the involved area.

4. *If signs and symptoms of neurovascular damage occur, notify the physician immediately.*

5. *Implement measures to prevent neurovascular damage* in the extremities:
– Maintain proper body alignment by logrolling (every 2 hours for the first 24 to 48 hours) and positioning with pillows.
– Use a firm mattress and a bed board.

6. *Maintain patency of the wound drainage system* if present.

7. Administer corticosteroids if ordered, and document their use.

8. *Implement measures to minimize neurovascular damage* if initial signs and symptoms of impairment occur.
– Assess for and correct improper body alignment.
– If footdrop is present, initiate passive range-of-motion exercises every 1 to 2 hours while the patient is awake.
– Stabilize the foot with ancillary equipment, such as a footboard, sandbags, pillows, foam boots, or foot positioners.

9. Prepare the patient for surgical intervention if evacuation of a hematoma at the surgical site is indicated. See the "Perioperative care" care plan, page 146.

10. Additional individualized interventions: _____

RATIONALES

1. Postoperative deficits may result from pressure on the spinal cord or spinal nerve roots caused by surgical trauma or hematoma. Early detection of altered function allows for prompt intervention.

2. Although preoperative numbness and pain in the lower back and affected leg will remain for some time after surgery, pain may increase from edema secondary to nerve compression. Early detection of nerve compression allows for prompt intervention.

3. An untreated hematoma at the surgical site may cause such irreversible neurologic damage as paraplegia or bowel and bladder dysfunction.

4. Prompt intervention may help minimize neurovascular damage.

5. These measures help reduce stress and pressure on the surgical site until healing occurs.

6. Maintaining drainage decreases pressure on the surgical site. A hematoma may cause serious neurovascular complications.

7. Corticosteroids decrease inflammation in the surgical area.

8. These measures help prevent further damage from uneven or excessive pressure on the operative site. Permanent disability may be prevented by careful attention to the occurrence and prompt treatment of motor and sensory deficits.

9. Prompt evacuation of a hematoma may minimize damage. Adequate preparation of the patient for surgical intervention helps allay anxieties. The "Perioperative care" care plan provides further details.

10. Rationales: _____

Neurologic disorders

Collaborative problem

Risk for cerebrospinal fistula associated with incomplete closure of the dura at the surgical site

NURSING PRIORITY

Detect any CSF leakage promptly.

PATIENT OUTCOME CRITERIA

Throughout the postoperative period, the patient will have:
- no CSF drainage from incision
- no signs or symptoms of meningitis.

INTERVENTIONS	RATIONALES
1. *Observe the patient carefully* every 2 to 4 hours for clear or slightly yellow drainage on or around the dressing or bulging at the incision site.	**1.** An abnormal opening between the subarachnoid space and the incision causes CSF to drain. Drainage on the dressing is an important sign of a fistula, usually a late postoperative complication occurring about a week after surgery. Bulging at the incision site may be due to a CSF leak or hematoma. Early detection of CSF leakage allows for prompt intervention and treatment. The patient is usually kept on flat bed rest 7 to 10 days to allow the dura tear to heal.
2. *Test the dressing with a reagent strip to check for glucose.*	**2.** Glucose is a CSF component whose presence indicates a fistula; it isn't normally present in serous wound drainage.
3. *Determine if the patient has a headache.*	**3.** A headache is a common symptom associated with CSF loss.
4. *Document any CSF drainage, and notify the physician immediately if it occurs.*	**4.** Untreated CSF leakage may be fatal.
5. *Implement measures to reduce stress on the surgical site.* See the "Acute pain" care plan, page 32, for details.	**5.** Decreasing stress on the surgical site, for example by logrolling and maintaining proper body alignment, promotes healing of the dura, which is incised during the surgical procedure. The "Acute pain" care plan contains specific details about stress reduction measures.
6. *Change the dressing when it becomes damp,* using strict sterile technique. *Assess for infection* at the incision site.	**6.** Microorganisms can pass through the fistula, multiply in the CSF, and infect the central nervous system. Changing a damp dressing immediately using sterile technique helps prevent infection at the site and reduces the risk of meningitis.
7. *Administer antibiotics as ordered,* and document their use.	**7.** Antibiotics help treat or prevent infection.
8. *Monitor temperature* every 4 hours for 48 to 72 hours after surgery. Monitor the white blood cell (WBC) count daily as ordered.	**8.** The temperature may be elevated to 102° F (38.9° C) for the first few postoperative days because of the body's normal response to tissue injury and inflammation. Temperature elevation from infection would normally be accompanied by an increased WBC count.
9. *Assess for signs and symptoms of meningitis:* headache, fever, chills, nuchal rigidity, photophobia, and positive Kernig's and Brudzinski's signs.	**9.** Meningitis is a common complication resulting from contamination of CSF. Undetected, it may be fatal within a short time.

10. If a fistula occurs and doesn't heal spontaneously, prepare the patient for surgical closure. See the "Perioperative care" care plan, page 146.

11. Additional individualized interventions: _____
_____

10. Adequate preparation before surgical closure of the dura helps allay patient anxiety. The "Perioperative care" care plan contains detailed information on preparation for surgery.

11. Rationales: _____
_____

Nursing diagnosis

Acute pain related to immobility, muscle spasm, and paresthesia secondary to surgical trauma and postoperative edema

NURSING PRIORITY

Relieve discomfort or pain.

PATIENT OUTCOME CRITERIA

Within 1 day of surgery, the patient will:
- describe pain as within tolerable limits (typically less than 3 on a 0 to 10 pain rating scale)
- verbalize decreased pain, numbness, and tingling.
  Within 2 days of surgery, the patient will:
- increase participation in activities (as allowed).
  Within 3 days of surgery, the patient will:
- tolerate prescribed activity.
  By the time of discharge, the patient will:
- use correct body mechanics and ambulate well.

INTERVENTIONS

1. *Refer to the "Acute pain" care plan, page 32.*

2. *Assess the lumbar laminectomy or spinal fusion patient every 2 to 4 hours for discomfort or pain* — specifically, muscle spasm and pain in the lower back, abdomen, and thighs as well as pain, numbness, or tingling in the affected leg or legs. For cervical surgery, assess for pain at the donor site as well as in the neck and arms. If pain is present at the donor site, apply an ice bag as needed and give ice chips for sore throat.

3. *Assess for associated signs and symptoms:* rubbing of the lower back and hips, guarding of the affected extremity, and showing reluctance to move. For cervical surgery, assess for pain at the donor site as well in the neck and arms.

4. *Administer muscle relaxants or anti-inflammatory agents as ordered,* and document their effects.

RATIONALES

1. The "Acute pain" care plan contains general information on pain as well as additional information specific to laminectomy.

2. Preoperative numbness and pain in the lower back and affected leg will remain for some time after surgery. (Some patients experience pain and muscle spasm throughout the hospital stay). Postoperative pain and muscle spasms are usually caused by irritation of nerve roots and muscles from edema and surgical trauma. Muscle spasms tend to occur on the 3rd or 4th postoperative day. Using a pain rating scale improves consistency of pain assessment. In cervical surgery, donor sites are typically more painful than the operative site.

3. The patient may not report pain, but nonverbal indicators may reveal its presence. Some patients are reluctant to request pain medication.

4. These drugs decrease pain and discomfort. Muscle relaxants (such as diazepam [Valium] or methocarbamol [Robaxin]) decrease muscle spasms; anti-inflammatory agents (such as dexamethasone [Decadron]) reduce edema and inflammation at the operative site.

Neurologic disorders

5. *Administer analgesics judiciously as ordered,* and document their use. Use patient-controlled analgesia (PCA) as ordered. Assess the patient for pain relief 30 minutes after giving medication and document findings.

5. Pain medication works best when it's given before the onset of severe pain. If the patient is accustomed to chronic back pain, he may wait to request medication until the pain is severe, when the medication may provide less relief. Medication administered per a PCA pump allows for continuous pain relief.

6. *To reduce the patient's discomfort,* take the following measures:
– Position the patient to maintain body alignment with his spine straight.
– Use a firm mattress or a bed board under the mattress.
– Avoid positioning the patient in the prone position.
– Logroll for the first 48 hours after surgery to avoid twisting, flexing, or hyperextending the spine.
– Elevate the head of the bed with the patient's knees slightly flexed or positioned as ordered.
– Turn the patient every 2 hours.
– Use a bed cradle over areas of paresthesia.
– Place personal items and the call bell within the patient's reach.
– Teach the patient to avoid coughing, sneezing, or straining at stool.

6. These measures help alleviate discomfort by reducing stress and strain on the surgical site and by reducing pressure on the spinal nerve roots.

7. *Maintain the patient on bed rest for 24 to 48 hours* or as ordered.

7. Bed rest promotes healing.

8. Use a trapeze bar if prescribed.

8. A trapeze bar will assist the patient in moving.

9. When increased activity is ordered, instruct the patient about getting out of bed using arm and abdominal muscles; limiting initial activity to sitting in a straight-backed chair for short intervals or ambulating; and avoiding slumping or limping.

9. Activity must be increased gradually and proper body alignment must be maintained at all times to prevent muscle spasm and spinal trauma. Although slumping and limping may be comfortable at first, they cause fatigue.

10. Consult with the physician about using antitussives, decongestants, laxatives, or stool softeners, as needed.

10. Use of these medications as indicated prevents pressure and associated stress on the surgical site.

11. Additional individualized interventions:_____

11. Rationales:_____

Suggested NIC Interventions
Medication management; Pain management; Analgesic administration

Suggested NOC Outcomes
Comfort level; Pain control; Pain: Disruptive effects; Pain level

---

Collaborative problem

Risk for paralytic ileus related to anesthesia, medications, retroperitoneal bleeding, or injury to the spinal nerve roots

NURSING PRIORITY

Prevent or promptly detect paralytic ileus.

PATIENT OUTCOME CRITERIA

Within 2 days of surgery, the patient will:
■ have bowel sounds and expel flatus.
  By the time of discharge, the patient will:
■ have normal bowel sounds.

INTERVENTIONS

1. *Perform a complete abdominal assessment every 4 hours for at least the first 48 hours after surgery, then in all four quadrants as needed.* Auscultate for bowel sounds and inspect, palpate, and percuss for abdominal distention. Measure abdominal girth if distention is present. Observe for passing of flatus.

2. *Assess for associated signs and symptoms of ileus,* such as nausea, vomiting, and increased back pain.

3. *Notify the physician of abdominal distention or absent bowel sounds.* See the "Perioperative care" care plan, page 146, for further management.

4. Allow the patient to sit for bowel movements, condition permitting. Otherwise, logroll the patient onto a fracture bedpan.

5. Additional individualized interventions: _____
_____

RATIONALES

1. Transient paralytic ileus is a common complication after laminectomy. Parasympathetic nervous system and sympathetic nervous system (SNS) innervation of the bowels originates in the lumbosacral spine. SNS stimulation contributes to loss of peristalsis and to decreased contraction of the internal sphincters, resulting in paralytic ileus. Normal bowel sounds (5 to 30 per minute) passing flatus, and a soft, tympanic, nondistended abdomen indicate normal bowel functioning.

2. If ileus is present, attempts to take fluids orally will cause nausea and vomiting. Back pain may worsen from increased pressure on the surgical site.

3. These signs may indicate ileus has developed. Immediate intervention is required. The "Perioperative care" care plan provides further details.

4. The sitting position helps the patient to expel flatus and stools while maintaining correct spinal alignment.

5. Rationales: _____
_____

Nursing diagnosis

Risk for deficient fluid volume related to blood loss during surgery, vascular injury, hemorrhage at the incision site, or retroperitoneal hemorrhage

NURSING PRIORITY
Prevent or minimize bleeding.

PATIENT OUTCOME CRITERIA
Within 4 hours of surgery, the patient will:
■ have no unusual bleeding or change in status.
  Within 24 hours of surgery, the patient will:
■ have stable vital signs, typically: heart rate, 60 to 100 beats/minute; systolic blood pressure, 90 to 140 mm Hg, and diastolic blood pressure 50 to 90 mm Hg
■ show no signs of bleeding
■ have normal hemoglobin level and hematocrit.

INTERVENTIONS

1. *Implement standard postoperative care related to potential deficient fluid volume:* monitor vital signs, clinical status, hemoglobin level and hematocrit, and surgical drainage. See the "Perioperative care" care plan, page 146, for details.

2. *Assess for flank pain, tenderness, and paresthesia* every 2 to 4 hours for the first 72 hours, then every 8 hours. Compare findings with previous assessments. Observe for bulging at the incision site.

3. *Monitor drainage from the surgical drain,* usually a Jackson-Pratt drain or closed drainage system.

RATIONALES

1. The "Perioperative care" care plan contains detailed measures that apply to any postoperative patient. This plan provides additional measures specific to laminectomy.

2. These symptoms may indicate retroperitoneal hemorrhage. Bulging at the incision site may be due to hematoma.

3. Drainage is usually minimal. Excessive drainage indicates bleeding.

4. *Notify the physician of any unusual bleeding or a change in status.*

5. Additional individualized interventions: _____

_____

4. Prompt intervention is essential to prevent shock.

5. Rationales: _____

_____

Suggested NIC Interventions
Acid-base management; Fluid and electrolyte management; Fluid monitoring; Hypovolemia management; intravenous (I.V.) therapy

Suggested NOC Outcomes
Electrolyte and acid-base balance; Fluid balance; Hydration

Nursing diagnosis

Ineffective tissue perfusion (renal) related to supine positioning, pain, anxiety, narcotics, anesthesia, decreased activity, cord edema, or injury to the spinal nerve roots innervating the bladder

NURSING PRIORITY

Prevent or minimize urine retention.

PATIENT OUTCOME CRITERIA

Within 8 hours of surgery, the patient will have:
- adequate urine output
- no complaints of urgency, fullness, or suprapubic discomfort
- no suprapubic distention.
  Within 2 days of surgery, the patient will:
- show balanced fluid intake and output
- void sufficiently at normal intervals.

INTERVENTIONS

1. *Assess for signs and symptoms of urine retention,* such as absence of voiding within 8 hours of surgery, frequent voiding of small amounts (50 ml or less), complaints of bladder fullness or urgency, pain on palpating bladder, and suprapubic distention.

2. *Implement standard postoperative measures to monitor fluid intake and output, facilitate voiding, and provide catheterization.* See the "Perioperative care" care plan, page 146, for details.

3. Administer bethanechol (Urecholine) as ordered.

4. Additional individualized interventions: _____

_____

RATIONALES

1. Pain and lying flat in bed make it difficult for the patient to void after surgery. Transient voiding problems caused by temporary loss of bladder tone from cord edema are common after lumbar laminectomy. Autonomic innervation of the bladder smooth muscle is from the thoracolumbar sympathetic outflow and the sacral parasympathetic outflow. Cervical surgery may affect the parasympathetic system. The micturition center is located in the lumbosacral area. An inability to void or incontinence may also indicate damage to the sacral spinal nerves controlling the detrusor muscle in the bladder.

2. These measures are the same for any postoperative patient and are explained further in the "Perioperative care" care plan.

3. Bethanechol stimulates the detrusor muscles of the bladder.

4. Rationales: _____

_____

> **Suggested NIC Interventions**
> *Urinary bladder training; Urinary catheterization: Intermittent; Urinary elimination management; Urinary retention care*

> **Suggested NOC Outcomes**
> *Urinary continence; Urinary elimination*

Nursing diagnosis

Deficient knowledge (home care) related to lack of exposure to information

NURSING PRIORITY

Increase knowledge about home care.

PATIENT OUTCOME CRITERIA

By the time of discharge, the patient will, upon request:
- list signs and symptoms of complications to report to the physician
- verbalize understanding of recommended follow-up home care
- list five ways to help prevent recurrent disk herniation.

INTERVENTIONS

1. *Tell the patient to report signs and symptoms to the physician,* including:
– change in movement, sensation, color, pain, or temperature in the extremities
– new onset of neurologic deficit or pain
– increased pain at the incision site
– difficulty standing erect
– persistent or severe headache
– drainage from the incision site
– bleeding from the incision
– swelling or redness around the incision site or odor from site
– elevated temperature
– loss of bowel or bladder function
– symptoms of graft dislodgment, such as dysphagia and feeling of "fullness" in the throat (for cervical fusion or laminectomy).

2. *Teach the patient about care of the incision including:*
– keeping sutures or staples clean and dry
– changing dressing when it becomes damp or soiled.

3. *Teach the patient about postsurgical restrictions* and when to resume activities (at approximately 6 to 12 weeks postsurgery), including:
– restricting driving and riding in cars
– avoiding pulling, bending, stooping, pushing, lifting, twisting, or stair climbing
– logrolling into or out of bed
– avoiding tub bathing
– refraining from sexual activity
– standing or sitting for only short periods
– resting after activities
– avoiding carrying or lifting anything heavier than 5 lb (2.3 kg)
– avoiding heavy work for 6 to 12 weeks after surgery

RATIONALES

1. Knowing what to observe for and report will help minimize complications.

2. These measures help prevent infection.

3. Patients may hesitate to ask questions about home activities. Providing information before discharge about activities that place stress on the spinal column and incision site may prevent complications.

– wearing a brace or collar for 6 weeks or as ordered for cervical laminectomy or fusion.

4. *Provide information about comfort measures,* including:
– lying with knees bent
– using stronger muscles, such as arm and leg muscles, to change positions
– shifting weight from one foot to the other when standing for long periods
– sitting with knees higher than hips
– using correct posture when sitting or standing
– sitting forward with knees crossed and with abdominal muscles tightened to flatten the back (if sitting for long periods)
– sleeping on one's side
– sleeping on one's back only if the knees are supported with a pillow
– using a heating pad as needed
– using prescribed muscle relaxants or analgesics
– avoiding fatigue and cold.

4. Muscle spasms and pain may persist for a time after surgery. Reducing pain, spasms, and stress on the lumbosacral spine will increase comfort.

5. *Provide information about recommended alterations in lifestyle to reduce back strain,* such as:
– sleeping on a firm mattress or a bed board
– sitting on firm, straight-backed chairs
– using proper body mechanics (for example, bending at the knees, rather than at the waist, and carrying objects close to the body)
– maintaining correct posture
– wearing supportive shoes with moderate heels
– avoiding lifting heavy objects
– using thoracic and abdominal muscles when lifting objects
– using assistive devices, such as long-handled brushes and shoe horns
– using proper techniques for prescribed exercises
– scheduling adequate rest periods
– reducing or stopping any activity that causes or aggravates discomfort
– maintaining optimal weight using a prescribed, progressive exercise program if necessary.

5. Disk herniation can recur in the same area or at other levels of the lumbosacral spinal cord, particularly if degenerative changes are present. Reducing back strain lessens the potential for disk herniation.

6. *Provide additional instructions for patients with spinal fusion,* such as:
– wearing a chairback brace or rigid device when not in bed
– putting on a device or brace when they're in bed by logrolling if ordered
– using proper body mechanics
– avoid sitting or standing for long periods of time.

6. These measures help maintain spinal alignment and stability and prevent stress on the operative site.

7. Additional individualized interventions:_____

7. Rationales: _____

Suggested NIC Interventions	Suggested NOC Outcomes
Teaching: Procedure/treatment	*Knowledge: Treatment regimen*

Discharge planning

DISCHARGE CHECKLIST

Before discharge, the patient shows evidence of:
- ❐ stable vital signs
- ❐ absence of fever
- ❐ absence of signs and symptoms of infection
- ❐ absence of cardiovascular or pulmonary complications, such as atelectasis and thrombophlebitis
- ❐ WBC count, hematocrit, and hemoglobin level within normal parameters
- ❐ decreasing pain, muscle spasm, numbness, and tingling in lower extremities (for lumbar surgery)
- ❐ decreasing pain in arm and neck and decreasing numbness or weakness of arm (for cervical surgery)
- ❐ ability to control pain using oral medications
- ❐ absence of bowel or bladder dysfunction
- ❐ wound drainage within expected parameters
- ❐ ability to perform wound care independently or with minimal assistance, using appropriate technique
- ❐ ability to tolerate adequate nutritional intake
- ❐ knowledge of activity restrictions
- ❐ ability to perform activities of daily living and to transfer and ambulate independently or with minimal assistance
- ❐ completion of initial physical therapy assessment and instructions
- ❐ adequate home support system or referral to home care if indicated by inadequate home support system or inability to perform self-care.

TEACHING CHECKLIST

Document evidence that the patient and his family demonstrate an understanding of:
- ❐ the purpose, dosages, administration schedule, and adverse effects of discharge medications (pain medications may be prescribed for continued pain and muscle spasm; laxatives may be prescribed to prevent constipation)
- ❐ infection prevention
- ❐ signs and symptoms of postoperative infection
- ❐ signs and symptoms of CSF drainage
- ❐ when and how to report signs and symptoms of complications
- ❐ recommended alterations in lifestyle to prevent recurrence of back problems
- ❐ comfort measures
- ❐ correct body mechanics
- ❐ use of pain-relief measures
- ❐ postsurgical activity restrictions
- ❐ date, time, and location of follow-up appointments

- ❐ how to contact the physician
- ❐ adequate nutritional intake.

DOCUMENTATION CHECKLIST

Using outcome criteria as a guide, document:
- ❐ patient's clinical status on admission
- ❐ significant changes in status, especially motor or sensory deficits, headaches, and weakness
- ❐ results of myelography, spine X-ray, CT scan, electromyography, MRI, and hemoglobin and hematocrit testing
- ❐ episodes of muscle spasms, severe pain at incision site or in extremities
- ❐ pain-relief measures
- ❐ nutritional intake
- ❐ elimination habits
- ❐ preoperative teaching
- ❐ patient and family teaching
- ❐ discharge planning.

Associated care plans

- ■ Acute pain
- ■ Anxiety
- ■ Impaired physical mobility
- ■ Ineffective individual coping
- ■ Knowledge deficit
- ■ Perioperative care
- ■ Pneumonia

References

Black, J., et al. *Medical-Surgical Nursing Clinical Management for Positive Outcomes,* 6th ed. Philadelphia: W.B. Saunders Co., 2001.

Hickey, J.V. *The Clinical Practice of Neurological and Neurosurgical Nursing,* 5th ed. Philadelphia: Lippincott Williams & Wilkins, 2002.

Ignatavicius, D.D., and Workman, M.L. *Medical-Surgical Nursing Critical Thinking for Collaborative Care,* 4th ed. Philadelphia: W.B. Saunders Co., 2002.

Lewis, S.M., et al. *Medical-Surgical Nursing Assessment and Management of Clinical Problems,* 5th ed. St. Louis: Mosby–Year Book, Inc., 2000.

Neurologic disorders

Multiple sclerosis

DRG INFORMATION
DRG 013   Multiple Sclerosis and Cerebellar Ataxia.
         Mean LOS = 5.4 days

Additional DRG information: Patients with multiple sclerosis (MS) are most commonly admitted to an acute care setting for complications, such as pneumonia or bowel or bladder dysfunction. However, in the past 5 years, some neurologists have been admitting MS patients for trials of various I.V. medications used to counteract MS symptoms. Only in these rare circumstances would MS be the principal diagnosis. More commonly, an MS patient would be diagnosed with another illness, and the DRG would be related to the principal diagnosis.

Introduction
DEFINITION AND TIME FOCUS
MS is a relatively common, chronic, degenerative disease causing demyelinization of the central nervous system (CNS). Approximately 500,000 cases occur in the United States each year. The disease is characterized by recurrent inflammatory reactions and the formation of sclerotic plaques throughout the CNS, which interfere with normal impulse conduction and eventually cause irreversible neurologic deficits. Exacerbations and remissions are common, with some symptoms appearing only briefly or intermittently. The prognosis is variable: Approximately one-third of patients experience minimal disability and can continue most normal activities; the remaining two-thirds have moderate to severe limitations and are susceptible to complications associated with relative or absolute immobility. MS affects about five times more women than men and typically is diagnosed in patients between ages 20 and 40. This care plan focuses on the patient admitted for diagnosis or management during an acute episode of MS. (See *Clinical snapshot: Multiple sclerosis*, page 220.)

ETIOLOGY AND PRECIPITATING FACTORS
Although the exact cause of MS isn't known, much scientific research indicates that several factors in combination are probably involved.
Immunologic
It's now generally accepted that MS involves an autoimmune process that causes the destruction of myelin, the fatty sheath that surrounds and insulates the nerve fibers. The demyelination causes nerve impulses to be slowed or halted, producing the symptoms of MS.

Environmental
The farther away from the equator, the greater the incidence of MS. Children who live in northern climates (high risk) and then move to a southern climate (low risk) before puberty, will greatly reduce their risk of developing MS in later life. However, teens and adults who similarly move aren't afforded the same protection.
Viral
Because some viruses are known causes of demyelination and inflammation, it's possible that a virus is the triggering factor in MS. Although measles, human herpes virus 6, and other viruses have been investigated to determine if they're involved in the development of MS, no definitive viral cause has yet been determined.
Genetic
Having a first-degree relative (parent or sibling) with MS increases the risk that one will develop the disease. Some neurologists theorize that persons are born with sensitivities to environmental agents, which trigger an autoimmune response.

Focused assessment guidelines
NURSING HISTORY
(FUNCTIONAL HEALTH PATTERN FINDINGS)
Health-perception–health-management pattern
■ Onset generally between ages 20 and 40
■ History of symptom-recovery cycles: mild, transient symptoms occurring in one body part, then subsiding, with the patient continuing to see himself as healthy until symptoms appear on another body part
■ Symptom-recovery cycles increasing in frequency and severity
Nutritional-metabolic pattern
■ Difficulty chewing food
■ Exhaustion from effort of eating
■ Choking (dysphagia) episodes from poor muscle control
Elimination pattern
■ Constipation, impaction, or incontinence (related to weakness or spasticity of the anal sphincter)
■ Urgency, frequency, or retention (from loss of bladder sphincter control)
Activity-exercise pattern
■ Spasticity and weakness of limbs
■ Weakness and fatigue with activity
Sleep-rest pattern
■ Initially, reduction of symptoms with rest
■ Later, spasticity that interrupts sleep

Cognitive-perceptual pattern
- Diplopia and eye pain
- Mentation disorders, such as impaired judgment and failure to comprehend or conceptualize

Self-perception–self-concept pattern
- Feelings of diminished self-worth as job performance becomes impaired (psychosocial disequilibrium)
- Emotional lability

Role-relationship pattern
- Increased dependence on others as disease progresses

Sexuality-reproductive pattern
- Occasional impotence in males
- Alterations in vaginal sensation in females
- Inability to achieve orgasm in females

Coping–stress tolerance pattern
- Difficulty adjusting to the disease if diagnosed in early to middle adult life
- Effective coping mechanisms if in remission phase early in the disease
- Ineffective coping mechanisms if exacerbation cycles become more frequent and symptoms more disabling

Value-belief pattern
- Neglect of mild, transient symptoms (denial), only to seek medical attention later when recurring symptoms become more severe

PHYSICAL FINDINGS
Gastrointestinal
- Impaction or incontinence

Neurologic
- Charcot's triad (classic): nystagmus, intention tremors, and scanning (slow, monotonous, slurred) speech
- Loss of coordination
- Ataxia
- Paralysis
- Cranial nerve impairment
- Evidence of optic neuritis with visual field deficits
- Presence of blind spot
- Dysarthria
- Dysphagia
- Loss of facial muscle control
- Lhermitte's sign (sudden "shock wave" down the body on forward neck flexion)
- Hyperreflexic deep tendon reflexes
- Sensory loss, including paresthesia
- Decreased vibratory sensation
- Decreased or absent proprioception

Musculoskeletal
- Spasticity
- Reduced mobility
- Contractures (related to immobility)

Genitourinary
- Incontinence
- Urine retention
- Combination of incontinence and retention

Integumentary
- Reddened pressure points, skin breakdown (effects of immobility)

DIAGNOSTIC STUDIES
- Electrophoresis — elevated oligoclonal banding of immunoglobulin G in 90% of patients (contributes evidence for differential diagnosis of MS)
- Hematology — gamma globulin levels abnormally high, reflecting increased immune system activity
- Evoked response potentials — delayed response after adequate stimulation of visual, auditory, or somatosensory mechanism suggests MS
- Computed tomography scan — may indicate lesion of CNS white matter, atrophy, or ventricular enlargement
- Lumbar puncture — increased protein and white blood cells in cerebrospinal fluid
- Core hyperthermia — increasing body core temperature to 102° F (38.9° C) causes marginal conduction to become incomplete or blocked; use as a diagnostic procedure is controversial because results may resemble symptoms of other CNS diseases; besides being diagnostically inconclusive, the test presents some risk to the patient
- Magnetic resonance imaging — may identify discrete lesion

POTENTIAL COMPLICATIONS
Those associated with immobility include:
- urinary tract infection (UTI)
- respiratory tract infection
- phlebitis or other thromboembolic phenomena.

CLINICAL SNAPSHOT ☀

Multiple sclerosis

Major nursing diagnoses	Key patient outcomes
Impaired physical mobility	Show no evidence of skin breakdown or other effects of immobility.
Constipation	Have satisfactory bowel elimination restored.
Sexual dysfunction	Identify sexual concerns.
Situational low self-esteem	Participate in care planning.
Compromised family coping	(The family will) participate in the patient's care.

Nursing diagnosis

Impaired physical mobility related to demyelinization

NURSING PRIORITIES
- Preserve maximum physical functioning.
- Protect patient from effects of immobility.

PATIENT OUTCOME CRITERIA
Within 3 days of admission, the patient will:
- recognize the need for rest
- show no evidence of skin breakdown or other effects of immobility.
  Within 5 days of admission, the patient will:
- verbalize the need for mobility assistance
- list three safety measures
- function at or above admission level.

INTERVENTIONS	RATIONALES
1. *Provide rest and prevent fatigue.**	1. Rest seems to alleviate symptoms; fatigue may worsen symptoms.
2. Begin a physical therapy program as ordered, including: – active and passive range-of-motion exercises – limb splints – gait training – use of leg weights and heavy shoes for balance during weight bearing – swimming.	2. Exercising prevents joint contractures and improves muscle tone. Circulation improves with exercise. As exercise endurance increases, the patient gains a sense of achievement.
3. *Administer medications as ordered* to control pain and muscle spasm. Observe precautions and watch for adverse reactions, as follows: – diazepam (Valium) — observe for increased fatigue, sedation, confusion, or depression – dantrolene (Dantrium) — monitor liver function studies (serum aspartate aminotransferase and serum alanine aminotransferase) as ordered, and observe for jaundice or other signs of liver damage as well as for drowsiness or increased weakness	3. Medications (antidepressants, analgesics, and antispasmodics) relax the patient by relieving pain and spasm, promoting comfort, and permitting physical activity. Adverse reactions to these medications may make their use questionable for some MS patients. Reduced muscle tone may contribute to increased weakness and risk of injury.

*Italics indicate key interventions.

– baclofen (Lioresal) — observe for increased fatigue, drowsiness, or dizziness.
– amitriptyline (Elavil) — observe for drowsiness or dry mouth
– tizanidine (Zanaflex) — observe for fatigue or drowsiness

4. *Assess breath sounds at least every 8 hours.* Report crackles, rhonchi, decreased breath sounds, or other abnormal findings promptly. Encourage incentive spirometer use as ordered, or other pulmonary hygiene measures.

5. *Teach the patient the need for specific mobility aids and how to use them,* such as a cane, a walker, crutches, or a wheelchair.

6. *Teach the patient safety measures to prevent injury* related to sensory loss, including:
– using a thermometer to test water temperature
– wearing gloves in inclement weather
– wearing an eye patch to alleviate eye disturbances
– using kitchen utensils with insulated handles to prevent burns.

7. *Frequently assess skin and bony prominences for pressure signs.* Reposition the patient to alleviate pressure effects. Teach the patient and his family how to assess skin and minimize pressure.

8. *Minimize the cardiovascular effects of immobility* by:
– using antiembolism stockings on the patient
– teaching the patient leg exercises to increase venous return
– checking indices of peripheral circulation — pulses, color, temperature, sensation, mobility, and capillary refill time
– looking for signs of dependent edema.

9. Administer the following medications as ordered, watching for adverse effects and providing appropriate patient teaching:
– The so-called "ABC" disease-modifying agents interferon beta-1a (Avonex), interferon beta-1b (Betaseron) and glatiramer acetate (Copaxone). Each medication has easy-to-understand and quite effective patient education materials. Some of the companies that produce these drugs have ongoing patient support systems.
– Corticosteroids — observe for hyperglycemia, excessive weight gain, and signs of bleeding, infection, or gastric distress. Caution the patient not to stop taking the medication abruptly without consulting the physician.

4. Immobility contributes to stasis of lung secretions, predisposing the MS patient to infections and other complications related to inadequate chest excursion.

5. Teaching the patient the importance of mobility aids helps the patient adjust to using them. Although adjusting to them may be difficult, aids can prevent injury and offer the mobile patient a sense of security.

6. Impaired sensory perception may cause injury. Especially significant is the effect of temperature changes: Increased core temperature has the potential to accentuate MS symptoms by blocking impulse conduction.

7. Frequent assessment and treatment of pressure areas is necessary because immobility predisposes the patient to circulatory impairment and resultant skin breakdown. Frequent position changes redistribute pressure. Teaching the patient and family may avert postdischarge problems.

8. Immobility influences all systems. Increasing venous return may reduce venous stasis and the risk of thromboembolism. Identifying arterial insufficiency helps ensure peripheral oxygenation. Edema suggests decreased peripheral circulation and the need for prompt limb elevation.

9. Medication therapy varies widely, depending on the patient's status and his physician's preference.

– With the success of these "ABC" disease-modifying agents, initiation of therapy is advised as soon as possible following a definite diagnosis of MS and determination of a relapsing-remitting course.

– Corticosteroids are commonly used for acute exacerbations in combination with disease-modifying agents. These drugs may reduce the length of exacerbations. Sudden withdrawal from corticosteroids may cause adrenal insufficiency.

Neurologic disorders

– Mitoxantrone (Novantrone), observe for seizures, heart failure, arrhythmias, renal failure, myelosuppression and sepsis. Tell the patient that his urine may appear blue-green for 24 hours after administration and sclera may appear bluish.

– Mitoxantrone, an antineoplastic agent, is approved for patients with progressive or worsening MS. Before its approval for use in MS, mitoxantrone was used only to treat certain forms of cancer. It acts in MS by suppressing the activity of immune cells that are thought to lead the attack on the myelin sheath. Because of the cardiotoxicity and adverse-effect profile of this chemotherapeutic drug, it's most safely administered in an oncology setting (outpatient chemotherapy clinic) with an oncologist on-site.

10. *Teach the patient to use stress-reduction techniques,* such as deep breathing, progressive relaxation, or visualization, when appropriate.

10. Stress may induce an acute episode.

11. Additional individualized interventions: _____

11. Rationales: _____

Suggested NIC Interventions
Exercise therapy: Ambulation; Exercise therapy: Balance; Exercise therapy: Joint mobility; Exercise therapy: Muscle control; Exercise promotion: Strength training

Suggested NOC Outcomes
Ambulation: Walking; Ambulation: Wheelchair; Joint movement: Active; Mobility level

---

Nursing diagnosis
Constipation related to demyelinization

NURSING PRIORITY
Maintain bowel function.

PATIENT OUTCOME CRITERIA
Within 5 days of admission, the patient will:
- comply with dietary recommendations
- have satisfactory bowel elimination restored
- list measures to maintain effective elimination, on request.

INTERVENTIONS

1. *Assess and record the patient's pattern of bowel and bladder function.* Identify any dysfunctional pattern.

2. *Evaluate dietary habits.* Determine the need for high-fiber, high-bulk foods, and foods low in saturated fat.

3. *Increase and record fluid intake* as appropriate.

4. *Initiate a bowel program,* as appropriate — for example, manual extraction and stimulation. Consult rehabilitation protocols for bowel retraining.

5. Administer laxatives, stool softeners, propantheline (Pro-Banthine), or polyethylene glycol (MiraLax) as ordered.

RATIONALES

1. MS may cause elimination problems from decreased peristalsis. Evaluating the patient's status helps identify elimination problems; for example, is the elimination problem constipation or retention?

2. A regulated diet high in fiber and bulk promotes normal peristalsis to move bowel contents through the alimentary canal. Foods low in saturated fat are thought to interrupt demyelinization.

3. Increased fluid intake promotes absorption and peristalsis.

4. Mechanical or manual assistance may be needed to overcome the effects of demyelinization on elimination. Protocols vary among institutions.

5. Medication may be required to adjust bowel absorption of metabolites and to reduce bowel spasticity problems.

6. *Teach the patient a bowel program for elimination management at home,* suggesting the following guidelines:
– Use suppositories as ordered.
– Maintain adequate fluid and fiber intake.
– Monitor times and consistency of bowel movements.

7. Additional individualized interventions:_____

6. In many cases, the patient can manage an effective elimination regimen at home, which can help reestablish a sense of independence and control.

7. Rationales: _____

Suggested NIC Interventions
Bowel management; Fluid and electrolyte management; Constipation and impaction management

Suggested NOC Outcomes
Bowel elimination; Hydration; Symptom control

Nursing diagnosis
Sexual dysfunction related to fatigue, decreased sensation, muscle spasm, or urinary incontinence

NURSING PRIORITIES
■ Promote healthy sexual identity.
■ Teach ways to minimize the effects of disease on sexual functioning.

PATIENT OUTCOME CRITERIA
■ During the admission interview, the patient will identify sexual concerns if desired.
■ Throughout the hospital stay, the patient will initiate affection, especially with partner or significant other if desired.
■ By the time of discharge, the patient will list three measures to minimize sexual dysfunction, on request.

INTERVENTIONS

1. *Assess the effects of MS on the patient's sexual function.* During the admission interview, ask the patient how the disease has affected his sexual performance.

2. *Encourage the patient and his spouse or partner to share sexual concerns.* Offer to be available as a resource, or refer the couple to another health care professional.

3. *Offer specific suggestions for identified problems,* such as teaching the patient to:
– initiate sexual activity when his energy levels are highest
– try different positions (for example, side-lying) if muscle spasm makes leg abduction difficult or if weakness limits activity
– empty the bladder before sexual activity and pad the bedding as necessary to protect against wetness
– try oral or manual stimulation if intercourse is difficult or unsatisfying.

RATIONALES

1. MS is extremely variable in its course and effects. The patient may be hesitant to broach the subject of sexuality. Gentle, matter-of-fact questioning during routine assessment provides the patient an opportunity to voice concerns.

2. Even couples who have no difficulty communicating in most areas may find it hard to verbalize feelings related to sexuality. Health professionals who are comfortable discussing sexual issues may be able to start and maintain a dialogue.

3. The patient needs concrete information on specific problems.
– Fatigue contributes to decreased libido.

– Muscle spasms commonly affect hip abductor and adductor muscles. Some positions require less energy expenditure.
– Urinary incontinence is more common during intercourse or masturbation.
– The MS patient may find intercourse less satisfying than before because decreased sensation makes orgasm more difficult to achieve.

Neurologic disorders

4. *Encourage expressions of affection between the patient and his partner.* If ongoing dysfunction has created anxiety about sexual encounters, suggest affectionate "play" sessions without intercourse as the goal.

5. *Emphasize the importance of discussing birth control and family planning with a physician.*

6. Additional individualized interventions: _____
_____

4. Sexuality involves more than the act of coitus. Emphasis on playful, affectionate exchanges between partners helps reduce anxiety, promotes trust, and improves the patient's body image and self-esteem.

5. An intrauterine device may be contraindicated because decreased sensation may cause complications to go undetected. Birth control pills may exacerbate MS symptoms. The familial tendency to develop MS and the lack of prenatal screening for the disease may be significant factors for the patient considering having a child.

6. Rationales: _____ .
_____

> **Suggested NIC Interventions**
> *Sexual counseling*

> **Suggested NOC Outcomes**
> *Sexual functioning*

Nursing diagnosis

Situational low self-esteem related to progressive, debilitating effects of disease

NURSING PRIORITY

Promote a healthy self-image and a realistic acceptance of limitations.

PATIENT OUTCOME CRITERIA

Throughout the hospital stay, the patient will:
- participate actively in care planning
- verbalize feelings related to losses
- participate in family activities as much as possible
- show interest in appearance and grooming
- initiate independent activities
- show an interest in others.

INTERVENTIONS

1. *Encourage the patient to participate in all decisions related to care planning.* Discourage overdependent behaviors. Help the patient set goals and work toward them.

2. *Promote the expression of feelings related to losses.* Avoid overly cheerful responses but still maintain a positive outlook. See the "Grieving" care plan, page 105, and the "Ineffective individual coping" care plan, page 124.

RATIONALES

1. Active participation fosters a sense of control and increases self-esteem. The patient with MS experiences loss of control in many areas; encouraging responsibility for self-care helps maintain dignity and independence. Goal setting helps maintain hope.

2. The patient suffering from a chronic debilitating disease may see each hospital stay as a further step in disease progression and loss of control. Healthy grieving is a realistic response to multiple losses and a normal part of acceptance. Overly cheerful responses indicate a lack of understanding of the profound changes MS entails for the patient. Empathy and realistic optimism, in contrast, show respect for the patient. The general care plans noted suggest other interventions that may be helpful for the patient with MS.

3. *Work with the family to promote maximum patient participation in familiar family roles and rituals or to identify new roles of value for the patient,* such as humorist, correspondent, or arbitrator.

4. During care activities, encourage the patient to touch affected body parts, perform self-lifting activities as much as possible, and participate in grooming and wardrobe selection.

5. *Provide recognition for goals achieved.* Acknowledge evidence of inner strengths and growth as well as external achievements; for example, notice difficult emotional issues the patient has dealt with positively as well as activity goals he has achieved.

6. Additional individualized interventions: _____

3. Disease progression and an increasing sense of helplessness are compounded by the inability to fulfill familiar family roles. Encouraging family recognition and support of these roles minimizes distress. Physical disability may nevertheless allow the patient to assume new roles within the family, thus helping the patient maintain a sense of self-worth.

4. Acceptance of altered body image and function is essential to a healthy self-concept. Touching one's body and becoming familiar with its limitations is the first step toward acceptance. Grooming promotes a positive self-concept.

5. Chronic progressive disease may narrow a patient's world view severely. Recognizing struggles and achievements decreases the sense of isolation. The patient can teach nurses much that may help them care for other patients. Acknowledging this gift may help provide a sense of meaning in difficult times and extend the patient's outlook toward others.

6. Rationales: _____

Suggested NIC Interventions
Decision-making support; Grief work facilitation; Anticipatory guidance; Coping enhancement; Self-esteem enhancement

Suggested NOC Outcomes
Decision making; Grief resolution; Psychosocial adjustment: Life change; Self-esteem

Neurologic disorders

Nursing diagnosis
Compromised family coping related to effects of progressive, debilitating disease on family members and resultant alteration in role-related behavior patterns

NURSING PRIORITY
Maintain family integrity while promoting a healthy adjustment to necessary role changes.

PATIENT OUTCOME CRITERIA
By the time of the patient's discharge, family members will:
- appear healthy and well rested
- participate actively in the patient's care
- participate in home care planning.

INTERVENTIONS

1. Assess the family system by observing family members' interaction with the patient, encouraging family participation in care activities and talking with family members individually or as a group about changes brought about by the disease. See the "Compromised family coping" care plan, page 67. Mention other resources for patients and families, such as the National Multiple Sclerosis Society, 733 Third Ave., New York, NY 10017, E-mail: info@nmss.org.

RATIONALES

1. Chronic diseases can be devastating for families as well as affected individuals. As the primary support for most patients, families must be considered in care planning. Open discussion among family members promotes mutual supportiveness and understanding. The "Compromised family coping" care plan provides interventions especially helpful for families in or at risk for crisis.

2. *Encourage family members to take turns in the caregiving role as necessary.*

2. As the disease progresses, the patient becomes more dependent on others for care. Sharing care responsibilities helps prevent burnout, provides variety in care routines, and allows for mutual understanding.

3. *Help the family understand and accept any mental changes that occur.*

3. From 40% to 60% of MS patients exhibit alterations in mental function, ranging from inattention and euphoria (early in the disease) to irritability, depression, disorientation, and loss of memory (later in the disease). Understanding that these symptoms are part of the disease and not intentional helps minimize distress for the patient and his family.

4. *Promote healthy habits for family members:* Urge adequate rest, proper dietary intake, exercise, and relaxation.

4. Adequate sleep, proper nutrition, exercise, and relaxation help family members remain strong, supportive, and capable of caring for the patient and each other. Guilt feelings may overpower an individual, preventing him from attending to his personal needs, such as hygiene, rest and relaxation, and nutrition and exercise. The health care provider can offer encouragement to help prevent guilt feelings.

5. *Help the family plan changes in the home environment* to make care easier, such as making structural changes (ramps, rails), rearranging furnishings and supplies to allow easy access for the patient, and having special supplies for incontinence available. Help the family arrange for transportation and obtain help with caregiving by providing a social services referral.

5. Without careful planning, the gradual progression of the disease may overwhelm the family with its new demands. Social services can offer many resources for patient and family support at home through volunteer, charitable, church, or public institutions.

6. Additional individualized interventions: _____

6. Rationales: _____

Suggested NIC Interventions
Coping enhancement; Family involvement promotion; Family mobilization; Family support

Suggested NOC Outcomes
Family coping; Family normalization

Discharge planning
DISCHARGE CHECKLIST
Before discharge, the patient shows evidence of:
- ❏ stable vital signs
- ❏ absence of fever
- ❏ absence of pulmonary or cardiovascular complications
- ❏ ability to manage bowel and bladder functioning independently or with minimal assistance
- ❏ absence of signs and symptoms of UTI
- ❏ ability to transfer and ambulate at prehospitalization levels or with minimal assistance, using appropriate assistive devices as ordered
- ❏ ability to tolerate adequate nutritional intake
- ❏ control of muscle spasms and pain with oral medications

- ❏ adequate home support system or referral to home care or a nursing home if indicated by inadequate home support system or inability to perform self-care.

TEACHING CHECKLIST
Document evidence that the patient and his family demonstrate an understanding of:
- ❏ the course and nature of MS
- ❏ the physical therapy program
- ❏ the purpose, dosage, administration schedule, and adverse effects of discharge medications (usual discharge medications include corticosteroids, antispasmodics, and stool softeners)
- ❏ mobility aids
- ❏ safety instructions for protection from injury related to sensory deficits

❏ information regarding problems associated with immobility
❏ stress reduction techniques
❏ specific suggestions for sexual problems
❏ community resources
❏ recommended therapeutic diet, including selection of
foods low in saturated fat
❏ bowel and bladder program
❏ the importance of avoiding exposure to infection
❏ the date, time, and location of follow-up appointments
❏ when to call the physician
❏ how to contact the physician.

DOCUMENTATION CHECKLIST
Using outcome criteria as a guide, document:
❏ the patient's clinical status on admission
❏ significant changes in clinical status
❏ pertinent laboratory data and diagnostic findings
❏ physical therapy program and activity tolerance
❏ medication administration
❏ nutritional intake
❏ fluid intake and output
❏ bowel and bladder function
❏ patient and family teaching
❏ discharge planning.

Associated care plans
■ Compromised family coping
■ Grieving
■ Ineffective individual coping

References
Lisak, D. "Overview of Symptomatic Management of Multiple
Sclerosis," *Journal of Neuroscience Nursing* 33(5):224-30,
October 2001.
Maloni, H.W. "Pain in Multiple Sclerosis: An Overview of its
Nature and Management," *Journal of Neuroscience Nursing*
32(3):139-44, June 2000.
The National Multiple Sclerosis Society. Etiology. Available:
www.nationalmssociety.org/sourcebook-etiology.asp.
Rudick R.A. "Contemporary Immunomodulatory Therapy
for Multiple Sclerosis," *Journal of Neuro-Ophthalmology*
21(4):284-91, December 2001.

Neurologic disorders

Seizures

DRG INFORMATION

DRG 024   Seizure and Headache with Complication or Comorbidity (CC). Age 17+.
Mean LOS = 5.0 days

DRG 025   Seizure and Headache without CC. Age 17+.
Mean LOS = 3.2 days

DRG 026   Seizure and Headache. Ages 0 to 17.
Mean LOS = 3.0 days

Introduction

DEFINITION AND TIME FOCUS

A seizure represents uncontrolled, paroxysmal, abnormal electrical discharge in the central nervous system (CNS). The precise mechanism involved isn't known, but a decreased neuronal firing threshold or excessive irritability is suspected.

Seizures are described as primary or secondary, depending on whether the cause can be identified. Primary (idiopathic) seizures appear without any identifiable cause, commonly arise in childhood, and may result from a congenital tendency. Secondary seizures are triggered by specific metabolic, structural, chemical, or physical abnormalities. Diagnostically, seizures are classified into two broad groups: partial and generalized. Partial seizures involve localized areas of brain irritability and are characterized by physical activity that corresponds to the affected area of the brain. Loss of consciousness may not occur. Generalized seizures involve both brain hemispheres and, usually, major bilateral muscle activity and loss of consciousness.

Seizures are commonly a sign of underlying abnormality, and any seizure, even in a patient with a preexisting seizure history, must be evaluated within the context of the patient's overall condition. In some patients, a single, brief seizure may be of minimal concern; in others, it may represent grave deterioration in the patient's neurologic status. Persistent or recurrent generalized seizures warrant immediate pharmacologic control and prompt identification and treatment of the underlying cause. Because seizures present such a wide range of physical manifestations, this care plan focuses on the patient exhibiting generalized tonic-clonic seizures; you should, however, be knowledgeable about and alert for more subtle types of seizures as well. (See *Clinical snapshot: Seizures*, page 230.)

ETIOLOGY AND PRECIPITATING FACTORS

- Metabolic conditions — hyperpyrexia, hypoxia, hypoglycemia, hyperglycemia, electrolyte imbalances, uremia, fluid overload
- Chemical or pharmacologic conditions — inadequate serum anticonvulsant levels, alcohol or drug overdose or toxicity, alcohol or drug withdrawal
- Infections — meningitis and encephalitis
- Structural or physical conditions — increased intracranial pressure (ICP), cerebral edema, cerebral or subdural hematoma, cerebral hemorrhage, eclampsia, malignant hypertension, tumor, congenital malformations
- Degenerative conditions — Alzheimer's disease, multiple sclerosis, systemic lupus erythematosus
- Reduced cardiac output — Stokes-Adams syncope, other arrhythmias
- Idiopathic origin

Focused assessment guidelines

The patient exhibiting generalized seizures can't always provide relevant historical information, so the nursing history (Functional Health Patterns) section of this care plan has been omitted. Instead, these guidelines for observing and documenting seizures can help in developing an accurate diagnosis and effective interventions.

Preictal phase

- Did an aura or warning precede seizure onset? What was the patient doing when the seizure began (or when the aura was noted)?

Tonic-clonic phases

- Did the patient give a shrill cry?
- Did the patient fall?
- What kind of movement was noted first?
- Where did the movement begin?
- Were other areas progressively involved? If so, in what pattern?
- If a tonic (rigid) phase occurred, how long did it last?
- If a clonic (jerking) phase occurred, how long did it last?
- How long did the entire seizure last?
- Did the patient lose bowel or bladder control?
- During the phases of the seizure, did the pupils react? Deviate?
- Did the patient lose consciousness? If so, when?

Postictal phase

- What was the patient's level of consciousness (LOC) after the seizure?

Physical findings in seizures

Body system	Tonic phase	Clonic phase	Postictal phase
Neurologic	• Shrill cry; then loss of consciousness • Pupils dilated and nonreactive	• Loss of consciousness • Pupils may remain dilated and nonreactive • Excessive salivation	• Deep sleep; then confusion, disorientation, amnesia • Reactive pupils
Musculoskeletal	• Opisthotonos • Rigidity • Jaw clenching • Extension of extremities • Clenched fists	• Violent, bilateral, rhythmic jerking • Facial grimacing	• Flaccidity
Pulmonary	• Apnea	• Stertorous, irregular respirations	• Deep, regular respirations
Renal/GI		• Fecal incontinence • Urinary incontinence	
Integumentary	• Cyanosis	• Profuse diaphoresis • Flushing	
Cardiovascular	• Bradycardia	• Bradycardia or tachycardia • Hypertension	

■ Did the patient exhibit amnesia, confusion, disorientation, or agitation when he regained consciousness?

■ Did the patient have motor, sensory, or perceptual deficits after the seizure?

■ How long did the postictal phase last?

PHYSICAL FINDINGS

Physical findings vary widely, depending on the type of seizure activity, the area of brain tissue involved, and the phase of the seizure (see *Physical findings in seizures*). Keep in mind that the range of physical manifestations is almost limitless.

DIAGNOSTIC STUDIES

Because a seizure represents a clinical sign, not a diagnosis, testing is usually needed to determine its cause. The following is a list of possible studies that may be ordered for this purpose.

■ Serum glucose tests — can rule out hypoglycemia or hyperglycemia as a cause of seizure

■ Serum phenytoin or serum phenobarbital levels — allow evaluation of adequacy of anticonvulsant dosage in the patient with a known seizure history

■ Blood urea nitrogen, creatinine studies — allow evaluation of renal function because uremia may induce seizures

■ Serum electrolytes — abnormal levels, particularly a calcium deficiency, may induce seizures

■ Arterial blood gas values — may indicate hypoxia, which can induce seizures or result from prolonged seizures or associated respiratory depression

■ Toxicology screening — may indicate drug ingestion as a cause of seizures

■ Blood cultures — can rule out sepsis as a cause of seizures

■ Computerized tomography scan — may identify cerebral abnormality, such as tumor, arteriovenous malformation, hemorrhage, or edema

■ Lumbar puncture — may identify infection, indicated by bacteria, increased white blood cell count, and decreased glucose level in cerebrospinal fluid; increased pressure may indicate a space-occupying lesion, or bleeding may indicate hemorrhage

■ EEG — may identify the lesion area. Increased electrical activity and spikes characterize generalized tonic-clonic seizures. Repeated studies may be necessary to record actual seizure activity

■ Magnetic resonance imaging — may reveal intracerebral abnormality

■ Skull X-rays — may indicate fractures or areas of calcification

■ Cerebral angiography — allows evaluation of cerebral circulatory status and identifies vascular abnormalities

■ ICP monitoring — allows for identification of possible increased ICP as cause of seizure

Neurologic disorders

POTENTIAL COMPLICATIONS

- Status epilepticus
- Airway obstruction
- Respiratory arrest
- Aspiration pneumonia
- Hyperthermia
- Hypoglycemia
- Renal failure
- Cerebral ischemia

CLINICAL SNAPSHOT ✳

Seizures

Major nursing diagnoses and collaborative problems	Key patient outcomes
ND: Ineffective airway clearance	Maintain a clear airway.
CP: Risk for status epilepticus	Maintain therapeutic drug levels.
ND: Risk for injury	Experience no injury related to muscle contraction.
ND: Deficient knowledge (seizure management)	Verbalize understanding of seizure management.

Nursing diagnosis

Ineffective airway clearance related to loss of consciousness, apnea, excessive secretions, jaw clenching, or airway occlusion by tongue or foreign body

NURSING PRIORITIES

- Maintain patent airway.
- Promote adequate oxygenation.

PATIENT OUTCOME CRITERION

Throughout the seizure, the patient will maintain a clear airway.

INTERVENTIONS	RATIONALES
1. *If the patient reports seeing an aura or if a warning phase occurs, turn the patient to the side and use the head-tilt–jaw-lift maneuver* as needed *to maintain an open airway.** Never try to force the jaw open or insert an oral airway during the seizure.	1. Turning the patient to the side promotes drainage of saliva from the mouth and reduces the risk of aspiration. Attempts to force the jaw open or insert objects during a seizure may cause damage to the teeth or injury to the caregiver. An apneic period of up to 60 seconds is usually followed by resumption of spontaneous respiration. If the airway becomes occluded during the tonic phase, significant hypoxia may ensue, so maintaining an open airway is essential.
2. *Suction the oropharynx as needed.* Provide supplemental oxygen via nasal cannula.	2. During the clonic and postictal phases, the patient who isn't fully conscious is at risk for aspirating saliva that has accumulated during the tonic phase. Vomiting may also occur. Supplemental oxygen is indicated because seizures cause increased oxygen demands. Also, some degree of respiratory depression commonly follows generalized seizures. A cannula is preferred because a mask may hamper airway clearance if vomiting occurs.

*Italics indicate key interventions.

3. *If seizures are persistent* (unresponsive to drug therapy) *or frequently recur, notify the physician immediately* and anticipate the need for endotracheal intubation and mechanical ventilation. See the "Mechanical ventilation" care plan, page 281.

3. Status epilepticus, in which seizure activity persists or recurs without the patient regaining consciousness, is a medical emergency. Irreversible brain damage may result from the prolonged apnea that occurs. Mechanical ventilation may be necessary to ensure adequate oxygenation while attempting to stop the seizures. The "Mechanical ventilation" care plan contains detailed interventions for the care of the patient on a ventilator.

4. After the seizure, insert a nasogastric (NG) tube and connect it to low suction, as ordered. Don't attempt to insert an NG tube during an active seizure.

4. Emptying the stomach of gastric contents prevents accidental aspiration should vomiting occur. Attempting to insert an NG tube during an active seizure could stimulate a gag reflex and vomiting.

5. Additional individualized interventions: _____

5. Rationales: _____

Suggested NIC Interventions
Airway management; Airway suctioning; Aspiration precautions; Positioning; Ventilation assistance

Suggested NOC Outcomes
Aspiration control; Respiratory status: Airway patency; Respiratory status: Gas exchange; Respiratory status: Ventilation

---

Collaborative problem

Risk for status epilepticus related to inadequate pharmacologic control or misidentification of underlying cause

NURSING PRIORITIES
- Stop seizures.
- Treat underlying cause.

PATIENT OUTCOME CRITERIA
Following onset of seizures, the patient will:
- be recognized as being at risk for status epilepticus
- receive appropriate anticonvulsants promptly
- have underlying causes identified and treated.
  Throughout the hospital stay, the patient will:
- maintain therapeutic drug levels
- receive appropriate therapy for the underlying cause of seizures.

INTERVENTIONS

1. *Administer I.V. antiseizure medication as ordered.* Commonly ordered medications for acute seizures include the following:

– diazepam (Valium), 5 to 10 mg I.V.; may repeat every 10 to 15 minutes, not to exceed 30 mg in an hour. Observe the patient closely for respiratory depression. Monitor for drug interactions, especially if the patient is also taking phenothiazines, barbiturates, narcotics, or monoamine oxidase inhibitors.

RATIONALES

1. Prolonged seizures may result in respiratory depression or arrest, cardiovascular insufficiency, or cerebral edema. Antiseizure medications suppress the ectopic focus.
– Diazepam is the initial drug of choice for generalized motor status epilepticus, although it's neither recommended nor sufficient for ongoing seizure control. It appears to act on the limbic system, thalamus, and hypothalamus to stop seizures. Respiratory depression is a common adverse reaction. The medications listed may potentiate the actions of diazepam and increase the risk of respiratory compromise.

Neurologic disorders

– phenobarbital (Luminal) and other barbiturate anticonvulsants. The usual dose of phenobarbital ranges from 60 to 400 mg/day. Observe the patient closely for respiratory depression, especially if the patient also received diazepam. Monitor carefully for drug interactions, especially if the patient is taking phenothiazines, warfarin (Coumadin), digoxin (Lanoxin), or disulfiram (Antabuse).

– phenytoin (Dilantin) the usual loading dose is 10 to 15 mg/kg, followed by 100 mg every 6 to 8 hours. Administer phenytoin slowly in normal saline solution, giving no more than 50 mg/minute. Observe the patient's electrocardiogram (ECG) during phenytoin administration. Monitor closely for adverse reactions or indications of possible toxicity, such as anemia, elevated serum glucose levels, GI upset, and diplopia with nystagmus.

– Monitor therapeutic blood levels as ordered.

– Monitor carefully for possible drug interactions. Drugs that may increase serum phenytoin levels include chloramphenicol (Chloromycetin), isoniazid (Laniazid), salicylates, sulfonamides, cimetidine (Tagamet), warfarin, and benzodiazepines; acute alcohol ingestion may also increase serum phenytoin levels. Phenytoin may increase metabolism of warfarin (Coumadin) and digoxin. Digoxin, reserpine (Diupres), prednisone (Deltasone), phenobarbital (Bellatal), and chronic alcoholism may decrease phenytoin levels.

2. Consider possible underlying causes. Assist with identification and treatment. Underlying causes include:

– head trauma

– electrolyte imbalance

– hypoxia

– hypoglycemia or hyperglycemia

– brain tumors

– As with diazepam, phenobarbital depresses the CNS. Its precise action is unclear, but it appears to reduce cerebral oxygen consumption and may help decrease ICP. It also potentiates phenothiazines. Phenobarbital may decrease warfarin absorption and digoxin metabolism. Disulfiram may increase the likelihood of toxicity.

– Phenytoin appears to act on the motor cortex to stabilize the threshold against neuronal hyperexcitability, possibly by aiding the efflux of sodium from neurons. Phenytoin must be administered in saline solution because it precipitates in glucose-containing solutions. ECG monitoring is essential; giving phenytoin too rapidly may cause arrhythmias or cardiac arrest.

– Assessing serum phenytoin levels allows the determination of the optimal dosage and minimizes the risk of toxicity.

– Phenytoin reacts with many other medications so controlling seizures may involve balancing phenytoin with other drugs. Watch for adverse reactions and signs of toxicity or inadequate therapeutic effect.

2. In a patient without a history of seizures, treating the underlying cause is crucial to seizure control.

– Secondary seizures are caused most commonly by head trauma. If the patient was admitted after an acute traumatic event, this link may be obvious. However, seizures may occur months or even years after head injury, as scar tissue creates a focus for abnormal neuronal activity, so careful history taking is needed.

– Electrolyte imbalances may induce seizures by altering cell membrane permeability, thus interfering with normal neuronal electrical conduction.

– Sufficient oxygen is essential for maintaining the normal neuronal ionic gradient. Any condition that lowers the level of oxygen delivered to sensitive brain tissue may contribute to seizure activity.

– Cerebral neurons are extremely sensitive to decreased glucose levels because glucose is their primary substrate. A sudden drop in blood glucose seems more likely to cause neurologic problems than a gradual decline. Hyperglycemia may contribute to a hyperosmolar crenation of brain cells, with resultant irritability and altered conduction pathways. Also, seizure activity increases cerebral metabolic needs and depletes stores of glucose and energy.

– Seizures are the major initial sign in as many as 18% of patients with undetected brain tumors. Tissue compression from tumor growth is usually the cause.

– infections

– cerebral hemorrhage

– toxins.

– Infections may contribute to seizures by leading to scarring (in response to inflammatory changes), cerebral edema (in acute infections), hyperpyrexia, abscesses, or autoimmune demyelinization (as in encephalomyelitis, for example).

– Localized ischemic damage to brain tissue may cause seizures.

– Toxins may cause seizures by interfering with the cell's metabolic processes, altering cell membrane function and integrity. Some hydrocarbons, lead, mercury, and arsenic may cause seizures in high concentrations. A hypersensitive patient may develop seizures in response to certain medications such as phenothiazines. Withdrawal from alcohol or barbiturates is a common cause of seizures because abrupt withdrawal from the CNS-depressant effects of either appears to increase neuronal irritability.

3. If seizures don't respond to drug therapy, anticipate possible preparation for neuromuscular blockade or general anesthesia, with mechanical ventilation.

3. Status epilepticus has a mortality of about 10% and causes one-third of seizure-related deaths. As seizures persist, cerebral vasodilation occurs, perfusion pressure drops, and irreversible cell damage follows from nutritional depletion and neuronal exhaustion. Neuromuscular blockade stops motor activity but doesn't directly interrupt brain electrical activity. General anesthesia causes global depression of cerebral function, interrupting the cycle of hyperexcitability at its source.

4. Additional individualized interventions: _____

4. Rationales: _____

Nursing diagnosis

Risk for injury (trauma or myoglobinuria) related to excessive uncontrolled muscle activity

NURSING PRIORITY
Prevent injury.

PATIENT OUTCOME CRITERION
During and after the seizure episode, the patient will experience no injury from muscle contractions.

INTERVENTIONS

1. *At the seizure's onset, ensure safe patient positioning.* Place pillows or padding around the patient and raise and pad the side rails. Don't restrain the patient's arms and legs. Maintain the bed in low position.

2. *During the seizure, stay with the patient.* Maintain a patent airway and suction secretions as needed. Provide privacy when possible.

RATIONALES

1. Violent muscle contractions may cause injury without protective measures. Padded side rails help prevent injury if the patient strikes the rails during the seizure. Restraining arms and legs may result in fractures during the clonic phase.

2. The seizing patient is extremely vulnerable to injury because of uncontrollable muscle activity. After the seizure, the patient is commonly embarrassed and ashamed of the loss of control. Providing privacy helps protect the patient's dignity.

Neurologic disorders

3. *After motor activity stops, place the patient in the side-lying position.* Perform a neurologic evaluation, noting pupil size and reactivity, LOC, responsiveness to stimuli, and respiratory status. Repeat the evaluation every 15 to 30 minutes until condition stabilizes. Inspect the oropharynx, tongue, and teeth for seizure-related injury.

4. *Avoid excessive environmental stimulation during the postictal period.*

5. *If the seizure was prolonged, monitor urine for possible myoglobinuria,* indicated by a red or cola color. Send urine specimen for myoglobin testing. Report findings to the physician promptly.

6. Additional individualized interventions:＿＿＿＿＿＿

＿＿＿＿＿＿＿＿＿＿＿＿＿＿＿＿＿＿＿＿＿

3. The side-lying position helps prevent aspiration. Careful monitoring of status during the postictal period is essential because respiratory depression is common. Violent seizure activity may result in mouth injury, and blood in the oropharynx and loose teeth may be aspirated.

4. Environmental stimulation (such as bright lights, abrupt movement, or loud, sudden noises) may reactivate neuronal irritability and stimulate further seizures.

5. Repeated, vigorous muscle contraction releases excess amounts of myoglobin into the bloodstream from muscle cell breakdown. If the quantity is sufficient, the accumulated myoglobin may occlude the kidneys and cause renal failure. Treatment involves flushing the renal system using fluids and diuretics.

6. Rationales: ＿＿＿＿＿＿＿＿＿＿＿＿＿＿＿

＿＿＿＿＿＿＿＿＿＿＿＿＿＿＿＿＿＿＿＿＿

Suggested NIC Interventions
Surveillance: Safety

Suggested NOC Outcomes
Safety status: Physical injury

Nursing diagnosis
Deficient knowledge (seizure management) related to lack of exposure to information

NURSING PRIORITY
Instruct the patient and family on seizure management.

PATIENT OUTCOME CRITERION
By the time of discharge, the patient and family will demonstrate and verbalize understanding of seizure management.

INTERVENTIONS

1. *Assess the patient's and his family's current level of understanding.* Refer to the "Knowledge deficit" care plan, page 129.

2. *Instruct the patient and his family about the disorder and the need to adhere to a medical regimen.*

3. *Instruct the patient and his family about medications and causes of seizures.*

4. Additional individualized interventions: ＿＿＿＿＿

＿＿＿＿＿＿＿＿＿＿＿＿＿＿＿＿＿＿＿＿＿

RATIONALES

1. Determining the level of understanding allows the nurse to individualize learning to meet patient needs. The "Knowledge deficit" care plan contains detailed information about this problem.

2. Understanding the disorder helps to increase compliance.

3. Teaching improves compliance. Failure to take medications is a common cause of recurrent seizures. Excessive stress, fatigue, and environmental factors may cause seizures in susceptible individuals.

4. Rationales: ＿＿＿＿＿＿＿＿＿＿＿＿＿＿＿＿

＿＿＿＿＿＿＿＿＿＿＿＿＿＿＿＿＿＿＿＿＿

Discharge planning

DISCHARGE CHECKLIST

Before discharge, the patient shows evidence that:
- ❏ cause of seizures is identified and treated
- ❏ seizures are controlled
- ❏ respiratory status is stable
- ❏ neurologic status is stable.

TEACHING CHECKLIST

Document evidence that the patient and his family demonstrate an understanding of:
- ❏ the cause and implications of seizures
- ❏ the treatments instituted
- ❏ signs of possible recurrence
- ❏ safety precautions.

DOCUMENTATION CHECKLIST

Using outcome criteria as a guide, document:
- ❏ the patient's clinical status on admission
- ❏ significant changes in status
- ❏ pertinent diagnostic test findings
- ❏ seizure episodes
- ❏ safety precautions instituted
- ❏ pharmacologic interventions
- ❏ patient and family teaching
- ❏ discharge planning.

Associated care plans

- Craniotomy
- Drug overdose
- Hypoglycemia
- Increased intracranial pressure
- Mechanical ventilation
- Multiple trauma

References

Hickey, J.V. *The Clinical Practice of Neurological and Neurosurgical Nursing*, 5th ed. Philadelphia: Lippincott Williams & Wilkins, 2002.

Jordan, K. (ed) *Emergency Nursing Care Curriculum.* Emergency Nurses Association. Philadelphia: W.B. Saunders, Co., 2000.

Lynn-McHale, D.J., and Carlson, K.K. American Association of Critical Care Nurses *AACN Procedure Manual,* 4th ed. Philadelphia: W.B. Saunders Co., 2001.

Phipps, W.J., et al. *Medical-Surgical Nursing, Health and Illness Perspective, 2003.* 7th ed. St. Louis: Mosby–Year Book, Inc., 2003.

Shoemaker, W.C., et al. *Textbook of Critical Care*, 4th ed. Philadelphia: W.B. Saunders Co., 2002.

Thompson, J.M., et al. *Mosby's Clinical Nursing*, 5th ed. St. Louis: Mosby–Year Book, Inc., 2002.

Neurologic disorders

Stroke

DRG INFORMATION

DRG 014 Specific Cerebrovascular Disorders. Except
transient ischemic attack.
Mean LOS = 5.9 days

Introduction
DEFINITION AND TIME FOCUS

Stroke, traditionally called a cerebrovascular accident, or
more recently, a brain attack, can take the form of any of
several pathophysiologic events that disrupt cerebral circulation. The cells at the site of the resulting infarction
then release chemicals that cause further damage and
compromise blood flow, resulting in ischemia in the surrounding area. If the ischemic damage continues, these
cells also may die, worsening the patient's cognitive and
functional deficits.

The most common causes of stroke include thrombosis, embolism, and hemorrhage. Rarely, stroke may stem
from arterial spasm or compression of cerebral blood
vessels that results from tumor growth or some other
cause. Regardless of the cause, the consistent factor in
all strokes is brain injury resulting from disrupted blood
circulation.

Deficits resulting from stroke may be temporary or
permanent, depending on the portion of the brain and
the vessels involved, the extent of injury, the patient's
preexisting physical and emotional health, and the presence of other diseases or injuries.

This care plan focuses on the care of the noncritical
patient who's admitted to a medical-surgical unit for diagnosis and nonsurgical treatment of a stroke. Surgical
interventions for stroke — such as carotid endarterectomy, extracranial-intracranial bypass, and craniotomy —
aren't discussed in this plan. For a sample clinical pathway, see *Clinical pathway: Nonhemorrhagic stroke,* pages
238 to 240. (See also *Clinical snapshot: Stroke,* page 241.)

ETIOLOGY AND PRECIPITATING FACTORS

■ Factors that cause occlusion of blood supply to cerebral tissue
– Cerebral thrombosis, such as from atherosclerosis,
inflammation from infection or other disease, mechanical constriction (for instance, from increased intracranial
pressure (ICP), prolonged vasoconstriction, systemic
hypotension, and hematologic disorders that increase
clotting tendencies
– Cerebral embolism, such as from cardiac disease (most
commonly atrial fibrillation), plaques or clots from elsewhere in the circulatory system, substances (such as air,
fat, or tumor particles) that enter the bloodstream, and
clotting disorders
■ Factors that contribute to intracerebral bleeding
– Hemorrhage, hypertension, ruptured aneurysm, trauma, ruptured arteriovenous malformations, bleeding
from the growth of a tumor, bleeding associated with a
disease (for example, leukemia, anemia, sickle cell disease, and hemophilia), anticoagulant therapy, and
edema
■ Factors causing cerebral ischemia
– Arterial spasm, systemic hypoxemia, and compression
of cerebral blood vessels
■ Factors that increase an individual's risk of stroke
– Hypertension, heart disease, smoking, diabetes, hypercholesterolemia, use of hormonal contraceptives, obesity, a family history of stroke, congenital anomalies, and
drug abuse

Focused assessment guidelines
NURSING HISTORY
(FUNCTIONAL HEALTH PATTERN FINDINGS)
Health-perception–health-management pattern
■ Symptoms that may have developed over several days
(thrombosis), minutes to hours (hemorrhage), or just a
few minutes (embolus)
■ Recent episodes of sudden weakness, vertigo, numbness or tingling in face or limbs, or speech or vision disturbances that resolved within 24 hours (transient ischemic attacks [TIAs]) or took longer than 24 hours to
resolve but left little or no deficit (reversible ischemic
neurologic deficits)
■ Use of hormonal contraceptives
■ Treatment of hypertension, heart disease, diabetes, or
other chronic condition
■ Noncompliance with antihypertensive regimen or fail-
ure to see a physician for many years
■ History of smoking for many years
Nutritional-metabolic pattern
■ Difficulty swallowing
■ Nausea and vomiting (usually associated with hemor-
rhage)
Elimination pattern
■ Urinary or fecal incontinence
Activity-exercise pattern
■ Inability to move one side of body (hemiplegia)
■ Fear of falling
■ Syncope

Sleep-rest pattern
- Symptoms (most commonly from thrombosis) that develop during sleep or shortly after awakening

Cognitive-perceptual pattern
- Inability to understand explanations of what has happened or to respond to questions
- Dizziness, drowsiness, headache, burning or aching in extremities, and stiff neck
- Slowed thinking, clumsiness

Self-perception–self-concept pattern
- Lack of awareness of affected side of body

Role-relationship pattern
- Emotional lability, behavioral changes, or altered speech or thinking abilities

PHYSICAL FINDINGS
Physical findings may be present, depending on the site of the stroke.

General appearance
- Facial droop
- Lateralized weakness or flaccidity on side opposite brain lesion

Cardiovascular
- Hypertension
- Hypotension
- Arrhythmia

Pulmonary
- Either increased or decreased respirations

Neurologic
- Seizures
- Altered level of consciousness (LOC)
- Nuchal rigidity
- Memory impairment
- Confusion
- Retinal hemorrhage
- Hemianesthesia
- Hemianopsia (visual field deficit in one or both eyes)
- Apraxia (inability to perform purposeful acts)
- Receptive aphasia (inability to understand words) or expressive aphasia (inability to say words)
- Agnosia (inability to recognize familiar objects)
- Disorientation
- Unequal pupil size
- Diplopia
- Disconjugate gaze
- Dysphagia
- Dysarthria (lack of muscle control to form words)
- Sensory deficits

Integumentary
- Flushing
- Pallor

Musculoskeletal
- Flaccidity
- Paralysis

DIAGNOSTIC STUDIES
Initially, the need for specific diagnostic studies depends on whether the stroke stems from a hemorrhagic or a nonhemorrhagic cause (treatment is significantly different for each). Laboratory data may show no significant abnormalities unless other conditions are present.

- Complete blood count — performed to establish a baseline; may reveal blood loss if stroke was caused by significant hemorrhage
- Chemistry panel — performed to establish a baseline; assesses renal function and electrolyte levels (these may be significant in a patient requiring fluid restriction); rules out hypoglycemia and hyperglycemia as contributors to the altered mental state
- Prothrombin time/international normalized ratio (PT/INR) and partial thromboplastin time (PTT) — performed to establish a baseline because the patient with a stroke caused by occlusion may need anticoagulants (INR expresses PT as a ratio to provide consistency for comparison from one laboratory to another)
- Urinalysis — rules out preexisting urinary tract infection (important because the patient is typically catheterized)
- Computed tomography (CT) scan of the head — differentiates infarction from hemorrhage and reveals extent of bleeding and brain compression (if present); may take several days for infarct to become visible
- Cerebral angiography — shows cerebral blood vessels and reveals the site of bleeding or blockage
- Positron emission tomography scan — computer interpretation of gamma ray emissions provides information on cerebral blood flow, volume, and metabolism
- Brain scan — cerebral infarction indicated by areas of radioisotope uptake; may not become positive for up to 2 weeks after a stroke
- EEG — reveals areas of abnormal brain activity and may help in diagnosing; however, a normal EEG doesn't rule out a pathologic condition
- Lumbar puncture — bloody cerebrospinal fluid may indicate intracerebral hemorrhage; used in fewer cases since CT scan became available
- Skull and cervical spine X-rays — rule out fractures, especially if the patient suffered a fall with the stroke
- Doppler ultrasonography — identifies abnormalities in blood flow in carotid, vertebral, basilar, and intracerebral arteries
- Echocardiology and transesophageal echocardiology reveal cardiac abnormalities contributing to stroke

POTENTIAL COMPLICATIONS
- Brain stem failure and cardiopulmonary arrest
- Brain compression
- Brain infarction
- Brain abscess
- Encephalitis

(Text continues on page 240.)

Neurologic disorders

Nonhemorrhagic stroke

Plan	Emergency department	Day 1
Laboratory studies	<ul><li>CBC</li><li>PT/PTT</li><li>Blood chemistry studies</li></ul>	<ul><li>PT/PTT every day if on anticoagulants</li><li>If lacunar infarct, sequential multiple analyzer with computer or VDRL test</li><li>Magnesium</li><li>Blood glucose testing q 6 hours</li></ul>
Tests	<ul><li>CT scan of brain</li><li>CXR</li><li>ECG</li><li>Telemetry if indicated</li><li>Pulse oximetry</li></ul>	<ul><li>Order CT scan for 48 hours after first CT scan if anterior, middle, or posterior cerebral artery stroke</li><li>Carotid duplex scan</li><li>ICU if meets criteria, based on test results and assessment findings</li><li>Telemetry</li><li>2-dimensional echocardiogram if ordered</li><li>MRI if lacunar or brain stem stroke suspected</li></ul>
Consultations		Consult if indicated:<ul><li>Neurology</li><li>Dietitian</li><li>Social worker</li><li>Swallowing team</li><li>Rehabilitation: PT, OT, speech therapist</li><li>Pastoral care</li><li>Psychiatric</li></ul>
Medications/I.V.	<ul><li>I.V.</li><li>Aspirin after CT</li></ul>	<ul><li>Aspirin or anticoagulants</li><li>Stool softeners or laxatives</li><li>I.V. normal saline lock</li><li>Heparin S.C., I.V.</li><li>Acetaminophen (Tylenol) if patient has fever</li></ul>
Treatments		
Nutrition		<ul><li>NPO until swallowing team or physician has cleared</li><li>Diet consistent with diagnosis or condition</li></ul>
Elimination		<ul><li>Assess normal pattern</li></ul>
Activity	<ul><li>HOB greater than 30 degrees</li></ul>	<ul><li>HOB greater than 30 degrees</li><li>High accident risk evaluation</li></ul>
Patient teaching		<ul><li>Telemetry</li><li>ICU orientation</li><li>Diagnostic testing</li><li>Stroke teaching materials</li><li>Stroke educator consulted</li></ul>
Discharge planning		<ul><li>Evaluate support systems and discharge needs</li></ul>

Day 2	Day 3
• Blood glucose testing q 6 hours	• CBC • Blood chemistry studies • Blood glucose testing q 6 hours
• Stop telemetry or discharge from ICU if patient stable	• CT scan/MRI repeat (48 hours after admission if anterior, middle, or posterior cerebral artery stroke)
• Rehabilitation unit • Functional independence measure score per rehabilitation	• Dietitian (if intake p.o. < 75% daily caloric requirements), if no previous consult
• Continue medications from Day 1	• Continue medications
• Diet recommendations followed • Calorie count if intake p.o.< 75% daily caloric requirement	
	• Administer laxatives if pattern abnormal
• Appropriate bed positioning • ADLs per PT or OT recommendation	• Progressive plan outlined by PT or OT
• PT education • OT education • Speech therapy education if needed Teaching materials include: • Stroke warning signs • Stroke effects • "Why Am I So Emotional?" (American Heart Association [AHA] handout) • "Why Am I So Depressed?" (AHA handout) • Resource list	• Diet • Swallowing team if involved • Teaching materials (AHA handouts): –"How Can I Reduce My Risk of Stroke?" –"How Can I Reduce High Blood Pressure?" –"Are There Complications from a Stroke?" • Smoking-cessation information
• Complete assessment • Continue to evaluate for discharge needs	• Rehabilitation unit evaluation by PT, OT, speech therapist • Discharge to home if transient ischemic attack

Neurologic disorders

(continued)

Nonhemorrhagic stroke *(continued)*

Plan	Day 4	Day 5	Day 6	Goals met
Laboratory studies	• Blood glucose testing q 6 hours	• Blood glucose testing q 6 hours	• Blood glucose testing q 6 hours	• Laboratory values return to baseline
Tests				• No further progression of stroke
Consultations	• Dietitian (if intake p.o. < 75% daily caloric requirements), if no previous consult			
Medications/ I.V.	• Continue medications from Day 1	• Continue medications	• Continue medications	• Tolerating medications
Treatment				• Plan arranged for continued therapy in an appropriate setting
Nutrition	• Institute enteral feedings per dietitian • Determine that calorie and protein intake is adequate	• Institute enteral feedings per dietitian • Determine that calorie and protein intake is adequate	• Institute enteral feedings per dietitian • Determine that calorie and protein intake is adequate	• Food and fluid intake meets caloric and protein needs
Elimination	• Administer laxatives if pattern abnormal	• Administer laxatives if pattern abnormal	• Administer laxatives if pattern abnormal	• WNL
Activity	• Progressive plan has been outlined per PT and OT			• Plan safely addresses current functional status
Patient teaching	• Nutrition or drug instructions • Medications • AHA teaching handouts: –"Can I Live At Home After My Stroke?" –"What Is Stroke Rehabilitation?"	• Review teaching materials with patient and family		• Patient and family verbalize: –Medications (name, dosage, adverse effects, purpose, schedule, nutrient and drug interactions) –Signs and symptoms of complications –Appropriate diet
Discharge planning	• Discharge to home, rehabilitation unit, or extended care facility as appropriate for condition (lacunar infarct) • Home care intervention considered if outcome goals not met	• Discharge plan in place, referrals made	• Discharge to home, rehabilitation unit, or extended care facility as appropriate for condition (anterior, middle, or posterior cerebral artery stroke) • Make referrals if discharged to home and outcome goals not met	• Ensure follow-up plan in place • Plan continued medical management if discharged to rehabilitation unit

- Pulmonary embolism
- Arrhythmias
- Heart failure
- Thrombophlebitis
- Pneumonia
- Dysfunctional limb contractures
- Pressure ulcers
- Malnutrition

CLINICAL SNAPSHOT ✳

Stroke

Major nursing diagnoses and collaborative problems	Key patient outcomes
ND: Ineffective airway clearance	Maintain a clear airway.
CP: Risk for further cerebral injury	Show stable or improving neurologic signs.
ND: Impaired physical mobility	Perform as much self-care as possible.
ND: Disturbed sensory perception	Demonstrate use of techniques to compensate for sensory loss.
ND: Impaired verbal communication	Establish some form of verbal or nonverbal communication.
ND: Deficient knowledge (stroke management)	Express understanding of the disease and the therapeutic regimen (patient and family).

Nursing diagnosis

Ineffective airway clearance related to hemiplegic effects of a stroke

NURSING PRIORITIES
- Maintain a patent airway.
- Prevent pulmonary complications.

PATIENT OUTCOME CRITERIA
Throughout the hospital stay, the patient will:
- maintain a clear airway
- cough and perform deep-breathing exercises every 2 hours while awake
- have clear breath sounds or prompt identification and treatment of pulmonary problems
- take food and fluids (as ordered) without aspirating or choking.

INTERVENTIONS

1. *Position the patient with his head turned to the side,* * supporting his trunk with pillows as needed. Elevate the head of the bed slightly. *Never leave the patient in the supine position while he's unattended. Provide a call bell within easy reach of his unaffected arm, or provide alternative means by which he can signal for help, as needed.*

2. *If hemiplegia is present, position the patient on the affected side for shorter periods (less than 1 hour) than on the unaffected side (2 hours).* Avoid positioning a patient's affected arm over his abdomen.

3. *Encourage the patient to cough and use deep breathing every 2 hours* while he's awake. Set up equipment for oral suctioning, and *suction accumulated secretions as necessary.*

RATIONALES

1. Hemiplegia, impaired cough reflex, or dysphagia may render the patient unable to clear his airway. If left in the supine position while unattended, the patient may aspirate; the supine position also increases the risk of airway obstruction from the tongue, especially if the patient is anesthetized. Providing the means to call for help is essential when the airway may become compromised.

2. Lying on the affected side may result in pooling of secretions, which are ineffectively cleared because of hemiplegia. The weight of an arm over the abdomen may further reduce the adequacy of thoracic expansion.

3. Accumulated secretions may obstruct the airway or predispose the patient to atelectasis or pneumonia. (Respiratory infection is one of the primary causes of death for stroke patients.)

---

*Italics indicate key interventions.

Neurologic disorders

4. *Assess breath sounds at least every 4 hours while the patient is awake. Also note the adequacy of his respiratory effort, the rate and characteristics of respirations, and his skin color. Investigate restlessness promptly,* especially in the aphasic patient. Report any abnormalities.

4. Many stroke patients have preexisting hypertension or heart disease, which may predispose them to heart failure. Abnormal breath sounds (crackles, gurgles) may be the first indicators of complications related to hypoventilation. Increased respiratory effort, tachypnea, ashen or cyanotic color, or restlessness may indicate hypoxemia. Early detection and reporting lead to prompt treatment.

5. *Allow nothing by mouth until the patient's ability to swallow is evaluated.* If the patient can swallow with minimum difficulty, help him eat or observe his eating, as needed. Place small bites of food in the unaffected side of his mouth. (Semisolid foods are usually handled better than thin liquids.)

5. Hemiplegia and associated dysphagia predispose the patient to aspiration. The patient may be better able to swallow if food is placed on his unaffected side. Small bites and thicker liquids decrease the risk of choking from aspiration.

6. Additional individualized interventions: _____
_____

6. Rationales: _____

Suggested NIC Interventions
Airway management; Airway suctioning; Acid-base monitoring; Aspiration precautions; Positioning; Respiratory monitoring; Ventilation assistance

Suggested NOC Outcomes
Aspiration control; Respiratory status: Airway patency; Respiratory status: Gas exchange; Respiratory status: Ventilation

---

Collaborative problem

Risk for further cerebral injury related to interrupted blood flow (embolus, thrombus, or hemorrhage)

NURSING PRIORITY

Improve cerebral tissue perfusion.

PATIENT OUTCOME CRITERIA

Within 2 days of admission, the patient will:
- show no further decrease in LOC
- show stable or improving neurologic signs.
  Throughout the hospital stay, the patient will:
- maintain fluid balance
- maintain electrolyte levels within normal limits.

INTERVENTIONS

1. *Assess the patient's neurologic status,* checking LOC, orientation, grip strength, drift, speech, leg strength, pupillary response, *and vital signs every hour until neurologic status is stable; repeat assessment at least every 4 hours thereafter. Promptly report abnormalities or changes,* especially decreasing alertness, progressing weakness, restlessness, unequal pupil size, widening pulse pressure, flexor or extensor posturing, seizures, severe headache, vertigo, syncope, or epistaxis.

2. *Elevate the head of the bed 30 degrees and provide supplemental oxygen as ordered.*

RATIONALES

1. When blood flow to and oxygenation of the brain are decreased, cerebral vasodilation and edema occur as the body attempts to compensate for the deficiency. Increasing cerebral edema causes increased ICP and may result in death if not treated promptly. Hemorrhage into enclosed intracranial spaces may also increase pressure. A decline in neurologic signs indicates progressive injury.

2. Elevating the head of the bed helps minimize cerebral edema, which can contribute to increased ischemia. The brain uses 20% of the oxygen normally available to the body. When a stroke causes cerebral ischemia, supplemental oxygen may help prevent brain tissue death.

3. *Administer anticoagulants, as ordered. Monitor appropriate laboratory findings* (PT/INR or PTT), *and check current results before giving each dose. Observe carefully for (and advise the patient or his family to report) melena, petechiae, epistaxis, hematuria, ecchymosis, oozing from wounds, or unusual bleeding. Observe for and report signs of intracranial bleeding* (headache, irritability, weakness, decreased LOC, or nuchal rigidity).

3. Use of anticoagulants can inhibit stroke progression and possibly reduce the number of thromboembolic events. Heparin inactivates thrombin, thus preventing fibrin clots. Therapeutic PTT should be 1 to $1^{1}/_{2}$ times the laboratory's normal value. Warfarin (Coumadin) interferes with vitamin K production, and thus decreases synthesis of several clotting factors. Therapeutic PT should be $1^{1}/_{2}$ to $2^{1}/_{2}$ times normal value. INR ranges vary depending on the reason for use. For all conditions that require anticoagulation therapy (except mechanical heart valve use or acute myocardial infarction), the recommended range is 2 to 3. Anticoagulants predispose the patient to systemic bleeding and may also cause intracranial bleeding.

4. *Administer antiplatelet aggregation medications as ordered.* Observe for gastric irritation.

4. Drugs, such as aspirin, clopidogrel (Plavix), dipyridamole and aspirin (Aggrenox), and ticlopidine (Ticlid), inhibit platelet aggregation and thus reduce the risk of embolus formation. Adverse effects include GI upset and bleeding, so these drugs may not be used if the patient has preexisting GI problems.

5. *Administer acetaminophen (Tylenol) as ordered for fever.*

5. Research suggests that even a 1-degree elevation may contribute to poor outcomes.

6. *Monitor the patient's blood glucose. Treat as ordered for hyperglycemia.*

6. Hyperglycemia is an independent risk factor predicting poor outcome.

7. *Administer medications to control blood pressure as ordered. Be alert for and immediately report signs of decreased cerebral perfusion. Check blood pressure at least every 4 hours while the patient is awake.*

7. Right after a stroke, the brain is in a hypermetabolic state and requires more blood flow to maintain perfusion, so blood pressure is allowed to run higher than normal. However, severe hypertension (systolic pressure greater than 200 mm Hg and diastolic pressure greater than 110 mm Hg) sustained over 30 to 60 minutes is treated because it may decrease perfusion to other organs and increase the risk of cerebral hemorrhage. Blood pressure should be brought down slowly because a sudden drop in cerebral blood flow may cause cerebral vasoconstriction, resulting in further ischemia.

8. Additional individualized interventions: _____
_____

8. Rationales: _____
_____

Nursing diagnosis
Impaired physical mobility related to damage to motor cortex or motor pathways

NURSING PRIORITY
Minimize effects of immobility and prevent associated complications.

PATIENT OUTCOME CRITERIA
Within 24 hours of admission, the patient will:
- begin passive range-of-motion (ROM) exercises
- have clean and dry skin
- have a patent urinary catheter or use a bedpan every 2 hours while awake with minimal incontinence.
  Throughout the hospital stay, the patient will:
- maintain functional alignment

Neurologic disorders

- perform as much self-care as possible
- maintain intact skin
- maintain adequate bowel and bladder elimination, with no signs of infection
- show no thromboembolic complications.

INTERVENTIONS

1. *Maintain functional alignment when positioning the patient at rest,* using a footboard, handroll, or trochanter roll as necessary. *Support the affected arm when the patient is out of bed.*

2. *Provide passive (and active, if appropriate) ROM exercise to all extremities at least four times per day, beginning upon admission. Increase activity levels as permitted and tolerated,* depending on the cause of the stroke. Collaborate with the physical therapist to plan a rehabilitation schedule with the patient and his family.

3. *When permitted, encourage the patient to perform as much self-care as possible.*

4. *Provide antiembolism stockings, leg compression devices, or low-dose heparin, as ordered. Assess the patient for signs of thromboembolic complications. Report immediately any chest pain, shortness of breath, calf pain, or redness or swelling in an extremity.*

5. *Protect skin integrity.* Turn the patient from side to side at least every 2 hours. Keep bedding clean and dry. Massage bony prominences. Watch for fragile, thin, or excoriated skin, which may shear during turning. Provide a special mattress or foam or other padding. Report any red or broken skin areas immediately.

6. *Maintain adequate elimination.* Avoid using an indwelling urinary catheter unless the patient is comatose or can't void. Begin bladder retraining as soon as possible, following an established protocol or medical order. If the patient isn't catheterized, offer a bedpan every 2 hours. Report cloudiness, excessive sediment, or the presence of white blood cells in the patient's urine. Provide stool softeners and laxatives as ordered, and monitor the frequency and characteristics of bowel movements. Reassure the patient that bowel and bladder control usually returns as rehabilitation progresses.

7. Additional individualized interventions:_____
_____

RATIONALES

1. A functional position prevents contractures and deformities that can further complicate recovery and can help reduce ICP. The weight of an unsupported arm may cause shoulder dislocation, joint inflammation, or both.

2. Even passive exercise helps maintain muscle tone and establish new impulse pathways and neuron regeneration. Adjacent brain cells may take up the function of damaged cells, new nerve cell fibers may develop collaterally, or alternative nerve pathways may take over. Learning and repetition appear to be key factors in the development of new neuronal connections. Establishing a schedule helps the patient set goals, maintain a sense of control, and measure progress.

3. Independence in self-care helps maintain self-respect and may improve motivation to increase mobility.

4. Antiembolism stockings and compression devices promote venous return, and low-dose heparin minimizes clotting, thus decreasing the risk of thrombus formation from immobility and venous stasis. The signs and symptoms listed may indicate pulmonary embolus or thrombophlebitis.

5. Impeccable skin care can prevent skin breakdown in the immobilized patient. Moisture promotes bacterial growth and increases skin friability. Turning and massage help prevent pressure sores from developing and promote circulation. An older patient is likely to have delicate skin, particularly if he's debilitated. If help didn't arrive quickly after the stroke, the patient's skin may be excoriated from the effects of urine, pressure, and dehydration. A special mattress or padding can help redistribute pressure. Prompt intervention can prevent serious skin problems that can interfere with recovery.

6. The interruption of neurosensory pathways that results from stroke may cause limited or altered sphincter control, either from actual brain damage or from stroke-related memory and inhibitory lapses. Incontinence and urinary stasis predispose the patient to infection. Bladder and bowel retraining reestablishes patterns and bolsters the patient's confidence in resuming activities as permitted. Reassuring the patient that incontinence is usually temporary helps decrease anxiety, embarrassment, and a sense of helplessness.

7. Rationales: _____
_____

Nursing diagnosis

Disturbed sensory perception related to cerebral injury

NURSING PRIORITY

Minimize the effects of deficits in perception and prevent related complications.

PATIENT OUTCOME CRITERIA

Throughout the hospital stay, the patient will:
- look at and touch the affected side of the body
- establish protective behavior for affected limbs
- demonstrate use of techniques to compensate for sensory loss.

INTERVENTIONS	RATIONALES
1. Use a calm and reassuring manner, eye contact, and touch to establish a relationship with the patient. Use the patient's preferred name, and approach the unaffected side.	**1.** Sensory-perceptual and communication deficits may contribute to profound isolation for the patient who has suffered a stroke. Use of nonverbal communication establishes contact and helps decrease anxiety. The patient may be unable to see or feel on the affected side of the body.
2. *Protect the patient from injury to the affected side.* Give regular reminders to look at and touch the affected side.	**2.** Hemiplegia may be accompanied by full or partial hemianesthesia, making the patient unaware of actual or impending injury. Relearning awareness and acceptance of the affected side by using that side helps move the patient toward functional recovery.
3. *If the patient has a visual field deficit, suggest frequent head-turning* to widen the visual field. Make sure that food and other objects at the bedside are placed well within the patient's visual field.	**3.** Visual field deficits may prevent the patient from observing the visual cues needed to prevent injury. Placing food and other objects in the patient's visual field helps prevent accidents and ensure adequate nutrition.
4. Additional individualized interventions:_____	**4.** Rationales: _____

Nursing diagnosis

Impaired verbal communication related to cerebral injury

Neurologic disorders

NURSING PRIORITY
Establish effective means of communication.

PATIENT OUTCOME CRITERION
Within 1 hour of admission, the conscious patient will establish some form of verbal or nonverbal communication.

INTERVENTIONS	RATIONALES
1. *Assess communication ability.* Explain to the patient that the stroke may have affected speech. Ask simple questions that evaluate the patient's ability to repeat words, interpret, follow directions, and express feelings. Allow ample time for responses.	1. Identifying speech problems (such as expressive or receptive aphasia) is the first step in planning rehabilitation. A patient with receptive aphasia may still be able to process information but is slower to interpret stimuli and form a response.
2. *Speak slowly and clearly, using short sentences;* never shout. Use simple explanations and gestures. Always include the patient in conversation when others are present. Avoid answering for the patient. Never use baby talk. Provide an alternative means of communication (such as a word board or pencil and paper) if needed.	2. Rapid or complex explanations may cause neurosensory overload, adding to the patient's frustration. Hearing usually isn't impaired, and shouting adds to the patient's distress over deficits. Answering for the patient, talking around the patient, and using baby talk are demeaning and contribute to the patient's sense of helplessness. Alternative means of communication may be needed while the patient relearns verbal skills.
3. *If significant speech deficits are present, arrange a referral to a speech therapist* for more comprehensive evaluation and rehabilitation services.	3. A speech therapist can pinpoint and treat specific speech problems.
4. *Reassure the patient that functional recovery is possible* with patience and consistent rehabilitation. Help the patient with repetition of verbal and physical exercises. Involve family members in the patient's exercises. If the patient uses inappropriate profanity, counsel the family.	4. A patient with severe deficits may despair of resuming normal activities; maintaining hope is vital for the fullest recovery. Over time, the brain can develop new pathways for functions; repetition aids this process. Family support helps maintain morale. Family members may be shocked by inappropriate profanity; advise them that this is typical in a patient whose speech has been affected by stroke.
5. Additional individualized interventions: _____	5. Rationales: _____

> **Suggested NIC Interventions**
> *Active listening; Communication enhancement: Hearing deficit; Communication enhancement: Speech deficit; Communication enhancement: Visual deficit*

> **Suggested NOC Outcomes**
> *Communication ability; Communication: Expressive ability; Communication: Receptive ability*

Nursing diagnosis
Deficient knowledge (stroke management) related to lack of exposure to information on self-care

NURSING PRIORITY
Provide thorough patient and family teaching.

PATIENT OUTCOME CRITERIA
By the time of discharge, the patient or family will, upon request:
- express understanding of what has happened
- name risk factors associated with a potential recurrence of stroke
- list and discuss all medications for use at home

- list four signs of bleeding (if the patient is taking an anticoagulant)
- list signs of TIA and stroke
- demonstrate understanding of the activity regimen and perform activities
- use mobility aids appropriately if needed
- name measures to protect the affected side
- verbalize understanding of the bowel and bladder control program
- express understanding of food and fluid intake recommendations
- tolerate frustration over speech deficits and use alternative measures to communicate
- express comprehension of the plan for ongoing rehabilitation
- express understanding of normal emotional responses.

INTERVENTIONS	RATIONALES
1. See the "Knowledge deficit" care plan, page 129.	**1.** The "Knowledge deficit" care plan provides general information for use in patient and family teaching. This care plan provides additional information specific to the stroke patient.
2. *Explain to the family that some emotional lability is typically associated with cerebral injury but that such behavior usually decreases over time.* Teach the family how to gently guide the patient back to appropriate emotional and physical responses. Encourage patience, affection, and the use of humor.	**2.** Family members may be confused and distressed by unexpected emotional outbursts, and they may be reassured to know that physiologic factors are at least partially responsible. The family may help the patient reestablish appropriate responses through supportive, gentle reminders. Family understanding and patience, with humor at appropriate moments, may defuse potentially volatile emotional outbursts.
3. Maintain an attitude of acceptance and understanding. Don't exacerbate emotional outbursts by reacting personally to them. Encourage normal expression of feelings related to lost abilities.	**3.** A patient who has suffered a stroke typically exhibits excessive or inappropriate emotions as a result of brain injury. The profound alteration such deficits as aphasia cause in the patient's relationship with the environment can also cause widely varied emotional reactions, ranging from rage to grief; expression of such feelings is part of coping. The patient may be unable to control emotional responses, and strong reactions on the part of family members or caregivers may add to the patient's isolation and distress.
4. *Instruct the patient and his family about medications to be taken at home,* including antihypertensive drugs, anticoagulants, and antiplatelet aggregation medication.	**4.** Understanding and complying with the drug regimen decreases the risk of a stroke recurring.
5. *If the patient will be receiving anticoagulant therapy at home, provide thorough instructions* about: – the action, dosage, and schedule of the medication – the need for frequent follow-up laboratory testing to determine dosage requirements – signs of bleeding problems (melena, petechiae, easy bruising, hematuria, epistaxis) and the need to report them – measures to control bleeding – dietary considerations – the need to avoid aspirin and other over-the-counter medications unless specifically approved by the physician – the need to avoid trauma	**5.** Because anticoagulant use may cause life-threatening bleeding, the patient and his family must understand the regimen completely. – Anticoagulants should be taken on a regular schedule in the prescribed dosage for maximum effectiveness. – Tests determine the need for dosage adjustments. – Excessive bleeding may indicate the need for a dosage adjustment, a therapeutic antidote, or both. – Uncontrolled hemorrhage can be fatal. – Vitamin K intake can affect dosage requirements. – Some drugs can augment the effects of anticoagulants. – Even minimal trauma may cause serious injury because of the effects of anticoagulants.

Neurologic disorders

– the importance of wearing a medical identification bracelet and of notifying other health care professionals (such as the dentist or optometrist) of anticoagulant therapy.

6. Teach the importance of lifestyle modifications to minimize the risk of stroke recurrence, including blood pressure control, weight control, cholesterol management, exercise, smoking cessation, diabetes control, diet modifications, and stress reduction.

7. *Teach the patient and his family to recognize and seek help for signs and symptoms associated with strokes:* vertigo, vision disturbances, sudden weakness or falls without loss of consciousness (drop attacks), paresthesia of the face or extremities, speech disturbances, lateralized temporary weakness, or sudden, severe, unexplained headache.

8. *Teach the patient and family about rehabilitation plans, and arrange for home care follow-up or in-home assistance, as needed.* Also teach the patient specific, individualized information on activities, safety measures, and proper positioning. Show how to use mobility aids (slings, braces, or walkers), and demonstrate airway maintenance and feeding techniques. Go over the patient's bowel and bladder control program. Reinforce the signs and symptoms of complications (decreasing neurologic status, infection, bleeding, or thromboembolic events). Make sure the patient and his family understand food and fluid intake recommendations, skin care measures, communication techniques, and how to cope with emotional lability.

9. Discuss with the family the advisability of learning cardiopulmonary resuscitation (CPR) techniques.

10. Additional individualized interventions: _____
_____

– Other health care providers must be aware of the patient's medication regimen so that they can adjust their care to prevent injury.

6. These lifestyle modifications may decrease the risk of a stroke recurring.

7. Recognizing the signs and symptoms of a stroke and quickly seeking medical help allows for medical interventions that can decrease the extent of brain tissue damage.

8. The rehabilitation level at discharge varies from patient to patient and may also depend on the availability of home care resources. Most stroke patients require some assistance at home after discharge, either from motivated and well-taught family members or from professional caregivers. Because of the impact of DRGs, a stroke patient may be discharged from the hospital early in the rehabilitation process. Discharge planning should always address ongoing rehabilitation.

9. Many risk factors for stroke—such as hypertension and atherosclerosis—also are risk factors for myocardial infarction and cardiac arrest. Cardiac arrest can also cause further stroke from ischemia.

10. Rationales: _____
_____

Suggested NIC Interventions Teaching: Procedure/treatment	*Suggested NOC Outcomes* Knowledge: Treatment regimen

---

Discharge planning
DISCHARGE CHECKLIST
Before discharge, the patient shows evidence of:
- ❑ absence of fever and pulmonary or cardiovascular complications
- ❑ stable vital signs
- ❑ absence of signs and symptoms indicating progression of neurologic deficit
- ❑ prothrombin level within acceptable parameters
- ❑ absence of skin breakdown and contractures
- ❑ ability to tolerate activity within expected parameters
- ❑ ability to transfer and ambulate
- ❑ ability to perform activities of daily living
- ❑ ability to compensate for neurologic deficit, such as paralysis, spasticity, or speech impairment
- ❑ ability to control bowel and bladder functions
- ❑ ability to tolerate nutritional intake
- ❑ participation in physical therapy and occupational therapy program with maximum benefit attained

- referral to home care if the patient is progressing toward maximum rehabilitation potential and home support system is adequate
- referral to a rehabilitation facility or nursing home for continued rehabilitation if the home support is inadequate or the patient needs continued rehabilitation outside the home
- referral form reflecting the patient's progress, potential, and goals and containing all other appropriate information necessary to provide continuity of care.

TEACHING CHECKLIST

Document evidence that the patient and his family demonstrate an understanding of:
- the injury or disease process and its implications
- the purpose, dosage, administration schedule, and adverse effects of all discharge medications (these may include anticoagulants, antiplatelet aggregation medications, and antihypertensives)
- the need for follow-up laboratory tests (if indicated)
- signs of cerebral impairment
- signs of infection
- signs of thromboembolic or other complications
- activity and positioning recommendations and mobility aids
- food and fluid intake recommendations
- the bowel and bladder control program
- risk factors
- safety measures
- use of medical identification bracelet
- the advisability of CPR classes for the family
- skin care
- communication measures
- verbal practice exercises
- expected emotional lability and coping methods
- community resources
- when and how to use the emergency medical system
- date, time, and location of follow-up appointment
- home care arrangements.

DOCUMENTATION CHECKLIST

Using outcome criteria as a guide, document:
- clinical status on admission
- significant changes in status
- neurologic assessments
- pertinent laboratory and diagnostic test findings
- medication therapy
- activity and positioning
- food intake
- fluid intake and output
- bowel and bladder control measures
- communication measures
- patient and family teaching
- discharge planning.

Associated care plans

- Compromised family coping
- Geriatric care
- Grieving
- Impaired physical mobility
- Ineffective individual coping
- Knowledge deficit
- Nutritional deficit
- Seizures
- Thrombophlebitis

References

Bogousslavsky, J., and Caplan, L., eds. *Stroke Syndrome*, 2nd ed. New York: Cambridge University Press, 2001.

Fisher, M. *Stroke Therapy*, 2nd ed. Boston: Butterworth-Heinemann, 2001.

Gilroy, J. *Basic Neurology*, 3rd ed. New York: McGraw Hill Book Co., 2000.

Kammersgaard, L.P. "Admission Body Temperature Predicts Associated Long-term Mortality After Acute Stroke," *Stroke* 33(7):1759-62, July 2002.

Parsons, M.W., et al. "Acute Hyperglycemia Adversely Affects Stroke Outcome: A Magnetic Resonance and Spectroscopy Study," *Annals of Neurology* 52(1):20-28, July 2002.

Saver, J. "Highlights from the 27th International Stroke Conference," Medscape *Neurology and Neurosurgery* 4(1), February 2002.

Sole, J.L., et al. *Introduction to Critical Care Nursing*, 3rd ed. Philadelphia: W.B. Saunders Co., 2001.

Victor, M., and Ropper, A. *Adams and Victor's Manual of Neurology*, 7th ed. New York: McGraw Hill Book Co., 2001.

Warlow, C.P., et al. *Stroke: A Practical Guide to Management*, 2nd ed. Oxford: Blackwell Science Pubs., 2001.

Neurologic disorders

Respiratory disorders

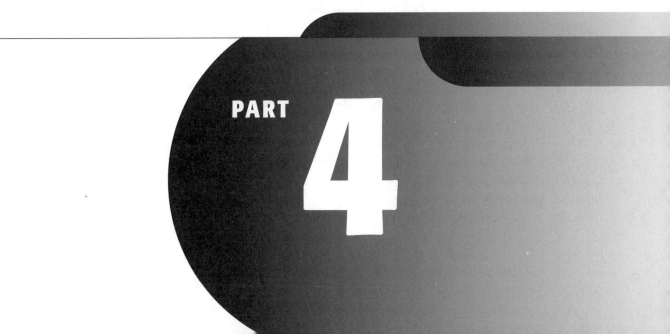

PART

4

Acute respiratory distress syndrome

DRG INFORMATION
DRG 099   Respiratory Signs and Symptoms with Complication or Comorbidity (CC).
Mean LOS = 3.2 days
DRG 100   Respiratory Signs and Symptoms without CC.
Mean LOS = 2.2 days
DRG 087   Pulmonary Edema and Respiratory Failure.
Mean LOS = 6.3 days
DRG 475   Respiratory System Diagnosis with Ventilator Support.
Mean LOS = 11.2 days

Introduction

DEFINITION AND TIME FOCUS
Acute respiratory distress syndrome (ARDS) is a complex, poorly understood syndrome of diffuse damage to the alveolar-capillary membrane. The most common cause of respiratory failure in the intensive care setting, ARDS may represent the ultimate manifestation of several unrelated physiologic insults that produce direct or indirect pulmonary injury. Key clinical features necessary for its diagnosis include a history consistent with ARDS, moderate to severe hypoxemia, bilateral diffuse infiltrates on chest X-ray, and exclusion of other causes of pulmonary congestion, specifically left-sided heart failure.

Known by many other names (such as noncardiogenic pulmonary edema, shock lung, and postpump lung), ARDS is characterized by interstitial and alveolar pulmonary edema resulting from increased permeability of the pulmonary microvasculature. Other key pathophysiologic features include a massive pulmonary shunt, decreased lung compliance, and increased alveolar dead space. On autopsy, lungs are heavy and wet, demonstrating congestive atelectasis, and marked by hyaline membrane formation and pulmonary fibrosis.

The chemical mediators involved in ARDS are complex and poorly understood. One theory is that in sepsis, bacteria stimulate granulocytes lodged in the lung. The resulting oxidative burst releases toxic metabolites (such as free radicals) and proteolytic enzymes, both of which can cause severe pulmonary injury. Other chemical mediators include histamine, serotonin, and prostaglandins. This care plan focuses on the critically ill patient with a diagnosis of ARDS. (See *Clinical snapshot: Acute respiratory distress syndrome.*)

ETIOLOGY AND PRECIPITATING FACTORS
- Gram-negative sepsis, *Pneumocystis carinii* pneumonia, bacterial or viral pneumonia, or other infections
- Aspiration of gastric contents, fresh or salt water (near drowning), or other liquids
- Pulmonary contusion, nonthoracic trauma, burns, or other types of trauma
- Inhalation of smoke, toxic levels of oxygen, corrosive chemicals, or other toxins
- Shock
- Fat embolism, cardiopulmonary bypass, massive transfusions, disseminated intravascular coagulation, transfusion reaction, or other hematologic causes
- Drug overdose, particularly heroin, methadone (Dolophine), and propoxyphene (Darvon)
- Pancreatitis, uremia, or miliary tuberculosis (rare)

Focused assessment guidelines

NURSING HISTORY (FUNCTIONAL HEALTH PATTERN FINDINGS)
Health-perception–health-management pattern
- History of catastrophic pulmonary insult followed by a lag time of several hours to several days and then progressive dyspnea

PHYSICAL FINDINGS
General appearance
- Restlessness

Pulmonary
- Tachypnea
- Hyperventilation
- Progressive dyspnea
- Fine, diffuse crackles
- Increased peak inspiratory pressure (if on ventilator)

Neurologic
- Deteriorating level of consciousness (LOC)

Integumentary
- Cyanosis

DIAGNOSTIC STUDIES
No single diagnostic test exists for ARDS.
- Arterial blood gas (ABG) values — reveal moderate to severe hypoxemia (partial pressure of arterial oxygen [Pao_2] less than 50 mm Hg), even when the inspired oxygen concentration is greater than 60%, and hypercapnia (partial pressure of arterial carbon dioxide [$Paco_2$] is greater than 50 mm Hg)

- Alveolar-arterial gradient — reveals increased gradient (greater than 15 mm Hg on room air or greater than 50 mm Hg on l00% oxygen)
- Shunt calculation — reveals pulmonary shunt in excess of 5%, typically 20% to 30%
- Bronchial fluid protein to serum protein ratio — greater than 0.5, indicating unusually high protein concentration in the bronchial fluid (implying that a damaged alveolar-capillary membrane is allowing proteins to leak through capillary walls)
- Chest X-ray — reveals bilaterally diffuse infiltrates
- Lung compliance — reduced below 50 ml/cm H_2O, typically 20 to 30 ml/cm H_2O

- Pulmonary artery wedge pressure — normal or only slightly elevated (less than 15 mm Hg), indicating that left-sided heart failure isn't causing pulmonary congestion
- Functional residual capacity — reduced

POTENTIAL COMPLICATIONS
- Respiratory arrest
- Respiratory failure
- Pulmonary fibrosis
- Disseminated intravascular coagulation
- Persistent pulmonary function abnormalities after recovery (such as mild restrictive disease, impaired gas transfer, or expiratory small-airway obstruction)

CLINICAL SNAPSHOT ☀

Acute respiratory distress syndrome

Major nursing diagnoses and collaborative problems	Key patient outcomes
CP: Hypoxemia	Exhibit arterial blood gas levels within normal limits, typically: pH, 7.35 to 7.45; Pao_2, 80 to 100 mm Hg; $Paco_2$, 35 to 45 mm Hg; and HCO_3^-, 22 to 26 mEq/L.
CP: Risk for complications	Maintain vital signs within normal limits, typically: heart rate, 60 to 100 beats/minute; systolic blood pressure, 90 to 140 mm Hg; and diastolic blood pressure, 50 to 90 mm Hg.
ND: Ineffective coping	Display effective coping skills.

Collaborative problem

Hypoxemia related to pulmonary shunt, interstitial edema, and alveolar edema

NURSING PRIORITIES
- Prevent further deterioration of lung function.
- Support the lung during healing.
- Maintain oxygenation.

PATIENT OUTCOME CRITERIA
Within 3 days of the initial insult and continuously thereafter, the patient will:
- display eupnea
- have a respiratory rate of 12 to 20 breaths/minute
- have clear breath sounds
- display an LOC equal to or better than that on admission
- have normal chest X-rays
- maintain ABG values within normal limits, typically: pH, 7.35 to 7.45; Pao_2, 80 to 100 mm Hg; $Paco_2$, 35 to 45 mm Hg; and HCO_3^-, 22 to 26 mEq/L
- have an arterial oxygen saturation (Sao_2) of 95% or better and a mixed venous oxygen saturation ($S\bar{v}o_2$) of 60% to 80% if oximetry is used.

INTERVENTIONS

1. *Monitor for clinical signs and symptoms:* *

– initial insult period — persistent unexplained mild tachypnea, breathlessness, air hunger, and normal breath sounds

– latent period — persistent moderate tachypnea; increasing dyspnea; neck, chest, or abdominal muscle use; fatigue; restlessness; confusion; and crackles
– progressive pulmonary insufficiency — severe tachypnea and hyperventilation, progressive dyspnea, gurgles, and deteriorating LOC

– terminal stage — depressed LOC, arrhythmias, and profound shock leading to asystole.

2. *Obtain chest X-rays daily as ordered, and monitor serial findings.* Be alert for reports indicating patchy infiltrates or "whiteout." Also note any other abnormal findings.

3. *Obtain ABG values at least every 4 hours as ordered.* Note degree of hypoxemia and any acid-base imbalance, typically:
– normal Pao_2, mild hypocapnia, and respiratory alkalosis during the insult period

– borderline hypoxemia during the latent period

– progressive hypoxemia, increasing hypercapnia, and worsening respiratory and metabolic acidosis as pulmonary insufficiency becomes more pronounced

– refractory hypoxemia, hypercapnia, and severe respiratory and metabolic acidosis during the terminal stage.

RATIONALES

1. Clinical signs and symptoms, when correlated with ABG values and chest X-ray results, indicate the syndrome's progression.
– The initial insult is followed by a variable lag period before signs and symptoms appear. About 60% of ARDS patients develop clinical indicators within 24 hours, 30% within 24 to 72 hours, and 10% after 72 hours. During the initial insult, signs and symptoms are mild and nonspecific. Tachypnea despite a normal Pao_2, the most characteristic finding, probably results from stimulation of juxtacapillary receptors in the alveolar interstitium.
– Signs and symptoms during the latent phase reflect borderline hypoxemia and interstitial edema.

– As the syndrome worsens, respiratory distress becomes marked. Increased dead space creates a need for high minute volumes at the same time as decreasing compliance creates a need for high inspiratory pressures. The continuing capillary leak produces frank alveolar edema, and the massive pulmonary shunt produces hypoxemia.
– In the terminal stage, hypoxemia refractory to therapy produces profound brain and heart dysfunction, terminating in cardiopulmonary arrest.

2. Chest X-rays are used to monitor the degree of edema and the development of complications. During the initial insult, the X-ray is typically normal. Patchy infiltrates appear during the latent period, worsen during pulmonary insufficiency, and culminate in a complete "whiteout" in the terminal stage.

3. ABG values provide a way to assess and document gas exchange abnormalities.

– During the insult period, tachypnea maintains a normal Pao_2, but the accompanying carbon dioxide blow-off produces hypocapnia and respiratory alkalosis.
– Borderline hypoxemia reflects early impairment of gas diffusion.
– Hypercapnia develops later because carbon dioxide is much more diffusible than oxygen. Carbon dioxide retention produces respiratory acidosis. The worsening oxygen deprivation causes cells to switch from aerobic to anaerobic metabolism, resulting in lactic acidosis.
– Refractory hypoxemia results from a massive pulmonary shunt. Interstitial edema compresses alveoli and alveolar edema fills them with fluid. In both cases, the alveoli can't oxygenate capillary blood flowing past them. The resulting perfusion without ventilation converts the alveolar-capillary units to shunt units. Without open alveoli, supplemental oxygen can't reach capillary blood.

*Italics indicate key interventions.

4. *Continuously monitor gas exchange status,* as ordered, by monitoring Sao_2 with a pulse oximeter or $S\bar{v}o_2$ with an $S\bar{v}o_2$ catheter. Monitoring the end-tidal carbon dioxide ($ETco_2$) level can also be helpful.

5. *Prepare for endotracheal (ET) intubation* if the respiratory rate exceeds 30 breaths/minute and the patient is elderly, chronically ill, suffering from preexisting pulmonary disease, fatigued, or exhibiting an increasing $Paco_2$.

6. *Implement mechanical ventilation as ordered.* See the "Mechanical ventilation" care plan, page 281.

7. Implement PEEP as ordered, typically if an inspired oxygen concentration greater than 50% is needed for more than 24 hours or if Pao_2 falls below 50 mm Hg even though oxygen concentration exceeds 60%. Place the patient with severe ARDS in the prone position for 24 hours. Then alternate to supine position for 24 hours.

8. Monitor compliance as described in the "Mechanical ventilation" care plan, page 281.

9. *Administer medications as ordered.* Document effectiveness and observe for adverse reactions.
– corticosteroids, typically methylprednisolone (Solu-Medrol)

– antibiotics

4. Conventional ABG sampling can't provide a continuous indication of gas exchange and results aren't immediately available. Continuous monitoring provides uninterrupted data, allowing early detection of impending deterioration and close monitoring of the effects of nursing interventions. It also permits assessment of the effects of multiple interventions that may have opposing effects on oxygenation and cardiac output—for instance, administration of dopamine (Intropin) and nitroprusside (Nitropress) to a patient on positive-pressure ventilation and positive end-expiratory pressure (PEEP). Pulse oximetry monitors oxygen supplied to tissues; $S\bar{v}o_2$ monitoring indicates tissue oxygen consumption. $ETco_2$ evaluates ventilation.

5. ET intubation is usually necessary to protect the airway and allow for delivery of high levels of oxygen and PEEP. Advanced age, chronic illness, or preexisting pulmonary disease increases the likelihood the patient will be unable to tolerate the rapid respiratory rate. Fatigue and increasing $Paco_2$ indicate inadequate spontaneous ventilation.

6. The widespread pulmonary congestion impairs alveolar expansion. Surfactant production decreases, making alveoli even more difficult to expand. The high inspiratory pressures required to expand alveoli and the high minute volume needed to compensate for increased physiologic dead space increase the work of breathing so markedly that the patient can't maintain spontaneous ventilation. Also, hypoxemia makes the patient prone to respiratory arrest. Mechanical ventilation conserves the patient's energy, prevents respiratory arrest, and allows time for the lung injury to heal.

7. PEEP, a mainstay in the treatment of ARDS, is believed to increase alveolar size and restore alveolar ventilation. It thus increases functional residual capacity, decreases shunting, improves ventilation-perfusion matching, and improves compliance. The prone position improves gas distribution to gravity-dependent areas of the lung.

8. Compliance objectively measures the ease of lung expansion. Decreasing compliance, implying increasing lung stiffness, indicates that ARDS is worsening. Interpreting compliance values is covered in the "Mechanical ventilation" care plan.

9. Medications have limited effectiveness in ARDS but may be prescribed empirically.
– Corticosteroid administration in ARDS is controversial. Although anecdotal reports and limited clinical and animal studies suggest possible effectiveness in certain types of ARDS such as radiation pneumonitis, no randomized, controlled study in humans has demonstrated its effectiveness.
– Antibiotics are usually prescribed for suspected or documented infection. Although many physicians prescribe them prophylactically in ARDS, such use hasn't been proven effective.

– sedatives

– Morphine, diazepam (Valium), and other sedatives can help control struggling, thus improving oxygenation and decreasing the risk of barotrauma. The patient's sedation level should be carefully monitored. If a paralytic agent such as pancuronium is used, the patient should also receive an amnesiac agent.

10. Additional individualized interventions:_____

10. Rationales:_____

Collaborative problem
Risk for complications related to single or multiple organ failure

NURSING PRIORITY
Minimize the effects of related organ failure.

PATIENT OUTCOME CRITERIA
Within 24 hours of the initial insult and then continuously, the patient will:
- maintain vital signs within normal limits, typically: heart rate, 60 to 100 beats/minute; systolic blood pressure, 90 to 140 mm Hg; and diastolic blood pressure, 50 to 90 mm Hg
- display normal sinus rhythm
- produce an hourly urine output greater than 30 ml
- show no signs of infection.

INTERVENTIONS

1. *Maintain adequate cardiac output.* Assist with pulmonary artery (PA) catheter insertion, if indicated. Monitor PA pressures, vital signs, electrocardiogram, and urine output according to appendix A, Monitoring standards.

2. *Administer packed red blood cells as ordered* to maintain the hemoglobin level between 12 and 15 g/dl.

3. *Administer crystalloid or colloid I.V. fluids as ordered.* Monitor fluid administration closely.

4. If the patient has gastric distention, a decreased LOC, or impaired airway protection reflexes, obtain an order to institute gastric drainage.

5. *Provide nutritional support as ordered.* See the "Nutritional deficit" care plan, page 138.

RATIONALES

1. Arterial oxygen transport (the amount delivered to the tissues) depends on cardiac output and oxygen content. Close monitoring of hemodynamic values is essential: Enough fluid must be given to maintain cardiac output, but too much fluid worsens the pulmonary capillary leak. A PA catheter also helps differentiate cardiac from noncardiac pulmonary edema.

2. Oxygen content depends on the hemoglobin level, hemoglobin saturation, and Pao_2. This hemoglobin level maintains normal oxygen transport.

3. The choice of appropriate fluid in ARDS remains controversial. Crystalloids readily cross from the vascular to the interstitial space, potentially worsening edema. Colloids also cross the leaky capillary membrane, move into the interstitial space, and draw water to the space by osmosis, also worsening edema. Close monitoring minimizes the potential for developing shock and fluid overload, two risk factors for ARDS.

4. Aspiration of gastric contents is a risk factor for ARDS. Gastric drainage can prevent such aspiration.

5. The protracted period of mechanical ventilation necessary for most ARDS patients requires total parenteral nutrition to maintain pulmonary muscle strength and immunologic defense mechanisms.

6. *Maintain strict asepsis.* Monitor for signs and symptoms of infection, and document and report them promptly to the physician. Institute aggressive treatment measures as ordered.

6. A major infection in an ARDS patient can readily lead to death if the source of the infection can't be identified. After the source is identified, prompt, aggressive treatment can save the patient's life.

7. *Observe for signs of single or multiple organ dysfunction syndrome,* especially central nervous system failure, renal failure, and GI dysfunction.

7. Failure or dysfunction of additional organ systems is linked with increased mortality in ARDS.

8. *Implement general supportive nursing measures to prevent the complications of immobility.* See the "Impaired physical mobility" care plan, page 111.

8. The patient on prolonged bed rest is at risk for many complications that worsen lung function, such as pneumonia, atelectasis, and pulmonary embolism. The "Impaired physical mobility" care plan contains detailed interventions for these and other potential complications.

9. Additional individualized interventions:_____
_____

9. Rationales:_____
_____

Nursing diagnosis

Ineffective coping related to abrupt onset of life-threatening illness

NURSING PRIORITY

Maximize the patient's and his family's coping skills.

PATIENT OUTCOME CRITERION

The patient will indicate increased ability to cope, if able to communicate.

INTERVENTIONS

1. *Implement the measures outlined in the "Ineffective individual coping" care plan,* page 124.

RATIONALES

1. Whether ARDS occurs after a catastrophic incident such as trauma or complicates an already critical illness, its onset places the patient and his family under severe stress. This stress is increased by the treatments the patient must undergo, particularly mechanical ventilation, which precludes oral communication at the time when the patient and his family most need it. Using the measures detailed in the "Ineffective individual coping" care plan makes the ordeal more bearable and decreases anxiety-induced oxygen requirements.

2. *Encourage the family to interact with the patient.*

2. Interaction with loved ones decreases the patient's sense of isolation and encourages a positive attitude toward treatment.

3. *Encourage the patient to express his feelings about treatments,* especially mechanical ventilation.

3. Becoming aware of feelings and expressing them clearly and appropriately are healthy coping behaviors.

4. *Provide another method of communication for the patient,* such as eye blinks or paper and pencil.

4. Intubation prevents the patient from speaking. Providing another means of communicating increases the patient's sense of security and promotes safety.

5. Additional individualized interventions: _____
_____

5. Rationales: _____
_____

Suggested NIC Interventions	*Suggested NOC Outcomes*
Coping enhancement; Family involvement promotion	*Coping; Social support*

Discharge planning

DISCHARGE CHECKLIST

Before discharge, the patient shows evidence of:
❐ vital signs within normal limits for the patient
❐ spontaneous respiratory rate of 12 to 24 breaths/minute
❐ patent airway without ET intubation
❐ discontinuation of PA catheter.

TEACHING CHECKLIST

Document evidence that the patient and his family demonstrate an understanding of:
❐ definition and pathophysiology of ARDS
❐ probable cause
❐ prognosis
❐ rationale for mechanical ventilation, PEEP, and other therapies.

DOCUMENTATION CHECKLIST

Using outcome criteria as a guide, document:
❐ the patient's clinical status on admission
❐ significant changes in status
❐ pertinent diagnostic test findings
❐ airway care
❐ tolerance of ventilator and PEEP
❐ response to medications
❐ fluid therapy
❐ nutritional support
❐ nursing care to combat effects of immobility
❐ psychological coping
❐ patient and family teaching
❐ discharge planning.

Associated care plans

- Compromised family coping
- Disseminated intravascular coagulation
- Grieving
- Hypovolemic shock
- Impaired physical mobility
- Ineffective individual coping
- Mechanical ventilation
- Multiple trauma
- Nutritional deficit
- Septic shock

References

American Lung Association Web site: *www.lungusa.org/diseases/ards_factsheet.html.*

Handbook of Diseases, 2nd ed. Springhouse, Pa.: Springhouse Corp., 2000.

Intelihealth Web site: *www.intelihealth.com.*

Jordan, K. (ed). *Emergency Nursing Care Curriculum.* Emergency Nurses Association. Philadelphia: W.B. Saunders Co., 2000.

Lynn-McHale, D.J., and Carlson, K.K. American Association of Critical Care Nurses *AACN Procedure Manual,* 4th ed. Philadelphia: W.B. Saunders Co., 2001.

Phipps, W.J., et al. *Medical-Surgical Nursing, Health and Illness Perspective,* 7th ed. St. Louis: Mosby–Year Book, Inc., 2003.

Shoemaker, W.C., et al. *Textbook of Critical Care,* 4th ed. Philadelphia: W.B. Saunders Co., 2002.

Thompson, J.M., et al. *Mosby's Clinical Nursing,* 5th ed. St. Louis: Mosby–Year Book, Inc., 2002.

Asthma

DRG INFORMATION

DRG 087   Pulmonary Edema and Respiratory Failure.
     Mean LOS = 6.3 days

DRG 088   Chronic Obstructive Pulmonary Disease.
     Mean LOS = 5.1 days

DRG 096   Bronchitis and Asthma with Complication or
     Comorbidity (CC). Age 17+.
     Mean LOS = 4.6 days

DRG 097   Bronchitis and Asthma without CC. Ages 17
     to 69.
     Mean LOS = 3.6 days

DRG 098   Bronchitis and Asthma. Ages 0 to 17.
     Mean LOS = 4.2 days

DRG 475   Respiratory System Diagnosis with Ventilator
     Support.
     Mean LOS = 11.2 days

Introduction

DEFINITION AND TIME FOCUS

Asthma is characterized by widespread narrowing of the airways (bronchoconstriction), increased mucus production, mucosal inflammation and edema, and airflow obstruction. These effects result from an increased responsiveness and hyperreactivity of the tracheal and bronchial smooth muscle to various stimuli and are reversible, either spontaneously or as a result of therapy. Between asthma attacks, the individual may remain symptom-free. Attacks vary in severity, from mild obstruction to profound respiratory failure. *Status asthmaticus* is a nonspecific term used when usual medical treatment fails to relieve severe obstruction.

Asthma is divided into two types:

- extrinsic asthma — begins in childhood and usually disappears in the adult; positive family history; usually seasonal; multiple, well-defined allergies; positive response to allergy skin testing (indicates an antigen-antibody response)
- intrinsic asthma — seen in adults after age 30; may be more severe in nature and continuous; associated with a history of recurrent respiratory tract infections; multiple nonspecific conditions can provoke an attack; negative response to allergy skin testing.

The adult patient admitted to the acute-care setting usually has intrinsic asthma and is in acute respiratory distress. This care plan focuses on the patient admitted after self-management or outpatient intervention has failed to stop an asthma attack. (See *Clinical snapshot: Asthma*, page 261.)

ETIOLOGY AND PRECIPITATING FACTORS

- Acute episode may have numerous causes:
- infection (viral or bacterial)
- environmental exposure to a nonspecific allergen (such as secondhand smoke, dust, or cleaning compounds)
- chronic sinusitis
- weather changes (such as heat, cold, fog, or wind)
- exercise
- gastroesophageal reflux disease
- psychogenic factors
- ingestion of aspirin (aspirin-sensitive individuals may also be sensitive to indomethacin [Indocin], mefenamic acid [Ponstel], or tartrazine [yellow dye found in many medications]).

Focused assessment guidelines

NURSING HISTORY
(FUNCTIONAL HEALTH PATTERN FINDINGS)

Health-perception–health-management pattern

- Increasing shortness of breath, stated as "can't catch breath," "can't inhale," or "hyperventilating"
- Chest tightness
- Feeling of panic or suffocation (typically resists oxygen mask)
- Increased coughing, usually dry and nonproductive, leading to shortness of breath
- Inability to move sputum out of lungs
- Attack in progress for some time before admission to acute-care setting
- Increasing fatigue and inability to handle the attack with usual measures
- Noncompliance with prescribed outpatient treatments
- Continual inhaler use (either prescription or nonprescription type) without benefit
- Identification of certain events or environmental factors as major contributors to the attack's development

Sleep-rest pattern

- Coughing that disturbs sleep

Nutritional-metabolic pattern

- Dehydration (from shortness of breath, mouth breathing, or reluctance to drink water)
- Lack of eating since the attack's onset because of preoccupation and shortness of breath; may complain of nausea, which may be related to medication use or abuse
- Weight gain (long-term corticosteroid users)

Activity-exercise pattern
- Ongoing exercise limitations because exercise can cause wheezing and shortness of breath
- Difficulty maintaining desired level of physical conditioning if exercise is limited

Cognitive-perceptual pattern
- Ability to describe complex strategies for self-management during an acute attack, but reported inability to put them into effect during an actual attack, when panic may overwhelm problem-solving skills and hypoxemia may impair thinking

Role-relationship pattern
- Avoidance of public events and activities because of embarrassment from severe dyspnea and cough
- Attack precipitated by laughing
- Attack precipitated by partner, family, or social group via such environmental irritants as cigarette smoke

Self-perception–self-concept pattern
- Changes in body image related to medication's cushingoid effects (if maintenance corticosteroid therapy is used)
- Discouragement with appearance and inability to prevent or alter physiologic changes

Coping–stress tolerance pattern
- Fluctuations in emotions, such as:
- denial of problem (may ignore potential irritants by refusing to give away a pet, stop smoking, or remove offending furniture; may refuse to learn medication routines and self-management strategies)
- anger (may blame others for causing attack; may describe asthma as a "kid's disease")

PHYSICAL FINDINGS
Physical parameters, which vary with the attack's severity, are good indicators of treatment outcomes.

General appearance
- Anxiety
- Maintenance of upright position
- Fever (if infection is present)

Neurologic
- Initially, hyperalert, awake, and oriented; may become progressively less alert, although awake and oriented, as fatigue progresses
- Restlessness (from hypoxemia)
- Lethargy (from increased carbon dioxide levels)

Integumentary
- Color initially good; may be flushed; cyanosis a late, unreliable sign
- Diaphoresis
- Dry mucous membranes from rapid oral breathing and dehydration

Cardiovascular
- Sinus tachycardia (related to bronchodilating medications and stress response)
- Mild to moderate hypertension (related to medications and anxiety)
- Paradoxical pulse becoming more pronounced (greater than 15 mm Hg) as air trapping increases
- Potential arrhythmias

Respiratory
- Accessory neck muscles used during breathing; becomes more pronounced as obstruction worsens
- Respiratory rate less than 30 breaths/minute, increasing as attack worsens but possibly lessening with fatigue
- Prolonged exhalations
- Wheezing; may be audible from a distance (timing varies with severity: initially expiratory wheezing, then inspiratory-expiratory, finally no wheezing — "silent" chest indicates critical airflow limitation)
- Cough, possibly decreased sputum production (increased production a positive sign; can be yellow, thick, or crusted)
- Monosyllabic speech with worsening airflow limitation

DIAGNOSTIC STUDIES
- Arterial blood gas (ABG) measurements — may be obtained only in severe or prolonged attack; hypoxemia always present; carbon dioxide level used to stage attack's progress
- Stage 1: decreased partial pressure of oxygen (Pao_2) and partial pressure of carbon dioxide ($Paco_2$) levels (hyperventilation)
- Stage 2: decreased Pao_2 level, normal $Paco_2$ level (increased fatigue)
- Stage 3: decreased Pao_2 level (less than 50 mm Hg), increased $Paco_2$ level (critical hypoventilation and fatigue)
- Sputum specimens — Gram stain is used to detect treatable organisms; eosinophil smear is done if allergens are suspected as primary cause; culture and sensitivity testing are difficult to obtain because mucus is initially thick, tenacious, and difficult to mobilize; casts and plugs are present when sputum is mobilized
- Complete blood count and differential — white blood cell (WBC) count is increased with infection; eosinophil count is increased with allergy
- Serum electrolyte levels — potassium level is invariably decreased
- Theophylline level — may be necessary in the acute phase if the patient treated himself extensively with nonprescription and prescription remedies; normal level is 10 to 20 mg/ml; an elevated level may indicate medication misuse; a decreased level may indicate noncompliance
- Chest X-ray — shows hyperinflation; air trapping decreases as airflow obstruction improves; between attacks, hyperinflation resolves; infiltrates are present if infection is a major cause
- Pulmonary function testing (PFT) — not usually performed during an acute attack; measures of airflow rate, peak expiratory flow rate (PEFR), and forced expiratory

flow rate in 1 second (FEV$_1$) are less than 25% of predicted value in severe obstruction; full PFT demonstrates dramatic response to bronchodilators; methacholine or histamine challenge provokes increased airway resistance

- Allergen skin test — negative; positive skin test doesn't necessarily indicate that exposure will trigger a respiratory response

POTENTIAL COMPLICATIONS

- Cardiopulmonary arrest
- Cardiac arrhythmias
- Rib fractures (from violent coughing)
- Pneumothorax
- Atelectasis
- Pneumonia
- Drug overdose related to noncompliance or knowledge deficit about medication use during an acute attack

---

CLINICAL SNAPSHOT ✳

Asthma

Major diagnoses and collaborative problems	Key patient outcomes
CP: Risk for status asthmaticus or pulmonary arrest	Exhibit stable vital signs within the patient's normal limits, typically: heart rate, 60 to 100 beats/minute; systolic blood pressure, 90 to 140 mm Hg; and diastolic blood pressure, 50 to 90 mm Hg.
ND: Deficient knowledge (treatment regimen)	Describe personal plan of treatment for variations in peak flow.

Collaborative problem

Risk for status asthmaticus or pulmonary arrest related to airway obstruction, hypoxemia, and progressive fatigue

NURSING PRIORITIES

- Maintain effective airway clearance.
- Promote an efficient breathing pattern.

PATIENT OUTCOME CRITERIA

Within 1 hour of beginning therapy, the patient will:
- show an improved flow rate (FEV$_1$ and PEFR)
- mobilize sputum
- exhibit reduced anxiety while maintaining a normal level of consciousness (LOC)
- have reduced hypoxemia, with Paco$_2$ level at or below normal.
  When stabilized, the patient will:
- have improved breath sounds
- decrease use of accessory muscles for breathing
- exhibit stable vital signs within the patient's normal limits, typically: heart rate, 60 to 100 beats/minute; systolic blood pressure, 90 to 140 mm Hg; and diastolic blood pressure, 50 to 90 mm Hg
- have improved ABG measurements.

INTERVENTIONS	RATIONALES
1. *Administer oxygen via nasal cannula, 2 to 3 L/minute or more, as ordered.* *	**1.** Hypoxemia is always present in an acute asthma attack because of ventilation-perfusion imbalance. Supplemental oxygen decreases the work of breathing and reduces the potential for cardiac dysfunction.

---

*Italics indicate key interventions.

2. *Administer fluid therapy orally or I.V. as ordered.* The usual fluid goal, eight to twelve 8-oz (237-ml) glasses every 24 hours, may vary with the patient's age and general status.

2. The patient is usually dehydrated on admission. Hydration promotes expectoration of thickened sputum and minimizes development of impacted mucus.

3. *Monitor the patient's status continually until it stabilizes. Parameters to monitor include LOC, skin color and moisture, speech pattern, use of accessory muscles for breathing, breath sounds, sputum production, respiratory rate, pulse, blood pressure, and paradoxical pulse.* Obtain ABG measurements as ordered, and expiratory flow rates. After baselines are established, use a pulse oximeter to monitor oxygenation. Thoroughly document findings. Report changes that indicate deteriorating status.

3. Parameters vary with the attack's severity, the patient's response to treatment, and patient fatigue. Because the patient is physiologically unstable during an attack, parameters may change rapidly.

4. *Be especially alert for signs of a potentially fatal attack,* and promptly report them to the physician. Such signs include:
– previous severe asthma attacks
– FEV_1 of less than 500 cc or PEFR of less than 35% of predicted
– little or no response to bronchodilator therapy in 1 hour, as evidenced by flow rate measurements
– altered LOC, gasping respirations, and no evidence of air movement on auscultation
– cyanosis
– Pao_2 less than 50 mm Hg
– $Paco_2$ greater than 45 mm Hg
– paradoxical pulse (a drop in systolic pressure of more than 10 mm Hg on inspiration)
– electrocardiogram abnormality
– pneumothorax
– sweating
– use of accessory muscles.

4. One or more of these signs may indicate a potentially fatal attack. Prompt, aggressive therapy is needed to prevent pulmonary arrest.

5. *Administer medications as ordered.* The medication regimen varies but typically includes:

– bronchodilators, such as beta-adrenergics and theophylline (Slo-Phyllin). Beta-adrenergics (such as epinephrine [Adrenalin], terbutaline [Brethaire], isoproterenol [Isuprel], and metaproterenol [Alupent]) are given subcutaneously, inhaled from a pressurized canister or nebulizer, or taken orally; observe for such adverse effects as nervousness or hypertension. Theophylline preparations such as aminophylline (Phyllocontin) are initially given I.V. and then orally; observe for and report arrhythmias, tachycardia, hypotension, vomiting, or other adverse effects.

5. Although some patients can control signs and symptoms with relaxation techniques, medication is usually necessary and is more effective when used before the attack becomes severe or prolonged.
– Cyclic adenosine monophosphate (cAMP) is a chemical mediator that controls bronchodilation. Beta-adrenergics and theophyllines stimulate production or prevent destruction of cAMP and thus produce bronchodilation. Effectiveness varies with blood level.
– Corticosteroids are initially given I.V., then orally, and tapered off as soon as possible. Aerosolized corticosteroids, with or without oral agents, may be given to some patients.
– I.V. and oral corticosteroids are believed to reduce inflammation, thereby reducing edema in bronchial mucosa. Aerosolized corticosteroids may provide beneficial effects with minimal adverse effects because they're delivered directly to the affected tissues.

6. *Take steps to alleviate panic, ensure safety, and promote relaxation. Place the patient in an upright position with adequate support; promote exhalation of trapped air* by instructing the patient to prolong exhalation and to exhale without force; maintain a calm, reassuring attitude; and reduce environmental stimulation if possible.

6. The acutely asthmatic patient experiences extreme anxiety and panic and may try to lessen discomfort with counterproductive posturing and breathing patterns and with restless activity. Characteristically, the harder the patient attempts to breathe, the less productive the effort and the greater the amount of air trapped. Prolonged exhalation promotes a relaxed expiratory effort and reduces air trapping.

7. *Assess therapeutic medication levels daily, watching for associated electrolyte and glucose imbalances,* as ordered. Report abnormal findings.

7. Establishing a therapeutic medication regimen requires monitoring of drug levels and electrolyte status as the patient is rehydrated and stabilized. Theophylline clearance may be impaired, or electrolyte or glucose levels may be altered, or both — especially in the patient who has cardiac or liver disease, is hypertensive, or uses other medications.

8. *Initiate measures to mobilize sputum, such as postural drainage and percussion, suctioning (if necessary), and controlled coughing.* Keep in mind that each of these measures can intensify hypoxemia. Use supplemental oxygen, temporarily increasing the liter flow if respiratory distress is observed.

8. After hydration is begun, the patient must mobilize the thick, crusty mucus rapidly to prevent bronchial plugging. The fatigued patient may need assistance.

9. *Monitor fluid balance, noting intake and output, weight, skin turgor, condition of mucous membranes, characteristics of sputum, presence or absence of edema, and urine specific gravity and hematocrit.* Document and report abnormalities.

9. During an asthma attack, profuse diaphoresis and tachypnea cause fluid loss. Because the patient is usually too dyspneic and panicked to take oral fluids, significant dehydration may quickly occur. I.V. fluid replacement must be tailored to each patient and monitored carefully; otherwise, aggressive hydration may lead to fluid overload in the patient with compromised cardiovascular status.

10. *Don't administer narcotics or sedatives for anxiety.*

10. Anxiety in the asthmatic patient stems from hypoxemia; sedation would worsen the situation by depressing the respiratory drive and worsening hypoventilation.

11. *Watch for indications that the patient needs intubation, including fatigue, further reduction in thoracic expansion, decreasing LOC, an increase in $Paco_2$ level of more than 10 mm Hg above the resting level, severe hypoxemia, and decreasing breath sounds.* Alert the physician immediately if any of these appear.

11. When the work of breathing becomes overwhelming, exhaustion results. If intubation and mechanical ventilation aren't started promptly, pulmonary arrest can occur.

12. Additional individualized interventions: _____

_____

12. Rationales: _____

_____

Nursing diagnosis

Deficient knowledge (treatment regimen) related to complexity of therapeutic regimen

NURSING PRIORITY

Improve the patient's ability to prevent or cope with breathing difficulties.

PATIENT OUTCOME CRITERIA

By the time of discharge, the patient will:
- demonstrate appropriate breathing techniques during activity-induced shortness of breath or coughing episodes
- describe proactive strategies for dealing with environmental irritants

Respiratory disorders

■ realistically describe body-image changes related to adverse effects of medications while continuing to comply with the medication regimen

■ identify factors that may trigger attacks.

INTERVENTIONS

1. *After the acute episode resolves, help the patient identify triggers that may cause or contribute to attacks* (see *Triggers of asthma attacks.*) Such triggers may stem from the patient's diet, medications, emotional states, and specific environment.

2. *Teach the patient how to use a peak flow meter (PFM) to assess his condition. Make sure the patient knows what to do when the PFM indicates a variation in flow,* including when to use bronchodilators, anti-inflammatory agents, or antibiotics and when to contact the physician, based on his specific plan of treatment.

3. *After the acute episode resolves, discuss and demonstrate (through role playing) proactive strategies the patient can use when confronted with an environmental irritant* (such as secondhand smoke). Have the patient return the demonstration.

4. *Teach the patient how to use a metered-dose inhaler. Discuss with the patient potential adverse effects the medications can cause,* such as anxiety and tremor from bronchodilators and moon face, loss of muscle tissue, and a tendency to bruise from corticosteroids. Encourage expression of frustration about the effects on socialization that can result from these adverse effects.

5. *Demonstrate strategies to be used during a coughing episode* (for example, controlled cough technique or "huff" coughing) and for acute shortness of breath during an activity (for example, upright and forward posturing, with shoulder relaxation and prolonged exhalation). Coach the patient in using these strategies.

6. *Demonstrate and have the patient practice relaxation and stress reduction exercises.*

7. *Teach the patient the symptoms of an attack* — pain or tightness in the chest, shortness of breath, an itchy chin or throat, and a dry mouth. *Review discharge and over-the-counter medications and bronchial hygiene measures,* including the purpose, dosage schedule, and adverse effects of medications, particularly effects that require medical attention. Explain that the patient will be taking two basic types of asthma medications — one to prevent an attack, usually taken daily, and one to relieve the symptoms of an attack, taken as soon as symptoms occur.

RATIONALES

1. When the patient knows what can cause an attack, he can take steps to reduce or eliminate his exposure to these triggers.

2. Used for patients with limited expiratory flow rates, a PFM measures peak expiratory flow, an indicator of lung function. It can be used in the morning and at night when the patient is at an increased risk for attacks. If readings are abnormal, the patient needs to know how to follow his plan of treatment and when to contact the physician, who may vary the dosage of the patient's medication or take other steps to prevent a major attack.

3. The patient will be more likely to implement an assertive, nonaggressive strategy for dealing with potentially hazardous situations if he has several alternative responses. The patient may not be aware of the right to request environmental changes or may not know how to make such requests.

4. The patient needs to understand how to use a metered dose inhaler to deliver asthma medications. Although adverse effects can't be eliminated, compliance with the prescribed regimen may be improved if the patient is given a chance to express feelings about such effects.

5. Breathing strategies reduce forceful exhalation, which occurs during coughing or acute shortness of breath and results in increased airway obstruction. Using these strategies as soon as possible during an attack will lessen the anxiety that shortness of breath can cause.

6. These exercises may help reduce the frequency of attacks.

7. Teaching helps the patient follow the daily care principles needed to help prevent attacks and ensures that he knows what steps to take (including seeking emergency care) should an attack occur.

8. Improve the patient's self-efficacy (a person's belief in his ability to produce or achieve goals). On a scale of 1 to 5 (1 = not at all; 5 = very much), have the patient rate his ability to:
– decrease asthma symptoms
– take medications appropriately
– use an asthma inhaler correctly
– avoid asthma attacks
– perform relaxation exercises.
Use teaching and return demonstration to improve the patient's confidence in his ability to perform these tasks.

9. Additional individualized interventions: _____

8. An improvement in self-efficacy correlates with an improvement in future success.

9. Rationales: _____

Suggested NIC Interventions
Teaching: Procedure/treatment

Suggested NOC Outcomes
Knowledge: Treatment regimen

Triggers of asthma attacks

The four categories below include examples of specific irritants that can cause or contribute to an asthma attack.

Allergic triggers	Chemical medication triggers	Irritant triggers	Physical triggers
• House dust and dust mites • Feathers and animal dander • Mold spores and mildew • Pollens • Infections	• Alcohol • Nose drops, sprays (Neo-Synephrine) • Aspirin • Reserpine (Serpalan) • Guanethidine (Ismelin) • Propranolol (Inderal) • Methyldopa (Aldomet) • Methantheline (Banthine) • Thioridazine (Mellaril)	• Smog • Smoke • Fumes (industrial, chemicals, household cleaners, paints, varnishes) • Strong odors (perfumes, cooking odors) • Dusts (sawdust, chalk dust) • Sprays (hair spray, insect spray)	• Sulfur dioxide (food additives) • Temperature and barometric pressure change • Humidity • Winds • Strenuous exercise • Menstruation, pregnancy, menopause, or other hormonal changes

Discharge planning
DISCHARGE CHECKLIST
Before discharge, the patient shows evidence of:
❐ WBC count within normal parameters
❐ oxygen and I.V. therapy discontinued for at least 24 hours
❐ stable vital signs
❐ ABG measurements within expected parameters
❐ absence of cardiovascular and pulmonary complications (such as arrhythmias or atelectasis)
❐ tolerance of and response to oral medication regimen
❐ absence of signs and symptoms of dehydration
❐ ability to tolerate adequate nutritional intake
❐ absence of acute shortness of breath on exertion
❐ ability to ambulate and perform activities of daily living at prehospitalization level

❐ adequate home support or referral to home care if indicated by inadequate home support system or patient's inability to perform self-care.

TEACHING CHECKLIST
Document evidence that the patient and his family demonstrate an understanding of:
❐ factors that trigger an asthma attack (specific to the patient if possible)
❐ how to assess home and work environments and how to modify them to counter potential irritants
❐ preventive measures for use when irritant exposure is unavoidable
❐ clinical indicators of an impending attack
❐ relaxation and breathing exercises to improve control during an attack

Respiratory disorders

❏ purpose, dosage, administration schedule, and adverse effects requiring medical attention of all discharge medications (usual discharge medications include bronchodilators and corticosteroids)

❏ purpose and use of over-the-counter medications (bronchodilators, expectorants, cough suppressants, cold remedies, or sleep remedies) as well as precautions to take when using them

❏ bronchial hygiene measures, including indications, schedule, and use

❏ use and cleaning of respiratory therapy equipment such as metered dose inhaler, PFM, and nebulizers

❏ self-management plan, including decision-making strategies for mild attacks or early stages of an attack and an emergency plan for severe or progressing attacks

❏ hydration requirements

❏ controlled cough techniques

❏ exercise recommendations and limitations, if any

❏ measures to control shortness of breath when performing activities

❏ need for flu and pneumococcus vaccine

❏ date, time, and location of follow-up appointment

❏ how to contact the physician.

DOCUMENTATION CHECKLIST

Using outcome criteria as a guide, document:

❏ clinical status on admission

❏ significant changes in status

❏ pertinent laboratory and diagnostic test findings

❏ treatments, including patient responses

❏ respiratory status (each shift)

❏ oxygen therapy

❏ medications

❏ hydration status and fluid intake and output

❏ patient and family teaching

❏ discharge planning.

Associated care plans

■ Ineffective individual coping
■ Knowledge deficit

References

American Lung Association Web site: *www.lungusa.org/diseases.*

Crapo, J.D. et al. *Baum's Textbook of Pulmonary Diseases,* Philadelphia: Lippincott Williams & Wilkins, 2003.

Handbook of Diseases, 2nd ed. Springhouse, Pa.: Springhouse Corp., 2000.

Intelihealth Web site: *www.intelihealth.com.*

Phipps, W.J., et al. *Medical-Surgical Nursing, Health and Illness Perspectives* 7th ed. St. Louis: Mosby–Year Book, Inc., 2003.

Thompson, J.M., et al. *Mosby's Clinical Nursing,* 5th ed. St. Louis: Mosby–Year Book, Inc., 2002.

Chronic obstructive pulmonary disease

DRG INFORMATION
DRG 079 Respiratory Infections and Inflammations with Complication or Comorbidity (CC); Age 17+.
Mean LOS = 8.5 days
DRG 088 Chronic Obstructive Pulmonary Disease (COPD).
Mean LOS = 5.1 days
DRG 089 Simple Pneumonia and Pleurisy with CC; Age 17+.
Mean LOS = 6.0 days

Introduction
DEFINITION AND TIME FOCUS
COPD is a diagnostic category applied to patients whose primary respiratory difficulty involves exhalation. This plan focuses on two diseases, emphysema and chronic bronchitis. (Asthma, another disorder sometimes included in COPD, is covered in a separate care plan.)

Emphysema is the permanent destruction of alveoli that results in dyspnea inappropriate for an individual's age and level of exertion. Chronic bronchitis (inflammation of the bronchi) is characterized by a chronic productive cough resulting from hyperplasia of mucus-producing cells and increased mucus production. Most patients experience a combination of symptoms.

Common features of the stable state include:
- difficulty exhaling because of airway collapse, especially with increased effort (the harder the patient tries to exhale, the more difficult it becomes)
- air trapping with hyperinflation
- dyspnea
- history of smoking
- airway hypersensitivity to various stimuli
- difficulty clearing secretions.

Common features of an exacerbation include those of the stable state plus ventilation perfusion imbalance resulting in:
- increased breathing work
- increased myocardial work
- hypoxemia
- carbon dioxide retention.

This care plan focuses on the COPD patient who is admitted to the acute care setting with an exacerbation of the disease and for whom prescribed therapies have failed to control the symptoms. (See *Clinical snapshot: Chronic obstructive pulmonary disease,* page 269.)

ETIOLOGY AND PRECIPITATING FACTORS
Exacerbation is usually caused by a viral or bacterial infection; other common causes include exposure to environmental pollutants (secondhand smoke, dust, or cleaning compounds), exercise, and weather changes (heat, cold, fog, or wind) (See *Clinical Pathway: Managing COPD*, pages 270 to 272.)

Focused assessment guidelines
NURSING HISTORY
(FUNCTIONAL HEALTH PATTERN FINDINGS)
Health-perception–health-management pattern
- Greater than normal shortness of breath, with inability to control symptoms with prescribed or nonprescribed therapies
- Increased fatigue and inability to cope with crisis
- Increasing anxiety and panic
- Increasing difficulty expectorating sputum

Nutritional-metabolic pattern
- Anorexia
- Inability to eat and digest without shortness of breath
- Nausea, possibly associated with medications
- Bloating, especially after eating foods known to cause flatulence
- Difficulty maintaining adequate fluid intake (at least eight 8-oz [237-ml] glasses per day)
- Symptoms of fluid and electrolyte disturbance, such as weakness, lethargy, confusion, weight changes, and muscle cramping

Activity-exercise pattern
- Shortness of breath with even minimal exertion or when performing activities of daily living (ADLs)
- Shortness of breath and panic controlled with breathing techniques

Sleep-rest pattern
- Sleep pattern disturbance
- Sleeping upright (usually in a reclining chair)
- Shortness of breath during the night, relieved by bronchial hygiene and expectoration of secretions
- Nervousness and difficulty falling asleep
- Chronic fatigue and sleepiness during the day
- Nocturia (possibly related to medications)
- Morning headache

Cognitive-perceptual pattern
- Fluctuating compliance with therapeutic regimen (patient may perceive regimen as complex and difficult to understand and follow)

Role-relationship pattern
- Multiple role changes, resulting in depression, isolation, and increased dependence
- Difficulty verbalizing feelings because emotions intensify shortness of breath

Sexuality-reproductive pattern
- Complex interpersonal role changes with spouse or partner, with decreased desire for and frequency of sexual activity because of actual or potential shortness of breath

Coping–stress tolerance pattern
- Difficulty expressing either positive or negative emotions because of shortness of breath
- Fluctuating behavior (alternately passive, angry, abusive, or manipulative)

Value-belief pattern
- Ambivalence about resuscitative measures that may be necessary during hospital stay but may not ultimately improve the quality of life

PHYSICAL FINDINGS
General appearance
- Apprehension and anxiety; maintenance of upright, tense posture
- Tendency to panic easily if activity is requested
- Cachexia (emphysema); plethora (chronic bronchitis)

Cardiovascular
- Typically, rapid pulse because of medications; expected upper limit for medication-induced tachycardia is 120 beats/minute
- Atrial fibrillation or multifocal atrial tachycardia (common arrhythmias of COPD)
- Signs of cor pulmonale and right-sided heart failure (edema, jugular vein distention, or crackles)

Pulmonary
- Accentuated accessory neck muscles
- Barrel chest from hyperinflation
- Decreased breath sounds bilaterally
- Prolonged expiratory phase
- Productive cough: tapioca-like plugs (hallmark of emphysema) or copious amounts of sputum (hallmark of chronic bronchitis)
- Gurgles if secretions are copious; crackles if heart failure or pneumonia is present (crackles aren't a common or expected finding in COPD)
- Chronic sinus drainage with accompanying sinus pain (may cause recurring infections)

Neurologic
- Anxiety
- Restlessness with hypoxemia
- Lethargy and sleepiness with increased partial pressure of arterial carbon dioxide ($Paco_2$) levels

Integumentary
- Skin that discolors (mottling and cyanosis) easily during coughing spells, strenuous activity, or episodes of acute shortness of breath

DIAGNOSTIC STUDIES
- Arterial blood gas (ABG) measurements — specific values vary with disease
- Hypoxemia: most common; more pronounced with exercise; in stable state, partial pressure of arterial oxygen (Pao_2) level should be between 55 and 65 mm Hg because the patient may have a reduced respiratory drive when Pao_2 level is greater than 65 mm Hg; in acute exacerbation, Pao_2 level commonly falls below 55 mm Hg
- Increased carbon dioxide level: in stable state, $Paco_2$ level should be maintained at 50 mm Hg or less; during exacerbation, $Paco_2$ level above 50 mm Hg is common
- Acid-base imbalance: in stable state, body compensates for respiratory acidosis; during exacerbation, both respiratory and metabolic acidosis may be present
- Sputum specimens — if infection is suspected, Gram stain and culture and sensitivity tests are done to determine appropriate antibiotic
- Theophylline level — normal is 10 to 15 µg/ml (normal may be 5 to 12 µg/ml if the patient is using other drugs); may be elevated if the patient has adjusted theophylline dose
- Alpha$_1$-antitrypsin assay — uncommon; performed to determine alpha$_1$-antitrypsin deficiency in young patients with suspected emphysema
- Other tests — white blood cell count, hematocrit, and serum electrolyte levels are performed, according to suspected cause
- Chest X-ray — shows hyperinflation, with flattening of the diaphragm caused by air trapping in the chest, which may worsen during exacerbation; may also show infiltrates, depending on the cause of the exacerbation
- Pulmonary function test — usually not performed in acute exacerbation; common findings in stable state include:
- reduced expiratory flow rates, especially with effort; airway obstruction more pronounced as the patient tries harder to exhale
- some response to bronchodilators in patients with chronic bronchitis; no response in patients with emphysema
- decreased diffusion capacity in patients with emphysema predominating.

POTENTIAL COMPLICATIONS
- Acute respiratory failure
- Cardiac arrhythmias
- Depressed brain function; permanent brain injury
- Other organ injury (such as kidney)
- Pneumonia
- Pneumothorax
- Cor pulmonale

Chronic obstructive pulmonary disease

Major nursing diagnoses	Key patient outcomes
Impaired gas exchange	Exhibit ABG levels within normal limits for the patient.
Ineffective breathing pattern	Display use of effective breathing techniques, especially when experiencing shortness of breath or during exercise.
Imbalanced nutrition: Less than body requirements	Eat meals without acute shortness of breath.
Activity intolerance	Demonstrate the method for gaining control of activity-related shortness of breath.
Disturbed sleep pattern	Report an improved sleep pattern.
Deficient knowledge	List four indicators of impending exacerbation.
Ineffective sexuality patterns	Describe ways to use therapies for maximum benefit in order to engage in sexual activity.

Nursing diagnosis

Impaired gas exchange (Pao_2 level less than 50 mm Hg, with or without $Paco_2$ level greater than 50 mm Hg) related to ventilation-perfusion imbalance

NURSING PRIORITIES
- Maintain adequate airway clearance.
- Reverse hypoxemia and carbon dioxide retention.
- Maintain optimum environment for adequate function of the patient's limited respiratory reserves.
- Resolve causative factors.

PATIENT OUTCOME CRITERIA
Within 48 hours of admission, the patient will:
- exhibit a Pao_2 level greater than 50 mm Hg, with or without supplemental oxygen
- exhibit a $Paco_2$ level within the patient's normal range, typically less than 50 mm Hg
- exhibit fewer and shorter periods of acute shortness of breath.
  By the time of discharge, the patient will:
- exhibit reduced evidence of infection or environmental irritation
- easily expectorate clear or white, thin sputum
- have lungs clear on auscultation, without gurgles or crackles.

INTERVENTIONS

1. *Obtain and report ABG measurements as needed** to determine the patient's baseline, to monitor the appropriateness of therapy, and to determine the effect of an acute episode (if the patient becomes somnolent or increasingly restless or has a sudden personality change).

RATIONALES

1. ABG evaluations are the only reliable way of assessing the patient's oxygenation and carbon dioxide status. No formula exists for determining the precise percentage of oxygen a patient needs because the appropriateness of the oxygen dosage can be evaluated only by serial ABG determinations.

(Text continues on page 273.)

*Italics indicate key interventions.

Managing COPD

Patient problem	1 to 4 hours/Direct admission only	Day 1
Pulmonary • Ineffective tissue perfusion (cardiopulmonary)	• Goal: Stable pulmonary function: RR 18 to 25 breaths/minute; effective airway clearance; no change in mental status or LOC; use of diaphragmatic muscles for breathing; no restlessness or anxiety; antibiotics and theophylline I.V. given within 45 minutes of admission • VS • O_2 by nasal cannula or mask • Unit dose nebulizer with bronchodilator • MDI • Antibiotic I.V. within 45 minutes of admission • Theophylline I.V. within 45 minutes of admission • Steroid I.V. within 45 minutes of admission • I.V. fluids and saline lock • Pharmacy to assess drug orders • Drug allergies assessment and notifying pharmacy	• Goal: Stable pulmonary function: RR 18 to 25 breaths/minute; effective airway clearance; no change in mental status or LOC; use of diaphragmatic muscles for breathing; no restlessness or anxiety • VS q 8 hours • Breath sounds assessment every shift • O_2, nasal or mask • Unit dose nebulizer with bronchodilator • MDI • I.V. fluids
Tests • Anxiety related to tests, procedures, and hospitalization	• Goal: Laboratory work and tests completed within 45 minutes of admission: sputum culture and sensitivity (collect within 45 minutes of admission; document attempts; if unable, RT to induce); blood chemistry; CBC; CXR; ABG values (collect within 45 minutes of admission); theophylline level; urinalysis; PBS (if indicated); ECG	• Goal: Laboratory work and tests within expected limits: sputum report for acceptability assessment; notifying physician to reorder, if unacceptable
Activity • Risk for activity intolerance • Impaired physical mobility related to illness	• Skin breakdown assessment and documentation	• Goal: Patient tolerates activity progression: stable BP and pulse and RR; patient performs self-care with assistance; patient feeds himself • Assisting with personal care daily • Active ROM exercises q 2 hours • Initiating skin care protocol
Gastrointestinal • Imbalanced nutrition: Less than body requirements • Constipation	• Goal: Stable GI function: active bowel sounds; abdomen nondistended • GI assessment	• Goal: Stable GI function: active bowel sounds; abdomen nondistended; normal bowel pattern • GI assessment q 8 hours • Goal: Nutritional intake meets body requirements: dietary intake > 50% per meal; P.O. intake ≥ 2,000 ml/day • Intake P.O. assessment (I&O q 8 hours) • Need for supplemental intake assessment q 8 hours
Teaching • Knowledge deficit related to disease process, medication, and preventive measures		• Goal: Patient and his family participate in identifying learning needs: They verbalize understanding of care plan; demonstrate ability to follow instructions • Knowledge of disease process assessment • Providing COPD and asthma patient booklets • Teaching pursed-lip breathing • Special needs assessment
Discharge planning • Risk for self-care deficit • Risk for impaired home maintenance management	• Goal: Patient and his family participate in identifying discharge needs: They verbalize needs; acknowledge discharge process • Notifying case manager • Discharge planning assessment	• Goal: Patient and his family participate in identification of discharge needs: They verbalize needs; acknowledge discharge process • Discharge planning nurse to see if indicated
Psychosocial-spiritual • Compromised family coping • Ineffective individual coping		• Goal: Patient and family demonstrate adequate coping: They verbalize fears and anxieties; demonstrate compliance with care; participate in care • Allowing time to verbalize concerns • Pastoral care p.r.n. • Response to care or treatment assessment • Support system assessment

Day 2	Day 3
• Goal: Stable pulmonary function: RR 18 to 25 breaths/minute; effective airway clearance; no change in mental status or LOC; use of diaphragmatic muscles for breathing; no restlessness or anxiety • VS q 8 hours • Breath sounds assessment q shift • O_2, nasal or mask • Unit dose nebulizer with bronchodilator • MDI • I.V. fluids • Pharmacy for medication review	• Goal: Stable pulmonary function: RR 18 to 25 breaths/minute; effective airway clearance; no change in mental status or LOC; use of diaphragmatic muscles for breathing; no restlessness or anxiety; VS WNL; $Sao_2 \geq 92\%$; breath sounds clear; weaning steroids • VS q 8 hours • Breath sounds assessment q shift • O_2, wean O_2 • MDI • Pulse oximetry (if on O_2) (Call the physician if < 90%.) • Changing to P.O. antibiotics • Changing I.V. to saline lock • Need to change I.V. site assessment
• Goal: Laboratory work or tests within expected limits: theophylline level; CBC; blood chemistry (repeat if abnormal previously); preliminary sputum results assessment; pattern blood glucose (if indicated)	• Goal: Laboratory work or tests WNL: theophylline level normal; CBC normal; survey 6 normal (if ordered); pattern blood glucose normal (if ordered) • Pattern blood glucose (if indicated)
• Goal: Patient tolerates activity progression: stable BP and pulse and RR; patient performs self-care; patient tolerates chair 1 hour t.i.d. • OOB in chair t.i.d. • Up in chair with meals • Skin care protocol	• Goal: Patient tolerates activity progression: stable HR, BP, and RR; patient performs self-care; patient tolerates ambulation t.i.d. • Patient ambulating with assistance t.i.d. • Up in chair with meals • Skin care protocol
• Goal: Stable GI function: active bowel sounds; abdomen nondistended; normal bowel pattern • GI assessment q 8 hours • Goal: Nutritional intake meets body requirements: dietary intake > 50% per meal; P.O. intake ≥ 2,000 ml/day • P.O. intake assessment • Need for supplemental intake assessment q 8 hours	• Goal: Stable GI function: active bowel sounds; abdomen nondistended; normal bowel pattern • GI assessment q 8 hours • Goal: Nutritional intake meets body requirements: dietary intake > 50% per meal; P.O. intake ≥ 2,000 ml/day • P.O. intake assessment • Need for supplemental intake assessment q 8 hours
• Goal: Identified learning needs met: Patient verbalizes understanding of care plan; demonstrates ability to follow instructions; verbalizes special needs • Providing smoking-cessation information as appropriate • Knowledge of disease process assessment • Encouraging questions • Teaching progression of activity, pulmonary care, and equipment needs	• Goal: Identified learning needs met: Patient verbalizes understanding of progression of care; demonstrates ability to follow instructions; verbalizes special needs • Assessing knowledge of measures to prevent infection and symptoms to report to the physician at home • Teaching progression of activity, pulmonary care, and equipment needs
• Goal: Patient and his family participate in identification of discharge needs: They verbalize needs; acknowledge discharge process; participate in decision making • Discharge planning nurse to see if indicated	• Goal: Patient and his family participate in identifying discharge needs: They verbalize needs; acknowledge discharge process; participate in decision making • Home health care and equipment needs assessment and arrangement • Need for skilled nursing unit assessment • Need for pulmonary rehabilitation assessment
• Goal: Patient demonstrates adequate coping: Patient verbalizes fears and anxieties; demonstrates compliance with care; participates in care • Allowing time to verbalize concerns • Pastoral care p.r.n. • Response to care and treatment assessment • Support system assessment	• Goal: Patient demonstrates adequate coping: Patient verbalizes fears and anxieties; demonstrates compliance with care; participates in care • Allowing time to verbalize concerns • Pastoral care p.r.n. • Response to care and treatment assessment • Support system assessment

(continued)

Respiratory disorders

Managing COPD *(continued)*

Patient problem	Day 4	Day 5
Pulmonary • Ineffective tissue perfusion (cardiopulmonary)	• Goal: Stable pulmonary function: RR 18 to 25 breaths/minute; effective airway clearance; no change in mental status/LOC; use of diaphragmatic muscles for breathing; no restlessness or anxiety; stable VS; $Sao_2 \geq 92\%$; breath sounds clear; weaning steroids • VS q 8 hours • Breath sounds assessment q shift • D/C O_2 • D/C unit dose nebulizer • MDI • Changing to P.O. theophylline • Changing to P.O. steroids • I.V. site care • Pharmacy to assess discharge medications	• Goal: Stable pulmonary function: respiratory rate 18 to 25 breaths/minute; effective airway clearance; no change in mental status or LOC; use of diaphragmatic muscles for breathing; no restlessness or anxiety; stable vital signs; $Sao_2 \geq 92\%$; breath sounds clear; weaning steroids • VS assessment q 8 hours • Breath sounds assessment every shift • MDI • D/C saline lock • Pulmonary discharge instructions review
Tests • Anxiety related to tests, procedures, and hospitalization	• Goal: Patient tolerates activity progression: stable HR, BP, and RR; patient performs self-care; patient tolerates ambulation • Patient ambulating independently q.i.d. • Skin care protocol	• Pattern blood glucose (if indicated)
Activity • Risk for activity intolerance • Impaired physical mobility related to illness	• Goal: Stable GI function: active bowel sounds; abdomen nondistended; normal bowel pattern • GI assessment q 8 hours	• Goal: Patient tolerates activity progression: stable HR, BP, and RR; patient performs personal care; increased activity time; independent ambulation • Up at will • Skin care protocol
Gastrointestinal • Imbalanced nutrition: Less than body requirements • Constipation	• Goal: Nutritional intake meets body requirements: dietary intake > 50% per meal; P.O. intake $\geq 2,000$ ml/day • P.O. intake assessment • Need for supplemental intake assessment q 8 hours	• Goal: Stable GI function: active bowel sounds; abdomen nondistended; normal bowel pattern • GI assessment q 8 hours • Goal: Nutritional intake meets body requirements: dietary intake > 50% per meal; P.O. intake $\geq 2,000$ ml/day • P.O. intake assessment • Need for supplemental intake assessment q 8 hours
Teaching • Knowledge deficit related to disease process, medication, and preventive measures	• Goal: Identified learning needs met: Patient verbalizes understanding of progression of care at home • Reinforcing prior instructions p.r.n. • Discharge instructions: COPD booklet; asthma booklet; medications; pulmonary care; pursed-lip breathing	• Goal: Identified learning needs met: Patient verbalizes understanding of progression of care at home • Reinforcing prior instructions • Discharge instructions review: COPD booklet; asthma booklet; medications; pulmonary care; pursed-lip breathing
Discharge planning • Risk for self-care deficit • Risk for impaired home maintenance management	• Goal: Patient and family participate in identifying discharge needs: They verbalize needs; acknowledge discharge process; participate in decision making • Discharge plans completed	• Goal: Identified discharge needs met: Patient and family describe home care plan; demonstrate ability to manage home care • Home care plan review • Discharge medications and instructions review
Psychosocial-spiritual • Compromised family coping • Ineffective individual coping	• Goal: Patient demonstrates adequate coping: Patient verbalizes fears and anxieties; demonstrates compliance with care; participates in care • Allowing time to verbalize concern • Pastoral care p.r.n. • Response to care and treatment assessment • Support system assessment	

2. *Administer oxygen as ordered,* generally 2 L/minute during the day and 3 L/minute at night or during activity.

2. The patient with COPD may have an altered respiration-regulating mechanism. Instead of responding to an elevated carbon dioxide level (normal response), the patient with COPD may respond only to a need for oxygen. Low percentages of oxygen are less likely to decrease the respiratory drive. Oxygen supply decreases at night (nocturnal desaturation) because of decreased intercostal muscle tone during sleep. Oxygen demand increases with activity.

3. *Administer pharmacologic agents and monitor therapeutic levels as ordered.*
– Bronchodilators (commonly self-administered by patient using metered-dose inhalers)

3. Pharmacologic agents are ordered according to the severity of the disease.
– Three main classes of bronchodilators used in the treatment of COPD include anticholinergic agents (such as ipratropium), beta agonists (such as albuterol), and methylxanthines (such as theophylline). The preferred route is by metered-dose inhaler. Proper use of the inhaler provides the maximum effective dosage; a spacer device or aerochamber can be used, especially by an elderly or very young patient, to ensure adequate dosing.

– Antibiotics
– Corticosteroids

– Expectorants

– Antibiotics are ordered for the specific organism.
– Corticosteroids (I.V. or oral) are believed to reduce inflammation.
– Expectorants may be used as an adjunct to fluid therapy.

4. *Perform bronchial hygiene measures as ordered.* Assess breath sounds before and after all treatments and at least every 4 hours when the patient is awake. Report and document the effectiveness of all of the following treatments that are used: aerosols, postural drainage and percussion, and suctioning (if the coughing mechanism is inadequate).

4. Ventilation-perfusion abnormalities are the major reason for respiratory failure in the patient with COPD. Bronchial hygiene measures open obstructed airways for more effective ventilation while conserving oxygen reserves.

5. *Maintain fluid intake at eight to twelve 8-oz (237-ml) glasses of water per day,* unless contraindicated.

5. Sputum viscosity is related to the patient's hydration status. Water is the most physiologically compatible expectorant.

6. *Monitor, document, and report signs of infection or further deterioration of respiratory status,* such as an increase or decrease of sputum, changes in the sputum's color or consistency, fever, increased shortness of breath, and changes in breath sounds.

6. Routine monitoring and accurate documentation allows early detection of subtle changes in the patient's condition that might signal illness progression.

7. *If possible, reduce or eliminate environmental irritants:* Encourage the patient who smokes to quit, and don't use (or allow roommates or visitors to use) hair, deodorant, or room-freshening sprays or strong fragrances near the patient.

7. Many environmental substances and sprays can cause airway irritation in the patient with COPD (especially when the airways are already compromised) and exacerbate the condition.

8. Additional individualized interventions: _____

8. Rationales: _____

_____   _____

Respiratory disorders

Nursing diagnosis

Ineffective breathing pattern related to emotional stimulation, fatigue, or blunting of respiratory drive

NURSING PRIORITY

Maintain an effective breathing pattern.

PATIENT OUTCOME CRITERIA

Immediately upon admission, after coaching by the nurse, the patient will:
- use effective breathing techniques, especially when experiencing shortness of breath or during exercise.
  Within 24 hours, the patient will:
- pace activities to coincide with periods of maximum bronchodilation and peak energy.

INTERVENTIONS

1. *Reduce the work of breathing, and lessen depletion of oxygen reserves* through teaching and by promoting relaxation as follows:
– Position the patient for comfort (an upright position may be best, with a pillow under the patient's elbows and the patient leaning on the overbed table).
– Remind the patient to relax the shoulders and neck muscles.
– Instruct the patient to prolong exhalation.
– Sit with the patient, and encourage rhythmic breathing.
– Use a calm, unhurried manner.

2. *Teach and help the patient to perform breathing exercises, and coordinate breathing with activity.*

3. *Pace all activities* according to periods of maximum bronchodilation and peak energy. Encourage energy conservation.

4. *Instruct the patient in breathing techniques to use when expressing feelings that may cause shortness of breath.*

5. *Avoid the use of sedatives or narcotics.*

6. Additional individualized interventions: _____
_____
_____

RATIONALES

1. Inhalation normally requires muscle work and energy expenditure. Exhalation is ordinarily passive, not requiring extra energy and oxygen, but because the patient with COPD in distress uses oxygen for both inhalation and exhalation, a large amount of oxygen from each inhalation is used to take and expel the next breath. Also, because shortness of breath causes anxiety, the patient tends to tighten muscle groups, thus using even more oxygen. Relaxation and easy, prolonged exhalation maximize lung expansion while minimizing energy and oxygen expenditures. Despite the value of breathing techniques, the patient with COPD may forget them in a crisis and need the nurse's assistance to regain control.

2. Breath holding during exertion dramatically increases shortness of breath.

3. Pacing allows activity while conserving energy reserves.

4. Any expression of emotion, such as happiness, anger, or sadness, affects respiratory patterns and may increase shortness of breath.

5. These agents further depress the respiratory centers and may provoke respiratory arrest.

6. Rationales: _____
_____
_____

> **Suggested NIC Interventions**
> *Airway management; Airway suctioning; Ventilation assistance; Respiratory monitoring; Vital signs monitoring*

> **Suggested NOC Outcomes**
> *Respiratory status: Airway patency; Respiratory status: Ventilation; Vital signs status*

Nursing diagnosis

Imbalanced nutrition: Less than body requirements related to shortness of breath during and after meals

NURSING PRIORITIES

- Maintain adequate caloric and nutritional intake.
- Reduce deterrents to eating.
- Optimize environmental conditions to increase appetite.

PATIENT OUTCOME CRITERIA

Within 48 hours of admission, the patient will:
- take meals without episodes of acute shortness of breath.
  By the time of discharge, the patient will:
- have a stable weight.

INTERVENTIONS

1. *Use supplemental oxygen during mealtimes* as ordered.

2. *Perform bronchial hygiene measures before meals.* Provide mouth care, and remove secretions from the eating area.

3. *Provide frequent, small meals.*

4. *Monitor the patient's weight and nutritional intake.*

5. *Obtain a dietary consultation as soon as the patient can take foods or fluids,* with special attention to needs for:
– high-protein, low-carbohydrate, high-fat supplements

– eliminating gas-producing foods from diet

– considering the patient's food preferences and adherence to any dietary restrictions such as limiting salt.

6. Additional individualized interventions: _____

_____

RATIONALES

1. The act of eating requires oxygen. Supplemental oxygen during meals bolsters oxygen reserves.

2. Performing hygiene measures before meals ensures maximum bronchodilation and reduces activity-related ventilation-perfusion imbalances that may cause hypoxemia. The presence of sputum may decrease appetite.

3. Small meals require less oxygen for eating and digestion than do large meals.

4. During periods of exacerbation, metabolic demands may increase, creating an increased demand for calories to maintain weight. A steady weight loss over weeks to months points to insufficient calories; a weight gain of 3 lb (1.4 kg) or more within 4 days may indicate fluid retention.

5. Early dietary consultation can prevent complications from further debilitation.

– The patient with COPD has an increased respiratory rate and increased work of breathing, resulting in greater metabolic demands. A diet with a low calorie-to-nitrogen ratio will meet metabolic demands without increasing carbon dioxide production.
– Abdominal distention can cause diaphragmatic compression, increasing the sensation of shortness of breath.
– The patient is more likely to follow a nutritional plan that includes favorite, familiar foods. Necessary restrictions must be observed to promote optimal health.

6. Rationales: _____

_____

Suggested NIC Interventions *Diet staging; Nutrition management; Weight gain assistance; Fluid monitoring; Nutritional monitoring*	**Suggested NOC Outcomes** *Nutritional status; Nutritional status: Food and fluid intake; Nutritional status: Nutrient intake; Weight control*

Nursing diagnosis

Activity intolerance related to shortness of breath, avoidance of physical activity with resultant muscle weakness, deconditioning, depression and, possibly, exercise-related hypoxemia

NURSING PRIORITY

Promote a gradual return to an optimal level of activity, with absent or controlled episodes of shortness of breath. (*Note:* Progress on this priority will depend on resolving the exacerbation and its causative factors.)

PATIENT OUTCOME CRITERIA

Throughout the hospital stay, the patient will:
■ increase the ability to ambulate over longer times and distances without shortness of breath, pulse changes (rate or rhythm), blood pressure drop, or a color change.
   By the time of discharge, the patient will:
■ demonstrate the method for gaining control of activity-related shortness of breath.

INTERVENTIONS

1. *Assess the patient's ability to perform household chores, movements, work, family and social activities, volunteer work, and recreation.* Help the patient identify barriers, and develop alternative approaches to activities.

2. *Instruct the patient in breathing techniques to use when performing ADLs:* slow and relaxed exhalation, avoidance of breath holding, and relaxation of accessory muscles. (For more information and pictures of these techniques for use during instruction, contact the local American Lung Association chapter.)

3. *Administer oxygen during activity as ordered.*

4. *Before recommending an activity level, assess for stable ABG measurements and fitness level* (the pulmonary function or respiratory therapy department can assist in determining an appropriate exercise level). Also assess for other factors that can contribute to inactivity (such as family relationships), concomitant diseases (such as arthritis), or environmental conditions.

5. *Develop and implement a daily walking schedule,* increasing time and distance as tolerated. Before beginning, teach the patient how to control shortness of breath. This includes telling the patient to stop, lean back, position his hips against a sturdy object or wall, and stand with his feet apart.

RATIONALES

1. An inability to cope psychologically with the disruptive effects of disease is significantly linked to increased mortality.

2. Breathing techniques make full exhalation easier, thereby promoting removal of stale air, increasing ventilatory efficiency, and permitting a wider range of physical activity.

3. Increased activity requires supplemental oxygen.

4. If undertaken prematurely, increased activity may worsen the patient's symptoms. The patient is unlikely to follow an activity prescription that doesn't take into account ABG measurements, level of fitness, and other deterrents to activity.

5. Implementation of a walking schedule should start in the hospital, if possible, so that the patient can be observed and coached in appropriate breathing techniques. Gaining control over shortness of breath improves the patient's confidence in walking independently.

6. *Before, during, and after walking, monitor the patient's response to exercise.* Along with the time and distance walked, document the following: blood pressure (before and after), pulse rate and rhythm, patient's color, respiratory rate, and degree of shortness of breath.

7. Additional individualized interventions: _____

6. If a patient experiences desaturation or acidosis during the walk, these events will be reflected in vital sign changes. More sophisticated exercise testing may be needed to determine the extent of disability and the appropriate therapy.

7. Rationales: _____

Suggested NIC Interventions
Activity therapy; Energy management; Exercise promotion: Strength training; Nutrition management; Self-care assistance; Home maintenance assistance

Suggested NOC Outcomes
Activity intolerance; Endurance; Energy conservation; Self-care: Activities of daily living (ADL); Self-care: instrumental activities of daily living (IADL)

Nursing diagnosis
Disturbed sleep pattern related to a bronchodilator's stimulant effect, shortness of breath, depression, and anxiety

NURSING PRIORITY
Minimize sleep disruption.

PATIENT OUTCOME CRITERIA
By the time of discharge, the patient will:
- report fewer episodes of nocturnal shortness of breath
- fall asleep easily at night
- sleep throughout the night, without early morning headache or excessive drowsiness during the day
- report an improved sleep pattern or more easily controlled episodes of nocturnal shortness of breath, or both.

INTERVENTIONS

1. *Identify the patient's normal sleep pattern as well as the abnormal pattern.*

2. *Consult with the physician about adjusting medications to optimize bronchodilation with minimal stimulant effects.*

3. *Teach the patient how to perform bronchial hygiene* before retiring and as needed for nocturnal dyspnea.

4. *Administer oxygen therapy during the night as ordered.*

5. *Monitor periods of sleeplessness,* including degree of shortness of breath, pulse rate and rhythm, respiratory rate, and breath sounds. Observe which treatments provide the most benefits.

RATIONALES

1. The patient may have misconceptions about normal and abnormal sleep patterns. Discussion may clarify factors contributing to sleep disturbance.

2. Bronchodilators vary in their stimulant properties. Stimulants may cause myocardial irritability, nervousness, and anxiety and may increase oxygen demand.

3. Nocturnal shortness of breath may be unavoidable, so the patient needs to know how to deal with such episodes effectively.

4. Pao_2 levels normally decrease at night. Although most people can tolerate the decrease, the already hypoxemic COPD patient can't because hypoxemia-induced pulmonary vasoconstriction can cause or exacerbate cor pulmonale.

5. Observing a sleeplessness episode and its resolution may provide clues for preventing or coping with future episodes.

Respiratory disorders

6. *Instruct the patient in relaxation techniques to be used at bedtime.* (A patient with COPD shouldn't use sleeping medications unless the physician specifically prescribes them.)

6. Relaxation techniques can promote sleep and minimize oxygen demands. Sleeping medications may depress respirations in the already compromised patient.

7. Additional individualized interventions:_____
_____

7. Rationales: _____
_____

Suggested NIC Interventions	*Suggested NOC Outcomes*
Energy management; Sleep enhancement; Coping enhancement	Rest; Sleep; Well-being

Nursing diagnosis

Deficient knowledge (illness care) related to complexity of disorder

NURSING PRIORITY

Teach the patient to recognize an impending infection or exacerbation and to seek appropriate treatment.

PATIENT OUTCOME CRITERIA

By the time of discharge, the patient will:
- list four indicators of an impending infection or exacerbation
- correctly identify the rationale for notifying the physician before adjusting the medication regimen.

INTERVENTIONS

1. *Teach the patient the signs and symptoms of an impending infection or exacerbation,* including:
– increased or decreased sputum production
– change in the color or character of sputum over a 24-hour period
– fever (based on baseline normal temperature)
– restlessness or inability to sleep for more than one night
– increased fatigue or sleepiness.

2. *Emphasize the need to notify the physician promptly if these symptoms occur* rather than altering the medication regimen without the physician's knowledge.

3. *Caution the patient to avoid overmedication* with prescription drugs or over-the-counter (OTC) remedies.

4. Additional individualized interventions: _____
_____

RATIONALES

1. Early detection and intervention increase the likelihood of successful reversal or control of the episode.

2. Appropriate intervention requires medical judgment.

3. Overuse of some medications such as bronchodilators may actually increase oxygen demands. OTC remedies may contain substances such as ephedrine that increase or counteract the therapeutic effects of prescribed medication.

4. Rationales: _____
_____

Suggested NIC Interventions	*Suggested NOC Outcomes*
Teaching: Procedure/treatment	Knowledge: Treatment regimen

Nursing diagnosis

Ineffective sexuality patterns related to shortness of breath, change in body image, deconditioning, change in relationship with spouse or partner, and adverse reactions to medications

NURSING PRIORITY

Help the patient and spouse (or partner) to discuss feelings, and determine realistic expectations.

PATIENT OUTCOME CRITERION

By the time of discharge, the patient will describe ways to use therapies for maximum benefit in order to engage in sexual activity.

INTERVENTIONS	RATIONALES
1. Establish rapport with the patient and his spouse (or partner). Discuss their feelings concerning changes in sexual functioning.	**1.** A sense of rapport makes discussion of this sensitive topic more comfortable. Discussion will help clarify the issues involved and the expectations held by the patient and spouse (or partner).
2. Help the patient learn or arrange for therapies to optimize sexual function as desired (including medication schedule, oxygen level, bronchial hygiene, and energy conservation).	**2.** As with other activities, the patient must learn to arrange therapies to accomplish desired goals.
3. Additional individualized interventions: _____	**3.** Rationales: _____

> **Suggested NIC Interventions**
> *Body image enhancement; Role enhancement; Self-esteem enhancement; Sexual counseling*

> **Suggested NOC Outcomes**
> *Body image; Role performance; Self-esteem; Sexual identity: Acceptance*

Discharge planning

DISCHARGE CHECKLIST

Before discharge, the patient shows evidence of:
- ❑ absence of fever and other signs of infection
- ❑ ABG levels within acceptable parameters
- ❑ absence of cardiovascular or pulmonary complications
- ❑ minimal shortness of breath
- ❑ breath sounds clear or normal for patient when not in exacerbated state
- ❑ ability to tolerate ambulation with minimal limitations, as before exacerbation and hospitalization
- ❑ ability to perform ADLs independently (or with minimal assistance) at preexacerbation level
- ❑ ability to tolerate diet with minimal shortness of breath
- ❑ stabilized weight (within 5 lb [2.3 kg] of normal weight)
- ❑ adequate home support system or referral to home care if indicated because of inadequate home support, inability to perform ADLs at preexacerbation levels, or need for continued assistance with bronchial hygiene measures.

Keep in mind that the patient with COPD won't be "normal" when discharged. Therefore, discharge evaluation should relate to the patient's condition before the exacerbation. The most important thing to document is the absence of acute infection, but also note ABG levels on discharge. ABG levels must be within acceptable parameters because abnormal levels on discharge commonly cause readmission within a short time.

TEACHING CHECKLIST

Document evidence that the patient and family demonstrate an understanding of:
- ❑ practical energy conservation and breathing techniques
- ❑ signs and symptoms of infection or exacerbation
- ❑ the purpose, dosage, administration schedule, and adverse reactions requiring medical attention of all discharge medications (usual discharge medications include bronchodilators, corticosteroids, antibiotics, and expectorants)
- ❑ bronchial hygiene measures
- ❑ the use, care, and cleaning of respiratory equipment

Respiratory disorders

- the need for drinking eight to twelve 8-oz glasses of water per day
- dietary restrictions
- twice-weekly weight monitoring
- the importance of avoiding exposure to infections and the need for flu vaccination
- the importance of avoiding lung irritants, such as cold air, secondhand smoke, sprays, and dust
- the importance of avoiding situations that increase the potential for infection
- exercise prescription
- a referral to community agencies as appropriate (such as Meals On Wheels, American Lung Association, Better Breathers Club, respiratory equipment company and name of representative, emergency response service, home care agency, and smoking-cessation group)
- the date, time, and location of the next appointment
- how to contact the physician.

DOCUMENTATION CHECKLIST
Using outcome criteria as a guide, document:
- the patient's clinical status on admission
- significant changes in status
- pertinent laboratory and diagnostic tests such as ABG levels
- episodes of shortness of breath, including physical assessment parameters during each episode, treatment administered, and treatment outcome
- respiratory status per shift, including breath sounds, character of cough, and character, color, and amount of sputum
- administration and outcome of therapies given
- nutritional intake
- fluid intake
- exercise ability and activity level
- patient and family teaching
- discharge planning.

Associated care plans

- Dying
- Grieving
- Ineffective individual coping
- Knowledge deficit
- Pneumonia

References

Gibbons, D. "A Nurse-Led Pulmonary Rehabilitation Program for Patients with COPD," *Professional Nurse* 17(3):185-88, November 2001.

Handbook of Diseases, 2nd ed. Springhouse, Pa.: Springhouse Corp., 1999.

Heffner, J.E. "Chronic Obstructive Pulmonary Disease: On an Exonential Curve of Progress," *Respiratory Care* 47(5):568-607, May 2002.

Marley, A.M. "A Care Pathway for COPD," *Professional Nurse* 16(1):821-23, October 2000.

McDermott, A. "Pulmonary Rehabilitation for Patients with COPD," *Professional Nurse* 17(9):553-56, May 2002.

Narvasage, G.L. "Factors Associated with Referral of Elderly Individuals with Cardiac and Pulmonary Disorders for Home Care Services Following Hospital Discharge," *Journal of Gerontology Nursing* 6(5):14-20, May 2000.

Patient Teaching Reference Manual. Springhouse, Pa.: Springhouse Corp., 2002.

Trudeau, M.E., and Solano-McGuire, S.M. "Evaluating the Quality of COPD Care," *AJN* 99(3):47-49, March 1999.

Mechanical ventilation

DRG INFORMATION

DRG 475   Respiratory System Diagnosis with Ventilator Support.
Mean LOS 5 11.2 days

Introduction

DEFINITION AND TIME FOCUS

Mechanical ventilation (providing gas volumes sufficient to maintain alveolar ventilation) is commonly required for patients with significant breathing abnormalities that may lead to apnea or respiratory failure. This care plan focuses on the patient receiving positive-pressure ventilation, the most common type of mechanical ventilation in critical care. (See *Clinical snapshot: Mechanical ventilation*, page 282.)

ETIOLOGY AND PRECIPITATING FACTORS

■ Central respiratory depression, from such factors as drug overdose, head trauma, stroke, anesthesia, or cardiac arrest
■ Airway diseases, such as asthma and bronchitis
■ Parenchymal diseases, such as acute respiratory distress syndrome (ARDS), pulmonary edema, pneumonia, and emphysema
■ Neuromuscular disorders, such as myasthenia gravis and Guillain-Barré syndrome
■ Chest wall injury, such as pneumothorax, flail chest, and major thoracic surgery

Focused assessment guidelines

NURSING HISTORY
(FUNCTIONAL HEALTH PATTERN FINDINGS)

Health-perception–health-management pattern
■ Sudden or progressive onset of abnormal ventilatory patterns or airway obstruction
■ Severe dyspnea or air hunger (if patient is able to speak)
■ History of motor vehicle accident, assault, or other head, chest, or orthopedic trauma
■ Treatment for long-standing chronic respiratory disease
■ Recent major surgical procedure involving the thorax or upper abdomen
■ History of drug or alcohol abuse
■ History of cardiac disease

PHYSICAL FINDINGS
Pulmonary
■ Labored breathing
■ Shallow breathing
■ Agonal breathing or other abnormal breathing pattern
■ Tachypnea
■ Intercostal retractions
■ Nasal flaring
■ Accessory muscle use
■ Decreased or absent breath sounds
■ Crackles, gurgles, or wheezes
■ Increased secretions
Neurologic
■ Restlessness
■ Confusion
■ Agitation
■ Somnolence
■ Unconsciousness
Cardiovascular
■ Tachycardia (early), bradycardia (late)
■ Arrhythmias
■ Hypertension or hypotension
Integumentary
■ Diaphoresis
■ Cyanosis (central or peripheral)

DIAGNOSTIC STUDIES

■ Arterial blood gas (ABG) levels — reveal hypercapnia (partial pressure of arterial carbon dioxide [$Paco_2$] greater than 50 mm Hg) in a patient who previously had normal levels (or greater than 10 mm Hg increase above usual value in a patient with chronic obstructive pulmonary disease). ABG levels also reveal hypoxemia with a partial pressure of arterial oxygen (Pao_2) less than 50 mm Hg on supplemental oxygen
■ Alveolar-arterial (A-a) gradient — may be greater than 300 mm Hg on 100% oxygen
■ Shunt — may be greater than 30%
■ Minute ventilation (MV) (spontaneous) — may be less than 5 L/minute, indicating insufficient ventilation to remove carbon dioxide adequately, or greater than 10 L/minute, indicating excessive work of breathing
■ Vital capacity (VC) — may be less than 15 ml/kg body weight, indicating poor ventilatory reserve
■ Maximum inspiratory pressure (MIP) — may be less than 20 cm H_2O, indicating weak respiratory drive or respiratory musculature
■ Dead space: tidal volume (V_D:V_T) ratio — may be greater than 0.6, indicating excessive wasted ventilation

POTENTIAL COMPLICATIONS

- Tension pneumothorax
- GI hemorrhage
- Shock
- Pneumonia
- Ventilator malfunction
- Airway obstruction
- Long-term ventilator dependency

CLINICAL SNAPSHOT ✷

Mechanical ventilation

Major nursing diagnoses and collaborative problems	Key patient outcomes
ND: Impaired gas exchange related to failure to maintain prescribed ventilator settings	Maintain ABG levels within expected limits for the underlying disorder.
ND: Impaired gas exchange related to insufficient oxygen levels or inadequate PEEP level	Maintain Pao_2 and Sao_2 within expected limits.
ND: Ineffective airway clearance	Maintain a patent airway.
ND: Risk for injury	Remain free from pulmonary infection and other complications.
ND: Fear	Communicate needs, if conscious.
CP: Risk for dysfunctional ventilatory weaning response	Maintain a spontaneous respiratory rate of 12 to 24 breaths/minute.

Nursing diagnosis

Impaired gas exchange related to failure to maintain prescribed ventilator settings

NURSING PRIORITY

Maintain settings as ordered.

PATIENT OUTCOME CRITERIA

Once placed on mechanical ventilation and continuously thereafter, the patient will:
- have bilaterally equal chest excursion and breath sounds
- manifest compliance values within usual limits for the underlying disorder
- maintain ABG levels within expected limits for the underlying disorder.

INTERVENTIONS	RATIONALES
1. *Confirm orders for mechanical ventilation,** particularly: – Ventilator type	1. Mechanical ventilation may be achieved with many combinations of modes and settings. – The type of ventilator is determined by how the machine controls inspiration. In the acute care setting, ventilators that can deliver a prescribed volume are indicated; these are volume-cycled ventilators. Other types include time-cycled and pressure-cycled ventilators, both of which can have variable V_Ts and are used only for special situations.

*Italics indicate key interventions.

Advances in technology and an increased need for equipment have resulted in a proliferation of different ventilators. The ventilator selected depends on the patient's ventilation requirements, type of monitoring desired, and weaning options.

– Inspiratory mode

– Inspiratory modes determine the type and degree of control over inspiration.

– Control

– The control mode provides complete ventilatory support by delivering a set number of breaths per minute, regardless of the patient's inspiratory efforts. The least-used mode, it's appropriate only for an apneic or paralyzed patient (such as a patient with central nervous system dysfunction or drug-induced paralysis), or in patients with chest trauma for whom negative inspiratory pressure would be harmful (such as in flail chest). Keep in mind that this mode prevents the patient from taking additional breaths.

– Assist-control

– Assist-control, the most common mode, is suitable for almost all initial ventilator setups. This mode ensures delivery of a preset minimum number of breaths per minute but allows the patient to initiate the breath and to breathe more rapidly if desired. If the patient initiates a breath, the machine delivers the desired volume; if the patient doesn't breathe, the machine supplies the breath. Because the ventilator delivers a preset volume even on patient-initiated breaths, it lessens the work of breathing while improving alveolar ventilation.

– Synchronized intermittent mandatory ventilation (SIMV)

– SIMV, once used only for the difficult-to-wean patient, is now considered a standard ventilatory mode for full or partial ventilatory support. The machine delivers a preset number of mandatory breaths. In between, the patient can breathe spontaneously through the ventilator circuit. The ventilator senses each breath and synchronizes the mandatory breaths in such a way as not to "stack" breaths on top of each other. Because these spontaneous breaths depend on the negative pressure the patient can generate, their V_T may vary significantly from the ventilator V_T. SIMV has several advantages; it maintains lower mean airway pressures (reducing the risk of barotrauma — lung damage from excessive pressure — and depression of cardiac output), reduces the risk of hyperventilation, helps maintain respiratory muscle strength, provides ventilatory support at rapid respiratory rates, and assures more even ventilation throughout the lung.

– Pressure support

– Pressure support uses small amounts of pressure at the end of inspiration to increase V_T in a spontaneously breathing patient. Similar to intermittent positive-pressure breathing machines, pressure support can be used in combination with SIMV or as a weaning mode for a patient with inadequate spontaneous volumes.

– Pressure control

– Pressure control uses peak pressure to limit the inspiratory cycle, although V_T will vary. Close monitoring is essential.

– Expiratory maneuvers

– Expiratory maneuvers determine the degree of resistance to expiration.

Respiratory disorders

– Positive end-expiratory pressure (PEEP)

– PEEP is used commonly with positive-pressure ventilation of the patient with alveolar collapse (from loss of surfactant, early small-airway closure, or atelectasis) or alveolar filling (as in pulmonary edema and ARDS). In such a patient, nonfunctioning alveoli, unable to oxygenate blood flowing through pulmonary capillaries, produce an abnormal pulmonary shunt and hypoxemia refractory to oxygen therapy. PEEP is thought to help keep alveoli from collapsing and to recruit nonfunctioning alveoli. It also increases functional residual capacity (FRC) and allows gas diffusion to take place throughout the respiratory cycle. Because PEEP improves ventilation-perfusion matching, oxygenation improves. PEEP permits lowering of inspired oxygen concentration, helpful in preventing lung damage from excessive oxygen exposure. However, care needs to be taken to prevent trauma from higher pressures.

– Continuous positive airway pressure (CPAP)

– Similar to PEEP, CPAP is used for a spontaneously breathing patient. It maintains positive airway pressure throughout the respiratory cycle. Its benefits are similar to those of PEEP. It can be applied through a ventilator during spontaneous respiration or via a special device, such as nasal CPAP, for a nonintubated patient.

2. *Collaborate with the respiratory therapist to monitor prescribed settings* when settings are changed, when arterial blood is drawn for ABG measurements, or when pulse oximetry or capnography is used.

2. Depending on the unit protocol, either the nurse or the respiratory therapist may be responsible for checking the ventilator. If the respiratory therapist checks, the nurse should confirm that ventilator settings are as ordered when first assuming responsibility for the patient. The nurse and the respiratory therapist must collaborate closely to provide the best patient care. Checking at the times indicated ensures that prescribed settings are accurate.

– Respiratory rate: Count the machine rate and the patient's rate for 1 minute each and compare. Check controls for proper settings.

– With all ventilatory modes, the ventilator may not actually deliver the number of breaths set. Also, with assist-control or SIMV, the patient can breathe above the set rate.

– V_T: Compare delivered V_T to desired V_T, typically 10 to 15 ml/kg. On newer models, read inspired V_T from the digital readout. On models with no readout, measure exhaled V_T with a Wright respirometer.

– V_T is the amount of air inspired. Measuring exhaled V_T indicates the volume actually received. Decreasing V_T may indicate a machine, cuff, or bronchopulmonary leak.

– MV: If the patient is on assist-control or SIMV, compare actual and desired MV. If the patient is on SIMV, also compare total and non-SIMV MV.

– MV, the product of the respiratory rate and the V_T, determines alveolar ventilation. MV is related inversely to $Paco_2$: As MV increases, $Paco_2$ decreases, and vice versa. Decreased MV is associated with carbon dioxide retention and respiratory acidosis, whereas increased MV is associated with carbon dioxide blow-off and respiratory alkalosis.

Comparing actual and desired MV indicates how well the machine meets the patient's ventilatory needs. Comparing total and non-SIMV MV indicates what amount the patient's spontaneous breaths are contributing to total MV; monitoring this amount can help the physician or respiratory therapist evaluate the patient's readiness for weaning.

– Inspiratory flow rate

– This rate is the speed of airflow per unit of time. Slower flow rates are preferred because they result in better gas flow characteristics: less turbulence, lower mean airway pressure, and better gas distribution within the lungs. It may be necessary to increase the flow rate so that the patient has time to exhale before the next breath is triggered or gas may be trapped in the lungs; this is called *autoPEEP*. Newer models contain demand valves so the patient can receive the flow needed.

– Inspiratory-expiratory (I:E) ratio (typically 1:2 or greater)

– Expiration should be longer than inspiration to avoid air trapping. In some situations, reversing the I:E ratio may help improve oxygenation. Inspiration is then controlled by inspiratory flow, and expiratory time is controlled by respiratory rate.

– Airway pressure (normally 20 to 40 cm H_2O and relatively constant): Monitor peak inspiratory pressure and inspiratory plateau pressure, noting sudden changes in airway pressures or a trend of increasing pressures.

– Peak inspiratory pressure is the pressure at peak inspiration. It reflects the maximum pressure needed to overcome resistance to flow and to lung and chest wall expansion. Increased peak inspiratory pressure implies increased airway resistance, from such factors as secretions or bronchospasm. Plateau pressure is the pressure at end-inspiration. It reflects the pressure necessary to hold the airways open and deliver the volume of gas. Increased plateau pressure implies stiffness of lung tissue, pneumothorax, or a decrease in chest wall mobility.

– Pressure limit

– This setting limits the amount of pressure that the machine can exert when delivering volume in order to prevent barotrauma. Once this level is reached, inspiration stops even if the desired V_T hasn't been delivered. The pressure limit may be reached occasionally if the patient is coughing or has excessive airway secretions or if the ventilator tubing is kinked. Consistently reaching the pressure limit suggests decreased compliance or a pneumothorax.

– Sensitivity (typically 2 cm H_2O below zero or PEEP level)

– The sensitivity knob controls the amount of negative inspiratory pressure the patient must generate in order to trigger an inspiration.

– Sigh

– A sigh is a periodic deep breath delivered by the ventilator. Thought to prevent atelectasis, sighing isn't commonly used. Instead, the patient is ventilated with large V_Ts to prevent atelectasis.

– Alarms and monitor

– Alarms need to be set for high airway pressure (usually the same as the pressure limit), low airway pressure (disconnect alarm), high and low volumes (to detect leaks), and high and low fraction of inspired oxygen (FIO_2). There are many other parameters that can be monitored and for which alarms can be set. Newer ventilators employ microprocessors that can simultaneously and continuously monitor almost all parameters related to the ventilators.

Respiratory disorders

3. In collaboration with the respiratory therapist, *monitor compliance every 8 hours:*

– Monitor static compliance (V$_T$ divided by end-inspiratory [plateau] pressure) or dynamic compliance (V$_T$ divided by peak inspiratory pressure). If PEEP is used, subtract PEEP value from pressure before dividing.

– Compare the patient's values to normal values (static: 100 ml/cm H$_2$O; dynamic: 50 ml/cm H$_2$O). Monitor compliance curves or note trend of values.

3. Compliance measures the resistance to expansion. It's determined by the amount of change in volume that results from a given change in pressure (volume in milliliters divided by pressure in centimeters of water pressure equals compliance [ml/cm H$_2$O]). Decreased lung compliance signifies that the lungs require more pressure to ventilate; they're stiffer than usual, as in ARDS. Increased compliance, rarely a clinical problem, indicates that the lungs are easier to ventilate than usual. For example, in emphysema, where elasticity is lost, lung compliance increases, even though airway obstruction may hinder ventilation.

– Static compliance indicates compliance when the lungs are at rest, whereas dynamic compliance indicates compliance when airflow is occurring. Static compliance values reflect lung compliance; dynamic compliance values also reflect airway resistance.

– Comparing static and dynamic values can help identify the source of difficulty in ventilating a patient. For example, a near-normal static compliance with a low dynamic compliance suggests that the problem is increased airway resistance, whereas both low static and low dynamic compliance suggest the problem is the lung itself, as occurs with ARDS. Compliance curves — serial plotting of pressure changes compared to volume changes — indicate trends graphically and may allow determination of the best combination of pressure and volume for a patient.

4. *Evaluate pulmonary status at least every 2 hours.* Note particularly the symmetry of chest excursion, bilateral breath sounds, and any adventitious sounds.

4. These factors provide data about adequacy of airflow throughout the pulmonary tree and about secretions or obstructions to flow.

5. Additional individualized interventions: _____

5. Rationales: _____

Suggested NIC Interventions
Acid-base management; Electrolyte management; Laboratory data interpretation; Oxygen therapy; Ventilation assistance; Airway management; Respiratory monitoring; Embolus care: Pulmonary; Hemodynamic regulation; Vital signs monitoring

Suggested NOC Outcomes
Electrolyte and acid-base balance; Respiratory status: Gas exchange; Respiratory status: Ventilation; Tissue perfusion: Pulmonary; Vital signs status

---

Nursing diagnosis

Impaired gas exchange related to insufficient oxygen levels or inadequate PEEP level

NURSING PRIORITY

Maintain optimal oxygenation.

PATIENT OUTCOME CRITERIA

Within 24 hours of onset of mechanical ventilation and then continuously, the patient will:
- maintain a Pao$_2$ and oxygen saturation within expected limits
- display no signs or symptoms of oxygen toxicity.

INTERVENTIONS

1. *Compare delivered oxygen percentage to the desired percentage*, typically 100% initially and thereafter adjusted according to Pao$_2$. With newer models, read the delivered oxygen percentage from the digital display of the built-in oxygen analyzer. With older models, use a hand-held oxygen analyzer. Initially, use pulse oximetry, if desired, to titrate the Fio$_2$. *Confirm the pulse oximetry readings with ABG oxygenation values.*

2. *Be aware if the Fio$_2$ is greater than 50%.*

– In conjunction with the physician, consider the risk of oxygen toxicity in relation to the need for oxygen therapy. If possible, implement ways to reduce the oxygen dose as ordered.

– If it isn't possible to reduce the oxygen dosage, observe the patient for sharp, pleuritic chest pain (typically after about 6 hours on 100% oxygen), decreased VC and decreased compliance (typically after 18 hours), and signs and symptoms of ARDS (typically after 24 to 48 hours). Document your observations, and promptly notify the physician if any of these signs or symptoms occur.

3. *Monitor PEEP,* typically ordered if the patient can't maintain a Pao$_2$ greater than 60 mm Hg on less than 50% oxygen.
– Visually monitor the PEEP level (usually 5 to 15 cm H$_2$O) on the PEEP gauge or inspiratory pressure gauge (instead of dropping to zero at the end of expiration, the needle drops to the PEEP level).
– Assist the respiratory therapist with titration of PEEP by correlating the PEEP level with inspired oxygen percentage, the resulting Pao$_2$ level, and hemodynamic values. Apply PEEP in increments of 3 to 5 cm H$_2$O to reach a maintenance level of 5 to 15 cm H$_2$O as ordered.

4. Additional individualized interventions: _____

RATIONALES

1. The machine may not deliver the set oxygen percentage. The oxygen analyzer evaluates the accuracy of oxygen delivery. Too low a percentage promotes hypoxemia, whereas too high a percentage promotes oxygen toxicity (see "Risk for injury," page 289).

2. Prolonged exposure to high alveolar oxygen tension promotes oxygen toxicity. Although an Fio$_2$ greater than 60% doesn't cause clinically significant parenchymal abnormalities in normal lungs, an Fio$_2$ greater than 50% may cause serious lung dysfunction in previously damaged or susceptible lung tissue.
– Signs and symptoms of oxygen toxicity reflect the progression from the initial phase of tracheobronchitis through the exudative phase of alveolar-capillary membrane damage. If unchecked, the syndrome progresses to a proliferative stage that results in pulmonary fibrosis. To assess for chest pain in an intubated patient, look for indications of pain such as grimacing and analyze pain characteristics by asking the patient questions that can be answered with a "yes" or "no" signal.
– Lowering the oxygen dose, as can be achieved through PEEP, helps decrease the risk of toxicity. However, the need to treat hypoxemia takes precedence over the potential danger of oxygen toxicity.

3. By increasing FRC and recruiting shunt units, PEEP improves oxygen transport and allows the use of a lower inspired oxygen concentration.
– Visual monitoring confirms that the prescribed PEEP level is being maintained.

– The optimal PEEP level for a given patient depends on several factors, including shunt reduction, lung compliance, and cardiac output. The desired goal is maintenance of an adequate Pao$_2$ level on less than 50% oxygen. PEEP levels above 15 cm H$_2$O are associated with increased barotrauma and depressed cardiac output.

4. Rationales: _____

Nursing diagnosis

Ineffective airway clearance related to presence of an endotracheal (ET) tube, increased secretions, and the underlying disease

NURSING PRIORITY

Maintain airway patency.

PATIENT OUTCOME CRITERIA

Continuously during mechanical ventilation, the patient will:
- maintain a patent airway
- have clear breath sounds bilaterally, as the underlying condition allows.

INTERVENTIONS

1. *Provide artificial airway care* according to unit protocol or as ordered, including the following:
– Support the ventilator tubing so it doesn't press on the edge of the patient's nose or mouth.

– Measure cuff pressures at least every 8 hours. Optimally, maintain cuff pressure at less than 20 mm Hg with a minimal leak.

2. *Monitor ET tube position.* When oral or nasal ET tube position is confirmed after intubation, mark the tube and trim excess. Check tube placement frequently by noting the relationship between the mark and the patient's lip or nostril. Also assess breath sounds every 1 to 2 hours.

3. *Keep a manual self-inflating bag and mask connected to 100% oxygen at the bedside.* If accidental extubation occurs, open the airway and ventilate with the bag and mask. Summon medical assistance.

4. *Change the patient's position every 1 to 2 hours,* including the prone position. Provide chest physiotherapy as indicated.

5. *Suction when needed, as indicated by dyspnea, coughing, gurgles, appearance of visible secretions in the tube, or a high-pressure alarm.* Follow these guidelines for suctioning:

RATIONALES

1. Meticulous airway care can prevent many potential complications associated with endotracheal intubation.
– Maintaining proper alignment prevents accidental extubation, tube advancement, or nasotracheal or orotracheal erosion.
– Monitoring cuff pressures permits early detection of pressures high enough to cause tracheal ischemia and necrosis.

2. An ET tube can migrate downward and rest against the carina, obstructing airflow and causing the patient to cough and fight the ventilator, or enter one of the bronchi (usually the right mainstem bronchi), preventing ventilation of the opposite lung. It also can migrate upward, increasing the risk of unintended extubation. Checking the tube position and assessing breath sounds allows for detection of tube movement and repositioning as needed. Trimming oral tubes decreases mechanical dead space.

3. The bag and mask allow for emergency ventilation in the event of accidental extubation or mechanical failure. Reintubation must be performed by someone skilled in the technique.

4. Position changes help drain secretions and promote ventilation of all lung areas. Placing the patient in a prone position may optimize ventilation and oxygenation in acute hypoxemia. Chest physiotherapy promotes secretion drainage.

5. Intubation prevents an effective cough reflex and subsequent airway clearance. Frequent suctioning decreases the risks of suction-induced hypoxemia, arrhythmias, bronchospasm, and loss of PEEP.

– Use a self-inflating bag to hyperoxygenate the patient with 100% oxygen before, during, and after suctioning. For suctioning, use a catheter with a diameter less than 50% of the ET tube diameter. Suction for no more than 15 seconds. Always reset the oxygen to its previous level after hyperoxygenation. Alternatively, use an in-line suction catheter to suction the trachea without disconnecting the patient from the ventilator. Hyperoxygenate the patient before, during, and after suctioning, and return the ventilator to its previous setting.

– If the patient is on PEEP, use a manual self-inflating bag with a PEEP valve or a closed suctioning system when suctioning.

– Suctioning causes arterial oxygen desaturation, the degree of which depends on the presuctioning Pao_2 level, catheter size in relation to ET tube size, duration of suctioning, and other factors. Following the recommended guidelines helps minimize hypoxemia. Resetting the oxygen level minimizes the risk of oxygen toxicity.

– A bag with a PEEP valve minimizes loss of PEEP support. A closed suctioning system maintains the ventilator connection, including PEEP, and may minimize hypoxemia. However, if suction flow is greater than the volume delivered by the ventilator, alveolar collapse may occur, producing arterial desaturation.

– Apply suction only while withdrawing the catheter.
– Monitor blood pressure, heart rate, and electrocardiogram (ECG) pattern during suctioning. If adverse reactions, such as bradycardia, hypotension, or arrhythmias occur, immediately remove the suctioning catheter and ventilate the patient with 100% oxygen.
– While suctioning, observe for paroxysmal coughing without deep breaths; remove the catheter if it occurs.

– This technique minimizes trauma to the endothelium.
– Bradycardia, hypotension, and arrhythmias may result from stimulation of vagal fibers at the carina, hyperinflation, or hypoxemia.

– Paroxysmal coughing mimics the effects of a sustained Valsalva's maneuver at pressures high enough to cause bradycardia and hypotension. Removing the catheter reduces airway obstruction.

– If the patient reacts adversely to traditional suctioning, consult with the physician about administering an anticholinergic agent such as atropine or an anesthetic such as lidocaine (Xylocaine) before suctioning.

– An anticholinergic agent will prevent bradycardia caused by vagal stimulation. Lidocaine decreases coughing and, in a patient with increased intracranial pressure (ICP), helps prevent further pressure increases.

6. Additional individualized interventions: _____

6. Rationales: _____

Suggested NIC Interventions
Airway management; Airway suctioning; Acid-base monitoring; Aspiration precautions; Positioning; Respiratory monitoring; Ventilation assistance

Suggested NOC Outcomes
Aspiration control; Respiratory status: Airway patency; Respiratory status: Gas exchange; Respiratory status: Ventilation

---

Nursing diagnosis

Risk for injury related to patient deterioration, mechanical breakdown, increased intrathoracic pressure, or bypassed defense mechanisms

NURSING PRIORITIES
- Prevent complications when possible.
- Respond appropriately if complications occur.

PATIENT OUTCOME CRITERIA
Throughout the period of mechanical ventilation, the patient will:
- maintain vital signs within acceptable limits, typically: heart rate, 60 to 100 beats/minute; systolic blood pressure, 90 to 140 mm Hg; and diastolic blood pressure, 50 to 90 mm Hg
- maintain a cardiac index of 2.5 to 4.0 L/minute/m²
- remain free from pulmonary infection and other complications.

Respiratory disorders

INTERVENTIONS	RATIONALES

Abrupt respiratory distress

1. *Keep ventilator alarms turned on at all times.*

1. The patient's life depends on this therapy, and alarms can warn of potentially fatal problems. Turning the alarms off places the patient at risk for unobserved disconnection, cardiac arrest, or other catastrophe.

2. *Be familiar with troubleshooting techniques before they're needed.*

2. Troubleshooting techniques are complex and vary among ventilators. Learning troubleshooting techniques in advance reduces anxiety and improves the likelihood of prompt, successful resolution of a problem.

3. *Continually observe whether the patient is breathing in synchrony with the ventilator.* If the patient develops sudden respiratory distress or the ventilator fails abruptly, take the following steps:

3. Breathing out of synchrony (sometimes called fighting the ventilator or breathing out of phase with the ventilator) markedly increases intrathoracic pressure; failure of mechanical ventilation places the patient's life in jeopardy.

– Immediately disconnect the ventilator, open the airway if necessary, and ventilate the patient using a manual self-inflating bag and 100% oxygen.

– Determining whether the cause of the respiratory distress is patient- or ventilator-related is crucial. Patient-related problems (such as airway obstruction or tension pneumothorax) require immediate intervention, while distress from ventilator malfunction can be relieved by ventilating the patient manually until the exact cause can be evaluated. Manual ventilation provides a quick way to distinguish between the two categories, supplies adequate emergency ventilation, and allows rapid detection of increased airway resistance or decreased compliance.

– Once ventilation is established, reevaluate the patient. If the distress has cleared, check the ventilator settings. Obtain ABG levels or evaluate oximetry readings.

– If the respiratory distress has cleared, the ventilator is at fault. ABG levels or oximetry readings may reveal hypoxemia or hypercapnia, possible indicators of inadequate mechanical ventilation. The ventilator may need to be replaced or adjusted to meet the patient's needs.

– If the distress continues, perform a rapid cardiopulmonary assessment, suction the airway if indicated, or obtain medical assistance.

– Your assessment may reveal the cause of the distress, such as airway obstruction or tension pneumothorax.

– Evaluate for signs of tension pneumothorax, such as a sudden unexplained increase in inspiratory pressure, shock, decreased or absent breath sounds on the affected side, tracheal deviation away from the affected side, air hunger, or intense anxiety. If any of these signs are present, anticipate immediate chest X-ray, needle thoracentesis, or chest tube insertion.

– Positive pressure ventilation increases the risk of barotrauma. Tension pneumothorax, a life-threatening emergency, may result from such factors as rupture of lung blebs, friable tissue, suture disruption, or central line insertion. Immediate chest decompression is needed to prevent cardiopulmonary arrest from mediastinal shift.

– If the problem's source can't be identified and you suspect patient panic, hand-ventilate at a rate faster than the patient's, gradually slow down to the ventilator rate, and then reconnect the ventilator, coaching the patient in a calm, reassuring tone to breathe with the ventilator. Sedate the patient as needed.

– The patient may panic about the need for mechanical ventilation or the sensations associated with it. Hyperventilation may worsen the panic. Adjusting the ventilatory rate as described helps the patient gain control over hyperventilation. Conveying calmness while coaching the patient in specific maneuvers helps build a sense of trust and provides reassurance that the situation is under control. Sedation lessens the patient's awareness of mechanical ventilation.

– If the problem persists, implement changes in ventilator settings, sedate the patient (usually with morphine), or paralyze the patient (for example, pancuronium [Pavulon]), as ordered. If paralysis is prescribed, make sure that sedation with an amnesic agent, such as diazepam (Valium) or midazolam (Versed), is also prescribed. Carefully monitor the level of sedation.

4. *Monitor the patient on PEEP* closely for barotrauma, decreased cardiac output, water retention and, if the patient has an ICP monitor, increased ICP.

5. Additional individualized interventions: _____
_____

Decreased cardiac output

1. *Monitor the patient for signs and symptoms of decreased cardiac output,* such as hypotension, tachycardia, deteriorating mental status, and arrhythmias. Report findings promptly to the physician. Administer I.V. fluid or vasopressors as ordered.

2. *Read pulmonary artery (PA) and wedge pressures at the end of expiration.*

3. *If the patient is on PEEP, consult the physician about the specific technique for reading wedge pressures.* In general, leave the patient on the ventilator and don't make any adjustments in response to the readings; instead, watch for trends.

4. Additional individualized interventions: _____
_____

– Persistent struggling may indicate the need for ventilator adjustments or pharmacologic support. Morphine reduces anxiety and respiratory drive. Pancuronium bromide induces apnea, eliminating the problem of "fighting" the ventilator, but doesn't blunt consciousness. Because paralysis can be terrifying for the fully conscious patient, sedation with an amnesic agent is indicated.

4. Because PEEP is superimposed on intrathoracic pressure already increased from mechanical ventilation, it further increases the risks of barotrauma and cardiovascular deterioration. The mechanism by which PEEP alters fluid imbalance is unclear, but it may be mediated by antidiuretic hormone, baroreceptors, renin production, or stimulation of the sympathetic nervous system. PEEP may increase pressure in the superior vena cava, impeding cerebral venous drainage and raising ICP.

5. Rationales: _____
_____

1. Increased intrathoracic pressure associated with mechanical ventilation diminishes venous return and may cause a right-to-left shift of the interventricular septum, impinging on left ventricular filling. Reducing the work required for breathing and administering oxygen, sedatives, or other therapies such as vasodilators can cause abrupt, significant decreases in the level of sympathetic tone supporting blood pressure. Most patients placed on mechanical ventilation develop hypotension, but it usually responds well to fluid and vasopressor support.

2. PA waveforms reflect fluctuations in intrathoracic pressure. Positive pressure ventilation causes the waveforms to rise during inspiration and drop during expiration. Reading pressures at the end of expiration minimizes the effects of respiratory variation.

3. Controversy exists over the extent to which PEEP affects wedge pressures. Usually, wedge pressures obtained on the ventilator are similar to those obtained with the ventilator disconnected (probably because poorly compliant lungs don't transmit airway pressures well to the heart and pulmonary capillary bed), so the benefit of maintaining PEEP argues in favor of reading pressures on the ventilator. If there's a discrepancy, the physician may wish to confirm by X-ray that the catheter tip lies in the basal third of the lung, where pulmonary vascular pressures may be least affected by alveolar pressure. A recently developed volumetric right-sided heart catheter, which measures blood volume rather than pressure, may eliminate this problem.

4. Rationales: _____
_____

Pulmonary infection

1. *Monitor the humidifier's water level and temperature,* usually set at body temperature.

1. Artificial airways bypass the upper-airway mechanisms for warming, humidifying, and purifying inspired air. Humidification is added to the ventilator to prevent mucosal dehydration and thickened secretions. The temperature is controlled to prevent loss of body heat or tracheal burns.

2. *Drain condensed fluid from the ventilator tubing.*

2. This condensation, from humidified air passed through the ventilator, must be discarded because it increases expiratory pressure and resistance in the ventilatory circuit. It could also be aspirated.

3. *Maintain sterile technique,* good oral care, and careful positioning, and observe for signs of pulmonary infection, such as fever, purulent secretions, or elevated white blood cell count.

3. Artificial airways provide a direct access through which contaminants can enter the lungs. Sterile technique, good oral care, and careful positioning help prevent nosocomial infections.

4. *If signs and symptoms of infection are present, consult with the physician.*

4. Pulmonary infections are a major contributor to mortality from mechanical ventilation. Because they usually occur in debilitated patients and are caused by virulent pathogens, pulmonary infections require prompt, aggressive therapy.

5. Additional individualized interventions: _____

5. Rationales: _____

Gastrointestinal bleeding

1. *Insert a nasogastric (NG) tube as ordered.*

1. NG intubation helps prevent gastric dilation and reduces the risk of aspiration.

2. *Administer antacids,* ranitidine (Zantac), or cimetidine (Tagamet) *as ordered,* spacing doses. *Implement additional measures from the "Gastrointestinal hemorrhage" care plan,* page 487, as appropriate.

2. GI hemorrhage may result from the development of a stress ulcer, a complication of prolonged mechanical ventilation. Although their exact causes aren't well understood, stress ulcers are thought to result from excess gastric acid secretion and decreased gastric mucosal resistance. Antacids neutralize gastric acid; cimetidine and ranitidine decrease gastric acid secretion. Antacids shouldn't be given concurrently with cimetidine because they may impair its absorption. The "Gastrointestinal hemorrhage" care plan contains detailed interventions for ulcer-related bleeding.

3. Additional individualized interventions: _____

3. Rationales: _____

Fluid retention

1. *Monitor for signs and symptoms of fluid retention.* If it's present, consult with the physician about treatment.

1. Fluid retention may result from the humidifier's interference with insensible water loss via the lungs, decreased lymphatic flow, or altered secretion of antidiuretic hormone.

2. Additional individualized interventions: _____

2. Rationales: _____

Tracheal trauma

1. *Monitor cuff pressure and the position of the ET tube.* Maintain cuff pressure well below diastolic blood pressure; a safe cuff pressure ranges from 15 to 20 mm Hg.

2. With the physician, consider tracheostomy for long-term ventilation.

3. Additional individualized interventions: _____
_____

1. An ET tube can damage vocal cords and tracheal mucosa, resulting in scarring and stenosis. Maintaining cuff pressure below diastolic blood pressure permits mucosal perfusion.

2. To prevent a range of upper airway problems, including sinusitis and tracheal stenosis, an ET tube should be replaced with a tracheostomy tube, which is better tolerated for long-term ventilation.

3. Rationales: _____
_____

Suggested NIC Interventions
Surveillance: Safety

Suggested NOC Outcomes
Safety status: Physical injury

Nursing diagnosis
Fear related to inability to speak and dependence on a machine for life support

NURSING PRIORITY
Promote acceptance of mechanical ventilation.

PATIENT OUTCOME CRITERIA
Within 2 hours of being placed on mechanical ventilation and then continuously, the patient will:
■ be able to communicate needs, if conscious
■ appear relaxed.

INTERVENTIONS

1. *Implement the general measures in the "Ineffective individual coping" care plan,* page 124, as appropriate.

2. *Establish a communication method,* such as eye blinks, magic slate, or paper and pencil. Make sure the call light is always within the patient's reach.

3. *Reduce the patient's need for communication by anticipating needs, providing consistency in staffing and routines, using frequent eye contact, and reassuring the patient that monitoring is constant.* Emphasize that a nurse is available immediately, if needed.

4. *Explain the reason for mechanical ventilation.* Briefly orient the patient and family to the ventilator's features, if appropriate, emphasizing features (such as alarms) that may be important to them. Encourage questions. Stress the temporary nature of ventilation, if applicable.

RATIONALES

1. Mechanical ventilation is a stressful experience for patients. The "Ineffective individual coping" care plan contains comprehensive information on ways to decrease the stress of critical illness and promote positive coping.

2. Intubation prevents use of the vocal cords. Needing to communicate and being unable to do so is extremely stressful. Providing alternative methods of communication increases security and promotes patient safety.

3. Although alternative communication methods do work, they're cumbersome and fatiguing. Reducing the need for communication helps reduce the patient's fatigue and frustration, and reassurance helps reduce fear.

4. Mechanical ventilation is commonly instituted under crisis conditions, when explanation and emotional preparation may not have been possible. Even if the patient and family were prepared, stress may have caused them to block or selectively filter information. Briefly reviewing the procedure and encouraging questions may relieve unstated anxiety about the device.

Respiratory disorders

5. Additional individualized interventions: _____

_____

5. Rationales: _____

_____

┌───┐
Suggested NIC Interventions
Anxiety reduction; Coping enhancement; Security enhancement
└───┘

┌───┐
Suggested NOC Outcomes
Anxiety control; Fear control
└───┘

Collaborative problem

Risk for dysfunctional ventilatory weaning response related to lack of physiologic or psychological readiness

NURSING PRIORITY
Promote a smooth transition to spontaneous ventilation.

PATIENT OUTCOME CRITERIA
During weaning and continuously thereafter, the patient will:
- maintain a clear airway
- maintain a spontaneous respiratory rate of 12 to 24 breaths/minute
- manifest ABG levels within normal limits
- display pulmonary function measurements within normal limits
- display normal sinus rhythm with no ectopic beats, or a benign variant such as sinus arrhythmia or a normal sinus rhythm with fewer than 4 premature ventricular contractions/minute
- remain alert and oriented.

INTERVENTIONS

1. *Anticipate weaning when the patient meets these criteria: improvement in respiratory status* (as evidenced by an A-a gradient less than 300 mm Hg on 100% oxygen, shunt less than 20%, $V_D:V_T$ less than 0.6, respiratory rate less than 24 breaths/minute, and MV 5 to 10 L), *stable hemodynamic status, and adequate muscle strength* (as evidenced by VC greater than 10 to 15 ml/kg and MIP greater than –20 cm H_2O).

2. *Make sure the patient is rested, well nourished, oriented, able to follow commands, and not receiving any respiratory depressants.*

3. *Explain weaning to the patient and family.* Mention that the patient may feel short of breath initially. Stress that the patient will be attended closely during the trial of spontaneous breathing and that if it isn't successful, it will be tried again later.

4. *Obtain baseline vital signs, ABG levels, and pulmonary function measurements. Suction the airway.*

RATIONALES

1. Many factors affect the success of weaning attempts. Premature attempts to wean impose unnecessary physiologic stress on the patient, jeopardizing recovery. Meeting the listed criteria increases the likelihood that weaning will be accomplished with few or no setbacks.

2. Reestablishing spontaneous ventilation is physically demanding, and the patient must have enough energy reserves to succeed. The ability to take a deep breath and cough on command helps prevent atelectasis and airway obstruction. A strong respiratory drive is crucial to resume spontaneous breathing.

3. Weaning is stressful psychologically. Thorough emotional preparation promotes a sense of security. Preparing the patient for the possibility of trying again later may reduce the sense of failure if the weaning attempt is unsuccessful.

4. These measurements provide a basis for comparison to evaluate the appropriateness of weaning. Suctioning the airway reduces the risk of aspiration because secretions may have accumulated above the cuff.

5. *Implement the weaning method ordered:* CPAP, SIMV, T-piece, or pressure support.

5. CPAP or pressure support may make weaning easier for the patient on PEEP by maintaining some positive pressure during the trial of spontaneous breathing. SIMV supplies periodic mandatory deep breaths; the rate can be decreased by two breaths at a time until the patient's breathing is completely spontaneous. A T-piece provides supplemental oxygen during weaning. Pressure support can increase V_T in a patient too weak to wean on a T-piece alone.

6. *Monitor the blood pressure, heart rate, pulse oximeter oxygen saturation, ECG rhythm, respiratory rate, ease of breathing, level of consciousness, and level of fatigue constantly for the first 20 to 30 minutes and every 5 minutes thereafter until weaning is complete.*

6. Frequent monitoring provides ongoing indications of the success or failure of the weaning attempt.

7. *In collaboration with the physician, terminate weaning if adverse reactions occur,* such as a heart rate increase greater than 20 beats/minute, systolic blood pressure increase greater than 20 mm Hg, arterial oxygen saturation less than 90%, respiratory rate less than 8 or greater than 24 breaths/minute, ventricular arrhythmias, labored or erratic breathing, fatigue, or panic.

7. Attempts to persist in weaning an unstable patient may cause cardiorespiratory arrest from hypoxia or arrhythmias.

8. *If weaning continues, measure the V_T, MV, and ABG values in 20 to 30 minutes.* Compare to desired values for the patient, determined in collaboration with the physician, typically: V_T, 300 to 700 ml; MV, 5 to 10 L; pH, 7.35 to 7.45; Pao_2 greater than 70 mm Hg; and $Paco_2$, 35 to 45 mm Hg.

8. Values at this point help determine the appropriateness of continuing weaning.

9. *If physiologic parameters indicate that weaning is feasible but the patient resists, consider the possibility of psychological dependence on the ventilator.* Consult with the physician, pulmonary nurse specialist, or psychiatric nurse clinician as appropriate.

9. Psychological dependence is a common problem after prolonged mechanical ventilation. Possible causes for dependency include fear of dying, depression from chronic illness, and secondary gains from the illness role. Consulting with other professionals may help to uncover causes and allow the formulation of appropriate interventions to resolve underlying fears or conflicts.

10. *Assist with extubation, when ordered.* Confirm that someone qualified to reintubate is present.

10. The same criteria used to evaluate readiness for weaning are used to determine readiness for extubation. A patient ventilated for short periods (24 to 48 hours) usually is ready for extubation after a 30-minute trial of spontaneous breathing, whereas those ventilated for longer periods may require days to weeks of gradual weaning. Availability of immediate reintubation is critical because postextubation airway obstruction can be sudden and fatal.

11. Additional individualized interventions: _____
_____

11. Rationales: _____
_____

Discharge planning

DISCHARGE CHECKLIST

Before discharge, the patient shows evidence of:

❏ stable respiratory status (after extubation) for more than 12 hours
❏ absence of significant arrhythmias (without I.V. antiarrhythmic drugs) for more than 12 hours
❏ stable level of consciousness for more than 12 hours
❏ vital signs within normal limits.

TEACHING CHECKLIST

Document evidence that the patient and family demonstrate an understanding of:

❏ the reason for mechanical ventilation
❏ communication measures
❏ alarms
❏ weaning.

DOCUMENTATION CHECKLIST

Using outcome criteria as a guide, document:

❏ the patient's clinical status on admission
❏ significant changes in status
❏ pertinent diagnostic test findings
❏ ventilator and patient checks
❏ ventilator alarm status
❏ airway care
❏ measures to prevent or detect and treat complications
❏ communication measures
❏ emotional support
❏ sedative or paralyzing pharmacologic agents, if used
❏ weaning
❏ patient and family teaching
❏ discharge planning.

Associated care plans

- Acute respiratory distress syndrome
- Confusion
- Impaired physical mobility
- Ineffective individual coping
- Nutritional deficit

References

American Heart Association in Collaboration with the International Liaison Committee on Resuscitation. "Guidelines 2000 for Cardiopulmonary Resuscitation and Emergency Cardiovascular Care," *Circulation* 102(8 Suppl):I1-384, August 2000.

Asselin, M.E., and Cullen, H.A. "What You Need to Know about the New ACLS Guidelines," *Nursing2001* 31(4):48-50, April 2001.

Kern, K.B., et al. "New Guidelines for Cardiopulmonary Resuscitation and Emergency Cardiac Care: Changes in the Management of Cardiac Arrest," *JAMA* 285(10):1267-69, March 2001.

Wong, E., et al. "Confirmation of Endotracheal Tube Placement: Analysis of 6,294 Emergency Department Intubations," *Annals of Emergency Medicine* 36(4 Part 2):S53, October 2000.

Pneumonia

DRG INFORMATION

DRG 079   Respiratory Infections and Inflammations with Complication or Comorbidity (CC); Age 171.
Mean LOS 5 8.5 days

DRG 080   Respiratory Infections and Inflammations without CC; Age 171.
Mean LOS 5 5.6 days

DRG 081   Respiratory Infections and Inflammations; Ages 0 to 17.
Mean LOS 5 Not available

DRG 089   Simple Pneumonia and Pleurisy with CC; Age 171.
Mean LOS 5 6.0 days

DRG 090   Simple Pneumonia and Pleurisy without CC; Age 171.
Mean LOS 5 4.1 days

DRG 091   Simple Pneumonia; Ages 0 to 17.
Mean LOS 5 4.4 days

Introduction

DEFINITION AND TIME FOCUS

Respiratory infections account for a significant number of hospitalizations each year, particularly among the two groups most susceptible to serious respiratory illness — the very old and the very young. Respiratory infections include bacterial pneumonias (most commonly caused by pneumococci), viral pneumonias (most commonly caused by influenza and other viral diseases), tuberculosis, lung abscesses, fungal infections, bronchitis from various causes, and pulmonary empyema resulting from another disorder.

Pneumonia is the second most common nosocomial infection in the United States and is linked with substantial morbidity and a mortality rate estimated at 30% to 70%. It's especially dangerous in elderly people and those with severe underlying diseases (such as cardiopulmonary disease).

Since the advent of antibiotic therapy, patients are hospitalized for treatment less commonly today than they were in the past. Although many patients still need hospitalization, a patient may receive treatment at home if he prefers, if he can drink fluids and take medications by mouth, if he has a willing and capable caregiver, and if he has no severe underlying medical conditions.

This care plan focuses on the patient with pneumonia who is admitted to the medical-surgical setting for diagnosis and treatment. Similar nursing interventions apply to most patients with respiratory infections of other types. (See *Clinical snapshot: Pneumonia,* page 299.)

ETIOLOGY AND PRECIPITATING FACTORS

For community-acquired disease

- Particularly virulent organism or high level of exposure in otherwise healthy person
- Chronic obstructive pulmonary disease, alcoholism, influenza, pulmonary neoplasms, heart failure, altered consciousness, or swallowing disorders in older person
- Viruses, pneumococci, or *Mycoplasma pneumoniae*

For nosocomial disease

- Presence in medical-surgical units and intensive care units
- Intubation, mechanical ventilation, recumbent position, increased risk for aspiration, incompetent lower esophageal sphincter, which allows gastric contents to flow back up
- Patient's age, severity of underlying disorder, primary diagnosis, and response to therapy
- Gram-negative bacteria, which colonize the oropharynx in hospitalized patients (the stress that typically occurs in hospitalized patients is believed to alter saliva composition, changing the resident flora in the mouth and thus increasing the risk of pneumonia if sufficient numbers of these organisms are aspirated into the lungs)

Focused assessment guidelines

The manifestations of pneumonia vary considerably, depending on the degree of inflammation, the disease stage, and the pathogenic organism involved.

NURSING HISTORY
(FUNCTIONAL HEALTH PATTERN FINDINGS)
Health-perception–health-management pattern

- Fatigue, malaise, and respiratory signs and symptoms, such as cough, pleurisy (chest pain with inspiration), and sputum production
- Recent upper respiratory infection or sinus disease if disease is community-acquired; self-treatment is common — patient may have used outdated antibiotics (prescribed for a previous illness), over-the-counter medications, or both
- History of smoking, alcohol abuse, or multiple stressors contributing to overall fatigue
- Multiple risk factors (with nosocomial disease), such as activity restriction, depressed inspiratory effort, depressed cough reflex, and use of respiratory equipment

or an artificial airway; patient may not have been admitted for a primary respiratory disorder

Nutritional-metabolic pattern

- Anorexia during illness; poor nutrition before onset of respiratory illness

Activity-exercise pattern

- Limited activity because of fatigue and shortness of breath

Sleep-rest pattern

- Fatigue with inability to "catch up" on needed rest
- Sleep disturbance if cough is present

Cognitive-perceptual pattern

- Community-acquired disease: questioning of why illness occurred despite good physical condition; failure to relate subtle increase in stress to present illness; possible delay in seeking medical attention because illness seemed like "just a little cold"
- Nosocomial disease: failure to understand connection between primary reason for hospitalization and present illness

PHYSICAL FINDINGS

General appearance

- Fever — low grade or with shaking chills, depending on pathogenic organism (if possible, compare it to patient's normal temperature because a low-grade fever may actually represent a significant elevation such as in an older patient)

Pulmonary

- Crackles
- Decreased breath sounds over area of infection
- Increased respiratory rate
- Shallow, labored breathing (may not report shortness of breath)
- Possible abnormal bronchial breath sounds heard on auscultation over area of consolidation
- Fremitus — normal or increased
- Possible cough
- Possible sputum production and rhinorrhea — character, color, and odor of secretions depend on pathogenic organism (generally, viral organisms produce clear secretions, whereas bacterial organisms produce discolored and purulent secretions)

Gastrointestinal

- Possible vomiting

Integumentary

- Warm, moist skin
- Possible cyanosis, pallor, or flushing

Lymphoreticular system

- Possible cervical lymphadenopathy or tenderness in salivary glands

Musculoskeletal

- Weakness

DIAGNOSTIC STUDIES

- Pulse oximetry — may show hypoxemia
- Arterial blood gas (ABG) measurements — may show hypoxemia; possible hypocapnia related to increased minute volume in response to hypoxemia
- Sputum specimen (Gram stain or culture and sensitivity testing or both) — performed to identify causative organisms; may be difficult to differentiate between colonization by an organism that isn't the primary cause of infection and the pathogenic organism; even isolation of a specific pathogen doesn't necessarily prove pneumonia's cause
- Transtracheal aspiration — may be performed in an attempt to obtain a sputum specimen free from saliva or mouth flora; an increased number of polymorphonuclear cells with few squamous cells indicates an acceptable specimen
- Blood culture — may match organism in sputum, increasing likelihood that organism is causative pathogen
- Bronchoscopy — may be performed to obtain a sputum specimen, identify the problem, or clear the airways
- Chest X-ray — shows pulmonary infiltrates in affected areas from the inflammatory process (occasionally clear); may show pleural effusion
- Thoracentesis — done to identify organism if significant pleural fluid is present on chest X-ray and sputum specimen is unobtainable
- Pulmonary function tests — forced vital capacity decreased
- White blood cell (WBC) count — may be elevated but doesn't contribute directly to diagnosis

POTENTIAL COMPLICATIONS

- Severe hypoxemia
- Acute respiratory distress syndrome (ARDS)
- Empyema
- Sepsis
- Lung abscess
- Pulmonary embolism
- Pneumothorax
- Pericarditis
- Meningitis

CLINICAL SNAPSHOT ※

Pneumonia

Major nursing diagnoses and collaborative problems	Key patient outcomes
ND: Risk for infection	Remain free from nosocomial infections.
CP: Risk for hypoxemia	Maintain Pao_2 levels within normal limits on room air, typically 80 to 100 mm Hg.
ND: Acute pain	Rate pain as less than 3 on a 0 to 10 pain rating scale.
ND: Deficient knowledge (treatment regimen)	Demonstrate effective pulmonary hygiene measures for home use.

Nursing diagnosis

Risk for infection related to stress and other risk factors

NURSING PRIORITY

Prevent nosocomial infection, if possible.

PATIENT OUTCOME CRITERION

Throughout the hospital stay, the patient is expected to remain free from nosocomial infections.

INTERVENTIONS	RATIONALES
1. *Wash hands between patients.* *	1. Oropharyngeal secretions on unwashed hands increase the risk of cross-contamination.
2. *Elevate the head of the patient's bed.*	2. An elevated head helps prevent the reflux of oropharyngeal secretions and endotracheal tube condensate.
3. *Consult the physician about administering sucralfate* in place of antacids to prevent stress-induced GI bleeding.	3. Antacids alkalinize the stomach; when aspirated, the high pH fosters overgrowth of gram-negative organisms.
4. Additional individualized interventions: _____	4. Rationales: _____

> **Suggested NIC Interventions**
> *Infection control; Infection protection; Incision site care; Wound care*

> **Suggested NOC Outcomes**
> *Infection status; Wound healing: Primary intention*

Collaborative problem

Risk for hypoxemia related to inflammatory response to pathogen and inadequate airway and alveolar clearance

NURSING PRIORITY

Optimize oxygenation and airway and alveolar clearance. (See *Clinical Pathway: Managing pneumonia,* pages 300 and 301.)

PATIENT OUTCOME CRITERIA

Within 2 days of admission, the patient will:

_____
*Italics indicate key interventions.

(Text continues on page 302.)

Managing pneumonia

Level of care	Day 1 (admission)	Day 2
Assessments	<ul><li>Breath sounds q 4 hours and p.r.n.</li><li>Respiratory effort – prevent fatigue</li><li>I&O</li><li>Skin care needs</li><li>Sputum</li><li>Daily weight</li><li>Immunization status for Pneumovax, flu shot, diphtheria or tetanus or both</li></ul>	<ul><li>Breath sounds</li><li>Respiratory effort</li><li>I&O</li><li>Skin care needs</li><li>Weight</li></ul>
Diagnostic testing	<ul><li>AA Chem</li><li>CBC</li><li>Sputum culture and sensitivity, Gram stain</li><li>Blood culture × 2</li><li>Sputum for acidfast bacilli smear and culture</li><li>Cold agglutinins</li><li>Urinalysis</li><li>ECG, if indicated</li><li>ABGs</li><li>CXR</li><li>Pulse oximetry</li></ul>	<ul><li>CBC</li><li>ABGs</li><li>Pulse oximetry</li></ul>
Treatments	<ul><li>O_2</li></ul>	<ul><li>O_2</li><li>D/C of O_2 per criteria</li></ul>
Activity	<ul><li>Active and passive ROM</li><li>Bed rest with bedside commode</li><li>HOB elevated</li><li>Turning, coughing, and deep breathing q 2 hours</li></ul>	<ul><li>Rest times postactivity</li><li>Chair b.i.d.</li></ul>
Consultations	<ul><li>Social services p.r.n.</li><li>Respiratory care assessment</li></ul>	<ul><li>Social services p.r.n.</li><li>Dietary p.r.n.</li></ul>
Medications and I.V.	<ul><li>I.V. fluids</li><li>Antibiotics</li><li>Antipyretics</li><li>Home medications</li></ul>	<ul><li>I.V. fluids</li><li>Antibiotics</li><li>Antipyretics</li><li>Home medications</li></ul>
Nutrition	<ul><li>Regular diet</li><li>Encouraging fluid intake</li></ul>	<ul><li>Regular diet</li><li>Encouraging fluid intake</li></ul>
Psychosocial, emotional, spiritual needs	<ul><li>Chaplain p.r.n.</li></ul>	<ul><li>Chaplain p.r.n.</li></ul>
Patient and family education	<ul><li>Orienting patient to unit</li><li>Calling nurse if the patient is dyspneic</li><li>Calling for assistance to bedside commode</li><li>Instituting isolation technique, if appropriate</li><li>Following proper hand-washing guidelines</li><li>Diet, medications, activity, safety</li></ul>	<ul><li>Cough technique</li><li>Fluid intake</li><li>Disease process, symptoms, and therapy prescribed (printed materials)</li></ul>
Discharge planning	<ul><li>Initial assessment</li><li>Advanced directives review</li><li>Pathway review</li></ul>	<ul><li>Facilitating team conference</li><li>Home O_2 or I.V. antibiotics or both, if indicated</li><li>Need for follow-up care assessment</li></ul>
Expected outcomes	<ul><li>Antibiotics initiated within 4 hours of order</li><li>Fluid intake > 2,000 ml/24 hours</li><li>Resting quietly</li></ul>	<ul><li>Temperature decreasing</li><li>Tolerating P.O. intake of 1,500 ml/24 hours</li><li>Tolerating activity</li><li>50% diet consumed</li></ul>

Day 3	Day 4	Day 5
• Breath sounds • Respiratory effort • I&O • Weight	• Breath sounds • I&O • Weight	• Breath sounds • I&O • Weight
• ABGs • Pulse oximetry	• CBC • CXR	
• O$_2$ • D/C of O$_2$ per criteria • Immunization as indicated		
• Ambulating in room at will • Chair t.i.d.	• Ambulating at will • Chair q.i.d.	• Activity at will • Chair q.i.d.
• Social services p.r.n. • Dietary p.r.n. • Home infusion p.r.n.	• Social services p.r.n. • Dietary p.r.n.	
• I.V. ➤ intermittent infusion device • P.O. antibiotics, if possible • Home medications	• Home medications • P.O. antibiotics or arrange for outpatient I.V. antibiotics	• I.V. discontinued • P.O. antibiotics • Home medications
• Regular diet • Encouraging fluid intake	• Regular diet • Encouraging fluid intake	• Regular diet • Encouraging fluid intake
• Chaplain p.r.n.	• Chaplain p.r.n.	• Chaplain p.r.n.
• Medications: dosage, frequency, precautions, potential adverse effects • Importance of taking all of the prescribed antibiotic • Signs and symptoms of pneumonia and importance of reporting them to the physician • Risks for recurring respiratory infections • Home care instructions	Same as Day 3	Same as Day 3
Same as Day 2	Same as Day 2	Same as Day 2
• Temperature decreasing • Dyspnea decreasing • O$_2$ D/C • ADLs with minimal assistance • 75% diet consumed • Effective cough	• CXR without progression • WBC ↓ by 50% • Temperature decreasing • Breath sounds without progression	• Rx reviewed • Room air • Temperature < 100.5° F (38° C) • Breath sounds without progression • Home support system in place • Discharged

- maintain partial pressure of arterial oxygen (Pao_2) levels within normal limits on room air, typically 80 to 100 mm Hg
- easily expectorate less purulent sputum
- exhibit decreased crackles
- perform pulmonary hygiene measures hourly while awake
- exhibit increased vigor and ability to perform self-care measures
- have no fever
- take oral fluids to recommended level
- have adequate dietary intake.

INTERVENTIONS	RATIONALES
1. *Administer oxygen therapy as ordered.* Document therapy on initiation and once per shift.	**1.** Until the airway and alveoli are clear, supplemental oxygen is necessary to reduce the system's need to maintain high minute volumes. Although high minute volumes help compensate for hypoxemia, they may contribute to respiratory fatigue and, ultimately, respiratory failure. Usual administration ranges from 1 to 6 L/minute by nasal cannula.
2. *Maintain oxygen therapy during activities* such as ambulation to the bathroom. Note activity tolerance, observing for increased fatigue, tachypnea, cyanosis, tachycardia, and other signs of impaired oxygenation.	**2.** Increased activity levels increase oxygen demands and further tax the already compromised system.
3. *Administer and document antibiotic therapy as ordered.* Monitor the results of indicated blood level studies. Monitor and document the antibiotic's adverse effects.	**3.** Specific treatments vary, depending on when the pneumonia developed, prior antibiotic therapy, and the specific flora that exist on the unit; the antibiotic of choice depends on the pathogen identified. Optimum antibiotic blood levels, necessary to achieve desired results, vary among individuals. Some adverse effects require changes in medication levels or therapy to prevent immediate or long-term complications.
4. *Evaluate the patient's progress, and document the respiratory parameters once per shift and as needed*, including level of consciousness (LOC), sputum character and color, presence or absence of cough, temperature, pulse, respiratory rate, skin color, breath sounds, and activity tolerance.	**4.** Changes in LOC, such as increased restlessness or lethargy, can indicate deterioration and impending respiratory failure. Other parameters should improve if antibiotic and airway clearance therapy is effective.
5. *Collect sputum specimens in the recommended manner.* Maintain a sterile collection cup. When the patient expectorates lower respiratory tract secretions, send the specimen to the laboratory immediately to prevent overgrowth of normal oral flora. If necessary, ask the respiratory therapy department to perform a sputum induction to collect an adequate specimen.	**5.** Appropriate antibiotic therapy depends on accurate pathogen identification.
6. *Perform noninvasive measures to promote airway clearance:* – If the patient can cooperate, have him breathe deeply and cough each hour and use an incentive spirometer as ordered. – If the patient can't cooperate, perform artificial sighing and coughing each hour, using a manual resuscitation bag. – Perform postural drainage and percussion with vibration every 4 hours or as ordered.	**6.** Noninvasive clearance measures move purulent, infectious secretions from the alveoli up toward the major airways, where they can be expectorated or suctioned.

7. *Perform nasotracheal suctioning if the patient can't cough effectively.* Suction as needed, as indicated by gurgles heard over the major airways. Consider the use of a nasal trumpet for frequent nasal suctioning. Follow standard precautions, including wearing eye protection and gloves.

7. Nasotracheal suctioning is effective only if secretions are within reach of the suction catheter, typically above the carina (at the level of the angle of Louis). Because nasotracheal suctioning can damage the tracheal mucosa, it should be performed only if secretions are within reach. Although a nasal trumpet can also cause some damage, it can reduce trauma in a patient who must undergo frequent nasal suctioning. Following standard precautions reduces exposure to infectious organisms.

8. *Use increased levels of supplemental oxygen before and during airway clearance procedures.*

8. Measures used to clear the airways may intensify hypoxemia while they're being performed, especially if the patient has concomitant cardiovascular disease. Supplemental oxygen can be maintained via nasal prongs during nasotracheal suctioning.

9. *Encourage the patient to increase fluid intake* to at least eight 8-oz (237-ml) glasses per day.

9. Sputum's viscosity is related to the patient's overall hydration status. Fever contributes to dehydration. Adequate fluid intake promotes thinner secretions that can be expectorated more easily, decreasing the risk of hypoxemia related to sputum plugs in airway.

10. *Encourage small, frequent, high-protein, high-calorie meals.* If the patient can't eat, begin total parenteral nutrition as ordered.

10. Protein and calorie malnutrition may contribute to impaired humoral and cell-mediated host defenses. Malnutrition also weakens the patient, contributing to a less vigorous respiratory effort.

11. *Monitor ABG levels as ordered and as needed,* if dyspnea increases or respiratory effort is inadequate. Report abnormalities immediately, and prepare the patient for possible ventilatory support.

11. Indications of severe hypoxemia and developing ARDS include a dropping Pao_2 level despite a stable or increasing level of supplemental oxygen.

12. Additional individualized interventions: _____

12. Rationales: _____

Nursing diagnosis

Acute pain related to fever and pleuritic irritation

NURSING PRIORITY

Minimize discomfort while promoting adequate oxygenation.

PATIENT OUTCOME CRITERIA

Within 24 hours of admission, the patient will:
- demonstrate splinting technique while performing pulmonary hygiene measures, if the patient is stable
- rate pain using oral medications as less than 3 on a 0 to 10 pain rating scale
- demonstrate adequate chest expansion during inspiration.

INTERVENTIONS

1. *See the "Acute pain" care plan,* page 32.

RATIONALES

1. The "Acute pain" care plan contains general interventions for the care of the patient in pain. This plan contains additional measures specific to pneumonia.

2. *Administer antipyretics, analgesics, or both, as ordered and as needed.* Use caution in administering sedatives or narcotics, if ordered. Document the patient's response.

2. Pleuritic pain and discomfort from fever may be so severe that the patient inhibits thoracic expansion to minimize pain, increasing the likelihood of atelectasis, hypoventilation, inadequate airway clearance, and hypoxemia. Sedatives or narcotics may cause respiratory depression.

3. *Teach the patient to splint the chest wall with his hands or pillows as needed,* while coughing, deep breathing, or performing other pulmonary hygiene measures.

3. Splinting may help reduce unnecessary chest wall movement, which contributes to pain. Supporting painful areas helps promote fuller chest expansion.

4. *Apply a heating pad or hot packs* to areas of chest wall discomfort as ordered.

4. Heat reduces inflammation and promotes muscle relaxation.

5. Additional individualized interventions: _____
_____

5. Rationales: _____
_____

Suggested NIC Interventions
Medication management; Pain management; Patient-controlled analgesia (PCA) assistance, Analgesic administration; Conscious sedation

Suggested NOC Outcomes
Comfort level; Pain control; Pain: Disruptive effects; Pain level

---

Nursing diagnosis
Deficient knowledge (treatment regimen) related to lack of exposure to information

NURSING PRIORITY
Teach home care and preventive measures.

PATIENT OUTCOME CRITERIA
By the time of discharge, the patient will:
- demonstrate effective pulmonary hygiene measures for home use
- list three preventive measures
- list three symptoms indicating possible recurrence.

INTERVENTIONS

1. *Emphasize the importance of an ongoing pulmonary hygiene regimen.* Teach the patient and family techniques for home use, based on the patient's condition and capabilities at discharge.

2. *Teach the patient the importance of rest* during convalescence at home.

3. *Teach the patient to avoid infections* by:
– avoiding respiratory irritants
– avoiding crowds and persons with known infections
– being aware of the mode of transmission of infection (usually airborne) and keeping in mind that saliva and sputum contain increased concentrations of pathogens
– getting an influenza vaccination, once he's stable, if the physician recommends it
– completing the entire course of antibiotics even if symptoms resolve.

RATIONALES

1. Deep-breathing exercises should be continued at home for at least 4 to 6 weeks to help reduce atelectasis and promote healing. Ongoing pulmonary hygiene measures may be indicated for the patient with a coexisting condition such as emphysema that's associated with a higher incidence of recurrence.

2. Respiratory infections place significant stresses on the body. Overexertion may further tax compromised defenses. Rest promotes healing.

3. Persons recovering from respiratory infections tend to be susceptible to other infections and are also at increased risk for recurrence after healing. Preventive measures may help the patient avoid further illness.

4. *Teach the patient and his family the importance of promptly reporting signs and symptoms that may indicate recurrence,* such as headache, fever, dyspnea, chest pain, and other signs and symptoms of a cold or the flu.

5. Additional individualized interventions: _____

4. Early and appropriate treatment of respiratory infections results in shorter periods of illness. In older patients and other high-risk groups, a delay in reporting symptoms is associated with higher mortality rate.

5. Rationales: _____

Suggested NIC Interventions	**Suggested NOC Outcomes**
Teaching: Procedure/treatment	*Knowledge: Treatment regimen*

Discharge planning

DISCHARGE CHECKLIST

Before discharge, the patient shows evidence of:

❑ absence of pulmonary or cardiovascular complications (dullness on auscultation may still be present)
❑ normal ABG levels and WBC count
❑ absence of fever for at least 24 hours
❑ clearing pleural effusion on chest X-ray
❑ decreasing sputum production
❑ ability to tolerate adequate dietary and fluid intake
❑ ability to control pain using oral medications
❑ ability to ambulate and perform activities of daily living at the same level as before hospitalization
❑ adequate home support system or referral to home care or a nursing home.

TEACHING CHECKLIST

Document evidence that the patient and family demonstrate an understanding of:

❑ purpose, dosage, administration schedule, and adverse effects requiring medical intervention of all discharge medications
❑ recommended dietary plan and need for ongoing fluid intake
❑ realistic plan for rest and activity
❑ care and use of oxygen equipment
❑ pulmonary hygiene measures
❑ preventive measures to avoid recurrence
❑ signs and symptoms requiring medical intervention
❑ date, time, and location of follow-up appointments
❑ how to contact the physician.

DOCUMENTATION CHECKLIST

Using outcome criteria as a guide, document:

❑ clinical status on admission
❑ significant changes in status
❑ pertinent diagnostic findings
❑ ABG test results
❑ pain-relief measures
❑ nutrition and fluid intake
❑ oxygen therapy
❑ airway clearance measures and results

❑ patient and family teaching
❑ discharge planning.

Associated care plans

■ Acquired immunodeficiency syndrome
■ Acute pain
■ Chronic obstructive pulmonary disease
■ Geriatric care
■ Ineffective individual coping
■ Knowledge deficit

References

American Thoracic Society. "ATS Releases New Pneumonia Guidelines," *AARC Times* 25(8):66, August 2001.

Handbook of Diseases, 2nd ed. Springhouse, Pa.: Springhouse Corp., 1999.

Fitzgerald, M.A. "Community-Acquired Pneumonia in Adults," *Nurse Practitioner* 26 (11):14-16, November 2001.

Murphy, M., et al. "A Multihospital Effort to Reduce Inpatient Lengths of Stay for Pneumonia," *Journal of Nursing Care Quality* (13)5:11-15, June 1999.

Respiratory disorders

Pulmonary embolism

DRG INFORMATION
DRG 07   Other Respiratory System or Procedure with
          Complication or Comorbidity.
          Mean LOS = 9.9 days

Introduction
DEFINITION AND TIME FOCUS
A pulmonary embolus (PE) is debris deposited in a
branch of the pulmonary artery that partially or completely obstructs blood flow. Venous thromboemboli are
the most common cause of obstruction, accounting for
approximately 95% of all cases; most arise from deep
vein thrombosis (DVT) in the lower extremities. Other
types of PE include air, fat, and amniotic fluid emboli,
septic emboli, and bone fragments.

The severity of the associated signs and symptoms
depends on the size of the embolus and amount of lung
affected by the altered perfusion. Emboli range in size
from small to massive. Small emboli usually lodge in the
peripheral pulmonary arterial bed and may cause cardiopulmonary compromise. A massive PE that obstructs
more than 50% of the pulmonary artery (PA) circulation
leads to severe cardiopulmonary compromise. The location and size of the embolus or emboli may vary; for instance, a single embolus may block the PA bifurcation (a
saddle embolus), or small emboli may be scattered
throughout pulmonary tissue, causing anywhere from no
symptoms to significant symptoms depending on the
amount of tissue affected. If the embolus isn't a venous
thromboembolus, other systems may be compromised
(for example, fat emboli may cause opthalmic complications, result in acute renal failure, or compromise perfusion to distal extremities).

This care plan covers all phases of care, from the initial diagnosis in the medical-surgical setting, through the
critical care phase, to readying the patient for discharge.
(See *Clinical snapshot: Pulmonary embolism*, page 308.)

ETIOLOGY AND PRECIPITATING FACTORS
■ Venous stasis, from such factors as DVT, immobility,
burns, varicose veins, heart failure, atrial fibrillation,
right ventricular infarction, or myocardial infarction (MI)
(diminished or absent ventricular motion)
■ Injury of the vascular endothelium, from such factors
as venipuncture of the legs, surgery (especially of the abdomen, pelvis, or hip), I.V. drug abuse, or trauma (particularly long-bone fractures or MI)

■ Hypercoagulability, from such factors as sepsis, dehydration, hormonal contraceptive use, blood dyscrasias,
pregnancy, or recent childbirth

Focused assessment guidelines
NURSING HISTORY
(FUNCTIONAL HEALTH PATTERN FINDINGS)
Health-perception–health-management pattern
■ Sudden shortness of breath (most common symptom)
Cognitive-perceptual pattern
■ A sense of impending doom
■ Chest pain that worsens with inspiration
■ Headache
Coping–stress tolerance pattern
■ Apprehension or fear
■ Anxiety

PHYSICAL FINDINGS
More than one-half of all patients who have DVT have
no signs or symptoms. If they do, signs and symptoms
may include the following.
General appearance
■ Restlessness
■ Acute distress
Neurologic
■ Altered (decreased) level of consciousness (LOC)
■ Confusion
■ Hallucinations
■ Euphoria
Cardiovascular
■ Tachycardia (in 60% to 75% of patients)
■ Arrhythmias (commonly atrial)
■ Murmur
■ Hypotension
■ Low-grade fever (with massive PE)
■ Accentuated heart sound (S_2)
■ Neck vein distention
■ S_3 gallop (rare)
Integumentary
■ Pallor
■ Cyanosis
■ Diaphoresis (with massive PE)
■ Petechiae of face, neck, and chest (especially with fat
embolism)
Renal
■ Oliguria
■ Altered electrolyte, creatinine, and blood urea nitrogen
levels

Pulmonary

- Tachypnea
- Localized crackles
- Wheezes
- Decreased breath sounds
- Pleural friction rub
- Cough (may be associated with pulmonary injury)
- Unexplained hemoptysis (may be associated with pulmonary injury)

Musculoskeletal

- Swelling (variation in calf size)
- Pain
- Warmth
- Erythema

DIAGNOSTIC STUDIES

Laboratory data are used to rule out other conditions or provide general confirming evidence.

- Ventilation-perfusion lung scan — typically performed in two stages; stage 1, perfusion, uses radioisotope-tagged albumin to identify perfusion defects in pulmonary vasculature; stage 2, ventilation, is performed if stage 1 is inconclusive and requires the patient to breathe radioactive gas in a closed system while lung fields are scanned with a special camera
- Pulmonary angiography — considered the gold standard test for detecting and confirming PE; it uses multiple films to reveal constant intraluminal filling defects and a sharp cutoff in vessels greater than 2.5 mm in diameter; this procedure can cause pulmonary vascular compromise
- Arterial blood gas (ABG) levels — may reveal partial pressure of arterial oxygen (Pao_2) less than 60 mm Hg, partial pressure of arterial carbon dioxide ($Paco_2$) less than 35 mm Hg, and an increased alveolar-arterial gradient
- Spiral computed tomography scanning — evolving to replace pulmonary angiography and ventilation-perfusion lung scans for rapid diagnosis of PE
- Echocardiography
- 12-lead electrocardiogram (ECG) — used to rule out MI; in PE, it shows ST-segment depression, right axis deviation, right bundle-branch block, peaked P waves, and Q waves in lead III.
- Chest X-ray — may be normal or may reveal:
  - elevated diaphragm on affected side
  - enlarged pulmonary arteries
  - sudden cutoff of a pulmonary shadow
  - cardiac enlargement with prominent right atrial border
  - right ventricular dilation
  - dilated superior vena cava or hump-shaped shadow on the affected side (if pulmonary infarction is present).
- Noninvasive vasculature ultrasonography — supports the diagnosis of PE if thrombosis present

- Baseline coagulation studies: prothrombin time/International Normalized Ratio (INR); partial thromboplastin time (PTT), D-dimer; fibrin split products

POTENTIAL COMPLICATIONS

- Recurrent embolism
- Right-sided heart failure
- Shock (cardiogenic or distributive)
- Arrhythmias
- Hypoxemia
- Pulmonary hemorrhage
- Pulmonary infarction
- Cardiopulmonary arrest

CLINICAL SNAPSHOT ☀

Pulmonary embolism

Major nursing diagnoses and collaborative problems	Key patient outcomes
ND: Risk for injury	Maintain stable vital signs: heart rate, 60 to 100 beats/minute; systolic blood pressure, 90 to 140 mm Hg; and diastolic blood pressure, 50 to 90 mm Hg.
ND: Impaired gas exchange	Maintain normal ABG levels: pH, 7.35 to 7.45; $Paco_2$, 35 to 45 mm Hg; HCO_3^-, 22 to 26 mEq/L; Pao_2, 80 to 100 mm Hg; and $Sao_2 > 90\%$.
CP: Risk for cardiogenic shock	Maintain normal hemodynamic values: PASP, 20 to 30 mm Hg; PADP, 10 to 15 mm Hg; and PAWP, 4 to 12 mm Hg.
CP: Risk for complications	Experience minimal, if any, bleeding.
ND: Deficient knowledge (treatment regimen)	Describe safety considerations while on anticoagulant therapy.
ND: Compromised family coping	Display effective coping methods.

Nursing diagnosis

Risk for injury related to presence of risk factors

NURSING PRIORITY

Provide early recognition of PE signs and symptoms in high-risk patients.

PATIENT OUTCOME CRITERIA

Within 24 hours of admission, the patient will:
- maintain stable vital signs, typically: heart rate, 60 to 100 beats/minute; systolic blood pressure, 90 to 140 mm Hg; and diastolic blood pressure, 50 to 90 mm Hg
- be alert and oriented
- have lungs clear on auscultation
- have no complaints of leg or chest pain
- maintain oxygen saturation greater than 90%
- remain free from respiratory distress.

INTERVENTIONS

1. *Identify patient at risk for vascular injury, venous stasis, or hypercoagulability.* *

2. *Perform a thorough physical assessment of the patient on admission, and review the patient's initial laboratory and diagnostic information.*

3. *Assess the patient for changes* every 2 hours and as necessary

RATIONALES

1. Early identification of patients at risk allows for close monitoring for initial indications of PE.

2. A thorough physical assessment and initial laboratory and diagnostic information establish a baseline that can be used to gauge changes in the patient's condition.

3. Regular assessment allows the detection of initial, subtle changes, such as restlessness, a feeling of apprehension, or a slight drop in oxygen saturation.

---

*Italics indicate key interventions.

4. *Take steps to help prevent thromboemboli:* Use anti-embolism stockings or sequential compression devices, perform passive range-of-motion exercises or have the patient perform active exercises, ensure adequate fluid intake, and avoid high-Fowler's position, knee gatching, and leg massages.

4. These measures help maintain peripheral venous blood flow by preventing stasis, hypercoagulability, and clot dislodgment and by minimizing clot formation.

5. *Help the patient mobilize as soon as possible.*

5. Early mobilization helps stimulate peripheral venous blood flow, minimizing clot formation.

6. *Collaborate with the appropriate health care professionals if the patient's condition starts to deteriorate.*

6. A team of health care professionals can provide the interventions necessary to prevent complications.

7. Additional individualized interventions: _____

7. Rationales: _____

Suggested NIC Interventions
Surveillance: Safety

Suggested NOC Outcomes
Safety status: Physical injury

Nursing diagnosis
Impaired gas exchange related to ventilation-perfusion mismatch

NURSING PRIORITIES
Maintain adequate spontaneous ventilation. Ensure adequate oxygen supplementation as indicated by pulse oximetry or ABG results.

PATIENT OUTCOME CRITERIA
Within 48 hours of onset, the patient will:
- maintain normal ABG levels, typically: pH, 7.35 to 7.45; $Paco_2$, 35 to 45 mm Hg; HCO_3^-, 22 to 26 mEq/L; Pao_2, 80 to 100 mm Hg; and Sao_2, greater than 90%
- have clear bilateral breath sounds
- display no dyspnea
- no longer require mechanical ventilation.

INTERVENTIONS

1. *Assess pulmonary status at least every hour.* Note the presence of:
– tachypnea and dyspnea

– wheezing

RATIONALES

1. Serial assessments indicate the disorder's severity and the effectiveness of interventions.
– Tachypnea, a cardinal sign, is a compensatory measure to increase oxygenation and is attributed to stimulation of intrapulmonary receptors in the alveolar-capillary wall. Dyspnea results from apprehension or the sudden increase in alveolar dead space from alveoli that are ventilated but not perfused. Ventilation without perfusion impairs gas exchange.
– Wheezing results from pneumoconstriction following hypocapnia and platelet degranulation. Local hypocapnia constricts bronchial smooth muscle, increasing airway resistance and redirecting ventilation to better perfused areas; the resulting reduction in wasted ventilation is a protective mechanism. The thromboembolus consists of fibrin, red blood cells, and platelets; platelet degranulation releases substances that provoke bronchoconstriction and vasoconstriction.

Respiratory disorders

– decreased or absent breath sounds

– crackles and gurgles

– mentation changes, such as restlessness, changes in LOC, or irritability.

2. *Monitor ABG levels or pulse oximeter readings (arterial oxygen saturation [SaO₂]) or both as ordered.*

3. *Administer supplemental oxygen as ordered.*

4. *Elevate the head of the bed 30 to 45 degrees.* Use pillows to support the patient in a comfortable position.

5. *Maintain strict bed rest.* Assist the patient with bathing, eating, and other activities that increase dyspnea.

6. *Implement a program of vigorous pulmonary hygiene,* including deep-breathing exercises, coughing, incentive spirometry, and frequent repositioning. Suction as necessary.

7. *Assist with intubation and mechanical ventilation with positive end-expiratory pressure (PEEP) as needed.* Refer to the "Mechanical ventilation" care plan, page 281, for guidelines.

8. Additional individualized interventions: _____

– Normally, surfactant reduces surface tension as alveoli deflate, preventing alveolar collapse and lessening the work necessary to reinflate alveoli. Decreased surfactant production leads to atelectasis, as evidenced by decreased or absent breath sounds.
– Normally, surfactant also minimizes leakage of capillary fluid into alveoli by controlling alveolar surface tension. Decreased surfactant increases surface tension and allows fluid leakage, resulting in interstitial edema, as evidenced by crackles and gurgles.
– Mentation changes reflect cerebral hypoxia.

2. Monitor ABG levels or pulse oximeter readings (SaO_2) or both as ordered. ABG levels and pulse oximeter readings provide objective evidence of the degree of hypoxemia, which is useful in evaluating the severity of the PE and the effectiveness of interventions.

3. Supplemental oxygen prevents the immediate consequences of hypoxemia, which may include arrhythmias, cerebral ischemia, and MI.

4. This position promotes respiratory excursion and reduces the cardiopulmonary workload.

5. Rest conserves energy needed for breathing.

6. Adequate alveolar ventilation can reduce elevated $PaCO_2$ levels. Restoring effective aeration may prevent the onset of pneumonia from retention of secretions in the atelectatic area.

7. If the above measures fail to control hypoxemia, intubation and mechanical ventilation with PEEP may reopen collapsed alveoli. The "Mechanical ventilation" care plan details the care involved in this therapy.

8. Rationales: _____

> **Suggested NIC Interventions**
> *Acid-base management; Electrolyte management; Laboratory data interpretation; Oxygen therapy; Ventilation assistance; Airway management; Respiratory monitoring; Embolus care: Pulmonary; Hemodynamic regulation; Vital signs monitoring*

> **Suggested NOC Outcomes**
> *Electrolyte and acid-base balance; Respiratory status: Gas exchange; Respiratory status: Ventilation; Tissue perfusion: Pulmonary; Vital signs status*

Collaborative problem

Risk for cardiogenic shock related to pulmonary hypertension and right-sided heart failure

NURSING PRIORITY

Maintain adequate cardiac output.

PATIENT OUTCOME CRITERIA

Within 48 hours of symptom onset, the patient will have:
- stable vital signs, typically: heart rate, 60 to 100 beats/minute; systolic blood pressure, 90 to 140 mm Hg; and diastolic blood pressure, 50 to 90 mm Hg
- cardiac rhythm within normal limits
- hemodynamic parameters within normal limits, typically: PA systolic pressure, 20 to 30 mm Hg; PA diastolic pressure, 10 to 15 mm Hg; PAWP, 4 to 12 mm Hg; and cardiac output, 4 to 6 L/minute
- warm and dry skin
- urine output greater than 60 ml/hour.

Within 72 hours of symptom onset, the patient will:
- have the PA catheter removed
- have no complications from PA catheter monitoring.

INTERVENTIONS	RATIONALES
1. *Institute constant ECG monitoring if it isn't already taking place.* Observe for arrhythmias, particularly paroxysmal atrial tachycardia (PAT) or right bundle-branch block.	**1.** The right ventricle may decompensate in response to the sudden elevation in pulmonary pressure. PAT or other atrial arrhythmias reflect atrial stretching from volume overload, whereas bundle-branch block probably reflects right ventricular strain. Other arrhythmias may result from cardiac ischemia or hypoxemia; cardiopulmonary arrest may occur in massive embolism.
2. *Maintain I.V. line patency and administer fluids as ordered.*	**2.** Although the PE patient isn't volume depleted, I.V. access is critical for medication administration.
3. *Assist with PA catheter insertion as ordered.* Monitor PA pressure and pulmonary artery wedge pressure (PAWP) as ordered, typically every hour until the patient is stable and then every 2 to 4 hours.	**3.** A PA catheter provides objective data useful in assessing hemodynamic function of the left and right sides of the heart.
4. *Monitor for signs and symptoms of right-sided heart failure,* such as neck vein distention and elevated central venous pressure readings. If any are present, notify the physician.	**4.** Mechanical obstruction from the embolus and release of vasoconstrictors, described above, elevate pulmonary vascular resistance. The increased resistance to right ventricular ejection may cause right-sided heart failure.
5. *Monitor for signs and symptoms of cardiogenic shock,* such as severe hypotension and elevated PAWP. If present, notify the physician and implement measures in the "Cardiogenic shock" care plan, page 382, as appropriate.	**5.** Major obstruction to ventricular ejection produces cardiogenic shock. The "Cardiogenic shock" care plan presents detailed assessment and interventions for this complication.
6. *If the above measures are ineffective or the PE is life-threatening, prepare the patient for emergency surgery,* if ordered.	**6.** Pulmonary embolectomy may be a lifesaving operation.
7. Additional individualized interventions: _____	**7.** Rationales: _____

Collaborative problem

Risk for complications related to thrombolytic or anticoagulant therapy

NURSING PRIORITY

Prevent or minimize complications.

PATIENT OUTCOME CRITERIA

Throughout the hospital stay, the patient will:
- experience minimal, if any, bleeding
- display no signs of recurrent emboli.

INTERVENTIONS

1. *Administer a continuous low-dose heparin infusion as ordered or following protocol.* Monitor the PTT or INR daily or following protocol. Maintain values within the therapeutic range (PTT is normally twice the control value, and INR is normally 2.0 to 3.0). If PTT exceeds 100 seconds, the infusion is generally stopped for a period of time. For anticoagulant overdosing, administer protamine as ordered.

2. *Administer thrombolytics* (streptokinase [Streptase] or urokinase [Abbokinase]) *according to unit protocol* as ordered. Protocols vary but generally include:
– contraindications, such as recent surgery or stroke, active bleeding, and severe hypertension
– administration via a PA catheter or systemic infusion
– a loading dose followed by constant infusion for several hours
– maintaining thrombin time at two to five times normal
– monitoring for bleeding episodes.

3. *Start a second vascular access site for collection of blood samples for laboratory tests.* Maintain the site with normal saline flushes. Minimize the risk of bleeding by avoiding I.M. injections when possible and collaborating with the physician or clinical pharmacist to limit interactions between anticoagulants, thrombolytic agents, and other medications. Monitor for apparent and occult bleeding, by observing for hematomas and by guaiac-testing gastric contents and stool.

4. *If emboli recur despite the above measures, prepare the patient for surgery as ordered.*

5. *Teach the patient and family about the prescribed anticoagulant therapy, clot formation, and safety considerations.*

6. Additional individualized interventions: _____
_____

RATIONALES

1. Heparin is a potent anticoagulant that inactivates thrombin and blocks further clot formation. It also inhibits platelet degranulation around the thrombus and limits the release of vasoconstrictors. Subtherapeutic values place the patient at continued risk for recurrent emboli; values beyond the therapeutic range place the patient at risk for bleeding episodes. Protamine counteracts the effects of heparin.

2. Streptokinase or urokinase therapy may be ordered for the unstable patient with massive embolism. These thrombolytic agents dissolve already formed clots, decreasing symptoms. Streptokinase, the enzyme from beta-hemolytic streptococci, converts plasminogen to plasmin, producing fibrinolysis and resulting in decreased blood viscosity, improved microcirculation, and improved oxygen delivery. Urokinase also converts plasminogen to plasmin, degrading fibrin clots, fibrinogen, and other plasma proteins. Unit protocols vary regarding details of administration.

3. Anticoagulation and thrombolytic therapies increase the risk of bleeding. The second access site allows the collection of blood samples without increasing the risk of bleeding from multiple venipunctures. Early detection of bleeding permits dosage adjustment before massive hemorrhage occurs.

4. Vena cava ligation or insertion of a vena cava umbrella can trap recurrent emboli, which fibrinolysis can then dissolve.

5. Such information will help prevent clotting and bleeding complications.

6. Rationales: _____
_____

Nursing diagnosis

Deficient knowledge (treatment regimen) related to complex disorder and therapy

NURSING PRIORITY

Teach the patient how to prevent complications.

PATIENT OUTCOME CRITERIA

By the time of discharge, the patient and family will:
■ describe the action, dosage, frequency, and adverse effects of the prescribed anticoagulant
■ describe activities that can cause or prevent clot formation
■ describe safety considerations while the patient is on anticoagulant therapy.

INTERVENTIONS	RATIONALES
1. *Teach the patient and his family about clot formation and anticoagulant therapy.* Explain what activities can trigger clot formation and what steps they can take to prevent clot formation; make sure the patient can describe the safety considerations he should follow while on anticoagulant therapy. These include using an electric razor, wearing shoes, taking safety precautions when using potentially dangerous mechanical equipment, preventing cuts, and avoiding trauma to extremities.	**1.** The patient and his family need to understand what activities are safe and how to prevent clots from forming.
2. *Make sure the patient and his family can describe the prescribed anticoagulant,* including dosage, frequency, actions, and adverse effects. Give the patient information about follow-up laboratory testing to monitor anticoagulant therapy.	**2.** The patient and his family need to understand how the patient should take discharge medications, what adverse effects to look for, and when to report for follow-up testing (usually at least three times per week initially and then as directed).
3. Additional individualized interventions: _____ _____	**3.** Rationales: _____ _____

> **Suggested NIC Interventions**
> Teaching: Procedure/treatment

> **Suggested NOC Outcomes**
> Knowledge: Treatment regimen

Nursing diagnosis
Compromised family coping related to potentially life-threatening situation

NURSING PRIORITY
Provide emotional support to the family.

PATIENT OUTCOME CRITERIA
By the time of discharge, the family will:
- verbalize increased ability to cope and participate in establishing a family action plan to cope with crisis.
  Should the patient die, the family will:
- meet the outcome criteria identified in the "Dying" care plan, page 78, such as making contact with support persons.

INTERVENTIONS	RATIONALES
1. *Implement measures in the "Ineffective individual coping" care plan,* page 124, and *"Compromised family coping" care plan,* page 67, as appropriate. If death is imminent, implement measures in the "Dying" care plan, page 78, as appropriate.	**1.** PE is a major psychological threat, evidenced by the classic finding of a sense of impending doom. The "Ineffective individual coping" and "Compromised family coping" care plans contain measures to help the patient and his family deal with the emotional aftermath of a PE. If therapeutic measures are ineffective and the patient's condition continues to deteriorate, measures in the "Dying" care plan may help the patient and his family cope with approaching death.
2. Additional individualized interventions: _____ _____	**2.** Rationales: _____ _____

Respiratory disorders

Discharge planning

DISCHARGE CHECKLIST

Before discharge, the patient shows evidence of:

❐ stable blood pressure, pulse, and respiratory rate
❐ ABGs within normal limits for patient.

TEACHING CHECKLIST

Document evidence that the patient and his family demonstrate an understanding of:

❐ underlying reasons for clot development
❐ rationale for therapy
❐ measures to prevent recurrence.

DOCUMENTATION CHECKLIST

Using outcome criteria as a guide, document:

❐ clinical status on admission
❐ significant changes in status
❐ pertinent diagnostic test findings
❐ oxygen therapy
❐ heparin therapy
❐ thrombolytic therapy
❐ patient and family teaching
❐ discharge planning.

Associated care plans

- Acute pain
- Cardiogenic shock
- Compromised family coping
- Dying
- Ineffective individual coping

References

Kelly, J., et al. "Plasma D-dimers in the Diagnosis of Venous Thromboembolism," *Archives of Internal Medicine* 162(7):747-56, April 2002.

Kinney, M.R., et al. *AACN's Clinical Reference for Critical Care Nursing,* 4th ed. St. Louis: Mosby–Year Book, Inc., 1998.

Wood, K.E. "Major Pulmonary Embolism: A Review of a Pathophysiologic Approach to the Golden Hour of a Hemodynamically Significant Pulmonary Embolism," *Chest* 121(3):877-905, March 2002.

Thoracotomy

DRG INFORMATION
DRG 075   Major Chest Procedures.
Mean LOS = 9.9 days

Introduction
DEFINITION AND TIME FOCUS

A thoracotomy is an incision into the chest wall (thorax); its location depends on the surgery's purpose. A posterolateral or anterolateral approach (through the ribs) is common with general thoracic surgery, whereas a median sternotomy (through the sternum) is commonly used for cardiothoracic surgery. The ribs or sternal halves are spread to gain access to the pleural cavities or the mediastinum. Common thoracotomy procedures on the lungs include exploratory thoracotomy, pneumonectomy (removal of a lung), lobectomy (removal of a lobe), segmental resection (removal of one or several lung segments), wedge resection (removal of part of a lung segment), decortication (removal of scarred, fibrous tissue over the pleura), and thoracoplasty (removal of ribs). Thoracotomies are also used to perform esophageal, diaphragmatic, aortic, or open-heart procedures. Used in patients who have accessible peripheral lesions, video or endoscopic thoracotomy involves inserting a fiber-optic camera and instruments through small, inch-size chest incisions to remove lesions. A full thoracotomy is a major surgical procedure that requires careful preoperative and postoperative patient management and may require mechanical ventilation and closed chest drainage. This care plan focuses on preoperative care, postoperative stabilization, and initial recovery of the thoracotomy patient. (See *Clinical snapshot: Thoracotomy*, page 317.)

ETIOLOGY AND PRECIPITATING FACTORS

■ Pulmonary conditions, such as cancer, benign tumors, tuberculosis, abscesses or infection, bronchiectasis, blebs caused by emphysema, or empyema
■ Cardiac conditions, such as arteriosclerotic coronary arteries, valvular disease, mural wall defects, aortic aneurysm, cardiomyopathy, or congenital heart disease
■ Hiatal hernias or esophageal problems
■ Chest trauma involving one or more of the vital chest structures (lungs, heart, aorta, trachea, esophagus, or superior or inferior vena cava)

Focused assessment guidelines
NURSING HISTORY
(FUNCTIONAL HEALTH PATTERN FINDINGS)
Health-perception–health-management pattern

■ Shortness of breath or labored breathing on exertion
■ Bloody or excessive sputum
■ Tiredness and less tolerance for exercise than usual
■ Swelling of feet and ankles
■ Family history of heart disease or lung conditions such as asthma
■ High-risk cardiac and respiratory health patterns, such as sedentary lifestyle, overeating, lack of exercise, stress, smoking, or exposure to respiratory toxins
■ Major traumatic accident with a blow to the chest

Nutritional-metabolic pattern

■ Loss of appetite (respiratory or cardiac problem)
■ Weight gain (cardiac problem)
■ Weight loss (respiratory problem)

Activity-exercise pattern

■ Difficulty in breathing at rest and during exercise
■ Weakness and fatigue

Cognitive-perceptual pattern

■ Fear about serious nature of illness and impending major surgery
■ Periods of dizziness

Self-perception–self-concept pattern

■ Fear of disfigurement and scarring

Role-relationship pattern

■ Fear of inability to return to work after surgical procedure
■ High-risk job that subjects patient to excessive stress or exposure to respiratory toxins

Sexuality-reproductive pattern

■ Fatigue and inability to sustain sexual activity

PHYSICAL FINDINGS

Physical findings may vary depending on the nature of the condition requiring the thoracotomy.

General appearance

■ Cardiac condition: possibly typical signs and symptoms of angina, acute myocardial infarction, or heart failure. See the "Angina pectoris" care plan, page 355, "Acute myocardial infarction" care plan, page 337, or the "Heart failure" care plan, page 411 for the general appearance of a patient with these problems.
■ Pulmonary condition: possibly respiratory distress or general debilitation, depending on whether the condition is rapidly progressing or more chronic

- Chest trauma: possibly respiratory and cardiac distress and obvious crushing or penetrating injuries to the chest

Cardiovascular
- Arrhythmias
- Classic angina (substernal pain radiating to the left shoulder and arm that's relieved by nitroglycerin or rest)
- Unstable angina (substernal and radiating pain that isn't relieved by nitroglycerin or rest and that's more serious, prolonged, and unpredictable than classic angina)
- Noncardiac chest pain
- Hypotension
- Tachycardia

Pulmonary
- Dyspnea
- Shortness of breath
- Tachypnea
- Use of accessory muscles
- Gurgles, wheezes, crackles
- Chest trauma: possible open sucking wound, flail chest, paradoxical asymmetrical chest movements, or orthopnea

Gastrointestinal
- Hiatal hernia or esophageal problem: may have regurgitation, heartburn 30 to 60 minutes after meals, substernal pain, dysphagia, or feelings of fullness
- Cardiac problem: may have nausea and vomiting

Integumentary
- Cyanosis
- Pallor
- Chest trauma: abrasions or open wounds

DIAGNOSTIC STUDIES

Because of the various conditions for which thoracotomy may be performed, no typical laboratory data exist. This section instead presents monitoring tests.
- Arterial blood gas (ABG) levels — monitor oxygenation, ventilation, and acid-base status
- Cardiac enzymes, creatine kinase, lactic acid dehydrogenase — may reveal cardiac tissue damage
- Complete blood count — monitors red blood cell count, white blood cell (WBC) count, and platelet count. (Altered hemoglobin level and hematocrit reflect any potential blood loss and the blood's oxygen-carrying ability. An elevated WBC count and an elevated sedimentation rate may reflect an inflammatory response.)
- Serum creatinine, blood urea nitrogen levels — monitor the adequacy of renal function
- Serum electrolyte panel — monitors fluid, electrolyte, and acid-base status
- Urinalysis — monitors renal status, including renal secretion and concentration abilities
- Sputum assessment — monitors for infection
- Blood coagulation studies — monitor clotting
- For all conditions:
– Chest X-ray — may reveal abnormalities of the chest structures and heart and lung tissues

– Electrocardiogram — may reveal changes associated with ischemia
– Fluoroscopy — may reveal mobility abnormalities of the intrathoracic structures
– Magnetic resonance imaging — may reveal abnormalities of the thoracic structures and organs
- For cardiac or pulmonary conditions:
– Computed tomography — may reveal abnormalities of the lung, such as tumors, calcium deposits, or cavities, and abnormalities of the heart such as enlargement
– Biopsy — may aid in definitive diagnosis of lung or heart problems
– Gallium scan — may reveal inflammation or tumors of the heart or lungs
- For pulmonary conditions:
– Ventilation-perfusion pulmonary scan — may reveal areas of nonventilation and nonperfusion
– Pulmonary function tests — monitor static and dynamic lung volumes and capacities
– Bronchoscopy — may reveal abnormalities of the pulmonary tree
– Sonogram of the lung — may reveal collections of fluid and may be used postoperatively to locate the best site for thoracentesis
– Thoracentesis — may reveal abnormal fluid or tissue specimens
– Bronchograms — may reveal abnormal airway structures or a tumor
- For cardiac conditions:
– Cardiac radionuclide imaging — may reveal areas of cardiac ischemia and necrosis
– Echocardiography — may reveal structural and motion abnormalities of the heart
– Cardiac catheterization — may reveal abnormalities of the coronary arteries (during left-sided heart catheterization) or pulmonary artery (PA) vasculature (during right-sided heart catheterization)
- For esophageal conditions:
– Barium swallow, esophagoscopy, motility studies — may reveal esophageal abnormalities

POTENTIAL COMPLICATIONS
- Cardiac arrhythmias
- Atelectasis
- Pleural effusion
- Pericardial effusion
- Tension pneumothorax
- Hemothorax
- Infection
- Pulmonary edema
- Pulmonary embolism
- Hemorrhage
- Cardiac arrest
- Shock
- Cardiac tamponade

CLINICAL SNAPSHOT ☀

Thoracotomy

Major nursing diagnoses and collaborative problems	Key patient outcomes
ND: Deficient knowledge (treatment regimen)	Verbalize or demonstrate understanding of preoperative and postoperative thoracotomy care.
ND: Impaired gas exchange	Maintain normal ABG and oximetry levels, typically: pH, 7.35 to 7.45; $Paco_2$, 35 to 45 mm Hg; HCO_3^-, 22 to 26 mEq/L; Pao_2, 80 to 100 mm Hg; and Sao_2, > 90%.
CP: Risk for acute respiratory distress	Have a normal respiratory status.
CP: Risk for complications	Display no signs of complications.
ND: Risk for infection	Have a clean, dry, and healing wound.

Nursing diagnosis

Deficient knowledge (treatment regimen) related to unfamiliarity with thoracotomy

NURSING PRIORITY

Prepare the patient and family preoperatively for surgery and postoperative care.

PATIENT OUTCOME CRITERIA

Within 2 hours after preoperative teaching, the patient will (on request):
- explain the purpose and goal of thoracotomy and describe the general procedure and specific points covered during teaching
- verbalize or demonstrate understanding of preoperative and postoperative thoracotomy care.

INTERVENTIONS	RATIONALES
1. *Refer to the "Knowledge deficit" care plan,* page 129.*	1. The "Knowledge deficit" care plan contains general assessments and interventions for teaching and learning. This plan provides additional information specific to thoracotomy.
2. *Provide information about the surgery.* Document teaching and the patient's and family's response. Include the following points: – purpose, goal, and general procedure	2. Preoperative teaching may allay fears and anxiety about the unknown and help the patient cooperate with care and summon energy for healing. – A general understanding of the purpose and goal of a thoracotomy and what the procedure will be like will help orient the patient to upcoming nursing and medical care.
– type of incision	– Knowing what the incision will look like beforehand helps reduce the patient's anxiety.
– usual scar	– Knowing that the incision will heal to a thin, white line helps reduce the patient's fear of major disfigurement.
– preoperative medication	– Knowing that preoperative sedation is available helps reduce the patient's anxiety.
– anesthesia	– Teaching about the methods and effects of anesthesia helps prepare the patient for possible adverse reactions after surgery.

*Italics indicate key interventions.

Respiratory disorders

– expected location for recovery in the immediate post-operative period

– I.V. and other lines

– oxygen therapy

– chest tubes and drainage system

– nasogastric (NG) tube

– indwelling urinary catheter.

3. *Describe endotracheal intubation and mechanical ventilation, if appropriate.* See the "Mechanical ventilation" care plan, page 281. Document teaching and patient response.

4. *Explain thoracotomy's general effects on the lungs and describe reexpansion methods.* Coach the patient on deep breathing, coughing, and using an incentive spirometer, if ordered. Describe measurement of vital capacity and maximum inspiratory pressures. Observe return demonstrations. Document teaching and patient response.

5. *Discuss methods to relieve postoperative pain,* including using pain medication and splinting the incision with a pillow during deep breathing and coughing. Document teaching and patient response. Explain that an epidural catheter may be used for management of pain during the initial postoperative period.

6. *Describe and document the expected level of postoperative activity,* including turning from side to side, as allowed, every 2 hours on the day of surgery; sitting in semi-Fowler's position and sitting on the side of the bed with legs dangling on the 1st day after surgery; getting into a chair with assistance on the 1st or 2nd day after surgery; and ambulating in the room and hallway on the 2nd or 3rd day after surgery. Emphasize the importance of activity despite postoperative discomfort.

7. *Explain and demonstrate the use of antiembolism stockings.* Document teaching.

– Telling the patient where recovery will take place helps reduce postoperative disorientation.

– A postoperative thoracotomy patient may have peripheral I.V., central I.V., and monitoring lines. The necessary tubing and equipment could be frightening without preoperative preparation.

– All thoracotomy patients require oxygen therapy after surgery because of the atelectasis and hypoxemia produced by opening the chest and by anesthesia. The specific type of oxygen therapy depends on the surgery. Preoperative explanation about the oxygen therapy to be used may increase postoperative cooperation, particularly with the patient who will be intubated and placed on mechanical ventilation.

– Explaining the need for chest tubes and a drainage system to help reexpand the lungs and hasten recovery may allay anxiety about the invasive nature of these tubes.

– Explaining that an NG tube reduces abdominal discomfort until the GI tract resumes function may increase patient tolerance.

– Explaining the need to closely monitor fluid intake and output, including urine, after surgery may reduce anxiety about the catheter.

3. Explaining intubation and mechanical ventilation, including the temporary loss of speech, may allay anxiety about this treatment. The "Mechanical ventilation" care plan includes detailed information about caring for a mechanically ventilated patient.

4. Explaining the effect that opening the chest wall has on the lungs and describing reexpansion methods provide an incentive for active patient involvement. The patient's postoperative efforts to reexpand the lungs, remove secretions, and participate in respiratory function measurements may be more successful if practiced preoperatively, when the patient is under less stress and is free from pain.

5. Most patients describe thoracotomy pain as severe. The patient may be reassured to learn that pain relief is an important part of therapy. Explanations about the timely use of pain medication and pillow splinting may increase the patient's willingness to initiate and perform coughing and deep-breathing exercises.

6. A thoracotomy patient is likely to resist activity because of pain, fatigue, and weakness. Knowledge of expected activity and its importance provides a foundation on which the nurse can build when implementing the activity schedule.

7. Antiembolism stockings aid venous return and help prevent thrombus formation in the lower extremities.

8. Additional individualized interventions: _____

8. Rationales: _____

Suggested NIC Interventions *Teaching: Procedure/treatment*	**Suggested NOC Outcomes** *Knowledge: Treatment regimen*

Nursing diagnosis

Impaired gas exchange related to hypoventilation from anesthesia, pain, and analgesic medications as well as arrhythmias, atelectasis, and thickened secretions

NURSING PRIORITY

Optimize ventilation and oxygenation.

PATIENT OUTCOME CRITERIA

Within 4 hours after surgery, the patient will:
- perform deep breathing and coughing
- use the incentive spirometer
- request pain medication when needed.
  Within 8 hours after surgery, the patient will:
- manifest stable vital signs, typically: heart rate, 60 to 100 beats/minute; systolic blood pressure, 90 to 140 mm Hg; and diastolic blood pressure, 50 to 90 mm Hg
- display usual level of consciousness (LOC); minimally diminished breath sounds and chest movements
- maintain trachea in normal position
- have pink mucous membranes
- have minimal dullness to percussion over operative side, except for pneumonectomy
- be free from subcutaneous emphysema and premature ventricular contractions (PVCs) or other arrhythmias
- turn every 2 hours with assistance.
  Within 2 days after surgery, the patient will:
- use a spirometer two to three times per hour while awake
- display minimal or absent crackles, gurgles, or wheezes
- maintain normal ABG levels and oximetry levels, typically: pH, 7.35 to 7.45; $Paco_2$, 35 to 45 mm Hg; HCO_3^-, 22 to 26 mEq/L; Pao_2, 80 to 100 mm Hg; Sao_2, greater than 90%
- display minimal pain and sit up in a chair.
  Within 3 days after surgery, the patient will:
- have nearly equal bilateral breath sounds, chest expansion, and resonance to percussion, as appropriate for type of surgery
- begin to ambulate.

INTERVENTIONS

1. *After surgery, assess respiratory status* as needed and according to unit protocol, typically every 15 minutes until stable, every 30 minutes for 2 hours, then every 1 to 2 hours. Document and notify the physician of abnormal findings:
– respiratory rate, depth, and pattern; pulse rate; and blood pressure
– LOC

RATIONALES

1. The patient usually returns from surgery with a PA catheter, arterial line, peripheral I.V. lines, and pleural or mediastinal chest tubes or both. Frequent assessments of the cardiopulmonary system may reveal problems and permit timely interventions.
– Hypoxemia is reflected in vital sign changes.

– Decreased oxygen delivery to the brain is reflected in changes in LOC and mentation.

– bilateral breath sounds and bilateral chest movements

– accessory muscle use
– tracheal position

– color of mucous membranes, circumoral skin, and earlobes.

2. *Assess percussion notes and vocal fremitus as well as the amount, color, and consistency of sputum* every 1 to 2 hours and as needed.

3. *Palpate the chest wall every 1 to 2 hours and as needed.* Note the presence of tenderness, pain, or subcutaneous emphysema.

4. *Monitor cardiac rhythm constantly.* Note and report to the physician atrial fibrillation, PVCs, or other cardiac arrhythmias. Refer to appendix A, Monitoring standards.

5. *Monitor ABG levels* every shift and as needed for suspected changes in respiratory status as ordered. Notify the physician and document results.

6. *Monitor and document arterial oxygen levels* using pulse oximetry twice per shift and as needed, as ordered.

7. *Provide humidified oxygen* for the first 1 to 2 days and as needed for respiratory distress. Document its use.

8. *Medicate for pain* every 1 to 4 hours and as needed, as ordered. Monitor respiratory status to prevent respiratory depression. Document findings. Refer to the "Acute pain" care plan, page 32, for further details.

9. *Show the patient how to support the incision* with his hands or a small, hard pillow as needed during deep-breathing and coughing efforts. Encourage deep breathing and coughing two to three times every hour while awake.

– After thoracotomy, sounds and chest movements may be diminished over the operative area. These findings usually lessen and then disappear as recovery progresses. Adventitious sounds or persistence or further diminishing or chest sounds and movements may reflect fluid accumulation, atelectasis, or other respiratory problems.
– Use of accessory muscles may reflect dyspnea.
– Tracheal deviation from midline may indicate increased intrathoracic pressure on the side opposite the deviation or lung collapse on the same side as the deviation.
– Cyanotic mucous membranes, circumoral skin, and earlobes may indicate hypoxemia.

2. Dullness to percussion and decreased vocal fremitus are common after surgery and reflect consolidation from atelectatic areas. Resonance to percussion and normal vocal fremitus should return gradually as recovery progresses, except in pneumonectomy. Sputum characteristics may reflect hydration status, bleeding or infection, or pulmonary edema.

3. Areas of increasing tenderness or pain imply infection or another complication. Subcutaneous emphysema may occur when an air leak increases intrapleural pressure and eventually results in air spreading throughout the surrounding tissues. Subcutaneous emphysema is usually self-limiting and reabsorbs in several days; however, it may indicate a need for increased pleural suction pressures.

4. Cardiac arrhythmias, including atrial fibrillation and PVCs, are common after a thoracotomy, particularly after open-heart surgery. Appendix A, Monitoring standards, includes specific assessments and interventions for arrhythmias.

5. ABG levels reflect general oxygenation levels. Low partial pressure of arterial oxygen levels may indicate a need for increased oxygen therapy and more vigorous pulmonary hygiene.

6. Oximetry monitors arterial oxygen levels without needle sticks.

7. Oxygen therapy may be required until the lungs are fully reexpanded and the breathing pattern and airway clearance are more effective.

8. Pain relief promotes effective deep breathing and coughing. Respiratory depressants such as morphine must be used cautiously to prevent inadequate ventilation, which would be counterproductive to deep breathing and coughing. The "Acute pain" care plan contains general assessments and interventions for pain.

9. Support over the incision may decrease pain during deep breathing and coughing. Regular deep breathing and coughing promotes reexpansion of the lungs, mobilizes secretions, and prevents atelectasis.

10. *Promote and document incentive spirometer use,* as ordered, several times per hour while the patient is awake.

11. *Provide adequate hydration.* Document fluid intake.

12. *Help the patient get in to the upright position for deep-breathing and coughing efforts.* Provide an overhead trapeze bar or hand pulls attached to the end of the bed frame.

13. *Implement and document a progressive activity program* as allowed, typically:
– turning from side to side every 2 hours on the day of surgery, and sitting in semi-Fowler's position and on the side of the bed with legs dangling on the 1st postoperative day

– getting into a chair with assistance on the 1st or 2nd postoperative day and ambulating in the room and hallway on the 2nd or 3rd postoperative day.

14. Additional individualized interventions: _____

10. Spirometers encourage deep inspiratory efforts, which are more effective in reexpanding alveoli than forceful expiratory efforts.

11. Adequate hydration promotes liquid, easily removed lung secretions. Other means of humidification, such as intermittent positive-pressure breathing, may be undesirable because of the danger of a pneumothorax.

12. An upright position promotes lung expansion by gravity. These devices provide better mobility than does pushing against the bed.

13. Progressive activity is important to restore optimal cardiopulmonary function.
– Frequent position changes reexpand the lungs and prevent atelectasis and pooling of secretions. A patient who has had a pneumonectomy can be turned slightly toward the operative side or onto the back. Turning toward the nonoperative side could collapse the remaining lung, drain secretions into that lung, or cause a dangerous mediastinal shift. Semi-Fowler's position may aid reexpansion of the lungs by gravity; leg dangling allows the neurovascular reflexes to adjust to the upright position.
– Early chair sitting and ambulation may prevent thrombus formation in the lower extremities and aid adjustment to the upright position.

14. Rationales: _____

Suggested NIC Interventions
Acid-base management; Electrolyte management; Laboratory data interpretation; Oxygen therapy; Ventilation assistance; Airway management; Respiratory monitoring; Embolus care: Pulmonary; Hemodynamic regulation; Vital signs monitoring

Suggested NOC Outcomes
Electrolyte and acid-base balance; Respiratory status: Gas exchange; Respiratory status: Ventilation; Tissue perfusion: Pulmonary; Vital signs status

---

Collaborative problem
Risk for acute respiratory distress related to pneumothorax, hemothorax, or mediastinal shift secondary to malfunction or removal of chest drainage system

NURSING PRIORITIES
- Maintain patency of chest drainage system.
- Observe for complications after chest tube removal.

PATIENT OUTCOME CRITERIA
On admission and continuously, the patient will:
- have a properly functioning chest drainage system.
  Within 3 to 4 days after surgery, the patient will:
- have fully expanded lungs
- be free from air and fluid in the pleural space

Respiratory disorders

- have chest tubes removed.

Within 1 week after surgery, the patient will:
- display no dyspnea
- have normal respiratory status.

INTERVENTIONS

1. *Maintain an intact water-seal drainage system, if used.* In the event of disconnection or a broken chamber, reattach the tube or submerge it in water while the patient exhales. If reattachment isn't possible or water is unavailable, leave the chest tube open to air until a new system can be attached. Notify the physician and document occurrence. Arrange for a chest X-ray.

2. *Inspect the chest tube insertion site* every 2 hours and as needed for the presence of:
– intact occlusive dressings

– blood or drainage on the dressing

– proper position of the chest tubes within the chest and attachment to the chest wall.

3. *Observe the drainage tubing and connectors* every 1 to 2 hours for proper connection and taping of connectors. Coil the tubing to prevent dependent loops.

4. *Milk the tubing* every 1 to 2 hours and as needed, as ordered, during the 1st postoperative day. Document these actions.

5. *Assess the drainage receptacle* every 1 to 2 hours and as needed for secure attachment to the drainage tubing. If bottle drainage is used, maintain the end of the tube in the water-seal chamber ³/₄″ (2 cm) below the water level.

6. *Observe for and document tidalling* (fluctuation of water level during respirations) in the submerged water-seal tube every 2 hours. To do this, turn off the suction or pinch the suction tubing temporarily.

RATIONALES

1. Although most thoracotomy patients have them, chest tubes aren't usually used after pneumonectomy because serous fluid collection promotes the development of fibrotic tissue in the empty space. If the patient does have a chest tube, disconnection may allow air to enter the pleural space and cause a pneumothorax. Exhalation during reattachment may force excess air from the pleural space. Leaving the tube open to air creates the potential for a small open pneumothorax but may be less harmful than clamping the tube and possibly causing a tension pneumothorax, especially in a patient with an air leak. A chest X-ray may be necessary to assess respiratory status.

2. Frequent inspection may reveal problems and allow for timely interventions.
– Occlusive dressings are used to prevent air from entering the pleural space around the chest tube insertion site and to prevent accidental dislodgment of the tubes.
– Blood or drainage on the dressing may indicate recent bleeding or infection.
– Dislodgment of the tubes can create a dangerous increase of air or drainage within the pleural space, which could cause the lung to collapse.

3. The closed drainage system must be sealed to prevent air from entering the pleural space. Taped connectors are less likely to disconnect or develop air leaks. Improperly looped tubing may inhibit gravity flow of drainage.

4. This procedure assists drainage by creating negative pressure and preventing clotting and plugging of the tubes.

5. Securely attaching the drainage tubing to the drainage receptacle and placing the end of the water-seal tube below the water level prevent air from entering the drainage system and the pleural space.

6. Tidalling indicates a functioning, airtight system between the pleura and the drainage receptacle. During spontaneous ventilation, inspiration creates negative pressure in the pleura and the drainage system, which pulls the water level upward in the tubing. The level moves downward on expiration. Fluctuations are the reverse for a patient on mechanical ventilation: the positive pressure applied during inspiration pushes the water level downward, whereas termination of the positive pressure on expiration allows the water level to move upward. Absence of tidalling may indicate a blocked chest tube or complete lung expansion.

7. *Observe the water-seal chamber for intermittent bubbling during respiration* every 2 hours and as needed. Document the amount of bubbling and where in the respiratory cycle it occurs.

7. Intermittent bubbling represents drainage of air from within the pleural spaces. Bubbling occurs normally during expiration with spontaneous ventilation or during inspiration with mechanical ventilation.

8. *If continuous bubbling occurs in the water-seal chamber, search for the source of the leak.* Briefly clamp consecutive parts of the system, beginning at the chest wall, until the bubbling stops. If the bubbling stops when the clamp is proximal to the chest wall, notify the physician. If the bubbling stops when the clamp is distal to the chest wall, replace the system beyond that point.

8. Continuous bubbling indicates an air leak within the patient or the drainage system. Clamping as described helps isolate the leak. Bubbling that stops when the clamp is proximal to the chest wall indicates an air leak within the patient, which requires medical evaluation. Bubbling that stops when the clamp is distal to the chest wall indicates a leak in the drainage system, which requires replacement of the system.

9. *Maintain and document the ordered amount of suction, if used.* With Emerson suction, check the pressure set on the dial and the pressure registering on the gauge. With a multiple-chamber system (such as Pleur-evac), check the water level in the suction control chamber to ensure that it equals the ordered amount of negative pressure.

9. Negative pressure may be required to remove secretions and air from the intrapleural space. Inadequate negative pressure may prevent drainage and reexpansion of the lungs, whereas excessive pressure may damage pleural tissue.

10. *Monitor the amount, color, and consistency of chest tube drainage* every 30 minutes for 2 hours, every hour for 6 hours, and then every 2 hours and as needed. Notify the physician if large amounts of drainage occur (more than 200 ml/hour for 3 hours). Document findings.

10. Large amounts of drainage may indicate bleeding and require immediate intervention to prevent shock. Absence of drainage, particularly in the immediate postoperative period, may indicate a plugged chest tube, which could cause a dangerous increase in intrapleural pressure. Chest tubes commonly drain up to 500 ml in the first 8 hours, decreasing to zero drainage 3 to 4 days after surgery as the pleurae realign and the lungs reexpand.

11. *Assist with removal of chest tubes* 3 to 4 days after surgery.
– Before removal, look for an absence of chest tube drainage, tidalling with respirations, and the return of breath sounds in the affected area.
– Medicate with an analgesic before removal as ordered.
– Place the patient in high-Fowler's position. Have the patient take a deep breath and cough vigorously. At maximum inspiration, assist in removing the tube and tightening the purse-string skin suture.

– Apply a sterile occlusive dressing.

– After chest tube removal, assess the patient for signs and symptoms of respiratory distress, including dyspnea, pain, absent breath sounds, uneven chest movement, dull percussion sounds, cardiac arrhythmias, or anxiety.

11. Chest tubes are removed when the lungs have reexpanded.
– These signs indicate lung reexpansion.

– An analgesic helps decrease pain during removal.
– High-Fowler's position, deep breathing, and vigorous coughing may prevent the development of a pneumothorax during tube removal and suture tightening by providing maximum lung expansion and positive intrapleural pressure.
– A sterile occlusive dressing may prevent infection and air leaks into the pleural space.
– Rarely, the patient may develop such complications as pneumothorax, hemothorax, or mediastinal shift, which may compromise the respiratory and cardiac systems. Careful assessment allows early identification and intervention.

12. If necessary, assist the physician with reinsertion of the chest tubes or thoracentesis. Document the procedure.

12. Rarely, the patient may accumulate fluid or air and may require reinsertion of chest tubes or thoracentesis.

13. Additional individualized interventions: _____

13. Rationales: _____

Collaborative problem

Risk for complications related to surgical procedure, such as hemorrhage, pneumothorax, pleural effusion, atelectasis, pulmonary edema, or pulmonary embolism

NURSING PRIORITY
Monitor for and promptly report signs and symptoms of complications.

PATIENT OUTCOME CRITERION
By 3 to 7 days after surgery, the patient will display no signs of complications, such as hemorrhage, cardiac arrhythmias, hemothorax, cardiac tamponade, pneumothorax, pleural effusion, atelectasis, subcutaneous emphysema, bronchopleural fistula, or mediastinal shift.

INTERVENTIONS

1. See the "Perioperative care" care plan, page 146.

2. *Monitor for signs and symptoms of hemorrhage.* If present, alert the physician immediately and document. Observe for:
– tachycardia, hypotension, low hemodynamic measurements, and excessive chest drainage
– decreasing or absent breath sounds, increasing dullness to percussion, or decreased or absent fremitus
– decreased heart sounds, paradoxical pulse greater than 10 mm Hg on inspiration, or high central venous pressure (CVP).

3. *Monitor for signs of pneumothorax,* including tachypnea, dyspnea, decreased or absent breath sounds, absent vocal fremitus, and hyperresonance. Notify the physician and document their occurrences.

4. *Monitor for signs of pleural effusion,* including decreased or absent breath sounds, decreased vocal fremitus, increased dullness, and tachypnea. Notify the physician and document their occurrences.

5. *Monitor for signs of increasing atelectasis,* including fever, tachypnea, tachycardia, increasing dullness, increased vocal fremitus, and bronchial or bronchovesicular breath sounds in the lung periphery. Notify the physician and document their occurrences.

6. *Monitor for signs and symptoms of pulmonary edema,* including tachypnea; tachycardia; dyspnea; shortness of breath; cough; crackles; wheezing; pink, frothy sputum; and anxiety. Notify the physician and document their occurrences.

RATIONALES

1. The "Perioperative care" care plan covers general postoperative problems and interventions. This plan focuses on thoracotomy.

2. Hemorrhage may result from surgical trauma, inadequate hemostasis, or other factors. It always requires immediate medical evaluation and intervention.
– These signs may indicate hemorrhage and require a return to surgery to ligate bleeding vessels.
– These signs may reflect a hemothorax. Thoracentesis or reinsertion of chest tubes may be necessary.
– These signs may indicate cardiac tamponade, which requires immediate pericardiocentesis.

3. A pneumothorax prevents reexpansion of the lungs and may require reinsertion of chest tubes.

4. A pleural effusion may compress the lungs, causing hypoxemia. Chest tube reinsertion may be necessary to remove the fluid and reexpand the lungs. Failure to remove the fluid may result in empyema.

5. Atelectasis commonly caused by poor bronchial hygiene, produces hypoxemia reflected in tachypnea and tachycardia. Dullness, increased fremitus, and abnormal breath sounds all result from consolidation.

6. Pulmonary edema is a life-threatening condition that requires immediate intervention, such as use of diuretics, inotropic agents, rotating tourniquets, and positive-pressure breathing. A patient with other problems, particularly cardiac problems, may be at high risk for this complication.

7. *Continuously monitor a pneumonectomy patient* for the following complications:

– Hemorrhage: If a patient has a sudden, large hemoptysis, place the patient in high-Fowler's position, turned toward the operative side; summon immediate medical assistance.

– Bronchopleural fistula: Observe for hemoptysis, an extensive air leak, subcutaneous emphysema, or fever.

– Subcutaneous emphysema: Observe for swelling, puffiness, or crepitation of the skin.

– Excessive mediastinal shift: Observe for excessive deviation of the trachea at the sternal notch, hypotension, tachycardia, weak peripheral pulses, and other signs of decreased cardiac output.

8. *Monitor for signs and symptoms of pulmonary embolism,* including chest pain, dyspnea, fever, hemoptysis, changes in vital signs, and increased CVP. Notify the physician and document. Refer to the "Pulmonary embolism" care plan, page 306, for further information.

9. Additional individualized interventions: _____

_____

7. A pneumonectomy, the most traumatic form of thoracotomy, has a high incidence of complications.

– Hemorrhage may result from inadequate surgical hemostasis, development of a bronchopleural fistula, or other factors. Placing the patient in high-Fowler's position toward the operative side may prevent drainage into the remaining lung.

– A bronchopleural fistula may develop after surgery, most commonly during the first week, causing bleeding, air leaks, or infection. Depending on the size and location of the fistula, it may require surgery (to close the bronchial stump) and antibiotics.

– A bronchial stump leak may cause a large amount of subcutaneous emphysema. An air leak usually resolves over 3 days to a week but may require surgery.

– After lung removal, the mediastinum isn't supported on one side and may shift. The residual pleural space should fill after surgery by a combination of mediastinal shift, diaphragm elevation, coagulation of serous drainage, and development of fibrotic tissue. If mediastinal shift is excessive, decreased cardiac output may occur, requiring mediastinal stabilization by fluid or air injection or thoracentesis.

8. Pulmonary embolism, a serious complication, may result from deep vein thrombosis and cause varying signs and symptoms depending on the size of the embolus. Prompt medical treatment is required to prevent further pulmonary tissue damage. The "Pulmonary embolism" care plan covers this disorder in detail.

9. Rationales: _____

_____

Nursing diagnosis

Risk for infection related to surgical incision and endotracheal intubation

NURSING PRIORITY
Prevent infection.

PATIENT OUTCOME CRITERIA
Within 3 days after surgery, the patient will:
- have a clean, dry, and healing wound
- display stable vital signs: heart rate, 60 to 100 beats/minute; systolic blood pressure, 90 to 140 mm Hg; and diastolic blood pressure, 50 to 90 mm Hg
- display a normal WBC count and sedimentation rate.
  By the time of discharge, the patient will:
- have clear breath sounds, normal fremitus, and normal resonance to percussion, as appropriate to type of surgery.

INTERVENTIONS

1. *Monitor for and document signs of pneumonia,* including fever, tachypnea, bronchial or bronchovesicular breath sounds in the periphery, increased vocal fremitus, increased dullness, and dyspnea. Notify the physician if any of these signs occur.

RATIONALES

1. Invasive chest surgery and endotracheal intubation place the patient at high risk for pneumonia. Treatment may require aggressive pulmonary hygiene, antibiotics, and positive-pressure breathing treatments.

Respiratory disorders

2. *Assess for signs and symptoms of wound infection* every 2 to 4 hours and as needed. When the incision can be seen directly, observe for redness and swelling. Monitor for elevated WBC count or sedimentation rate as ordered.

3. *Monitor culture and sensitivity test results* for wound drainage as ordered.

4. *Reinforce or change dressings as needed,* using *sterile technique.*

5. Additional individualized interventions: _____
_____

2. Regular assessments may provide early warning of infection. Occlusive dressings may remain over the incision sites for 1 to 3 days, making direct observation of the sites difficult.

3. Culture and sensitivity tests help identify the infective organism and the most effective antibiotic treatment.

4. The dressing is usually reinforced, not changed, during the first 1 to 2 days after surgery to prevent exposure to microorganisms.

5. Rationales: _____
_____

Suggested NIC Interventions
Infection control; Infection protection; Incision site care; Wound care

Suggested NOC Outcomes
Infection status; Wound healing: Primary intention

Discharge planning

DISCHARGE CHECKLIST
Before discharge, the patient shows evidence of:
❏ stable vital signs and monitoring parameters
❏ clear breath sounds, bilateral lung expansion, and bilateral resonance to percussion as appropriate
❏ absence of major complications
❏ healing surgical incision.

TEACHING CHECKLIST
Document evidence that the patient and family demonstrate an understanding of:
❏ surgical procedure, including expected postoperative course
❏ deep breathing, coughing, and spirometer use
❏ comfort measures
❏ range-of-motion (ROM) and other exercises
❏ purpose and mechanism of chest drainage system.

DOCUMENTATION CHECKLIST
Using outcome criteria as a guide, document:
❏ the patient's clinical status on admission
❏ significant changes in status
❏ pertinent diagnostic test findings
❏ chest drainage (amount, consistency, and color)
❏ functioning of chest drainage equipment
❏ complications such as subcutaneous emphysema
❏ deep breathing, coughing, and spirometer efforts
❏ oxygen therapy
❏ pain and effects of medication
❏ activity levels and ROM
❏ patient and family teaching discharge planning.

Associated care plans

■ Acute pain
■ Mechanical ventilation
■ Pulmonary embolism

References
Ballantyne, J.C., et al. "The Comparative Effects of Postoperative Analgesic Therapies on Pulmonary Outcome: Cumulative Meta-analyses of Randomized, Controlled Trials," *Anesthesia and Analgesia* 86(3):598-612, March 1998.

Black, J.M., et al. *Medical Surgical Nursing: Clinical Management for Positive Outcomes,* 6th ed. Philadelphia: W.B. Saunders Co., 2001.

Handbook of Diseases, 2nd ed. Springhouse, Pa.: Springhouse Corp., 1999.

Mentzer, S.J., et al. "Mediastinoscopy, Thoracoscopy, and Video-Assisted Thoracic Surgery in the Diagnosis and Staging of Lung Cancer," *Chest* 112(4 suppl):239S-41S, October 1997.

Peeters-Asdourian, C., and Gupta, S. "Choices in Pain Management Following Thoracotomy," *Chest* 115(5 suppl):122S-24S, May 1999.

Cardiovascular disorders

PART

5

Abdominal aortic aneurysm repair

DRG INFORMATION
DRG 110   Major Cardiovascular Procedures with Complication or Comorbidity (CC).
          Mean LOS = 9.2 days
DRG 111   Major Cardiovascular Procedures without CC.
          Mean LOS = 4.7 days

Introduction
DEFINITION AND TIME FOCUS
The arterial wall consists of three tissue layers: the intima, the media, and the adventitia. In abdominal aneurysm, degeneration of the media causes the aorta to dilate, usually distal to the renal arteries. The vessel wall progressively weakens, increasing the risk of life-threatening rupture. In traditional abdominal aortic aneurysm repair, the diseased portion of the artery (aneurysm) is surgically replaced with a synthetic polyester (Dacron) graft. The graft may be tubular and straight or bifurcated (split into two branches), depending on the segment involved. Although cardiopulmonary bypass isn't performed, the aorta is cross-clamped to prevent forward flow of blood during repair. The graft is then placed in the lumen of the aneurysm so that the outer layers of the arterial wall will close over and protect the graft.

One alternative technique to an aneurysm repair is endovascular stenting. In this procedure, a large catheter is inserted through a femoral incision to place expandable synthetic polytetrafluoroethylene balloon stents into the lumen of the aneurysm. The stents may also be used with Dacron grafts. The Dacron graft is sutured to hold the stent in place. Instead of the aneurysm being resected, blood flow is diverted from the aneurysm through the lumen of the stent; the aneurysm tissue eventually adheres to the outer wall of the stent. Another technique under investigation in some medical centers involves endoscopic aneurysm repair. The technique is similar to traditional aneurysm repair but is performed using endoscopic equipment and techniques. Both endovascular stenting and endoscopic techniques require shorter hospital stays, and patients typically can ambulate within 24 hours of surgery.

The abdominal aortic aneurysm patient typically spends 24 to 48 hours in the intensive care unit (ICU). Most patients are elderly and have one or more comorbidities, such as cardiovascular disease, diabetes, renal failure, and pulmonary disease. This care plan focuses on preoperative care as well as the management of potential multisystem complications during the initial recovery period in the ICU and the medical-surgical unit. (See *Clinical snapshot: Abdominal aortic aneurysm repair*.)

ETIOLOGY AND PRECIPITATING FACTORS
The most common cause of aneurysm is atherosclerosis. Risk factors for atherosclerosis include:
- cigarette smoking
- hypercholesterolemia
- hypertension
- diabetes mellitus
- obesity
- hypertriglyceridemia
- sedentary lifestyle
- stress
- family history of cardiovascular disease.
  Other causes of aneurysm include:
- congenital disorders such as Marfan syndrome
- bacterial or fungal infections that invade the vessel wall (mycotic aneurysm)
- syphilitic aortitis
- blunt or sharp trauma
- chronic aortitis related to Takayasu's arteritis or rheumatic spondylitis.

Focused assessment guidelines
NURSING HISTORY
(FUNCTIONAL HEALTH PATTERN FINDINGS)
Health-perception–health-management pattern
- Abdominal or back discomfort
- Feeling of heartbeat in the abdomen
- History of exercise intolerance
- Family history of atherosclerosis
- Cardiac and respiratory risk factors, such as cigarette smoking; high-fat, high-cholesterol diet; or sedentary lifestyle

Activity-exercise pattern
- Intermittent claudication or pain at rest
- Shortness of breath if a heavy smoker

Sexuality-reproductive pattern
- Impotence

Cognitive-perceptual pattern
- Fear about impending surgery

PHYSICAL FINDINGS
Cardiovascular
- Hypertension
- Arrhythmias

- Diminished peripheral pulses, claudication or pain at rest, trophic changes (if associated with atherosclerosis)
- Palpable abdominal mass above or at the umbilicus, extending toward the epigastrium
- Carotid, femoral, or abdominal aortic bruits

Integumentary
Integumentary changes are associated with atherosclerotic changes or distal embolization:
- Cyanosis of lower extremities
- Dependent rubor, with pallor on elevation
- Thickened toenails
- Decreased hair growth on lower extremities
- Coolness of lower extremities

DIAGNOSTIC STUDIES
- Arterial blood gas (ABG) levels — monitor oxygenation, ventilation, and acid-base status
- Complete blood count — monitors red blood cell, white blood cell (WBC), and platelet counts. Altered hemoglobin levels and hematocrit reflect any blood loss and the oxygen-carrying ability of the blood. An elevated WBC count reflects an inflammatory response.
- Serum electrolyte panel — monitors fluid, electrolyte, and acid-base status
- Serum creatinine and blood urea nitrogen (BUN) levels — monitor renal function
- Blood coagulation studies — monitor clotting
- Urinalysis—monitors renal status, including secretion and concentration

- Blood typing and crossmatching — necessary for blood replacement
- Electrocardiography (ECG) — may reveal cardiac changes associated with ischemia
- Chest X-ray — may reveal abnormalities of the chest, heart, and lungs
- Abdominal X-ray — may reveal calcium in the aneurysm wall
- Abdominal ultrasound — may reveal the aneurysm's size
- Abdominal computed tomography scan — may reveal a leaking aneurysm
- Aortic arteriogram — may show aberrant renal arteries, mesenteric artery patency, and iliac artery involvement
- Magnetic resonance angiography — form of magnetic resonance imaging that may give information on blood flow within the aneurysm

POTENTIAL COMPLICATIONS
- Myocardial infarction
- Hemorrhage
- Microembolization
- Respiratory failure
- Lower limb ischemia
- Renal failure
- Bowel ischemia
- Spinal cord ischemia
- Infection
- Impotence

CLINICAL SNAPSHOT ✸

Abdominal aortic aneurysm repair

Major nursing diagnoses and collaborative problems	Key patient outcomes
ND: Deficient knowledge	Verbalize understanding of perioperative routines.
ND: Decreased cardiac output	Maintain stable vital signs, typically: heart rate, 60 to 100 beats/minute; systolic blood pressure, 90 to 140 mm Hg; and diastolic blood pressure, 50 to 90 mm Hg.
ND: Ineffective breathing pattern	Maintain ABGs within normal limits, typically: pH, 7.35 to 7.45; $Paco_2$, 35 to 45 mm Hg; HCO_3^-, 22 to 26 mEq/L; Pao_2, 80 to 100 mm Hg; and Sao_2, > 90%.
CP: Risk for bleeding	Remain free from signs and symptoms of bleeding.
CP: Risk for complications	Have any complication immediately detected, reported, and treated as appropriate.
ND: Acute pain	Rate pain with oral medication as less than 3 on a 0 to 10 pain rating scale.

Nursing diagnosis

Deficient knowledge (preoperative and postoperative care) related to unfamiliarity with aortic surgery

NURSING PRIORITY
Prepare the patient and family for the impending surgery.

PATIENT OUTCOME CRITERIA
Within 2 hours after preoperative teaching, the patient will (on request):
- verbalize understanding of perioperative routines
- demonstrate the ability to cough; breathe deeply; use an incentive spirometer, if applicable; and splint the incision.

INTERVENTIONS	RATIONALES
1. *See the "Knowledge deficit" care plan,* page 129.*	1. The "Knowledge deficit" care plan provides general patient teaching information. This plan focuses specifically on abdominal aortic aneurysm repair.
2. *See the "Perioperative care" care plan,* page 146.	2. The "Perioperative care" care plan describes what to teach the patient about perioperative routines.
3. *Describe endotracheal intubation and mechanical ventilation.* Refer to the "Mechanical ventilation" care plan, page 281.	3. The patient undergoing abdominal aortic aneurysm repair may require intubation and mechanical ventilation for the first 8 hours after surgery. Intubation time may be shorter with endoscopic or endovascular repair. Explaining mechanical ventilation and weaning may allay the patient's anxiety. The "Mechanical ventilation" care plan provides detailed information about teaching a mechanically ventilated patient.
4. *Explain to the patient and family the need for close monitoring after surgery and the expected length of stay in ICU,* usually 24 to 48 hours.	4. Explaining the expected postoperative course may minimize the patient's and his family's anxieties. The length of time spent in ICU varies among facilities.
5. *Explain the need for frequent vascular checks* to assess graft patency and peripheral vascular status.	5. Peripheral pulses are checked hourly for the first 24 hours. Assessing capillary refill time and the appearance of skin on the feet can lead to early detection of micro-embolization. A Doppler ultrasound stethoscope may also be used. Knowing that frequent assessment is normal may allay the patient's fears that the surgery failed.
6. *Review activities that may prevent graft kinking or compression and postoperative edema in the lower extremities,* such as reclining while sitting in a chair, avoiding leg crossing or dangling the legs over the bedside, elevating the foot of the bed, and keeping the head of the bed at an angle of less than 45 degrees. The reverse Trendelenburg position may benefit a patient who has pulmonary complications.	6. Reclining positions may prevent pressure on the graft site and kinking of an aortobifemoral graft in the groin. Preventing leg crossing or dangling the legs over the bedside and elevating the foot of the bed may prevent or decrease lower extremity edema.
7. Additional individualized interventions: _____	7. Rationales: _____

*Italics indicate key interventions.

| **Suggested NIC Interventions**
Teaching: Procedure/treatment | **Suggested NOC Outcomes**
Knowledge: Treatment regimen |

Nursing diagnosis

Decreased cardiac output related to changes in intravascular volume, third space fluid shift, and increased systemic vascular resistance

NURSING PRIORITY

Promptly detect changes in cardiac status.

PATIENT OUTCOME CRITERIA

Within the first 24 hours after surgery, the patient will:
- maintain stable vital signs, typically: heart rate, 60 to 100 beats/minute; systolic blood pressure, 90 to 140 mm Hg; and diastolic blood pressure, 50 to 90 mm Hg
- be free from cardiac complications
- maintain graft patency.

INTERVENTIONS	**RATIONALES**
1. *After surgery, monitor the patient's vital signs* according to unit protocol and nursing judgment (typically every 15 minutes until stable, then every hour for the first 12 hours, then every 2 hours until discharge to the medical-surgical unit, then every 4 hours until discharge from the hospital).	**1.** Decreased cardiac output is the major complication that leads to morbidity following aortic surgery.
2. *Monitor hemodynamic parameters* (central venous pressure [CVP], pulmonary artery wedge pressure [PAWP], cardiac output, and cardiac index) according to ICU protocol or physician's orders until the pulmonary artery (PA) catheter is removed.	**2.** The patient usually returns from surgery with an arterial line, peripheral I.V. lines, and an indwelling urinary catheter. The patient may also have a PA catheter. Hemodynamic monitoring provides an accurate evaluation of myocardial sensitivity and guides drug and fluid therapy to prevent cardiac complications.
3. *Continuously monitor heart rate and ECG* for arrhythmias, particularly atrial fibrillation, and ST-segment elevation until the patient is discharged to the medical-surgical unit. Document and report abnormalities to the physician. Obtain a 12-lead ECG if ST-segment elevation or chest pain develops.	**3.** Frequent cardiopulmonary assessments may reveal problems and allow for timely interventions. (Thromboembolism from atrial fibrillation may interfere with vital arterial blood flow.)
4. Monitor effectiveness of antihypertensive or vasopressor medications, if prescribed.	**4.** Hypertension and hypotension affect graft patency.
5. *Monitor for fluid and electrolyte imbalances.* See appendix C, Fluid and electrolyte imbalances.	**5.** The Fluid and electrolyte imbalances appendix addresses assessment parameters and interventions.
6. Additional individualized interventions: _____	**6.** Rationales: _____

Suggested NIC Interventions
Cardiac care; Cardiac care: Acute; Hemodynamic regulation; Shock management: Cardiac; Circulatory care: Arterial insufficiency; Circulatory care: Venous insufficiency; Intravenous (I.V.) therapy; Vital signs monitoring

Suggested NOC Outcomes
Cardiac pump effectiveness; Circulation status; Tissue perfusion: Abdominal organs; Tissue perfusion: Peripheral; Vital signs status

---

Nursing diagnosis

Ineffective breathing pattern related to endotracheal intubation, physiologic changes associated with aging, effects of general anesthesia, and presence of an abdominal incision

NURSING PRIORITY

Optimize ventilation and oxygenation.

PATIENT OUTCOME CRITERIA

Within 4 hours after surgery, the patient will:
- exhibit bilaterally clear breath sounds
- have minimal endotracheal secretions
- maintain ABG levels within normal limits, typically: pH, 7.35 to 7.45, $Paco_2$, 35 to 45 mm Hg; HCO_3^-, 22 to 26 mEq/L; Pao_2, 80 to 100 mm Hg; and Sao_2, greater than 90%
- maintain oxygen saturation greater than or equal to 95%.
   Within 4 hours of extubation, the patient will:
- perform incentive spirometry without difficulty
- have bilaterally clear anterior and posterior breath sounds
- maintain Sao_2 greater than or equal to 95%.

INTERVENTIONS

1. *Assess the patient's vital signs* on admission to the ICU and every hour for 24 hours, then every 2 hours until the patient is returned to the medical-surgical unit, then every 4 hours. Note respiratory effort and the amount and character of sputum. Provide routine suctioning according to unit protocol while the patient is intubated. Document and report abnormalities.

2. *See the "Mechanical ventilation" care plan,* page 281.

3. *After the patient is extubated, provide supplemental oxygen as ordered.* Have the patient turn, cough, and deep breathe with an incentive spirometer every 2 hours. Instruct the patient on how to splint the incision with a pillow while coughing and deep breathing. Monitor oxygen saturation through pulse oximetry or ABG levels or both as ordered. See the "Mechanical ventilation" care plan, page 281.

4. *Administer analgesics for pain as ordered. Monitor for signs and symptoms of respiratory depression.* See the "Acute pain" care plan, page 32.

RATIONALES

1. A patient undergoing abdominal aortic aneurysm repair may be intubated overnight after surgery. Elevated temperature may indicate atelectasis. Respiratory effort may be minimal immediately after surgery. Suctioning promotes airway clearance.

2. The "Mechanical ventilation" care plan provides specific information on assessments and interventions for the intubated patient.

3. Supplemental oxygen may be ordered to promote adequate tissue oxygenation. Position changes, deep breathing, and coughing exercises clear the airway and prevent atelectasis. The "Mechanical ventilation" care plan provides detailed information on pulse oximetry.

4. Pain medications may be necessary to increase the force of coughing. However, some narcotic analgesics exacerbate respiratory depression, particularly in the older patient. The "Acute pain" care plan provides detailed information on assessing and managing this problem.

5. Additional individualized interventions: _____

5. Rationales: _____

> **Suggested NIC Interventions**
> *Airway management; Airway suctioning; Ventilation assistance; Respiratory monitoring; Vital signs monitoring*

> **Suggested NOC Outcomes**
> *Respiratory status: Airway patency; Respiratory status: Ventilation; Vital signs status*

Collaborative problem

Risk for bleeding related to extensive retroperitoneal dissection and vascular anastomosis

NURSING PRIORITY

Promptly detect signs and symptoms of bleeding.

PATIENT OUTCOME CRITERIA

Within 24 hours after surgery, the patient will:
- remain free from signs and symptoms of bleeding
- have a dry, intact dressing
- maintain stable vital signs, typically: heart rate, 60 to 100 beats/minute; systolic blood pressure, 90 to 140 mm Hg; and diastolic blood pressure, 50 to 90 mm Hg.

INTERVENTIONS

1. *Monitor and document intake and output and vital signs* every hour for 24 hours; *monitor and document CVP, PAWP,* and laboratory values according to protocol or physician's orders. *Measure abdominal girth every 2 hours* for 12 hours, then once every shift. Be alert for decreased urine output, tachycardia, hypotension, decreased CVP or PAWP, decreased hematocrit, increased girth, and back pain. Document and report abnormalities.

2. *Assess the dressings* when the patient is admitted to the unit and every hour for 8 hours, then every 4 hours. Be alert for an expanding pulsatile groin mass.

3. *Monitor and document the amount and character of nasogastric (NG) tube drainage* every 2 hours for 12 hours, then every 8 hours.

4. Additional individualized interventions: _____

RATIONALES

1. These signs may indicate intra-abdominal bleeding.

2. Frequent assessments allow for prompt detection of hemorrhage. An expanding pulsatile groin mass may indicate hemorrhage at the distal anastomosis of a bifurcated graft.

3. Bloody NG tube drainage may indicate intra-abdominal bleeding.

4. Rationales: _____

Collaborative problem

Risk for complications related to surgical procedure and atherosclerosis

NURSING PRIORITY

Promptly detect complications.

PATIENT OUTCOME CRITERIA

Within 24 to 48 hours after surgery, the patient will:
- have adequate perfusion to the upper and lower extremities, kidneys, bowel, and spinal cord, as evidenced by palpable 3 + pulses, urine output 60 ml/hour or more, normal-appearing bowel movements, spontaneous movement of extremities, and warm, dry skin
- have any complications immediately detected, reported, and treated as appropriate.
  Before discharge, the patient will:
- have clean, dry, and intact incision lines
- be afebrile, with a WBC count within normal limits.

INTERVENTIONS	RATIONALES

1. *Monitor for decreased peripheral tissue perfusion:* check peripheral pulses (upper and lower extremities) immediately upon admission and every hour for the first 12 hours, then every 4 hours until discharge.
 	
Document the location and character of the pulse using this scale:
  0 = absent
  1 = detectable by Doppler ultrasound stethoscope only
  2 = weakly palpable
  3 = strong.
Document evidence of capillary refill and signs of cyanosis and mottling. Notify the physician of changes.
	1. A decrease in peripheral tissue perfusion in the legs may result from graft thrombosis or distal embolization of atherosclerotic plaque. An arterial line may cause distal embolization as well as arterial dissection, arteriovenous fistula, false aneurysm, and hematoma formation. Accurate assessment of perfusion is crucial in the early postoperative period to detect early thrombosis formation and prevent limb loss.

2. *Monitor for signs and symptoms of acute renal failure.* Record hourly urine output until the indwelling urinary catheter is removed. Monitor BUN and creatinine levels as ordered. Be alert for a urine output of less than 30 ml/hour for 2 consecutive hours and elevated BUN and creatinine levels, and notify the physician if they occur.	2. Renal failure may result from atheromatous embolization to the renal arteries or prolonged cross-clamping of the aorta. A low urine output associated with elevated serum creatinine and BUN levels may indicate renal failure. (Creatinine clearance may be a better indicator of renal failure in the older patient.)
3. *Monitor for signs and symptoms of bowel ischemia,* including diarrhea (may be positive for occult bleeding), abdominal tenderness, fever, prolonged ileus, sepsis, shock, leukocytosis, and metabolic acidosis.	3. Approximately 2% of patients undergoing abdominal aortic aneurysm repair develop mesenteric artery ischemia, with a 50% mortality. This complication is related to low flow states, thrombosis, embolization, and fibrillatory cardiac disease. Signs and symptoms are most likely to occur in the first 48 hours after surgery.
4. *Monitor for signs and symptoms of spinal cord or cerebral ischemia.* Monitor sensory and motor function of the lower extremities as well as temperature, color, and pulses every hour for the first 24 hours. Assess the patient's level of consciousness (LOC) and orientation every hour for 12 hours, then every 4 hours.	4. The incidence of spinal cord ischemia after abdominal aortic aneurysm repair is quite low but warrants monitoring. Interruption of the arterial supply to the spinal cord may result from hypotension or embolus to the artery, causing lower extremity paraplegia. A decreased LOC or change in mental status may indicate cerebral ischemia.
5. *Monitor for intra-abdominal graft infection* by noting temperature elevations, leukocytosis, or prolonged ileus.	5. Unexplained fevers, leukocytosis, or prolonged ileus may indicate graft infection (a late complication).
6. *Monitor for local wound infection* by inspecting incision lines for erythema and edema, and observe the amount, color, and odor of any drainage every 4 hours and as needed until discharge. Document and notify the physician of any changes.	6. Regular assessments may provide early warning of local wound infection.
7. Additional individualized interventions: _____	7. Rationales: _____

Nursing diagnosis

Acute pain related to surgical tissue trauma or ischemia

NURSING PRIORITY
Relieve pain.

PATIENT OUTCOME CRITERIA
Within 1 hour of complaint of pain, the patient will:
- rate pain (with oral medication) as less than 3 on a 0 to 10 pain rating scale
- appear relaxed.

INTERVENTIONS	RATIONALES
1. *Assess patency and stability of the epidural catheter, if used.* Monitor effectiveness of epidural analgesia and watch for adverse reactions.	**1.** Epidural analgesia may be used to manage pain after abdominal aortic aneurysm repair.
2. *See the "Acute pain" care plan,* page 32.	**2.** The "Acute pain" care plan specifically addresses pain assessment and management.
3. Additional individualized interventions: _____	**3.** Rationales: _____

> ### Suggested NIC Interventions
> *Medication management; Pain management; Patient-controlled analgesia (PCA) assistance; Analgesic administration; Conscious sedation*

> ### Suggested NOC Outcomes
> *Comfort level; Pain control; Pain: Disruptive effects; Pain level*

Discharge planning

DISCHARGE CHECKLIST
Before discharge, the patient shows evidence of:
- ❏ stable vital signs
- ❏ normal body temperature
- ❏ absence of pulmonary and cardiovascular complications
- ❏ ability to tolerate oral intake
- ❏ ability to void and defecate same as before surgery
- ❏ healing wound free from signs of infection
- ❏ ability to ambulate according to progressive activity plan
- ❏ pain controlled with oral medication
- ❏ knowledge of activity and position restrictions
- ❏ adequate home support or referral to home health care or skilled care facility if indicated by lack of home support or by self-care limitations.

TEACHING CHECKLIST
Document evidence that the patient and family demonstrate an understanding of:
- ❏ progressive activity and ambulation plan
- ❏ incision care
- ❏ signs and symptoms of wound infection and graft thrombosis
- ❏ purpose, dosage, administration, and adverse effects of all discharge medications
- ❏ risk factors for atherosclerosis and how to reduce them
- ❏ available community resources
- ❏ date, time, and location of follow-up appointments.

DOCUMENTATION CHECKLIST
Using outcome criteria as a guide, document:
- ❏ clinical status on admission
- ❏ significant changes in status
- ❏ pertinent diagnostic test findings
- ❏ presence or absence of peripheral pulses
- ❏ pain-relief measures
- ❏ wound site appearance and amount, color, and consistency of any drainage
- ❏ activity tolerance and the patient's response to progressive ambulation
- ❏ patient and family teaching
- ❏ discharge planning.

Associated care plans

- Acute pain
- Knowledge deficit
- Mechanical ventilation
- Perioperative care

References

Berne, R.M., and Levy, M.N. *Cardiovascular Physiology,* 8th ed. St. Louis: Mosby–Year Book, Inc., 2001.

Edwards J.Z., and Weiner, S.D. "Chronic Back Pain Caused by an Abdominal Aortic Aneurysm: Case Report and Review of the Literature," *Orthopedics* 26(2):191-92, February 2003.

Frazier, M.S., and Drzymkowski, J.W. *Essentials of Human Diseases and Conditions,* 2nd ed. Philadelphia: W.B. Saunders Co., 2000.

Groer, M. *Advanced Pathophysiology: Application to Clinical Practice.* Philadelphia: Lippincott Williams & Wilkins, 2001.

Porth, C. *Pathophysiology: Concepts in Altered Health States,* 6th ed. Philadelphia: Lippincott Williams & Wilkins, 2002.

Acute myocardial infarction

DRG INFORMATION
DRG 121 Circulatory Disorders with Acute Myocardial Infarction (AMI) and Major Complications, Discharged Alive.
Mean LOS = 6.4 days
DRG 122 Circulatory Disorders with AMI, without Major Complications, Discharged Alive.
Mean LOS = 3.7 days
DRG 123 Circulatory Disorders with AMI, Expired.
Mean LOS = 4.6 days

Introduction
DEFINITION AND TIME FOCUS
AMI is the death of myocardial tissue, usually resulting from coronary artery occlusion or spasm. It may present as subendocardial infarction, involving the inner myocardial layer, or transmural infarction, involving the full thickness of the myocardium. Mortality depends on the extent and location of the infarct, the patient's preexisting health status, and the speed and effectiveness of therapy.

This care plan focuses on the critically ill patient admitted for diagnosis and management during an attack of severe crushing chest pain, the classic presentation in AMI. (See *Clinical snapshot: Acute myocardial infarction,* page 338.)

ETIOLOGY AND PRECIPITATING FACTORS
- Coronary artery disease, coronary artery spasm, hypotension, hypoxemia, severe bradycardia or tachycardia (especially with poor cardiac reserve), or other factors decreasing myocardial oxygen supply
- Exercise, emotional stress, exposure to extreme heat or cold, eating, tachycardia, or other factors increasing myocardial oxygen demand

Focused assessment guidelines
NURSING HISTORY
(FUNCTIONAL HEALTH PATTERN FINDINGS)
Health-perception–health-management pattern
- Sudden onset of severe chest pain — heavy, tight, crushing, or constricting quality; usually retrosternal; usually radiates to the left arm but may radiate to the right arm, back, epigastrium, jaw, or neck; lasts longer than 30 minutes; unrelieved by rest or nitroglycerin; however, AMI is painless in some instances

- Treatment for angina, atherosclerosis, hyperlipidemia, hypertension, heart failure, arrhythmias, stroke, peripheral vascular disease, or diabetes mellitus
- History of previous AMI, cardiac surgery, or oral contraceptive use
- Coronary artery disease risk factors, such as obesity or cigarette smoking
- Other high-risk categories (such as male over age 40 or postmenopausal female)

Nutritional-metabolic pattern
- Indigestion, nausea, or vomiting
- Diet high in calories, fat, and salt (common)

Elimination pattern
- Feeling of fullness or bowel movement coinciding with onset of chest pain

Activity-exercise pattern
- Shortness of breath
- Sporadic exercise or sedentary lifestyle (common)

Sleep-rest pattern
- Sleep disturbances

Cognitive-perceptual pattern
- History of recurrent chest pain

Self-perception–self-concept pattern
- Great concern about ability to return to work as soon as possible

Role-relationship pattern
- Description of self as someone upon whom others depend
- Family history of death from AMI (especially before age 50)

Coping–stress tolerance pattern
- Anxiety, tension, type A personality (aggressive, competitive, impatient)
- Fear of death or of the unknown

Value-belief pattern
- Delayed pursuit of medical attention or expressed disbelief over condition (denial)

PHYSICAL FINDINGS
Cardiovascular
- Hypotension or hypertension
- Tachycardia or, uncommonly, bradycardia
- Other arrhythmias
- S_3 or S_4
- Slowed capillary refill time (in shock)

Pulmonary
- Crackles (if heart failure present)

Gastrointestinal
- Vomiting
- Abdominal distention

Neurologic
- Restlessness
- Irritability
- Confusion

Integumentary
- Diaphoresis
- Cool, clammy skin
- Variable skin color (may be normal, pale, ashen, or cyanotic)

Musculoskeletal
- Pained or anxious facial expression
- Tense posture

DIAGNOSTIC STUDIES

Initial laboratory data may reflect no significant abnormalities; subsequent tests may reveal the following:
- Cardiac isoenzymes — show characteristic trends, particularly elevated CK-MB
- Positive troponin I or increased myoglobin levels or both
- Arterial blood gas (ABG) levels — may reveal hypoxemia and acid-base abnormalities
- Electrolyte panel — used to rule out disturbances affecting cardiac conduction and contractility (such as hypokalemia, hyperkalemia, hypocalcemia, hypercalcemia, or hypomagnesemia)
- White blood cell count and sedimentation rate — usually rise on 2nd day because of inflammatory response
- Blood urea nitrogen levels and creatinine clearance — may rise, indicating diminished renal perfusion
- Serum cholesterol and triglyceride levels — may be elevated, indicating increased risk of atherosclerosis
- Serum drug levels — may indicate subtherapeutic or toxic levels of antiarrhythmic agents such as cardiac glycosides
- 12-lead electrocardiography (ECG) — with transmural infarction, elevated ST segment and upright T waves in hyperacute phase, progressing to deeply inverted T waves and pathologic Q waves in leads overlooking the infarcted area; with subendocardial infarction, depressed ST segment and inverted T waves
- Chest X-ray — may show cardiac enlargement produced by heart failure
- Myocardial imaging (radionuclide) studies — demonstrate areas of poor or absent perfusion, wall motion abnormalities, and reduced ejection fraction
- Echocardiography — may illustrate structural or functional cardiac abnormalities

POTENTIAL COMPLICATIONS
- Arrhythmias
- Sudden death
- Cardiogenic shock
- Heart failure
- Pulmonary edema
- Papillary muscle dysfunction or rupture
- Ventricular rupture
- Pericarditis
- Pulmonary embolism
- Ventricular aneurysm
- Cardiac tamponade

(See *Clinical pathway: Acute myocardial infarction*, pages 340 to 342.)

CLINICAL SNAPSHOT ☀

Acute myocardial infarction

Major nursing diagnoses and collaborative problems	Key patient outcomes
CP: Risk for cardiogenic shock	Maintain vital signs within normal limits, typically: heart rate, 60 to 100 beats/minute; systolic blood pressure, 90 to 140 mm Hg; diastolic blood pressure, 50 to 90 mm Hg.
ND: Impaired gas exchange	Maintain $Pao_2 > 80$ mm Hg; maintain Sao_2 on pulse oximetry $> 90\%$.
ND: Acute pain (chest)	Rate pain as 0 on a 0 to 10 pain rating scale.
ND: Ineffective coping	Verbalize feelings appropriate to initial stage of coping.
ND: Risk for constipation	Resume a regular bowel elimination pattern.
ND: Risk for injury	Show no signs of complications.
ND: Deficient knowledge	Begin to identify long-range learning needs.

Collaborative problem

Risk for cardiogenic shock related to arrhythmias, impaired contractility, or thrombosis

NURSING PRIORITY

Optimize cardiac output and cellular perfusion.

PATIENT OUTCOME CRITERIA

Within 24 hours of admission, the patient will:
- maintain vital signs within normal limits, typically: heart rate, 60 to 100 beats/minute; systolic blood pressure, 90 to 140 mm Hg; and diastolic blood pressure, 50 to 90 mm Hg
- show normal skin color
- have a capillary refill time less than 3 seconds.
  Within 3 days of admission, the patient will:
- experience no life-threatening arrhythmias

INTERVENTIONS	RATIONALES
1. *Institute and document continuous ECG monitoring** on admission, with alarms on at all times. Preferably, monitor lead MCL_1 or MCL_6. See "Risk for injury," page 347, for details about specific arrhythmias.	**1.** Arrhythmias are the primary cause of death in the first 24 hours after infarction. MCL_1 and MCL_6 best differentiate supraventricular aberration from ventricular ectopy.
2. *Record and analyze rhythm strips,* following unit protocol and as needed for significant variations. Mount strips in chart.	**2.** Systematic analysis may warn of impending problems with impulse initiation or conduction.
3. *Obtain serial 12-lead ECGs* on admission, daily, and as needed for chest pain. If percutaneous transluminal coronary angioplasty (PTCA) or other interventions are done, obtain ECG postprocedure.	**3.** The ECG obtained on admission provides a baseline for infarct localization. Serial ECGs monitor changes. Revascularization can promote resolution of ECG changes.
4. *Evaluate and document clinical status* every hour or as needed, including level of consciousness (LOC), pulse, blood pressure, heart sounds, breath sounds, urine output, skin color and temperature, and capillary refill time.	**4.** LOC is a sensitive indicator of cerebral ischemia. Pulse rate may indicate fluid deficit, pulse rhythm may indicate ectopic beats, and pulse volume may indicate fluid deficit or overload. A systolic blood pressure reading more than 20 mm Hg below the patient's normal value or a systolic blood pressure of 80 mm Hg or less indicates shock. Abnormal heart sounds indicate various problems: S_3 or S_4 indicate heart failure, murmurs indicate incompetent or stenotic valves, and pericardial friction rub indicates pericarditis. Abnormal breath sounds (particularly crackles that don't clear with coughing) suggest heart failure. A urine output of less than 60 ml/hour suggests decreased renal perfusion. Pale, cyanotic, mottled, or cool skin indicates decreased peripheral perfusion, as does a capillary refill time greater than 3 seconds.
5. *Establish and maintain a patent I.V. line* on admission. Document cumulative fluid intake and output hourly.	**5.** An I.V. line is necessary for emergency fluid and drug administration. Intake and output records provide clues to developing fluid imbalances.
6. *Administer aspirin as ordered.*	**6.** Aspirin is commonly used to decrease platelet aggregation.

(Text continues on page 342.)

*Italics indicate key interventions.

Acute myocardial infarction

Plan	Day 1 (ED, Cath Lab, ICU/Interventional Unit)	Day 2
Assessments	• History and physical examination • Nursing admission assessment • Systems reassessment every shift and p.r.n	• 24-hour summary and progress note • Systems assessment every shift and p.r.n. • Plan for cardiac catheterization if not already done
Consultations	• Cardiology • Cardiology interventionalist • Social service	• Social service or case management • Cardiac rehabilitation if postintervention
Diagnostics	• CK with ISO q 8 hours until peak • Troponin I • PTT, PT • Chemistry studies including magnesium • CBC • ECG daily and p.r.n. with pain • Echocardiogram day 1 or 2	• PTT if on heparin drip • CBC, PT if warfarin (Coumadin) is indicated • Lipid profile (fasting) • Chemistry studies • Magnesium • ECG and p.r.n. if pain or arrhythmia • Echocardiogram (if not obtained day 1)
Interventions	• Continuous ECG monitoring • VS monitoring q 2 hours and p.r.n. • Pulse oximetry continuous or every 2 hours with VS • Rhythm strip q shift and p.r.n. • I&O • Chest pain protocol • Guaiac stools if on anticoagulation • I.V. site care • No I.M. injections • May need emergency cardiac catheterization based on clinical assessment, CK with ISO and troponin levels, and ECG changes • Refer to PTCA section, page 432	• Continuous ECG monitoring • VS q 4 hours and p.r.n. • Pulse oximetry q 4 hours and p.r.n. • Rhythm strip q shift and p.r.n. • I&O • Chest pain protocol • Guaiac stool if on anticoagulation • I.V. site care • If postcatheterization: follow PTCA care plan protocol with site checks for hematoma and bleeding along with vascular checks for pulse quality, extremity temperature, and color.
Medications and I.V.s	As indicated: • NTG infusion • Heparin infusion • Aspirin, antiarrhythmics • IIB, IIIA inhibitors • Beta-adrenergic blockers, calcium channel blockers • ACE inhibitors • Analgesics and sleeping aids • Stool softeners • O_2 • p.r.n. medications: antiemetics, sedatives, antacids	If post-PTCA with interventions (as prescribed by physician): • Aspirin, antiarrhythmics • IIB, IIIA inhibitors • Cardiac medications • Analgesics PRN medications: • Sleep aids • Stool softeners • Sedatives • Antacids If no PTCA, may continue: • NTG drip • Heparin infusion plus above medications
Diet	• NPO if catheterization required • No catheterization ➤ low-fat, low-salt diet • ADA diet	• Low-fat, low-cholesterol diet • ADA diet • May be NPO for cardiac catheterization
Activity	• Bed rest with bathroom or commode privileges as tolerated • If pain free, OOB to chair b.i.d.	• OOB to chair as needed or as necessary • Ambulating in room and hall • Assistance with grooming needs
Teaching and discharge planning	• Procedural information as needed • Pain rating scale	• If PTCA done, initiation of postteaching site care, activity, lifting precautions • If no PTCA, cardiac teaching • Risk factor modification • Home assessment, if necessary • Continued cardiac teaching, including diet, activity, and medications
Key indicators	• Chest pain? Y_ N_ • Chest pain protocol effective in resolving chest pain? Y_ N_ • $Sao_2 > 90\%$ without O_2? Y_ N_ • Does patient have symptomatic arrhythmia? Y_ N_ • Is patient hemodynamically stable? Y_ N_ • Is patient OOB at least t.i.d. for meals? Y_ N_ • Is patient weaned off I.V. infusions? Y_ N_	• Does the patient have chest pain? Y_ N_ • Was the chest pain protocol effective in resolving chest pain? Y_ N_ • $Sao_2 > 90\%$ without O_2? Y_ N_ • Does patient have symptomatic arrhythmia? Y_ N_ • Is patient hemodynamically stable? Y_ N_ • Is patient OOB for 1 hour t.i.d.? Y_ N_ • Did patient comply with postcatheter interventions and instructions? Y_ N_ • Is groin site free from hematoma, ecchymosis, and infection? Y_ N_ • Are distal pulses present in affected extremity? Y_ N_

Day 3

- 24-hour summary and progress note
- Systems assessment every shift and p.r.n.
- Discharge potential assessment and discharge plan on Day 4

- Cardiac rehabilitation
- Dietary, if needed
- Continued social service, if needed

- CBC
- Repeating chemistry studies if abnormal laboratory values corrected
- PT if Coumadin therapy indicated
- ECG with pain of onset of arrhythmia

- Continuous ECG monitoring
- VS q 4 hours and p.r.n.
- Pulse oximetry q shift, if normal
- Rhythm strip q shift and p.r.n.
- I&O
- Chest pain protocol
- Guaiac stool if on anticoagulation
- I.V. site care
- Postcatheterization site care and assessment for hematoma or ecchymosis q 4 hours
- Vascular check of accessed extremity q 4 hours

As indicated and prescribed by physician:
- Aspirin
- Antiarrhythmics
- IIB, IIIA Inhibitor
- Beta-adrenergic blockers
- ACE inhibitors
- Calcium channel blockers
  PRN medications as previously listed:
- I.V. nitrates should be weaned or changed to oral, patch, or paste
- Heparin drip possibly continuing with introduction of Coumadin as indicated

- Continued ordered diet

- Ambulating independently
- Self-grooming

- Continuing post-PTCA and intervention teaching
- Identifying modifiable risk factors, and providing information for successful adaptation
- Continuing medication teaching
- Planning for any durable medical products such as home O_2

- Can patient perform ADLs independently? Y_ N_
- Can patient ambulate in hallway independently? Y_ N_
- Did patient comply with postcatheter or intervention instructions and activity restrictions? Y_ N_
- Is site free from signs and symptoms of hematoma, hemorrhage, infection? Y_ N_
- Are distal pulses present in affected extremity? Y_ N_
- Urine output > 600 ml per shift? Y_ N_
- Postintervention only:
  – Does the patient have chest pain? Y_ N_
  – Was chest pain protocol effective in resolving chest pain? Y_ N_
  – Is patient without significant ECG changes after procedure? Y_ N_
  – Was bleeding noted from puncture sites or other source? Y_ N_ Note source _____

(continued)

Acute myocardial infarction *(continued)*

Plan	Day 4
Assessments	● 24-hour summary, progress and discharge plan ● Discharge plan to include: – Medications and prescriptions as indicated – Activity - Return to work, if applicable - Exercise-schedule with cardiac rehabilitation - Sexual activity - Driving ● Follow-up appointments ● Risk factor modification: – Diabetic teaching or reinforcement – Smoking cessation – Weight reduction – Alcohol consumption
Consultations	● As previously mentioned
Diagnostics	● Discharge ECG, PT if on Coumadin
Interventions	● D/C cardiac monitoring upon discharge ● VS q shift ● Rhythm strip prior to removal of monitoring ● D/C I.V. upon discharge order ● Catheterization site assessment q shift or prior to discharge ● Vascular check of accessed extremity q shift or prior to discharge
Medications and I.V.s	● As previously indicated and as prescribed by physician: – Aspirin, IIB, IIIA, cardiac medications, Coumadin, stool softeners
Diet	As ordered
Activity	● Ambulation as necessary ● Self-grooming
Teaching and discharge planning	● Reference to physician's discharge plan ● Reviewing medications – Include dose, time of administration, action, adverse effects, and monitoring of laboratory values, such as PT and Coumadin ● Reviewing activities and limitations ● Reviewing appointment schedule ● Identifying modifiable risk factors and supportive solutions
Key indicators	● Is patient hemodynamically stable per standards? Y_ N_ ● Is patient free from chest pain, heart failure, ischemia, or significant arrhythmia? Y_ N_ ● Can patient perform ADLs? Y_ N_ ● Can patient demonstrate knowledge of discharge instructions? Y_ N_

7. *Administer heparin as ordered.*

7. Heparin commonly is ordered prophylactically to minimize the risk of thromboembolism from arrhythmias or immobility. It may also be used to limit extension of a thrombus that produced an AMI.

8. *Prepare the patient for aggressive treatment measures as ordered,* which may include:
– emergency coronary arteriography

– PTCA intracoronary stenting and atherectomy

– thrombolytic therapy with alteplase (Activase); usually used in facilities that don't have cardiac catheterization laboratories

8. Infarctions that are impending, in progress, or complicated may require immediate aggressive interventions.
– Coronary arteriography is the most accurate way to determine the extent of coronary artery disease.
– PTCA, intracoronary stenting, and atherectomy may increase coronary artery blood flow by compressing occluding lesions and dilating the vessel lumen. The resulting increase in luminal cross-sectional area improves blood flow to ischemic tissue.
– Thrombolytic therapy may be administered to lyse fresh clots, thus relieving the occlusion and reestablishing perfusion to the damaged area.

– coronary artery bypass grafting.

9. Additional individualized interventions: _____
_____

– Emergency surgery may be necessary to bypass life-threatening lesions.

9. Rationales: _____
_____

Nursing diagnosis

Impaired gas exchange related to ventilation-perfusion imbalance

NURSING PRIORITIES
- Optimize myocardial oxygen demand-supply ratio.
- Minimize the risk of further infarction.

PATIENT OUTCOME CRITERIA

Within 24 hours of admission, the patient will:
- show no dyspnea
- maintain partial pressure of arterial oxygen greater than 80 mm Hg
- maintain arterial oxygen saturation (Sao_2) greater than 90% on pulse oximetry
- display normal sinus rhythm or controlled arrhythmias
- have normal skin color
- rest comfortably.

INTERVENTIONS	RATIONALES
1. *Observe for signs of hypoxemia,* such as tachycardia, restlessness, irritability, or tachypnea. Monitor Sao_2 by pulse oximetry and ABG values as ordered.	**1.** Cellular hypoxia commonly results from impaired coronary artery perfusion, decreased systemic perfusion, and respiratory depressant effects of analgesics and sedatives. Sao_2 and ABG values provide objective evidence of the degree of hypoxemia. Prompt treatment minimizes ischemic damage.
2. *Administer and document oxygen therapy* on admission, according to medical protocol and nursing judgment — typically 2 to 5 L/minute by nasal cannula for the first 24 to 48 hours.	**2.** Supplemental oxygen will elevate arterial oxygen content and may relieve myocardial ischemia.
3. *If blood pressure is stable within normal limits, place the patient in semi-Fowler's position.*	**3.** The semi-upright position facilitates breathing.
4. *During the period of acute instability, place the patient on bed rest or chair rest.* Once stabilized, increase activity as tolerated. See "Activity intolerance," page 389, in the "Cardiogenic shock" care plan.	**4.** Rest reduces myocardial oxygen demands. Controlling oxygen demands helps limit infarct extension. Gradual resumption of activity helps promote a sense of well-being. "Activity intolerance" contains detailed information on assessing activity tolerance and promoting safe resumption of physical activity.
5. *Provide adequate rest periods.* Set priorities for care and group procedures.	**5.** Sleep deprivation, common in the critical care setting, can lead to increased irritability, confusion, increased sensitivity to pain, and other problems.
6. Additional individualized interventions: _____ _____	**6.** Rationales: _____ _____

Nursing diagnosis

Acute pain (chest) related to myocardial ischemia

NURSING PRIORITY

Relieve chest pain.

PATIENT OUTCOME CRITERIA

Within 1 to 2 hours of admission, the patient will:
- rate pain as 0 on a 0 to 10 pain rating scale
- display no associated signs and symptoms of pain
- assume a relaxed posture
- have a relaxed facial expression.

INTERVENTIONS

1. *Teach the patient to report immediately any unusual chest sensation,* such as chest pain, tightness, heaviness, or burning.

2. *Monitor continually for indications of chest pain,* such as complaints of discomfort, sternal rubbing, tense posture, emotional withdrawal, facial grimacing, shortness of breath, diaphoresis, or restlessness.

3. *Document pain episodes:* Analyze pain characteristics (including value on pain rating scale), record a monitor rhythm strip, and obtain a 12-lead ECG.

4. *Administer medication promptly at the onset of pain* and document its use, according to medical protocol or orders. Administer oxygen when pain occurs. Evaluate and document blood pressure, pulse, and respirations before and after administration. Assess pain relief after 30 minutes. (See *Medication therapy after AMI.*)

5. *During the initial period of cardiovascular instability, titrate I.V. medications as ordered:* morphine — give typically in 2- to 5-mg doses, according to the level of pain and vital signs. Withhold morphine and contact the physician if the respiratory rate is less than 12 breaths/minute or the systolic blood pressure is less than 90 mm Hg (for a previously normotensive patient), or more than 20 mm Hg below the baseline value (for a previously hypertensive patient). If blood pressure decreases, notify the physician.

RATIONALES

1. Symptoms other than obvious pain may indicate ischemia. Awareness of more subtle symptoms suggesting ischemia promotes early intervention.

2. The patient may not report pain, but astute observation may detect associated signs and symptoms and allow for early intervention. Shortness of breath and diaphoresis may result from sympathetic stimulation; restlessness may reflect cerebral ischemia.

3. Careful analysis of characteristics allows for differential diagnosis of pain. The rhythm strip can document new arrhythmias and the 12-lead ECG can document infarct extension.

4. Pain medication is more effective when given before severe pain develops. Pain may stimulate the sympathetic nervous system and increase myocardial workload. Supplemental oxygen may relieve pain and plays a role in reducing infarct size. Vital sign measurements before medication administration provide objective indicators of the degree of physiologic stress imposed by pain; those taken afterward indicate relief of such stress.

5. I.V. medications titrated to relieve signs and symptoms act more rapidly and reliably than by the I.M. route because poorly perfused muscles absorb medication erratically. I.M. injections also elevate creatine kinase levels, obscuring their diagnostic value. Morphine is the drug of choice for pain associated with AMI because it's a potent analgesic and causes peripheral vasodilation (lessening venous return and myocardial workload) and euphoria. The vital sign parameters listed indicate respiratory depression and excessive vasodilation, both possible adverse reactions to morphine.

Medication therapy after AMI

Drug	Action	Administration	Patient teaching	Possible adverse reactions
Vasodilator (such as nitroglycerin or long-acting nitrates)	Primarily dilates peripheral blood vessels, reducing myocardial workload	Can be given by mouth before meals; sublingual: one tablet every 5 minutes up to a maximum of three tablets; if no relief, call physician; dermal: patch or cream	Take prophylactically before activities as prescribed or at onset of chest pain. Take sitting or lying down to prevent orthostatic hypotension. If no relief after three tablets, don't drive yourself to hospital: Call an ambulance. Record number of tablets taken. Check expiration date. Carry nitroglycerin at all times. Wear medical alert bracelet. Avoid alcohol, which has additive vasodilating effects. Replace tablets at 4 months. If ointment or patch is prescribed, follow guidelines for correct application, skin care, site rotation, and frequency of change.	Transient headache, flushing, faintness, dizziness, or hypotension
Beta-adrenergic blocker (such as atenolol [Tenormin], metoprolol [Lopressor], or propranolol [Inderal])	Blocks beta-adrenergic receptors to decrease blood pressure, heart rate, and contractility; also decreases automaticity to slow sinus rate, suppress ectopic beats, and improve myocardial oxygenation	Initially given I.V., then by mouth	Monitor pulse rate and blood pressure; report rate under 60 beats/minute and irregular or changed pulse rate. Don't stop drug abruptly — may cause chest pain or myocardial infarction.	Bradycardia, hypotension, dizziness, nausea, vomiting, diarrhea, bronchoconstriction, or impotence
Calcium channel blocker (such as diltiazem [Cardizem], nifedipine [Procardia], verapamil [Calan])	Blocks transport of calcium across cell membrane, resulting in vasodilation and decreased contractility; verapamil also increases refractory period of atrioventricular node and decreases sinoatrial node rate	By mouth, 1 hour before meals or 2 hours after meals	Monitor pulse rate and blood pressure; report pulse rate under 50 beats/minute.	Orthostatic hypotension, bradycardia, headache, dizziness, syncope, nausea, edema, or constipation
Aspirin	Antiplatelet action; decreases aggregation	By mouth daily, or every other day, usually with food	Report ongoing GI upset or burning, dark tarlike stool, or easy bruising or bleeding; avoid aspirin and OTC aspirin-containing products.	GI upset and irritation; GI bleeding; increased bruising
GPIIb/IIIa receptors Tirofiban hydrochloride injection (Aggrastat) Eptifibatide injection (Integrilin) Abciximab (ReoPro) Clopidogrel (Plavix)	Inhibits platelet function by its ability to inhibit adenosine phosphate (ADP) induced platelet aggregation and prolonged bleeding time in patients with coronary artery disease	Aggrastat, Integrilin, and ReoPro are weight-based. I.V. bolus followed by infusion with time determined by physician; used in preparation for cardiac catheterization; Plavix is a 300-mg loading dose poststent placement; followed by a maintenance dose of 75 mg orally daily for 1 month	Monitor for signs of bleeding and bruising, such as bleeding gums when brushing teeth, hematuria, black stools. If undergoing elective surgery or procedures. Inform physician so Plavix can be stopped 7 days prior to procedure or physician preference.	Decrease platelet count Bleeding

– Nitroglycerine — titrate (3 to 100 mcg/minute) until patient is free from chest pain. Monitor for hypotension (blood pressure as with morphine or symptomatic). Monitor for headache, and medicate to relieve it as needed.
– Weight-based heparin infusion

– I.V. beta-adrenergic blockers

– Nitrates decrease myocardial oxygen demands by causing vasodilatation, which reduces preload and afterload and thus decreases cardiac workload and oxygen consumption.

– Administering heparin can reduce platelet aggregation at the site of an unstable atherosclerotic plaque.
– Beta-adrenergic blockers reduce the cardiac workload by reducing oxygen demand through decreasing heart rate and blood pressure.

6. *Remain with the patient until pain is relieved.*

6. The presence of a competent, confident caregiver may reassure the patient, relieving anxiety and thus lessening sympathetic stimulation.

7. Position the patient comfortably. *Use noninvasive pain-relief measures* as appropriate. See the "Acute pain" care plan, page 32, for details.

7. Comfortable positioning and noninvasive pain-relief measures, such as rhythmic breathing, distraction, and relaxation, may reduce the perception of pain and promote endorphin release. The "Acute pain" care plan discusses numerous alternative pain-relief strategies.

8. Additional individualized interventions: _____

8. Rationales: _____

Suggested NIC Interventions
Medication management; Pain management; Analgesic administration

Suggested NOC Outcomes
Comfort level; Pain control; Pain: Disruptive effects; Pain level

---

Nursing diagnosis

Ineffective coping related to fear of death, anxiety, denial, or depression

NURSING PRIORITY
Promote healthy coping.

PATIENT OUTCOME CRITERIA
Within 24 hours, the patient will:
- display feelings appropriate to initial stage of coping.
  Within 24 to 48 hours, the patient will:
- display the first signs of effective coping.

INTERVENTIONS

1. Implement measures in the "Ineffective individual coping" care plan, page 124, as appropriate.

2. Administer tranquilizers, as ordered, typically a benzodiazepine, such as alprazolam (Xanax), diazepam (Valium), or lorazepam (Ativan).

3. Additional individualized interventions: _____

RATIONALES

1. AMI is a major threat to psychological equilibrium and may provoke various protective responses. The "Ineffective individual coping" care plan contains comprehensive information on evaluating and promoting healthy responses.

2. Minor tranquilizers may be used to keep anxiety at a tolerable level and avoid the harmful physiologic effects of anxiety-triggered catecholamine release.

3. Rationales: _____

> **Suggested NIC Interventions**
> *Coping enhancement; Family involvement promotion*

> **Suggested NOC Outcomes**
> *Coping; Social support*

Nursing diagnosis
Risk for constipation related to diet, bed rest, immobility, or medications

NURSING PRIORITY
Prevent or minimize constipation.

PATIENT OUTCOME CRITERIA
Within 3 days, the patient will:
- resume a regular bowel elimination pattern
- experience no straining during defecation
- have soft stool.

INTERVENTIONS

1. Encourage the patient to follow the prescribed diet, which is usually low in calories, salt, and fat. Limit intake of caffeine. Document intake, likes, and dislikes.

2. Allow for bathroom privileges only if the patient's condition permits. If the patient's condition is questionable, have him use a bedside commode. Provide adequate toiletries (such as toilet paper, room deodorizer, and hand soap and towels.)

3. Administer stool softeners as ordered, and document their use. Use alternatives and supplements to stool softeners, such as increased dietary fiber and prune juice. Encourage increased fluid intake, if appropriate to medical status. Give laxatives as necessary.

4. Additional individualized interventions: _____
_____

RATIONALES

1. Dietary prescriptions vary with the patient's needs. Caffeine is avoided because it's a cardiac stimulant. The patient is more likely to adhere to a diet plan that respects personal food preferences.

2. Use of a bathroom allows for privacy and a more natural means of elimination. When necessary, a bedside commode requires less energy to use than does a bedpan, so elimination can be achieved without excessive myocardial oxygen demand.

3. Straining to defecate produces Valsalva's maneuver, which can cause bradycardia and decrease cardiac output. Rebound tachycardia and myocardial ischemia may follow. Dependence on laxatives diminishes the urge for spontaneous defecation.

4. Rationales: _____
_____

> **Suggested NIC Interventions**
> *Bowel management; Fluid and electrolyte management; Constipation and impaction management*

> **Suggested NOC Outcomes**
> *Bowel elimination; Hydration; Symptom control*

Nursing diagnosis
Risk for injury related to myocardial ischemia, injury, necrosis, inflammation, or arrhythmias

NURSING PRIORITY
Monitor for complications.

PATIENT OUTCOME CRITERIA
Within 24 hours of admission, the patient will:
- display normal sinus rhythm or a controlled arrhythmia with a ventricular rate of 60 to 100 beats/minute
- manifest strong, bilaterally equal peripheral pulses

- show no signs of complications.
  Within 3 days of admission, the patient will:
- have normal blood pressure for his condition
- have nonlabored respirations
- have clear breath sounds
- have clear heart sounds with decreasing or no S_3 or S_4, rub, or new murmurs
- experience no further chest pain
- show decreasing or no neck vein distention.

INTERVENTIONS	RATIONALES
1. *Monitor constantly for general complications of AMI:*	**1.** Several complications can impair recovery from AMI. Many occur with any type of infarct and are associated less with the infarct's location than with the extent of myocardial damage and degree of the underlying coronary artery disease. Other complications have a pathophysiologic correlation with a specific type of infarct.
Arrhythmias – *Observe constantly for ventricular arrhythmias:* ventricular premature beats, accelerated ventricular rhythm, ventricular tachycardia, and ventricular fibrillation.	– Ventricular arrhythmias are the most common complication of AMI. In the first few hours after infarction, they probably result from an ischemia-induced reentry mechanism, whereas later arrhythmias probably result from increased automaticity.
– *Observe constantly for supraventricular arrhythmias:* premature atrial or junctional beats; atrial tachycardia, flutter, or fibrillation; or supraventricular tachycardia.	– Supraventricular arrhythmias may result from ischemia, heart failure, catecholamine stimulation, and other factors. Although less serious than ventricular arrhythmias, they may contribute to an unstable physiologic status or to thromboembolism. Tachycardias increase myocardial oxygen demand, reduce left ventricular filling time, and reduce coronary artery perfusion time. The loss of atrial "kick" (normally coordinated atrial contraction) also may reduce cardiac output.
– *Administer and document antiarrhythmic agents as ordered.* Monitor effectiveness and adverse effects. Typical agents include:	– Arrhythmias may impair cardiac output or progress to cardiac arrest. Antiarrhythmic agents are classified according to their electrophysiologic properties.
- class IA agents, such as disopyramide (Norpace), procainamide (Pronestyl), and quinidine (Quinora)	- Class IA drugs, used for both atrial and ventricular arrhythmias (particularly reentrant ones), decrease automaticity, conduction, and repolarization.
- class IB agents, such as lidocaine (Xylocaine), ordered prophylactically or as needed for warning ventricular premature beats (more than 6 beats/minute, sequential, multifocal, or close to the preceding T wave), ventricular tachycardia, or ventricular fibrillation	- Class IB agents, used to prevent and treat ventricular arrhythmias, inhibit ventricular automaticity. Lidocaine also increases the threshold for fibrillation. Prophylactic lidocaine may be ordered because of AMI's high incidence of ventricular fibrillation, which commonly occurs without warning.
- class II agents, such as atenolol (Tenormin), metoprolol (Lopressor), and propranolol (Inderal)	- Class II agents, beta-adrenergic blockers, are used to control supraventricular arrhythmias. Their complex mechanisms include suppressing sinus node automaticity and decreasing atrioventricular (AV) conduction.
- class III agents, such as amiodarone (Cordarone) and bretylium (Bretylol)	- Bretylium suppresses reentrant ventricular arrhythmias and elevates the threshold for ventricular fibrillation. Amiodarone increases the refractory period and is useful in life-threatening ventricular tachyarrhythmias.
- class IV agents, such as diltiazem (Cardizem), nifedipine (Procardia), and verapamil (Calan).	- Class IV drugs, calcium channel blockers, inhibit sinoatrial (SA) and AV automaticity and prolong AV conduction. They're particularly useful in treating supraventricular tachycardias.

– Implement and document emergency measures as needed, based on medical protocol and nursing judgment.

Heart failure and cardiogenic shock
– Implement measures in the "Cardiogenic shock" care plan, page 382, and *"Heart failure" care plan,* page 411.

Infarct extension
– Monitor for new, increased, or persistent chest pain. Obtain a 12-lead ECG reading and administer oxygen and pain medication as ordered. Notify the physician about the pain and any new indicators of infarction on the ECG reading.

Pericarditis
– Observe for pericardial chest pain, typically stabbing, localized pain that worsens on deep inspiration and with movement. Also monitor for fever, tachycardia, and pericardial friction rub.
– Administer anti-inflammatory agents as ordered, typically aspirin, corticosteroids, or non-steroidal anti-inflammatory agents.
– Monitor for indicators of pericardial effusion: weak peripheral pulses, paradoxical pulse greater than 10 mm Hg, or a decreased LOC. If present, notify the physician promptly.

– Monitor for indicators of cardiac tamponade, including Beck's triad (elevated central venous pressure [CVP], profound hypotension, and distant heart sounds), neck vein distention, tachycardia, decreased pulse pressure, paradoxical pulse, and pericardial friction rub. If you observe these signs, summon immediate medical assistance and prepare for emergency pericardial aspiration.

Ventricular aneurysm
– Observe for indications of a ventricular aneurysm, which include signs and symptoms of heart failure, thromboembolism, and persistent ectopy. Alert the physician.

– Protocols usually allow for emergency treatment of warning and lethal arrhythmias (ventricular premature beats, tachycardia, fibrillation, asystole; symptomatic sinus bradycardia; and Mobitz II second- and third-degree AV blocks).

– Varying degrees of myocardial failure, such as heart failure or cardiogenic shock, are common during the first week after the infarction. Several factors place the AMI patient at risk for myocardial failure, including myocardial ischemia, hypoxemia, acidosis, hypotension, and paradoxical movement of the injured myocardial wall.

– Infarct extension may result from progressive ischemia of the myocardium secondary to swelling of damaged cells and inflammatory responses that compress surrounding tissue. Other factors that may cause extension of the infarct include hypoxemia and microemboli.

– Pericardial sac inflammation is a relatively benign complication. Focal pericarditis usually develops within 5 days; generalized pericarditis (Dressler's syndrome) typically develops within 14 days.
– Anti-inflammatory agents reduce inflammation, relieving signs and symptoms and reducing the risk of pericardial effusion.
– In pericardial effusion, fluid leaks across the walls of inflamed cells. The degree of leakage may vary from mild to major. Left untreated, an effusion may produce a cardiac tamponade large enough to induce cardiac arrest.
– Cardiac tamponade is a medical emergency. Because it impinges on ventricular expansion, it severely limits ventricular filling and therefore cardiac output. Immediate removal of the pericardial fluid permits ventricular filling and prevents cardiac arrest.

– Ventricular aneurysm is thought to occur in about 10% of AMI patients. Dilation most commonly occurs in the anterolateral area, although it may also occur in the posterior or septal walls or the apical area. The systolic outward bulging of the area weakened by the infarction decreases stroke volume. In addition, clots may occur in the dilated area and embolize to other organs. Aneurysmectomy removes the bulging, weakened area and prevents potentially fatal myocardial rupture.

Rupture

– *Monitor for signs and symptoms of papillary muscle rupture* — sudden shock, a loud holosystolic murmur radiating from the apex to the left axilla, and signs of severe left-sided heart failure. If these signs and symptoms occur, call for immediate medical assistance. Assist with treatment of cardiogenic shock or prepare the patient for surgery as ordered.

– *Observe for signs and symptoms of potential septal rupture* — severe chest pain, severe heart failure, a loud holosystolic murmur at the apex and lower left sternal border, or sudden cardiac death. If they occur, initiate cardiopulmonary resuscitation (CPR), if necessary, and call for immediate medical assistance. Implement measures to treat cardiogenic shock or prepare the patient for surgery as ordered.

– *Be alert for signs and symptoms of an impending myocardial rupture,* especially in a patient with a transmural infarction who is on anticoagulant therapy — persistent chest pain without ECG changes, persistent hypertension after the infarction, M-shaped QRS complexes, or pericardial blood or fluid detected by an echocardiogram. Notify the physician of such signs and symptoms immediately. Assist with emergency pericardiocentesis and treatment of cardiogenic shock as ordered.

2. *Monitor constantly for complications of particular types of AMI as appropriate:*

Anterior, anteroseptal, or anterolateral infarct

– *Monitor for signs or symptoms of potential bundle-branch block.* Constantly monitor QRS complex width and the pattern of deflections in V_1 and V_6 (or MCL_1 and MCL_6). On serial ECGs, note axis deviation.

– Document and alert the physician to the presence of any of the following:
  - Right bundle-branch block (RBBB): QRS greater than 0.12 seconds, RSR′ pattern in V_1

  - Left bundle-branch block (LBBB): QRS greater than 0.12 second, absent Q wave, and large monophasic R wave in V_6

– Papillary muscle rupture results from necrosis of the muscles that anchor the chordae tendineae of the mitral valve. It occurs most commonly with inferior infarction involving the posterior papillary muscle, although the anterior papillary muscle may be damaged with an anteroseptal infarct. The resulting acute mitral insufficiency may severely limit cardiac output. Definitive treatment is mitral valve replacement.

– Septal rupture, a rare but life-threatening emergency, results from necrosis of the interventricular septum. It may occur in inferior or anteroseptal infarcts and is most likely if significant disease is present in the right and left anterior descending coronary arteries. CPR and measures to combat cardiogenic shock may keep the patient alive until the ventricular septal defect can be repaired surgically.

– A devastating complication, rupture of the free ventricular wall occurs most commonly in the anterior or lateral walls. It may occur anywhere from 3 days to 3 weeks after the infarction during the healing stage when leukocytic removal of myocardial debris thins the myocardial wall. Hypertension, anticoagulation, and full-thickness infarction increase the risk of rupture. The resulting massive cardiac tamponade leads to death. The invariable mortality from rupture emphasizes the urgency of action when any signs and symptoms of impending rupture are detected.

2. Certain complications correlate with a particular type of infarct because they stem from a common pathophysiologic cause.

– Because the left anterior descending coronary artery nourishes the ventricular septum, where the bundle branches are located, an anterior infarct may produce septal ischemia or necrosis with resulting bundle-branch block (BBB). BBB widens the QRS complex beyond the normal limit because it disrupts the usual sequence or speed of depolarization. Because V_1 (MCL_1) is oriented to the right ventricle and V_6 (MCL_6) to the left, the pattern of deflections in these leads best indicates the timing and sequence of bundle-branch conduction.

– Untreated, certain blocks increase risk of mortality from AMI.
  - RBBB produces delayed right ventricular stimulation, prolonging the QRS duration. It also alters the usual sequence of deflections, in which septal depolarization is followed by simultaneous depolarization of both ventricles. Instead, RBBB produces a small positive wave of septal depolarization, a large negative wave of left ventricular depolarization, and a large positive wave of right ventricular depolarization.
  - LBBB disrupts the depolarization pattern to a greater extent than RBBB. It causes loss of the normal septal Q waves in leads oriented to the left ventricle and allows the right ventricle to depolarize before the left ventricle.

- Left anterior hemiblock or left posterior hemiblock

– *Observe closely for development of Mobitz II second-degree AV block or complete heart block,* particularly if RBBB with left anterior hemiblock or left posterior hemiblock is present. Prepare for prophylactic pacemaker insertion as ordered.

Inferior infarct
– *Monitor for sinus bradycardia and AV block,* particularly first-degree AV block and Mobitz I second-degree AV block.

- Correlate rhythm with clinical status, noting the presence of hypotension, altered LOC, chest pain, or increased ventricular premature beats.
- If the patient is symptomatic, administer atropine as ordered and according to unit protocol. Notify the physician and document the episode.
– *Observe for indicators of right ventricular infarction,* such as:

- jugular vein distention, positive hepatojugular reflux, positive Kussmaul's sign (increased neck vein distention on inspiration), or elevated CVP or right atrial pressure with normal or mildly elevated pulmonary artery wedge pressure (PAWP).
- widely split S_2, right ventricular S_3 or S_4 (audible at the third to fourth intercostal space at the left sternal border), or tricuspid insufficiency murmur

- bradycardia, AV blocks, and hypotension.

– *If the patient is dehydrated on admission, be especially alert for the above signs after I.V. hydration.*

- Hemiblocks are blocks of one fascicle of the left bundle branch. Left anterior hemiblock is more common than left posterior hemiblock because the anterior fascicle is thinner and has a more vulnerable blood supply. Left anterior hemiblock is considered relatively benign, whereas left posterior hemiblock is more serious because it implies extensive infarction.
– Progression to a more advanced blockage is possible at any time. RBBB with hemiblock indicates a blockage of two of the three fascicles responsible for ventricular conduction, leaving the patient dependent on a single fascicle. Mobitz II block is an ominous sign because it indicates intermittent blockage of all three fascicles, implies extensive myocardial necrosis, and commonly heralds complete heart block. Prophylactic pacemaker insertion prevents ventricular asystole if complete heart block occurs.

– Although these rhythms may occur with any type of infarct from excess vagal stimulation, they're most common in inferior infarction. An inferior infarct typically results from occlusion of the right coronary artery, which nourishes the SA node in about 90% of the population and the AV node in about 55%. Ischemia of the SA node produces sinus arrhythmias; AV nodal ischemia above the bundle of His produces progressive slowing of impulse conduction through the AV node. Such ischemia usually is transient and responds promptly to administration of atropine.
- These signs indicate that the arrhythmia is decreasing cardiac output.

- Atropine blocks vagal stimulation, thereby increasing SA node impulse formation and AV node conduction.

– Right ventricular infarction may occur with inferior or posterior left ventricular infarction because all these areas are perfused by the right coronary artery. Right ventricular infarction occurs in about 30% of inferior AMIs.
- These signs reflect the increased venous pressure that results from impaired right ventricular compliance and inability to pump blood effectively.

- The wide S_2 split reflects delayed pulmonary valve closure, the result of prolonged right ventricular ejection caused by the increased right ventricular volume and pressure. The S_3 or S_4 sound indicates decreased right ventricular compliance, and the tricuspid insufficiency murmur reflects a functional valvular insufficiency secondary to right ventricular dilation.
- Bradycardia probably reflects SA nodal ischemia, AV blocks indicate AV nodal ischemia, and hypotension results from impaired right ventricular stroke volume.
– Because the patient with AMI may be dehydrated from nausea, vomiting, and diaphoresis, signs of right ventricular infarction may appear only after rehydration.

– When recording 12-lead ECGs on a patient with suspected inferior or posterior infarction, routinely record right ventricular leads such as V_{4R}.

– The routine 12-lead ECG isn't helpful in detecting right ventricular infarction, although it will reveal signs of concomitant inferior or posterior infarction. Right ventricular leads typically reveal Q waves, ST-segment elevation, and T-wave inversion with acute right ventricular infarction.

– If indicators of right ventricular infarction are present, alert the physician. Obtain a chest X-ray and other non-invasive diagnostic studies as ordered.

– A chest X-ray and other diagnostic studies provide objective evidence of right ventricular infarction. With right ventricular infarction alone, the chest X-ray typically is clear. An echocardiogram helps differentiate right ventricular infarction from cardiac tamponade, whereas radionuclide studies identify areas of infarction or decreased right ventricular ejection fraction. Diagnostic studies also help differentiate hypotension resulting primarily from right ventricular dysfunction from that resulting from left ventricular dysfunction — an important distinction because the therapy for each is quite different.

– If right ventricular infarction is confirmed, collaborate with the physician to modify therapy.

– Although the treatment of right ventricular infarction differs from that for left ventricular infarction, the goal is the same: to improve left ventricular filling pressure and thereby optimize cardiac output.

- Avoid diuretics. Administer fluid boluses as ordered, typically to maintain right atrial pressure at 20 to 25 mm Hg and PAWP at 15 to 18 mm Hg.

- Because strong right ventricular contraction is absent with right ventricular infarction, blood flow from the right to the left side of the heart becomes passive and dependent on preload. Diuretics lower preload. Fluid is administered, rather than limited as in left ventricular infarction, to improve preload-dependent right ventricular systolic ejection, thereby increasing left ventricular filling pressure and cardiac output.

- Administer inotropes and vasodilators judiciously as ordered.

- Inotropes may increase right ventricular contractility. Vasodilators may be used to decrease pulmonary vascular resistance; the resulting right ventricular afterload reduction may improve left ventricular filling; the simultaneous left ventricular afterload reduction may improve left ventricular systolic emptying.

– Monitor hemodynamic parameters and clinical indicators of the effectiveness of therapy closely.

– The association of right ventricular infarction with left ventricular infarction can be confusing to interpret and a challenge to manage. The treatment of right ventricular infarction described above must take into consideration the therapy for left ventricular infarction. Continual surveillance is necessary to make sure that therapies are modified as necessary to achieve optimal cardiac output.

3. Additional individualized interventions:_____

_____

3. Rationales: _____

_____

Suggested NIC Interventions
Surveillance: Safety

Suggested NOC Outcomes
Safety status: Physical injury

Nursing diagnosis

Deficient knowledge (diagnostic procedures, therapeutic interventions, and long-range implications for lifestyle changes) related to complex diagnosis and therapeutic regimen

NURSING PRIORITY
Educate the patient and family about health status as appropriate.

PATIENT OUTCOME CRITERIA
Within 48 hours of admission, the patient and family will:
- provide feedback indicating an adequate knowledge base for immediate needs (for example, by asking appropriate questions and by respecting dietary restrictions)
- begin to identify long-range learning needs, on request.

INTERVENTIONS	RATIONALES
1. Implement measures in the "Knowledge deficit" care plan, page 129, as appropriate.	**1.** The "Knowledge deficit" care plan contains detailed information helpful in assessing and meeting learning needs for all patients. This plan focuses on information specific to AMI.
2. *Consult with cardiac rehabilitation staff for monitored exercise program.*	**2.** Participation in a cardiac rehabilitation program is an important adjunct to recovery due to continued monitoring during activity, educational benefits, and group support.
3. Capitalize on teachable moments:	**3.** Capitalizing on unexpected teaching opportunities provides a way to assess learning needs and meet immediate concerns.
– Establish rapport. Use eye contact, reflective listening, and nonverbal communication. Emphasize and display consistency as much as possible.	– Excessive anxiety interferes with learning. Establishing rapport through consistent, caring contact helps promote trust and relaxation, which can help the patient and family retain new information.
– Assess immediate learning needs, encourage questions, and provide brief explanations, correcting any misconceptions; repeat as necessary.	– AMI usually raises major questions for the patient and family about health and lifestyle. Responding to expressed needs displays sensitivity to the patient and family. Brief, repeated explanations may be necessary because high anxiety levels or medication effects may cause the patient to screen out information unintentionally. – Careful selection of initial teaching content helps prevent information overload.
– As appropriate, provide brief information about the pathophysiology of AMI, risk factor reduction, medications, dietary recommendations, activity restrictions, rehabilitation programs, community agencies, and support groups. – Note and document long-range learning needs. Communicate these needs to the rehabilitation program's staff.	– Documentation and communication of long-range learning needs allow continuity of care and personalization of ongoing educational efforts.
4. Additional individualized interventions: _____	**4.** Rationales: _____

Suggested NIC Interventions *Surveillance: Safety*	**Suggested NOC Outcomes** *Safety status: Physical injury*

Discharge planning

DISCHARGE CHECKLIST

Before discharge, the patient shows evidence of:
- ❑ stable blood pressure within normal limits without I.V. inotrope or vasodilator support
- ❑ stable cardiac rhythm with arrhythmias (if any) controlled by oral, sublingual, or transdermal medications or by permanent pacemaker
- ❑ spontaneous ventilation.

TEACHING CHECKLIST

Document evidence that the patient and family demonstrate an understanding of:
- ❑ extent of infarction
- ❑ activity restrictions
- ❑ recommended dietary modifications
- ❑ smoking-cessation program as needed
- ❑ common emotional changes
- ❑ community resources for lifestyle modification support and cardiac rehabilitation.

DOCUMENTATION CHECKLIST

Using outcome criteria as a guide, document:
- ❑ clinical status on admission
- ❑ significant changes in status
- ❑ pertinent diagnostic test findings
- ❑ chest pain
- ❑ pain-relief measures
- ❑ rhythm strip analyses
- ❑ use of emergency protocols
- ❑ hemodynamic trends and other data
- ❑ I.V. line patency
- ❑ oxygen therapy
- ❑ other therapies
- ❑ nutritional intake
- ❑ patient and family teaching, especially dose, route, action, and adverse effects of prescribed discharge medications
- ❑ discharge planning.

Associated care plans

- ■ Acute pain
- ■ Cardiogenic shock
- ■ Compromised family coping
- ■ Grieving
- ■ Heart failure
- ■ Impaired physical mobility
- ■ Ineffective individual coping
- ■ Knowledge deficit
- ■ Percutaneous transluminal coronary angioplasty

References

American Heart Association: *www.americanheart.org.*

Braunwald, E., et al., eds. *Harrison's Principles of Internal Medicine,* 15th ed. New York: McGraw-Hill Book Co., 2001.

Dakik, H.A., and Nasrallah, A. "Repeated Doses of Tissue Plasminogen Activator for Failed Thrombolysis: Case Report and Review of the Literature," *Heart Disease* 3(6): 362-64, November-December 2001.

DeBusk, R.F. "Sildenafil and Physical Exertion in Men with Coronary Artery Disease," *JAMA* 287(18):2359, May 2002.

HeartPoint: *www.heartpoint.com.*

Kinney, M.R., American Association of Critical-Care Nurses (et al.). *AACN's Clinical Reference for Critical Care Nursing,* 4th ed. St. Louis: Mosby–Year Book, Inc., 1998.

Lauer, M.S., "Clinical Practice, Aspirin for Primary Prevention of Coronary Events," *New England Journal of Medicine* 346(19):1468-74, May 2002.

Myocardial Infarction: An Incredibly Easy Miniguide, Springhouse Pa.: Springhouse Corp., 2000.

PDR 2000, 1st ed. *Antiplatelet and Antithrombotic Prescribing Guide.* Montvale, N.J.: Merck Medical Economics Co., 2000.

Angina pectoris

DRG INFORMATION
DRG 132   Atherosclerosis with Complication or Comorbidity.
Mean LOS = 3.0
DRG 140   Angina Pectoris.
Mean LOS = 2.7 days

Introduction
DEFINITION AND TIME FOCUS
Angina pectoris is transient insufficient coronary blood flow caused by obstruction, constriction, or spasm of the coronary arteries. Angina is characterized by brief episodes of substernal or retrosternal chest pain, commonly felt beneath the middle and upper third of the sternum. In men, angina pain usually radiates to the left shoulder, left arm, neck, jaw, or upper abdomen. Angina pain typically presents differently in women. Women don't always experience chest pain associated with angina. Instead, they frequently have vague chest pain, back pain, loss of appetite, fatigue, or shortness of breath. The cells within the heart muscle don't die in angina as they do in acute myocardial infarction (AMI) because the ischemia is transient.

Angina may be classified as stable or unstable. Unstable angina, along with AMI, is now recognized as part of a group of clinical diseases called acute coronary syndrome. The patient may also experience nocturnal angina, which occurs during sleep, or angina decubitus, which occurs only when the patient is supine, disappearing when the patient stands. Variant (Prinzmetal's) angina occurs during rest, usually during the same time each day, and may be caused by coronary artery spasm. These categories differ according to cause, precipitating factors, descriptions of pain, and electrocardiography (ECG) findings. This care plan focuses on the patient admitted for diagnosis and medical management during an initial acute attack. (See *Clinical snapshot: Angina pectoris,* page 357.)

ETIOLOGY AND PRECIPITATING FACTORS
Classic angina
- Any condition that decreases oxygen delivery by the coronary arteries, increases the cardiac workload, or increases myocardial need for oxygen, such as atherosclerosis, severe aortic stenosis, mitral stenosis or regurgitation, hypotension, hyperthyroidism, marked anemia, ventricular arrhythmias, early menopause, oral contraceptive use, or hypertension

- Classic coronary artery disease (CAD) risk factors, such as physical or emotional stress, physical inactivity, obesity, smoking, increased serum cholesterol level (above 200 mg/dl), or diabetes mellitus
- Genetic factors, such as hypertension or type II familial hyperlipoproteinemia
Prinzmetal's angina
- Coronary artery spasm

Focused assessment guidelines
NURSING HISTORY
(FUNCTIONAL HEALTH PATTERN FINDINGS)
Health-perception–health-management pattern
- Sudden onset of substernal chest pain, pressure, or both; not sharply localized — pain may radiate to arms, shoulders, neck, jaw, upper abdomen and usually lasts 2 to 5 minutes but not more than 30 minutes
- Pain described as "pressure," "tightness," "aching," or "squeezing"; rest or nitroglycerin provides relief
- Recent emotional stress, heavy exercise, a large meal, or exposure to cold (classic angina)
- Cyclic pain in absence of precipitating factors (Prinzmetal's angina)
- Treatment for hypertension, hyperlipidemia, or diabetes mellitus
- Left ventricular hypertrophy
- Obesity or cigarette smoking
- History of chronic stress, type A behavior, or sedentary lifestyle
- Increased risk among White males older than age 40, White females older than age 50, or Black males or females younger than age 45 with hypertension
Nutritional-metabolic pattern
- Nausea or indigestion
- Feeling of fullness
- Diet high in calories, cholesterol, saturated fat, and caffeine
- Pain episode after a large, heavy meal
Activity-exercise pattern
- Shortness of breath during chest pain episode
- Sedentary lifestyle with only sporadic exercise reported by patient (when stable)
- Transient chest pain episodes during increased activity, alleviated by rest
Sleep-rest pattern
- Sleep disturbance such as chest pain during dreams or when lying flat

Cognitive-perceptual pattern
- Feeling of impending doom during chest pain

Self-perception–self-concept pattern
- Difficulty believing something is physically wrong during pain-free intervals

Role-relationship pattern
- Family history of CAD
- Perception of responsibility for others
- Involvement in multiple high-stress roles, such as business executive, president of community group, and parent of teenager
- Concern that hospitalization will prevent resumption of occupation and lifestyle

Sexuality-reproductive pattern
- History of oral contraceptive use
- Previous chest pain episodes during sexual activity
- Concern over resuming normal sexual relations

Coping–stress tolerance pattern
- Type A personality traits are typical, such as overreaction to stress, exaggerated sense of urgency, excessive aggressiveness, and competitiveness
- Involvement in high-stress occupation
- Delay in seeking medical attention because chest pain subsided with rest (denial)

Value-belief pattern
- Compulsive striving for achievement

PHYSICAL FINDINGS
Cardiovascular
- Increased or decreased heart rate
- Elevated blood pressure at onset of pain
- Arrhythmias
- S_3 and S_4 gallop
- Transient jugular venous pressure elevations

Pulmonary
- Shortness of breath during chest pain episode
- Abnormal breath sounds, particularly crackles

Neurologic
- Anxiety
- Restlessness

Integumentary
- Cool, clammy skin
- Diaphoresis

Musculoskeletal
- Pained facial expression
- Clenched fists
- Tense, rigid posture

DIAGNOSTIC STUDIES
- Cardiac enzyme and isoenzyme levels — no elevations, or minor elevations without pattern characteristic of AMI
- Serum cardiac markers — troponin T or, if troponin T is elevated, troponin I normal (troponin T may be elevated in cases of angina, whereas troponin I isn't and therefore can be used to rule out AMI), myoglobin levels remain within normal limits
- Complete blood count — may show decreased hemoglobin level, hematocrit, and red blood cell level, suggesting anemia-induced angina
- Serum cholesterol, lipid profile, and homocysteine levels — may be elevated, indicating increased risk of CAD
- Serum electrolyte levels — used to determine imbalances, particularly in potassium and magnesium levels, that can cause arrhythmias
- Serum drug levels — may indicate toxic or subtherapeutic levels of cardiotonics or antiarrhythmics
- 12-lead ECG — resting ECG is usually normal in angina, with ischemic changes during chest pain: Classic angina causes T-wave inversion and ST-segment depression; Prinzmetal's angina causes ST-segment elevation
- Treadmill or exercise test — may reveal chest pain and ECG signs of ischemia on exertion, especially ST-segment and T-wave changes, ventricular arrhythmias, and downsloping or horizontal ST-segment depression
- Myocardial perfusion studies — may show ischemic areas of the myocardium (imaged with thallium-201) as "cold spots"
- Echocardiogram — may illustrate structural problems such as valvular disease or stenosis
- Cardiac catheterization and angiography — used to visualize blockage and to demonstrate coronary artery patency and ability to adequately perfuse myocardium

POTENTIAL COMPLICATIONS
- Sudden death
- AMI
- Intractable, unstable, or crescendo angina
- Arrhythmias, especially ventricular arrhythmias
- Decreased ventricular function

CLINICAL SNAPSHOT ✳

Angina pectoris

Major nursing diagnoses and collaborative problems	Key patient outcomes
ND: Acute pain	Rate chest pain as 0 on a 0 to 10 pain rating scale.
CP: Risk for arrhythmias or acute myocardial infarction	Maintain a normal sinus rhythm on ECG or have arrhythmia controlled by medications.
ND: Activity intolerance	Increase activity according to activity prescription.
ND: Risk for ineffective therapeutic regimen management	Indicate specific plans for appropriate lifestyle modifications.
ND: Deficient knowledge (cardiac procedures)	Verbalize knowledge of cardiac procedures.

Nursing diagnosis

Acute pain related to myocardial ischemia

NURSING PRIORITY

Identify and relieve chest pain.

PATIENT OUTCOME CRITERIA

Within 30 minutes of chest pain onset, the patient will:
- rate pain as 0 on a 0 to 10 pain rating scale
- display relaxed facial expression and body posture
- display normal depth and rate of respirations
- show no restlessness, grimacing, or other signs and symptoms of pain.
   Within 1 hour of chest pain onset, the patient will:
- display vital signs within normal limits, typically: heart rate, 60 to 100 beats/minute; systolic blood pressure, 90 to 140 mm Hg; and diastolic blood pressure, 50 to 90 mm Hg
- increase participation in appropriate activities
- show no life-threatening arrhythmias.

INTERVENTIONS

1. *Assess and document chest pain episodes** according to the following criteria: location, duration, quality (on a pain scale), causative factors, aggravating factors, alleviating factors, and associated signs and symptoms.

2. *Assess the patient for nonverbal signs of chest pain:* restlessness; clenched fists; rubbing of the chest, arms, or neck; chest clutching; and facial flushing or grimacing.

3. *Obtain a 12-lead ECG immediately during acute chest pain.*

RATIONALES

1. Many conditions can produce chest pain. The nurse must carefully assess the chest pain to differentiate angina from pain related to other causes, such as pleuritic, gastric, or musculoskeletal disorders.

2. Each patient differs in the ways he expresses pain and in the meaning pain has for him. Denial of cardiac symptoms is common initially. An increase or change in the degree or intensity of pain may indicate increasing myocardial ischemia.

3. Resting ECGs are usually normal in myocardial ischemia. Ischemic changes may be noted only during periods of actual chest pain.

---

*Italics indicate key interventions.

4. *Administer sublingual nitroglycerin promptly* at the onset of pain, as ordered. (The typical protocol is one 0.4-mg tablet every 5 minutes to a maximum of three tablets.) Assess pain relief after 15 to 20 minutes. Evaluate and document blood pressure, pulse rate, respirations, and pain before and after medication administration. If the pain is unrelieved after 15 to 20 minutes (or after three tablets), notify the physician immediately.

4. Nitrates decrease myocardial oxygen demands by causing vasodilation, which reduces preload and afterload and thus decreases cardiac workload and oxygen consumption. Pain unrelieved by nitroglycerin suggests extended ischemia or myocardial cell death.

5. *Implement measures to improve myocardial oxygenation:* Institute oxygen therapy, place the patient on bed rest in semi-Fowler's to high-Fowler's position with his shoulders pulled slightly back if possible, and minimize environmental noise and distractions.

5. These measures reduce the heart's oxygen demand and help alleviate chest pain and ensuing anxiety. Chest and head elevation eases lung ventilation. Sitting with the shoulders pulled slightly back allows unrestricted movement of the diaphragm. Decreasing anxiety reduces circulating catecholamine levels, thus decreasing blood pressure and myocardial oxygen consumption.

6. *Stay with the patient during chest pain episodes.*

6. The presence of a competent caregiver may decrease anxiety and promote patient comfort. It also allows for immediate intervention if problems occur.

7. Monitor and document the therapeutic effects of beta-adrenergic blockers, calcium channel blockers, vasodilators, platelet activation inhibitors, antihyperlipidemic agents, and glycoprotein (GP) inhibitors. Monitor for bradycardia, hypotension, arrhythmias, signs and symptoms of heart failure, constipation, and exacerbation of ischemic symptoms from medication therapies. (See *Drugs used to treat angina.*)

7. Beta-adrenergic blockers cut off the myocardial response to sympathetic stimulation, thus decreasing oxygen demand and preventing or relieving anginal pain. They also decrease heart rate, blood pressure, and myocardial contractility. Calcium channel blockers dilate the coronary arteries, thus decreasing coronary artery spasm and improving myocardial perfusion. Vasodilators that act on the arterial system may lessen the hypertensive response to exertion, which may prevent anginal attacks. Platelet activation inhibitors prevent platelet clumping, thus decreasing ischemia from platelet obstruction and decreasing the risk of coronary artery occlusion by platelet thrombi. Antihyperlipidemic agents interfere with cholesterol reabsorption and lower triglyceride levels, which impact favorably on the progression of atherosclerotic buildup in the coronary arteries. GP inhibitors block protein sites on platelets, which prevents platelet aggregation.

8. *Establish and maintain I.V. access.*

8. I.V. access is necessary for possible emergency medication administration.

9. Additional individualized interventions:_____

9. Rationales: _____

Suggested NIC Interventions
Physical comfort promotion: Pain management

Suggested NOC Outcomes
Pain: Psychological response

Collaborative problem

Risk for arrhythmias or AMI related to myocardial hypoxia and ischemia

NURSING PRIORITIES

- Optimize cardiac oxygenation and perfusion.
- Decrease myocardial oxygen demands.

Drugs used to treat angina

Drug class	Examples
Beta-adrenergic blockers	Propranolol (Inderal) Metoprolol (Lopressor) Nadolol (Corgard)
Calcium channel blockers	Verapamil (Calan) Nifedipine (Procardia)
Vasodilators	Hydralazine (Apresoline) Prazosin (Minipress)
Platelet activation inhibitors	Aspirin Dipyridamole (Persantine) Ticlopidine (Ticlid) Sulfinpyrazone (Anturane)
Antihyperlipidemic agents	Simvastatin (Zocor) Pravastatin (Pravachol) Lovastatin (Mevacor)
Glycoprotein inhibitors	Abciximab (ReoPro) Tirofiban (Aggrastat) Eptifibatide (Integrilin)

PATIENT OUTCOME CRITERIA

Within 30 minutes of chest pain onset, the patient will:

■ have stable vital signs, typically: heart rate, 60 to 100 beats/minute; systolic blood pressure, 90 to 140 mm Hg; and diastolic blood pressure, 50 to 90 mm Hg.

Within 24 hours of admission, the patient will:

■ display a heart rate of 60 to 100 beats/minute
■ maintain a normal sinus rhythm on ECG or have arrhythmias controlled with medications
■ have no syncope, palpitations, or skipped beats
■ have no pulse deficit.

Within 2 days of admission, the patient will:

■ have no elevating or decreasing cardiac enzyme levels
■ have a resting ECG negative for ST-segment elevation and Q waves
■ have normal blood pressure, pulse, and respirations
■ display clear lungs
■ maintain normal urine output.

INTERVENTIONS

1. *Monitor, report, and document signs and symptoms of arrhythmias,* such as irregular apical pulse, pulse deficit, pulse rate below 60 beats/minute or above 100 beats/minute, syncope, dizziness, palpitations, chest "fluttering," or abnormal configurations on rhythm strips or 12-lead ECGs.

2. *Administer antiarrhythmic medications,* as ordered, noting and documenting their effectiveness and adverse effects.

RATIONALES

1. Ventricular irritability secondary to myocardial ischemia can lead to life-threatening ventricular arrhythmias. Prompt arrhythmia identification is essential for stabilizing the patient's cardiovascular condition.

2. Common antiarrhythmic medications for ventricular arrhythmias include amiodarone (Cordarone), lidocaine (Xylocaine), and procainamide (Pronestyl). Lidocaine or amiodarone may be given for dangerous premature ventricular contractions (more than 6 per minute, sequential or multifocal), which are common with myocardial hypoxia and ischemia.

Atropine is the drug of choice for symptomatic brady-cardia. Diltiazem (Cardizem) is used for rate reduction in rapid atrial arrhythmias and to assist in the conversion to normal sinus rhythm. Adenosine (Adenocard) is used to convert paroxysmal supraventricular tachycardia to a normal sinus rhythm.

3. *Decrease myocardial oxygen demands* by restricting activity (based on the arrhythmia's severity), maintaining oxygen therapy, and providing a calm, supportive environment.

3. Activities that increase myocardial oxygen demands may trigger arrhythmias by promoting increased automaticity and impeding electrical conduction through the myocardium.

4. *Monitor, report, and document signs and symptoms of inadequate tissue perfusion,* such as decreasing blood pressure; cool, clammy skin; cyanosis; diminished peripheral pulses; decreased urine output; increased restlessness and agitation; and respiratory distress.

4. Arrhythmias may lead to decreased cardiac output, resulting in inadequate tissue perfusion. Prompt recognition can help minimize damage and complications.

5. *Monitor and report signs and symptoms of developing AMI,* such as chest pain lasting longer than 30 minutes and unrelieved by a short-acting nitrate, elevation of creatine kinase isoenzymes, elevated troponin and myoglobin levels, and ST-segment elevation and pathologic Q wave on a 12-lead ECG.

5. When myocardial ischemia is severe or prolonged, irreversible injury (tissue necrosis) occurs. Chest pain that doesn't respond to nitroglycerin within 30 minutes and positive diagnostic indications strongly suggests AMI.

6. If pain persists despite interventions and symptoms of AMI continue, the patient may require emergency cardiac catheterization and interventions.

6. Persistent pain can indicate complete blockage of the vessels. Percutaneous transluminal coronary angioplasty (PTCA) would open the vessels, thus promoting blood flow and diminishing myocardial muscle injury.

7. Additional individualized interventions: _____

7. Rationales: _____

Nursing diagnosis
Activity intolerance related to development of chest pain on exertion

NURSING PRIORITY
Promote gradual activity restoration, balancing myocardial oxygen supply and demand.

PATIENT OUTCOME CRITERIA
Within 24 hours of admission, the patient will:
- adhere to activity restrictions
- avoid Valsalva's maneuver.
  Within 48 hours of admission, the patient will:
- increase activity according to activity prescription
- have normal bowel elimination without straining.

INTERVENTIONS

1. *Instruct the patient to stop immediately any activity that causes chest pain.* If chest pain occurs, maintain the patient in Fowler's position, and administer oxygen therapy, as ordered.

RATIONALES

1. Pain may be relieved when the patient stops the physical activity that preceded its onset. Changing from a supine to a sitting position decreases central blood volume because blood pools in the extremities, reducing the heart's oxygen demand. Fowler's position allows maximum lung expansion; oxygen therapy decreases the heart's workload.

2. *Instruct the patient to avoid Valsalva's maneuver* by not straining at bowel movements and avoiding heavy lifting.

3. Document activity tolerance, and instruct the patient to increase activity gradually; monitor his pulse rate before and after activity; stop activity when he feels chest pain, fatigue, or marked tachycardia; and pace activities to avoid sudden demands on the heart.

4. Promote physical rest and emotional comfort.

5. Additional individualized interventions: _____
_____

2. Valsalva's maneuver induces parasympathetic stimulation, which can cause bradycardia and decrease cardiac output, leading to increased ischemia.

3. Physical activity increases myocardial oxygen demand and can cause chest pain. An activity prescription is determined for each patient to maintain cardiovascular stability and prevent fatigue.

4. Fear and anxiety increase sympathetic nervous system responses, increasing myocardial oxygen demand. Relaxation increases the patient's ability to cooperate and participate in therapeutic activities.

5. Rationales: _____
_____

> ### Suggested NIC Interventions
> *Activity therapy; Energy management; Exercise promotion: Strength training; Nutrition management; Self-care assistance; Home maintenance assistance*

> ### Suggested NOC Outcomes
> *Activity tolerance; Endurance; Energy conservation; Self-care: Activities of daily living (ADL); Self-care: Instrumental activities of daily living (IADL)*

Nursing diagnosis
Risk for ineffective therapeutic regimen management related to the impact of the complexity of cardiovascular risk factors

NURSING PRIORITY
Minimize the development of complications from modifiable risk factors.

PATIENT OUTCOME CRITERIA
Within 3 days of admission, the patient will:
- verbalize knowledge of diet, lifestyle, and health-habit modifications
- eliminate smoking
- indicate specific plans for appropriate lifestyle modifications.

INTERVENTIONS

1. *Teach the patient about factors that may cause anginal attacks after discharge,* such as strenuous exercise, changes in sexual habits or partners, exposure to extreme cold, strong emotions, stress, and smoking. Teach him ways to decrease the risk of chest pain, such as using sublingual nitroglycerin prophylactically, monitoring pulse rate before and after activity, and stopping activity if chest pain, dyspnea, or palpitations ensue. Use the patient's experience as a basis for teaching. Document his response to teaching.

RATIONALES

1. Teaching the patient ways to avoid anginal attacks will decrease anxiety and may increase his participation in self-care. Controlling risk factors may minimize disease progression and lessen its impact on the patient's lifestyle. Relating instruction to the patient's experience capitalizes on the principle that adults learn better when material is relevant to their needs and integrated with previous experience.

2. Instruct the patient to maintain a heart-healthy diet. The recommended diet is to limit foods high in saturated fat, trans fatty acids, cholesterol, fatty meats, tropical oils, partially hydrogenated vegetable oils, and egg yolks and to include a balanced intake of fruits, vegetables, whole grain products, fish, poultry, and lean meats. Inform the patient that the desired range for cholesterol is less than 200 mg/dl; for low-density lipoproteins, less than 100 mg/dl; and for high-density lipoproteins, 35 mg/dl or higher.

2. Exacerbation of CAD may be related to increased dietary intake of cholesterol, which contributes to increased plaque formation and narrowing of coronary arteries.

3. Document the patient's current height and weight. Teach him about the benefits of achieving and maintaining ideal body weight. Instruct him to limit intake of refined and processed sugars.

3. Obesity elevates blood pressure and places a greater demand on cardiac output. Obesity may also lead to hyperglycemia, which increases the patient's risk of developing CAD. A calorie-controlled, low-fat diet is a healthy way to reduce weight and maintain ideal body weight.

4. Provide six light meals per day rather than three heavy meals.

4. Although a subject of debate, large meals are believed to require an increased blood supply to the GI tract for digestion, increasing myocardial work. An anginal attack may be caused by a large, heavy meal. Small meals prevent epigastric fullness or indigestion that might be mistaken for anginal pain. In addition, small meals place less demand on myocardial oxygen consumption during digestion, reducing the risk of angina.

5. Tell the patient to avoid foods and beverages high in caffeine.

5. Coffee, tea, chocolate, and colas contain varying amounts of caffeine, a myocardial stimulant that increases myocardial oxygen consumption.

6. Discourage cigarette smoking and provide information on smoking-cessation resources, such as community self-help groups, nicotine patches, and gum.

6. Nicotine from inhaled smoke increases the blood carbon monoxide level, limiting oxygen supply and causing increased cardiac workload and platelet adhesion. The nicotinic acid in tobacco products increases the release of catecholamines, thus compromising blood flow.

7. Instruct the patient about the importance of maintaining normal blood pressure and a diet restricted to no more than 4 g per day of sodium.

7. Hypertension is a known risk factor that contributes to CAD. Commonly, the patient is asymptomatic until a complication occurs. Taking antihypertensive medications and eating a low-sodium diet are imperative to maintain a healthy blood pressure.

8. Instruct the patient in stress-reduction techniques.

8. Unresolved anxiety and a stressful lifestyle increase myocardial oxygen demands, so they are risk factors for cardiovascular disease. By decreasing stress levels, the patient may decrease circulating catecholamine levels and thus decrease blood pressure and overall myocardial oxygen consumption.

9. Start the patient on a cardiovascular fitness regimen when approved by the physician. Teach him how to check his own pulse and instruct him to stop exercising if his pulse increases more than 20 beats per minute from his normal resting pulse. Remind the patient to avoid overexertion and to stop when he becomes tired. Refer him to an outpatient cardiac rehabilitation program, as appropriate.

9. Supervised exercise enhances cardiovascular fitness while minimizing the chance of another cardiac event.

10. Additional individualized interventions:_____

10. Rationales: _____

> **Suggested NIC Interventions**
> *Behavior modification; Mutual goal setting; Patient contracting; Self-modification assistance; Teaching: Procedure/treatment; Decision-making support; Health system guidance; Self-responsibility facilitation; Teaching: Disease process*

> **Suggested NOC Outcomes**
> *Compliance behavior; Knowledge: Treatment regimen; Participation: Health care decisions; Treatment behavior: Illness or injury*

Nursing diagnosis
Deficient knowledge (cardiac procedures) related to unfamiliarity with diagnostic or therapeutic procedures

NURSING PRIORITY
Teach the patient about upcoming procedures.

PATIENT OUTCOME CRITERIA
Before a cardiac procedure, the patient will, on request, verbalize knowledge of the procedure, the risks and benefits, preprocedure and postprocedure care, possible complications, and postprocedure activity restrictions.

INTERVENTIONS	RATIONALES
1. See the "Knowledge deficit" care plan, page 129.	**1.** The "Knowledge deficit" care plan provides helpful interventions for patient teaching. This plan contains additional specific information for the patient undergoing an invasive diagnostic or corrective procedure.
2. *Explain hospital protocol for cardiac catheterization* to the patient and his family. Include procedural steps, the risks and benefits, preprocedure and postprocedure care, possible complications, and postprocedure activity restrictions.	**2.** Currently, the most accurate way to determine the extent of CAD is through cardiac catheterization. A special catheter is inserted through a distal vein or artery (usually the femoral) and advanced into the right or left chambers of the heart. During angiography, radiopaque contrast dye is injected through the catheter to trace coronary artery blood flow. Teaching the patient about the procedure will decrease anxiety and enhance cooperation.
3. Based on the results of cardiac catheterization, the patient may require PTCA, intracoronary stenting, or atherectomy. If the vessels aren't amenable to these procedures, coronary artery bypass graft (CABG) surgery may be necessary. If the patient isn't a candidate for invasive or surgical interventions, enhanced external counterpulsation (EECP) may be used.	**3.** When the coronary arteries are significantly blocked, when the patient develops intractable angina, or when medical management no longer controls anginal attacks, the physician usually recommends further interventions. PTCA is an invasive, nonsurgical procedure in which a balloon-equipped catheter is passed under fluoroscopy into a partially blocked coronary artery. When the balloon is inflated, it stretches the artery, opening the lumen and relieving the blockage. In intracoronary stenting, a mesh tube is inserted into the artery to hold it open. Atherectomy uses a catheter with a rotating cutting blade to scrape off and remove the atherosclerotic plaque and reopen the blocked coronary artery. CABG is indicated for the patient who isn't a candidate for interventional therapy due to more significant blockage. CABG uses a saphenous or mammary vein or a radial artery to bypass one or more blocked coronary arteries.

EECP is a noninvasive method of treating myocardial ischemia in patients who aren't candidates for invasive or surgical interventions. EECP treatment consists of sequential pneumatic compression and decompression of the lower extremities through inflation and deflation of large cuffs. The sequence is linked to the ECG cycle so that blood is pushed into the coronary arteries to open collateral circulation.

4. *For the patient undergoing PTCA, see the "Percutaneous transluminal coronary angioplasty" care plan, page 432.*

4. The "Percutaneous transluminal coronary angioplasty" care plan contains detailed information on this procedure.

5. *For the patient undergoing CABG, see the "Cardiac surgery" care plan, page 366.*

5. The "Cardiac surgery" care plan specifies nursing care for the patient undergoing cardiac surgery.

6. Additional individualized interventions: _____

6. Rationales: _____

Suggested NIC Interventions
Teaching: Procedure/treatment

Suggested NOC Outcomes
Knowledge: Treatment regimen

Discharge planning

DISCHARGE CHECKLIST
Before discharge, the patient shows evidence of:
❑ absence of chest pain, or angina controlled by oral or sublingual medications
❑ stable vital signs for at least 48 hours
❑ absence of fever and pulmonary or cardiovascular complications
❑ ability to perform activities of daily living and ambulate without chest pain
❑ blood chemistry studies within expected parameters
❑ normal sinus rhythm or arrhythmias controlled with drugs
❑ ability to tolerate activity at prescribed levels
❑ ability to tolerate diet and dietary restrictions
❑ normal voiding and bowel movements
❑ ability to list activities that may cause angina
❑ referral to outpatient cardiac programs (if applicable).

TEACHING CHECKLIST
Document evidence that the patient and his family demonstrate an understanding of:
❑ angina's pathophysiology and implications
❑ recommended modifications of risk factors (smoking, stress, obesity, lack of exercise, diet high in fat and cholesterol)
❑ prescribed dietary modifications
❑ resumption of daily activities
❑ purpose, dosage, administration schedule, adverse effects, and toxic effects of all discharge medications
❑ common emotional adjustments
❑ community resources for lifestyle and risk-factor modification, such as stress- and weight-reduction groups, cardiac exercise programs, and smoking-cessation programs
❑ signs and symptoms indicating need for medical attention, such as chest pain unrelieved by three nitroglycerin tablets within 20 minutes, new pattern of anginal attacks, palpitations or skipped beats, syncope, dyspnea, or diaphoresis
❑ date, time, and location of follow-up appointments
❑ how to contact the physician.

DOCUMENTATION CHECKLIST
Using outcome criteria as a guide, document:
❑ clinical status on admission
❑ significant changes in status
❑ chest pain episodes — precipitating, aggravating, and alleviating factors
❑ pertinent laboratory and diagnostic test results
❑ pain-relief measures
❑ oxygen therapy
❑ I.V. therapy
❑ use of protocols
❑ nutritional intake
❑ response to medications
❑ emotional response to illness; coping skills
❑ activity tolerance
❑ patient and family teaching
❑ discharge planning.

Associated care plans

- Acute myocardial infarction
- Acute pain
- Cardiac surgery
- Ineffective individual coping
- Knowledge deficit
- Percutaneous transluminal coronary angioplasty

References

Amsterdam, E., et al. "Immediate Exercise Testing to Evaluate Low-Risk Patients Presenting to the Emergency Department with Chest Pain," *Journal of the American College of Cardiology* 40(2):251-56, July 2002.

Braunwald, E., ed. *Heart Disease: A Textbook of Cardiovascular Medicine, Vol. 2,* 6th ed. Philadelphia: W.B. Saunders Co., 2001.

Braunwald, E. "ACC/AHA Guidelines for the Management of Patients with Unstable Angina and Non-ST-segment Elevation Myocardial Infarction: Executive Summary and Recommendations: A Report of the American College of Cardiology/American Heart Association Task Force on Practice Guidelines," *Circulation 2000* 102(10):1193-209, September 2000.

Canobio, M. *Mosby's Handbook of Patient Teaching,* 2nd ed. St. Louis: Mosby–Year Book, Inc., 2002.

Granger, B., and Miller, C. "Acute Coronary Syndrome," *Nursing2001* 31(11):36-43, November 2001.

Halm, M. "Heart Disease in Women," *AJN* 99(4):26-31, April 1999.

McAvoy, J. "Cardiac Pain: Discover the Unexpected," *Nursing2000* 30(3):34-39, March 2000.

Pearson, T., et al. "AHA Guidelines for Primary Prevention of Cardiovascular Disease and Stroke: 2002 Update," *Circulation 2002* 106(3):388-91, July 2002.

Ryan, D. "Is It an MI?" *RN* 63(1):27-30, January 2000.

Sole, M., Lamborn, M., and Hartshorn, J. *Introduction to Critical Care Nursing,* 3rd edition, St. Louis: Mosby–Year Book, Inc. 2001.

Stillwell, S. *Mosby's Critical Care Nursing Reference,* 3rd ed. St. Louis: Mosby–Year Book, Inc., 2002.

Swearingen, P., and Keen, J. *Manual of Critical Care Nursing: Nursing Interventions and Collaborative Management*, 4th ed. St. Louis: Mosby–Year Book, Inc., 2001.

Thompson, J., et al. *Mosby's Clinical Nursing.* 5th ed. St. Louis: Mosby–Year Book, Inc., 2002.

Tresch, D. "Diagnosis and Management of Myocardial Ischemia (Angina) in the Elderly Patient," *American Journal of Geriatric Cardiology* 10(6):337-44, November 2001.

Cardiac surgery

DRG INFORMATION

Cardiac surgery may be classified under several DRGs, depending on the principal operating room procedure and whether cardiac catheterization was performed.

DRG 104   Cardiac Valve and Other Major Cardiothoracic Procedures with Cardiac Catheterization.
Mean LOS = 11.3 days

DRG 105   Cardiac Valve Procedure and Other Major Cardiothoracic Procedures without Cardiac Catheterization.
Mean LOS = 9.3 days

DRG 106   Coronary Bypass with Percutaneous Transluminal Coronary Angioplasty
Mean LOS = 11.5 days

DRG 107   Coronary Bypass with Cardiac Catheterization
Mean LOS = 10.4 days

DRG 108   Other Cardiothoracic Procedures
Mean LOS = 10.2 days

    Additional DRG information: Hundreds of additional vascular operating room procedures also are classified under DRG 108. The above list details only coronary procedures. Other cardiac surgical procedures not addressed in the following plan (such as permanent pacemaker insertion) have still other DRG numbers.

Introduction

DEFINITION AND TIME FOCUS

Cardiac surgery can correct many structural and physiologic problems. During surgery, the surgical team stops the heart and collapses the lungs; cardiopulmonary bypass (CPB) maintains systemic perfusion and gas exchange during this time. CPB causes some predictable physiologic and hemodynamic changes during the early postoperative period; more recently developed, minimally invasive techniques may not require the use of CPB. Nursing care during this period focuses on assessing for anticipated changes, maintaining organ function, preventing complications, and providing emotional support to the patient and his family. This care plan focuses on the patient in the critical care unit during the first 12 to 24 hours after coronary artery bypass graft (CABG) or valve repair or replacement. It assumes that a cardiovascular nurse specialist or a similarly qualified person provided preoperative teaching and that a formal postoperative teaching and rehabilitation program has been planned. (See *Clinical snapshot: Cardiac surgery*, page 368.)

ETIOLOGY AND PRECIPITATING FACTORS

- Severe coronary artery disease (CAD) of one or more vessels, particularly the left anterior descending coronary artery
- Acute myocardial infarction (AMI), especially if complicated by cardiogenic shock, infarct extension, uncontrollable failure, papillary muscle rupture, or septal rupture
- Unstable or crescendo angina pectoris
- Previous bypass grafting with recurrent angina or angiographic evidence of graft closure
- Ventricular aneurysm
- Valvular stenosis or insufficiency with hemodynamic compromise

Focused assessment guidelines

NURSING HISTORY
(FUNCTIONAL HEALTH PATTERN FINDINGS)

Health-perception–health-management pattern

- History of acute or chronic CAD or valvular dysfunction
- Existence of a condition refractory to less invasive therapies such as medication. *Note:* Remaining health pattern findings are those of the underlying disease; refer to the "Acute myocardial infarction" care plan, page 337; "Heart failure" care plan, page 411; and "Cardiogenic shock" care plan, page 382 for examples.

PHYSICAL FINDINGS

Because the preoperative physical findings are those of the underlying disorder, they aren't repeated here; instead, this section presents typical postoperative findings.

General appearance

- Increase of 2 to 18 lb (1 to 8 kg) above preoperative weight

Cardiovascular

- Blood pressure variable
- Arrhythmias
- Heart sounds variable; may have early flow murmur or audible clicking after valve replacement
- Chest tube drainage variable
- Peripheral pulses usually equal bilaterally
- Slow capillary refill

Pulmonary

- Variable rate and depth, depending on ventilator settings

- Breath sounds usually diminished in left base
- Crackles or gurgles
- Persistent atelectasis

Neurologic
- Level of consciousness (LOC) variable (patient usually can be awakened)
- Confusion
- Disorientation

Integumentary
- Cool, dry skin
- Pallor
- Generalized edema
- Serosanguineous oozing from incisions

Gastrointestinal
- Absent bowel sounds
- Nasogastric tube drainage variable
- Pain may be increased or paralytic ileus prolonged with use of abdominal arterial bypass conduits (gastroepiploic or inferior epigastric arteries)

Renal
- Polyuria

DIAGNOSTIC STUDIES
The following tests are performed before surgery for baseline data. Common early postoperative findings include:

- hemoglobin level and hematocrit — decreased because of hemodilution; hematocrit is usually about 25% or lower
- coagulation panel — may reveal prolonged prothrombin time/international normalized ratio (PT/INR) and partial thromboplastin time (PTT), reflecting intraoperative heparinization; decreased platelet level, reflecting history of antiplatelet medication (aspirin, clopidogrel [Plavix], and eptifibatide [Integrilin]); and platelet destruction by CPB equipment, especially roller and filtration unit
- serum glucose level — elevated from stress-induced glycogenolysis and decreased insulin production
- serum electrolyte levels — vary, depending on preoperative status, replacement during surgery, fluid shifts, and other factors
- cardiac isoenzymes — may be elevated if AMI is present (slight elevation normal after surgery)
- 12-lead electrocardiography (ECG), resting and stress — findings vary, depending on preexisting disorders (such as AMI), acid-base status, electrolyte status, or medications
- chest X-ray — reveals cardiac size, mediastinal position, and pulmonary status; postoperatively, it confirms endotracheal tube, chest tube, central venous pressure line, and pulmonary artery (PA) catheter placement
- preoperative cardiac catheterization and coronary arteriography — reveal critical coronary artery occlusion, poor or normal left ventricular function, or hemodynamically significant valve stenosis or insufficiency (mani-

fested by elevated left ventricular end-diastolic and pulmonary pressures, cardiac index less than 2.5 L/minute/m^2, tight valve areas, increased valvular gradients, occlusive lesions, or shunts)
- echocardiography — compares preoperative and postoperative function (especially for valve repairs)

POTENTIAL COMPLICATIONS
- Cardiogenic shock
- Hypovolemic shock
- AMI
- Heart failure
- Endocarditis
- Graft occlusion
- Thromboembolism
- Atelectasis
- Stroke
- Hemorrhage
- Renal failure
- Infection

Cardiac surgery

Major nursing diagnoses and collaborative problems	Key patient outcomes
CP: Risk for low cardiac output syndrome	Maintain cardiac output and other hemodynamic values within desired limits, typically: cardiac output, 4 to 6 L/minute; PASP, 20 to 30 mm Hg; PADP, 10 to 15 mm Hg; and PAWP, 4 to 12 mm Hg.
CP: Risk for endocarditis or other infection	Display no signs or symptoms of endocarditis.
CP: Interstitial edema	Return to preoperative weight.
ND: Deficient fluid volume	Experience no signs or symptoms of excessive bleeding.
ND: Impaired gas exchange	Maintain ABG levels within normal limits, typically: pH, 7.35 to 7.45; $Paco_2$, 35 to 45 mm Hg; HCO_3^-, 22 to 26 mEq/L; Pao_2, 80 to 100 mm Hg; and Sao_2, greater than 90%.
ND: Acute confusion	Display a level of mentation within the patient's normal limits.
ND: Deficient knowledge (postoperative care)	Verbalize questions and concerns (patient and family).

Collaborative problem

Risk for low cardiac output syndrome related to hypothermia, excessive vasoconstriction, myocardial depression, arrhythmias, cardiac tamponade, or graft occlusion

NURSING PRIORITY

Maintain optimal cardiac output.

PATIENT OUTCOME CRITERIA

Within 24 hours after surgery, the patient will:
- have a mean arterial pressure (MAP) of 70 to 90 mm Hg
- have a regular supraventricular rhythm with a ventricular rate of 60 to 100 beats/minute (normal sinus rhythm is ideal)
- have peripheral pulses bilaterally equal and full
- have warm, dry arms and legs
- have a temperature of 98.6° to 101° F (37° to 38.3° C)
- display no signs of cardiac tamponade
- maintain right atrial pressure (RAP), pulmonary artery diastolic pressure (PADP), pulmonary artery systolic pressure (PASP), and pulmonary artery wedge pressure (PAWP) within desired limits, typically: RAP, 2 to 6 mm Hg; PASP, 20 to 30 mm Hg; PADP, 10 to 15 mm Hg; and PAWP, 4 to 12 mm Hg.

INTERVENTIONS

1. *Monitor blood pressure continuously** with an arterial catheter. Maintain MAP within desired limits; determine limits in consultation with the surgeon. In general, report a systolic blood pressure less than 80 mm Hg or greater than 150 mm Hg, a diastolic blood pressure greater than 100 mm Hg, or a MAP less than 60 mm Hg or greater than 90 mm Hg. Report any value abnormal for the patient.

2. *Measure cardiac output (CO) and cardiac index*, as ordered, typically every hour until normal and then every 2 hours. If you aren't using a computerized monitoring system, calculate cardiac index by dividing CO by body surface area (obtain value from a chart or nomogram); calculate systemic vascular resistance (SVR) by subtracting the RAP from the MAP and dividing the result by the CO:

$$\frac{(SVR = MAP - RAP \times 80)}{CO}$$

Follow the trend of cardiac index and SVR values, comparing them with normal ranges and previous values.

3. *Monitor PADP continuously* until stable. Monitor RAP, PASP, and PAWP, as ordered, typically every hour until stable. Compare with preoperative values and desired limits; determine limits in consultation with the surgeon.

4. *Provide constant ECG monitoring*. Observe for indicators of possible myocardial damage (such as ST-segment deviation, T-wave inversion, or pathologic Q waves) and for preexisting arrhythmias, new ventricular arrhythmias, and arrhythmias associated with the specific surgical procedure. (See *Arrhythmias associated with cardiac surgery*, page 370.) If present, assess for underlying causes, treat according to standing orders (usually with medications or temporary pacing), and document their occurrence.

RATIONALES

1. Low cardiac output syndrome, a potential postoperative problem, may result from preexisting abnormalities or the stress of surgery. Arterial monitoring provides the most direct and accurate blood pressure measurements. Because perfusion is directly related to blood pressure, maintaining optimal MAP ensures adequate organ perfusion. Hypothermia, used during surgery to lower metabolic demand and protect organs from ischemia, induces vasoconstriction, which increases SVR and the risk of hypertension. Stress triggers the release of catecholamines, antidiuretic hormone (ADH), and aldosterone, which may also produce hypertension. Persistent hypertension can cause leaking or rupture of suture lines. The causes of hypotension are discussed later in this plan.

2. Cardiac output may drop in the postoperative period because of decreased preload from a fluid volume deficit (discussed below), increased afterload from elevated SVR, or impaired contractility (discussed below). Any of these factors may cause the already stressed heart to fail. Cardiac output measurements and cardiac index calculations provide objective data on the adequacy of output, and SVR values show the degree of resistance to ventricular ejection. Increased afterload and hypertension increase myocardial workload. SVR values typically are elevated in the early postoperative period. SVR and blood pressure values should return to normal gradually as rewarming occurs.

3. PADP is a useful indirect indicator of left ventricular performance. RAP reflects CVP; PASP, the force of right ventricular ejection; and PAWP, left ventricular function. These values provide objective data for assessing the patient's fluid volume, cardiovascular function, and pulmonary status.

4. Constant monitoring provides early warning of possible myocardial damage or arrhythmias. Underlying causes may include pain, anxiety, hypokalemia, preexisting conditions (such as chronic atrial fibrillation), hypoxemia, and volume depletion. Arrhythmias usually respond to standard protocols, such as beta-adrenergic blockers or amiodarone administration for premature ventricular beats. In many patients, pacing wires are inserted during surgery and brought out through the chest wall. If necessary, they can be connected to a pacemaker to provide a stable rhythm until cardiac irritability or the underlying cause resolves.

---

*Italics indicate key interventions.

Arrhythmias associated with cardiac surgery

Certain cardiac procedures place the patient at risk for arrhythmias related to the underlying pathophysiology of the disorder or to the procedure itself.

Surgery	Possible ECG changes	Significance
Coronary artery bypass grafting	• ST-segment (ischemic) changes	• Related to myocardial ischemia, residual air in the coronary arteries, or an occluded graft
	• Ventricular ectopy	• Related to surgical manipulation, ischemia, or hypoxemia
	• New Q waves	• Indicate perioperative myocardial infarction
	• Atrial fibrillation	• Related to surgical manipulation of the atrium
Aortic valve replacement	• ST-segment (ischemic) changes	• Related to embolization of valve debris (such as calcium or tissue)
	• Left bundle-branch block	• Related to left ventricular hypertrophy
Mitral valve repair or replacement	• Atrial fibrillation	• Related to preoperative left atrial enlargement
	• ST-segment (ischemic) changes	• Related to embolization of valve debris
	• Heart block	• Usually associated with valve disease
Tricuspid valve repair or replacement	• Heart block	• Related to surgical manipulation of the bundle of His

5. *Monitor for indicators of myocardial ischemia* caused by graft occlusion: ECG changes, angina pectoris (must be differentiated from sternal incision pain), or cardiac enzymes (CK-MB) elevated above expected postoperative level (consult surgeon for acceptable level). Expect slight elevations 4 to 7 hours after CABG and higher elevations after valve replacement or repair than after CABG. Immediately report an elevation greater than 50 U/L or other significant changes. (See *Clinical pathway: Managing the CABG patient,* pages 372 to 374.)

6. *Monitor perfusion indicators* every 15 minutes to 1 hour until normal and stable. Specifically, monitor LOC; apical pulse rate; skin color, warmth, and temperature; peripheral pulse rates; and urine output. Report abnormalities to the surgeon promptly.

7. *Monitor core body temperature continuously* (via bladder or rectal probe or PA catheter) or every hour (with a rectal thermometer) until normal and then every 4 hours.

5. Early graft occlusion results from thrombus formation caused by poor runoff, graft injury, or faulty anastomosis. Late graft closure is related to subintimal thickening of the graft. The normal stress of surgery causes a slight CK-MB elevation a few hours after CABG. An elevation greater than 50 U/L after 18 to 30 hours may indicate a perioperative AMI. Higher CK-MB levels are normal after valve surgery because of greater tissue trauma.

6. These parameters indicate the adequacy of central and peripheral perfusion. Abnormalities may signal the development of several complications, such as graft occlusion and cardiac arrhythmias, and warrant medical evaluation.

7. The patient's body temperature is usually low after surgery from induced hypothermia and heat loss from the open chest. The temperature then typically rises somewhat above normal (because of the inflammatory response after surgery) and gradually returns to normal in approximately 3 days or less.

8. *Monitor body temperature.* If it's low, cover the patient with warmed blankets until it returns to normal. As his temperature rises, monitor him for signs of deficient fluid volume. If the temperature rises above 101° F (38.3° C), assess for underlying causes; administer antipyretics, such as acetaminophen (Tylenol), as ordered; and use a hypothermia blanket, as ordered, for high fever. Don't give the patient aspirin.

8. Gradual rewarming gives the heart time to adjust to the expanded vascular bed as vasoconstriction lessens. As body temperature rises, vasodilation may unmask a previously hidden fluid volume deficit. Temperatures above 101° F suggest a cause other than the normal inflammatory response, such as dehydration or sepsis. Because fever increases cardiac workload, reducing the patient's body temperature will reduce the stress on his heart. Aspirin is frequently given 12 to 24 hours after surgery to prevent graft occlusion.

9. *Administer vasodilators,* such as nitroprusside sodium (Nipride), as ordered. Refer to the "Heart failure" care plan, page 411, for details regarding administration. Correlate vasodilator administration with body temperature and rewarming.

9. Vasodilators control dilation of the vascular bed and reduce hypertension. Because afterload reduction lessens resistance to ventricular ejection, it also lessens myocardial workload. The "Heart failure" care plan covers vasodilator administration. Vasodilators, fever, and rewarming all cause vasodilation; therefore, their combined effects must be taken into account to avoid excessive vascular bed expansion.

10. *Administer positive inotropic agents,* as ordered, typically dopamine (Intropin), dobutamine (Dobutrex), or milrinone (Primacor). Refer to the "Heart failure" care plan, page 411, for details on administration.

10. Mild, transient depression of contractility is common because of hypothermia and myocardial edema. Dopamine improves contractility through its $beta_1$-adrenergic effects, but may cause tachycardia and arrhythmias. Dobutamine also increases contractility, but is less likely to cause tachycardia and arrhythmias. An inotropic may be used for the first 12 to 24 hours in an uncomplicated recovery; in cases of preoperative myocardial depression or intraoperative infarction, it may be used for a longer period. The "Heart failure" care plan covers administration of inotropic agents.

11. *Monitor for indicators of cardiac tamponade,* even when mediastinal chest tubes are draining freely. Observe for rapid hypotension, marked central venous pressure (CVP) elevation, jugular vein distention, muffled heart sounds, paradoxical pulse, or decreased QRS voltage on ECG; also observe for a sudden decrease in chest tube drainage.

11. Cardiac tamponade results when blood or fluid accumulates in the pericardium. Clotted chest tubes can produce tamponade; however, patent tubes don't necessarily reduce the risk of tamponade because fluid can accumulate in areas not drained by the tubes. Tamponade can rapidly interfere with ventricular filling and cardiac output.

12. *If tamponade with cardiac decompensation occurs, immediately notify the physician and prepare for emergency intervention.* Assemble supplies and equipment for open chest massage and maintain fluid replacement.

12. Cardiac decompensation is a medical emergency. Opening the chest allows evacuation of blood or fluid while cardiac massage perfuses the brain and other vital organs.

13. Additional individualized interventions: _____

13. Rationales: _____

Collaborative problem
Risk for endocarditis or other infection related to perioperative contamination

NURSING PRIORITIES
- Promote wound healing.
- Prevent nosocomial infection.

PATIENT OUTCOME CRITERION
After surgery, the patient will display no signs or symptoms of endocarditis or another infection.

(Text continues on page 374.)

Managing the CABG patient

Level of care	Preop	Day of surgery
Intermediate progression toward discharge	• Open heart preop workup complete • Informed consent complete • Patient/family state expected LOS and postop activities via CP	• Patient extubated w/adequate oxygenation • Patient hemodynamically stable • Patient verbalizes pain relief on I.V. meds • Patient/family state path expectations for DOS
Consults	• Cardiac surgery • Cardiology • Anesthesia	
Tests and diagnostic studies	• CBC with differential and platelet count, Chem 7, PT/INR • 12-lead ECG • Blood bank per protocol • CXR	• On admission: –12-lead ECG (hold if 100% paced); portable CXR – CPK with ISO, CBC/plt, Chem panel, ABG analysis • PRN labs: Coag panel for chest tube bleeding, additional HCT and K+ (per protocol) • Repeat ABG analysis: on CPAP, postextubation per protocol
Medications, I.V.s, blood work	• D/C Coumadin 3 days before admission • D/C aspirin 5 days before admission • Preop meds per attending physician	• Analgesics (I.V.) as ordered • Antibiotics as ordered • Titrate vasoactive meds as ordered • K+ replacement per protocol • Aspirin as ordered • Volume replacement per protocol; D/C after extubation • Autotransfuse MCT drainage per protocol
Treatments and interventions	• Betadine shower • Preop weight and height on chart • Shave/prep	• Monitor VS/hemodynamic parameters q 30 min × 2 then q 1 hr • Systemic rewarming to 96.8° F (36° C) • Pacemaker as ordered • Chest tube @ −20 cm, Foley to gravity • Monitor I&O q 1 hr • Wean FIO_2 to 40% using SaO_2, $S\bar{v}O_2$ and $ETCO_2$; initiate early extubation protocol if criteria met • Postextubation: – Titrate O_2 via FM/NC; keep SaO_2 > 92% – ICS q 1 hr when awake
Activity and mobility	• Ad lib	• When hemodynamically stable: – Turn q 2 hr and elevate HOB 30 degrees • Postextubation: – Dangle at side of bed
Nutrition	• NPO after midnight	• NPO: ice chips postextubation
Patient and family education	• Review preop teaching video/booklet • Review CABG recovery path with patient and family • Ask if patient has or wants information about advance directives	• Reorient patient upon reawakening • Instruct patient about: – CPAP/extubation and ICS procedures – Request pain meds p.r.n. • Instruct family/significant others about: – ICU routines, patient care updates
Case management and discharge planning	• Identify support systems and home situation	• Review CP expectations with patient/family

Postop day 1	Postop day 2	Postop day 3
• Patient extubated w/adequate O₂ on nasal oxygen; is hemodynamically stable w/o I.V. meds; tolerates ambulation to chair b.i.d.; responds to p.r.n. diuretic therapy; obtains pain relief on oral medication; states CP expectations for POD 1	• Oxygenation WNL for patient on RA • Cardiac rhythm/BP WNL for patient • Patient tolerates ambulation in room/hall b.i.d.; verbalizes pain relief on oral medication; tolerates oral intake without causing nausea/vomiting; states CP expectations for POD 2	• Oxygenation WNL for patient • Cardiac rhythm/BP WNL for patient • Patient tolerates ambulation in hall >5 min t.i.d.; verbalizes pain relief on oral medication; tolerates oral intake without nausea/vomiting; states CP expectations for POD 3
• Cardiac rehabilitation	• Cardiac rehabilitation	• Case management (p.r.n. for DC planning needs)
• a.m.: – Chem panel, CBC/plt, CPK with ISO – 12-lead ECG – Portable CXR	• Electrolytes, CBC	• K+ p.r.n. for continued diuresis
• Analgesics: start oral meds; I.V. for breakthrough pain • D/C vasoactive meds as tolerated • Diuresis/K+ replacement p.r.n. wt >preop • Enteric aspirin PO, multivitamin, stool softener daily • Restart needed preop meds • Start heparin lock before D/C central line	• Analgesics: Offer meds q 3 to 4 hr • Diuresis/K+ p.r.n. for wt >preop • Multivitamin daily • Enteric aspirin daily • Stool softener daily • Preop meds as needed • Peripheral heparin lock	• Analgesics: Offer meds q 3 to 4 hr • Diuresis/K+ p.r.n. for wt >preop • Multivitamin daily • Enteric aspirin daily • Stool softener daily • Preop meds as needed • Peripheral heparin lock
• D/C CVP/PA/A line per protocol • Monitor VS q 1 to 2 hr ➤ q 4 hr post-transfer • Weight in a.m. • Monitor I&O q 1 hr ➤ qs after transfer • Change dressings per protocol • D/C NG tube and Foley (unless diuresing) • Deliver O₂ via NC/RA to maintain Sao₂ >92% • ICS q 1 hr when awake • Cap pacer wires if unused • D/C chest tube per protocol	• Monitor VS q 4 hr • Weight in a.m. • Monitor I&O q shift • D/C dressings if not oozing • D/C O₂ if Sao₂ >92% on RA • ICS q 1 to 2 hour when awake • Cap pacer wires if unused • D/C remaining Foley or chest tube	• Monitor VS q 4 hr • Weight in a.m. • Monitor I&O q shift • Incisions open to air; wash daily • D/C O₂ if Sao₂ >92% on RA • Encourage independent ICS use • D/C pacer wires if unused
• Nursing: – OOB for meals with donor extremity elevated – Bath/grooming at bedside and BRP with assist	• OOB t.i.d. for meals with left extremity elevated • Bath/grooming with assist • Bathroom privileges with assist • Assist to ambulate b.i.d., distance as tolerated	• OOB t.i.d. for meals with left extremity elevated • Bath/grooming unassisted • Bathroom privileges unassisted • Ambulate t.i.d. >5 min, distance as tolerated • Assess for needed assistance
• Clear liquid, advance as tolerated	• LSF as tolerated (diabetic diet p.r.n.)	• LSF (diabetic diet p.r.n.)
• ICU: – Prepare patient/family for transfer – Reinforce pulmonary care – Provide patient care updates • Telemetry: – Introduce patient education materials – Begin cardiac rehab instruction	• Reinforce pulmonary care • Provide patient care progress updates • Review patient education booklets and videotapes • Cardiac rehab	• Reinforce pulmonary care • Provide patient care progress updates • Review patient education booklets and videotapes • Cardiac rehab
• Review CP expectations with patient/family	• Review CP expectations with patient and family • Assess home care situation and available resources	• Review CP expectations with patient and family • Notify case manager if home care or placement anticipated

(continued)

Managing the CABG patient *(continued)*

Level of care	Postop day 4	Postop day 5
Intermediate progression toward discharge	• Cardiac and respiratory status stable off telemetry • Patient tolerates ambulation in hall >5 min q.i.d. • Patient verbalizes pain relief on oral medication • Dietary intake and elimination normal for patient • Patient/family finalize plans for discharge per CP	• Cardiac and respiratory status stable • Independent with activity and ADLs • Scripts for home meds including pain Rx written • Dietary intake and elimination normal for patient • Patient/family education for home care completed
Consults	• Case management (p.r.n. for discharge planning needs)	• Outpatient cardiac rehab • SNF/Visiting Nurses p.r.n.
Tests and diagnostic studies	• PA and lateral CXR before discharge • PRN for abnormal pulmonary exam	

Medications, I.V.s, blood work	• Physician to write pain med prescription
	• Multivitamin daily
	• Enteric aspirin daily
	• Stool softener daily
	• Physician to write discharge prescriptions
	• D/C heparin lock if off telemetry/I.V. med
		• Home with discharge meds and instructions, continue after discharge:
		  – multivitamin daily
		  – enteric aspirin daily
		  – stool softener as needed
		• D/C heparin lock

Treatments and interventions	• Monitor VS q 8 hr • Weight in a.m. • D/C monitoring I&O • Incisions open to air; wash daily • D/C O_2 if Sao_2 > 92% on RA • Encourage independent ICS use • D/C remaining pacer wires	• VS q shift before discharge • Weight in a.m. • D/c chest tube sutures and cover sites with steri-strips • Continue ICS use at home
Activity and mobility	• OOB t.i.d. (minimum of 4 hr/day) • Independent self-care • Independent ambulation at slow pace q.i.d.; increase distance as tolerated • Up/down stairs with assist	• Home transport arranged • Walk 5 to 10 min, 4 to 5 × day unassisted • Up/down stairs • Independent with ADLs
Nutrition	• LSF (diabetic diet p.r.n.)	• LSF (diabetic diet p.r.n.)
Patient and family education	• Continue rehab education and begin home instructions • Review appropriate diet with patient and family, including meal preparer at home	• Home care instructions given and reviewed with patient and family • Teaching booklet sent home with patient • Home exercise plan reviewed • Discharge meds reviewed with patient and family
Case management and discharge planning	• Finalize plans for discharge with patient/family per CP • Consult case manager if home care or placement pending	• Discharge orders written in a.m. • Outpatient follow-up with physicians' offices scheduled

INTERVENTIONS

1. *Identify conditions that place the patient at risk for endocarditis or another infection*: previous endocarditis; valvular heart disease; rheumatic heart disease; Marfan syndrome; congenital heart disease; presence of foreign bodies, such as a pacemaker or prosthetic valves or grafts; or presence of invasive lines or a urinary catheter.

RATIONALES

1. These conditions increase the risk of endocarditis and other infections.

2. *Administer prophylactic antibiotics,* as ordered.

3. *Use strict sterile technique* during wound care and dressing changes.

4. *Assess for signs and symptoms of endocarditis* or another infection: elevated temperature; elevated white blood cell count; red, tender, or draining incision; changes in urine color, odor, clarity, or amount; malaise, weakness, diaphoresis, or easy fatigability; new murmur after valve surgery; or positive wound, blood, or urine cultures.

5. *If signs and symptoms of endocarditis or another infection develop, notify the physician promptly.* Obtain wound cultures and administer antibiotics as ordered. See the "Perioperative care" care plan, page 146, for further details.

6. Additional individualized interventions: _____

_____

2. Antibiotics are routinely administered for 24 hours after surgery (until invasive lines are removed).

3. Sterile technique prevents cross-contamination and transmission of bacteria to incision sites.

4. These are common findings for endocarditis or another infection.

5. Because of the high mortality rate associated with postoperative endocarditis and other infections, prompt, aggressive treatment is indicated. Cultures help to identify specific sites of infection, and antibiotics fight the organism involved. The "Perioperative care" care plan contains general information on infection control.

6. Rationales: _____

_____

Collaborative problem

Interstitial edema related to hemodilution, excessive fluid replacement, and stress adaptation syndrome

NURSING PRIORITY

Restore normal fluid volume.

PATIENT OUTCOME CRITERION

Within 24 hours after surgery, the patient will have a 24-hour fluid output greater than intake.

INTERVENTIONS

1. *Expect signs and symptoms of interstitial fluid overload; monitor degree of overload and speed of resolution:*

– Monitor generalized edema and tissue turgor.

– Monitor the patient's weight daily. Compare with preoperative and the previous day's values.

– Monitor for jugular vein distention and S_3 heart sounds; if present, notify the physician.

RATIONALES

1. During CPB, hemodilution is achieved with I.V. crystalloid solution. Because hemodilution decreases blood viscosity and peripheral vascular resistance, it minimizes microcirculatory sludging, thus protecting organs from ischemia during surgery.
– Hemodilution lowers plasma oncotic pressure, which allows fluid to shift from the vascular to interstitial spaces, producing generalized edema.
– Weight gain from hemodilution may approach 18 lb (8 kg). Daily weight comparisons provide objective evidence of the degree of fluid retention and the speed with which fluid is mobilized and excreted after surgery.
– Although most of the excess fluid is in the interstitial space, central blood volume may increase. These findings may reflect such an increase or may result from cardiac dysfunction (described below) and require medical evaluation.

2. *Administer I.V. solutions,* as ordered. Unless the patient is hypovolemic, limit fluid intake from all sources to 100 ml/hour or less.

2. Early hypovolemia is common, and I.V. fluids may be needed initially to compensate for interstitial fluid shifts, to increase plasma volume, and to optimize preload. Hemodilution during bypass pushes fluids to the interstitial space; however, this fluid shifts back into the vascular space between the second and fifth postoperative day. This, in addition to the large number of I.V. lines, can cause fluid overload unless total intake is monitored.

3. *Monitor intake and output measurements,* usually hourly on the first postoperative day and then every 8 hours.

3. The stress reaction triggered by surgery causes the release of ADH, the secretion of aldosterone, and sympathetic stimulation of the kidneys, all of which result in fluid retention. Monitoring intake and output records provides objective data on which to gauge fluid retention and base therapeutic decisions.

4. *Administer I.V. diuretics,* such as furosemide (Lasix), if ordered.

4. Aggressive diuresis may be used to eliminate excess interstitial fluid.

5. *Monitor for signs and symptoms of electrolyte imbalance,* particularly hypokalemia. See appendix C, Fluid and electrolyte imbalances for details. If hypokalemia is present:
– observe for arrhythmias
– add potassium to I.V. fluids, as ordered
– monitor serum levels closely, typically every 4 hours in the first 24 hours
– monitor for hyperkalemia.

5. Hypokalemia is common after surgery. It may result from preoperative diuretic administration, hemodilution, or postoperative diuresis. Supplemental I.V. potassium usually is necessary. Close monitoring of serum potassium levels is essential to guide replacement and to avoid hyperkalemia from potassium administration and potassium release from hemolyzed blood cells.

6. Additional individualized interventions: _____

6. Rationales: _____

Nursing diagnosis
Deficient fluid volume related to bleeding or diuresis

NURSING PRIORITY
Maintain normal fluid volume.

PATIENT OUTCOME CRITERIA
Within 3 hours after surgery, the patient will:
- have chest tube drainage of less than 200 ml/hour and declining.
  Within 4 hours after surgery, the patient will:
- have a urine output greater than 0.5 ml/kg/hour.
  Within 24 hours after surgery, the patient will:
- display minimal drainage from incisions
- have vital signs within normal limits, typically: heart rate, 60 to 100 beats/minute; systolic blood pressure, 90 to 140 mm Hg; and diastolic blood pressure, 50 to 90 mm Hg
- show hemoglobin levels, hematocrit, PT/INR, PTT, and platelet levels returning to normal
- experience no signs or symptoms of excessive bleeding.

INTERVENTIONS

1. *Monitor PT/INR, PTT, and platelet counts,* as ordered. Consult the surgeon about reportable values, particularly prolonged PT/INR, prolonged PTT, low platelet level, or other coagulation deficiencies. Note any use of aprotinin (Trasylol) during surgery, and monitor activated clotting time.

2. *Monitor hemoglobin levels and hematocrit.* Consult the surgeon about reportable values, particularly those that are declining. Have blood and blood products available.

3. *Measure and document chest tube drainage.* If drainage is constant or increasing, bright red, or exceeds 200 ml/hour, notify the surgeon. Also assess dressings for signs of drainage.

4. *Maintain the autotransfusion system, if used.*

5. *Observe for other signs of bleeding,* such as excessive oozing from incisions, petechiae, and ecchymoses. If hemoglobin levels, hematocrit, or coagulation values are abnormal, test urine, feces, and vomitus for occult blood.

6. *Monitor vital signs for tachycardia or hypotension.*

7. *Administer protamine, platelet concentrate, fresh frozen plasma, or red blood cells (RBCs),* as ordered.

8. *Monitor urine output and glucose serum levels.* Observe for urine output greater than 1 L/hour for the first 4 hours or increasing output thereafter. Also observe for urine output less than 0.5 ml/kg/hour. Monitor urine specific gravity every 2 hours for the first 24 hours. Report abnormal urine output and specific gravity values. Monitor serum glucose levels, as ordered. Correlate glucose values with urine output.

RATIONALES

1. Blood loss has multiple causes during and after surgery. During surgery, some blood loss is inevitable, and heparin is used to prevent clotting in the extracorporeal circuit. This anticoagulation is reversed with protamine sulfate, but inadequate reversal may result in bleeding. Heparin rebound also may occur from the release of heparin stored in the tissues. The CPB equipment, especially the roller pump and filtration unit, damages platelets. Finally, the patient may have a history of antiplatelet medication use. All of these factors may alter normal coagulation, so abnormal values are expected after surgery. Aprotinin is used to reduce bleeding during surgery by decreasing clotting time, as measured by activated clotting time. Reportable values vary among surgeons.

2. Hemoglobin levels and hematocrit are low after surgery as a result of hemodilution. As postoperative diuresis occurs, the values should return to normal. Failure to do so suggests continued bleeding. Usually, the patient will be transfused when the hematocrit drops below 25%.

3. Postoperative bleeding includes oozing of incisions, suture disruption, and chest tube drainage. Excessive or bloody drainage warrants surgical exploration.

4. Conserving the patient's blood avoids allergic reactions and the risks associated with blood from a blood bank.

5. Although laboratory tests provide valuable objective data of bleeding tendencies, they're no substitute for astute clinical assessment. Signs of frank or occult bleeding may be the first indication of abnormal coagulation.

6. Vital signs changes are usually nonspecific, relatively late indicators of bleeding; however, tachycardia is a compensatory response to hypovolemia, and hypotension can reflect significant blood loss or cardiac depression.

7. Protamine treats anticoagulation from inadequate heparin reversal. Platelet concentrate restores missing platelets, and fresh frozen plasma replaces platelets, clotting factors, and volume. RBCs provide hemoglobin.

8. Mannitol (Osmitrol), commonly administered during surgery to maintain cardiac output, produces osmotic diuresis. Diuretics may also be administered after surgery to eliminate retained fluid. Urine output may be as much as 1 L/hour for the first 4 hours. Oliguria with high specific gravity may indicate hypovolemia, whereas oliguria with low specific gravity may indicate renal damage. Hyperglycemia results from stress-induced glycogenolysis and decreased insulin production, producing osmotic diuresis. Correlating glucose levels with urine output may identify hyperglycemia as the cause of excessive diuresis.

9. Additional individualized interventions: _____

9. Rationales: _____

> **Suggested NIC Interventions**
> *Acid-base management; Fluid and electrolyte management; Fluid monitoring; Hypovolemia management; Intravenous (I.V.) therapy*

> **Suggested NOC Outcomes**
> *Electrolyte and acid base balance; Fluid balance, Hydration*

Nursing diagnosis

Impaired gas exchange related to alveolar collapse, increased pulmonary shunt, increased secretions, capillary leak, or pain

NURSING PRIORITY
Maintain oxygenation and ventilation.

PATIENT OUTCOME CRITERIA
Within 24 hours after surgery, the patient will:
- have a spontaneous respiratory rate of 12 to 24 breaths/minute
- maintain arterial blood gas (ABG) levels within normal limits, typically: pH, 7.35 to 7.45; partial pressure of arterial carbon dioxide, 35 to 45 mm Hg; bicarbonate, 22 to 26 mEq/L; partial pressure of arterial oxygen, 80 to 100 mm Hg; oxygen saturation (Sao_2), greater than 90%.

INTERVENTIONS

1. *Monitor pulmonary status and provide conscientious postoperative care to prevent pulmonary complications.* Refer to the "Perioperative care" care plan, page 146.

2. *Monitor mixed venous oxygen saturation* through a fiber-optic PA catheter to assess oxygen supply-demand balance.

3. *Monitor Sao_2 with pulse oximetry.*

4. *Provide care according to the "Mechanical ventilation" care plan,* page 281.

RATIONALES

1. Many factors place the patient undergoing cardiac surgery at risk for impaired gas exchange. Lung collapse during CPB results in atelectasis, and reduced surfactant production makes the lungs more difficult to expand after surgery. Hemodilution promotes interstitial fluid accumulation. CPB also activates complement and kinin systems, creating a capillary leak syndrome. Microcirculatory clotting increases pulmonary shunt. Anesthesia irritates the airways, increasing production of secretions, and depressed ciliary action impairs secretion removal. After surgery, lingering anesthetic effects and narcotics cause respiratory depression, and pain and splinting reduce lung expansion. As a result, close observation of pulmonary status and aggressive pulmonary hygiene are important after surgery. The "Perioperative care" care plan details the nursing measures used to achieve these goals.

2. Fiber-optic oximetry allows continuous monitoring of oxygen balance.

3. Monitoring Sao_2 alerts the clinician to potential hypoxemia.

4. The patient undergoing cardiac surgery usually is mechanically ventilated for several hours after surgery to reexpand collapsed alveoli and decrease cardiopulmonary workload. The "Mechanical ventilation" care plan details appropriate nursing care.

5. Additional individualized interventions: _____
_____

5. Rationales: _____
_____

> **Suggested NIC Interventions**
> *Respiratory management: Airway management; Airway suctioning; Oxygen therapy; Respiratory monitoring*

> **Suggested NOC Outcomes**
> *Respiratory status: Gas exchange; Respiratory status: Ventilation; Tissue perfusion: Cardiac; Tissue perfusion: Pulmonary*

Nursing diagnosis

Acute confusion related to sensory overload or deprivation from unit environment, anesthesia, cerebral ischemia or infarction, or prolonged CPB

NURSING PRIORITY
Optimize sensory-perceptual processing.

PATIENT OUTCOME CRITERION
Within 48 hours, the patient will be awake, alert, and oriented, if so preoperatively.

INTERVENTIONS	RATIONALES
1. *Implement measures in the "Confusion" care plan,* page 71, *as appropriate.*	**1.** The "Confusion" care plan describes interventions to reduce or eliminate sensory-perceptual dysfunction in an acutely ill patient.
2. *Assess for indicators of confusion for the first 12 to 24 hours postoperatively. Assess every 4 hours while the patient is awake or more frequently if the patient is disoriented. If indicators are present, reassure the patient and his family that these alterations are usually transient, continue implementing the measures in the "Confusion" care plan, and arrange for early transfer to a telemetry unit, if the patient's condition allows.*	**2.** Confusion may result from many factors in the critical care setting, including anxiety, sensory deprivation or overload, and sleep disruption; personality also plays a role. In addition, prolonged CPB, decreased cardiac output, hypotension, and vasoactive medications can contribute to disorientation. It usually resolves by the time the patient is transferred from the unit. Measures in the "Confusion" care plan are helpful, as is early transfer to a less hectic environment.
3. *Assess for indicators of cerebral ischemia or infarction:* a change in mental status or LOC (compare with preoperative status), motor weakness, hemiparesis, change in pupil size, or slurred speech.	**3.** Stroke is one of the most serious complications of open-heart surgery. It's more common in older patients, who are more likely to have atherosclerotic disease of the aorta or carotid and vertebral arteries. Possible causes include carotid disease and emboli from the heart (thrombi, calcium fragments from diseased valves, or air remaining in the cardiac chambers).
4. Additional individualized interventions:_____ _____	**4.** Rationales: _____ _____

> **Suggested NIC Interventions**
> *Cognitive stimulation; Mood management; Reality orientation; Anxiety reduction; Decision-making support; Family involvement promotion; Cognitive restructuring*

> **Suggested NOC Outcomes**
> *Cognitive ability; Cognitive orientation; Concentration; Decision making; Distorted thought control; Identity; Information processing; Memory; Neurologic status; Consciousness*

Nursing diagnosis

Deficient knowledge (postoperative care) related to complex, unfamiliar therapeutic regimen

NURSING PRIORITY

Educate the patient and his family about the early postoperative period, as needed.

PATIENT OUTCOME CRITERION

Throughout the unit stay, the patient (after extubation) and his family will verbalize questions and concerns.

INTERVENTIONS	RATIONALES
1. *Refer to the "Knowledge deficit" care plan,* page 129.	**1.** The "Knowledge deficit" care plan contains general information on assessing and meeting learning needs.
2. Ascertain whether preoperative teaching was provided. If the patient and family did receive preoperative teaching, reinforce explanations, as necessary. If emergency surgery was performed, provide explanations as the opportunity arises.	**2.** Before elective cardiac surgery, the patient and family usually receive extensive teaching. However, anxiety may limit retention of information and, for the patient, pain and medications affecting consciousness further limit recall. In emergency cardiac surgery, preoperative preparation is minimal, so teaching should be done as the opportunity arises.
3. Encourage questions.	**3.** Questions provide an opportunity for dealing with initial concerns, clarifying misconceptions, and eliminating knowledge gaps.
4. Begin discharge planning. Evaluate needs for discharge teaching. Explain to the family that detailed discharge education will be done after discharge to the telemetry unit. Document and communicate needs to staff members on the new unit when the patient is transferred.	**4.** Discharge planning is most effective when awareness of its importance pervades all phases of the hospital stay. Detailed discharge education is most appropriate after the patient is physiologically stable. Early identification of needs sets the stage for later teaching; documentation and communication enhance continuity of care.
5. Tailor education to the nature of the patient's surgery. For CABG, teach about risk factors; lifestyle modifications related to diet, exercise, and stress; and antiplatelet medication regimen (aspirin and dipyridamole). For valve repair or replacement, teach about signs and symptoms of infection, antibiotic prophylaxis before invasive procedures, anticoagulation medication (in patients with mechanical valves or history of chronic atrial fibrillation), signs and symptoms of valve failure, and signs and symptoms of thromboembolism.	**5.** An adult is more likely to learn information specific to personal needs. Coronary artery disease is progressive; knowledge of risk factors and potential lifestyle changes may retard disease progression. Antiplatelet medications decrease risk of thrombus formation and may maintain graft patency. The success of valve repair or replacement depends on both patient-related and prosthetic valve-related factors.
6. Additional individualized interventions: _____	**6.** Rationales: _____

> ### Suggested NIC Interventions
> *Teaching: Disease process; Teaching: Individual; Teaching: Prescribed medication*

> ### Suggested NOC Outcomes
> *Knowledge: Disease process; Knowledge: Health behavior; Knowledge: Treatment regimen*

Discharge planning
DISCHARGE CHECKLIST
Upon the patient's discharge, documentation shows evidence of:
❏ blood pressure within normal limits for 12 hours without I.V. drugs
❏ normal sinus rhythm or acceptable variant for 12 hours without I.V. antiarrhythmic drugs
❏ cardiac index, SVR, and other hemodynamic values within desired limits
❏ removal of PA catheter, arterial line, chest tubes, and indwelling urinary catheter
❏ spontaneous ventilation within normal limits for at least 12 hours
❏ ABG, hemoglobin, and electrolyte levels; hematocrit; and coagulation panel within normal limits.

TEACHING CHECKLIST
Document evidence that the patient and his family demonstrate an understanding of:
❏ signs and symptoms of prosthetic valve malfunction, if appropriate
❏ need for follow-up laboratory studies (PT/INR, if taking anticoagulants)
❏ signs and symptoms of endocarditis
❏ surgical procedure
❏ anticipated postoperative course
❏ rationale for interventions
❏ common emotional reactions
❏ medications (warfarin [Coumadin], antiplatelet therapy)
❏ discharge planning.

DOCUMENTATION CHECKLIST
Using outcome criteria as a guide, document:
❏ clinical status on admission
❏ significant changes in status
❏ pertinent diagnostic test findings
❏ cardiac index, SVR, and other hemodynamic parameters
❏ diuretic, inotropic, or vasodilator administration
❏ routine postoperative care
❏ emotional response
❏ fluid and electrolyte status
❏ pulmonary care
❏ complications, if any, and related interventions
❏ patient and family teaching
❏ discharge planning.

Associated care plans
■ Acute pain
■ Cardiogenic shock
■ Confusion
■ Grieving
■ Heart failure
■ Hypovolemic shock
■ Impaired physical mobility
■ Ineffective individual coping
■ Knowledge deficit
■ Mechanical ventilation
■ Perioperative care

References
Finklemeier, B. *Cardiothoracic-Surgical Nursing,* 2nd ed. Philadelphia: Lippincott Williams & Wilkins, 2000.

Lytle, B. "Coronary Bypass Surgery," in Hurst's *The Heart,* 10th ed. Edited by Furstes, V., et al. New York: McGraw-Hill Book Co., 2001.

Seifert, P.C. "Advances in Myocardial Protection," *Journal of Cardiovascular Nursing* (in press).

Seifert, P.C. *Cardiac Surgery: Perioperative Patient Care.* St. Louis: Mosby–Year Book, Inc., 2002.

Seifert, P.C. "Cardiac Surgery," in *Alexander's Care of the Patient in Surgery,* 11th ed. Edited by Meeker, M., and Rothrock, J. St. Louis: Mosby–Year Book, Inc. (in press).

Cardiogenic shock

DRG INFORMATION
DRG 121   Circulatory Disorders with Acute Myocardial Infarction (AMI) and Major Complications, Discharged Alive.
Mean LOS = 6.4 days

DRG 123   Circulatory Disorders with AMI, Expired.
Mean LOS = 4.6 days

DRG 127   Heart Failure and Shock.
Mean LOS = 5.3 days

Introduction
DEFINITION AND TIME FOCUS
Cardiogenic shock occurs when the heart fails to produce a cardiac output sufficient to meet metabolic demands, producing hypotension, vasoconstriction, and peripheral hypoperfusion. A major problem in critical care, cardiogenic shock usually results from a loss of 40% or more of functional myocardium, although it may be due to heart failure from any cause. Signs and symptoms result from fluid backup behind the failing ventricle (backward failure) or from decreased stroke volume (forward failure). When cardiac output is significantly decreased and physiologic compensatory mechanisms are ineffective, cardiogenic shock results. Because cardiogenic shock is associated with an 80% mortality rate, this plan focuses on the patient with acute heart failure and the interventions necessary to prevent or decrease the complications of cardiogenic shock. (See *Clinical snapshot: Cardiogenic shock.*)

ETIOLOGY AND PRECIPITATING FACTORS
- Increased preload, such as in severe valvular stenosis or insufficiency, ruptured interventricular septum, papillary muscle rupture, or rupture of chordae tendineae
- Decreased myocardial contractility, such as in massive AMI, cardiomyopathy, ventricular aneurysm, myocarditis, or cardiac tamponade
- Increased afterload, such as in systemic hypertension, pulmonary hypertension, or massive pulmonary embolism
- Severely abnormal heart rate, such as in severe tachycardia, bradycardia, or conduction disturbances

Focused assessment guidelines
NURSING HISTORY (FUNCTIONAL HEALTH PATTERN FINDINGS)
Health-perception–health-management pattern
- Fatigue, weakness, or shortness of breath
- Failure to comply with low-salt diet or medication regimen, if under treatment for chronic heart failure

Nutritional-metabolic pattern
- Anorexia, nausea, or vomiting

Activity-exercise pattern
- Dyspnea on exertion or at rest
- Palpitations
- Dizziness or fainting (syncope)

Sleep-rest pattern
- Insomnia, paroxysmal nocturnal dyspnea, or nocturia
- Use of several pillows to elevate head (orthopnea)

Coping–stress tolerance pattern
- Marked anxiety, apprehension, or sense of impending doom

PHYSICAL FINDINGS
Cardiovascular
- Hypotension
- Tachycardia or other arrhythmias
- S_3 or S_4 heart sounds or both
- Weak or irregular pulses
- Decreased pulse pressure

Pulmonary
- Crackles, usually bibasilar
- Air hunger
- Hyperventilation

Gastrointestinal
- Decreased bowel sounds

Integumentary
- Cyanosis
- Diaphoresis
- Pallor

Renal
- Oliguria

DIAGNOSTIC STUDIES
- Arterial blood gas (ABG) analysis — may reveal respiratory alkalosis (early stage) or hypoxemia and respiratory acidosis (late stage)
- Serum cardiac glycoside level — may reveal subtherapeutic range
- 12-lead electrocardiography (ECG) — reveals sinus tachycardia, frequent premature ventricular contractions, atrial fibrillation, or other arrhythmias

- Pulmonary artery pressures (PAPs) — reveal elevated pulmonary artery diastolic pressure (PADP) and pulmonary artery wedge pressure (PAWP)
- Chest X-ray — reveals pulmonary infiltrates or cardiac enlargement
- Complete blood count — may reveal dilutional changes
- Gated blood pool imaging — may reveal reduced ejection fraction

- Echocardiography — may reveal chamber enlargement, ventricular dyskinesia, or valvular abnormalities

POTENTIAL COMPLICATIONS
- Cardiac arrest
- Pulmonary edema
- Fluid and electrolyte imbalance

CLINICAL SNAPSHOT ☀

Cardiogenic shock

Major nursing diagnoses	Key patient outcomes
Impaired gas exchange	Display ABG values within acceptable range for individual.
Decreased cardiac output	Manifest cardiac index greater than 2.2 L/minute/m² and PAWP less than 18 mm Hg.
Activity intolerance	Show no activity intolerance during self-care activities.

Nursing diagnosis
Impaired gas exchange related to pulmonary congestion, decreased systemic perfusion, or both

NURSING PRIORITY
Maintain optimal gas exchange.

PATIENT OUTCOME CRITERIA
Within 3 days, the patient will:
- show no signs or symptoms of hypoxemia
- have ABG levels within acceptable range for individual
- display a level of consciousness (LOC) similar to or better than that before admission
- be free from restlessness, irritability, confusion, and somnolence
- have a PAWP within normal limits
- have lungs essentially clear to auscultation
- have an acceptable chest X-ray.

INTERVENTIONS	RATIONALES
1. *Monitor pulmonary status as needed,** typically every 15 minutes until stable and then every 2 hours. Observe for:	1. Baseline and ongoing monitoring of pulmonary status provides data to guide priorities and interventions.

*Italics indicate key interventions.

– crackles, gurgles, wheezes, dyspnea, orthopnea, shallow respirations, accessory muscle use, cough, or S_3 or S_4 heart sounds

– tachypnea, cyanosis, restlessness, irritability, confusion, somnolence, or slow or irregular respirations

– elevated PAWP.

2. *Monitor ABG values as needed or as ordered, typically every 4 hours until stable.* Obtain chest X-rays, as ordered.

3. *If pulmonary congestion is present, place the patient in semi-Fowler's or high Fowler's position.*

4. *Administer supplemental oxygen, as ordered,* typically by nasal cannula at 6 L/minute.

5. *Monitor arterial oxygen saturation (Sao_2) continuously by pulse oximetry.*

6. *Suction as needed.*

– Left ventricular end-diastolic pressure (LVEDP) most directly determines the strength of left ventricular contraction and the resulting adequacy of stroke volume. As the heart fails, decreased ventricular compliance raises LVEDP beyond the optimal stretch of myocardial fibers and, according to the Frank-Starling mechanism, optimal contractility. The elevated LVEDP is transferred to the pulmonary capillary bed and increases hydrostatic pressure in pulmonary capillaries, producing pulmonary congestion (backward failure). Elevated pulmonary capillary hydrostatic pressure causes fluid to shift across capillary walls into the interstitium and eventually into the alveoli. Crackles may result when pulmonary interstitial fluids accumulate in or compress the alveoli. Gurgles and wheezes indicate fluid accumulation in the large airways. Interstitial edema produces dyspnea, shallow respirations, and accessory muscle use, whereas alveolar edema produces orthopnea and cough. S_3 and S_4 heart sounds reflect decreased ventricular compliance or volume overload.

– Fluid-filled alveoli can't oxygenate the capillary blood flowing past them, producing a pulmonary shunt and hypoxemia. Tachypnea is an early compensatory mechanism for hypoxemia, whereas cyanosis is a late sign. Decreased cardiac output (forward failure) produces cerebral ischemia, resulting in an altered LOC. Ischemia of medullary and pontine respiratory centers causes altered breathing patterns.

– PAWP correlates with the degree of pulmonary congestion. Usually, a PAWP of 18 to 20 mm Hg correlates with the onset of congestion, 20 to 25 mm Hg with moderate congestion, 25 to 30 mm Hg with severe congestion, and more than 30 mm Hg with pulmonary edema.

2. ABG values provide evidence of hypoxemia and accompanying respiratory and metabolic acidosis, and chest X-rays provide evidence of pulmonary fluid infiltration.

3. Elevating the head of the bed improves diaphragmatic excursion, facilitating ventilation.

4. Supplemental oxygen helps saturate hemoglobin, raising arterial oxygen content and improving oxygen transport. A cannula is less likely to produce the feelings of suffocation that an air-hungry patient experiences with a mask.

5. Continuous pulse oximetry is a safe, noninvasive method for early detection of hypoxemia. Sao_2 trends provide important information about the effects of therapy.

6. In heart failure, the lungs may produce sputum so rapidly that the patient can't clear it spontaneously. Prompt suctioning not only improves gas exchange, but also lessens the patient's anxiety.

7. *Assist with insertion of a pulmonary artery (PA) catheter, as ordered.* A fiber-optic PA catheter for continuous venous oxygen saturation ($S\overline{v}o_2$) monitoring may be indicated.

7. The multiple therapies used in cardiogenic shock can affect the determinants of cardiac output. Interpreting these effects based on clinical signs alone can be confusing. A PA catheter allows objective cardiac output measurement and PAWP monitoring. PAWP monitoring is particularly important because it provides the most direct bedside indication of left ventricular function. In mitral valve or pulmonary disease, however, PAWP doesn't necessarily reflect left ventricular performance. $S\overline{v}o_2$ monitoring continuously reflects cardiac output and helps determine if the body's oxygen supply can meet tissue oxygen demand. Evaluation of tissue oxygenation provides early identification of hemodynamic changes and immediate evaluation of therapeutic interventions.

8. *Measure hemodynamic values according to unit protocol and as needed.* Typically, monitor PAP every hour, PAWP every 2 hours, and cardiac index every 4 hours. Note individual values and trends.

8. Objective measurements of PAWP and PADP provide a means of evaluating left ventricular filling pressure, whereas cardiac index indicates cardiac output adequacy. (Cardiac index equals cardiac output divided by body surface area, determined from a DuBois nomogram.) Cardiac index takes the patient's size into consideration, so it provides a more precise indication of the adequacy of cardiac output than does cardiac output alone. Isolated values provide immediate data, while trends indicate whether cardiogenic shock is resolving or worsening over time.

9. *Determine the presence and severity of heart failure* according to the PAWP and cardiac index. (See *Classification of heart failure by hemodynamic subsets,* page 387.)

9. Classification by hemodynamic status is used to distinguish disease patterns and plan therapy.

10. *Anticipate medical therapy and administer as ordered.*

10. Anticipation of therapy allows systematic planning and adequate patient preparation. Goals and therapeutic measures follow logically from the characteristics of each subset.

– For patients with no signs of failure (Subset I), observe for its development.

– Patients in Subset I have acceptable PAWP and cardiac index. However, because critically ill patients decompensate rapidly, continued observation is warranted.

– For patients with pulmonary congestion only (Subset II), administer medication, as ordered.

– Patients in Subset II have an elevated PAWP and a good cardiac index. Drug therapy is designed to decrease circulating blood volume, thereby relieving pulmonary congestion.

– If blood pressure is normal, administer diuretics, typically furosemide (Lasix) or bumetanide (Bumex). Document effectiveness and monitor for adverse effects, especially excessive diuresis or electrolyte imbalances (particularly hypokalemia).

– Diuretics reduce preload rapidly and effectively, improving ventricular compliance. Because diuretics block renal fluid reabsorption and increase renal tubular flow, potassium excretion increases. Excessive diuresis and hypokalemia are exaggerations of diuretics' therapeutic effects.

– If blood pressure is elevated, administer vasodilators, typically:

– When blood pressure is high enough to cause pulmonary congestion and reduce oxygenation, the patient's condition is too serious to wait for the action of diuretics. By expanding the vascular bed, vasodilators allow the vessels to accommodate the same amount of fluid in a larger area, thus lowering pressure. Vasodilation also lowers preload, which improves left ventricular performance.

– venodilators, such as nitroglycerin or morphine. Observe for and report adverse effects, especially hypotension and, with morphine, respiratory depression.

– arteriolar dilators, such as nitroprusside (Nipride). Monitor for and report adverse effects, especially hypotension, signs of hypoxemia, and thiocyanate and cyanide toxicity.

11. *If administering morphine, titrate doses to achieve desired effects without causing respiratory depression.* Observe for and report hypotension, nausea, and vomiting.

12. *Alert the physician immediately if the patient develops severe dyspnea, pink frothy sputum, or marked neck vein distention or describes a sense of impending doom.*

13. Additional individualized interventions: _____

– Nitroglycerin produces significant venodilation and relatively little arteriolar dilation. Used primarily for its venodilating properties, it decreases preload and pulmonary congestion. It also redistributes myocardial blood flow, causing greater dilation of large vessels than of small vessels, thus increasing flow to ischemic areas. As myocardial perfusion improves, more efficient contraction increases cardiac output. Morphine, the drug of choice in pulmonary edema, also induces vasodilation. The resulting reductions in preload, afterload, and myocardial work all improve cardiac output. Morphine also induces euphoria, particularly helpful in lessening the severe anxiety present with pulmonary edema.

– Although nitroprusside sodium dilates arteriolar and venous beds, it's used primarily for its arteriolar effects. Because it reduces afterload, systolic emptying is improved and myocardial work decreases. As a result, it produces a greater increase in cardiac output than nitroglycerin. Hypotension results from excessive dosage. Hypoxemia may result from reversal of pulmonary vasoconstriction, a compensatory mechanism that shunts blood to better-aerated alveoli. Thiocyanate and cyanide toxicity may develop from accumulation of toxic metabolites with long-term use, high dosage, or impaired liver or renal perfusion.

11. Morphine decreases pain, anxiety, catecholamine stimulation, and tachypnea, lessening the work of breathing. In a patient with respiratory center depression, however, it causes further depression and may trigger respiratory arrest. Titrating doses minimizes the risk of adverse effects. Morphine decreases the brain's oxygen requirement by nearly 50%, thereby decreasing the arterial blood flow needed to oxygenate the brain. Antiemetics may be administered with morphine to control nausea and vomiting.

12. These findings indicate pulmonary edema, a life-threatening condition. Immediate medical intervention is crucial.

13. Rationales:_____

Suggested NIC Interventions
Acid-base management; Electrolyte management; Laboratory data interpretation; Oxygen therapy; Ventilation assistance; Airway management; Respiratory monitoring; Embolus care: Pulmonary; Hemodynamic regulation; Vital signs monitoring

Suggested NOC Outcomes
Electrolyte and acid-base balance; Respiratory status: Gas exchange; Respiratory status: Ventilation; Tissue perfusion: Pulmonary; Vital signs status

Classification of heart failure by hemodynamic subsets

Subset	Classification
• Subset I: pulmonary artery wedge pressure (PAWP) 18 mm Hg and cardiac index 2.2 L/minute/m² (no failure)	• A PAWP of 18 mm Hg is the level above which signs of pulmonary congestion appear and a cardiac index of 2.2 L/minute/m² is the level below which signs of peripheral hypoperfusion appear. Increased PAWP and depressed cardiac index are the final common pathways for almost all signs of heart failure. In Subset I, a relatively normal PAWP and cardiac index indicate the absence of heart failure.
• Subset II: PAWP greater than 18 mm Hg and cardiac index greater than 2.2 L/minute/m² (pulmonary congestion)	• In Subset II, PAWP is elevated, but cardiac index is relatively normal. Clinically, the patient shows signs of pulmonary congestion.
• Subset III: PAWP less than 18 mm Hg and cardiac index less than 2.2 L/minute/m² (peripheral hypoperfusion)	• In Subset III, PAWP is relatively normal, but cardiac index is depressed. Clinically, the patient shows signs of peripheral hypoperfusion.
• Subset IV: PAWP greater than 18 mm Hg and cardiac index less than 2.2 L/minute/m² (pulmonary congestion and peripheral hypoperfusion)	• In Subset IV, PAWP is elevated and cardiac index is depressed. Clinically, the patient presents with pulmonary congestion and peripheral hypoperfusion.

Nursing diagnosis

Decreased cardiac output related to heart rate abnormalities or diminished contractility

NURSING PRIORITY

Maintain adequate cardiac output.

PATIENT OUTCOME CRITERIA

Within 3 days, the patient will have:
- blood pressure within acceptable limits
- heart rate within normal limits, ideally 60 to 80 beats/minute
- cardiac index greater than 2.2 L/minute/m² and PAWP less than 18 mm Hg
- strong, bilaterally equal peripheral pulses.

INTERVENTIONS

1. *Observe for signs and symptoms of decreased cardiac output,* such as:

– arterial hypotension, tachycardia, increased systemic vascular resistance (SVR), narrowed pulse pressure, weak peripheral pulses

– restlessness, irritability, confusion, somnolence

RATIONALES

1. Cardiogenic shock is considered a form of heart failure because of several interrelated mechanisms. Decreased contractility makes the heart unable to move blood efficiently. The resulting distention causes ventricular fibers to exceed optimal stretch according to the Frank-Starling curve, so the ejection fraction falls and systemic perfusion suffers. Failure of the left ventricle affects all body systems.

– SVR increases initially in an attempt to maintain mean arterial pressure. Pulse pressure narrows because the decreased cardiac output lowers systolic pressure, while the increased SVR elevates diastolic pressure. Tachycardia, although a compensatory response to decreased cardiac output, may actually impair it further by limiting ventricular filling time.

– Changes in LOC or mentation reflect cerebral hypoxemia or ischemia.

– weakness and fatigue

– cool, mottled, or cyanotic skin

– decreased urine output.

2. *Monitor the ECG continuously.* Document and report significant findings. (See appendix A, Monitoring standards for details.)

3. *For patients with hypoperfusion only (Subset III), provide the following care, as ordered:*

– If heart rate is elevated, administer fluids. Document effectiveness and observe for adverse effects, especially fluid overload.

– If heart rate is depressed, assist with pacemaker insertion. Document effectiveness, and observe for pacemaker malfunction.

4. *For patients with pulmonary congestion and peripheral hypoperfusion (Subset IV), administer medications, as ordered.*
– If blood pressure is depressed, administer positive inotropics, typically:

– cardiac glycoside preparations. Observe for and report signs of toxicity, including GI distress, bradycardia, atrioventricular block, premature beats, and atrial tachycardia with block.
– dopamine (Intropin). Observe for and report hypotension, tachyarrhythmias, ectopic beats, vasoconstriction with high doses, and I.V. fluid infiltration.

– dobutamine (Dobutrex). Monitor for and report adverse effects, especially tachycardia and arrhythmias.

– Weakness and fatigue result from diminished skeletal muscle perfusion, excessive work of breathing, and sleep disturbances.
– Skin changes reflect shunting away from skeletal muscles as the body attempts to preserve perfusion of core organs.
– Decreased urine output reflects diminished renal perfusion resulting from decreased circulating blood volume and intense sympathetic vasoconstriction of afferent arterioles.

2. Because cardiac output depends on the heart rate and stroke volume, arrhythmias can affect cardiac output significantly; a dramatic drop in cardiac output can cause cardiac arrest. Continuous monitoring allows for prompt treatment of arrhythmias.

3. Measures for patients in Subset III are designed to increase cardiac output, thereby increasing peripheral perfusion.
– Tachycardia is a primary compensatory response to hypovolemia. Administering fluid increases preload and thus increases cardiac output. The resulting increase in circulating blood volume restores peripheral perfusion and relieves tachycardia because as stroke volume increases, heart rate returns to normal.
– Because heart rate is a primary determinant of cardiac output, bradycardia with hypoperfusion indicates a need to restore the normal heart rate. Pacemaker insertion provides an immediate way to increase the heart rate while the underlying problem, such as heart block, is identified and resolved.

4. Patients in Subset IV have an elevated PAWP and depressed cardiac index, so the treatment goals are to lower PAWP and improve cardiac index.
– Elevated PAWP, depressed cardiac index, and depressed blood pressure strongly suggest depressed myocardial contractility. Positive inotropic agents increase myocardial contractility, thus improving cardiac index and lowering PAWP as fluid is moved efficiently through the heart.
– Cardiac glycosides improve contractility, but they also slow heart rate and cardiac conduction. They may also provoke various arrhythmias by increasing automaticity.

– Dopamine has complex dose-related pharmacologic actions. In heart failure, midrange doses (2 to 10 mcg/kg/minute) increase renal perfusion via dopaminergic effects and increase heart rate and contractility via beta$_1$-adrenergic stimulating effects.
– Dobutamine, primarily a direct beta$_1$ stimulator, is a potent inotropic agent that exerts less effect on heart rate than dopamine. As such, it significantly improves contractility with less tendency to cause arrhythmias than dopamine.

– combined inotropic and vasodilator therapy, such as dopamine and nitroprusside sodium or amrinone (Inocor). With dopamine and nitroprusside, monitor for and report adverse reactions, especially chest pain or increased ventricular arrhythmias. With amrinone, observe for and report adverse reactions, including arrhythmias, hypotension, and GI distress.

–Two synergistic drugs improve cardiac output better and more safely than either agent used alone. For example, dopamine and nitroprusside in combination reduce preload, augment contractility, and reduce afterload better than if used alone. However, both agents may decrease myocardial oxygen supply. Amrinone has inotropic and vasodilating properties that lessen pulmonary congestion and improve cardiac output. It's used commonly for short-term management of patients with heart failure who are unresponsive to other therapies.

– If blood pressure is normal, administer vasodilators. See "Impaired gas exchange," page 383, for details.

– Patients with congestion, hypoperfusion, and normal blood pressure may benefit from afterload reduction achieved through vasodilation.

5. *For patients in Subsets III and IV who don't respond to fluid and drug therapy, assist with intra-aortic balloon pump (IABP) counterpulsation, as ordered.* Monitor augmentation as necessary, every 15 minutes until stable and then every hour. Document the effectiveness of counterpulsation, and observe for complications and IABP malfunction.

5. IABP counterpulsation increases coronary artery perfusion, contractility, and vital organ perfusion and reduces afterload and myocardial oxygen demand. Balloon inflation during diastole displaces blood from the aorta, augmenting coronary artery and peripheral perfusion by increasing the diastolic pressure. Balloon deflation at the end of diastole decreases pressure in the ascending aorta, thus reducing LVEDP and workload.

6. Additional individualized interventions: _____

6. Rationales: _____

Suggested NIC Interventions
Cardiac care; Cardiac care: Acute; Hemodynamic regulation; Shock management: Cardiac; Circulatory care: Arterial insufficiency; Circulatory care: Mechanical assist device; Circulatory care: Venous insufficiency; Intravenous (I.V.) therapy; Embolus care: Peripheral; Vital signs monitoring

Suggested NOC Outcomes
Cardiac pump effectiveness; Circulation status; Tissue perfusion: Abdominal organs; Tissue perfusion: Peripheral; Vital signs status

---

Nursing diagnosis

Activity intolerance related to hypoxemia, weakness, or diminished cardiovascular reserve

NURSING PRIORITY
Promote rest.

PATIENT OUTCOME CRITERION
By the time of discharge, the patient will show no signs or symptoms of activity intolerance during self-care activities.

INTERVENTIONS

1. *Assess for signs and symptoms of activity intolerance,* such as heart rate increase greater than 25%, blood pressure increase greater than 25%, any heart rate or blood pressure decrease, chest pain, arrhythmias, decreased LOC, or complaints of weakness or fatigue.

RATIONALES

1. A dysfunctional myocardium may be unable to adjust stroke volume and oxygen during exertion. The unmet oxygen needs may cause tachycardia and myocardial or cerebral ischemia. Anaerobic metabolism resulting from impaired skeletal muscle perfusion results in weakness or fatigue.

2. *Place the patient on complete bed rest.* Assist with activity, as needed. Implement measures in the "Impaired physical mobility" care plan, page 111, as appropriate.

2. Bed rest decreases myocardial workload. Assisting with activity conserves cardiovascular and energy reserves. The "Impaired physical mobility" care plan contains measures to counteract the complications of immobility.

3. *Pace nursing care to promote rest.* If possible, allow at least 90 minutes of uninterrupted sleep at a time.

3. The numerous medical and nursing measures necessary to treat heart failure and cardiogenic shock may interrupt rest and exhaust the patient. The average sleep cycle lasts 90 minutes. Providing at least this much uninterrupted rest at a time allows the patient to progress through rapid eye movement (REM) sleep, which helps restore psychological equilibrium, and non-REM sleep, which helps restore physiologic well-being.

4. When the patient's condition stabilizes, increase activity gradually, as ordered.
– Maintain supplemental oxygen.

4. A gradual activity increase allows neurovascular compensatory mechanisms to adjust to increased demands.
– Supplemental oxygen helps meet increased tissue oxygen demands during exercise.

– Monitor the patient's response to increased activity. Slow or discontinue activity progression if the patient shows signs of intolerance.

– Close monitoring allows the nurse to match exercise level with energy resources.

5. Additional individualized interventions: _____

5. Rationales: _____

Suggested NIC Interventions
Activity therapy; Energy management; Exercise promotion: Strength training; Nutrition management; Self-care assistance; Home maintenance assistance

Suggested NOC Outcomes
Activity tolerance; Endurance; Energy conservation; Self care: Activities of daily living (ADL); Self-care: Instrumental activities of daily living (IADL)

Discharge planning
DISCHARGE CHECKLIST
Before discharge, the patient shows evidence of:
- ❏ blood pressure within 30 mm Hg of normal value for at least 12 hours without I.V. vasodilators
- ❏ no significant arrhythmias for at least 12 hours without I.V. antiarrhythmic agents
- ❏ stable hemodynamic status for at least 12 hours without IABP counterpulsation
- ❏ absence of arterial and PA line
- ❏ stable respiratory status for at least 12 hours without mechanical ventilation.

TEACHING CHECKLIST
Document evidence that the patient and his family demonstrate an understanding of:
- ❏ cause and implications of cardiogenic shock
- ❏ purpose of medications
- ❏ rationales for other therapeutic interventions
- ❏ need for continued treatment of underlying cause, including lifestyle modifications if appropriate.

DOCUMENTATION CHECKLIST
Using outcome criteria as a guide, document:
- ❏ clinical status on admission
- ❏ significant changes in status
- ❏ pertinent laboratory and diagnostic test findings
- ❏ hemodynamic measurements
- ❏ oxygen therapy
- ❏ response to cardiac assist devices, such as a pacemaker or IABP
- ❏ fluid therapy or restrictions
- ❏ response to inotropics, vasodilators, or other drugs
- ❏ dietary modifications
- ❏ activity restrictions
- ❏ patient and family teaching
- ❏ discharge planning.

Associated care plans
- ▪ Acute myocardial infarction
- ▪ Knowledge deficit
- ▪ Hypovolemic shock
- ▪ Impaired physical mobility

References

Menon, V., and Fincke, R. "Cardiogenic Shock: A Summary of the Randomized SHOCK Trial," *Congestive Heart Failure* 9(1):35-39, January-February 2003.

Picard, M.H., et al. "Echocardiographic Predictors of Survival and Response to Early Revascularization in Cardiogenic Shock," *Circulation* 107(2):279-84, January 2003.

Velmahos, G.C., et al. "Normal Electrocardiography and Serum Troponin I Levels Preclude the Presence of Clinically Significant Blunt Cardiac Injury," *Journal of Trauma* 54(1):45-51, January 2003.

Carotid endarterectomy

DRG INFORMATION
DRG 005   Extracranial Vascular Procedures.
        Mean LOS = 3.2 days
    Includes Carotid Endarterectomy (CEA) with synthetic or tissue patch graft.

Introduction
DEFINITION AND TIME FOCUS
CEA is the most commonly performed noncardiac vascular procedure and is considered the gold-standard treatment for carotid artery stenosis. A potential alternative to CEA is carotid angioplasty with stent placement. This plan focuses primarily on the patient undergoing CEA — the surgical removal of atherosclerotic plaque from the inner lining of the carotid artery to widen the vessel lumen. Endarterectomy increases cerebral blood flow and reduces the risk of stroke.

The surgical incision is made along the anterior sternocleidomastoid muscle to expose the carotid bifurcation, the most common site of plaque formation. The diseased artery is dissected away from surrounding tissue and nerves and clamped above and below the obstruction. After the plaque is removed, the artery is sutured or closed with a vein or synthetic polyester (Dacron) patch graft.

CEA is generally viewed as preventive surgery and is best performed before the patient shows significant neurologic loss. He may have had transient ischemic attacks (TIAs) or a stroke with minimal reversible ischemic neurologic deficits (RINDs). Symptoms usually occur when the artery is 70% occluded.

Carotid angioplasty with stenting is used for narrowed internal and external carotid arteries and its bifurcation and is particularly useful for the patient who doesn't meet the inclusion criterion for CEA, is considered at higher risk for endarterectomy, or who has surgically inaccessible lesions. Instead of being removed, the carotid atheroma is pushed into the arterial wall with an endovascular balloon. A stent may be inserted to keep the arterial vessel open. The procedure is usually performed using local anesthesia at the femoral artery region. After the procedure, the patient may be monitored for 12 to 24 hours in the critical care unit. This care plan focuses primarily on the immediate postoperative care of a patient undergoing elective CEA for an atherosclerotic lesion of an internal carotid artery. (See *Clinical snapshot: Carotid endarterectomy*, page 394.)

ETIOLOGY AND PRECIPITATING FACTORS
Atherosclerosis is the underlying cause in 90% of extracranial carotid disease, resulting in partial or complete occlusion. Indicators for surgery include:
- TIAs or RINDs with arteriographic evidence of an atherosclerotic carotid lesion. TIAs and RINDs usually affect the face and extremities (on the side opposite the involved cerebral hemisphere) as a result of temporarily insufficient blood supply to focal brain areas. TIAs resolve in 24 hours or less with no residual deficits, while RINDs last from 24 to 72 hours.
- stroke from a carotid lesion with severe stenosis of the internal carotid artery and a good recovery (mild or no residual neurologic deficits) at least 5 weeks after the stroke. A stroke is characterized by hemiplegia and sensory loss on the side of the body opposite the involved hemisphere and visual-field defects on the same side as the involved hemisphere.
- asymptomatic carotid bruits with severe stenosis of one internal carotid artery and total occlusion of the opposite carotid artery, bilateral stenosis, a markedly ulcerated plaque, or stenosis in the artery to the dominant hemisphere.
- recurrence of stenosis after endarterectomy.

Focused assessment guidelines
NURSING HISTORY
(FUNCTIONAL HEALTH PATTERN FINDINGS)
Health-perception–health-management pattern
- History of TIAs, RINDs, or completed stroke
- Treatment of hypertension or diabetes mellitus
- History of atherosclerosis elsewhere, such as coronary artery disease (CAD), angina or peripheral arterial occlusive disease (intermittent claudication)
- History of acute myocardial infarction (AMI)
- Risk factors, such as smoking, obesity, and sedentary lifestyle; high stress levels; high serum cholesterol, lipoprotein, and triglyceride levels; vasospasms of cerebral arteries; clotting abnormalities; polycythemia; or substance abuse
- At increased risk, if a black male
- At increased risk if older than age 45; if older than age 65, risk increases further
- Noncompliance with antihypertensive regimen; may not have sought medical attention for many years

Nutritional-metabolic pattern
- Diet high in calories, fat, cholesterol, and salt
- Transient or ongoing difficulty swallowing

Elimination pattern
- Transient or ongoing bowel or bladder incontinence

Activity-exercise pattern
- Sedentary lifestyle and lack of regular exercise (with history of TIAs, RINDs, or stroke) because of transient visual deficits (blurred vision, diplopia, blindness in one eye, or tunnel vision), motor deficits (contralateral weakness or paralysis in arm, hand, or leg), or vertigo (less common); may have minimal residual deficits that interfere with activity and exercise
- Fear of falling because of previous TIAs, RINDs, or stroke

Cognitive-perceptual pattern
- Dizziness
- Slowed mentation or clumsiness associated with previous TIAs or stroke

Sleep-rest pattern
- History of TIAs, RINDs, or stroke as a result of thrombosis; symptoms may have developed during sleep or shortly after awakening

Self-perception–self-concept pattern
- Altered self-concept, particularly if residual neurologic deficits are present

Role-relationship pattern
- Fear of inability to perform usual roles because of residual neurologic deficits or fear that TIA or stroke will occur during role performance

PHYSICAL FINDINGS

Clinical manifestations will vary depending on the extent of the disease at the bifurcation and the adequacy of collateral blood supply to the affected area. The patient may remain asymptomatic if there's sufficient collateral blood supply.

General appearance
- Some residual facial drooping from stroke

Neurologic
- Change in level of consciousness (LOC), such as confusion and syncope
- Transient motor and sensory deficits, such as numbness, weakness, or paralysis of the face, hand, arm, or leg on the side opposite the lesion (contralateral); less commonly, gait disturbance (ataxia)
- Visual deficits, such as transient scotoma (area of poor vision surrounded by normal vision), tunnel vision, diplopia, blurred vision, or amaurosis fugax (transient blindness in one eye, lasting 10 minutes or less) on same side as affected carotid artery
- Speech difficulties, such as transient motor or expressive aphasia if the dominant hemisphere is involved
- Vertigo

Cardiovascular
- Hypertension
- Carotid bruit localized to site of carotid bifurcation: characteristically loud, harsh, high-pitched systolic murmur that extends into diastole, associated with a de-

creased carotid pulse (no bruit is heard in about 20% of patients with significant obstruction of internal carotid artery)
- Decreased facial and superficial temporal pulses on side of lesion

Gastrointestinal
- Dysphagia

Musculoskeletal
- Minimal residual weakness on side opposite lesion

DIAGNOSTIC STUDIES

Screening tests are recommended before arteriography. Commonly used noninvasive tests include:
- oculoplethysmography — reveals significant disruption of blood flow to the ophthalmic artery, an important branch of the internal carotid artery, when carotid stenosis is present
- duplex B-mode ultrasonography — determines percentage of stenosis in the vessel lumen
- carotid Doppler ultrasound — differentiates thrombotic from ulcerative plaques in the stenosed carotid artery
- Doppler imaging — detects abnormal carotid blood flow and ulcerative plaques within carotid arteries; highly accurate
- carotid phonoangiography — identifies origin of bruits and estimates severity of stenosis
- magnetic resonance angiography — evaluates arterial vessels, particularly helpful for patients allergic to contrast media or those with renal insufficiency
- computed tomography (CT) scan — reveals ischemia and hemorrhage and identifies other causes of signs (such as tumors, hematomas, or cerebral aneurysms); discovery of a cerebral infarction may alter timing of surgery and indicate need for an intraluminal shunt during surgery; serves as baseline in event of perioperative neurologic deficit. CT or magnetic resonance imaging also are used for angioplasty, to establish a baseline of the brain

Commonly used invasive tests include:
- digital subtraction angiography (DSA) — provides anatomic detail of the aortic arch, subclavian and vertebral arteries, and extracranial carotid arteries; identifies moderate to severe carotid artery stenosis; may be used in place of standard angiography for the asymptomatic patient in whom noninvasive tests demonstrate a significant stenosis; if DSA appears normal in symptomatic patients, standard angiography should be performed because minor stenoses and small ulcerations may be overlooked
- cerebral arteriography — identifies exact location and extent of atherosclerotic lesions; indicated if noninvasive screening reveals severe obstruction with harsh, bilateral bruits or progressive atherosclerosis elsewhere (recommended for all patients being considered for surgery)

- blood urea nitrogen and creatinine levels — monitor renal function before and after angiography or DSA because dyes used in these tests may affect renal function
- hemoglobin level and hematocrit — provide baseline for comparison with postoperative values to detect bleeding
- coagulation panel — may be increased if the patient takes antiplatelet medications such as aspirin; before surgery, provides a baseline for comparison with postoperative values to detect clotting abnormalities
- electrolyte panel — provides a baseline for comparison with postoperative values because electrolyte imbalances may occur after surgery (existing electrolyte imbalances are corrected before surgery)
- arterial blood gas (ABG) analysis — provides a baseline for comparison because hypoxemia is a major concern after surgery
- electrocardiography (ECG), treadmill exercise test, myocardial perfusion scans, and coronary angiography — screen for cardiac disease

POTENTIAL COMPLICATIONS

- Blood pressure lability (hypertension most common, hypotension less common)
- AMI
- Cerebral ischemia or stroke (major and minor strokes with angioplasty)
- Cranial nerve injury
- Airway obstruction secondary to hemorrhage and hematoma formation
- Acute respiratory insufficiency
- Hyperperfusion syndromes (rare), such as ipsilateral vascular type headaches, seizures, or intracerebral hemorrhage
- Increased intracranial pressure (ICP) secondary to cerebral hemorrhage
- Rarely, vocal cord paralysis
- Infection
- Seizures
- With angioplasty or stenting, poststenting restenosis

CLINICAL SNAPSHOT ✳

Carotid endarterectomy

Major nursing diagnoses and collaborative problems	Key patient outcomes
CP: Blood pressure lability	Maintain stable blood pressure within desired limits.
CP: Risk for ineffective tissue perfusion (cerebral)	Exhibit signs of adequate cerebral blood flow.
CP: Risk for cranial nerve injury	Manifest no signs or symptoms of cranial nerve injury.
CP: Risk for AMI	Have an ECG with no evidence of infarction.
ND: Impaired gas exchange	Have ABG values within normal limits.

Collaborative problem

Blood pressure lability related to carotid sinus dysfunction, manipulation of the carotid bulb, hypovolemia secondary to intraoperative or postoperative bleeding or fluid imbalance, AMI, or hypoxia

NURSING PRIORITY

Maintain blood pressure within prescribed limits.

PATIENT OUTCOME CRITERIA

Within 24 hours after surgery, the patient will:

- maintain stable systolic or diastolic blood pressure or mean arterial pressure (MAP) within desired limits without antihypertensive or vasopressor drugs, typically: heart rate, 60 to 100 beats/minute; systolic blood pressure, 90 to 140 mm Hg; and diastolic blood pressure, 50 to 90 mm Hg
- exhibit fluid balance, as evidenced by approximately equal intake and output, blood pressure within desired limits, and pulmonary artery pressures within normal limits
- have ABG values within normal limits: pH, 7.35 to 7.45; partial pressure of arterial carbon dioxide ($Paco_2$), 35 to 45 mm Hg; and bicarbonate (HCO_3^-), 22 to 28 mEq/L
- exhibit little or no bleeding from the surgical site.

INTERVENTIONS

1. *Assess blood pressure** every 15 minutes for the first hour, then every hour or as needed for the first 24 hours after surgery. Ideally, use an arterial line for the first 24 hours or until blood pressure stabilizes. If medication is needed to control blood pressure, assess it every 15 to 30 minutes and as needed.

2. *Implement measures to control hypertension:*
– Administer antihypertensive medications, such as nitroprusside (Nipride), to maintain a systolic blood pressure at no more than 120 to 150 mm Hg, diastolic blood pressure at 70 to 90 mm Hg, or MAP at 86 to 110 mm Hg, or as ordered. (Diltiazem [Cardizem] I.V. may be used postangioplasty). Notify the physician immediately if the medication can't maintain blood pressure within this range.
– Administer pain medication as ordered.
– Provide a quiet, restful environment.
– Maintain activity restrictions as ordered, usually bed rest for the first 24 hours.
– Maintain fluid restrictions as ordered.

3. *Implement measures to control hypotension:*

– Assess fluid intake and output every hour or as needed for the first 24 hours. If a pulmonary artery (PA) catheter is in place, assess cardiac output, pulmonary artery wedge pressure (PAWP), and central venous pressure (CVP) every hour or as needed for the first 24 hours.
– If hypotension results from fluid loss, replace fluids as ordered.
– Assess for evidence of AMI (ECG changes, elevated creatine kinase [CK] and CK_2-MB isoenzymes, elevated troponin level and chest pain); if hypotension is caused by an AMI, see the "Acute myocardial infarction" care plan, page 337, for further interventions.
– Administer vasopressors, such as dopamine (Intropin), dobutamine (Dobutrex), or phenylephrine (Neo-Synephrine), to maintain blood pressure within the limits specified above, as ordered.

– Administer pain medications judiciously.

– Monitor the incision and drainage system for bleeding and drainage.

*Italics indicate key interventions.

RATIONALES

1. Baroreceptors at the carotid bifurcation normally control blood pressure. Surgical manipulation of these baroreceptors may impair carotid sinus reflexes, causing blood pressure instability. Additionally, hypovolemia and hypoxia contribute to fluctuating blood pressure. If uncontrolled, extreme hypertension or hypotension can cause a stroke. Blood pressure is most accurately measured with an arterial line.

2. Surgical trauma may render the carotid sinus insensitive to increasing blood pressure, resulting in hypertension. Because surgery increases blood supply to the cerebrum, capillaries are more prone to rupture when hypertension occurs, causing intracerebral bleeding and cerebral infarction. As blood pressure exceeds the limits of cerebral autoregulation (MAP of 60 to 160 mm Hg), increased pressure forces more blood into the cerebrum, leading to increased ICP and cerebral ischemia. (See the "Increased intracranial pressure" care plan, page 190.) Research shows that stimuli (particularly noxious stimuli), hypervolemia, pain, and stress increase blood pressure. Hypertension increases the risk of bleeding at the suture line and may also cause the graft site to rupture. With angioplasty, a MAP of 10% to 20% below baseline may help prevent reperfusion injury.

3. Hypotension is less common after surgery than hypertension. The carotid sinus may be hypersensitive after surgery if the removed plaque had been dampening pressure signals. Frequent checks of the indicated parameters alert the nurse to hypotension and help differentiate between two common causes, hypovolemia and AMI.
– Frequent assessment provides early warning of developing problems.

– Fluid volume replacement increases cardiac output, thus increasing blood pressure and cerebral perfusion.
– Hypotension may result from fluid deficit or myocardial dysfunction.

– Hypotension, whether caused by hypovolemia or decreased contractility with an AMI, results in decreased cerebral perfusion, decreased oxygenation, cerebral ischemia, and possible neurologic deficits and infarction. Short-acting drugs, such as dopamine or dobutamine, increase cardiac contractility, thus increasing cardiac output and blood pressure.
– Pain medications keep the patient comfortable while maintaining blood pressure within desired limits.
– Excessive bleeding or drainage indicates the need for prompt intervention to prevent hypovolemia.

4. *Maintain oxygenation* as ordered, usually 2 to 5 L by nasal cannula after extubation. Assess oxygenation levels by continuous pulse oximetry or ABG levels, as needed.

4. Hypoxemia contributes to blood pressure fluctuations because the heart rate increases to supply additional oxygen to vital organs, thus increasing cardiac output and blood pressure. Conversely, if the carotid body has been damaged, there may be a loss of the normal circulatory response to hypoxia. Because hypoxia causes the cerebral arteries to dilate, blood flow to the cerebrum increases, potentially increasing ICP and causing ischemia.

5. Additional individualized interventions: _____
_____

5. Rationales: _____
_____

Collaborative problem
Risk for ineffective tissue perfusion (cerebral) related to multiple factors

NURSING PRIORITY
Prevent or minimize cerebral ischemia.

PATIENT OUTCOME CRITERIA
Within 24 hours after surgery, the patient will:
- exhibit signs of adequate cerebral blood flow as evidenced by alertness and orientation, intact motor and sensory function, and normal pupil reactions
- maintain stable vital signs, typically: heart rate, 60 to 100 beats/minute; systolic blood pressure, 90 to 140 mm Hg; and diastolic blood pressure, 50 to 90 mm Hg
- have hemoglobin levels, hematocrit, and bleeding times within prescribed limits
- exhibit little or no bleeding.

INTERVENTIONS

1. *Assess neurological status* hourly or as needed for the first 24 hours. Assess LOC, orientation, pupillary reaction, and motor and sensory function. Document and report immediately a decreased LOC; change in orientation; pupillary changes, such as unequal pupils, a sluggish or absent pupillary reaction to light, or pupil deviation from midline position; motor and sensory deficits, such as paresthesia, motor weakness, or contralateral hemiparesis; and slurred speech or seizures. When the patient is fully recovered from anesthesia, report any visual disturbances (such as blurred or dimmed vision, diplopia, or ipsilateral change in visual field) or headache.

2. *Assess blood pressure, pulse, and respiratory rate* hourly or as needed for the first 24 hours after surgery. Report increased or decreased pulse rate, marked fluctuations in blood pressure, and changes in respiratory rate and pattern (refer to "Blood pressure lability," page 394).

3. *Assess for internal carotid artery patency* by lightly palpating the superficial temporal and facial arteries hourly or by monitoring vital signs. Document and report any change from the baseline assessment.

RATIONALES

1. Cerebral ischemia or infarction is a major concern after endarterectomy. It may result from carotid artery clamping during surgery or vasospasm from clamping and manipulating cerebral vessels, hypovolemia secondary to blood loss, cerebral vessel compression from hematoma or edema, cerebral embolization from manipulation of the arteries, marked fluctuations in blood pressure, or thrombosis at the endarterectomy site. Depending on the extent of ischemia, signs vary from mild ischemia to stroke. Assessing frequently for signs of decreased cerebral perfusion reduces the risk of permanent damage, as appropriate action can be taken immediately.

2. Such changes as increased pulse and respiratory rates and decreased blood pressure may indicate hypovolemia caused by fluid deficit or bleeding. Hypovolemia leading to decreased cardiac output, hypertension, and hypoxia increases the risk of cerebral ischemia. Bradycardia contributes to decreased cardiac output and may be caused by vagal nerve stimulation and baroreceptor stimulation during surgery.

3. Strong palpable pulses indicate good flow through the carotid artery and are a useful adjunct to other assessments.

4. *Assess for signs of bleeding:* increased neck circumference, bright red blood on the dressing, deviated trachea and respiratory distress (see "Impaired gas exchange," page 400), or increased drainage in the collection system, if used. Monitor vital signs. Document and immediately report any changes from baseline. Assess hemoglobin levels, hematocrit values, and bleeding times, as ordered, and report changes that indicate bleeding, such as decreasing hemoglobin level and hematocrit and increased bleeding times.

5. *If bleeding is present, prepare the patient for corrective procedures,* such as noninvasive or invasive testing, surgery to correct a suture line bleed, or arteriotomy and thrombectomy to remove a thrombus. Consult the "Perioperative care" care plan, page 146, for details.

6. *Implement measures to promote adequate cerebral blood flow,* as ordered:
– Detect and treat hypovolemia.
– Maintain drain patency by keeping tubing free from kinks and emptying the collection device as necessary.
– Change or reinforce the dressing as necessary.
– Apply an ice pack at the incision line, as ordered.
– Support the patient's head and neck during position changes and maintain alignment.
– Position the patient on the unoperated side.
– Avoid neck flexion.
– Administer corticosteroids, if ordered, and monitor for therapeutic and nontherapeutic effects.
– Control hypertension with antihypertensive medications such as nitroprusside sodium.
– Control hypotension with fluid replacement or vasopressors, such as dopamine or dobutamine.
– Maintain activity restrictions.

7. *Implement measures to minimize injury* if signs and symptoms of cerebral ischemia occur:
– Continue the measures above to promote cerebral blood flow.
– Assess and report progression of sign and symptoms.

– Maintain the patient on bed rest with the head of the bed flat, unless contraindicated. The head of the bed may be elevated 30 degrees, or as ordered, when vital signs are stable.
– Initiate seizure precautions.
– Provide emotional support to the patient and his family.

8. Additional individualized interventions: _____
_____

4. The patient undergoing carotid endarterectomy usually receives aspirin before surgery, sometimes up until the time of surgery, as well as heparin during surgery. Immediate detection of increased bleeding is therefore a high priority because decreased circulating blood volume increases the potential for cerebral ischemia. In addition to compromising cerebral blood flow, hematomas may cause tracheal compression, obstructing the airway. The patient may require further surgery to detect the cause of bleeding.

5. Prompt detection and correction of the cause of cerebral ischemia may minimize damage. Adequate patient preparation for testing or surgery helps allay anxieties. The "Perioperative care" care plan provides detailed information for this problem.

6. These measures promote cerebral circulation, help prevent hematoma formation, or reduce edema and stress at the suture line, reducing the risk of bleeding.

7. Minimizing injury reduces the risk of permanent neurologic damage.
– Promoting cerebral blood flow reduces the risk of further injury.
– The progression of signs and symptoms alerts the nurse to the need for more aggressive intervention. Continued deterioration, bleeding, hematoma formation, or increased ICP may require further surgery.
– The supine position improves blood flow to the brain, while elevation of the head of the bed decreases edema in the operative site.

– Cerebral ischemia may trigger seizures.
– Keeping the family informed about what's happening may help to reduce anxiety and secure their cooperation in the patient's care.

8. Rationales: _____
_____

Collaborative problem

Risk for cranial nerve injury (particularly cranial nerves III, VII, IX, X, XI, and XII) related to surgical trauma or blood accumulation and edema in the surgical area

NURSING PRIORITY

Detect and minimize neurologic impairment.

PATIENT OUTCOME CRITERIA

Within 24 hours after surgery, the patient will:
- manifest no signs and symptoms of cranial nerve damage.
  If damage has occurred, within 72 hours after surgery, the patient will:
- experience beginning resolution of cranial nerve damage as evidenced by a gradual improvement in facial muscle tone, movements and sensation, ability to chew and swallow, speech, and shoulder movements
- begin therapy for more severe cranial nerve damage, such as speech therapy or physical therapy.

INTERVENTIONS	RATIONALES
1. *Assess cranial nerve function* hourly for the first 24 hours after surgery or as needed. Check for the following:	1. The cranial nerves lie close to the endarterectomy site. Clamping of or trauma to the nerves during surgery can impair their normal function. Nerves also may be severed accidentally during dissection to access the carotid artery.
– full extraocular movements (EOMs)	– Normal EOMs indicate that the oculomotor nerve (cranial nerve III) is intact.
– ability to smile and clench teeth symmetrically; general facial symmetry present	– These findings demonstrate normal facial nerve (cranial nerve VII) function.
– swallows easily, uvula in the midline position, gag reflex intact, speaks clearly with normal tones, symmetrical movements of vocal chords and soft palate	– These findings demonstrate normal glossopharyngeal (cranial nerve IX) and vagus nerve (cranial nerve X) function (these two nerves are tested together).
– shoulders symmetrical; able to rotate head to side and shrug shoulders against resistance (may be contraindicated for the first 24 hours because both maneuvers exert pressure on the operative site)	– These movements indicate normal spinal accessory nerve (cranial nerve XI) function.
– tongue midline, able to protrude tongue in the midline position and move it laterally with normal movements; able to speak, eat, and swallow without difficulty	– These capacities demonstrate hypoglossal nerve (cranial nerve XII) function.
– facial sensation, particularly in the earlobe and over the mastoid process.	– These sensations show normal greater auricular nerve function.
2. *Compare cranial nerve assessment to preoperative or recovery room baseline. Immediately report deviations:* incomplete EOMs, ipsilateral facial drooping (loss of nasolabial fold, drooping of corner of mouth or lower eyelid), difficulty swallowing, absent or diminished gag reflex, hoarse speech, early voice fatigue, unilateral shoulder sag, difficulty raising arm on affected side to horizontal position or raising shoulder against resistance, ipsilateral tongue deviation, dysphagia, tongue biting while eating, or loss of facial sensation.	2. An awareness of preexisting deficits facilitates prompt detection of cranial nerve damage. Dysfunction may be caused by stretching of the nerves during retraction, pressure from blood accumulation, or edema in the surrounding tissues. Prompt detection of cranial nerve damage facilitates appropriate interventions to minimize complications and injury to the patient.
3. *Implement measures to reduce edema or accumulation of fluid in the surgical area:* – Elevate the head of the bed as prescribed. – Maintain patency of surgical drains, if present. – Keep the head and neck in the midline position when the patient is supine. Support his head and neck when turning.	3. Reducing edema and fluid accumulation in the surgical area minimizes pressure on the cranial nerves, reducing the potential for dysfunction. Corticosteroids are used to reduce edema.

– Keep the head and neck in correct alignment with pillows or rolls when the patient is turned to the side. Position on the unoperated side.
– Apply an ice pack at the incision line, as ordered.
– Monitor for therapeutic and nontherapeutic effects of corticosteroids, if administered.

4. *If nerve damage occurs, implement measures to prevent injury to the patient,* particularly to the facial, hypoglossal, vagus, or glossopharyngeal nerves:
– Keep suctioning equipment at the bedside and perform oral, pharyngeal, or tracheal suctioning as needed.

– Withhold oral fluids and food until the gag reflex returns.
– Assess the patient's ability to chew and swallow before offering fluids or food.
– Place the patient in high Fowler's position, unless contraindicated, during and after oral intake.
– Instill isotonic eyedrops or tape the eyelids shut if the patient's blink reflex is decreased or absent.

5. *Implement measures to facilitate communication if the vagus or glossopharyngeal nerve is damaged* (as shown by hoarseness, difficulty speaking clearly, or asymmetrical movement of vocal cords). Maintain a quiet environment; establish a means of communication with the eyes (blinking for yes and no); provide pencil and paper, magic slate, flash cards, or pictures; and pay close attention when the patient communicates.

6. If nerve damage occurs, provide emotional support to the patient and his family by listening and providing information as appropriate.

7. Initiate appropriate referrals for follow-up care when cranial nerve damage persists.

8. Additional individualized interventions: _____

_____

4. Compensating for nerve deficits reduces the risk of injury.

– Suctioning excess secretions reduces the risk of aspiration and subsequent aspiration pneumonia. This is particularly important for the endarterectomy patient, who should avoid hypoxemia.
– Withholding fluids and food when the gag reflex is absent prevents aspiration.
– Assessing the ability to chew and swallow helps the nurse gauge the risk of aspiration.
– Placing the patient in this position facilitates swallowing and decreases the risk of aspiration.
– Artificial tears and taping help prevent corneal irritation and permanent eye damage.

5. The inability to communicate effectively can be stressful, if not terrifying. Providing the patient with a means of communication or signaling helps reduce anxiety.

6. The effects of cranial nerve damage can be frightening for the patient and his family. Providing the opportunity to express concerns and giving appropriate information can relieve anxiety and stress.

7. Nerve damage usually isn't permanent, but the symptoms may take months to resolve. Working with such health care team members as the speech pathologist, physical therapist, or dietitian facilitates recovery and should begin as soon as the deficits are discovered.

8. Rationales: _____

_____

Collaborative problem
Risk for AMI related to atherosclerosis and trauma of surgery

NURSING PRIORITY
Promptly detect and treat AMI.

PATIENT OUTCOME CRITERION
Within 24 hours after surgery, the patient will exhibit stable cardiac status as evidenced by vital signs within normal limits and an ECG with no evidence of further infarction.

INTERVENTIONS

1. *Assess for chest pain (see the "Acute myocardial infarction" care plan,* page 337). Also evaluate laboratory and diagnostic tests specific to cardiac function: 12-lead ECG, arrhythmia monitoring, CK and CK isoenzymes, and troponin. Document and immediately report ECG changes consistent with AMI — elevated CK, CK_2-MB, and troponin 1 levels; elevated ST segment; and premature ventricular contractions during continuous monitoring. Compare to baseline values.

2. *Assess hemodynamic measurements* (blood pressure, pulse rate, CVP, and urine output) hourly, or as ordered. If a PA catheter is used, assess PAWP every 2 hours and cardiac output or cardiac index every 4 hours, or as ordered. Correlate abnormal findings with laboratory and diagnostic test results.

3. *Administer nitroglycerin,* as ordered, until preoperative cardiac medications can be resumed.

4. *Implement the measures in the "Acute myocardial infarction" care plan,* page 337 *for the patient with AMI.*

5. Additional individualized interventions: _____
_____

RATIONALES

1. Because generalized atherosclerosis is common in patients undergoing endarterectomy, CAD is usually present. AMI is the leading cause of death after endarterectomy. Continuous cardiac monitoring after surgery may detect ischemia and arrhythmias. Early detection of ischemia or an AMI facilitates prompt treatment and may help prevent cardiovascular complications.

2. Decreased blood pressure, cardiac output, and cardiac index, along with increased pulse and respiratory rates, PAWP, and CVP help to differentiate an AMI from other postoperative complications. Laboratory and diagnostic test results also help rule out other complications. Urine output is one of the best indicators of cardiac output, particularly if a PA catheter isn't in place.

3. Nitroglycerin may be ordered for the patient with known CAD to increase blood flow and decrease cardiac workload by vasodilation.

4. The "Acute myocardial infarction" care plan provides detailed information about the care of the patient with an AMI.

5. Rationales: _____
_____

Nursing diagnosis

Impaired gas exchange related to airway obstruction from tracheal compression or aspiration

NURSING PRIORITIES
- Minimize or prevent airway obstruction and aspiration.
- Maintain oxygenation.

PATIENT OUTCOME CRITERIA
Within 24 hours after surgery, the patient will:
- have a patent airway as evidenced by normal respiratory rate and effort, normal breath sounds, and appropriate LOC
- have ABG values within normal limits, typically: pH, 7.35 to 7.45; $Paco_2$, 35 to 45 mm Hg; and HCO_3^-, 22 to 28 mEq/L
- produce minimal drainage from the incision
- display trachea in the midline position.

INTERVENTIONS

1. *Assess airway patency* every 15 minutes for the first hour after surgery and then hourly, as needed, for 24 hours. Assess respiratory rate and effort, respiratory pattern, chest excursion, position of trachea, breath sounds, LOC, and color. Document and immediately report increased respiratory rate, accessory muscle use, unequal chest excursion, altered LOC (such as lethargy, restlessness, or confusion), pale to cyanotic color, shortness of breath, tracheal deviation, stridor, wheezing, or labored respirations.

2. *Assess oxygenation levels* by continuous pulse oximetry or ABG levels, as needed. Also, monitor ABG levels to ensure that pH and $Paco_2$ stay within normal limits. Document and report oxygen saturation below 95%, or as ordered, and ABG values outside the prescribed limits.

3. *If airway obstruction occurs, prepare to assist with immediate medical intervention,* endotracheal (ET) intubation, tracheostomy, or drainage of an incisional hematoma. Anticipate intubation even if signs of hypoxemia haven't yet developed. A tracheostomy tray should be available at the bedside or in the critical care unit.

4. *Assess for bleeding and hematoma formation:*

– Assess neck size closely every 15 minutes for the first hour, then hourly, as needed, for the first 24 hours after surgery. To maintain accuracy, mark the point at which the circumference is measured on the dressing. Observe for blood on the dressing. Document and immediately report excessive bleeding or a sudden increase in the neck's circumference.
– Check for bleeding behind the neck of the supine patient. If a bulky neck dressing makes inspection difficult, use the quality of respirations and ability to swallow as guidelines.
– Monitor hemoglobin levels and hematocrit as ordered and report decreases.
– If a drain is present, maintain patency, and note the amount of drainage. Document and report excessive drainage.

5. *Evaluate the patient's ability to swallow.*

6. *Assess for laryngeal nerve function:* an intact gag reflex, ability to swallow and speak clearly with normal tones, and symmetrical movements of the vocal cords and soft palate.

RATIONALES

1. Maintaining a patent airway is essential. The most common cause of acute postoperative airway obstruction is compression of the trachea by a hematoma or edema at the surgical site. Tracheal deviation and signs of hypoxemia, including altered LOC, labored respirations, and wheezing or stridor, are key assessment findings for the obstructed airway.

2. Pulse oximetry provides ongoing noninvasive monitoring of arterial oxygen saturation. ABG values provide objective documentation of acid-base status and are a helpful adjunct to observations of respiratory status. Acidosis, hypoxemia, or hypercapnia may increase cerebral edema.

3. Although usually done in the operating room, emergency drainage of a life-threatening hematoma in the neck may be performed at the patient's bedside. Drainage may be necessary before an ET tube can be inserted. The postoperative CEA patient must avoid hypoxemia because sufficient damage to the carotid body impairs ventilatory and circulatory responses to hypoxia. Therefore, the patient may be intubated before hypoxemia develops. If the physician is unable to intubate, a tracheostomy may be performed.

4. Bleeding can lead to hypovolemia, whereas hematoma formation may compress the airway.
– Neck size increases with a developing hematoma. Closely observing neck size, ensuring consistency in measurements, and monitoring for bleeding promotes early detection of hypoxia.

– Blood may pool, promoting hematoma formation posterior to the incision.

– Decreasing hemoglobin levels and hematocrit may indicate slow bleeding.
– Excessive bleeding through a drain may lead to hypovolemia and hypotension.

5. Edema that exerts pressure on the trachea and esophagus makes swallowing difficult and increases the risk of airway obstruction.

6. Damage to the laryngeal branches of the vagus nerve prevents closure of the glottis, which can lead to aspiration and subsequent aspiration pneumonia. Pneumonia may cause hypoxia, a potentially dangerous condition after carotid endarterectomy.

7. *Keep suctioning equipment at the bedside* for oral, pharyngeal, or ET suctioning, as needed.

8. *Implement measures to increase gas exchange and prevent hypoxemia:*
– Elevate the head of the bed as ordered, as soon as vital signs are stable.
– Encourage deep breathing every 2 hours. Remind the patient to yawn and sigh periodically. Provide frequent position changes after vital signs have stabilized, minimizing stress on the operative site by supporting the head and maintaining proper alignment when turning and positioning the patient. Suction secretions as necessary.
– Discourage the patient from coughing during the first 24 hours after surgery.
– Evaluate respiratory rate and effort before administering analgesics or sedation.
– Maintain supplemental oxygen as ordered.

9. Additional individualized interventions: _____

7. Prompt suctioning can prevent aspiration.

8. Facilitating gas exchange helps prevent hypoxemia and the complications associated with it.
– An upright position facilitates diaphragmatic excursion.

– These measures lessen postoperative atelectasis.

– Coughing during the first 24 hours can exert excessive pressure on the incision and may cause it to rupture.
– Analgesics and sedatives can depress the respiratory center, promoting hypoxemia.
– Supplemental oxygen increases blood oxygen content.

9. Rationales: _____

Suggested NIC Interventions
Acid-base management; Electrolyte management; Laboratory data interpretation; Oxygen therapy; Ventilation assistance; Airway management; Respiratory monitoring; Embolus care: Pulmonary; Hemodynamic regulation; Vital signs monitoring

Suggested NOC Outcomes
Electrolyte and acid-base balance; Respiratory status: Gas exchange; Respiratory status: Ventilation; Tissue perfusion: Pulmonary; Vital signs status

---

Discharge planning
DISCHARGE CHECKLIST
Before discharge, the patient shows evidence of:
❒ patent airway
❒ stable blood pressure within normal limits without I.V. inotropic or vasodilator support
❒ ABG measurements or oxygenation saturation within normal limits
❒ no bleeding from incision
❒ stable neurologic function
❒ absence of cardiovascular, respiratory, or neurologic complications
❒ normal fluid and electrolyte balance
❒ absence of infection
❒ absence or control of seizures
❒ absence of headaches.

TEACHING CHECKLIST
Document evidence that the patient and his family demonstrate an understanding of:
❒ extent of surgery
❒ extent of neurologic deficits, if any

❒ incision care
❒ no heavy lifting, exercising, straining, or driving
❒ with angioplasty, avoid vigorous neck manipulation or deep massage
❒ rehabilitation, if needed
❒ risk factors for atherosclerosis
❒ need for lifestyle modifications
❒ recommended dietary modifications
❒ lifestyle modification programs, such as stress management, cardiovascular fitness, weight loss, and smoking-cessation and alcohol rehabilitation programs, as needed
❒ community resources for lifestyle modification support
❒ all discharge medications' purpose, dosage, schedule, and adverse effects
❒ signs and symptoms to report to the health care provider after surgery
❒ signs and symptoms of impending stroke to report to the health care provider
❒ follow-up care.

DOCUMENTATION CHECKLIST

Using outcome criteria as a guide, document:

❐ clinical status on admission
❐ significant changes in status, especially regarding motor, sensory, or visual deficits or episodes of hypertension or hypotension
❐ wound condition
❐ pertinent laboratory and diagnostic test findings
❐ episodes of headaches or seizures
❐ respiratory support measures
❐ pain-relief measures
❐ nutritional status
❐ preoperative teaching
❐ patient and family teaching
❐ rehabilitation needs
❐ discharge planning.

Associated care plans

■ Acute myocardial infarction
■ Acute pain
■ Anxiety
■ Knowledge deficit
■ Geriatric care
■ Impaired physical mobility
■ Increased intracranial pressure
■ Ineffective individual coping
■ Mechanical ventilation
■ Perioperative care

References

Black, J.M., et al. *Medical-Surgical Nursing, Clinical Management for Positive Outcomes*, 6th ed. Philadelphia: W.B. Saunders Co., 2001.

Cundy, J.B. "Carotid Artery Stenosis and Endarterectomy," *AORN Journal* 75(2):310-24, February 2002.

Kirkpatrick, P.J. "Carotid Artery Disease: Should Angioplasty be Considered an Alternative to Open Carotid Surgery?" *Journal of Neurosurgical Anesthesiology* 13(3):270-73, July 2001.

Lewis, S.M., et al. *Medical-Surgical Nursing Assessment and Management of Clinical Problems*, 5th ed. St. Louis: Mosby–Year Book, Inc., 2000.

Phatouros, C.C., et al. "Carotid Artery Stent Placement for Atherosclerotic Disease: Rationale, Technique, and Current Status," *Radiology* 217(1):26-39, October 2000.

Urden, L.D., et al. *Thelan's Critical Care Nursing Diagnosis and Management*, 4th ed. St. Louis: Mosby–Year Book, Inc., 2002.

Femoral popliteal bypass

DRG INFORMATION
DRG 478 Other Vascular Procedures with Complication or Comorbidities (CC).
Mean LOS = 7.3 days
DRG 479 Other Vascular Procedures without CC.
Mean LOS = 3.5 days

Introduction
DEFINITION AND TIME FOCUS
Femoral popliteal bypass is one of several surgical revascularization techniques used to relieve symptoms of acute or chronic ischemia of the lower extremities. It involves using an autologous graft (usually the saphenous vein) or synthetic graft (polytetrafluoroethylene or Dacron) to route arterial blood from the femoral artery around a blocked popliteal artery, thus reestablishing blood flow in the tibial arteries. If revascularization fails, amputation is the treatment of last resort.

Femoral popliteal bypass may be the primary treatment or an adjunct to other revascularization techniques, such as angioplasty or intravascular stent placement. These newer, less-invasive approaches to revascularization are associated with problems characteristic of any evolving technology, such as unsuitable design, insufficient technical guidance, and operator inexperience. These new techniques also carry a higher reported incidence of rapid thrombus formation, vessel perforation, vessel dissection, and rapid reocclusion of the manipulated vessel.

This care plan focuses on postoperative care for the patient undergoing femoral popliteal bypass surgery. (See *Clinical snapshot: Femoral popliteal bypass*, page 406.)

ETIOLOGY AND PRECIPITATING FACTORS
Acute occlusion
- Traumatic transection or occlusion
- Disorders associated with embolus formation, such as endocarditis, aneurysms of the left ventricle or aorta, and atrial fibrillation
- Collagen diseases and vasospastic disorders such as thromboangiitis obliterans (Buerger's disease)
- Diagnostic procedures such as angiography
  (*Note:* Acute occlusion is usually treated with anticoagulants, antiplatelet agents, vasodilators, embolectomy, or plasty repairs. Femoral popliteal bypass may be used when these approaches fail or if the vessel is destroyed.)

Chronic occlusion
- Atherosclerosis, especially in a person older than age 60 with a coexisting vascular disorder
- Aneurysm of the popliteal artery
- Chronic infection
- Restenosis of previous grafts
  (*Note:* Chronic occlusion may present with signs and symptoms of long-term ischemia or with evidence of acute limb-threatening ischemia. A stenosis of 60% or greater will produce significant symptoms. The typical blockage ranges in length from $1\frac{1}{4}''$ to $9\frac{1}{4}''$ [3 cm to 23.5 cm].)

Focused assessment guidelines
NURSING HISTORY
(FUNCTIONAL HEALTH PATTERN FINDINGS)
Nutritional-metabolic pattern
- Obesity
- Type 1 or type 2 diabetes mellitus
- Adherence to a low-salt, low-cholesterol diet to control cardiovascular disease
- Severe nutritional deficit related to multisystem vascular insufficiency or advanced age

Elimination pattern
- Sudden onset of severe abdominal distress if ischemia is associated with multiple emboli and infarction of mesenteric vessels
- Symptoms of acute renal failure if ischemia is associated with multiple emboli and infarction of the renal or arcuate arteries
- Symptoms of chronic renal failure associated with hypertension and diabetes
- Neurosensory impairment of bowel function (constipation or diarrhea) associated with long-term diabetes
- Constipation associated with decreased physical activity
- Inability to perform activities of daily living (ADLs)

Activity-exercise pattern
- Sedentary lifestyle typical before onset of symptoms
- Limited mobility related to the onset of ischemic muscle pain with physical activity typically reported
- Leg muscle weakness associated with ischemic changes
- Sports- or work-related injury (dislocation of the knee)
- Fractures resulting from muscle weakness and sensory loss

- Inability to perform ADLs
- Unilateral or bilateral intermittent claudication

Sleep-rest pattern
- Sleep disturbance related to ischemic pain occurring at rest

Cognitive-perceptual pattern
- Low self-esteem as a result of inability to exercise or perform usual activities
- Depression
- History of stroke with residual neurologic damage

Role-relationship pattern
- Diminished social interaction related to inability to maintain usual activities
- History of chronic alcohol abuse
- Diminished cognitive abilities associated with previous stroke

Sexuality-reproductive pattern
- Decreased libido if diabetic
- Impotence, if diabetic male
- Developing symptoms after menopause, if female
- Atrophy of secondary sex characteristics, if age 60 or older
- Hormonal contraceptive use or the recent birth of a child (uncommon)

Coping–stress tolerance pattern
- History of cigarette smoking
- History of chronic alcohol abuse

PHYSICAL FINDINGS
Cardiovascular
- Hypertension
- Decreased or absent peripheral pulses
- Bruits over abdominal aorta, femoral artery, or popliteal artery
- Increased capillary refill time
- Dependent rubor or cyanosis
- Atrial fibrillation
- Ventricular, aortic, or popliteal aneurysm

Renal
- Chronic renal failure
- Acute renal failure

Pulmonary
- Symptoms of heart failure or chronic obstructive pulmonary disease

Gastrointestinal
- Diarrhea or constipation
- Paralytic ileus

Neurologic
- Decreased sensory perception (heat, cold, pressure, vibration, and pain) in affected extremities
- Decreased proprioception in affected extremities
- Altered cognitive function

Integumentary
- Thinning
- Hair loss

- Paresthesia
- Ulcerations that fail to heal
- Skin cool or cold to touch
- Gangrene

Musculoskeletal
- Weakness
- Atrophy

DIAGNOSTIC STUDIES
- Multiplane (retrograde femoral or translumbar) arteriography — visualizes abdominal aorta and vessels in the lower extremities
- Ultrasound Doppler and duplex waveform analyses — demonstrate direction and velocity of arterial flow
- ^{99m}Tc-hexametazime-labeled leukocyte imaging — radioactive scan, localizes infection in grafts from previous bypass procedures
- Ankle-brachial index (ABI) — noninvasive hemodynamic study, estimates the degree of arterial occlusion (a normal ABI is 1.0; single vessel occlusion, 0.5 to 1.0; multiple vessel occlusion, below 0.5)
- Toe-ankle index — noninvasive hemodynamic study, estimates degree of occlusion (normal toe-ankle index is above 0.65)
- Stress tests — estimate the degree of disease based on development of claudication
- Serum cholesterol — may be elevated if arterial occlusion is related to systemic vascular disease
- Serum triglycerides — may be elevated if symptoms are related to systemic vascular disease
- Blood glucose — may be elevated because diabetes mellitus is commonly associated with peripheral vascular disease
- Blood urea nitrogen — may be elevated if hypertension has affected renal function
- Liver function tests — may be altered in the patient with a history of alcohol abuse

POTENTIAL COMPLICATIONS
- Hematoma formation
- Infection
- Emboli or thrombi
- Gangrene
- Skin ulcers

CLINICAL SNAPSHOT ✳

Femoral popliteal bypass

Major nursing diagnoses and collaborative problems	Key patient outcomes
CP: Arterial insufficiency	Have bilaterally equal peripheral pulses.
ND: Impaired skin integrity	Display no signs of infection.
ND: Impaired physical mobility	Comply with activity restrictions.
ND: Acute pain	Report pain, if any (controlled by oral medications), as less than 3 on a 0 to 10 pain rating scale.

Collaborative problem

Arterial insufficiency related to arterial graft occlusion, reperfusion injury, or coexisting microangiopathy associated with diabetes or microemboli

NURSING PRIORITY
Maintain arterial flow.

PATIENT OUTCOME CRITERIA
Within 24 hours after surgery and then continuously, the patient will have:
- no ischemic pain
- bilaterally equal peripheral pulses.

INTERVENTIONS	RATIONALES
1. *Assess and document appearance of surgical site.** Include type of dressing, extent of drainage, and any drainage devices (such as a Hemovac).	1. Baseline assessment permits later comparison of data. A surgical drain may be in place to remove lymph or blood. Drainage should be minimal and bright red initially, becoming serous within 24 hours.
2. *Note the contours of the surgical site and compare with the opposite side.* Observe for masses, ecchymoses, and skin changes. Monitor hemoglobin levels and hematocrit.	2. Disruption of graft anastomosis, hemorrhage of soft tissues, or drainage from severed lymph vessels can produce enough fluid to occlude the graft. Fluid collection causes the skin at the site to become taut, with a dimpled appearance. A mass will be palpable. Surgical fluid removal is necessary if graft occlusion is imminent. Ecchymoses indicate arterial bleeding and possible disruption of the anastomoses. Decreased hemoglobin levels and hematocrit may indicate bleeding also.
3. *Measure calf circumference* hourly for the first 24 hours, then as condition warrants. Observe for increased capillary refill time; diminished or absent pulses; mild pain beginning in the feet and lateral to the tibia, progressing to pain unrelieved by narcotics; decreased range of motion (ROM) and ABI; or cold, cyanotic skin. Document findings.	3. These signs and symptoms suggest anterior compartment syndrome caused by tissue edema and hemorrhage. Emergency fasciotomy may be necessary to relieve signs and symptoms.
4. *Position the leg to avoid hyperextension and undue pressure on the graft site.*	4. Hyperextension of the knee or pressure from body weight can retard venous flow, increasing tissue edema. Pressure also can diminish arterial flow through the graft. The resulting thrombosis calls for an emergency embolectomy.

---

*Italics indicate key interventions.

5. *Observe for symptoms of deficient fluid volume or hypotension.* Document findings.

6. Administer ordered drugs and monitor for adverse reactions. If the antiplatelet medication will be continued after discharge, teach the patient about administration and possible adverse effects.

7. *Observe for signs and symptoms of reperfusion injury* (same as for severe hypoxia — cyanosis, coldness, and pain — with pulses still present). Maintain adequate hydration. If cyanosis, coldness, or pain occurs, check for presence of peripheral pulses using a Doppler waveform analysis. Notify the physician of findings promptly and administer treatment as ordered, typically mannitol (Osmitrol).

8. Additional individualized interventions: _____
_____

5. The patient is at greatest risk for shunt occlusion immediately after surgery. Factors that decrease blood pressure could cause shunt collapse.

6. Antiplatelet drugs, such as dipyridamole (Persantine), ticlopidine (Ticlid), and aspirin; and anticoagulant drugs, such as heparin and warfarin (Coumadin), are usually ordered. Urokinase (Abbokinase) or streptokinase (Streptase) may be used to reverse shunt occlusion. The patient is usually continued on antiplatelet therapy after discharge.

7. In reperfusion injury, reperfused tissues typically demonstrate initial improvement, only to undergo severe hypoxic changes within 2 hours after surgery. Reperfused cells produce high levels of free oxygen radicals, which injure cells. Adequate hydration lessens the risk of reperfusion injury. The presence of peripheral pulses differentiates arterial reocclusion (in which pulses are absent) from reperfusion injury. Mannitol helps control reperfusion injury by acting as a free-radical scavenger.

8. Rationales: _____
_____

Nursing diagnosis
Impaired skin integrity related to surgical incision and possible preexisting stasis ulcers

NURSING PRIORITIES
■ Promote wound healing.
■ Prevent infection.

PATIENT OUTCOME CRITERIA
By the time of discharge, the patient will:
■ demonstrate evidence of wound healing by primary intention
■ display no signs or symptoms of infection.

INTERVENTIONS

1. *Maintain strict sterile technique* in caring for the surgical wound, drains, and stasis ulcers of the feet and legs.

2. *Don't administer injections on the affected side.*

3. *Assess for signs and symptoms of infection:* fever, chills, malaise, increased pain at the surgical site, signs of arterial insufficiency distal to the site, incisional edema, drainage, and redness. Instruct the patient to observe for signs and symptoms of infection daily for 90 days after surgery.

4. *Administer antibiotics* and observe for adverse reactions.

RATIONALES

1. The arterial graft lies close to the skin surface. As a result, infection at the surgical site can extend quickly to the shunt. In addition, lymph channels are severed during surgery, so debris from infected stasis ulcers drains into the surgical site, fostering infection at the graft.

2. Edema, tissue swelling, and the severing of lymph channels all slow circulation on the affected side, resulting in unpredictable drug absorption.

3. Tissue hypoxia before surgery increases the risk of infection. Infection with shunt occlusion can occur as late as 90 days after surgery.

4. Antibiotics are prescribed routinely because the risk of infection with subsequent shunt loss is high.

5. *Reposition the patient and perform skin care every 2 hours.* Consider using a specialty bed or mattress for the patient with a chronic mobility problem, such as a multisystem disorder, obesity, or advanced age. Document your actions.

5. The skin, particularly on bony prominences, is prone to breakdown. Ulcers may already be present.

6. *Monitor and document fluid and food intake.*

6. Adequate hydration and nutrition are necessary for wound healing and prevention of skin breakdown.

7. Additional individualized interventions: _____
_____

7. Rationales: _____

Suggested NIC Interventions
Pressure management; Pressure ulcer care; Skin surveillance; Incision site care; Wound care

Suggested NOC Outcomes
Tissue integrity: Skin and mucous membranes; Wound healing: Primary intention; Wound healing: Secondary intention

---

Nursing diagnosis

Impaired physical mobility related to surgery and preexisting disability

NURSING PRIORITY

Help the patient return to highest level of self-care and mobility possible.

PATIENT OUTCOME CRITERIA

By the time of discharge, the patient will:
- demonstrate no complications associated with immobility
- demonstrate improved mobility
- verbalize an understanding of the prescribed treatment regimen
- comply with activity restrictions.

INTERVENTIONS

1. *Before surgery, instruct the patient about positioning the affected extremity:* avoiding hyperextension of the knee, leg-crossing, any position that puts pressure on the popliteal space, sitting for more than 20 minutes, or wearing clothing that restricts arterial flow.

2. *After surgery, maintain the patient on bed rest as ordered,* usually for 24 to 48 hours. Position the affected joint as ordered.

3. *Encourage active ROM exercises of all unaffected joints* 3 to 4 times daily or, if the patient is unable, perform passive ROM exercises.

4. Collaborate with the health care team to design an appropriate rehabilitation program. Instruct the patient accordingly.

5. Additional individualized interventions: _____
_____

RATIONALES

1. Preoperative teaching helps the patient avoid positions that could cause shunt occlusion.

2. Bed rest is usually maintained until shunt patency is ensured. Positioning depends on the type of surgery.

3. Exercise maintains joint flexibility and prevents postoperative complications associated with bed rest.

4. Extensive reconditioning may be necessary for the patient with long-term hypoxic injury to muscles and nerves or a history of myocardial infarction or stroke. Patient compliance with the rehabilitation regimen depends on an understanding of the prescribed treatment.

5. Rationales: _____
_____

Suggested NIC Interventions
Exercise therapy: Ambulation; Exercise therapy: Balance; Exercise therapy: Joint mobility; Exercise therapy: Muscle control; Exercise promotion: Strength training

Suggested NOC Outcomes
Ambulation: Walking; Ambulation: Wheelchair; Joint movement: Active; Mobility level

---

Nursing diagnosis
Acute pain related to the surgical incision

NURSING PRIORITY
Control pain.

PATIENT OUTCOME CRITERION
Upon discharge, the patient will report pain (controlled with oral medication) as less than 3 on a 0 to 10 pain rating scale.

INTERVENTIONS	RATIONALES
1. *See the "Acute pain" care plan,* page 32.	**1.** General interventions for pain control are detailed in the "Acute pain" care plan.
2. *Identify and document the source and degree of pain,* using a pain rating scale. Instruct the patient to report unrelieved pain.	**2.** Prolonged or increasing pain could indicate hematoma or seroma formation at the surgical site. Unrelieved pain distal to the surgical site indicates anterior compartment syndrome, described under "Arterial insufficiency," page 406, or shunt occlusion.
3. *Elevate the affected extremity.*	**3.** Moderate elevation, so as to not impair arterial flow, helps decrease tissue edema and swelling associated with surgical trauma.
4. *Administer pain medication, as necessary, and observe for adverse reactions.*	**4.** Narcotic analgesics are used judiciously in the early postoperative period.
5. Additional individualized interventions: _____	**5.** Rationales: _____

Suggested NIC Interventions
Pain management

Suggested NOC Outcomes
Pain; Psychological response

Discharge planning
DISCHARGE CHECKLIST
Before discharge, the patient shows evidence of:
❑ wound healing
❑ vital signs within normal limits for age and coexisting disorders
❑ absence of infection
❑ shunt patency
❑ absence of or minimal reports of pain
❑ restored arterial flow.

TEACHING CHECKLIST
Document evidence that the patient and his family demonstrate an understanding of:
❑ medication regimen
❑ proper positioning
❑ desirable lifestyle changes such as smoking cessation
❑ rehabilitation regimen
❑ dates and times of follow-up care
❑ symptoms of infection
❑ symptoms of arterial insufficiency
❑ symptoms requiring medical intervention.

DOCUMENTATION CHECKLIST

Using outcome criteria as a guide, document:

❏ clinical status on admission
❏ significant changes in the preoperative state
❏ completion of preoperative checklist
❏ preoperative teaching
❏ clinical status on admission from postanesthesia unit
❏ amount and character of drainage from wounds or drains
❏ tube patency
❏ pain-relief measures
❏ activity tolerance
❏ nutritional intake
❏ elimination status
❏ pertinent laboratory findings
❏ patient and family teaching
❏ discharge planning
❏ clinical status upon discharge.

Associated care plans

▪ Acute pain
▪ Amputation
▪ Perioperative care

References

Brewster, D. "Evaluation of Arterial Insufficiency of the Lower Extremities," *Primary Care Medicine.* Philadelphia: Lippincott Williams & Wilkins, 2002.

DeFrang, R.D., et al. "Repeat Leg Bypass After Multiple Prior Bypass Failures," *Journal of Vascular Surgery* 19(2):268-76, February 1994.

Desgranges, P., et al. "Acute Occlusion of Popliteal and/or Tibial Arteries: The Value of Percutaneous Treatment," *European Journal Vascular & Endovascular Surgery* 20(2):138-45, August 2000.

Scott, M. Graft Type for Femoro-Popliteal Bypass Surgery, *www.update-software.com/abstracts/ab001487.htm*.

Heart failure

DRG INFORMATION

DRG 127   Heart Failure and Shock.
         Mean LOS = 5.3 days
DRG 127 is one of the most prevalent DRGs in the United States; however, heart failure frequently accompanies other diagnoses, particularly other cardiovascular diagnoses. In these instances, one of the other diagnoses is likely to be the principal diagnosis.

Introduction

DEFINITION AND TIME FOCUS

Heart failure is the end result of several disease states in which cardiac output fails to meet the body's metabolic demands, resulting in pulmonary and systemic congestion. Inadequate cardiac output stimulates the sympathetic nervous system, resulting in increased heart rate, myocardial contractility, vasoconstriction, and salt and water retention. Cardiac and peripheral oxygen demands also increase. If the underlying problem can't be corrected, these compensatory mechanisms lead to progressive fluid retention and further deterioration of cardiac efficiency. This care plan focuses on the care of the patient admitted for treatment of an acute exacerbation of chronic heart failure or treatment of heart failure resulting from an acute event (such as acute myocardial infarction [AMI]). (See *Clinical snapshot: Heart failure,* page 413.)

ETIOLOGY AND PRECIPITATING FACTORS

■ Conditions that reduce myocardial *contractility,* such as cardiomyopathies, ischemic cardiac disease, ventricular aneurysms, or constrictive pericarditis
■ Conditions that increase fluid volume and lead to circulatory overload (increased preload), such as too-rapid infusion of I.V. fluids, increased sodium intake, or inadequate diuretic therapy
■ Conditions that alter cardiac rhythm, such as severe bradycardia in the presence of decreased contractility or tachycardia severe enough to decrease cardiac filling time and diminish cardiac output
■ Conditions that increase resistance to blood flow out of the heart (increased afterload), such as arteriosclerotic heart disease, hypertensive heart disease, or pulmonary hypertension
■ Conditions that interfere with blood flow through the heart such as valvular insufficiency or stenosis
■ Conditions that increase oxygen demands beyond the heart's capabilities, such as hyperthyroidism, fever, pregnancy, or anemia

Focused assessment guidelines

NURSING HISTORY (FUNCTIONAL HEALTH PATTERN FINDINGS)

Health-perception–health-management pattern
■ Long-term treatment for heart failure or a precipitating disease such as hypertensive heart disease
■ No experience with signs and symptoms if episode occurs in response to an acute event such as an AMI
■ Noncompliance with prescribed diet, medications, or activity restrictions
■ Peripheral edema or fatigue (common)

Nutritional-metabolic pattern
■ Anorexia (common); occasionally, nausea or vomiting from congested peripheral circulation or from medication adverse effects
■ Weight loss and cachexia from decreased calorie intake and poor nutrient absorption

Elimination pattern
■ Altered urinary patterns (from diuretic treatment or decreased renal blood flow)
■ Constipation (from edema of the GI tract)

Activity-exercise pattern
■ Inability to participate in exercise or leisure activities (common)
■ Difficulty participating in activities of daily living (ADLs) because of fatigue or shortness of breath

Sleep-rest pattern
■ Disturbed sleep patterns from dyspnea and nocturia (common)
■ Use of 2 or 3 pillows during sleep because of orthopnea (common)
■ Paroxysmal nocturnal dyspnea

Cognitive-perceptual pattern
■ Failure to understand problem and treatment protocols (if heart failure is an acute event)
■ Headaches, confusion, or memory impairment

Self-perception–self-concept pattern
■ Body image disturbances related to edema and decreased activity level

Role-relationship pattern
■ Difficulty fulfilling role responsibilities because of fatigue, weakness, or decreased activity tolerance (common)

Sexuality-reproductive pattern
■ Decreased libido and impotence or orgasmic dysfunction related to fatigue or medications

Coping–stress tolerance pattern
■ Anxiety related to shortness of breath
■ Anxiety related to chronic illness

- Grief over loss of former level of health and loss of former roles and function
- Anticipation of premature death

PHYSICAL FINDINGS
Cardiovascular
- Tachycardia
- S_3
- S_4 with summation gallop (with tachycardia)
- Atrial and ventricular arrhythmias
- Jugular vein distention
- Systolic murmur (in advanced heart failure)
- Decreased peripheral pulses
Pulmonary
- Dyspnea
- Crackles
- Nonproductive cough
- Progressive bilateral diminishing of breath sounds, beginning at bases
Neurologic
- Increased irritability
- Impaired memory
- Confusion (rare)
Gastrointestinal
- Abdominal distention
- Vomiting
- Tenderness over liver
- Liver enlargement
Renal
- Decreased urine output
Integumentary
- Dependent edema such as in feet and sacrum
- Cyanosis
- Clubbing of fingers (in chronic heart failure)
Musculoskeletal
- Weakness and easy fatigability
- Muscle wasting (rare)

DIAGNOSTIC STUDIES
- Serum electrolyte levels — electrolyte imbalances may occur from fluid shifts, diuretic therapy, or response of organ systems to decreased oxygen and increased congestion
 – Hyponatremia: volume overload causes dilutional hyponatremia; sodium restriction and diuretics may also lead to low serum sodium level
 – Hypokalemia: most commonly used diuretics cause potassium loss
 – Hyperkalemia: can occur with oliguria or anuria or excess potassium replacement
- Arterial blood gas (ABG) measurements
 – Lowered partial pressure of arterial oxygen related to pulmonary congestion
 – Elevated partial pressure of arterial carbon dioxide (respiratory acidosis) may be from pulmonary edema or hypoventilation

- Prothrombin time/international normalized ratio (PT/INR), partial thromboplastin time (PTT) — obtained to determine baseline before beginning anticoagulant therapy or to evaluate clotting status during anticoagulant therapy
- Blood urea nitrogen (BUN) and creatinine levels — elevated, reflecting decreased renal function
- Bilirubin, aspartate aminotransferase, lactate dehydrogenase levels — elevated, indicating decreased liver function
- Urinalysis — reveals proteinuria and elevated specific gravity
- Chest X-ray — may reveal enlarged cardiac silhouette (common), distended pulmonary veins from redistribution of pulmonary blood flow, and interstitial and alveolar edema (common)
- Electrocardiogram — nonspecific diagnostically, but useful in identifying rhythm disturbances, conduction defects, axis deviations, and hypertrophy
- Echocardiography — can identify valvular abnormalities, chamber enlargement, abnormal wall motion, hypertrophy, pericardial effusion, and mural thrombi
- Multigated blood pool imaging scan — demonstrates decreased ejection fraction and abnormal wall motion

POTENTIAL COMPLICATIONS
- Cardiogenic shock
- Pulmonary edema
- AMI
- Arrhythmias
- Thrombolytic complications
- Renal failure
- Liver failure

CLINICAL SNAPSHOT ✳

Heart failure

Major nursing diagnoses	Key patient outcomes
Decreased cardiac output	Display signs of normal cardiac output.
Excess fluid volume	Have fluid intake and output in approximate balance.
Activity intolerance	Perform ADLs independently.
Imbalanced nutrition: Less than body requirements	Meet daily calorie requirements.
Deficient knowledge (treatment regimen)	Give name, purpose, dosage, schedule, and possible adverse effects for all discharge medications.
Ineffective therapeutic regimen management	Identify areas of potential ineffective management.

Nursing diagnosis

Decreased cardiac output related to decreased contractility, altered heart rhythm, fluid volume overload, or increased afterload

NURSING PRIORITY

Maintain optimum cardiac output.

PATIENT OUTCOME CRITERIA

By the time of discharge, the patient will:
- exhibit heart rate under 100 beats/minute
- exhibit optimal cardiac output, as manifested by capillary refill time of less than 3 seconds, minimal or absent peripheral edema, normal peripheral pulses, and warm, dry skin
- have no S_3
- have stable cardiac rhythm with any life-threatening arrhythmias under control
- have lungs clear to auscultation
- perform ADLs without incapacitating dyspnea
- have mental status within normal limits.

INTERVENTIONS

1. *Monitor and document cardiovascular status:** heart rate and rhythm, heart sounds, blood pressure, pulse pressure, and the presence or absence of peripheral pulses. Compare to the baseline assessment. Report abnormalities to the physician, particularly tachycardia, a new S_3 heart sound or systolic murmur, hypotension, decreased pulse pressure or pulse loss, or increased arrhythmias.

2. *Administer cardiac medications, as ordered,* and document the patient's response. Observe for therapeutic and adverse effects:

RATIONALES

1. One of the earliest signs of worsening heart failure is increased heart rate. A new S_3 heart sound or a systolic murmur may reflect increased fluid volume, leading to increased cardiac congestion and failure. Hypotension can reflect decreased cardiac output from impaired myocardial contractility or overdiuresis. Diminished pulse pressure or peripheral pulse loss can indicate a decrease in cardiac output. Increased arrhythmias can reflect an increased number of premature atrial or ventricular contractions — signs of increasing failure or medication toxicity.

2. Pharmacotherapeutic agents may relieve heart failure by altering preload, contractility, or afterload — major determinants of cardiac output. However, many of these agents have narrow therapeutic ranges or adverse effects that can worsen the underlying disease.

*Italics indicate key interventions.

– Angiotensin-converting enzyme (ACE) inhibitors, such as captopril (Capoten) and enalapril (Vasotec), and angiotensin II receptor antagonists, such as losartan (Cozaar), monitor for hypotension, hyperkalemia, and cough.

– The renin-angiotensin-aldosterone system is activated by low cardiac output and decreased renal blood flow. Stimulation of the system results in the production of angiotensin II (a vasoconstrictor) and contributes to sympathetic nervous system stimulation and aldosterone production. The physiologic result of these substances is increased renal sodium retention and fluid retention. ACE inhibitors are the foundation of medical treatment for heart failure and relieve symptoms, improve exercise capacity, and reduce mortality.

– Inotropic agents (cardiac glycoside derivatives) monitor for anorexia, pulse rate less than or above 100 beats/minute, irregular heart rate, nausea, vomiting, and vision disturbances. Withhold the dose and contact the physician if these signs or symptoms occur.

– Inotropic agents increase contractility, but can also increase myocardial oxygen consumption and cardiac workload, increasing heart failure. Cardiac glycosides, one of the most common medications used, have a narrow therapeutic range. (Therapeutic range via immunoassay is 0.5 to 2.0 ng/ml.) Early toxic adverse effects include anorexia; later, severe bradyarrhythmias, tachyarrhythmias, and irregular cardiac rhythms can compromise cardiac output. Cardiac glycoside toxicity is more common in patients with compromised renal function and in the elderly.

– Diuretics, such as hydrochlorothiazide (Esidrix) and furosemide (Lasix), monitor for hypovolemia and hypokalemia. (See appendix C, Fluid and electrolyte imbalances for details.)

– Diuretics decrease preload, but can cause true hypovolemia from excessive fluid loss or hypokalemia from potassium loss.

– Nitrates, such as isosorbide dinitrate (Isordil), monitor for signs of hypovolemia.

– Nitrates cause venodilation, reducing preload but also increasing the risk of relative hypovolemia from redistribution of blood volume to the periphery.

– Afterload reducers (vasodilators), such as hydralazine (Apresoline), monitor for hypotension.

– Afterload reducers lower resistance to ventricular ejection, but may lower blood pressure enough to compromise organ perfusion.

3. *Observe for signs and symptoms of hypoxemia,* such as confusion, restlessness, dyspnea, arrhythmias, tachycardia, and cyanosis. Ensure adequate oxygenation with proper positioning (semi-Fowler's or upright) and supplemental oxygen, as ordered.

3. Prompt detection of hypoxemia allows timely intervention. The semi-Fowler's position prevents abdominal organs from pressing on the diaphragm and interfering with its movement. An upright position permits a severely dyspneic patient to use accessory muscles for breathing; it also redistributes blood to dependent areas, decreasing blood return to the heart and reducing preload in a patient with volume overload. A patient who has difficulty maintaining an arterial oxygen level above 60 mm Hg may benefit from supplemental oxygen.

4. *Ensure adequate rest* by monitoring the noise level, limiting visitors, grouping diagnostic tests (such as by ordering multiple blood tests on one blood sample, when possible), and spacing therapeutic interventions.

4. Rest reduces myocardial oxygen consumption.

5. *Monitor fluid status:* Obtain accurate daily weight.

5. Fluid volume may be increased from the heart's inability to maintain adequate flow and pressure through the kidneys.
– Rapid weight gain (1 to 2 lb [0.5 to 1 kg] a day) indicates fluid retention and the need for increased diuresis.
– Maintain an accurate intake and output record.
– Assess the lungs for crackles, decreased sounds, and a change from vesicular to bronchial breath sounds.
– Assess for dependent edema and increasing dyspnea.

– Assess for signs of dehydration.
– Accurate intake and output records can warn of early fluid excess.
– Crackles, decreased sounds, and bronchial breath sounds indicate fluid in the lungs and signal increasing left-sided heart failure.
– Dependent edema and dyspnea are signs of increasing right-sided and left-sided heart failure, respectively.
– Fluid volume may be decreased from excessive diuresis.

6. *Assess for increasing confusion.*

6. When cardiac output is decreased, cerebral perfusion suffers, producing confusion.

7. Decrease the patient's fear and anxiety by providing information and by eliciting concerns and responding to them. See the "Ineffective individual coping" care plan, page 124, for details.

7. Fear and anxiety activate the sympathetic nervous system and increase heart rate, myocardial contractility, and vasoconstriction. All these factors increase myocardial oxygen consumption. The "Ineffective individual coping" care plan contains general interventions to reduce anxiety.

8. Additional individualized interventions: _____

8. Rationales: _____

Suggested NIC Interventions
Cardiac care; Cardiac care: Acute; Hemodynamic regulation; Shock management: Cardiac; Circulatory care: Arterial insufficiency; Circulatory care: Mechanical assist device; Circulatory care: Venous insufficiency; Intravenous (I.V.) therapy; Embolus care: Peripheral; Vital signs monitoring

Suggested NOC Outcomes
Cardiac pump effectiveness; Circulation status; Tissue perfusion: Abdominal organs; Tissue perfusion: Peripheral; Vital signs status

---

Nursing diagnosis

Excess fluid volume related to decreased myocardial contractility, decreased renal perfusion, and increased sodium and water retention

NURSING PRIORITY

Optimize and monitor volume status and electrolyte balance.

PATIENT OUTCOME CRITERIA

By the time of discharge, the patient will:
- have fluid intake and output in approximate balance
- exhibit sodium, potassium, creatinine, and BUN levels within expected parameters.

INTERVENTIONS

1. *See appendix C, Fluid and electrolyte imbalances.*

2. *Monitor fluid balance:* hourly fluid intake and output and 24-hour fluid balance. Weigh the patient daily.

RATIONALES

1. The Fluid and electrolyte imbalances appendix describes the causes, signs and symptoms, laboratory findings, and treatments of these disorders.

2. Intake and output monitoring provides an objective method of tracking fluid gains or losses, while 24-hour summaries indicate net fluid balance. Daily weight measurements are a rough measure of fluid status; a weight change of 2.2 lb (1 kg) corresponds with a 1 L change in fluid balance.

3. *Administer I.V. solutions, as ordered.* Avoid saline solutions.

3. The type and amount of I.V. fluid ordered depends upon the patient's current condition and the cause of heart failure. Saline solutions can cause water retention.

4. *Implement fluid restriction if ordered:*
– explain the rationale to the patient and his family

4. Fluid restriction helps limit excessive preload.
– The patient and his family are more likely to comply with fluid restriction if they understand the reasons behind it. Thirst is a powerful need, and restricting fluids may cause the patient to feel deprived or punished. Explaining the rationale may help him view the situation positively.
– Regular fluid intake, consistent measurements, and use of microdrip tubing or infusion devices help ensure maintenance of fluid restrictions.

– establish a fluid intake schedule, teach the patient how to record oral fluids, and use microdrip tubing or an infusion pump to control I.V. intake.

5. *Monitor BUN and creatinine level* and report increasing values.

5. BUN and creatinine levels reflect decreased renal perfusion from worsening heart failure. The BUN level rises disproportionately; the BUN-creatinine level ratio can increase from the normal of 10:1 to as high as 40:1.

6. *Monitor sodium and potassium levels.* Report abnormal values and signs of imbalances.

6. Hyponatremia can cause decreased blood pressure, confusion, headache, and seizures; hypokalemia, weakness, fatigue, ileus, and ventricular fibrillation; and hyperkalemia, bradycardia, and ventricular asystole.

7. Additional individualized interventions: _____

7. Rationales: _____

Suggested NIC Interventions
Tissue perfusion management: Fluid management; Fluid monitoring; Hemodynamic regulation

Suggested NOC Outcomes
Fluid balance; Hydration

Nursing diagnosis

Activity intolerance related to bed rest and decreased cardiac output

NURSING PRIORITIES
■ Prevent complications of bed rest.
■ Increase activity level without exceeding cardiac energy reserves.

PATIENT OUTCOME CRITERIA
By the time of discharge, the patient will:
■ exhibit no evidence of thrombophlebitis or pulmonary embolism
■ maintain a normal bowel pattern
■ perform ADLs (feeding, bathing, and dressing) independently, with no significant change in heart rate or blood pressure
■ walk in hall with no significant change in heart rate and blood pressure and no complaints of chest pain or profound fatigue.

INTERVENTIONS

1. *Determine cardiac stability* by evaluating blood pressure, heart rhythm and rate, and indicators of oxygenation, such as level of consciousness (LOC) and skin color.

RATIONALES

1. Activity increases myocardial contractility, heart rate, blood pressure, and myocardial oxygen consumption. If cardiac output is already compromised (as in tachycardia or severe arrhythmias), activity will reduce it further.

2. *When the patient is stable, institute a graduated activity program* according to unit protocol. Begin with regular position changes and range-of-motion (ROM) exercises during bed rest. Then, as tolerated, progress to active ROM exercises, chair sitting, and ambulation.

2. Bed rest has many detrimental effects, including cardiac deconditioning, increased risk of atelectasis and pneumonia, and skin breakdown. It also promotes venous stasis, further increasing the risk of thromboembolism from depressed myocardial contractility and atrial fibrillation — an arrhythmia common in heart failure because of atrial distention. Position changes and exercises that involve a change in muscle length (such as active or passive limb flexion) improve peripheral circulation and reduce the risks associated with immobility.

3. *Evaluate patient tolerance to new activities.* Monitor blood pressure and pulse; respiratory rate, pattern, and depth; LOC and coordination; and patient reports of energy and strength. Discontinue activity, and resume it later at a slower pace, if any of the following occur:
– pulse rate greater than 30 beats/minute above resting level (or greater than 15 beats/minute if taking beta-adrenergic blockers)
– systolic blood pressure 15 mm Hg or more below resting level
– diastolic blood pressure 10 mm Hg or more above resting level
– new or increased pulse irregularity
– dyspnea, slowed respiratory rate, or shallow respirations
– decreased LOC or loss of coordination
– chest or leg pain
– fatigue disproportionate to activity level
– profound weakness.

3. A too-rapid activity increase can exacerbate heart failure, myocardial ischemia, or peripheral vascular insufficiency. It also may cause hypotension, syncope, or cardiovascular collapse. At the least, activity goals that exceed the patient's capabilities may cause a psychological setback.

4. *Alternate activity with rest periods.*

4. Bed rest and inactivity cause cardiac and muscle deconditioning. Initially, even short periods of activity can induce symptoms of cardiac compromise. Regular rest prevents depletion of cardiac reserves.

5. *Administer anticoagulants, as ordered.* Monitor appropriate coagulation studies and report results that exceed set limits.

5. Heparin inactivates thrombin, preventing fibrin clot formation. Warfarin (Coumadin) interferes with vitamin K production, decreasing synthesis of several clotting factors. The therapeutic PT and PTT should be $1\frac{1}{2}$ to 2 times normal. The therapeutic level of INR depends on why the patient is taking warfarin and other risk factors. To prevent deep vein thrombosis, the therapeutic range of INR is 2.0 to 3.0.

6. *Teach the patient how to avoid Valsalva's maneuver* (forced expiration against a closed glottis), such as by exhaling when changing position, and to increase fiber intake to promote bowel elimination.

6. Valsalva's maneuver increases intrathoracic pressure and decreases blood return to the heart. When the breath is released, venous return increases by reflex. Valsalva's maneuver has been associated with syncope and premature ventricular contractions.

7. Additional individualized interventions: _____

7. Rationales: _____

Nursing diagnosis

Imbalanced nutrition: Less than body requirements related to decreased appetite and unpalatability of low-sodium diet

NURSING PRIORITY

Ensure adequate intake of nutrients needed for healing and increased energy requirements.

PATIENT OUTCOME CRITERION

By the time of discharge, the patient will meet daily calorie requirements.

INTERVENTIONS	RATIONALES
1. *Consult the "Nutritional deficit" care plan,* page 138. Keep a daily record to monitor calorie intake. Consult with the dietitian to identify the patient's calorie needs.	**1.** The "Nutritional deficit" care plan contains detailed information on assessing and meeting a patient's nutritional needs. Calorie needs vary with the patient's illness stage, activity level, and weight.
2. *Assess the patient's food preferences,* and honor them when appropriate.	**2.** A low-sodium diet reduces cardiac preload by decreasing water retention. Unfortunately, low-sodium diets may be unpalatable to the patient accustomed to seasoned foods. The patient may be more compliant if food preferences are considered whenever possible.
3. Additional individualized interventions: _____ _____	**3.** Rationales: _____ _____

Nursing diagnosis

Deficient knowledge (treatment regimen) related to lack of exposure to information

NURSING PRIORITY

Prepare the patient to implement necessary lifestyle modifications to prevent recurrent episodes of heart failure, if possible.

PATIENT OUTCOME CRITERIA

By the time of discharge, the patient will:
- state intent to follow dietary recommendations
- demonstrate correct method for measuring pulse rate
- list five signs or symptoms of activity intolerance, on request

- give name, purpose, dosage, schedule, and possible adverse effects for all discharge medications
- verbalize understanding of when to seek emergency medical care
- have made first appointment for follow-up care
- verbalize understanding of daily weight measurement and weight gain requiring notification of the physician.

INTERVENTIONS	RATIONALES
1. *After the patient is stable, institute a structured teaching plan* only as the condition allows. See the "Knowledge deficit" care plan, page 129, for details.	**1.** The acutely ill patient usually is unable to tolerate sustained teaching. Planned teaching is more efficient and effective than haphazard instruction. The "Knowledge deficit" care plan describes assessing readiness to learn and selecting teaching methods.
2. *Briefly explain the pathophysiology of heart failure.* Relate the explanation to the patient's signs and symptoms.	**2.** Although extensive teaching should be deferred until the patient is stable, a brief explanation may help the patient understand the rationales for therapy. An adult learns best when the information relates directly to personal experience. Relevant information is helpful, but excessive detail can overwhelm and confuse him.
3. *Emphasize the patient's role in controlling the disease and the importance of medical follow-up.*	**3.** Heart failure commonly becomes chronic or recurrent. The patient's active participation in implementing and monitoring treatment can be instrumental in limiting the disease's progression.
4. *With the dietitian, instruct the patient and his family about the prescribed diet,* which is usually low in sodium, fat, cholesterol, and (if the patient is overweight) calories. Explain the rationale for such dietary restrictions as reducing sodium intake. Provide a list of high-sodium foods to avoid and suggest alternatives to salt such as seasoning foods with lemon juice and herbs. Recommend low-sodium cookbooks. Stress the importance of family support in making the necessary lifestyle changes.	**4.** Many of the therapies for chronic or recurrent heart failure involve lifestyle modifications, such as a low-sodium diet, that may affect other family members. Other changes may involve habits the patient finds pleasurable such as smoking. In either case, family support can smooth the transition to a more healthful lifestyle. Successful management of heart failure requires lifelong lifestyle modifications — changing eating habits is one of the most difficult. Understanding the reason for restrictions may help motivate the patient to establish and maintain the prescribed diet.
5. *Explain the rationale for activity restrictions.* Provide specific information about recommended activities. Teach the patient to monitor activity tolerance by measuring his pulse rate before and after activity and by watching for symptoms of overexertion. (See "Activity intolerance," page 416, for details.)	**5.** Vague instructions to "take it easy" leave the patient confused and may impair adjustment to an altered lifestyle. Providing information specific to the patient's condition lessens uncertainty and facilitates adjustment to recommended activity levels.
6. *Teach about discharge medications* — typically ACE inhibitors, inotropic agents, diuretics, vasodilators, or anticoagulants. Provide information sheets, and review the medications' purpose, dosage, schedule, adverse effects, and toxic effects. Stress the importance of taking doses on time. Suggest labeling a pillbox with days and times for doses.	**6.** Successful heart failure management typically involves a long-term, complex drug regimen. Information about these medications better equips the patient and his family to manage therapy at home. Understanding the drugs' purpose may increase the patient's motivation to take them; understanding dosage may increase accuracy. A properly labeled pillbox may decrease confusion and improve compliance.

7. *Emphasize the importance of self-monitoring for signs and symptoms of increasing heart failure,* such as ankle or leg swelling, breathlessness, tachycardia, and new or increased pulse irregularity. Teach the patient about the importance of measuring his weight daily on the same scale at the same time of day. Instruct him to contact the physician based on specified weight parameters, such as when a 2-lb (1-kg) or greater weight gain occurs in 1 day or when a 4-lb (2-kg) weight gain occurs over 1 week.

7. An alert, informed patient and family are the first line of defense against recurrence or aggravation of heart failure. Knowing what to observe for and what measures to take increases the likelihood that the patient will receive prompt treatment. Early detection of increasing heart failure allows prompt adjustment of the therapeutic regimen. The patient is best able to identify subtle physiologic changes.

8. *Discuss with the patient and his family an emergency plan,* if needed, including:
– a medical alert bracelet
– circumstances that warrant emergency medical care, such as severe chest pain, marked difficulty breathing, and cessation of breathing
– access to emergency care
– cardiopulmonary resuscitation classes for the family.

8. The patient with heart failure is at increased risk for other cardiovascular complications, such as AMI or cardiac arrest. Planning increases the likelihood of prompt, appropriate action in an emergency.

9. *Review the plan for follow-up care* — the physician's name and telephone number and the date, time, and location of the next appointment.

9. Management of heart failure requires consistent follow-up care.

10. Additional individualized interventions: _____

10. Rationales: _____

Suggested NIC Interventions
Teaching: Procedure/treatment

Suggested NOC Outcomes
Knowledge: Treatment regimen

Nursing diagnosis

Ineffective therapeutic regimen management related to health beliefs, a negative relationship with caregivers, or the complexity of the regimen

NURSING PRIORITY

Maximize likelihood of effective management.

PATIENT OUTCOME CRITERIA

Within 2 days of admission, the patient will:
- identify areas of potential ineffective management
- identify reasons for potential ineffective management
- verbalize willingness and ability to follow modified therapeutic plan, when possible.

INTERVENTIONS

1. *Observe for indicators of ineffective management,* such as exacerbation of signs and symptoms, development of complications, failure to keep follow-up appointments, reports of behavior contrary to health recommendations, failure to seek health care when indicated, despairing remarks about health status, or belligerent exchanges with caregivers.

RATIONALES

1. Ineffective management can have serious repercussions. Early identification of a problem increases the likelihood of its successful resolution.

2. *Evaluate the extent and result of ineffective management.*

2. If ineffective management is limited to areas of minor consequence in the overall care plan, no further action may be necessary.

3. Differentiate possible causes of ineffective management, such as knowledge deficit, lack of family support, memory deficits, adverse effects of treatment, transportation difficulties, denial, poor self-esteem, or self-destructive behavior. Consult the "Ineffective individual coping" care plan, page 124, and the "Knowledge deficit" care plan, page 129, for possible interventions. Take appropriate steps, such as providing information or making necessary referrals, as indicated.

3. Identifying problems accurately increases the likelihood of appropriate intervention and resolution.

4. *Initiate discussion of the situation with the patient and family,* involving a psychiatric clinician or other health care team members as needed.

4. Open discussion can help reveal the reasons for ineffective management. The patient, his family, and health care team members all can contribute insights and observations helpful in reevaluating the care plan.

5. Express concern for the patient as a person.

5. Expression of human caring and warmth may help break a cycle of negativity, if present, and free emotional energy for improved self-care. Nurturing behavior also may help establish rapport and trust.

6. *Emphasize the seriousness of heart failure and the importance of self-care.* Use the patient's situation to explain how ineffective management affects health, and emphasize the positive outcomes of effective management.

6. Failure to accept an illness's seriousness can be linked to ineffective management. Discussion that incorporates the patient's experiences is most effective in making points "come alive."

7. *Discuss possible influencing factors with the patient:*
– life priorities
– perception of prognosis
– feelings about the illness's duration
– complexity of treatment
– degree of confidence in caregivers
– health care beliefs.

7. Apparent deliberate ineffective management may actually reflect preoccupation with more pressing needs, such as food and shelter. The patient's perception of expected outcomes may be overly pessimistic. Prolonged illness, complex treatment, lack of confidence in caregivers, and health care beliefs that differ from caregivers' beliefs increase the likelihood of ineffective management.

8. Consider the patient's cultural and spiritual heritage.

8. The patient is less likely to accept treatment that clashes with cultural or spiritual beliefs.

9. Ask the patient about satisfaction with caregivers. Also, examine caregivers' attitudes: if nontherapeutic, either help establish more positive attitudes or assign other caregivers to the patient.

9. The patient's level of dissatisfaction with caregivers influences management of the therapeutic regimen. A caregiver's negative attitude that results from frustration may be changed through expression and peer support. A negative attitude that results from burnout or personality clashes, however, may be best handled by removing the caregiver from the situation.

10. Validate conclusions about reasons for behavior with the patient and his family.

10. Obtaining feedback about the accuracy of conclusions helps avoid erroneous assumptions and inappropriate interventions.

11. Collaborate with other caregivers to reevaluate the goals and implementation of care. Consider possible modifications.

11. Insisting on a plan to which the patient objects may create a power struggle between the patient and caregivers. Flexibility and adaptability are more likely to achieve the desired ends.

12. Search for alternative solutions. Ask what the patient wants or is willing to do to bring about agreement to the care plan.

12. Focusing on what the patient wants or is willing to do interrupts negativism and recasts the situation in a positive light. Such refocusing may free energy for creative problem solving and increase the patient's sense of control.

13. Use creative negotiation strategies to set goals with the patient. Consider changing the agreement's scope, shortening its length, or making trade-offs.

13. If full agreement isn't possible, partial or temporary agreement may be. The patient may be willing to trade compliance in one area (such as medications) for greater freedom in another (such as food intake).

14. Maintain open communication if the patient makes an informed choice not to follow the recommendations. If negotiation isn't possible:
– avoid punitive responses and accept the decision

14. Patients have the right of self-determination.

– keep open the option for treatment

– respect the patient's readiness to die.

– Exhibiting rejecting or other punitive behavior is disrespectful and may provoke the patient to terminate contact with health care resources.
– As the patient's condition changes, resistance may soften.
– Every person has the right to die with dignity. The patient's decision to refuse care may be a rational choice to live out the remaining period of life in a meaningful way.

15. Additional individualized interventions: _____

15. Rationales: _____

Suggested NIC Interventions
Behavior modification; Mutual goal setting; Patient contracting; Self-modification assistance; Teaching: Procedure/treatment; Decision-making support; Health system guidance; Self-responsibility facilitation; Teaching: Disease process

Suggested NOC Outcomes
Compliance behavior; Knowledge: Treatment regimen; Participation: Health care decisions; Treatment behavior: Illness or injury

---

Discharge planning
DISCHARGE CHECKLIST
Before discharge, the patient shows evidence of:
- ❐ stable vital signs
- ❐ absence of fever and pulmonary or cardiovascular complications
- ❐ ability to tolerate adequate nutritional intake
- ❐ stable cardiac rhythm with arrhythmias controlled
- ❐ shortness of breath that's no worse than usual
- ❐ peripheral edema within acceptable limits or no worse than usual
- ❐ ABG measurements within acceptable parameters
- ❐ clear lung fields shown on chest X-ray within 48 hours of discharge
- ❐ absence of supplemental oxygen for at least 48 hours before discharge
- ❐ absence of signs and symptoms of dehydration
- ❐ mental status within normal limits
- ❐ laboratory values within expected parameters
- ❐ absence of urinary or bowel dysfunction
- ❐ ability to perform ADLs and ambulate the same as before admission
- ❐ adequate home support system, or referral to home care if indicated by inadequate home support or inability to perform ADLs
- ❐ referral to community heart failure support group.

TEACHING CHECKLIST
Document evidence that the patient and his family demonstrate an understanding of:
- ❐ cause and implications of heart failure
- ❐ signs and symptoms of increasing heart failure
- ❐ all discharge medications' purpose, dosage, administration schedule, and adverse effects requiring medical attention (usual discharge medications include inotropic agents, diuretics, vasodilators, or anticoagulants)
- ❐ need for lifestyle modifications
- ❐ dietary restrictions
- ❐ activity restrictions
- ❐ plan for follow-up care
- ❐ plan for emergency care
- ❐ how to contact the physician.

DOCUMENTATION CHECKLIST
Using outcome criteria as a guide, document:
- ❐ clinical status on admission
- ❐ significant changes in clinical status
- ❐ pertinent laboratory and diagnostic findings
- ❐ intake and output
- ❐ nutritional intake
- ❐ response to activity progression
- ❐ response to illness and hospitalization
- ❐ family's response to illness

❏ patient and family teaching
❏ discharge planning.

Associated care plans

- Acute myocardial infarction
- Chronic renal failure
- Dying
- Grieving
- Ineffective individual coping
- Knowledge deficit
- Nutritional deficit

References

Brewster, D. "Evaluation of Arterial Insufficiency of the Lower Extremities," *Primary Care Medicine*. Philadelphia: Lippincott Williams & Wilkins, 2000.

DeFrang, R.D., et al. "Repeat Leg Bypass After Multiple Prior Bypass Failures, *Journal of Vascular Surgery* 19(2):268-76, February 1999.

Desgranges, P., et al. "Acute Occlusion of Popliteal and/or Tibial Arteries: The Value of Percutaneous Treatment," *European Journal Vascular and Endovascular Surgery* 20(2):138-45, August 2000.

Scott, M. Graft Type for Femoro-Popliteal Bypass Surgery, *www.update-software.com/abstracts/ab001487.htm*.

Hypovolemic shock

DRG INFORMATION
DRG 127   Heart Failure and Shock.
      Mean LOS = 5.2 days

Introduction
DEFINITION AND TIME FOCUS

Hypovolemic shock is a complex, life-threatening process of microcirculatory dysfunction and altered cellular metabolism resulting from decreased circulating blood volume. Sympathetic stimulation mediates hypovolemic shock's systemic effects, which include constriction of precapillary sphincters and venules. The resulting low capillary pressure promotes an interstitial-to-intravascular fluid shift that temporarily compensates for diminished circulating blood volume and maintains capillary flow. As shock progresses, however, this powerful compensatory mechanism fails. Decompensation results in capillary hypoxemia and acidosis, which promote sphincter relaxation, allowing capillary pressure to rise. Increased capillary permeability permits fluid to leak into the tissues, and the resulting decreased circulating blood volume increases hypoxemia and acidosis, creating a vicious cycle that ultimately causes irreparable damage.

On a cellular level, shock disrupts vital processes. Delicate sodium-potassium transport mechanisms are paralyzed, allowing sodium to accumulate inside the cell and produce swelling. Mitochondrial depression impairs energy production; oxygen deprivation causes cells to switch from aerobic to anaerobic metabolism. Anaerobic metabolism, an inefficient energy-generating process, also depletes glucose stores and produces lactic acid, creating metabolic acidosis. As cells die, lysosomal destruction releases proteases, enzymes, and cellular debris. These materials wreak havoc on surrounding cells' integrity and trigger the release of vasoactive substances, including myocardial depressant factor, that cause myocardial depression and severe vasodilation, further accelerating the vicious cycle. This care plan focuses on recognizing the patient in the medical-surgical setting who's at risk for developing hypovolemic shock as well as the critically ill patient with hypovolemic shock. (See *Clinical snapshot: Hypovolemic shock*.)

ETIOLOGY AND PRECIPITATING FACTORS
- Hemorrhage
- Excessive GI fluid losses through emesis and diarrhea
- Severe dehydration
- Excessive diuresis
- Burns
- Trauma
- Diabetes mellitus or diabetes insipidus
- Surgical interventions

Focused assessment guidelines
NURSING HISTORY
(FUNCTIONAL HEALTH PATTERN FINDINGS)
Health-perception–health-management pattern
- History of diabetes mellitus, heart failure, pancreatitis, hypertension, hemorrhage (internal or external), or other factors affecting fluid balance
- Recent invasive procedure performed, especially any major surgical procedure, such as open-heart surgery, abdominal resection, or massive trauma repair
- History of recent trauma (particularly to the chest, abdomen, or spinal cord) or burns

Nutritional-metabolic pattern
- Intense thirst
- Inability to verbalize need for fluids

Elimination pattern
- Increased urination or severe diarrhea (early) or oliguria (late)

Activity-exercise pattern
- Weakness and fatigue typical

Cognitive-perceptual pattern
- Reduced alertness, restlessness or anxiety

PHYSICAL FINDINGS
Cardiovascular
- Orthostatic hypotension (early)
- Supine hypotension (late)
- Tachycardia
- Arrhythmias
- Decreased or thready peripheral pulses
- Capillary filling time greater than 3 seconds

Neurologic
- Altered level of consciousness (LOC), ranging from confusion, irritability, or restlessness (early) to coma (late)

Integumentary
- Altered skin temperature, ranging from coolness (early) to coldness (late)
- Altered skin tone, ranging from pallor to mottling to cyanosis

Gastrointestinal
- Pale or cyanotic oral mucous membranes

Renal
- Oliguria or anuria

DIAGNOSTIC STUDIES

No laboratory tests are diagnostic for hypovolemic shock. Values will change reflecting end-organ deterioration. Such changes may include:

- complete blood count (CBC) — may vary, depending on shock stage; may be decreased with blood loss; typically, decreased hemoglobin level and increased hematocrit
- blood glucose level — elevated, reflecting stress-induced sympathetic stimulation
- blood urea nitrogen (BUN) and creatinine levels — elevated, reflecting decreased renal perfusion
- serum electrolyte levels — may vary, depending on the underlying problem and shock stage. Commonly, hypernatremia reflects increased renal sodium retention in response to volume losses; hypokalemia reflects urinary potassium losses in exchange for sodium; and hyperkalemia reflects acidosis, decreased glomerular filtration, and cell necrosis
- arterial blood gas (ABG) levels — reveal increased pH level and decreased partial pressure of arterial oxygen (Pao_2) in early shock, reflecting respiratory alkalosis caused by hyperventilation that progresses to decreased pH level, increased partial pressure of arterial carbon dioxide ($Paco_2$), and decreased bicarbonate (HCO_3^-) level in late shock, reflecting respiratory acidosis caused by hypoventilation and metabolic acidosis caused by anaerobic metabolism
- clotting profile — may reveal coagulopathy, shown by decreased platelet level, decreased fibrinogen level, and increased fibrin split products or altered D-dimer results
- serum osmolality — may increase, reflecting fluid loss
- urine osmolality or specific gravity — may increase, reflecting volume loss
- 12-lead electrocardiogram (ECG) — may reveal arrhythmias or changes reflecting myocardial ischemia, acute myocardial infarction (AMI), or electrolyte imbalances
- chest X-ray — may reveal pneumothorax or hemothorax.

POTENTIAL COMPLICATIONS

- Acute renal failure
- Acute respiratory distress syndrome (ARDS)
- Disseminated intravascular coagulation (DIC)
- Cardiogenic shock
- Cerebral anoxia
- Multiple organ dysfunction syndrome

CLINICAL SNAPSHOT ✸

Hypovolemic shock

Major nursing diagnoses and collaborative problems	Key patient outcomes
ND: Risk for deficient fluid volume	Maintain stable vital signs, typically: heart rate, 60 to 100 beats/minute; systolic blood pressure, 90 to 140 mm Hg; and diastolic blood pressure, 50 to 90 mm Hg.
CP: Hypovolemic shock	Have warm, dry extremities, indicating sufficient tissue perfusion.
ND: Impaired gas exchange	Show pulse oximetry and ABG levels within expected limits.
ND: Risk for injury	Show no signs of end-organ failure.
ND: Ineffective coping	Use support offered by caregivers.

Nursing diagnosis

Risk for deficient fluid volume related to disease processes, surgical interventions, or iatrogenic interventions

NURSING PRIORITIES

- Recognize patients at high risk for developing hypovolemia.
- Monitor patient status and prevent progression to shock state.

PATIENT OUTCOME CRITERIA

Within 48 hours, the patient will:

- show stable vital signs, typically: heart rate, 60 to 100 beats/minute; systolic blood pressure, 90 to 140 mm Hg; and diastolic blood pressure, 50 to 90 mm Hg

- have adequate urine output (greater than 30 ml/hour)
- have strong peripheral pulses
- have normal skin temperature
- display level of consciousness normal for patient.

INTERVENTIONS	RATIONALES
1. *Identify patients at risk for development of hypovolemic shock.**	**1.** Early intervention may prevent progression of hypovolemia to a hypovolemic shock state that may result in end-organ damage. Hemorrhage is the primary reason for development of hypovolemia; excessive GI losses are the second reason.
2. *If patient is actively bleeding, apply direct continuous pressure and elevate the area, if possible.*	**2.** Direct pressure to bleeding sites mechanically controls hemorrhage and aids in clot formation.
3. *Assess as accurately as possible the volume of loss* from emesis, diarrhea, drainage tubes, ostomies, fistulas, dressings, and other sources.	**3.** Measurement of volumes from these sources is commonly inaccurate, leading to inadequate fluid volume replacement therapy.
4. *Assess for changes in vital signs:* –pulse quality –blood pressure –tachypnea –urine output	**4.** These changes may indicate a potential problem: –Thin and thready pulse indicates hypovolemia; bounding pulse indicates hypervolemia. –Orthostatic (postural) changes indicate hypovolemia. –Increased respiratory rate indicates attempt to increase circulating oxygen. –A rate of less than 30 ml/hour indicates decreased cardiac output.
5. *Obtain orders for fluid volume replacement, if indicated.* Monitor for indications of normalizing volume status, such as normalizing blood pressure, slowing of heart rate to within normal range, and increased urine output.	**5.** Early replacement of lost volume with either crystalloids or colloids may prevent progression of hypovolemia to shock.
6. Additional individualized interventions: _____	**6.** Rationales: _____

Suggested NIC Interventions
Acid-base management; Fluid and electrolyte management; Fluid monitoring; Hypovolemia management; Intravenous (I.V.) therapy

Suggested NOC Outcomes
Electrolyte and acid-base balance; Fluid balance; Hydration

Collaborative problem

Hypovolemic shock related to blood loss, diuresis, dehydration, or third-space fluid shift

NURSING PRIORITY
Restore fluid volume.

PATIENT OUTCOME CRITERIA
Within 48 hours, the patient will:
- show stable vital signs, typically: heart rate, 60 to 100 beats/minute; systolic blood pressure, 90 to 140 mm Hg; and diastolic blood pressure, 50 to 90 mm Hg
- be hemodynamically stable and no longer require hemodynamic monitoring
- show no signs of fluid overload

---

*Italics indicate key interventions.

■ have warm, dry extremities indicating sufficient tissue perfusion
■ have stable neurologic status — ideally, alert and oriented.

INTERVENTIONS	RATIONALES
1. *Observe for signs and symptoms of fluid loss:*	**1.** Signs and symptoms correlate with the approximate percentage of volume loss. (The percentage of volume loss varies with reference source.)
– minimal volume loss: slight tachycardia; normal supine blood pressure; positive postural vital signs (systolic blood pressure decrease greater than 10 mm Hg or pulse increase greater than 20 beats/minute); capillary refill time greater than 3 seconds; urine output greater than 30 ml/hour; cool, pale extremities; and anxiety	– Powerful compensatory mechanisms produce these signs, which correlate with blood volume loss between 10% and 15%. Medullary vasomotor center stimulation via the baroreceptor reflex causes tachycardia and vasoconstriction. Also, antidiuretic hormone and aldosterone release causes the kidneys to retain sodium and water. All of these mechanisms help to maintain blood volume and normal supine blood pressure. However, postural vital signs are positive because homeostatic mechanisms can't compensate for the added stress of a position change. Prolonged capillary refill time and slight oliguria reflect decreased circulating volume. Cool, pale skin and normal mental status reflect shunting of blood away from the periphery to preserve function of the brain and heart.
– moderate volume loss: rapid, thready pulse; supine hypotension; cool truncal skin; urine output 10 to 30 ml/hour; severe thirst; and restlessness, confusion, or irritability	– These signs correlate with a volume loss of approximately 25%. As circulating blood volume drops to this level, compensatory mechanisms are no longer sufficient, and decompensation occurs. Oliguria reflects decreased renal perfusion, whereas mental changes indicate decreased cerebral perfusion.
– severe volume loss: marked tachycardia and hypotension; weak or absent peripheral pulses; cold, mottled, or cyanotic skin; urine output less than 10 ml/hour; and unconsciousness.	– These signs reflect a volume loss of at least 40% and severely decreased vital organ perfusion.
2. *Elevate the patient's legs above heart level,* unless contraindicated by active bleeding from the head and neck or suspected increased intracranial pressure or cardiogenic shock.	**2.** Elevation promotes venous drainage from the legs and increases circulating blood volume as much as 800 ml. This measure will exacerbate the conditions indicated, however.
3. *Obtain initial and serial diagnostic tests,* including CBC, blood typing and crossmatching, serum electrolyte levels, ABG levels, urinalysis, 12-lead ECG, and chest X-ray.	**3.** Serial data provide objective evidence of the disorder's severity and the effectiveness of interventions.
4. *Insert and maintain the following, as ordered:* – *two or more large-bore I.V. lines* – *indwelling urinary catheter.*	**4.** These invasive measures will combat shock. – Large-bore I.V. lines allow rapid infusion of large fluid volumes. – An indwelling catheter facilitates urine output monitoring, the most easily assessed indicator of renal perfusion as well as an indicator of cardiac output.
5. *Assist with insertion of a central venous pressure (CVP) catheter or pulmonary artery (PA) catheter, if ordered.* Monitor CVP or pulmonary artery wedge pressure (PAWP) hourly or according to protocol. Determine the frequency of measurement according to the depth of shock and rapidity of its progression.	**5.** CVP measurements can be used to guide fluid volume replacement and may be ordered for patients with lesser degrees of shock. For patients with severe shock, a PA catheter is preferred because it allows measurement of PAWP, which reflects left ventricular filling pressures more accurately than CVP does. Frequent measurements help determine the degree of shock and evaluate the effectiveness of interventions.

6. *Administer a fluid challenge, if ordered.*

6. A fluid challenge involves administration of a fluid bolus over a limited period. It allows assessment of hemodynamic response to rapid volume administration, which helps identify hypovolemic shock.

7. *Administer blood products and crystalloid or colloid I.V. solutions, as ordered.*

7. Various I.V. solutions may be used; their advantages and drawbacks remain controversial. Blood products should be given to replace direct losses. Colloids — solutions containing protein — help expand intravascular volume through osmosis; however, proteins may leak into the interstitial space, causing complications such as pulmonary edema. Crystalloid solutions — solutions containing salt, sugar, or both — require relatively large volumes because they leave the vascular space quickly. They also move into interstitial and intracellular spaces, potentially causing edema as well.

8. *Monitor blood pressure, particularly mean arterial pressure (MAP).*
– If an arterial line isn't in place, measure cuff blood pressure every 5 to 15 minutes until stable, then every hour. Monitor MAP electronically or calculate it by adding one-third of pulse pressure to diastolic pressure or by using this formula:

$$\frac{SP + (DP \times 2)}{3}$$

where SP equals systolic pressure and DP equals diastolic pressure.
– Assist with insertion of an arterial line, if ordered. Monitor MAP electronically.

– Maintain MAP within the desired range — usually at least 70 mm Hg. Consult with the physician about the appropriate range for the patient.

8. MAP reflects the average pressure at which organs are perfused.
– Cuff blood pressure measurements and arithmetic MAP calculation, though less desirable than intra-arterial measurement, provide valuable data. MAP is closer to diastolic blood pressure than to systolic blood pressure because diastole is about twice as long as systole in the cardiac cycle.

– Direct blood pressure measurement is preferred because it provides more accurate data than cuff measurements.
– Maintaining MAP within the desired range provides for adequate organ perfusion. In most cases, MAP must be maintained above 70 mm Hg in a previously normotensive patient. A higher MAP is appropriate for the patient with chronic hypertension. An MAP that's too low promotes ischemia; one that's too high contributes to such complications as cerebral and pulmonary edema.

9. *During all fluid administration, monitor the trend of hemodynamic measurements and urine output.* Observe for signs of fluid overload, such as crackles, jugular vein distention, or a third heart sound.

9. Because the patient in shock is hemodynamically unstable and has compromised compensatory mechanisms, volume administration may cause rapid progression from fluid depletion to fluid overload. If not detected promptly, fluid overload may cause pulmonary edema, heart failure, or cerebral edema.

10. Additional individualized interventions: _____

10. Rationales: _____

Nursing diagnosis
Impaired gas exchange related to ventilation-perfusion imbalance

NURSING PRIORITY
Maintain ventilation and oxygenation.

PATIENT OUTCOME CRITERIA

Within 48 hours, the patient will:

- maintain a patent airway
- have clearing breath sounds bilaterally
- have ABG values within normal limits: pH, 7.35 to 7.45; $Paco_2$, 35 to 45 mm Hg; HCO_3^-, 23 to 28 mEq/L; Pao_2, more than 60 mm Hg; and Sao_2, greater than 90%.

INTERVENTIONS	RATIONALES
1. *Provide standard nursing care related to impaired gas exchange:* maintain airway patency; monitor respiratory status; suction as necessary; provide supplemental oxygen, as ordered; and assist with intubation and mechanical ventilation, if indicated.	**1.** Numerous factors may cause ventilation-perfusion imbalance in shock, including atelectasis, microemboli, pulmonary congestion, and impaired capillary perfusion. The general measures listed apply to the care of any critically ill patient.
2. *Monitor Sao_2 through continuous pulse oximetry.* Monitor ABG levels, as ordered — typically at least every 4 hours.	**2.** Pulse oximetry determines Sao_2 rapidly, continuously, and noninvasively. ABG results indicate oxygenation status and degree of acid-base imbalance at the time the sample was drawn. Hyperventilation, a compensatory response to hypoxemia, is common in early hypovolemic shock and can lead to respiratory alkalosis. Combined metabolic acidosis (lactic acid production in anaerobic metabolism from increased capillary perfusion time) and respiratory acidosis (due to hypercarbia) characterize late hypovolemic shock.
3. Additional individualized interventions: _____	**3.** Rationales: _____

> **Suggested NIC Interventions**
> *Acid-base management; Electrolyte management; Laboratory data interpretation; Oxygen therapy; Ventilation assistance; Airway management; Respiratory monitoring; Hemodynamic regulation; Vital signs monitoring*

> **Suggested NOC Outcomes**
> *Electrolyte and acid-base balance; Respiratory status: Gas exchange; Respiratory status: Ventilation; Tissue perfusion: Pulmonary; Vital signs status*

Nursing diagnosis

Risk for injury due to complications related to ischemia

NURSING PRIORITY

Prevent or minimize complications.

PATIENT OUTCOME CRITERIA

By the time of discharge, the patient will show no signs of end-organ failure of the following systems:

- neurologic
- cardiac
- pulmonary
- mesenteric and hepatic
- renal
- hematologic.

INTERVENTIONS

1. *Prevent paralytic ileus and stress ulcers.* Withhold food and fluids; insert a nasogastric tube connected to suction, as ordered. Administer proton pump inhibitors (omeprazole [Prilosec] or esomeprazole [Nexium]), H_2 blockers (cimetidine [Tagamet] or ranitidine [Zantac]), or anti-ulcer medications (sucralfate [Carafate] or antacids). Monitor bowel sounds.

2. *Observe for signs and symptoms of ARDS,* such as tachypnea, progressive dyspnea, increased inspiratory pressure (if the patient is mechanically ventilated), deteriorating ABG or pulse oximetry values, or lung compliance less than 50 ml/cm H_2O. If you detect these problems, document them and alert the physician. Implement measures described in the "Acute respiratory distress syndrome" care plan, page 252, as appropriate.

3. *Observe for signs and symptoms of AMI,* such as severe chest pain, shortness of breath, hypotension, diaphoresis, pained facial expression, elevated cardiac isoenzymes, or ECG showing ST-segment displacement, T-wave inversion, or pathologic Q waves. See the "Acute myocardial infarction" care plan, page 337, for more details.

4. *Observe for signs and symptoms of DIC,* such as blood oozing from multiple sites, repeated bleeding episodes, oral cyanosis, petechiae, ecchymoses, hematomas, prolonged prothrombin time (PT), prolonged partial thromboplastin time, decreased fibrinogen level, decreased platelet count, elevated fibrin split products level, or altered D-dimer results. See the "Disseminated intravascular coagulation" care plan, page 764, for details.

5. *Observe for signs and symptoms of acute renal failure,* such as oliguria or anuria, weight gain, neck vein distention, crackles, dependent edema, or elevated BUN and serum creatinine levels. As appropriate, implement measures described in the "Acute renal failure" care plan, page 668.

6. *Observe for signs and symptoms of liver failure,* such as drowsiness, intellectual deterioration, personality changes, septicemia, fever, hyperkinetic circulation, jaundice, hepatomegaly, ascites, easy bruising, increased PT, elevated serum aspartate aminotransferase level, or increased bilirubin level. See the "Liver failure" care plan, page 533.

7. Additional individualized interventions: _____

RATIONALES

1. Paralytic ileus may result from mesenteric ischemia. The resulting gastric distention provokes vomiting, which can lead to chemical pneumonitis if aspiration occurs. Withholding food and fluids reduces stress on the stomach. Nasogastric drainage decompresses the stomach. The medications listed reduce the risk of stress ulcers by decreasing hydrochloric acid secretion, coating the gastric mucosa, or inhibiting gastric acid secretion.

2. Shock ranks as a major potential complication of ARDS because of such factors as decreased perfusion, hypoxemia, increased capillary permeability, and high oxygen levels used in treatment. The "Acute respiratory distress syndrome" care plan describes this ominous development and related care.

3. Decreased perfusion, catecholamine stimulation, hypoxemia, and increased afterload all may cause AMI. The "Acute myocardial infarction" care plan gives details on this complication.

4. Shock is a major risk factor for DIC because of such factors as capillary sludging, acidosis, sepsis, trauma, or other underlying causes. The "Disseminated intravascular coagulation" care plan describes this devastating development in depth.

5. Constriction of renal blood vessels is an early compensatory mechanism in shock. Although this constriction limits glomerular filtration, thus conserving fluid volume, it impairs renal perfusion, which may result in acute renal failure. The "Acute renal failure" care plan describes this complication in detail.

6. Although shock may damage hepatic cells, prompt correction of shock may allow these cells to regenerate. Early detection of liver failure may prevent severe damage to this critical organ. The "Liver failure" care plan presents the pathophysiology of this disorder and related care.

7. Rationales: _____

Suggested NIC Interventions
Surveillance: Safety

Suggested NOC Outcomes
Safety status: Physical injury

Nursing diagnosis

Ineffective coping related to threat to life

NURSING PRIORITY

Provide emotional support to the patient and his family.

PATIENT OUTCOME CRITERIA

By the time of discharge, the patient will verbalize increased coping ability and establish a family action plan to cope with this crisis.

INTERVENTIONS	RATIONALES
1. Implement measures described in the "Ineffective individual coping" care plan, page 124, as appropriate.	**1.** Alert patients are aware that shock is life-threatening, and they react to the possibility of death in various ways. Measures to help them cope with their realistic fear and other emotional responses are described in the "Ineffective individual coping" care plan.
2. Additional individualized interventions: _____	**2.** Rationales: _____

> **Suggested NIC Interventions**
> *Coping enhancement*

> **Suggested NOC Outcomes**
> *Coping; Social support*

Discharge planning

DISCHARGE CHECKLIST

Before discharge, the patient shows evidence of:
- ❑ blood pressure within normal limits without I.V. inotropic or vasopressor support
- ❑ pulse and respirations within normal limits
- ❑ ABG levels within expected limits for recovery stage
- ❑ urine output within normal limits
- ❑ no evidence of major complications.

TEACHING CHECKLIST

Document evidence that the patient and his family demonstrate an understanding of:
- ❑ cause and significance of shock
- ❑ expectations for recovery
- ❑ purpose of monitoring devices
- ❑ rationales for therapeutic interventions.

DOCUMENTATION CHECKLIST

Using outcome criteria as a guide, document:
- ❑ clinical status on admission
- ❑ significant changes in status
- ❑ pertinent diagnostic test findings
- ❑ care for invasive monitoring lines
- ❑ fluid administration
- ❑ use of inotropic agents, vasopressors, or other pharmacologic agents

- ❑ measures to support ventilation and oxygenation
- ❑ emotional support
- ❑ patient and family teaching
- ❑ discharge planning.

Associated care plans

- ■ Acute respiratory distress syndrome
- ■ Compromised family coping
- ■ Disseminated intravascular coagulation
- ■ Impaired physical mobility
- ■ Ineffective individual coping
- ■ Liver failure
- ■ Major burns
- ■ Mechanical ventilation
- ■ Multiple trauma
- ■ Pulmonary embolism

References

Jordan, K. (ed). *Emergency Nursing Core Curriculum.* Emergency Nurses Association. Philadelphia: W.B. Saunders Co., 2000.

Lynn-McHale, D.J., and Carlson, K.K. American Association of Critical Care Nurses *AACN Procedure Manual for Critical Care,* 4th ed. Philadelphia: W.B. Saunders Co., 2001.

Shoemaker, W.C., et al. *Textbook of Critical Care,* 4th ed. Philadelphia: W.B. Saunders Co., 2002.

Percutaneous transluminal coronary angioplasty

DRG INFORMATION

DRG 116   Other Permanent Cardiac Pacemaker Implant or Percutaneous Transluminal Coronary Angioplasty (PTCA) with Coronary Artery Stent Implant.
Mean LOS = 3.6 days

DRG 112   Percutaneous Cardiovascular Procedures.
Mean LOS = 3.7 days

The differentiation in the above selections is whether a coronary artery stent is implanted when performing PTCA. It's important to note, however, that if PTCA is performed during heart catheterization using only intracoronary thrombolytics (such as tissue plasminogen activator or heparin), it isn't grouped to DRG 112. DRG 112 is acquired only when a coronary atherectomy or balloon angioplasty is performed. To reiterate, the placement of a coronary artery stent moves the patient to DRG 116.

If the patient fails angioplasty or stent placement and is taken for cardiac surgery, the cardiac surgery performed would then take precedence in DRG selection.

Introduction

DEFINITION AND TIME FOCUS

PTCA is a therapeutic alternative to coronary artery bypass surgery for patients with coronary artery disease (CAD). Over the past 20 years, PTCA has become an effective, widely used treatment for patients with coronary ischemia. In the past decade alone, the number of PTCAs performed has increased more than tenfold. PTCA has several advantages over cardiac surgery: shorter hospital stay, less discomfort for the patient, fewer potential complications, faster convalescence, and lower cost.

The procedure is performed in the cardiac catheterization laboratory and lasts 1 to 4 hours. The cardiac surgical team is on standby in the event of a complication and the need for open-heart surgery. Patients are admitted the evening before or the morning of the procedure and are discharged an average of 28 hours after it.

During PTCA, a cardiologist places an expandable dilatation balloon in the partially obstructed coronary artery and then inflates it to widen the lumen of the vessel. Most PTCAs are performed percutaneously via the femoral artery, which requires insertion of an arterial introducer sheath at the access site in the groin. This approach allows for left-sided heart catheterization, angiog-

raphy, and angioplasty. A venous sheath is placed only if right-sided heart catheterization is performed. At the end of the procedure, the sheaths are flushed with heparin and capped. The sheaths are then sutured in place. Most patients are admitted to an intensive care unit or telemetry unit after PTCA. Sheaths commonly remain in place several hours or sometimes overnight; they then are removed by a physician or specially trained nurse.

This care plan focuses on the patient undergoing routine (nonacute myocardial infarction [MI]) PTCA from the preprocedure stage to discharge. (See *Clinical snapshot: Percutaneous transluminal coronary angioplasty*.)

ETIOLOGY AND PRECIPITATING FACTORS

- CAD
- Angina poorly controlled or refractory to conventional medical therapy
- Objective evidence of ischemia
- Good left ventricular function
- Candidate for coronary artery bypass surgery
- Coronary artery lesions amenable to dilatation
- One or more coronary vessels
- Proximal lesion
- Discrete
- Concentric
- Noncalcified

Focused assessment guidelines

NURSING HISTORY
(FUNCTIONAL HEALTH PATTERN FINDINGS)

Because PTCA is performed to relieve angina, findings are the same as in the "Angina pectoris" care plan, page 355.

POTENTIAL COMPLICATIONS

- Rupture of coronary artery
- Major bleeding at access site
- Abrupt closure of the treated vessel
- MI
- Arterial occlusion

Percutaneous transluminal coronary angioplasty

Major nursing diagnoses and collaborative problems	Key patient outcomes
ND: Anxiety	Verbalize fears and concerns, if desired, about diagnosis and treatment.
CP: Risk for femoral artery occlusion	Have palpable pedal pulses greater than 2+ on a scale of 0 to 4.
ND: Risk for injury	Display no evidence of excessive bleeding or significant hematoma.
CP: Risk for hypovolemia	Have stable vital signs, typically: heart rate, 60 to 100 beats/ minute; systolic blood pressure, 90 to 140 mm Hg; and diastolic blood pressure, 50 to 90 mm Hg.
ND: Acute pain	Rate pain as less than 3 on a pain rating scale of 0 to 10.
ND: Deficient knowledge (postdischarge care)	Be able to correctly describe site care and what to do for signs and symptoms of complications.

Nursing diagnosis

Anxiety related to known risks associated with PTCA and to fear of the unknown

NURSING PRIORITY

Relieve anxiety and foster effective coping.

PATIENT OUTCOME CRITERIA

Before PTCA, the patient will:
- if desired, verbalize fears and concerns related to diagnosis and treatment
- exhibit effective coping behavior, such as asking questions and responding calmly to questions from staff.

INTERVENTIONS

1. If the patient is admitted to the unit before PTCA, *assess his level of knowledge about the procedure and his level of anxiety.* *

2. *Provide preprocedure teaching or reinforce knowledge.* Discuss the following with the patient:
– preoperative routine, including nothing by mouth 12 hours before the procedure, allergies, need to empty bladder on call, and premedication
– appearance of cardiac catheterization laboratory, such as staff in surgical scrub suits and monitoring equipment and fluoroscope
– preparation in catheterization laboratory, including use of cardiac monitor, I.V. lines, site preparation, and pretest sedative
– expected sensations with PTCA, especially flushing with dye or chest discomfort with balloon inflation

RATIONALES

1. In some cases, preprocedure teaching will be accomplished on an outpatient basis.

2. The patient may have detailed teaching before admission. Describing activity and what to expect can lessen fear of the unknown.

*Italics indicate key interventions.

– description of how to obtain pain medication and how to cope with need to urinate
– intraprocedure and postprocedure monitoring for complications
– explanation of physician's requests to cough and breathe deeply during procedure
– postprocedure care, including need for bed rest, importance of keeping leg straight, and sheath removal
– where family can wait and how they will be kept informed during procedure.

3. Additional individualized interventions: _____

3. Rationales: _____

Suggested NIC Interventions
Anxiety reduction

Suggested NOC Outcomes
Acceptance: Health status; Coping

Collaborative problem
Risk for femoral artery occlusion related to indwelling sheath

NURSING PRIORITY
Promptly detect and report femoral artery occlusion.

PATIENT OUTCOME CRITERION
Throughout the post-PTCA period, the patient will have palpable pedal pulses greater than 2 + on a scale of 0 to 4.

INTERVENTIONS

1. With each assessment of vital signs, *check bilateral distal pulses* (dorsalis pedis or posterior tibial). Mark pulse locations on feet with a marker for easy identification. *Use Doppler ultrasound to verify pulses if they are weak or nonpalpable.* If a dorsalis pedis pulse is absent, assess posterior tibial pulses. *If pulses are absent or diminished in the catheterized limb, alert the physician immediately.*

2. *Maintain the heparin infusion,* as ordered. To determine dose, use a heparin nomogram dosing chart, such as a heparin dosing flowchart based on weight or partial thromboplastin time (PTT) values. Keep PTT values within limits specified by the cardiologist, typically 60 to 90 seconds.

3. Discontinue heparin 2 to 4 hours before removal of the sheath, if ordered.

4. Additional individualized interventions: _____

RATIONALES

1. Femoral artery occlusion may occur in the catheterized extremity as a complication of PTCA due to thrombus formation on the catheter or a possible embolism. Presence of normal distal pulses indicates adequate blood flow. Pulses should be equal bilaterally. The dorsalis pedis pulse may be absent bilaterally as a normal variant. Otherwise, a diminished or absent pulse requires prompt medical intervention to restore flow.

2. A national survey of PTCA care practices (Juran et al., 1996) revealed wide variability in heparin administration post-PTCA. About 41% of the 70 hospitals surveyed maintain a heparin infusion for 12 to 18 hours postprocedure, but 31% don't infuse heparin at all. Using a flowchart helps determine appropriate doses of heparin based on PTT measurement. Doses are titrated to the patient's coagulation status.

3. Nationally, 54% of hospitals using heparin post-PTCA discontinue it 2 to 4 hours before sheath removal; the remaining 46% discontinue it either before 2 hours or after 4 hours.

4. Rationales: _____

Nursing diagnosis

Risk for injury related to break in skin and presence of foreign body

NURSING PRIORITY

Protect the patient from injury.

PATIENT OUTCOME CRITERION

Throughout the post-PTCA period, the patient will adhere to activity limitations.

INTERVENTIONS	RATIONALES
1. *Maintain complete bed rest, with the head of the bed flat or elevated up to 30 degrees* for prescribed time, usually 8 to 24 hours. Consult the physician about acceptability of logrolling to the side-lying position.	**1.** The femoral sheath, venous sheath, or both are left in place for several hours after the procedure. Most physicians will allow logrolling, as long as the affected leg is maintained straight and no hip flexion occurs.
2. *Instruct the patient to report to the nurse bleeding at the site or a warm, wet feeling at the groin site. Also teach the patient to keep the affected leg straight and to avoid straining with turning or bowel movement for 12 to 24 hours.*	**2.** The patient can serve as a monitor of the integrity of the groin site. If the patient flexes at the groin or strains, the rigid sheath might injure the vessel, triggering bleeding.
3. Additional individualized interventions: _____	**3.** Rationales: _____

> **Suggested NIC Interventions**
> *Skin/wound management: Incision site care; Skin surveillance; Wound care*

> **Suggested NOC Outcomes**
> *Wound healing: Primary intention*

Collaborative problem

Risk for hypovolemia related to bleeding or diuresis

NURSING PRIORITIES

- Promptly detect bleeding.
- Restore fluid volume.

PATIENT OUTCOME CRITERIA

Immediately following PTCA and thereafter, the patient will:
- have normal vital signs, typically: heart rate, 60 to 100 beats/minute; systolic blood pressure, 90 to 140 mm Hg; and diastolic blood pressure, 50 to 90 mm Hg.
    Within 1 to 2 hours before discharge, the patient will:
- ambulate without assistance, without excessive pain (less than 3 on a 0 to 10 pain rating scale), and with no bleeding.

INTERVENTIONS	RATIONALES
1. Measure pulse and blood pressure four times every 15 minutes, four times every 30 minutes, every hour while the sheath is in place, and then every 4 hours and as necessary. Monitor cardiac rhythm continuously.	**1.** The contrast agent used during angiography causes an osmotic diuresis. Frequent vital signs checks allow prompt detection of hypovolemia, which may result from diuresis or internal bleeding. Continuous cardiac monitoring is necessary to detect arrhythmias, a complication of PTCA.

2. *With each vital sign check, assess the access site for bleeding, swelling, or discoloration.*

2. The patient usually receives one or more boluses of heparin or a continuous infusion during the procedure for anticoagulation. Hemorrhage is a constant danger. Swelling and discoloration are indicators of hematoma formation.

3. *If bleeding occurs at the insertion site while the sheath is in place, remove the dressing and evaluate the amount of blood. Apply a sterile dressing over the access site and apply manual pressure above the introducer until bleeding stops. Notify the cardiologist and administer a transfusion, if ordered.*

3. Removing the dressing allows for adequate observation of the site. Manual pressure stops the bleeding and allows clotting to occur. A transfusion may be needed to replace blood volume.

4. Assist with sheath removal according to unit protocol. (See *Sheath removal after percutaneous transluminal coronary angioplasty.*)

4. In two-thirds of the hospitals surveyed, a specially trained nurse pulls the sheath; in the remaining hospitals, a physician performs this action.

5. After sheath removal, *maintain dressing per unit protocol.*

5. About two-thirds of all hospitals surveyed apply a pressure dressing after sheath removal. The remainder use a plain dressing, adhesive bandages, or no dressing at all. Sandbags are used by 83% of those surveyed, although they don't decrease bleeding. Sandbags also increase pain.

6. Maintain the I.V. line, as ordered.

6. An I.V. line provides emergency access for medication administration, fluid to promote excretion of the contrast medium, and a ready source of additional volume if the patient becomes hypovolemic.

7. Encourage the patient to drink water freely.

7. Oral intake of water replaces water lost during osmotic diuresis. Also, the contrast medium is nephrotoxic and may cause renal tubular necrosis and subsequent renal failure.

8. Monitor urine output.

8. Urine output is an indicator of renal perfusion and should measure at least 30 ml/hour.

9. *Assess for orthostatic hypotension before allowing the patient out of bed for the first time.* Measure blood pressure and pulse while the patient is supine; then have the patient sit up and promptly repeat measurement. Compare values, looking for a systolic blood pressure drop of 10 mm Hg or more or a pulse increase of 20 beats or more per minute. If these symptoms are present, keep the patient in bed and increase I.V. fluids as ordered until the supine and sitting blood pressure values are within 10 mm Hg of each other and the pulse rates are within 20 beats of each other.

9. Internal hemorrhage and internal bleeding may also occur, especially retroperitoneal bleeding from perforation of the iliac artery. Orthostatic vital signs can identify hidden hypovolemia. Although blood pressure and pulse may be normal in the supine position because of compensatory mechanisms for volume loss, the body may be unable to compensate for the additional stress of position change. If blood pressure drops 10 mm Hg or more or pulse increases 20 beats/minute or more, positive orthostatic vital signs are present, indicating an inadequate blood volume.

10. Additional individualized interventions: _____

10. Rationales: _____

Sheath removal after percutaneous transluminal coronary angioplasty

A specially trained nurse or physician takes the following steps to remove a sheath. In addition to the person removing the sheath, an additional nurse is needed to monitor the patient's tolerance of the procedure.

Before pulling the sheath	Pulling the sheath	After pulling the sheath
• Discontinue the heparin drip, as ordered. • Confirm nothing by mouth status for 1 to 2 hours. • Explain the procedure to the patient, including the need to avoid holding his breath while intense pressure is exerted on the site after the catheter is removed (to avoid a vasovagal response with bradycardia and hypotension). • Premedicate the patient, as ordered, usually with morphine. • Evaluate the patient's vital signs, cardiac rhythm, and quality of pedal pulses every 5 minutes during removal.	• Remove the dressing. • Check the groin for ecchymosis and hematoma. • Instill a local anesthetic per protocol. • Remove sutures, if any. • Remove the sheath.	• Immediately apply pressure until hemostasis is established (typically 15 to 30 minutes manual pressure, or use a mechanical pressure device, such as a C-clamp or other device). Remind the patient to breathe freely. • Assess the patient for chest, back, and site pain. • Apply a pressure dressing per unit protocol. • Remind the patient to keep the leg straight and remain on bed rest another 6 to 8 hours. • Instruct the patient to call the nurse for any pain or sense of wetness at the groin. • Document the sheath removal and vital signs, site, and circulatory assessments. • Maintain complete bed rest for 6 to 8 hours. • Consult the clinical plan for additional measures for monitoring vital signs and for complications.

Nursing diagnosis

Acute pain related to restrictions on mobility and percutaneous puncture at the groin site

NURSING PRIORITY
Promptly detect and relieve pain.

PATIENT OUTCOME CRITERIA
Throughout the post-PTCA period, the patient will:
- experience no chest pain
- rate other pain (such as back pain) as less than 3 on a 0 to 10 pain rating scale.

INTERVENTIONS

1. *On admission to the unit, ask whether the patient has leg or back pain.* Also specifically ask about the presence of chest discomfort. Instruct the patient to report pain or other discomfort to you promptly.

2. *If back or leg pain is present, reposition the patient within accepted limits.* Use other nonpharmacologic nursing measures, such as back rubs, massage, relaxation, music, or imagery. If necessary, administer pain medication, as ordered.

RATIONALES

1. During PTCA, the patient must lie on a hard table for 1 to 4 hours. Following the procedure, bed rest is necessary while the sheaths are in place (4 to 12 hours) and for an additional 6 to 8 hours after a sheath is removed. As a result, the patient may spend as much as 24 to 36 hours on complete bed rest. The primary discomforts that the patient may report after PTCA are back and leg pain from prolonged bed rest and restricted mobility.

2. Recent studies suggest that the head of the bed can safely be elevated up to 60 degrees. A flexible sheath has recently become available, allowing for more liberal positioning. Various nursing measures may help to reduce the patient's perception of pain. Pain medication should successfully control pain that can't be relieved by other measures.

3. *If chest pain is present, assess and treat it according to unit protocol for chest pain.* Notify the cardiologist immediately.

4. Additional individualized interventions: _____
_____

3. Chest pain may recur as a result of the underlying pathologic condition or from abrupt reocclusion of a coronary artery from vasospasm or thrombus. Angina occurs as a result of decreased coronary blood flow to the myocardium. Prolonged ischemia may result in an MI.

4. Rationales: _____
_____

Suggested NIC Interventions
Pain management

Suggested NOC Outcomes
Pain: Psychological response

Nursing diagnosis

Deficient knowledge (postdischarge care) related to lack of exposure to information

NURSING PRIORITY

Teach the patient and his family about postdischarge care.

PATIENT OUTCOME CRITERIA

Before discharge, the patient will:
- describe site care at home
- describe signs and symptoms of complications and what to do
- verbalize a commitment to reduce risk factors.

INTERVENTIONS

1. Before discharge, discuss with the patient and his family and evaluate their comprehension of:
- need for follow-up care
- site care and signs and symptoms of infection
- pain management
- signs and symptoms to report to the physician, such as pain, numbness, tingling, bleeding, and difficulty breathing
- discharge medications
- date, time, and place of next appointment
- risk factor modification — including diet, exercise, and smoking cessation.

2. Additional individualized interventions: _____
_____

RATIONALES

1. The patient and his family are more likely to follow through with postprocedure care if they are taught what they need to know and if their understanding of the care is assessed before discharge.

2. Rationales: _____
_____

Suggested NIC Interventions
Teaching: Disease process; Teaching: Individual; Teaching: Prescribed medication

Suggested NOC Outcomes
Knowledge: Disease process; Knowledge: Health behaviors; Knowledge: Treatment regimen

Discharge planning

DISCHARGE CHECKLIST

Before discharge, the patient shows evidence of:
- ❏ vital signs within normal limits
- ❏ pain controllable with oral medication
- ❏ affected leg warm, dry, and of normal color
- ❏ pulses same as on admission
- ❏ no signs or symptoms of complications.

TEACHING CHECKLIST

Document evidence that the patient and his family demonstrate an understanding of:
- ❏ diagnosis
- ❏ insertion site care
- ❏ measures for pain control
- ❏ activity restrictions
- ❏ symptoms to report to the physician
- ❏ all discharge medications
- ❏ activity resumption.

DOCUMENTATION CHECKLIST

Using outcome criteria as a guide, document:
- ❏ clinical status on admission
- ❏ significant changes in status
- ❏ pertinent diagnostic test findings
- ❏ heparin therapy
- ❏ adherence to positioning limitations
- ❏ patient and family teaching
- ❏ discharge planning.

Associated care plans

- ■ Acute myocardial infarction
- ■ Acute pain
- ■ Angina pectoris
- ■ Compromised family copying
- ■ Impaired physical mobility
- ■ Ineffective individual coping
- ■ Knowledge deficit

References

D'Epiro, N.V. "Advances in Imaging Technology," *Patient Care 2000* 34(3):206, February 2000.

Silva, J.A. "Percutaneous Coronary Intervention of Thrombotic Lesions: Still Challenging!" *Catheterization and Cardiovascular Interventions* 56(1):8-9, April 2002.

Wiley, J.M., et al. "Noncoronary Complications of Coronary Intervention," *Catheterization and Cardiovascular Interventions* 57(2):257-65, September 2002.

Yoon, S.C., et al. "Assessment of Contemporary Stent Deployment Using Intravascular Ultrasound," *Catheterization and Cardiovascular Interventions* 57(2):150-54, September 2002.

Permanent pacemaker insertion

DRG INFORMATION

DRG 115   Permanent Cardiac Pacemaker Implant with Acute Myocardial Infarction, Heart Failure, or Shock or Automatic Implantable Cardioverter-Defibrillator Lead or Generator Procedure. Mean LOS = 8.1 days

DRG 116   Other Permanent Cardiac Pacemaker Implant or Percutaneous Transluminal Coronary Angioplasty with Coronary Artery Stent Implant. Mean LOS = 3.6 days

Introduction

DEFINITION AND TIME FOCUS

Permanent pacemaker insertion may be required when the patient experiences symptoms of decreased cardiac output secondary to irreversible or uncontrolled arrhythmias. Irreversible bradycardia results from atrioventricular (AV) heart block (typically Mobitz type II second- or third-degree), sinus bradycardia, sinus arrest, or sinoatrial (SA) block. Some tachyarrhythmias unresponsive to other treatments may also benefit from a permanent pacemaker, as may sick sinus (bradycardia-tachycardia) syndrome. This care plan focuses on managing the patient who has had a permanent pacemaker inserted transvenously. The lead is inserted through a vein — commonly the cephalic, jugular, or subclavian — and positioned with fluoroscopy in the right atrium or ventricle. Lead attachment to the endocardium is either passive, with fibrosis occurring at the contact point, or active, with the lead screwed into the muscle. A subcutaneous pocket is made in the submammary area, upper chest, or abdominal region, and the pulse generator box is placed in it. The distal end of the lead is connected under the skin to the generator box. The procedure is commonly done on a patient under local anesthesia who's given some additional sedation and pain relief. (See *Clinical snapshot: Permanent pacemaker insertion*.)

ETIOLOGY AND PRECIPITATING FACTORS

- Idiopathic sclerotic degeneration of the SA node
- Coronary artery disease, especially with significant disease or infarction involving the artery to the SA node (right coronary artery in 55% of the population, circumflex in 45%) or the AV node (right coronary artery in 90%, circumflex in 10%)
- Rheumatic heart disease
- Cardiomyopathy
- Congenital heart disease, such as ventricular septal defect or transposition of the great vessels
- Surgical trauma or edema affecting the cardiac conduction system
- Myocarditis
- Hypersensitive carotid sinus syndrome

Focused assessment guidelines

NURSING HISTORY (FUNCTIONAL HEALTH PATTERN FINDINGS)

Note: Findings vary, depending on the underlying condition.

Health-perception–health-management pattern
- Treatment of arrhythmias
- Treatment of angina, atherosclerosis, hypertension, or heart failure
- History of myocardial infarction, congenital heart disease, or cardiac surgery

Nutritional-metabolic pattern
- Swelling of extremities and weight gain

Activity-exercise pattern
- Shortness of breath, fatigue, activity intolerance, and paroxysmal nocturnal dyspnea

Cognitive-perceptual pattern
- Chest pain
- Palpitations
- Syncope, dizziness, and light-headedness (Adams-Stokes disease)

Self-perception–self-concept pattern
- Concern over anticipated changes in body image and functioning
- Concern over follow-up care and restrictions

PHYSICAL FINDINGS

Physical findings before pacemaker insertion appear below.

Cardiovascular
- Arrhythmias — bradycardia, irregular rhythms, or (uncommonly) tachycardia
- Hypotension
- Venous engorgement or jugular vein distention
- Third or fourth heart sounds
- Decreased peripheral pulses
- Increased capillary refill time

Pulmonary
- Crackles
- Shortness of breath
- Orthopnea

Neurologic
- Dizziness
- Syncope

- Seizures
- Transient ischemic attacks

Integumentary
- Cool, clammy skin
- Edema

Renal
- Weight gain (from fluid retention)

Gastrointestinal
- Liver enlargement
- Positive hepatojugular reflux

DIAGNOSTIC STUDIES

- Electrolyte panel — deviations from normal in potassium, magnesium, and calcium may affect cardiac conduction and contractility
- Serum drug levels — may reveal subtherapeutic or toxic medication levels that may affect heart rate and rhythm (medications that may affect heart rate or rhythm include digoxin [Lanoxin], quinidine (Quinalan), procainamide (Procanbid), narcotics, and some psychotropics)
- Blood urea nitrogen and creatinine levels — may reflect low renal perfusion from low cardiac output
- Triiodothyronine and thyroxine levels — may be low, indicating that hypothyroidism may be depressing cardiac impulse formation or conduction

- 12-lead electrocardiogram (ECG) — may reveal electrical activity not obvious in a single-lead rhythm strip and may help identify the arrhythmia
- Holter monitor — may be used to confirm sick sinus syndrome or other transient arrhythmias
- Chest X-ray — may show cardiac enlargement and respiratory status
- Electrophysiology studies — may allow induction and identification of symptom-causing arrhythmias

POTENTIAL COMPLICATIONS

- Arrhythmias
- Infection
- Thrombosis or embolism
- Tamponade or perforation of myocardium
- Hematoma or hemorrhage
- Lead fracture
- Pneumothorax
- Hiccups (diaphragmatic pacing)
- Tricuspid insufficiency
- Painful subcutaneous pocket or pocket erosion
- Pacemaker syndrome (shortness of breath, dizziness, chest pain resulting from suboptimal pacing mode or inappropriate pacing parameters)

CLINICAL SNAPSHOT ☀

Permanent pacemaker insertion

Major nursing diagnoses and collaborative problems	Key patient outcomes
CP: Risk for arrhythmias	Display ECG evidence of appropriate pacer sensing, firing, and capturing.
ND: Risk for infection	Show no signs of infection.
ND: Bathing or hygiene self-care deficit	Resume normal self-care activities.
ND: Deficient knowledge (self-care after discharge)	Demonstrate accurate pulse rate measurement.
ND: Disturbed body image	Ask appropriate questions and show interest in learning about the pacemaker.

Collaborative problem

Risk for arrhythmias related to pacemaker malfunction or lead or electrode displacement

NURSING PRIORITY

Maintain optimal cardiac rhythm.

PATIENT OUTCOME CRITERIA

Immediately after surgery and throughout the hospital stay, the patient will:
- display a cardiac rate no less than pacemaker setting
- display ECG evidence of appropriate pacer sensing, firing, and capturing.

Within 3 days after surgery, the patient will:
- have decreased or no signs and symptoms of low cardiac output (if present before surgery)
- visit the pacemaker clinic for a definitive check of pacemaker functioning.

INTERVENTIONS

1. *Initiate constant ECG monitoring until discharged or as ordered.** Keep alarms on at all times. Set the low limit at 3 beats/minute less than the pacer setting. Set the high limit 10 beats/minute above the anticipated maximum cardiac rate. Place monitoring electrodes 2″ (5 cm) away from the generator box. Change the monitoring electrode sites to obtain another perspective if the pacer appears to be malfunctioning.

2. *Document in the care plan the patient's intrinsic rate and rhythm.* Also, indicate the pacemaker type and rate. (See *Generic pacemaker code.*)

3. *Record and document rhythm strips every shift* and mount them in the patient's chart. Analyze the strips: Appropriately paced beats will show a pacer spike artifact followed by a depolarization wave that differs from the intrinsic waveform. Notify the physician promptly if problems occur with impulse initiation, conduction, or sensing.
– failure to sense — pacer spikes occur despite the presence of the patient's intrinsic beat

– failure to capture — pacing spikes not followed by cardiac depolarization

– failure to pace — absence of pacing spikes when the intrinsic rate is below the pacer setting.

4. *Maintain standby transdermal pacing equipment.*

5. *Obtain 12-lead simultaneous ECG recordings,* as ordered.

RATIONALES

1. Continuous monitoring facilitates early problem detection. If the pacemaker is functioning properly, the cardiac rate shouldn't go below the pacer setting. The risk of tachyarrhythmias can't be ignored. Monitoring electrodes placed near the generator box or in lead locations where the ECG amplitude is small may result in failure to record intrinsic beats.

2. This information is necessary for correct ECG interpretation.

3. Systematic documentation provides an objective, organized means of analyzing pacer activity. Waveforms of paced and intrinsic beats differ because of independent conduction paths.

– The sensitivity setting may be such that the pacemaker undersenses and doesn't consistently detect intrinsic low-amplitude cardiac electrical activity. Failure to sense may also result from fibrosis at the lead tip, lead fracture, or a dislodged lead. Failure to sense may result in inappropriate, unnecessary pacing and may cause R-on-T phenomenon, in which a pacer spike falls on the downslope of the preceding T wave, triggering ventricular tachycardia or ventricular fibrillation.
– Failure to capture results when the voltage of the pacemaker stimulus is insufficient to trigger depolarization. It may result from fibrosis at the lead-myocardial junction, a weak battery, the effect of cardiac drugs, electrolyte imbalance, or a dislodged or malpositioned lead.
– Failure to pace may result from a fractured leadwire, malfunction at the lead-generator connection, power source depletion, or oversensing — the sensing of noncardiac electrical activity, such as muscle activity near the generator box, power lines, other sources of electrical noise, or crosstalk in dual chamber pacemakers.

4. Alternative emergency pacing may be needed.

5. A 12-lead ECG recording shows pacer function and cardiac electrical activity more accurately than a single-lead rhythm strip. Simultaneous tracings help to confirm pacing spikes and intrinsic beats that may vary in amplitude in different leads and therefore may not be obvious in one particular lead.

---

*Italics indicate key interventions.

Generic pacemaker code

The North American Society of Pacing and Electrophysiology and the British Pacing and Electrophysiology Group have recommended a sequence of five letters to designate pacemaker capabilities. Note that the first three positions are used for antibradyarrhythmia function exclusively.

Chamber paced (Position I)	Chamber sensed (Position II)	Response to sensing (Position III)	Programmability, rate modulation (Position IV)	Antitachyarrhythmia function (Position V)
O = none A = atrium V = ventricle D = dual (A and V)	O = none A = atrium V = ventricle D = dual (A and V)	O = none T = triggered I = inhibited D = dual (T and I)	O = none P = simple programmable M = multiprogrammable C = communicating R = rate modulation	O = none P = pacing (antitachy - arrhythmia) S = shock D = dual (P and S)

Adapted from Bernstein, A.D., et al. "The NASPE/BPEG Generic Pacemaker Code for Antibradyarrhythmia and Adaptive Rate Pacing and Antitachyarrhythmia Devices," *PACE* 10:794-99, July-August 1987. Used with permission.

---

6. *Administer cardiac medications,* as ordered, and document their effectiveness and adverse effects.

6. Cardiac medications may be indicated for treatment of underlying cardiac problems, such as coronary artery or valvular disease.

7. *Observe for signs and symptoms of decreased cardiac output.* Monitor blood pressure, apical pulse, and respirations.

7. Deviation from postoperative baseline vital signs may indicate pacemaker failure or other complications.

8. *Maintain and document I.V. line patency,* as ordered.

8. The I.V. line may be needed to administer emergency medications.

9. Maintain the patient on bed rest with turning limitations and with the head of the bed elevated 30 to 45 degrees, as ordered.

9. With passive lead placement, activity and positioning limitations may be needed temporarily to maintain lead placement until fibrosis develops around the electrode tip and anchors it in place. Limitations may be less restrictive with active lead attachment.

10. If use of the affected arm is restricted, perform limited passive range-of-motion (ROM) exercises with the arm every hour during the first 24 hours after surgery.

10. Movement restrictions may be ordered to reduce the chance of lead displacement. Passive ROM exercises may prevent frozen shoulder.

11. Make sure that chest X-ray is performed, as ordered.

11. Chest X-ray may be used to confirm lead placement.

12. Additional individualized interventions: _____

12. Rationales: _____

Nursing diagnosis
Risk for infection related to surgical disruption of skin barrier

NURSING PRIORITIES
- Promote incisional healing by primary intention.
- Prevent or promptly detect infection.

PATIENT OUTCOME CRITERIA
Within 1 day after surgery and throughout the hospital stay, the patient will:
- have a dry and intact incision
- experience no fever.
  By the time of discharge, the patient will:

- have a white blood cell (WBC) count within normal limits
- show no signs of infection.

INTERVENTIONS	RATIONALES
1. *Check the primary dressing for drainage.* Circle any drainage, and write the date and time when first discovered.	**1.** This is an objective method of monitoring for bleeding and incisional drainage.
2. *Reinforce the primary dressing as needed for 24 hours.* Don't change the primary dressing without an order from the physician.	**2.** Reinforcement protects the incision and aids hemostasis while providing a protective barrier against microorganisms. Removing the primary dressing increases the risk of accidentally disrupting the incision and causing bleeding.
3. *After removal of the primary dressing, check the incision for excessive redness, swelling, warmth, and drainage.*	**3.** These signs may reflect infection.
4. *Perform wound care,* as ordered.	**4.** The pacemaker pocket is the most common entry site for infectious organisms, which can migrate along the pacing wires to the heart. A clean, dry incision promotes healing.
5. *Administer antibiotics,* as ordered.	**5.** Antibiotics may be prescribed prophylactically because pacemaker insertion is an invasive procedure that involves implanting a foreign object into the heart. Also, the disruption of the skin barrier provides a potential portal of entry for infectious organisms into the heart.
6. *Monitor body temperature,* as ordered. Notify the physician if the patient's oral temperature exceeds 100° F (37.8° C).	**6.** Commonly, elevated temperature is a systemic response to infection.
7. *Monitor the WBC count,* as ordered.	**7.** The WBC count increases in response to infectious organisms.
8. *Culture purulent drainage,* if present, as ordered.	**8.** WBCs and cellular debris accumulate locally in response to infectious organisms. Proper treatment requires identifying the causative agent and its medication sensitivity.
9. Additional individualized interventions: _____	**9.** Rationales: _____

Suggested NIC Interventions
Infection control; Infection protection; Incision site care; Wound care

Suggested NOC Outcomes
Infection status; Wound healing: Primary intention

Nursing diagnosis
Bathing or hygiene self-care deficit related to bed rest and activity limitations

NURSING PRIORITY
Assist with bathing and toileting when bed rest is required.

PATIENT OUTCOME CRITERIA

While on bed rest, the patient will:
- accept self-care assistance
- observe activity restrictions.
  Within 3 days after surgery, the patient will:
- resume normal self-care activities
- perform normal bowel elimination without straining.

INTERVENTIONS	RATIONALES
1. Assist with bathing and oral hygiene daily, as needed.	1. Bed rest and arm movement limitations prevent the patient from sitting up and using bathing and oral hygiene supplies.
2. Assist the patient at mealtime. Elevate the head of the bed, as ordered.	2. The patient may be unable to reach or manipulate items on the meal tray while on bed rest. Raising the head of the bed facilitates swallowing and minimizes the risk of aspiration.
3. Assist the patient with a bedpan and urinal, as needed.	3. The patient will be unable to use the bathroom.
4. Administer stool softeners and laxatives judiciously, as ordered, and document their use. Encourage alternatives or supplements to stool softeners and laxatives, such as increased dietary fiber (if possible) and prune juice.	4. Straining to defecate requires considerable energy and may produce vagal-mediated arrhythmias. Laxative dependence diminishes the urge for normal defecation.
5. If arm use isn't restricted, encourage the patient to move the arm and resume self-care.	5. The patient may be hesitant to use the arm initially for fear of dislodging the electrode.
6. Additional individualized interventions: _____	6. Rationales: _____

> **Suggested NIC Interventions**
> *Self-care assisstance: Bathing/hygiene; Self-care assisstance: Dressing/grooming*

> **Suggested NOC Outcomes**
> *Self-care: Bathing; Self-care: Eating; Self-care: Toileting*

Nursing diagnosis

Deficient knowledge (self-care after discharge) related to unfamiliar therapeutic intervention

NURSING PRIORITY

Teach the information and skills necessary for optimal self-care.

PATIENT OUTCOME CRITERIA

By the time of discharge, the patient will:
- demonstrate accurate pulse rate measurement
- list significant, reportable signs and symptoms
- verbalize activity expectations, limitations, and environmental hazards
- reinforce initial follow-up arrangements or appointments
- state the purpose, dosage, administration schedule, and adverse effects of medications
- verbalize understanding of the need to inform health care providers about the pacemaker.

INTERVENTIONS	RATIONALES
1. *Explain potential signs and symptoms of decreased cardiac output* that should be reported to the physician, such as shortness of breath, low or erratic pulse, light-headedness, chest pains, decreased exercise tolerance, prolonged fatigue or weakness, or recurrence of preimplant symptoms.	**1.** These signs and symptoms may indicate pacemaker malfunction.
2. *Discuss signs and symptoms of extraneous stimulation* that should be reported, such as muscle, arm, or skin twitching near the generator box or prolonged and rapid hiccups.	**2.** These signs and symptoms may result from electrode or lead malposition and adjacent tissue stimulation.
3. *Teach the patient to recognize and report signs and symptoms of pocket infection,* such as fever or chills and incisional drainage, redness, swelling, or pain.	**3.** Infection may not be apparent until after discharge.
4. *Teach the patient to check the radial pulse* for a full minute at the same time daily after resting for 5 minutes; reinforce guidelines for reporting significant changes, particularly a decrease of 3 to 5 beats/minute below the pacer setting or an erratic, persistent high rate.	**4.** Changes in pacemaker function may be detected by regular assessment.
5. *Emphasize the importance of complying with the follow-up monitoring regimen* (by in-person appointments or a telephone monitoring device).	**5.** Pacemaker function can be evaluated most accurately by an ECG. Periodic checks using a donut-shaped magnet help determine when a new battery is needed.
6. *Emphasize the need to inform health care providers about the pacemaker.* The patient should wear a medical alert bracelet and carry a wallet identification card with pacemaker specifications.	**6.** Certain procedures, such as electrocautery, diathermy, lithotripsy, radiation treatment, transcutaneous epidermal nerve stimulation, and nuclear magnetic resonance imaging, may be contraindicated. A medical identification bracelet and pacemaker specifications will help ensure faster treatment if an emergency occurs.
7. *Discuss potential environmental hazards,* such as power plants, high-voltage power lines, radio and television transmitters, and electromagnetic power fields. Potential hazards include antitheft devices, airport security systems, close proximity to the generator of a running car engine, and use of cellular phones close to the pacemaker site. Encourage the patient to discuss limitations and hazards with the physician.	**7.** Exposure to electromagnetic power sources has the potential to interfere with some pacemakers, depending on the age of the pacemaker, mode of action, and type of lead. Most home electrical appliances, including microwave ovens, aren't a problem if in proper working order.
8. Gradual resumption of activities according to patient tolerance generally is encouraged. Activities involving abrupt, forceful arm movement (such as tennis and golf) that may cause lead fracture may be limited for several weeks. Contact sports typically aren't allowed. Tight clothing over the incision may impair healing. Activities involving arm pushing create myopotentials that may be interpreted by some pacemakers as intrinsic heartbeats.	**8.** As specified by the physician, instruct the patient about resuming activity and about any limitations on travel, exercise, bathing and showering, tight clothing, and sexual activity.
9. *Teach the purpose, dosage, administration schedule, and adverse effects of all medications.*	**9.** Knowledge may increase compliance.
10. *Provide written material for all patient-teaching topics.*	**10.** Written material reinforces and serves as a reference for this detailed information.
11. Additional individualized interventions: _____	**11.** Rationales: _____

> **Suggested NIC Interventions**
> *Teaching: Disease process; Teaching: Individual;*
> *Teaching: Procedure/treatment*

> **Suggested NOC Outcomes**
> *Knowledge: Treatment procedures; Knowledge: Treatment regimen; Knowledge: Disease process*

Nursing diagnosis
Disturbed body image related to dependence on pacemaker

NURSING PRIORITY
Promote positive incorporation of the pacemaker into the patient's body image.

PATIENT OUTCOME CRITERIA
By the time of discharge, the patient will:
- participate actively in self-care
- ask appropriate questions and show interest in learning about the pacemaker
- show no evidence of maladaptive coping.

INTERVENTIONS	RATIONALES
1. *Assess the patient's adaptation to change,* including perceptions and personal meaning of limitations.	**1.** The changes caused by pacemaker implantation will vary in significance among patients. Many patients welcome the increased activity tolerance and show signs of improved self-image. For others, however, loss of a body function may trigger the grieving process.
2. Encourage the patient to ask questions and verbalize feelings.	**2.** Verbalization enables the nurse to listen to, assess, and validate the patient's feelings, thus facilitating adjustment to change.
3. Encourage the patient to look at the incision and the pacemaker site.	**3.** Willingness to view the incision and site may reflect beginning acceptance and adjustment.
4. *Assess for maladaptive coping behaviors,* such as manipulating the generator box, verbalizing an inability to make lifestyle or health-promoting changes, crying or a flat affect, lack of participation and interest in activities, or anxiety.	**4.** These behaviors may indicate that the patient is having difficulty adjusting to the physical change and the need for pacemaker dependence.
5. If indicated, consult the "Grieving" care plan, page 105 and "Ineffective individual coping" care plan, page 124.	**5.** These care plans contain generalized interventions related to these problems.
6. Additional individualized interventions: _____	**6.** Rationales: _____

> **Suggested NIC Interventions**
> *Body image enhancement; Grief work facilitation;*
> *Anticipatory guidance; Coping enhancement; Self-*
> *esteem enhancement*

> **Suggested NOC Outcomes**
> *Body image; Grief resolution; Self-esteem*

Discharge planning

DISCHARGE CHECKLIST

Before discharge, the patient shows evidence of:

❏ normal body temperature

❏ absence of angina and arrhythmias

❏ ECG within expected parameters, indicating appropriate pacemaker settings, sensing, firing, and capturing

❏ vital signs within acceptable parameters

❏ absence of pulmonary and cardiovascular complications

❏ absence of redness, swelling, and drainage at incision site

❏ WBC count within normal parameters

❏ ability to transfer, ambulate, and perform activities of daily living (ADLs) in the same manner as before hospitalization or better

❏ adequate home support system or referral to home care if indicated by inadequate support system and the patient's inability to perform ADLs.

TEACHING CHECKLIST

Document evidence that the patient and his family demonstrate an understanding of:

❏ symptoms of pacemaker failure or complications

❏ signs and symptoms of infection

❏ type of pacemaker and rate

❏ need for daily pulse rate measurement

❏ how to obtain a wallet pacemaker specification card and medical alert bracelet

❏ need to inform other health care providers about the pacemaker

❏ plan for resuming activities

❏ limitations and precautions

❏ all discharge medications' purpose, dosage, administration schedule, and adverse effects requiring medical attention

❏ follow-up monitoring

❏ how to contact the physician.

DOCUMENTATION CHECKLIST

Using outcome criteria as a guide, document before surgery:

❏ clinical status on admission

❏ 12-lead ECG reading

❏ chest X-ray and results

❏ urinalysis results

❏ blood chemistry studies and complete blood counts

❏ Prothrombin time/international normalized ratio and partial thromboplastin time

❏ patient teaching

❏ surgical skin preparation

❏ I.V. line patency and site condition

❏ nothing-by-mouth status.

Using outcome criteria as a guide, document after surgery:

❏ clinical status

❏ telemetry findings

❏ 12-lead ECG reading

❏ incision status and care

❏ I.V. line patency and site condition

❏ chest X-ray and results

❏ pacemaker clinic check completed or a clinic appointment

❏ patient and family teaching

❏ discharge planning.

Associated care plans

■ Acute myocardial infarction

■ Acute pain

■ Angina pectoris

■ Geriatric care

■ Grieving

■ Heart failure

■ Ineffective individual coping

■ Perioperative care

■ Thrombophlebitis

References

Espiritu, J.D., and Keller, C.A. "Pneumomediastinum and Subcutaneous Emphysema from Pacemaker Placement," *Pacing Clinics Electrophysiology* 24(6):1041-42, June 2001.

Essebag, V. et al. "Amiodarone and the Risk of Bradyarrhythmia Requiring Permanent Pacemaker in Elderly Patients with Atrial Fibrillation and Prior Myocardial Infarction," *Journal of the American College of Cardiology* 41(2):249-54, January 2003.

Jordan, K. (ed). *Emergency Nursing Core Curriculum.* Emergency Nurses Association. Philadelphia: W.B. Saunders Co., 2000

Lynn-McHale, D.J., and Carlson, K.K. American Association of Critical Care Nurses *AACN Procedure Manual for Critical Care,* 4th ed. Philadelphia: W.B. Saunders Co., 2001.

Shoemaker, W.C., et al. *Textbook of Critical Care,* 4th ed. Philadelphia: W.B. Saunders Co., 2002.

Septic shock

DRG INFORMATION

DRG 415   Operating Room Procedure for Infectious and
           Parasitic Diseases.
           Mean LOS = 14.4 days
DRG 416   Septicemia; Age 18 + .
           Mean LOS = 7.4 days
DRG 417   Septicemia; Ages 0 to 17.
           Mean LOS = 5 days

Introduction

DEFINITION AND TIME FOCUS

Septic shock is one of three forms of distributive shock.
It's a complex, life-threatening process of microcirculatory dysfunction and altered cellular metabolism resulting
from altered blood flow and capillary permeability at the
microcirculatory level. Septic shock usually starts with
an infection that progresses to bacteremia (when the infectious agents enter the vascular compartment) and
then to sepsis with a systemic response (tachycardia,
tachypnea, pyrexia, and leukocytosis). The condition
advances to shock when the immune system is overwhelmed and hypotension and altered tissue perfusion
are present. Although any type of bacteria (gram-positive
and gram-negative), virus, parasite, or fungus may precipitate the condition, septic shock in adults is typically
due to the gram-negative organism.

Much of the shock state is caused by chemical mediators and immunologic responses to the infectious agent.
The responses and mediators include significant elevations of white blood cells (WBCs), cytokines, tumor
necrosis factor, and interleukins 1 and 6; activation of
the complement system with prostaglandins and their
metabolites; and other endogenous mediators that exacerbate vasodilation and vascular permeability. As the
shock state progresses, the changes in vascular permeability allow the development of edema, which may
mask hypovolemia. With cytokine release, the patient
commonly has a temperature greater than 101° F
(38.3° C). Changes in systemic vascular resistance (SVR)
and blood pressure may cause flushed skin that can lead
to the false assumption that the body is sufficiently perfused, although the cells actually have significant increases in oxygen demand (hypermetabolism). With
activation of the complement system, microvascular
damage leads to fibrin and platelet clumping in the capillary beds. The development of disseminated intravascular coagulation (DIC) occurs rapidly. Following release of
the prostaglandins, blood flow stagnates because of the
zones of vasoconstriction and vasodilation, further inhibiting tissue perfusion and allowing for the development of ischemia. With the body under such significant
stress, changes in glucose, cortisol, and glucagon occur,
resulting in elevated serum glucose levels. The infection
overwhelms the body's defenses, and a vicious cycle of
destruction occurs as additional systems are activated.
This care plan focuses on recognizing the patient in the
medical-surgical setting who's at risk for or develops
septic shock as well as the critically ill patient with septic shock. (See *Clinical snapshot: Septic shock,* page 451.)

ETIOLOGY AND PRECIPITATING FACTORS

See *Risk factors for nosocomial infection*, page 450.

Focused assessment guidelines

NURSING HISTORY
(FUNCTIONAL HEALTH PATTERN FINDINGS)
Health-perception–health-management pattern
■ History of heart failure, diabetes mellitus, malnutrition, burns, or other factors affecting fluid balance
■ Recent invasive procedure, especially any major surgi-
cal procedure, such as abdominal surgery, massive trau-
ma repairs, or placement of invasive hemodynamic mon-
itoring lines or urinary catheters
■ Recent history of an infection — bacterial, viral, fun-
gal, or parasitic
■ History of recent antibiotic use
Nutritional-metabolic pattern
■ History of elevated serum glucose levels unresponsive
to treatment
■ Altered or decreased intake
■ Temperature elevation
Elimination pattern
■ History of recent urinary tract infection (UTI)
■ Diarrhea or alterations in bowel pattern
■ Severe abdominal pain
Activity-exercise pattern
■ Weakness and fatigue
Cognitive-perceptual pattern
■ Restlessness, anxiety, or altered level of consciousness
(LOC)

PHYSICAL FINDINGS
Neurologic
■ Altered LOC, ranging from subtle changes (early),
restlessness, anxiety, irritability, disorientation, and
lethargy to coma (late)

Risk factors for nosocomial infection

The table below lists endogenous and exogenous risk factors for nosocomial infection.

Endogenous	Exogenous
• Age over 70	• Abdominal or thoracic surgery
• Alcoholism	• Conditions favoring aspiration
• Cardiopulmonary disease (for example, heart failure or chronic obstructive pulmonary disease)	– Endotracheal intubation
	– Nasogastric intubation
• Depressed level of consciousness	– Supine positioning
• Diabetes	• Immobility
• Malnutrition	• Prolonged mechanical ventilation
• Severe underlying disease (for example, acquired immunodeficiency syndrome or cancer)	• Use of antibiotics
	• Use of histamine₂ blockers or antacids
	• Use of immunosuppressive drugs (such as steroids)
	• Lapses in sterile technique
	• Burns
	• Trauma
	• Invasive catheters

Adapted from Tasota, F., et al. "Protecting ICU Patients from Nosocomial Infections: Practical Measures for Favorable Outcomes," *Critical Care Nurse* 18(1):54-65, February 1998.

■ Possible slight decrease in Glasgow Coma Scale score

Cardiovascular
■ Hypotension that doesn't respond to vasopressors
■ Tachycardia
■ Arrhythmias
■ Temperature greater than 101° F (38.3° C)
■ Altered hemodynamic parameters (markedly increased cardiac output, decreased ejection fraction, decreased SVR in early stage; decreased cardiac output, ejection fraction, and SVR in late stage)
■ Increased capillary refill time (greater than 3 seconds)
■ Decreased or thready peripheral pulses

Pulmonary
■ Tachypnea (usually greater than 36 breaths/minute)
■ Hyperventilation (respiratory alkalosis)
■ Altered or decreased oxygen saturation levels
■ Dyspnea on exertion
■ Increasing presence of crackles

Gastrointestinal
■ Abdominal tenderness or pain, especially over right upper quadrant
■ Pale or cyanotic oral mucous membranes

Hematologic
■ Presence of slow bleeding from mucous membranes
■ Bleeding from puncture sites, incisions, or the GI or genitourinary tract

Renal
■ Oliguria to anuria

Integumentary
■ Altered skin temperature: warm progressing to cool
■ Progression from flushed to mottled to pallor to cyanosis

DIAGNOSTIC STUDIES

No laboratory tests are diagnostic for septic shock. Microbiology studies will support the diagnosis.

Values will change, reflecting end-organ deterioration. Possible changes include:
■ complete blood count — may vary, depending on shock stage; significant elevation of WBC count (greater than 15,000/ml); red blood cells may be decreased with blood loss; decreased hemoglobin levels and increased hematocrit
■ serum osmolality — may increase, reflecting fluid loss
■ urine osmolality or specific gravity — increased, reflecting volume loss
■ elevated serum lactate levels — reflect change by cells from aerobic to anaerobic metabolism; the higher the level, the greater the switch
■ blood urea nitrogen (BUN) and creatinine levels — increased, reflecting decreased renal perfusion
■ glucose level — increased, reflecting stress-induced sympathetic stimulation
■ serum electrolyte levels — may vary, depending on the underlying problem and shock stage. Commonly, hypernatremia reflects increased renal sodium retention in response to volume losses, hypokalemia reflects urinary potassium losses in exchange for sodium, and hyperkalemia reflects acidosis, decreased glomerular filtration, and cell necrosis.
■ arterial blood gas (ABG) levels — reveal increased pH level and decreased partial pressure of arterial carbon dioxide ($Paco_2$) in early shock, reflecting respiratory alkalosis caused by hyperventilation and stimulation of the hypothalmic respiratory center by the endotoxin. ABG

results progress to decreased pH level, increased $Paco_2$, and decreased bicarbonate (HCO_3^-) level in late shock, reflecting respiratory acidosis caused by hypoventilation and metabolic acidosis caused by anaerobic metabolism.
■ clotting profile — may reveal coagulopathy, shown as decreased platelet level, decreased fibrinogen level, increased fibrin split products, or altered D-dimer results
■ 12-lead electrocardiogram (ECG) — may reveal arrhythmias or changes reflecting myocardial ischemia, acute myocardial infarction (AMI), or electrolyte imbalances.

POTENTIAL COMPLICATIONS
■ Acute renal failure
■ Acute respiratory distress syndrome (ARDS)
■ DIC
■ Cardiogenic shock
■ Cerebral anoxia
■ Pancreatitis
■ Hepatic failure
■ Multiple organ dysfunction syndrome

CLINICAL SNAPSHOT ✷

Septic shock

Major nursing diagnoses and collaborative problems	Key patient outcomes
ND: Risk for infection	Show no signs of infection such as elevated temperature.
CP: Risk for hypovolemic shock	Have normal ABG values: pH, 7.35 to 7.45; $Paco_2$, 35 to 45 mm Hg; and HCO_3^-, 23 to 28 mEq/L.
ND: Impaired gas exchange	Maintain stable vital signs, typically: heart rate, 60 to 100 beats/minute; systolic blood pressure, 90 to 140 mm Hg; and diastolic blood pressure, 50 to 90 mm Hg.
ND: Risk for injury	Display normal organ function of neurologic, cardiovascular, pulmonary, and renal systems, as evidenced by normal LOC, vital signs, capillary refill, ABG values, and urine output.
ND: Ineffective coping	Describe his emotional state to the nurse.

Nursing diagnosis
Risk for infection related to increased exposure to pathogens, inadequate defenses, multiple invasive lines, surgical interventions, or multiple other risk factors

NURSING PRIORITIES
■ Prevent infection when possible.
■ Recognize patients at high risk for infection.
■ Prevent progression to shock.

PATIENT OUTCOME CRITERIA
Within 48 to 72 hours of onset of infection, the patient will:
■ maintain a normal temperature for him, ideally 98.6° F (37° C) or less
■ maintain a LOC normal for him, ideally alert and oriented to person, place, and time
■ maintain vital signs within normal limits, typically: heart rate, 60 to 100 beats/minute; systolic blood pressure, 90 to 140 mm Hg; and diastolic blood pressure, 50 to 90 mm Hg
■ display a WBC count between 5,000 and 10,000/µl.

INTERVENTIONS

1. *Be aware of the major sites for infection and constantly protect patients and staff.** For example, ensure that invasive devices are removed promptly, following facility or Centers for Disease Control and Prevention (CDC) guidelines.

2. *Be vigilant in applying standard precautions and other infection control measures.* Routinely follow principles of medical asepsis, especially hand washing. Teach the patient and his family the value of hand washing. Implement strategies to prevent nosocomial pneumonia (such as using sterile technique to suction secretions, providing meticulous mouth care, and elevating the head of the bed for a patient with a nasogastric [NG] tube), nosocomial UTI (such as using sterile technique to insert a urinary catheter and maintaining a closed drainage system), and I.V. catheter nosocomial infection (such as replacing peripheral catheters and dressings according to facility or CDC guidelines). Also, consult facility policy, the CDC's *Guidelines for Isolation Precautions in Hospitals,* and the latest CDC guidelines for further details.

3. *Identify patients at risk for bacteremia, sepsis, or septic shock.* Be on the alert for impending infections. Obtain orders to culture suspicious sites, secretions, or drainage. Also consider the need to obtain cultures when the patient has a fever of unknown origin or fails to improve despite antimicrobial therapy.

4. *Be meticulous in obtaining specimens for culture and sensitivity testing.* For example, obtain blood cultures, as ordered, before instituting antimicrobial therapy. Ideally, obtain blood cultures from different sites. When obtaining a urine specimen from a patient with a urinary catheter, obtain it from the sampling port. If no sampling port is present, obtain the specimen from the catheter rather than the drainage tubing or bag. Disinfect the catheter, and aspirate the sample with a needle and syringe.

RATIONALES

1. In the acute care setting, the three major sites for patient infection are the respiratory system, the urinary tract, and the bloodstream. Pneumonia, UTIs, and septicemia are common diagnoses for infections in these sites. The most important factor related to infections associated with invasive lines is the time that catheters are left in place.

2. Because of the high mortality for septic shock, prevention remains the most important strategy. The patient may develop infections from exogenous sources (outside the patient) or from endogenous sources (the patient's normal flora). Routine application of infection control measures is critical because an estimated 33% of nosocomial (hospital-acquired) infections are preventable. People are the major source of nosocomial infection. Pathogens on the hands may survive for several hours, and the spread of most infections can be prevented by simple hand washing. Lapses in sterile technique allow the introduction of organisms into the patient. The CDC's guidelines specify types of precautions appropriate to specific situations.

3. Bacteremia is the asymptomatic presence of bacteria in the bloodstream. Sepsis is present when a systemic inflammatory response occurs, producing systemic signs such as fever. Septic shock is present when a septic patient develops profound hypotension and markedly abnormal tissue perfusion. Early recognition and intervention may prevent infection from progressing to bacteremia, sepsis, or septic shock. Mortality from septic shock may be as high as 60% with aggressive early treatment and as high as 90% if early subtle signs are missed.

4. A contaminated specimen will produce inaccurate results. Treatment may then be inappropriate, and identification and treatment of an appropriate organism will be delayed. Starting antimicrobial therapy before obtaining blood cultures will lessen the number of pathogens in the bloodstream, thus masking infection. Having specimens from different sites increases the physician's ability to differentiate contaminants from pathogens. Using the urinary sampling port or aspirating from the catheter provides a fresh sample for testing.

---

*Italics indicate key interventions.

5. *Observe for local signs and symptoms of infection,* such as erythema and edema at a particular skin site or coughing or altered breath sounds. Monitor the patient for classic systemic signs and symptoms, such as fever or an increased WBC count. Consult with the physician about which level of increased temperature should be treated. Be alert for patients who can't mount a normal response to infection, such as those who are neutropenic or elderly. Monitor these patients for subtle signs of infection, such as confusion, fatigue, or restlessness.

5. Elderly patients are at risk because aging impairs numerous defense mechanisms. For example, in the pulmonary system, ciliary action decreases, respiratory excursion lessens, and the cough reflex becomes diminished, placing the patient at increased risk for respiratory infections. Protein malnutrition — common in the elderly — depletes energy reserves; it's linked to bacterial movement from the gut by bacterial translocation (movement of bacteria through an intact mucosal barrier) and disruption of the intestinal mucosal lining, which allows bacteria to move through the disrupted barrier. Fever, a protective response in a patient with normal immunity, creates a hostile environment for pathogens.

6. *Administer antimicrobial drugs empirically, as ordered.* When culture and sensitivity reports arrive, make sure the organism is sensitive to the drug in the dose ordered. Consult with the physician for definitive drug therapy.

6. Commonly, infection is suspected based on clinical evidence. Before the infecting organism is identified, a broad-spectrum antibiotic usually is used. The choice of drug is based on clinical judgment and experience as well as on the suspected organism and organisms usually found in similar clinical situations in the unit or facility. Common infecting organisms include *Pseudomonas aeruginosa, Staphylococcus aureus, Candida, Enterobacter,* and *Enterococcus.*

When the culture and sensitivity report arrives, check which body area the specimen came from (which will help you distinguish normal flora from pathogens), the colony count (number of organisms), and the identification of a specific pathogen. Then check the drugs to which the organism is sensitive, and double-check the dosage against the dosage the patient is receiving. The physician may wish to change the empiric medication to one or more specific to the organism.

7. Monitor closely for expected and adverse effects. Alert the physician if the drug seems ineffective, as evidenced by continuing or increasing signs of infection, deterioration in vital signs, or other indicators.

7. Monitoring drug effects is important not only for the patient but for all patients because of concern about the emergence of drug-resistant organisms. Drug resistance occurs when a specific pathogen no longer is killed by an antimicrobial to which it used to be effective. Among the greatest concerns are methicillin-resistant *S. aureus* and vancomycin-resistant *Enterococcus.* Overuse and misuse of antibiotics allows drug-resistant organisms to emerge.

8. Additional individualized interventions: _____

_____

8. Rationales: _____

_____

Suggested NIC Interventions
Infection control; Infection protection; Incision site care; Wound care

Suggested NOC Outcomes
Infection status; Wound healing: Primary intention

Collaborative problem

Risk for hypovolemic shock related to inflammatory mediators

NURSING PRIORITIES

- Identify the stage of septic shock.
- Intervene to maintain cardiac output.

PATIENT OUTCOME CRITERIA

Within 48 hours of developing septic shock, the patient will:
- maintain stable vital signs, typically: heart rate, 60 to 100 beats/minute; systolic blood pressure, 90 to 140 mm Hg; and diastolic blood pressure, 50 to 90 mm Hg
- display normal hemodynamic values (cardiac output, 4 to 6 L/minute; SVR, 800 to 1,200 dynes/sec/cm^{-5}; and pulmonary artery wedge pressure, 4 to 12 mm Hg)
- produce a normal urine output (60 to 150 ml/hour)
- have warm, dry skin and a capillary refill time of less than 3 seconds, indicating sufficient tissue perfusion
- display a stable neurologic status, ideally alert and oriented.

INTERVENTIONS	RATIONALES
1. *Be alert for the signs and symptoms of early stage septic shock:* flushed skin, tachycardia, tachypnea, and fever or reduced temperature.	**1.** Septic shock may progress from an early stage to a late stage. Early-stage septic shock is characterized by hyperdynamic cardiovascular function, peripheral vasodilation, systemic edema, and relative hypovolemia. These changes result from excessive vascular mediators released from the cell wall of dying cells. These mediators produce widespread vasodilation, characterized by warm, dry, flushed skin; tachycardia; and good urine output. Hemodynamic values typically reveal decreased SVR, markedly increased cardiac output, hypotension, and widened pulse pressure. The decreased SVR results in decreased resistance to cardiac ejection and shunting of blood to the peripheral tissues, producing the warm, flushed skin. Despite the increased cardiac output, myocardial function decreases, probably due to the release of myocardial depressant factor. Increased vascular permeability results in fluid movement from the vascular system to the interstitium, producing systemic edema and relative hypovolemia. Other signs seen during this early stage are tachypnea and a subtly decreased LOC, which appears as confusion, restlessness, or agitation. Fever may be present if the patient has been able to mount an immune response to the organism. If not, hypothermia is present. This can be misleading because the patient who formerly had a decreased temperature may now have a temperature within the normal range, which represents an increased temperature for him.
2. *Implement therapy, as ordered,* including fluid administration and antimicrobial drugs. See "Risk for infection," page 451, for further information on drug administration. Assist the physician with removal of the infection's source, if possible (for example, abscess drainage or wound debridement).	**2.** Early, aggressive treatment is key to intervening in septic shock. Because of marked vasodilation and increased vascular permeability, fluid shifts from the vascular system to the periphery, producing relative hypovolemia. Therefore, treatment of early septic shock includes generous fluid replacement and administration of vasopressors to counteract the decreased SVR as well as administration of antimicrobials presumed effective against the suspected pathogen.

3. *Be alert for signs of late-stage septic shock:* severe hypotension, cold mottled extremities, poor peripheral pulses, markedly decreased LOC, systemic and pulmonary edema, and oliguria or anuria. Monitor hemodynamic values for decreased cardiac output and SVR. As ordered, implement standard hypovolemic shock measures, as detailed in the "Hypovolemic shock" care plan, page 424.

4. Additional individualized interventions: _____
_____

3. The late stage of septic shock is decompensation. Hypodynamic cardiac function produces decreased cardiac output, responsible for such signs as severe hypotension and oliguria or anuria. Treatment of this stage is similar to that of hypovolemic shock, with increased emphasis on monitoring the patient for signs of fluid overload and cautious titration of vasopressors to maximize cardiac output. The "Hypovolemic shock" care plan details further management of this stage.

4. Rationales: _____
_____

Nursing diagnosis

Impaired gas exchange related to ventilation-perfusion imbalance and diffusion defects

NURSING PRIORITY
Maintain ventilation and oxygenation.

PATIENT OUTCOME CRITERIA
Within 48 hours, the patient will:
- show ABG levels within expected limits
- have clearing breath sounds bilaterally
- show no or limited signs of ARDS progression.
  By discharge, the patient will:
- maintain a patent airway
- be free from mechanical ventilation support
- have normal ABG results and pulmonary function values
- have stabilized oxygen consumption values.

INTERVENTIONS

1. *Provide standard nursing care related to impaired gas exchange.* Maintain airway patency and monitor respiratory status. Suction as necessary. Provide supplemental oxygen, as ordered, and assist with intubation and mechanical ventilation if indicated.

2. *Monitor oxygen saturation* through continuous pulse oximetry. Monitor ABG levels, as ordered, typically at least every 4 to 12 hours.

3. *Observe for signs and symptoms of ARDS,* such as tachypnea, progressive dyspnea, increasing inspiratory pressure, lung compliance less than 50 ml/cm H_2O (if mechanically ventilated), deteriorating ABG or pulse oximetry values, or hypoxemia. If you detect these problems, document them and alert the physician. Implement measures described in the "Acute respiratory distress syndrome" care plan, page 252, as appropriate.

RATIONALES

1. Numerous factors may cause ventilation-perfusion imbalance in shock, including atelectasis, microemboli, pulmonary congestion, and impaired capillary perfusion. The general measures listed apply to the care of any critically ill patient.

2. Pulse oximetry determines oxygen saturation rapidly, continuously, and noninvasively. ABG results indicate oxygenation status and degree of acid-base imbalance. Hyperventilation, a compensatory response to hypoxemia, is common in early septic shock and can lead to respiratory alkalosis. Late septic shock is characterized by combined metabolic acidosis from decreased capillary perfusion (lactic acid production and anaerobic metabolism) and respiratory acidosis (due to hypercarbia).

3. Septic shock ranks as a major risk factor for ARDS due to such factors as decreased perfusion, hypoxemia, increased capillary permeability, and high oxygen levels used in treatment. The "Acute respiratory distress syndrome" care plan describes this ominous complication and related care.

4. *Assist with pulmonary artery catheter insertion, if ordered. Monitor hemodynamic parameters* as well as oxygen delivery and oxygen consumption (VO_2).

4. With the progression of septic shock, there are changes in the hemodynamic parameters as well as in cellular VO_2 and oxygen delivery. The tissues have increased demand, yet altered cellular metabolism prevents the cells from extracting sufficient oxygen to meet metabolic needs; therefore, mixed venous saturation is greater than 80% (normal is 60% to 80%).

5. Additional individualized interventions: _____

5. Rationales: _____

Suggested NIC Interventions
Acid-base management; Electrolyte management; Laboratory data interpretation; Oxygen therapy; Ventilation assistance; Airway management; Respiratory monitoring; Embolus care: Pulmonary; Hemodynamic regulation; Vital signs monitoring

Suggested NOC Outcomes
Electrolyte and acid-base balance; Respiratory status: Gas exchange; Respiratory status: Ventilation; Tissue perfusion: Pulmonary; Vital signs status

---

Nursing diagnosis
Risk for injury due to complications related to ischemia or bleeding

NURSING PRIORITY
Prevent or minimize complications.

PATIENT OUTCOME CRITERIA
By the time of discharge, the patient will:
■ be alert and oriented to person, place, and time, moving all extremities spontaneously
■ maintain stable vital signs, typically: heart rate, 60 to 100 beats/minute; systolic blood pressure, 90 to 140 mm Hg; diastolic blood pressure, 50 to 90 mm Hg; and normal perfusion (evidenced by capillary refill less than 3 seconds)
■ have normal ABG values: pH, 7.35 to 7.45; $Paco_2$, 35 to 45 mm Hg; and HCO_3^-, 23 to 28 mEq/L
■ have a urine output of 60 to 150 ml/hour.

INTERVENTIONS

1. *Prevent paralytic ileus and stress ulcers.* Withhold food and fluids; insert an NG tube connected to suction, as ordered. Administer cimetidine (Tagamet), ranitidine (Zantac), sucralfate (Carafate), or antacids, as ordered. Monitor bowel sounds.

2. *Administer antibiotics, as ordered,* by mouth or NG tube if indicated. Attempt enteral feedings if the patient is able to tolerate food and there's adequate bowel motility. If not, use parenteral feedings to provide nutrients. See the "Nutritional deficit" care plan, page 138, for further details.)

RATIONALES

1. Paralytic ileus may result from mesenteric ischemia. The resulting gastric distention provokes vomiting, which can lead to chemical pneumonitis if aspiration occurs. Withholding food and fluids reduces stress on the stomach. NG drainage decompresses the stomach. The medications listed reduce the risk of stress ulcers by decreasing hydrochloric acid secretion or coating the gastric mucosa.

2. This antibiotic regimen may prevent translocation of GI bacteria from the lumen of the gut into the vascular compartment, thereby limiting an additional source of infection. Food in a mobile gut is thought to prevent translocation of bacteria. If the patient is unable to tolerate enteral feedings, use parenteral feedings to support hypermetabolic tissue demands. The "Nutritional deficit" care plan provides detailed information on this problem.

3. *Observe for signs and symptoms of AMI,* such as severe chest pain, shortness of breath, hypotension, diaphoresis, pained facial expression, elevated cardiac isoenzymes, or ECG showing ST-segment displacement, T-wave inversion, or pathologic Q waves. See the "Acute myocardial infarction" care plan, page 337.

4. *Observe for signs and symptoms of DIC,* such as blood oozing from multiple sites, repeated bleeding episodes, oral cyanosis, petechiae, ecchymoses, hematomas, prolonged prothrombin time (PT), prolonged partial thromboplastin time, decreased fibrinogen level, decreased platelet count, or elevated fibrin split products level. Refer to the "Disseminated intravascular coagulation" care plan, page 764, for further information.

5. *Observe for signs and symptoms of acute renal failure,* such as oliguria or anuria, weight gain, neck vein distention, crackles, dependent edema, or elevated BUN and serum creatinine levels. As appropriate, implement measures described in the "Acute renal failure" care plan, page 668.

6. *Observe for signs and symptoms of liver failure,* such as drowsiness, intellectual deterioration, personality changes, septicemia, fever, hyperkinetic circulation, elevated serum ammonium levels, jaundice, hepatomegaly, ascites, easy bruising, increased PT, elevated serum aspartate aminotransferase level, or increased bilirubin level. See the "Liver failure" care plan, page 533.

7. Additional individualized interventions: _____
_____

3. Decreased perfusion of the heart, catecholamine stimulation, hypoxemia, and increased afterload all may cause AMI. Decreased perfusion of the pancreas may release myocardial depressant factor, which may also cause AMI. The "Acute myocardial infarction" care plan gives details on this complication.

4. Shock is a major risk factor for DIC because of such factors as capillary sludging, acidosis, sepsis, trauma, or other underlying causes. The "Disseminated intravascular coagulation" care plan describes this devastating development in-depth.

5. Renal blood vessel constriction is an early compensatory mechanism in shock. Although this constriction limits glomerular filtration, thus conserving fluid volume, it impairs renal perfusion, which may result in acute renal failure. The "Acute renal failure" care plan describes this complication in detail.

6. Although shock may damage hepatic cells, prompt correction of shock may allow these cells to regenerate. Early detection of liver failure may prevent severe damage to this critical organ. The "Liver failure" care plan presents the pathophysiology of this disorder and related care.

7. Rationales: _____
_____

Suggested NIC Interventions
Surveillance: Safety

Suggested NOC Outcomes
Safety status: Physical injury

Nursing diagnosis
Ineffective coping related to threat to life

NURSING PRIORITY
Provide emotional support to the patient.

PATIENT OUTCOME CRITERIA
By the time of discharge, the patient will meet outcome criteria identified in the "Ineffective individual coping" care plan, page 124.

INTERVENTIONS	**RATIONALES**
1. Provide standard nursing care related to ineffective individual coping and compromised family coping. Implement measures described in "Ineffective individual coping," page 124, and "Compromised family coping" page 67, as appropriate.	1. Families (and alert patients) are aware that shock is life-threatening, and they react to the possibility of death in various ways. These care plans describe measures to help them cope with their realistic fear and other emotional responses.
2. Additional individualized interventions: _____	2. Rationales: _____

> **Suggested NIC Interventions**
> *Decision-making support; Emotional support*

> **Suggested NOC Outcomes**
> *Coping; Fear control*

Discharge planning
DISCHARGE CHECKLIST
Before discharge, the patient shows evidence of:
- ❏ blood pressure within normal limits without I.V. inotropic or vasopressor support
- ❏ pulse and respirations within normal limits
- ❏ ABG levels within expected limits for recovery stage
- ❏ urine output within normal limits
- ❏ freedom from infection
- ❏ freedom from major complications.

TEACHING CHECKLIST
Document evidence that the patient and his family demonstrate an understanding of:
- ❏ cause and significance of shock
- ❏ expectations for recovery
- ❏ purpose of monitoring devices
- ❏ rationales for therapeutic interventions.

DOCUMENTATION CHECKLIST
Using outcome criteria as a guide, document:
- ❏ clinical status on admission
- ❏ significant changes in status
- ❏ pertinent diagnostic test findings
- ❏ care for invasive monitoring lines
- ❏ fluid administration
- ❏ use of inotropic agents, vasopressors, or other pharmacologic agents
- ❏ measures to support ventilation and oxygenation
- ❏ emotional support
- ❏ patient and family teaching
- ❏ discharge planning.

Associated care plans
- Acute myocardial infarction
- Acute renal failure
- Acute respiratory distress syndrome
- Cardiogenic shock

- Compromised family coping
- Disseminated intravascular coagulation
- Gastrointestinal hemorrhage
- Hypovolemic shock
- Impaired physical mobility
- Ineffective individual coping
- Liver failure
- Major burns
- Mechanical ventilation
- Multiple trauma
- Pulmonary embolism

References
Balcl, C., et al. "Usefulness of Procalcitonin for Diagnosis of Sepsis in the Intensive Care Unit," *Critical Care* 7(1):85-90, February 2003.

Dellinger, R.P. "Cardiovascular Management of Septic Shock," *Critical Care Medicine* 31(3):946-55, March 2003.

Jordan, K. (ed). *Emergency Nursing Core Curriculum.* Emergency Nurses Association. Philadelphia: W.B. Saunders Co., 2000.

Lynn-McHale, D.J., and Carlson, K.K. American Association of Critical Care Nurses *AACN Procedure Manual for Critical Care,* 4th ed. Philadelphia: W.B. Saunders Co., 2001.

Shoemaker, W.C., et al. *Textbook of Critical Care,* 4th ed. Philadelphia: W.B. Saunders Co., 2002.

Thrombophlebitis

DRG INFORMATION
DRG 128   Deep Vein Thrombophlebitis.
              Mean LOS = 5.6 days
DRG 130   Peripheral Vascular Disorders with Complication or Comorbidity (CC).
              Mean LOS = 5.7 days
DRG 131   Peripheral Vascular Disorders without CC.
              Mean LOS = 4.2 days

Introduction
DEFINITION AND TIME FOCUS
Thrombophlebitis is the severe, acute inflammation of small- and medium-sized veins associated with secondary thrombus formation. It can occur in superficial or deep veins. The most common site of superficial thrombophlebitis is the saphenous vein; the most common sites of deep vein thrombosis are the iliofemoral vein, popliteal veins, and small calf veins. This care plan focuses on the patient admitted for diagnosis and management of acute lower-extremity thrombophlebitis. (See *Clinical snapshot: Thrombophlebitis,* page 460.)

ETIOLOGY AND PRECIPITATING FACTORS
- Venous stasis from prolonged bed rest, sitting, or standing; varicose veins; low cardiac output; obesity; or limb paralysis
- Hypercoagulability from dehydration or oral contraceptive use
- Vessel wall trauma from venipunctures, leg injury, venous disease, infection, or chemical irritants, such as I.V. antibiotics or potassium chloride
- Vascular narrowing or degeneration from hypertension, hypercholesterolemia, diabetes, kidney disease, stroke, or smoking

Focused assessment guidelines
NURSING HISTORY
(FUNCTIONAL HEALTH PATTERN FINDINGS)
Health-perception–health-management pattern
- Acute onset of local pain (relieved by elevation of extremity), tenderness, edema, erythema, warmth, induration, or febrile reaction
- Known risk factors for thrombophlebitis such as prolonged bed rest
- History of recent vessel cannulation or vessel trauma

Activity-exercise pattern
- Sedentary lifestyle or occupation that requires standing for long periods
- Recent prolonged bed rest or immobility

Role-relationship pattern
- Family history of cardiac risk factors

PHYSICAL FINDINGS
Cardiovascular
- Local edema
- Engorged vessel
- Positive Homans' sign

Integumentary
- Local erythema
- Warmth
- Local induration
- Ulceration

DIAGNOSTIC STUDIES
- Complete blood count — white blood cell count may reflect inflammatory response and systemic infection
- Partial thromboplastin time (PTT) and prothrombin time/international normalized ratio (PT/INR) — may be prolonged, indicating clotting defects or hypercoagulability
- Cholesterol or triglyceride levels — may be elevated, suggesting increased risk of atherosclerosis
- Serum glucose levels — may be elevated, reflecting stress response or diabetes
- Doppler ultrasound blood flow detector test — determines venous return, may identify thrombolic occlusion
- Plethysmography — may show segmental occlusion
- Venography — may indicate loss of significant venous return
- ^{125}I fibrinogen leg scanning — may reflect vascular insufficiency

POTENTIAL COMPLICATIONS
- Venous ulcer
- Pulmonary embolus
- Phlegmasia cerulea dolens (sudden, marked leg swelling and cyanosis related to iliofemoral venous thrombosis)

CLINICAL SNAPSHOT ✴

Thrombophlebitis

Major nursing diagnoses and collaborative problems	Key patient outcomes
CP: Acute venous insufficiency	Show improved color and temperature of affected area.
ND: Acute pain	Rate pain as less than 3 on a 0 to 10 pain rating scale.
CP: Risk for thromboembolism	Show no signs of pulmonary embolism.
ND: Deficient knowledge (treatment regimen)	Be able to correctly describe details of anticoagulant administration, if prescribed, and how to minimize bleeding risk.

Collaborative problem

Acute venous insufficiency related to obstruction and stasis

NURSING PRIORITY

Promote venous blood flow.

PATIENT OUTCOME CRITERIA

Within 3 days of admission, the patient will:
- show normal color and temperature (for example, pink and warm for a white patient) of affected area
- have decreased measurement of calf
- show no evidence of bleeding
- rate pain as less than 3 on a 0 to 10 pain rating scale.

INTERVENTIONS	RATIONALES
1. *Assess calves and thighs daily for signs and symptoms of thrombophlebitis.* ✴ Early signs include swelling, erythema, edema, tenderness, venous patterning, or engorgement along the vein. Later signs include pain, cording (vein has a cordlike feeling), and a positive Homans' sign (not always present). Avoid deep palpation. If swelling is suspected or present, measure and record calf circumference, placing a reference mark on the leg. Repeat the measurement daily, comparing the latest measurement with previous values.	1. Early signs and symptoms result from vessel wall inflammation; later signs and symptoms from thrombus formation. Homans' sign (pain in the calf on dorsiflexion of the foot), commonly believed to indicate deep vein thrombosis, is an unreliable indicator. Absent in many cases of deep vein thrombosis, Homans' sign can be produced in any painful calf condition. Deep palpation may dislodge a clot. Leg circumference monitoring provides an objective method to evaluate swelling; using a reference mark ensures consistency.
2. *Notify the physician immediately if new signs and symptoms develop or existing ones worsen,* such as onset of new pain or increased swelling.	2. New or worsening signs of thrombophlebitis require prompt medical attention. Superficial thrombophlebitis, although not dangerous, is painful. Untreated deep vein thrombophlebitis can be life-threatening if the thrombus moves to the lungs.
3. *Implement activity restrictions:* – Maintain complete bed rest, usually for 3 to 7 days. – Elevate the extremity at least 30 degrees continuously, unless contraindicated. – Avoid using the knee gatch, pillows under the knees and, when the patient is allowed out of bed, leg crossing and prolonged sitting.	3. Bed rest and elevation improve venous flow by using gravity to reduce the pressure gradient between the extremity and the heart. Also, bed rest reduces oxygen requirements, limits the risk of thrombus dislodgement, and promotes fibrinolytic breakdown and clot absorption. The remaining measures avoid increased popliteal pressure, which compresses veins and impedes venous return.

─────────
*Italics indicate key interventions.

4. *Encourage the patient to perform gentle foot and leg exercises every hour.* Consult the physician about appropriate exercises, which may include isometric exercises (quadriceps setting or plantar flexion against a footboard) or isotonic exercises (active or passive foot and leg flexion and extension and ankle rotation).

4. The pumping effect of muscle action promotes venous return. Gentle exercise minimizes further thrombus formation, but overly vigorous exercise may dislodge clots. Isometric exercises, generally recommended after surgery, increase venous flow, but may also increase blood pressure. Because this effect may be detrimental — particularly to the patient with cardiovascular disease — some physicians prefer isotonic exercises, which cause a more desirable cardiovascular response.

5. *Increase fluid intake* to eight 8-oz glasses (1,900 ml) a day, unless contraindicated.

5. Increased fluid intake increases vascular volume and reduces viscosity, thus improving blood flow.

6. *Consult the physician about using antiembolism stockings or an intermittent pneumatic compression device.*

6. Superficial veins may be dilated and tortuous, particularly in the older patient. Antiembolism stockings or intermittent pneumatic compression devices may support venous return by compressing superficial veins and redirecting blood flow to deeper veins.

7. Teach the patient stress-control measures, as needed, such as progressive relaxation techniques, breathing exercises, and visualization. Encourage smoking cessation, and refer the patient to appropriate resources for help.

7. Stress-related catecholamine release and smoking induce vasoconstriction.

8. Administer medications, as ordered: anti-inflammatory agents, such as ibuprofen (Advil) and indomethacin (Indocin), and anticoagulants, such as heparin, warfarin (Coumadin), or aspirin.

8. Anti-inflammatory agents are the primary treatment for superficial thrombophlebitis. Anticoagulants may be used if a superficial thrombus extends or threatens the deep venous system in the groin. Anticoagulants are the mainstay of treatment for deep venous thrombophlebitis. Heparin interferes with platelet aggregation, conversion of prothrombin to thrombin, and conversion of fibrinogen to fibrin, thereby minimizing further clot formation. Warfarin interferes with the vitamin K activity necessary for clotting. Aspirin interferes with platelet aggregation.

9. *Monitor clotting studies, as ordered:* PTT if the patient is receiving heparin, PT/INR if the patient is receiving warfarin. Report values outside the desired range to the physician before the next scheduled anticoagulant dose.

9. Dosages are adjusted to maintain PT/INR and PTT within a therapeutic range. The typical ranges desired are $1\frac{1}{2}$ to 2 times control values for PT and PTT and 2 to 3 times control value for INR.

10. *Observe for signs of bleeding,* such as oozing at I.V. or I.M. injection sites, epistaxis, bleeding gums, ecchymoses, hematuria, or melena.

10. Excessive anticoagulant dosages increase the risk of bleeding.

11. *Increase the patient's activity level, as ordered.*

11. Muscle movement compresses vessels, improving venous return.

12. *Observe for signs of chronic venous insufficiency:* dependent ankle edema, induration, shiny skin, varicosities, and stasis ulcers. Consult the physician if these signs are present.

12. Repeated episodes of deep vein thrombosis can cause chronic venous insufficiency from venous valvular destruction.

13. Additional individualized interventions: _____

13. Rationales: _____

Nursing diagnosis
Acute pain related to vessel obstruction, inflammation, and edema

NURSING PRIORITY
Relieve pain.

PATIENT OUTCOME CRITERION
Within 1 hour of reporting pain, the patient will rate pain level as less than 3 on a 0 to 10 pain rating scale.

INTERVENTIONS	RATIONALES
1. *See the "Acute pain" care plan,* page 32.	1. The "Acute pain" care plan contains multiple interventions for pain relief.
2. *Implement measures to promote venous flow* (such as bed rest and leg elevation), as described in the previous problem.	2. Eliminating the pain's cause is the most effective relief measure.
3. *Handle the affected extremity gently.* Use a bed cradle.	3. The thrombophlebitic extremity is extremely sensitive; even slight pressure or movement may be painful. A bed cradle keeps the weight of linens off the extremity.
4. *Apply warm, moist heat to the affected area, as ordered.*	4. Heat is soothing and causes vasodilation, improving blood flow.
5. *Administer analgesics, as ordered,* observing for therapeutic and adverse effects. Question the use of indomethacin or aspirin if the patient is receiving an anticoagulant.	5. The appropriate type and amount of analgesic depends on the degree of pain and the use of anticoagulants. Indomethacin and aspirin, which may be used to control pain, increase anticoagulant activity and may be inappropriate for the patient taking heparin or warfarin.
6. *Administer anti-inflammatory agents, as ordered.*	6. Reducing inflammation and edema reduces stimulation of nerve fibers and thus reduces pain.
7. Additional individualized interventions: _____	7. Rationales: _____

> **Suggested NIC Interventions**
> *Medication management; Pain management; Patient-controlled analgesia (PCA) assistance; Analgesic administration; Conscious sedation*

> **Suggested NOC Outcomes**
> *Comfort level; Pain control; Pain: Disruptive effects; Pain level*

Collaborative problem
Risk for thromboembolism related to dislodged thrombus

NURSING PRIORITY
Prevent or promptly detect thromboembolism.

PATIENT OUTCOME CRITERION
Within 24 hours of thrombophlebitis onset, the patient will show no signs of pulmonary embolism, (as evidenced by absence of tachypnea, cyanosis, dyspnea or chest pain).

INTERVENTIONS

1. *Monitor for signs and symptoms of a pulmonary embolism,* either a massive pulmonary embolism (profound shock, cyanosis, diaphoresis, and a sense of impending doom) or a lesser pulmonary embolism (tachypnea, dyspnea, pleuritic chest pain [sharp, stabbing pain that worsens on inspiration or coughing], and restlessness).

2. *Alert the physician promptly if any signs or symptoms of pulmonary embolism appear. If signs of massive pulmonary embolism occur, take emergency measures:* place the patient in the high Fowler position, administer oxygen at 6 L/minute by nasal prongs, monitor vital signs, and summon immediate medical assistance. Refer to the "Pulmonary embolism" care plan, page 306.

3. *During acute thrombophlebitis, maintain bed rest as ordered.* Request an order for graduated compression stockings or an intermittent pneumatic compression device for patients at risk for thrombophlebitis.

4. *Caution the patient against rubbing the painful area.*

5. *Help the patient avoid Valsalva's maneuver.* Teach the patient to exhale during defecation and provide fluid, high-fiber foods, prune juice, or other measures to promote passage of soft stool.

6. *Observe for persistent or recurrent thrombophlebitis.* If present, consult with the physician about further treatment.

7. Additional individualized interventions: _____
_____

RATIONALES

1. Pulmonary embolism is the most common pulmonary complication in hospitalized patients. Deep venous thrombosis is the primary risk factor for embolus development.

2. Pulmonary emboli can cause local areas of pulmonary dysfunction and increase the risk of massive embolism. Massive pulmonary embolism, in which 50% or more of the pulmonary vascular bed is occluded, is a medical emergency. Treatment may include full cardiopulmonary support, surgical intervention, I.V. streptokinase (Streptase), and heparin. The "Pulmonary embolism" care plan contains further details on this disorder.

3. Bed rest decreases the likelihood that muscle contractions will dislodge a clot, while compression improves venous flow.

4. Rubbing may cause the clot to break free and embolize.

5. A sudden increase in intrathoracic pressure, such as that produced by Valsalva's maneuver, may dislodge the clot.

6. Persistent or recurrent thrombophlebitis increases the risk of pulmonary embolism. Treatment may include prolonged anticoagulant therapy or insertion of an inferior vena caval umbrella to trap clots.

7. Rationales: _____
_____

Nursing diagnosis
Deficient knowledge (treatment regimen) related to lack of exposure to information

NURSING PRIORITY
Educate the patient and family about continuing therapy and preventing recurrence.

PATIENT OUTCOME CRITERIA
By the time of discharge, the patient will:
- be able to list personal risk factors
- be able to list the signs and symptoms of thrombophlebitis
- be able to identify five ways to improve venous flow
- be able to correctly describe the details of anticoagulant administration, if prescribed, and how to minimize bleeding risk
- verbalize the importance of regular medical follow-up
- verbalize intent to obtain a medical identification bracelet or necklace.

INTERVENTIONS

1. *Teach the patient and family about factors that may increase the risk of recurrence.* Discuss measures that may reduce or eliminate risk factors, including weight control through diet and exercise, smoking cessation, drug therapy for hypertension, and careful diabetes control.

2. *Teach the patient ways to improve venous flow:* exercising feet and legs hourly while awake; increasing fluid intake to at least eight 8-oz giasses (1,900 ml) a day (unless contraindicated); elevating the extremity when sitting or lying down; participating in prescribed activity program; avoiding girdles, garters, knee-high stockings, and other constricting clothing; using antiembolism stockings; avoiding leg crossing; and avoiding oral contraceptives.

3. *Teach the patient and family to observe for signs and symptoms of recurrence.*

4. *Teach the patient how to care for extremities:* maintaining clean, dry skin; carefully monitoring any skin lesions; and protecting skin from injury.

5. *Teach the patient and family about oral anticoagulant therapy,* if prescribed. Also teach ways to minimize the risk of bleeding, such as using an electric shaver and avoiding aspirin. See the "Stroke" care plan, page 236, for further details.

6. *Emphasize the importance of following the physician's recommendations* for regular medical follow-up, including laboratory test monitoring. Also stress the value of wearing a medical alert bracelet or necklace, and tell the patient how to obtain one.

7. Additional individualized interventions: _____

RATIONALES

1. Thrombophlebitis commonly recurs, particularly if risk factors aren't eliminated. Teaching measures to eliminate or reduce risk factors may avert further problems.

2. These methods prevent the classic causes of thrombophlebitis: venous stasis, vessel trauma, and hypercoagulability.

3. Early detection promotes early treatment.

4. Impaired circulation in the extremities predisposes the patient to stasis ulcers.

5. A patient with uncomplicated deep venous thrombophlebitis usually takes warfarin for 4 to 6 weeks after discharge. Complications may warrant lifelong anticoagulant therapy. The "Stroke" care plan contains further details related to anticoagulant therapy.

6. Thrombophlebitis may recur or develop into chronic venous insufficiency. Conscientious medical follow-up provides the greatest protection against future life-threatening episodes or chronicity. Monitoring laboratory parameters, such as PT/INR for the patient taking warfarin, helps the physician maintain a therapeutic dosage. A medical alert bracelet or necklace increases the likelihood of appropriate treatment should the patient be unable to communicate in a medical emergency.

7. Rationales: _____

> ### Suggested NIC Interventions
> *Teaching: Procedure/treatment*

> ### Suggested NOC Outcomes
> *Knowledge: Treatment regimen*

Discharge planning
DISCHARGE CHECKLIST
Before discharge, the patient shows evidence of:
- ❏ absence of heat, pain, swelling, or inflammation at affected site
- ❏ PTT or PT/INR within acceptable parameters
- ❏ absence of pulmonary or cardiovascular complications
- ❏ absence of fever
- ❏ vital signs within normal parameters
- ❏ absence of bowel or bladder dysfunction
- ❏ heparin therapy discontinued for 24 hours
- ❏ anticoagulation controlled with oral medication

❏ presence of bilateral pedal pulses

❏ absence of pain and pallor in the affected lower extremity

❏ ability to perform activities of daily living (ADLs), transfers, and ambulation same as before hospitalization

❏ adequate home support system, or referral to home care or a nursing home if indicated by lack of home support system or inability to perform ADLs, transfers, and ambulation.

TEACHING CHECKLIST

Document evidence that the patient and his family demonstrate an understanding of:

❏ signs and symptoms of recurring thrombophlebitis

❏ continued use of antiembolism stockings

❏ all discharge medications' purpose, dosage, administration schedule, all food and drug interactions, and adverse effects requiring medical attention (usual discharge medications include oral anticoagulants and anti-inflammatory medications)

❏ allowable activity level

❏ importance of wearing medical alert identification if the patient remains on anticoagulant therapy

❏ need to modify risk factors

❏ procedure for obtaining follow-up laboratory tests such as PT

❏ date, time, and location of follow-up appointments

❏ reportable signs and symptoms (such as those of pulmonary embolism) and how to contact the physician.

DOCUMENTATION CHECKLIST

Using outcome criteria as a guide, document:

❏ clinical status on admission

❏ significant changes in status

❏ pertinent laboratory data and diagnostic test findings

❏ pain-relief measures

❏ effect of position changes and extremity elevation

❏ application and effect of warm, moist compresses

❏ anticoagulant administration

❏ any change in clotting studies

❏ any bleeding tendencies

❏ administration of other pharmacologic agents, such as an anti-inflammatory, antibiotic, or fibrinolytic medication (such as streptokinase or urokinase)

❏ level of activity and the patient's response to progressive ambulation

❏ patient and family teaching

❏ discharge planning.

Associated care plans

- Acute pain
- Ineffective individual coping
- Knowledge deficit

- Perioperative care
- Pulmonary embolism
- Stroke

References

Black, J.M., et al. *Medical Surgical Nursing: Clinical Management for Positive Outcomes,* 6th ed. Philadelphia: W.B. Saunders Co., 2001.

Chernecky, C.C., and Berger, B.J. *Laboratory Tests and Diagnostic Procedures,* 3rd ed. Philadelphia: W.B. Saunders Co., 2001.

Handbook of Diseases, 2nd ed. Springhouse, Pa.: Springhouse Corp., 2000.

Gastrointestinal disorders

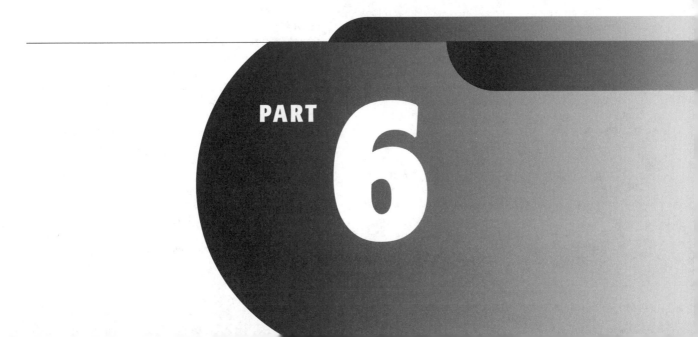

PART

6

Colostomy

DRG INFORMATION
DRG 146   Rectal Resection with Complication or Comorbidity (CC).
Mean LOS = 10.3 days
DRG 147   Rectal Resection without CC.
Mean LOS = 6.4 days
DRG 148   Major Small and Large Bowel Procedure with CC.
Mean LOS = 12.2 days
DRG 149   Major Small and Large Bowel Procedure without CC.
Mean LOS = 6.5 days

Introduction

DEFINITION AND TIME FOCUS

A colostomy is a surgically created opening (stoma) between the abdominal wall and the colon that permits fecal diversion. A colostomy may be created because of trauma, inflammation, or obstruction of the distal bowel or when the distal bowel is resected, as in proctocolectomy (excision of colon and rectum) or abdominoperineal resection (APR; removal of rectum).

The stoma's location in the GI tract determines stool consistency and frequency and affects selection of a management approach. With a descending or sigmoid colostomy, output is soft to solid, frequency is similar to preoperative patterns, and output may be regulated by irrigation. With a transverse colostomy, output is mushy, occurs after meals and unpredictably, and can't be regulated by irrigation.

Colostomies may be designated according to location (ascending, transverse, descending, sigmoid) or duration (temporary, permanent). (See *Clinical snapshot: Colostomy,* page 470).

Location

Although a colostomy may be constructed anywhere in the large bowel, the two most common locations are the transverse colon and the descending colon.

Construction

Common surgical construction methods include:
- end colostomy (bowel is divided; proximal bowel is brought out as a stoma and distal bowel is either removed — as in APR of the distal colon and rectum — or "oversewn" and left in place — as in Hartmann's procedure)
- double-barreled colostomy (bowel is divided and both ends are brought out as stomas; the proximal stoma drains stool and the distal stoma drains only mucus)
- loop colostomy (entire loop of bowel is brought out through the abdominal wall and stabilized over a rod, bridge, or catheter until granulation to the abdominal wall occurs; the bowel's anterior wall is opened to provide fecal diversion; the posterior bowel wall remains intact).

Duration

A colostomy is classified as permanent (no potential for reversal) if the rectum and anus are removed or as temporary (potential for reversal) if the rectum and anus remain.

This care plan focuses on preoperative assessment of teaching needs and on the postoperative phase, the "active teaching" phase, between initial recovery or stabilization and discharge.

ETIOLOGY AND PRECIPITATING FACTORS

- Disease conditions requiring removal of the distal bowel (for example, colorectal cancer or pelvic malignancies)
- Infectious or inflammatory conditions of the distal bowel requiring fecal diversion (for example, diverticulitis or Crohn's disease)
- Trauma to the distal bowel (as in a gunshot or stab wound)
- Extensive surgery of the distal bowel (for example, low anterior colon resection)
- Obstruction of the distal bowel (as in obstructing tumor)

Focused assessment guidelines

NURSING HISTORY
(FUNCTIONAL HEALTH PATTERN FINDINGS)

Because a colostomy may be performed for widely varied conditions, no typical presenting picture exists; therefore, the nursing history and physical findings sections are omitted in this care plan. The following are guidelines for preoperative assessment.

Health-perception–health-management pattern

- Determine the diagnosis or reason for colostomy. Determine the planned procedure, prognosis, and the patient's potential for independence as a basis for discharge planning and teaching.
- Explore the patient's perceptions concerning colostomy and its impact on health status and lifestyle. (*Note:* Previous contact with a person with an ostomy will affect the patient's expectations and adaptation.)

■ Identify any allergies, particularly to topical agents such as tape; the patient with such allergies may react to colostomy products.

Nutritional-metabolic pattern

■ Assess diet and fluid intake when planning patient teaching. Assess the home diet for adequate fiber and fluid intake and for consumption of gas-producing foods.

■ Assess nutritional status (skin turgor, mucous membranes, hair condition, height and weight, and recent weight loss). Be alert to signs of nutritional deficiency that may predispose the patient to postoperative complications, such as wound infection or delayed healing.

Elimination pattern

■ Determine usual bowel patterns. Assess the preoperative frequency and character of bowel movements as a basis for colostomy management and patient teaching (particularly important in selecting a management approach for a descending or sigmoid colostomy).

Activity-exercise pattern

■ Assess independence and any limitations in activities of daily living (ADLs). The amount of independence is significant in planning for colostomy management and patient-family teaching. The patient's manual dexterity and coordination are particularly significant in selecting appropriate equipment, such as a pouch system or clip.

Cognitive-perceptual pattern

■ When planning teaching, assess the patient's understanding of the diagnosis, prognosis, surgical procedure, and management of colostomy.

■ Assess for any sensory deficits, such as in visual and auditory acuity, when planning self-care instruction; most patients requiring colostomy are older than age 60, so sensory loss is common.

Self-perception–self-concept pattern

■ Self-concept and self-esteem correlate with adaptation potential; be alert to consistent self-derogatory statements or inappropriate affect, which may indicate low self-esteem.

■ Emotional response is variable. It's common for a patient to have negative feelings regarding colostomy.

■ Openness in expressing feelings is affected by the patient's personality and the nurse's communication skills.

Role-relationship pattern

■ Assess areas of concern about roles and relationships. Patients commonly express concern about a colostomy's effect on relationships, with major concern relating to spouse or partner reaction.

■ Young and middle-aged adults commonly express concern about their ability to resume preoperative roles and responsibilities.

■ Older adults commonly express concern about their ability to maintain independence and to manage the cost of ostomy supplies.

■ Assess family dynamics, particularly dependence-independence issues. Older patients may desire the involvement of a spouse or a family member in their care,

while younger adults may value independence and privacy.

Sexuality-reproductive pattern

■ Assess the patient's and partner's openness with each other and in discussing sexuality, preoperative sexual patterns, and other major concerns.

■ A common concern is how the colostomy affects intimate relationships — that is, sexual attractiveness and function.

Coping–stress tolerance pattern

■ The patient's and family's responses to colostomy are highly variable and reflect coping patterns.

■ Assess the patient's feelings about support groups to determine the appropriateness of referral to the United Ostomy Association.

Value-belief pattern

■ Response to colostomy is affected by cultural beliefs and the family's response to illness, surgery, and elimination.

DIAGNOSTIC STUDIES

Studies vary according to the patient's condition and the underlying disorder; they may include:

■ complete blood count — may reveal low hemoglobin level or hematocrit that indicate continuing or unreplaced blood loss; may also reveal elevated white blood cell count indicating infection, usually intra-abdominal

■ electrolyte panel — detects or rules out electrolyte abnormalities that affect fluid balance (for example, hyponatremia or hypernatremia) and GI tract function (for example, hypokalemia or hyperkalemia)

■ chemistry panel — detects electrolyte imbalances and nutritional deficits that affect wound healing (for example, hypoproteinemia) and monitors liver and kidney function, which may be affected by underlying disease, such as metastatic disease, or by treatment, such as antibiotic therapy

■ serum drug levels — peak and trough levels may detect toxic or subtherapeutic levels of prescribed antibiotics or other drugs

■ carcinoembryonic antigen (CEA) levels — may be done before and after surgery for comparison; if elevated before surgery, effective surgical resection should result in decreased CEA level

■ flat plate or upright abdominal X-ray — may be done before surgery to rule out colon perforation (in a trauma patient) or colon obstruction (in a patient with suspected malignancy); done after surgery as needed to differentiate postoperative ileus (visualized as air-filled loops of bowel) from mechanical obstruction (visualized as air-fluid levels and dilated proximal bowel)

■ transrectal ultrasound — may be done before surgery to determine lymph node involvement, tumor depth, and adhesions to adjacent structures

■ computed tomography scan of abdomen — may be used before or after surgery to rule out intra-abdominal abscess or to detect metastatic lesions

■ stool guaiac (Hemoccult) test — preliminary study to rule out GI bleeding; positive study requires further workup to rule out malignancy, hemorrhoidal bleeding, inflammatory bowel disease, or upper tract bleeding;

negative study inconclusive because of high incidence of false-negative results

■ barium enema with air and contrast — rules out diverticular disease and detects filling defects that indicate colon lesions (such as polyps and tumors)

■ sigmoidoscopy or colonoscopy — rules out colon lesions and allows removal of polyps or biopsy of suspicious lesions.

CLINICAL SNAPSHOT ☀

Colostomy

Major nursing diagnoses and collaborative problems	Key patient outcomes
CP: Risk for stomal necrosis	Display a pink and viable stoma.
CP: Risk for stomal retraction	Display a stoma granulated to the abdominal wall.
ND: Risk for impaired skin integrity	Display peristomal skin free from breakdown.
ND: Deficient knowledge (care of descending or sigmoid colostomy	Select a preferred bowel management approach.
ND: Disturbed body image	Discuss feeling about stoma.
ND: Sexual dysfunction	Describe any alteration in sexual function (if applicable).

Collaborative problem

Risk for stomal necrosis related to the surgical procedure, bowel wall edema, or traction on the mesentery

NURSING PRIORITIES
■ Optimize blood flow to the bowel wall.
■ Prevent complications related to circulatory impairment.

PATIENT OUTCOME CRITERION
Within the first 4 days after surgery, the patient will display a pink and viable stoma.

INTERVENTIONS	RATIONALES
1. *Assess and document stoma color** every 8 hours during the first 4 days after surgery (or until the stoma remains pink for 3 days).	1. Healthy bowel tissue is pink; a dusky blue color indicates ischemia; a brown or black color indicates necrosis. Ischemia may or may not progress to necrosis.
2. *If the stoma is ischemic or necrotic, check the viability of the proximal bowel* by inserting a test tube into the stoma and using a flashlight to assess the mucosa for ischemia. Document your findings.	2. A distal stoma is most likely to necrose because it's farthest from the mesenteric blood supply. Stomal necrosis doesn't necessarily represent a surgical emergency (the stoma may be allowed to "slough" as long as the proximal bowel is viable).
3. *Notify the physician promptly if necrosis extends to the end of the test tube* (see above).	3. Necrosis extending to the fascia represents a surgical emergency because of the threat of perforation and peritonitis.

---

*Italics indicate key interventions.

4. *Implement measures to minimize abdominal distention:* – Examine the abdomen for distention every 8 hours during the first 4 days after surgery. – If distention is present, monitor its degree by measuring abdominal girth at the umbilicus. – If distention is present, notify the physician and request an order to insert a nasogastric (NG) tube. – If an NG tube is present, irrigate as needed to maintain patency.	**4.** Severe abdominal distention may cause mesenteric stretching, which places blood vessels under tension; this stress may decrease blood flow to the distal bowel and stoma. Using the umbilicus as the reference point for measuring abdominal girth promotes consistency and accuracy of measurements.
5. Additional individualized interventions: _____	**5.** Rationales: _____

Collaborative problem

Risk for stomal retraction related to mucocutaneous separation

NURSING PRIORITIES
- Optimize wound healing and granulation of the stoma to the abdominal wall.
- Prevent stomal retraction.

PATIENT OUTCOME CRITERIA
By the time of discharge, the patient will:
- display a stoma granulated to the abdominal wall
- exhibit a healed mucocutaneous suture line
- show no stomal retraction.

INTERVENTIONS	**RATIONALES**
1. *Assess and document the integrity of the mucocutaneous suture line* at each pouch change.	**1.** Breakdown of the stoma or skin suture line is a major contributing factor to stomal retraction.
2. *Initiate and document nutritional support measures for the patient at risk for nutritional deficiency* based on the recommendations of a nutritional resource nurse or dietitian.	**2.** Nutritional deficiency causes negative nitrogen balance. Because wound repair depends on adequate protein stores, the suture line may break down.
3. Request vitamin A supplements for the patient receiving steroids.	**3.** Vitamin A partially compensates for the negative effects of corticosteroids on wound healing; by supporting macrophage activity and wound repair, vitamin A helps prevent suture line breakdown.
4. For the patient with a loop colostomy stabilized by a rod or bridge, expect that the loop support won't be removed until the stoma granulates to the abdominal wall.	**4.** Loop support removal before abdominal wall attachment may cause stomal retraction.
5. *If mucocutaneous separation occurs, alter the pouch system* to prevent fecal contamination of exposed subcutaneous tissue. Fill the separated area with absorptive powder or granules; cover with tape strips, then pectin-based paste. Apply a pouch sized to fit closely around the stoma.	**5.** An optimal environment for healing includes protection from secondary infection, absorption of exudate, and maintenance of a clean, moist surface. The absorptive agent and tape strips prevent fecal contamination and absorb exudate. Using paste and a pouch sized for the stoma provides a secure seal.
6. Additional individualized interventions: _____	**6.** Rationales: _____

Nursing diagnosis

Risk for impaired skin integrity: Peristomal breakdown related to fecal contamination of skin

NURSING PRIORITIES
- Maintain an intact pouch seal.
- Prevent peristomal skin breakdown.

PATIENT OUTCOME CRITERIA
- Throughout the postoperative phase, the patient will display peristomal skin free from breakdown.
- By the time of discharge, the patient will have had an intact pouch for 2 days.

INTERVENTIONS	RATIONALES
1. *Have an enterostomal therapy nurse mark the optimal stoma site before surgery, if possible.*	**1.** For best results, the stoma should be located in an area free from creases or folds, within the patient's view, and within the rectus muscle. Site selection is best done before surgery, when the patient can be evaluated lying down, sitting, and standing.
2. *Assess the patient's abdominal contours and select a pouch system that matches those contours:* for example, try an all-flexible system for a stoma in a crease or fold.	**2.** Accurately matching the pouch system to abdominal contours optimizes the pouch-to-skin seal and minimizes leakage.
3. *Use the appropriate principles in preparing and applying the pouch:* – Use a drainable pouch. – Remove peristomal hair with safety razor and shaving cream. Rinse and dry skin. – Use a skin sealant (such as Skin Prep) under the tape. – Use a pouch with a barrier ring sized to fit closely around the stoma; apply a thin layer of barrier paste (such as Stomahesive) around the stoma to fill in gaps and prevent leakage. – If an adhesive-only pouch is used, size it to clear the stoma by 1/8″ (3 mm); use a pouch with a barrier ring and paste.	**3.** Good technique provides maximum security and skin protection. – A drainable pouch can be emptied as needed without being removed. – Hair removal prevents folliculitis. – The copolymer film prevents epidermal stripping with pouch removal. – This procedure prevents fecal material from contacting skin and causing breakdown. – Inflexible pouch edges placed too close to the stoma can damage it during peristalsis. Exposed skin must be protected.
4. *Change the pouch routinely* every 5 to 7 days and as needed if there's leakage or if the patient complains of peristomal burning or itching occur.	**4.** Routine changes before leaks can occur protect skin and provide the patient with a sense of control. Burning or itching may indicate fecal contamination of skin.
5. *Inspect the skin at each pouch change,* and treat any denudation by dusting the area with absorptive powder (such as Stomahesive). Seal the area by blotting it with water or sealant (such as Skin Prep).	**5.** Powder provides an absorptive protective layer over the area of breakdown; sealing provides a surface for pouch adherence.
6. Additional individualized interventions: _____	**6.** Rationales: _____

> **Suggested NIC Interventions**
> *Pressure management; Pressure ulcer care; Skin surveillance; Incision site care; Wound care*

> **Suggested NOC Outcomes**
> *Tissue integrity: Skin and mucous membranes; Wound healing: Primary intention; Wound healing: Secondary intention*

Nursing diagnosis

Deficient knowledge (care of descending or sigmoid colostomy) related to unfamiliarity with altered bowel

NURSING PRIORITY
Help the patient select options most appropriate for personal physical status and lifestyle.

PATIENT OUTCOME CRITERION
By 2 days before discharge, the patient will describe options considered and select a preferred approach.

INTERVENTIONS	RATIONALES
1. *Assess the patient's candidacy for bowel function regulation by irrigation.* Consider the following factors: – Is the colostomy permanent? – Are there stomal complications, such as hernia or prolapse? – Is the patient mentally and physically able to learn and perform the procedure? – What were the preoperative bowel patterns? – Is the patient to receive radiation? – Does the patient have adequate home facilities?	**1.** Irrigation is usually contraindicated if: – the colostomy is temporary (because of the time factor and potential for bowel dependence) – the patient has a peristomal hernia (potential for perforation) or prolapse (potential for worsening of prolapse) – the patient has coordination problems or learning difficulties – the patient has a preoperative history of diarrhea (less likely to achieve control than the patient with a preoperative history of regular stools or constipation) – the patient is to receive radiation therapy (because diarrhea is a usual adverse effect) – the patient has no running water or indoor plumbing in the home.
2. *If the patient meets feasibility criteria, discuss management options:* – wearing a pouch continuously, emptying as needed, and changing every 5 to 7 days – daily or every-other-day irrigations to stimulate bowel movements, wearing a security pouch between irrigations.	**2.** Colostomy irrigations aren't necessary because peristalsis and bowel movements continue; however, regular irrigations induce evacuation and promote colonic "dependence" on their stimulating effects, providing increased control over bowel function. Thus, regulation by irrigation is a management option.
3. *Help the patient explore the options* based on personal priorities such as tolerance of the pouch versus the time required for regular irrigations.	**3.** Exploring the pros and cons of various options and discussing the patient's concerns and priorities facilitates decision making and increases the patient's sense of self-control.
4. *Establish a teaching plan based on the patient's decision.* Base teaching strategies on the patient's learning style and sensory strengths; for example, if a patient with diminished visual acuity learns best by doing, self-care instruction should involve much practice (with a magnifying mirror) but minimal reading.	**4.** The patient must be able to perform colostomy care before discharge.
5. Additional individualized interventions: _____	**5.** Rationales: _____

Suggested NIC Interventions *Teaching: Procedure/treatment*	***Suggested NOC Outcomes*** *Knowledge: Treatment regimen*

Gastrointestinal disorders

Nursing diagnosis

Disturbed body image related to loss of control over fecal elimination

NURSING PRIORITIES

- Prevent or minimize alteration in body image.
- Enhance the patient's sense of control over bowel functions.

PATIENT OUTCOME CRITERIA

By 2 days before discharge, the patient will:
- observe and perform stoma care
- discuss feelings about the stoma.
  By the time of discharge, the patient will:
- describe the colostomy as manageable
- describe plans for resuming preoperative lifestyle.

INTERVENTIONS

1. *Teach the patient measures for odor control,* such as performing regular pouch care; using an odor-proof pouch; using pouch deodorant, if desired; using a room deodorant when the pouch is emptied; altering diet to reduce fecal odor, if desired; and using over-the-counter internal deodorants, if desired, such as bismuth subgallate.

2. *Teach the patient measures to reduce and control flatus,* such as identifying gas-forming foods; understanding the "lag time" between ingestion and flatulence; muffling sounds of flatus; and using pouch filters that deodorize flatus.

3. *Teach the patient how to conceal the pouch* under clothing; wearing a knit or stretchy layer next to the skin holds the pouch close to the body and helps conceal large or bulky stomas.

4. *Discuss the normal emotional response to colostomy* with the patient and his family. Allow them to explore their feelings about the colostomy. Assess the patient's usual coping strategies. Present helpful coping strategies, such as discussing feelings and seeking information.

5. *Discuss colostomy management* during occupational, social, and sexual activity. Help the patient to role-play difficult situations such as telling someone about the stoma.

6. Offer information on the United Ostomy Association; arrange for an ostomy visitor if the patient wishes.

7. Additional individualized interventions: _____
_____

RATIONALES

1. Odor control is a major concern of most patients; instruction in odor-control methods increases feelings of control and confidence and reduces feelings of embarrassment and shame. Onions, garlic, beans, and cabbage generally increase odor; orange juice, buttermilk, and yogurt may decrease odor. Bismuth reduces flatus and odor and thickens stool; it's contraindicated in the patient with renal failure or on anticoagulant therapy.

2. Inability to control flatus may lead to social embarrassment and self-deprecation. The patient can time the intake of any gas-forming foods so that flatulence occurs during "safe" periods. Filters keep the pouch flat by allowing flatus to escape and prevent odor by first deodorizing flatus.

3. The ability to dress normally and look the same as before surgery diminishes alterations in body image and enhances self-concept.

4. Discussing the normal emotional response and accepting negative feelings gives the patient and his family permission to explore their feelings. Accepting feelings enhances self-concept and promotes adaptation. Discussing various coping strategies may provide the patient with new or more effective ways to handle emotions.

5. Preparing for such activities increases coping skills and the likelihood that the patient will manage them successfully. Role playing helps the patient prepare for difficult situations, which increases the sense of control and enhances self-concept.

6. Contact with others who have ostomies reduces isolation and increases perception of the colostomy as manageable, thus enhancing the patient's sense of control.

7. Rationales: _____
_____

> **Suggested NIC Interventions**
> *Body image enhancement; Grief work facilitation; Anticipatory guidance; Coping enhancement; Self-esteem enhancement*

> **Suggested NOC Outcomes**
> *Body image; Grief resolution; Self-esteem*

Nursing diagnosis

Sexual dysfunction related to change in body image or damage to autonomic nerves (applies to the patient with rectal resection, particularly wide resection for cancer treatment)

NURSING PRIORITIES
- Facilitate the resumption and maintenance of intimate relationships.
- Minimize alteration in sexual function.

PATIENT OUTCOME CRITERIA
By the time of discharge, the patient will:
- share feelings about stoma with his spouse or partner
- describe any alteration in sexual function (if applicable)
- describe measures for pouch management during sexual activity (if applicable).

INTERVENTIONS

1. *Discuss with the patient (and spouse or partner, if possible) the importance of openness and honesty as well as the fact that both must adapt to the ostomy.*

2. *Teach the patient measures for securing and concealing the pouch during sexual activity,* such as using a small pouch or wearing a pouch cover, or a cummerbund around the midriff, or crotchless panties for a female patient.

3. *For a female with a wide rectal resection, discuss the possible need for artificial lubrication.*

4. *For a male with a wide rectal resection, explain potential interference with erection and ejaculation;* explain that no loss of sensation or orgasmic potential will occur; explore alternatives to intercourse as indicated; explain the availability of penile injections, urethral inserts, penile prostheses, and vacuum devices to restore erectile function. Reinforce the importance of intimacy, whether or not it involves intercourse.

5. Additional individualized interventions: _____

RATIONALES

1. Both the patient and spouse (or partner) may have concerns and negative feelings that can affect their sexual relationship. Openness in discussing feelings may help resolve these.

2. The stoma and pouch affect overall body image and feelings of sexual attractiveness. Securing and concealing the pouch help prevent leakage and allow the patient to focus on sexuality and sharing rather than on the pouch and stoma.

3. Wide rectal resection may damage parasympathetic nerves thought to mediate vaginal lubrication.

4. Wide rectal resection may damage parasympathetic nerves controlling erection and sympathetic nerves controlling ejaculation. Sensation and orgasm, mediated by the pudendal nerve, remain intact. Intimacy — emotional closeness — is a human need separate from the desire for sexual expression. It can be met in ways other than sexual behavior, such as sharing feelings and affectionate touching. A number of medical and surgical interventions are now available that restore erectile function.

5. Rationales: _____

> **Suggested NIC Interventions**
> *Sexual counseling*

> **Suggested NOC Outcomes**
> *Sexual functioning*

Discharge planning

DISCHARGE CHECKLIST

Before discharge, the patient shows evidence of:
- ❏ absence of fever
- ❏ stable vital signs
- ❏ absence of pulmonary or cardiovascular complications
- ❏ healing wound with no signs of redness, swelling, or drainage
- ❏ ability to change and empty pouch using proper technique
- ❏ ability to tolerate diet
- ❏ absence of skin problems around stoma
- ❏ absence of bladder dysfunction
- ❏ absence of abdominal distention
- ❏ restored bowel function
- ❏ ability to perform ADLs and ambulate same as before surgery
- ❏ ability to control pain with oral medications
- ❏ adequate home support system or referral to home care if indicated by inadequate home support system or inability to manage colostomy care at home.

TEACHING CHECKLIST

Document evidence that the patient and family demonstrate an understanding of:
- ❏ reason for colostomy
- ❏ colostomy's impact on bowel function
- ❏ normal stoma characteristics and function
- ❏ pouch-emptying procedure
- ❏ pouch-changing procedure
- ❏ peristomal skin care
- ❏ colostomy irrigation procedure (if applicable)
- ❏ management of mucous fistula stoma (if applicable)
- ❏ flatus and odor control
- ❏ management of diarrhea and constipation
- ❏ normal adaptation process and feelings after colostomy
- ❏ community resources available for support
- ❏ recommendations affecting resumption of preoperative lifestyle
- ❏ potential alteration in sexual function (if applicable)
- ❏ sources of colostomy supplies and reimbursement procedures
- ❏ signs and symptoms to report to the physician
- ❏ need for follow-up appointment with the physician (and enterostomal therapy nurse, if available)
- ❏ how to contact the physician.

DOCUMENTATION CHECKLIST

Using outcome criteria as a guide, document:
- ❏ clinical status on admission
- ❏ significant changes in clinical status
- ❏ GI tract function (bowel sounds, NG tube output, and colostomy output)
- ❏ stoma color and status of mucocutaneous suture line
- ❏ oral intake and tolerance
- ❏ episodes of abdominal distention, nausea, and vomiting
- ❏ incision status (any signs of infection)
- ❏ stoma location and abdominal contours
- ❏ management plan, including pouch system selected (and decision about irrigation for the patient with a descending or sigmoid colostomy)
- ❏ peristomal skin status
- ❏ emotional response to colostomy and discussion of coping strategies
- ❏ patient and family teaching
- ❏ discharge planning.

Associated care plans

- Acute pain
- Compromised family coping
- Grieving
- Ineffective individual coping
- Knowledge deficit
- Perioperative care

References

Ghali, P., and Bitton, A. "The Role of Endoscopy in the Evaluation of Pouches and Ostomies," *Gastrointestinal Endoscopy Clinics of North America* 12(3):605-19, July 2002.

Jordan, K. (ed). *Emergency Nursing Core Curriculum.* Emergency Nurses Association. Philadelphia: W.B. Saunders Co., 2000

Lynn-McHale, D.J., and Carlson, K.K. American Association of Critical Care Nurses *AACN Procedure Manual for Critical Care,* 4th ed. Philadelphia: W.B. Saunders Co., 2001.

Marquis, P., et al. "Quality of Life in Patients with Stomas: The Montreux Study," *Ostomy Wound Management* 49(2):48-55, February 2003.

Shoemaker, W.C., et al. *Textbook of Critical Care,* 4th ed. Philadelphia: W.B. Saunders Co., 2002.

Turnbull, G.B. "A Look at the Purpose and Outcomes of Colostomy Irrigation," *Ostomy Wound Management* 49(2):19-20, February 2003.

Duodenal ulcer, esophagitis, and gastroenteritis

DRG INFORMATION

DRG 174 GI Hemorrhage with Complication or Comorbidity (CC).
Mean LOS = 4.8 days

DRG 175 GI Hemorrhage without CC.
Mean LOS = 2.9 days

DRG 182 Esophagitis, Gastroenteritis, and Miscellaneous Digestive Disorders; Age 17+ with Complication or Comorbidity (CC).
Mean LOS = 4.3 days

DRG 183 Esophagitis, Gastroenteritis, and Miscellaneous Digestive Disorders; Ages 0 to 17 without CC.
Mean LOS = 2.9 days

DRG 184 Esophagitis, Gastroenteritis, and Miscellaneous Digestive Disorders; Ages 0 to 17.
Mean LOS = 2.9 days

Introduction

DEFINITION AND TIME FOCUS

Duodenal ulcer results from an inflammatory and ulcerative process that affects the first portion of the duodenum within 1⅛ (3 cm) of the gastroduodenal junction. This care plan focuses on the duodenal ulcer patient admitted with signs and symptoms that haven't been controlled through outpatient management. Long-term maintenance medication therapy is generally recommended instead of surgical treatment; therefore, the plan focuses on medical treatment.

Esophagitis and gastroenteritis are nonspecific inflammatory conditions of the mucosa of the esophagus and the stomach and small bowel, respectively. Esophagitis is usually related to inadequate cardiac sphincter tone, resulting in gastric reflux and subsequent irritation. Gastroenteritis is most commonly caused by bacteria or viruses that produce severe vomiting, diarrhea, and abdominal cramping. Both conditions may cause temporary discomfort (which can be treated on an outpatient basis) or serious, even life-threatening, illness if the patient is elderly, debilitated, or otherwise at increased risk. This care plan focuses on the patient admitted for diagnosis and treatment of acute esophagitis or gastroenteritis. (See *Clinical snapshot: Duodenal ulcer, esophagitis, and gastroenteritis,* page 480.)

ETIOLOGY AND PRECIPITATING FACTORS

Duodenal ulcer

Gastric acid secretion is necessary for duodenal ulcers to develop. Pathophysiologic abnormalities that influence gastric acid secretion are:
- increased parietal cell and chief cell mass (related to gastrinomal gastrin-secreting tumor or familial or genetic factors)
- increased basal secretory or postprandial secretory drive (related to gastrinoma or antral G cell hyperfunction)
- rapid gastric emptying (related to familial or genetic factors)
- *Helicobacter pylori* infection (present in 90% of all duodenal peptic ulcers and 70% of all gastric ulcers)
- impaired mucosal defense (related to ingestion of aspirin, corticosteroids, or phenylbutazone and to other factors, such as stress or infectious agents).

Esophagitis and gastroenteritis

- Infectious agents — fungal (candidiasis), viral (herpes simplex), and bacterial (staphylococcus, *H. pylori*)
- Drugs and chemical agents — gastric acid reflux; bile reflux; ingestion of caustic substances (such as lye); medications such as aspirin, steroids, indomethacin (Indocin), or antibiotics
- Dietary factors — excessive ingestion of alcohol, spicy foods, mint, coffee, or caffeine-containing products; cigarette smoking; ingestion of very hot or cold substances
- Physical or trauma factors — hiatal hernia; obesity; nasogastric (NG) intubation; radiation therapy; severe physical stress from surgery, sepsis, burns, accidents, or heavy weight-lifting; excessive emotional stress

Focused assessment guidelines

NURSING HISTORY
(FUNCTIONAL HEALTH PATTERN FINDINGS)
Duodenal ulcer

Health-perception–health-management pattern

- Steady, gnawing, burning, aching, or hungerlike discomfort high in the right epigastrium; pain occurs 2 to 4 hours after meals, usually doesn't radiate, and is relieved by food or antacids
- Increased risk if male, ages 40 to 60, with type O blood, a cigarette smoker, or with chronic emotional stress

- Ingestion of certain drugs that contribute to duodenal ulceration, such as aspirin-containing compounds, corticosteroids, phenylbutazone, or indomethacin (Indocin)
- Family history of ulcers

Nutritional-metabolic pattern
- History of excessive alcohol consumption
- Nausea (vomiting not common)
- Appetite usually good

Elimination pattern
- Feeling of fullness, gaseous indigestion, or constipation

Activity-exercise pattern
- Fatigue
- Exacerbation of pain following unusual physical exertion
- Orthostatic hypotension if actively bleeding

Sleep-rest pattern
- Sleep disturbances from pain, commonly occurring between 12 a.m. and 3 a.m.

Coping–stress tolerance pattern
- Stressful life events — such as occupational, educational, or financial problems or family illness — preceding development or exacerbation of signs and symptoms
- Denial of signs and symptoms during pain-free periods (symptoms commonly disappear for weeks or months and then recur)

NURSING HISTORY (FUNCTIONAL HEALTH PATTERN FINDINGS)
Esophagitis and gastroenteritis
Health-perception–health-management pattern
- Various nonspecific symptoms; may be acute (as from infection or ingestion of a caustic substance) or gradual (reflux esophagitis)
- Delay in seeking medical attention because of vagueness of symptoms (reflux esophagitis)
- Tendency to self-medicate with multiple over-the-counter remedies for GI upset
- Radiation therapy for scleroderma or other disease that makes esophageal or gastric mucosa more susceptible to infection and inflammation
- Treatment of sepsis, trauma, burns, immunologic disorder, endocrine disorder, liver disease, pancreatitis, or pulmonary disease

Nutritional-metabolic pattern
- With esophagitis, may report heartburn, dysphagia, or odynophagia (pain on swallowing); with gastroenteritis, typically complains of epigastric or abdominal discomfort, nausea, vomiting, diarrhea, or fever
- Hematemesis and food regurgitation
- Eructation and epigastric fullness after meals
- Anorexia or weight loss
- Swollen and inflamed mouth
- History of excessive alcohol consumption, aspirin ingestion, cigarette smoking, or ingestion of caustic substance

- Habitually eating excessive amounts of spicy foods, consuming very hot or cold substances, and eating late at night

Elimination pattern
- Cramping, abdominal distention, diarrhea, increased flatus, or melena

Activity-exercise pattern
- Sudden or chronic fatigue

Sleep-rest pattern
- Restlessness
- Awakening at night because of pain or with regurgitated food on pillow

Cognitive-perceptual pattern
- Pain of varying intensity, depending on cause of problem (for example, acute gastritis may cause epigastric discomfort and abdominal cramping, and caustic chemical ingestion may cause immediate localized pain and odynophagia)
- Morning hoarseness (laryngitis)
- Salty salivary secretions (water brash)
- Altered taste (from damage of salivary glands) if symptoms result from ingestion of caustic substance

Coping–stress tolerance pattern
- High levels of stress at work or home

PHYSICAL FINDINGS
Duodenal ulcer
Gastrointestinal
- Localized tenderness in epigastrium over ulcer site

PHYSICAL FINDINGS
Esophagitis and gastroenteritis
Gastrointestinal: Esophagitis
- Hematemesis
- Eructation
- Dysphagia

Gastrointestinal: Gastroenteritis
- Vomiting
- Diarrhea
- Eructation
- Hyperactive bowel sounds
- Flatulence
- Hematemesis
- Melena

Cardiovascular
(if hypovolemia is present)
- Hypotension
- Tachycardia

Neurologic
(if hypovolemia is present)
- Dizziness
- Restlessness
- Irritability

Integumentary
(if hypovolemia is present)
- Pallor

- Cool, clammy skin
- Poor skin turgor

Musculoskeletal

(when in pain)

- Tense posture
- Facial grimacing

DIAGNOSTIC STUDIES

Duodenal ulcer

- Routine laboratory studies — add little to the workup
- More sophisticated GI studies, such as serum pepsinogen I or fasting gastrin levels — may be ordered based on the suspected cause of the duodenal ulcer; a high serum pepsinogen I level and a high fasting gastrin level provide evidence for gastrinoma or antral G cell hyperfunction
- Endoscopy — reveals the ulcer's location and allows for biopsy and cytology
- Abdominal films — reveals free air due to perforation
- Screening test for *H. pylori* — likely to be positive
- Single-or double-contrast radiography — may be ordered along with endoscopy to locate ulcer
- Hemoglobin level and hematocrit if bleeding is occurring

Esophagitis

- Complete blood count (CBC) — may show decreased hemoglobin level or hematocrit, possibly indicating GI blood loss; elevated white blood cell count may indicate infection or inflammation
- Serum electrolyte levels — may be studied to detect signs of fluid imbalance from blood loss, vomiting, or diarrhea (hypokalemia common with significant vomiting or diarrhea)
- Serum amylase and lipase levels — elevations indicate pancreatitis as cause of symptoms
- Cultures — may be taken to identify specific causative organism (especially for immunocompromised patients)
- Barium swallow — detects inflammation, ulceration, esophageal strictures, and gastric reflux
- Esophagoscopy — allows direct visualization of the esophagus to detect inflammation, ulceration, strictures, and hiatal hernia; biopsy of mucosa or brushing for cytology may be used for tissue diagnosis
- Esophageal manometry — may reveal decreased esophageal sphincter pressure, as seen with gastroesophageal reflux; may detect peristaltic abnormalities responsible for infections or inflammatory changes in the esophagus
- Acid perfusion test (Bernstein test) — if the patient has pain or burning during perfusion of acid (via a tube) into esophagus, may indicate esophagitis
- pH reflux test — a pH less than 4 may indicate gastroesophageal reflux (normal esophageal pH is greater than 5)

Gastroenteritis

- CBC — may show decreased hemoglobin level or hematocrit, possibly indicating GI blood loss; elevated white blood cell count may indicate infection or inflammation
- Serum electrolyte levels — may be studied to detect signs of fluid imbalance from blood loss, vomiting, or diarrhea (hypokalemia common with significant vomiting or diarrhea)
- Serum amylase and lipase levels — elevations indicate pancreatitis as cause of symptoms
- Cultures — may be taken to identify specific causative organism (especially for immunocompromised patients)
- Esophagogastroduodenoscopy — allows direct visualization of esophagus, stomach, and duodenum; biopsy of mucosa or brushing for cytology may be performed for tissue diagnosis; *Campylobacter*-like organism test may be performed to detect the urease enzyme of *H. pylori*
- Upper GI series — radiographically visualizes lining of esophagus, stomach, and duodenum; may detect inflammation, ulcerations, or strictures
- Guaiac test — occult blood in stool may indicate blood loss

POTENTIAL COMPLICATIONS

Duodenal ulcer

- Duodenal obstruction
– Gastric atony
– Mechanical obstruction
- Perforation

Esophagitis

- Ulcerative esophagitis
- Esophageal bleeding
- Hemorrhage
- Esophageal stricture
- Aspiration pneumonia
- Barrett's epithelium — columnar (gastric) epithelium in the esophagus resulting from chronic gastroesophageal reflux; places the patient at great risk for adenocarcinoma of the esophagus
- Esophageal carcinoma
- Inflammatory polyps of the vocal cords
- Lung abscess

Gastroenteritis

- Hemorrhage
- Ulceration — gastric or duodenal
- Gastric outlet obstruction
- Perforation of the GI lumen

Gastrointestinal disorders

CLINICAL SNAPSHOT ✳

Duodenal ulcer, esophagitis, and gastroenteritis

Major nursing diagnoses	Key patient outcomes
Risk for deficient fluid volume	Show stable vital signs, typically: heart rate, 60 to 100 beats/minute; systolic blood pressure, 90 to 140 mm Hg; and diastolic blood pressure, 50 to 90 mm Hg.
Chronic pain	Rate pain as less than 3 on a 0 to 10 pain rating scale.
Imbalanced nutrition: Less than body requirements	Discuss nutritional needs with the dietitian.

Nursing diagnosis

Risk for deficient fluid volume related to vomiting, diarrhea, or GI hemorrhage

NURSING PRIORITIES

- Observe for, prevent, or promptly treat hemorrhage.
- Reestablish and maintain fluid and electrolyte balance.

PATIENT OUTCOME CRITERIA

Within 2 hours of admission, the patient will:
- show stable vital signs, typically: heart rate, 60 to 100 beats/minute; systolic blood pressure, 90 to 140 mm Hg; and diastolic blood pressure, 50 to 90 mm Hg
- experience no vomiting
- maintain adequate urine output (greater than 60 ml/hour).

INTERVENTIONS

1. *Monitor and record the patient's vital signs every 15 minutes if bleeding or every 4 hours if stable.* ✱ Unless the patient is syncopal, frankly hypotensive, or severely tachycardic when supine, assess for orthostatic blood pressure and pulse rate changes every 8 hours: Take the patient's blood pressure and pulse while he is supine; then have the patient sit up and measure blood pressure and pulse rate again. Document your findings.

2. *Withhold oral foods and fluids until vomiting has subsided.* Administer I.V. fluids and blood transfusions, as ordered, and provide oxygen at 2 to 6 L/minute via nasal cannula. Monitor CBC and serum electrolyte levels, as ordered, and report abnormalities. See appendix C, Fluid and electrolyte imbalances.

3. Administer antiemetics, antidiarrheals, and anticholinergics, as ordered.

RATIONALES

1. Tachycardia and hypotension may indicate hypovolemia or shock. Orthostatic changes (a blood pressure decrease of 10 mm Hg or more or a pulse rate increase of 20 beats/minute or more) may indicate hypovolemia.

2. Allowing the patient to eat and drink may cause more vomiting and lead to metabolic alkalosis, hypokalemia, or hyponatremia. The Fluid and electrolyte imbalances appendix provides details related to specific abnormalities. Restoring intravascular volume and supplementing oxygen transport reduce the effects of blood loss on tissues until bleeding can be controlled.

3. Antiemetics, such as prochlorperazine (Compazine), promethazine (Phenergan), and chlorpromazine (Thorazine), prevent activation of the vomiting center in the brain stem. Adverse reactions include sedation, blurred vision, and restlessness.

✱Italics indicate key interventions.

Antidiarrheals, such as diphenoxylate with atropine (Lomotil), loperamide (Imodium), and kaolin and pectin (Kaopectate), may be used to decrease fluid loss from diarrhea. Diphenoxylate with atropine and loperamide are synthetic opium alkaloids that decrease intestinal motility, thereby decreasing diarrhea. They're contraindicated in patients with obstruction or diarrhea caused by infectious agents. Because kaolin and pectin act by adsorbing liquids, bacteria, toxins, nutrients, and drugs, loss of essential nutrients may occur with prolonged use.

Anticholinergics, such as dicyclomine (Bentyl) and propantheline (Pro-Banthine), decrease gastric acid secretion and GI tone and motility and effectively control nausea and vomiting in acute gastritis. Adverse reactions include urine retention, dryness of mucous membranes (including dry mouth), dizziness, flushing, and headache.

4. Monitor and record the effectiveness of medications.

4. Lack of effectiveness may indicate the need to reevaluate the pharmacologic regimen.

5. *Assess the patient's skin for signs of dehydration*—poor skin turgor, dry skin and mucous membranes, and pallor. Also assess for thirst, especially in the elderly or debilitated patient.

5. Poor skin turgor, dry skin and mucous membranes, and increased thirst may indicate hypovolemia resulting from decreased extracellular fluid volume.

6. *Monitor and record intake and output each shift.* Include all vomitus, diarrhea, tube drainage, and blood loss in output, and all blood products and I.V. fluids in input. Record hourly urine outputs in the unstable patient. Record daily weights. Test all GI output with guaiac reagent strips (Hemoccult).

6. Accurate monitoring of intake and output alerts caregivers to imbalances that may cause hypovolemic shock. Oliguria (less than 30 ml of urine per hour) indicates decreased glomerular filtration rate; this may result from decreased blood flow, as in hypovolemia. Weight loss may reflect fluid loss. Checking GI output for occult blood may provide early detection of bleeding.

7. *Assess and record the patient's level of consciousness (LOC), muscle strength, and coordination at least every 8 hours.* Report changes promptly.

7. Confusion, dizziness, or stupor may indicate hypovolemia and electrolyte imbalance. A decreased LOC reflects cerebral hypoxemia caused by decreased circulating blood volume. Vomiting and diarrhea can cause electrolyte loss. Sodium loss may cause confusion and delirium; potassium loss may cause muscle weakness.

8. *Observe for and report signs of GI hemorrhage.* Describe any hematemesis, melena, or other signs of intestinal bleeding, including amount, consistency, and color. Test all stools and vomitus with a guaiac reagent strip (Hemoccult). See the "Gastrointestinal hemorrhage" care plan on page 487.

8. Hematemesis of frank red blood indicates active bleeding, while coffee-ground vomitus indicates old bleeding. Guaiac testing unmasks occult bleeding. The "Gastrointestinal hemorrhage" care plan covers this disorder in detail.

9. *Institute NG intubation,* if ordered. Keep the tube patent by instilling 30 ml of saline solution every 2 to 4 hours, then removing the same amount by mechanical suction.

9. NG intubation reveals the presence or absence of blood in the stomach, helps assess the rate of bleeding, and provides a route for saline lavage. If the tube isn't patent, the patient may vomit stomach contents.

10. *Institute continuous saline lavage, if ordered.* Instill aliquots of room-temperature fluid (500 to 1,000 ml); then remove the same amount by gentle suction and gravity drainage.

10. Continuous lavage indicates the rapidity of bleeding and cleans the stomach should endoscopy be necessary. Iced saline may impair coagulation. Experimental evidence suggests that room-temperature water lavage may be as effective as iced saline lavage.

11. *If the patient is bleeding actively, check vital signs hourly* (more frequently if unstable). Alert the physician immediately to any deterioration, as indicated by decreasing alertness, dropping systolic blood pressure, tachycardia, narrowing pulse pressure, restlessness or agitation, or decreasing hemoglobin level.

11. Loss of blood volume leads rapidly to hypovolemic shock. Untreated, shock may progress to irreversible tissue ischemia; death follows quickly. Early detection of active bleeding and aggressive fluid replacement are essential to prevent shock.

12. Prepare the patient for surgery, if indicated.

12. Surgery may be indicated if bleeding continues longer than 48 hours, recurs, or is associated with perforation or obstruction. The preferred surgery is parietal cell vagotomy.

13. *Maintain the patient on bed rest after the bleeding episode.* Begin the prescribed medication regimen, as ordered.

13. Rest aids hemostasis and decreases GI tract activity. A medication regimen (as in the following nursing diagnosis) is the usual therapy before surgery is considered.

14. Additional individualized interventions: _____

14. Rationales: _____

> **Suggested NIC Interventions**
> *Acid-base management; Fluid and electrolyte management; Fluid monitoring; Hypovolemia management; Intravenous (I.V.) therapy*

> **Suggested NOC Outcomes**
> *Electrolyte and acid-base balance; Fluid balance; Hydration*

Nursing diagnosis
Chronic pain related to increased hydrochloric acid secretion; increased spasm, intragastric pressure, motility of upper GI tract, inflammation of the esophagus, stomach, and duodenum

NURSING PRIORITIES
- Relieve pain.
- Promote stomach and intestinal healing.
- Teach about risk factors and measures to prevent recurrence.

PATIENT OUTCOME CRITERIA
Within 2 days of admission, the patient will:
- rate pain as less than 3 on a 0 to 10 pain rating scale
- identify dietary intolerances
- observe dietary recommendations in menu selection
- identify personal stressors, on request
- demonstrate interest in stress-reduction measures
- list signs and symptoms of ulcer recurrence and bleeding
- state understanding of prescribed medications.

INTERVENTIONS
Duodenal ulcer

1. *Administer ulcer-healing medications and document their use,* as ordered. Medications may include one or a combination of the following:
– histamine (H$_2$)-receptor antagonists (cimetidine [Tagamet], ranitidine [Zantac], famotidine [Pepcid], and nizatidine [Axid]), usually given with meals and at bedtime
– antacids, given after meals and at bedtime unless otherwise ordered
– anticholinergics
– sucralfate (Carafate)
– anti-infectives.

2. *Provide bed rest and a quiet environment,* minimizing visitors and telephone calls.

3. *Teach and reinforce the role of diet in ulcer healing.* Help the patient identify specific foods that may increase discomfort.

4. *Encourage adequate caloric intake* from the basic food groups at regular intervals. Encourage frequent small meals.

5. *Teach and reinforce required lifestyle changes* to reduce physical and emotional stress. Help the patient identify specific personal stressors and recognize the relationship between increased stress and ulcer pain. As appropriate, present information on relaxation techniques, exercise, priority setting, time management and personal organization, building and nurturing relationships, the importance of "play" time, and assertiveness techniques.

6. Encourage the patient who smokes to quit.

7. *Teach the patient signs and symptoms indicating ulcer recurrence* and bleeding, including pain, hematemesis, dark or tarry stools, pallor, increasing weakness, dizziness, or faintness.

8. Additional individualized interventions:_____

Esophagitis and gastroenteritis

1. *See the "Chronic pain" care plan,* page 63.

RATIONALES

1. Increased hydrochloric acid secretion results in edema and inflammation of gastric mucosa. H$_2$-receptor antagonists inhibit gastrin release, antacids buffer hydrochloric acid, anticholinergics decrease hydrochloric acid secretion, and sucralfate binds to proteins at the base of the ulcer to form a protective barrier against acid and pepsin. An effective treatment for *H. pylori* in duodenal peptic ulcer disease is a 14-day regimen of bismuth subsalicylate, metronidazole tetracycline hydrochloride, and omeprazole. It's important for the patient to complete the entire therapy to eradicate the *H. pylori* infection. Eradication of *H. pylori* normally results in healing of a duodenal peptic ulcer and resolution of gastritis.

2. Ulcer symptoms are usually reduced by rest and a quiet environment.

3. Dietary restrictions other than avoidance of excessive alcohol and caffeine aren't currently recommended. Promotion of specific diets is highly controversial; none has been scientifically proved to promote healing. Identifying personal food intolerances aids diet planning.

4. Food itself acts as an antacid, neutralizing stomach acid 30 to 60 minutes after ingestion.

5. Stressful life situations, such as occupational, financial, or family problems, are reported more commonly in patients with duodenal ulcers that require longer than 6 weeks to heal. Identifying cause-and-effect relationships helps the patient make necessary lifestyle changes.

6. Research indicates that patients who smoke have impaired ulcer healing and a higher mortality when compared to nonsmokers.

7. Early identification of ulcer recurrence and bleeding may permit intervention before bleeding becomes severe.

8. Rationales: _____

1. Pain associated with esophagitis and gastroenteritis may be subtle, as in abdominal cramping or heartburn, or may be more acute such as sharp substernal pain similar to angina. The "Chronic pain" care plan provides general interventions for pain. This care plan contains additional information related to esophagitis and gastroenteritis.

2. *Assess and document the pain's characteristics:* onset, location, duration, and severity; radiation to back, neck, or shoulder; relationship to activity or position changes; relationship to eating patterns and bowel movements; and relationship to ingestion of spicy foods, coffee, alcohol, hot or cold liquids, or certain medications. Notify the physician of any findings. Assess and document pain-relief measures.

2. Accurate assessment is important in determining the pain's cause and formulating a medical diagnosis. Substernal burning pain (heartburn) and odynophagia are commonly associated with esophagitis. Epigastric pain while eating and abdominal cramping and tenderness are associated with acute gastritis.

3. Administer antacids (typically hourly and 1 hour after meals), H_2-receptor antagonists (1 hour before meals and at least 30 minutes before sucralfate (Carafate) administration), sucralfate, antibiotics, and antifungal medication, as ordered. In cases of severe pain, analgesics, such as viscous lidocaine or other topical agents, may be used. More potent analgesics may also be required.

3. Antacids are effective for about 30 minutes in the fasting stomach and should be given hourly for optimum neutralization of gastric acid. In case of severe pain, antacids may be given every 30 to 60 minutes. Antacids are most effective if given 1 hour after meals to neutralize increased gastric acid secretion stimulated by food ingestion.

H_2-receptor antagonists decrease gastric acid secretions and lower gastric pH by blocking H_2. They're poorly absorbed if given with meals, antacids, or sucralfate.

Sucralfate provides a protective coating for the gastric lining and isn't absorbed. It may be ordered crushed and mixed with water to form a slush that coats the esophagus.

Antibiotics should be given after meals. Combination therapy (two different antibiotics and bismuth salt) is given to treat *H. pylori* infection.

4. Monitor and record the effectiveness of medications.

4. Lack of effectiveness may indicate improper administration, inadequate dosage, the need to change medications, or new or complicating factors.

5. *Assist and instruct the patient to rest, physically and emotionally.* Help the patient identify personal stressors and ways to minimize their effects. Limit the number of visitors. Coordinate patient care to minimize interruptions. Keep room lights low. Teach stress-relieving techniques, such as deep-breathing and relaxation exercises.

5. Stress stimulates the vagus nerve, which increases gastric mucosal blood flow, gastric acid secretion, and gastric motility. These factors may increase pain and inhibit healing.

6. *Instruct the patient and family about pain-prevention measures.* If pain causes the patient to awake at night or if the pain is worse on awakening, instruct the patient to sleep with the head of the bed elevated and to avoid eating for 3 hours before bedtime. Advise the patient to avoid bending, lifting heavy objects, and wearing constrictive clothing. Administer stool softeners, if prescribed, to avoid straining during bowel movements. Assess the patient's diet and habits to identify known causes of pain, such as spicy foods, alcohol, caffeinated products, aspirin, and smoking.

6. Eating stimulates gastric acid secretion. The patient with esophagitis should avoid eating for 3 hours before bedtime and elevate the head of the bed to prevent gastric reflux during sleep. Bending, lifting, wearing constrictive clothing, and straining decrease esophageal pressure and increase intra-abdominal pressure. Spicy foods, alcohol, caffeinated products, and aspirin irritate the gastric lining, increasing discomfort, and should be avoided. Cigarette smoking stimulates increased gastric secretion, which may contribute to further inflammation.

7. Additional individualized interventions: _____

_____

7. Rationales: _____

_____

Suggested NIC Interventions
Medication management; Pain management; Analgesic administration; Patient-controlled analgesia (PCA) assistance; Conscious sedation

Suggested NOC Outcomes
Comfort level; Pain control; Pain: Disruptive effects; Pain level

Nursing diagnosis

Imbalanced nutrition: Less than body requirements related to nausea and vomiting, dysphagia, and mouth soreness

NURSING PRIORITY
Reestablish nutritional balance.

PATIENT OUTCOME CRITERIA
Within 2 hours of admission, the patient will:
- verbalize relief of nausea and vomiting.
  Within 24 hours of admission, the patient will:
- discuss nutritional needs with the dietitian.

INTERVENTIONS

1. *Assess the patient's ability to retain oral food and fluids,* noting any nausea, vomiting, or regurgitation; dysphagia for solids, liquids, or both; and complaints of mouth pain or soreness. Record all observations.

2. *Monitor intake and output.* Withhold oral foods and fluids until vomiting subsides. If parenteral nutrition (PN) is ordered, infuse the solution at the prescribed rate. (See the "Parenteral nutrition" care plan, page 510.) Administer oral nutritional and vitamin supplements as ordered. Record daily weights and calorie counts.

3. Explain the dilatation procedure, if ordered, for dysphagia, and assist when needed.

4. Help the dietitian teach the patient how to plan a well-balanced, nutritious diet. Teach the patient with esophageal strictures who can't eat solids to puree foods and drink nutritional supplements. Instruct the patient with acute gastritis to eat frequent small meals instead of three large meals per day. Tell the patient to restrict or avoid spicy foods, alcohol, and caffeinated products, if necessary. Record all patient teaching.

5. Additional individualized interventions: _____

RATIONALES

1. Careful assessment of symptoms aids differential diagnosis. Mouth pain or soreness may indicate fungal infection or occur after ingestion of a caustic substance. Dysphagia may result from stricture formation from reflux esophagitis or ingestion of a caustic substance.

2. Food and fluids may cause further vomiting, increasing the risk of such complications as Mallory-Weiss tears (tearing of the esophageal mucosa, usually after forceful or prolonged vomiting). PN may be necessary if oral intake is contraindicated for an extended period. The "Parenteral nutrition" care plan contains details about this therapy. Nutritional supplements are indicated for the patient with esophageal strictures who can't swallow solid foods or for the patient who can't maintain metabolic balance because of anorexia, nausea, or mouth soreness.

3. Esophageal strictures, a common cause of dysphagia in esophagitis, can result from ingestion of a caustic substance, gastric reflux, or chronic infection (such as candidiasis). Carefully explaining the dilatation procedure helps alleviate the patient's anxiety. (Because dilatation procedures vary widely, consult institution protocol for details.)

4. Dietary instruction aims to establish a balanced diet and ultimately return the patient's weight to normal. Thorough teaching may prevent subsequent problems and complications. Careful documentation of teaching provides a record for other caregivers so that reinforcement and review may be provided, as appropriate.

5. Rationales: _____

Suggested NIC Interventions
Diet staging; Nutrition management; Weight gain assistance; Fluid monitoring; Nutritional monitoring

Suggested NOC Outcomes
Nutritional status; Nutritional status: Food and fluid intake; Nutritional status: Nutrient intake; Weight control

Gastrointestinal disorders

Discharge planning

DISCHARGE CHECKLIST
Before discharge, the patient shows evidence of:
- ❏ stable vital signs
- ❏ absence of signs and symptoms of GI hemorrhage
- ❏ hemoglobin level within expected parameters
- ❏ absence of pain
- ❏ ability to tolerate nutritional intake as ordered
- ❏ ability to verbalize diet and medication instructions
- ❏ ability to perform activities of daily living and ambulate as before hospitalization
- ❏ adequate home support system or referral to home care if indicated by inadequate home support system or inability to perform self-care.
- ❏ absence of pulmonary or cardiovascular complications.

TEACHING CHECKLIST
Document evidence that the patient and family demonstrate an understanding of:
- ❏ nature and implications of disease
- ❏ pain-relief measures
- ❏ all discharge medications' purpose, dosage, administration schedule, and adverse effects requiring medical attention (usual discharge medications include antacids or H_2-receptor antagonists, or both)
- ❏ recommended dietary modifications
- ❏ need for smoking-cessation program (if applicable)
- ❏ stress-reduction measures
- ❏ signs and symptoms of ulcer recurrence and GI bleeding
- ❏ date, time, and location of follow-up appointment
- ❏ how to contact the physician.

DOCUMENTATION CHECKLIST
Using outcome criteria as a guide, document:
- ❏ clinical status on admission
- ❏ significant changes in status
- ❏ description of pain
- ❏ description of stools, vomitus, and episodes of nausea
- ❏ bleeding episodes
- ❏ pain-relief measures
- ❏ nutritional intake and intolerances
- ❏ pertinent diagnostic test findings
- ❏ medication administration
- ❏ patient and family teaching
- ❏ discharge planning.

Associated care plans
- ▪ Chronic pain
- ▪ Gastrointestinal hemorrhage
- ▪ Ineffective individual coping
- ▪ Knowledge deficit

References
Jordan, K. (ed). *Emergency Nursing Core Curriculum.* Emergency Nurses Association. Philadelphia: W.B. Saunders Co., 2000.

Lynn-McHale, D.J., and Carlson, K.K. American Association of Critical Care Nurses *AACN Procedure Manual for Critical Care,* 4th ed. Philadelphia: W.B. Saunders Co., 2001.

Shoemaker, W.C., et al. *Textbook of Critical Care,* 4th ed. Philadelphia: W.B. Saunders Co., 2002.

Urakami, Y., and Sano, T. "Long-term Follow-up of Gastric Metaplasia after Eradication of *Helicobacter pylori,*" *The Journal of Medical Investigation* 50(1-2):48-54, February 2003.

Gastrointestinal hemorrhage

DRG INFORMATION

DRG 174   Gastrointestinal Hemorrhage with Complication or Comorbidity (CC).
        Mean LOS 5 4.8 days

  Principal diagnoses include:
- GI hemorrhage — site or etiology unspecified
- hemorrhage of anus or rectum
- acute ulcer (gastric, peptic, duodenal, jejunal, or a combination of sites) with hemorrhage
- esophageal varices with hemorrhage.

DRG 175   Gastrointestinal Hemorrhage without CC.
        Mean LOS = 2.9 days

  Principal diagnoses include selected principal diagnoses listed under DRG 174. The distinction is that patients grouped under DRG 175 have no CC.

Introduction

DEFINITION AND TIME FOCUS

In the acute care setting, severe GI bleeding is most commonly associated with upper GI pathology; although bleeding can occur anywhere in the GI tract, lower GI bleeding is usually less severe. Bleeding may result from an underlying condition, such as ulcers, invasive tumors, or esophageal varices. (Gastritis and gastric ulcers are estimated to account for up to 80% of all GI bleeding episodes.) Bleeding may also develop as an untoward effect of therapeutically administered medications, such as anti-inflammatory drugs or anticoagulants. Trauma, burns, sepsis, and other conditions may cause stress ulcers, which usually manifest as sudden, severe, and painless bleeding. Regardless of the cause, acute GI bleeding may be life-threatening without prompt diagnosis and treatment. Delay in diagnosis is associated with a higher mortality and increased complications. (See *Clinical snapshot: Gastrointestinal hemorrhage,* page 488.) This care plan focuses on the patient experiencing an acute episode of upper GI bleeding. (See *Clinical pathway: Managing GI hemorrhage,* pages 495 and 495.)

ETIOLOGY AND PRECIPITATING FACTORS

- Gastric irritation or altered gastric pH, as with medication use (for example, salicylates, steroids, or other anti-inflammatory drugs), alcohol or caffeine abuse, toxic or allergic reactions, ingestion of corrosive substances, peptic or gastric ulcer, gastritis, and stress reactions
- Altered gastric function or circulation, as with tumors, portal hypertension or esophageal varices, or Mallory-Weiss laceration of gastric mucosa
- Altered blood coagulation, as with anticoagulant use, blood dyscrasias, cancer, shock, sepsis, uremia, and disseminated intravascular coagulation (DIC)

Focused assessment guidelines

NURSING HISTORY
(FUNCTIONAL HEALTH PATTERN FINDINGS)
Health-perception–health-management pattern
- History of gastric ulcer or gastritis
- History of heavy alcohol intake or cigarette smoking (associated with gastritis and esophageal varices)
- History of long-term steroid, salicylate, or other anti-inflammatory therapy

Nutritional-metabolic pattern
- Nausea
- Fullness in the abdomen
- Thirst
- Heartburn

Elimination pattern
- Dark or tarry stools
- History of coffee-ground vomitus

Activity-exercise pattern
- Weakness and easy fatigability

Cognitive-perceptual pattern
- With bleeding related to ulcer disease: gnawing, aching, or burning abdominal pain, which may be relieved by eating
- With bleeding related to stress ulcer: no pain

Coping–stress tolerance pattern
- Extreme fear in reaction to sight of own blood

PHYSICAL FINDINGS
General appearance
- Frightened or anxious facial expression

Cardiovascular
- Tachycardia
- Orthostatic hypotension
- Weak, thready peripheral pulse

Gastrointestinal
- Melena
- Hematemesis (associated with upper GI bleeding)
- Coffee-ground vomitus (indicates slower upper GI bleeding)
- Hematochezia (bright, bloody stools — usually indicates lower GI bleeding but may occur with rapid upper GI hemorrhage)

Pulmonary
- Hyperventilation

Neurologic
- Restlessness

- Decreased alertness (with shock)

Integumentary
- Pallor
- Diaphoresis

DIAGNOSTIC STUDIES

- Blood urea nitrogen (BUN) levels — elevated because of digestion of blood proteins in the GI tract and accumulated blood breakdown by-products
- Complete blood count (CBC) — obtained for baseline; may reflect minimal abnormalities for up to 36 hours if bleeding is slow. Eventually, reduced hemoglobin level, hematocrit, and red blood cell (RBC) count reflect overall blood loss; reticulocyte count may be elevated in response to bleeding
- Blood typing and crossmatching — obtained in anticipation of blood replacement; in acute bleeding, type-specific, noncrossmatched blood may be administered as an emergency measure
- Prothrombin time/international normalized ratio, activated partial thromboplastin time — obtained for baseline and for evaluation of altered coagulation status as cause of bleeding; further clotting studies may also be obtained if coagulation defects are suspected
- Gastric aspiration — provides information regarding amount and time of bleeding; results are used to guide further intervention (for example, a small aspiration of

material resembling coffee grounds may indicate old bleeding that warrants only close observation of the patient); aspiration of fresh bright red blood is evidence of active hemorrhage and demands prompt intervention
- Endoscopic examination, including flexible fiber-optic endoscopy — provides visualization of bleeding site and associated pathology; may permit tissue biopsy or direct coagulation of bleeding sites via endoscope
- Abdominal angiography — allows visualization of abdominal vasculature; used to locate bleeding sites and may be used for localized treatment by infusion of vasopressin (Pitressin) or injection of clot formation material (embolization)
- Computed tomography scan — may be used to detect tumors or polyps
- Barium studies — may be used to identify gastric erosions or tumors as bleeding source if angiography isn't available; used as a last resort in patients with active bleeding because barium obscures the field for subsequent endoscopic or angiographic assessment

POTENTIAL COMPLICATIONS

- Shock
- Renal failure
- DIC
- Hepatic encephalopathy
- Myocardial ischemia or myocardial infarction (MI)

CLINICAL SNAPSHOT ✳

Gastrointestinal hemorrhage

Major nursing diagnoses and collaborative problems	Key patient outcomes
CP: Risk for hypovolemic shock	Show stable vital signs, typically: heart rate, 60 to 100 beats/minute; systolic blood pressure, 90 to 140 mm Hg; and diastolic blood pressure, 50 to 90 mm Hg.
ND: Risk for injury	Remain alert and oriented.
ND: Fear	Verbalize feelings related to the condition, if desired.
ND: Deficient knowledge (potential recurrent bleeding)	Describe signs and symptoms of possible recurrent bleeding.

Collaborative problem
Risk for hypovolemic shock related to blood loss

NURSING PRIORITIES
- Assess amount of blood loss.
- Restore blood and fluid volume.
- Help identify the source or cause and provide treatment.

PATIENT OUTCOME CRITERIA
Within 24 hours of detection of bleeding, the patient will:
- show stable vital signs, typically: heart rate, 60 to 100 beats/minute; systolic blood pressure, 90 to 140 mm Hg; and diastolic blood pressure, 50 to 90 mm Hg

- show no orthostatic changes in vital signs
- have urine output of at least 60 ml/hour
- show no signs of frank bleeding
- have warm, dry skin
- exhibit gastric pH greater than 4.

INTERVENTIONS	RATIONALES
1. *Provide standard nursing care related to hypovolemic shock.** See the "Hypovolemic shock" care plan, page 424.	**1.** The "Hypovolemic shock" care plan provides detailed interventions for assessment and treatment of the patient in actual or impending shock.
2. *Assess the amount of blood loss* using the following procedures: – Maintain accurate intake and output records, including precise measurement of all vomitus and stools. Unless output is visibly bloody, perform a guaiac test.	**2.** Prevention of shock depends on accurate status assessment. – Direct measurement of bloody output is essential to guide replacement therapy. Guaiac testing provides objective assessment for the presence of occult blood. Careful monitoring of urine output is vital because a drop in hourly urine output (less than 60 ml/hour) may signal the development of shock.
– Evaluate vital signs every 4 hours, or more frequently if indicated; include evaluation of orthostatic changes unless the patient is syncopal, frankly hypotensive, or severely tachycardic when supine. Note and report promptly to the physician a systolic blood pressure decrease of more than 10 mm Hg or a pulse increase of more than 20 beats/minute.	– Compensatory neurovascular mechanisms may be able to maintain normal supine blood pressure when blood loss is less than 500 ml. Moving from a supine to a sitting position adds an orthostatic stress that may unmask hidden hypotension. A pulse increase of 20 to 30 beats/minute with no change in blood pressure correlates with a blood loss of 500 ml, while a pulse increase of more than 30 beats/minute and systolic blood pressure drop of more than 10 mm Hg may indicate a blood loss of 1,000 ml or more. Although many critically ill patients are too unstable to tolerate orthostatic assessment, it may provide useful data in the stable patient. However, when clear evidence of hypotension already exists, the test may accelerate shock progression.
– If the patient is in a critical care unit, evaluate hemodynamic pressures and electrocardiography (ECG) findings according to appendix A, Monitoring standards, or unit protocol.	– These parameters provide additional data useful in judging the degree of shock present.
– Obtain appropriate laboratory studies, as ordered, including CVC, BUN, and creatinine for baseline and ongoing monitoring.	– Hemoglobin level and hematocrit reflect blood volume status but may show no changes initially. BUN and creatinine levels are of greater diagnostic value. An elevated BUN level in the presence of normal creatinine level indicates a likely blood loss of more than 1,000 ml.
– Assess the patient frequently for clinical signs of hypovolemia. Note constellations of signs and symptoms, such as those of mild shock (for example, anxiety, perspiration, or weakness); moderate shock (for example, hyperactive bowel sounds, tachycardia, or thirst); or severe shock (for example, pallor, cool and clammy skin, decreased level of consciousness [LOC], decreased urine output, and thready pulse).	– Clinical parameters help define stages of blood loss. Signs and symptoms of mild shock (less than 500 ml blood loss) are nonspecific. Signs of moderate shock (500 to 1,000 ml blood loss) reflect progressive activation of sympathetic nervous system compensatory mechanisms and other homeostatic mechanisms. Signs of severe shock (more than 1,000 ml blood loss) reflect ischemia of core organ systems.

*Italics indicate key interventions.

Gastrointestinal disorders

– Insert and maintain a gastric tube, as ordered, and check drainage for blood.

– Gastric intubation permits removal and accurate measurement of accumulated blood from the stomach. It's also therapeutic because blood in the stomach may stimulate vomiting and excess gastric acid secretion, both of which may cause or accelerate bleeding. Finally, blood that passes into the intestines is broken down into ammonia, which may have toxic metabolic effects.

3. *Replace blood loss, as ordered,* by:

3. Replacement therapy is essential to prevent hypovolemia and hypoxemia related to reduced hemoglobin level.

– establishing and maintaining I.V. access with one or two large-bore cannulas
– rapidly administering I.V. crystalloid solution (such as lactated Ringer's solution)
– administering and monitoring the response to transfusion of packed RBCs, fresh frozen plasma, or other blood components as well as volume expanders, such as plasma protein fraction (Plasmanate) or albumin.

– A large-bore cannula is necessary for rapid infusion of blood and fluids.
– Crystalloid solutions effectively expand plasma volume. Rapid administration averts cardiovascular collapse.
– Restoration of circulating volume and replacement of blood components are essential to minimize cell death from hypoxemia. If heart failure is present, packed cells may be administered with minimal additional fluid to avert fluid overload. The hematocrit should increase with each unit of packed cells administered. Persistent bleeding is present if hematocrit doesn't improve. For other patients, volume expanders may be indicated. Albumin, for example, provides an osmotically induced fluid expansion equal to five times its volume. Blood that has been stored for a period of time may be deficient in some clotting factors, so the administration of fresh frozen plasma or other components may be needed.

– Prepare the patient for emergency surgery if blood pressure doesn't increase in response to 1 L of fluid given over 10 minutes or if hemoglobin level and hematocrit fail to increase in response to blood product administration.

– Emergency surgery is indicated to identify and correct the cause of massive bleeding.

4. *Initiate measures to stop bleeding, as ordered,* such as:

4. As many as 90% of upper GI hemorrhages cease spontaneously, but severe bleeding constitutes a medical or surgical emergency, and prompt corrective treatment is warranted.

– maintaining activity restrictions, which usually include strict bed rest.
– performing gastric lavage, usually with room temperature or iced normal saline solution, with or without addition of norepinephrine (Levophed) to the solution. If norepinephrine is used, the usual dilution is 2 ampules to 1,000 ml normal saline solution in a continuous irrigation.

– Activity may increase intra-abdominal pressure and accelerate bleeding.
– Gastric lavage removes accumulated blood and clots and clears the stomach for endoscopic examination. Iced lavage, which was traditionally ordered based on the theory that gastric cooling decreased blood flow, has become controversial as a therapeutic measure. Some studies have demonstrated prolonged clotting times in response to iced irrigation. Norepinephrine may be added for its local vasoconstrictive effects, although its value hasn't been proved. Systemic effects are minimized when norepinephrine is administered in this way because the drug is metabolized in the liver immediately after gastric absorption.

– administering vasopressin I.V., unless the patient has a history of coronary artery disease or other vascular problems. The dose range is 0.02 to 0.06 mcg/minute I.V. or through an arterial catheter placed near the bleeding site. Monitor the ECG during administration.

– Vasopressin causes vasoconstriction and contraction of smooth muscle in the GI tract. It also increases reabsorption of water in the renal tubules. However, its use may cause myocardial ischemia, MI, or hypertension, particularly in a patient with cardiovascular disease.

– preparing the patient with uncontrollably bleeding esophageal varices, if a poor surgical risk, for injection sclerotherapy; after injection, observe for rebleeding, chest pain, fever, and other complications

– preparing the patient for laser therapy, if ordered

– assisting with insertion, monitoring, and maintaining the placement of a Sengstaken-Blakemore tube or other compression tubes. Elevate the head of the bed. Suction the oropharynx, nasopharynx, and upper esophagus frequently. Irrigate the tube at least every 2 hours. Maintain proper balloon pressures. Maintain proper positioning by verifying balloon placement by X-ray, as ordered, and maintaining traction on the balloon. Cut and remove the tube immediately if airway compromise occurs.

– as an alternative to sclerotherapy, administering somatostatin in a 250-mg bolus followed by an I.V. infusion of 250 mg/hour or octreotide 50 mcg I.V. bolus followed by an I.V. infusion of 25 to 50 mcg/hour over 1 to 5 days.
– administering vitamin K_1 (phytonadione, AquaMEPHYTON) intramuscularly, as ordered

– preparing the patient for surgery if medical treatment is unsuccessful (bleeding requires more than 2 units of blood per hour to maintain blood pressure, requires more than 6 to 8 units of blood within 24 hours, exceeds more than 2,500 ml in the first 24 hours, or recurs during therapy).

– Injection sclerotherapy is a definitive treatment involving injection of a coagulating substance into a bleeding vessel. This produces intense inflammation and scarring, and stops bleeding in approximately 80% of cases. Hemorrhage may recur, requiring multiple treatments. Chest pain and fever (typically appearing within 6 hours and lasting 3 days) result from the inflammatory process.
– Laser coagulation therapy may be used when endoscopy indicates active bleeding, fresh clots, or a duodenal ulcer or gastric erosion with a visible vessel.
– Compression balloon tubes, such as the Sengstaken-Blakemore tube, may be used to control hemorrhage temporarily in patients with esophageal varices. However, the high rebleeding rate, significant discomfort, and risk of aspiration limit the tubes' usefulness. The balloon applies direct pressure against bleeding vessels, while the gastric tube permits continued decompression and aspiration. Elevating the head of the bed helps prevent esophageal reflux and associated irritation. When the tube is in place, the patient is unable to swallow salivary secretions. Also, nasal secretions may be increased because of local irritation from the tube. Irrigation ensures patency of the tube and prevents gastric distention.

Excessive pressure may result in perforation, inflammation, or ulceration of the esophagus or gastric mucosal lining, while insufficient pressure may render the tube ineffective or contribute to its displacement.

X-ray verification and maintenance of traction help ensure correct positioning. If the tube becomes displaced, it may obstruct the airway. Cutting the tube deflates the gastric and esophageal balloons and permits immediate removal.
– Somatostatin and octreotide are as effective as vasopressin with fewer systemic complications. Patients with known ischemic heart disease, peripheral vascular disease or cardiac arrhythmias will benefit from somatostatin or octreotide.
– The patient receiving I.V. feedings or multiple antibiotics for a prolonged period may develop vitamin K deficiency because this catalyst for clotting factor production is either obtained through a normal diet or synthesized by intestinal bacteria. Replacement therapy may be necessary to restore normal clotting status.
– If bleeding doesn't stop, surgery is indicated to identify and correct the problem.

Gastrointestinal disorders

5. *Administer medications to control gastric acidity,* typically histamine (H_2)-blockers such as cimetidine (Tagamet) or ranitidine (Zantac) I.V. during acute bleeding episodes. Monitor gastric aspirate pH and adjust dosage, as ordered, to maintain a pH greater than 4.0. Observe for drug interactions, especially if the patient is also receiving theophylline (Slo-Phyllin), procainamide (Pronestyl), or warfarin (Coumadin). Observe for signs of toxicity if cimetidine and lidocaine (Xylocaine) are administered concurrently.

5. Gastric hyperacidity, indicated by a low pH, is a primary contributor to ulcer development and the need for dosage increases. H_2-blockers inhibit the action of histamine, raising gastric pH. Cimetidine and ranitidine reduce theophylline clearance, increasing the risk of theophylline toxicity; impair metabolism of procainamide, possibly producing toxicity; and impair metabolism of warfarin, increasing the risk of bleeding. Cimetidine reduces liver clearance of lidocaine.

6. *Prepare the patient and family for and assist with diagnostic procedures, as ordered,* such as endoscopic examination, angiography, or other studies.

6. Identification of the site and cause of the bleeding is essential because delay in diagnosis is associated with a higher mortality.

7. Additional individualized interventions: _____
_____

7. Rationales: _____
_____

Nursing diagnosis

Risk for injury: Complications related to undetected bleeding, inadequate organ perfusion, accumulation of toxins, electrolyte imbalance, release of procoagulants, or ulcer perforation

NURSING PRIORITY
Prevent or promptly detect and treat complications.

PATIENT OUTCOME CRITERIA
Throughout the hospital stay, the patient will:
- exhibit decreasing BUN and normal creatinine values
- display electrolyte levels within normal limits
- maintain urine output greater than 60 ml/hour
- remain alert and oriented.

INTERVENTIONS

1. *Continue to perform guaiac tests* on all gastric contents and stools at least daily, even after the patient's condition has stabilized.

2. *Immediately report and thoroughly investigate any complaint of chest pain,* particularly in a patient with preexisting cardiac disease.

3. *Monitor renal and hepatic function,* including hourly urine output, LOC every 2 hours, daily BUN and creatinine levels, and daily weight. Note daily serum electrolyte values, including serum calcium, particularly if the patient has received multiple blood transfusions.

4. *Observe for bleeding from other sites,* such as epistaxis or petechiae. See the "Disseminated intravascular coagulation" care plan, page 764.

RATIONALES

1. As much as 200 ml of blood may be lost daily without detectable clinical signs. Early detection allows prompt treatment.

2. Blood loss reduces the level of circulating hemoglobin, thus compromising normal delivery of oxygen to tissues. If coronary circulation is already impaired, this reduction may cause ischemic changes or an acute myocardial infarction.

3. Hemorrhage and the resulting hypovolemia may cause renal and hepatic hypoperfusion, eventually leading to kidney or liver failure. Liver dysfunction, commonly associated with esophageal varices, contributes to elevated blood ammonia levels and can result in hepatic encephalopathy. Hypocalcemia is a common adverse effect of multiple transfusions because calcium binds with the preservative in stored blood.

4. Bleeding from other sites may signal the development of DIC, a grave complication of hemorrhage. The "Disseminated intravascular coagulation" care plan contains detailed interventions.

5. *Immediately report any complaint of sudden, severe abdominal pain or rigidity,* and prepare the patient for surgery if these occur.

6. Additional individualized interventions: _____
_____

5. These signs and symptoms may indicate gastric perforation, which causes peritonitis, sepsis, and shock unless promptly treated. Immediate surgical intervention is warranted to remove gastric contents from the peritoneal cavity.

6. Rationales: _____
_____

Suggested NIC Interventions
Surveillance: Safety

Suggested NOC Outcomes
Safety status: Physical injury

Nursing diagnosis
Fear related to sight of blood and distressing physical symptoms

NURSING PRIORITY
Reduce the patient's fear.

PATIENT OUTCOME CRITERION
After initial stabilization, the patient will verbalize feelings related to the condition, if desired.

INTERVENTIONS	RATIONALES
1. *Provide care promptly, explaining all interventions to the patient in simple terms.* Avoid expressing dismay or revulsion at the sight of bleeding; assume a calm, confident, matter-of-fact manner. Acknowledge the patient's fear by saying, for example, "I know it must be pretty scary to see all this blood, but we treat this condition often. We will be replacing your blood by giving you transfusions and extra fluids."	**1.** The sight of blood is extremely threatening to the patient, who justifiably may fear bleeding to death. Anxiety may interfere with the patient's ability to comprehend, but simple explanations about what's happening may reassure the patient that needed care is being given. Recognizing the normalcy of the patient's fear reduces the patient's sense of isolation. Patients typically are quite concerned about bloody excreta and losing bowel control. Calm acceptance may minimize shame related to these losses of bodily control.
2. *Encourage verbalization of feelings* by using active listening skills. See the "Ineffective individual coping" care plan, page 124.	**2.** Verbalizing feelings helps the patient identify specific fears and begin to mobilize coping strategies. The "Ineffective individual coping" care plan details interventions that may be helpful in promoting coping behaviors.
3. *Accept expressions of anxiety related to the possibility of death.* See the "Dying" care plan, page 78.	**3.** Issues of death are always of acute importance for the patient with a critical condition. The "Dying" care plan contains specific interventions useful in caring for patients and families confronting issues of mortality.
4. Additional individualized interventions: _____	**4.** Rationales: _____

Suggested NIC Interventions
Anxiety reduction; Coping enhancement; Security enhancement

Suggested NOC Outcomes
Anxiety control; Fear control

(Text continues on page 496.)

Managing GI hemorrhage

Patient problem	Day 1
Tests and procedures Risk of increased instability of condition related to delay in tests or procedures	● Goal: Tolerates tests and procedures; endoscopy/colonoscopy completed – Type and screen – PT/PTT – CBC – Hct q 6 hr – Renal profile – Upper endoscopy – Colonoscopy – Patient preparation as ordered
Medications and treatments Risk of recurrence of GI bleeding related to irritation or ulceration of site	● Goal: Exhibits appropriate therapeutic response to drugs; no adverse reactions – I.V. H_2-blockers – Transfuse per physician's orders – I.V. fluids
GI problem Risk for altered bowel function	● Goal: Stable GI function; no active bleeding; NG tube patent – NG tube – Document color, amount, character of aspirate, vomitus, stool – Collect specimens as ordered
Nutrition Risk for imbalanced nutrition: Less than body requirements	● Goal: Stable digestive processes; no vomiting, diarrhea – NPO
Activity Risk for activity intolerance related to weakness	● Goal: Compliant with activity restriction – Bed rest
Cardiovascular Risk for fluid volume deficit related to GI blood loss	● Goal: Stable CV function; adequate fluid balance, stable LOC, skin warm and dry, urine output > 60ml/hr, stable VS (SBP > 90, HR 60 to 100) – VS q 4 hr – I&O q shift – Indwelling urinary catheter
Psychosocial and spiritual needs Risk for ineffective coping related to illness or bleeding	● Goal: Effective coping patterns; patient and family verbalize thoughts and feelings about illness and demonstrate compliance with care – Allow the patient and his family to verbalize thoughts and feelings about illness – Assess response to care and treatment
Patient teaching Deficient knowledge related to illness, procedures, or preventive measures	● Goal: Patient and family participate in identification of learning needs and verbalize understanding of procedure, prep, and postprocedure care ● Assess deficient knowledge and begin teaching as indicated: – Procedures – Treatments – Medications
Discharge planning	● Goal: Discharge planning needs identified and addressed – Discharge planning assessment – Consult case manager to evaluate discharge needs

Day 2	Day 3	Day 4
• Goal: Tests normal; Hct stable, no hematemesis, melena, or rectal bleeding – Hct q 8 hr	• Goal: Tests normal: Hct normal or at baseline × 48 hr; no hematemesis, melena, or rectal bleeding – Hct q a.m.	• Goal: Tests normal
• Goal: Exhibits appropriate therapeutic response to drugs; no adverse reactions – I.V. H$_2$-blockers – I.V. fluids	• Goal: Exhibits appropriate therapeutic response to drugs; no adverse reactions – Change to P.O. meds – D/C I.V. fluids – Change I.V. to S.L.	• Goal: Exhibits appropriate therapeutic response to drugs; no adverse reactions – D/C saline lock
• Goal: Stable GI function; no active bleeding – D/C NG tube – Collect specimens as ordered	• Goal: Stable GI function; normal bowel pattern	• Goal: Stable GI function; normal bowel pattern; benign abdomen
• Goal: Stable digestive processes; tolerates P.O. intake; no vomiting, diarrhea – Clear liquids, advance as tolerated	• Goal: Stable digestive processes: P.O. intake ≥ 50% of meals; no nausea, vomiting, diarrhea – Advance diet as tolerated	• Goal: Stable digestive processes; tolerates 100% of meals; nutritional intake meets body requirements – Diet as tolerated
• Goal: Tolerates activity progression – Chair t.i.d.	• Goal: Tolerates activity progression – Up in room	• Goal: Patient and family or significant other able to manage care – Up ad lib
• Goal: Stable CV function: adequate fluid balance, stable LOC, skin warm and dry, urine output > 60 ml/hr, stable VS (SBP > 90, HR 60 to 100) – VS q 8 hr – I&O q shift – D/C indwelling urinary catheter	• Goal: Stable CV function: adequate fluid balance, stable LOC, skin warm and dry, urine output > 60 ml/hr, stable VS (SBP > 90, HR 60 to 100) – VS q 8 hr – I&O q shift	• Goal: Stable CV function; adequate fluid balance, stable LOC, skin warm and dry, urine output > 60 ml/hr, stable vital VS (SBP > 90, HR 60 to 100) – VS q 8 hr – I&O q shift
• Goal: Effective coping patterns: patient and family verbalize thoughts and feelings about illness and demonstrate compliance with care – Allow patient and family to verbalize thoughts and feelings about illness – Assess their response to care and treatment	• Goal: Effective coping patterns: the patient and his family verbalize thoughts and feelings about illness and demonstrate compliance with care – Allow patient and family to verbalize thoughts and feelings about illness – Assess their response to care and treatment	• Goal: Effective coping patterns; patient and family verbalize thoughts and feelings about illness and demonstrate compliance with care – Allow patient and family to verbalize thoughts and feelings about illness – Assess response to care and treatment
• Goal: Identified learning needs met; patient and family verbalize understanding of progression of care • Continue teaching: – Diet – Medications – Activity – Assessment and preventive measures	• Goal: Identified learning needs met; the patient and his family verbalize understanding of progression of care – Continue/reinforce teaching	• Goal: Identified learning needs met; patient and family verbalize understanding of: – _____ – _____ – _____
• Goal: Discharge planning needs identified and addressed; discharge planning assessment completed	• Goal: Discharge planning completed, needs identified, arrangements completed	• Goal: Discharge planning completed, needs identified, arrangements completed

Nursing diagnosis
Deficient knowledge (potential recurrent bleeding) related to unfamiliarity with disorder

NURSING PRIORITY
Teach assessment techniques and preventive measures.

PATIENT OUTCOME CRITERIA
Before discharge, the patient will (as condition allows):
- list any precipitating or contributing factors identified
- describe signs and symptoms of possible recurrence of bleeding
- verbalize understanding of any dietary recommendations.

INTERVENTIONS

1. *Provide standard care related to knowledge deficit.* See the "Knowledge deficit" care plan, page 129.

2. *Defer detailed teaching until the patient is alert and physiologically stable.* Then, as indicated by condition, discuss with the patient:
– precipitating or contributing factors of bleeding episode (for example, alcohol consumption or medication use)

– signs and symptoms indicating possible recurrence (for example, melena, coffee-ground vomitus, weakness, or dizziness)
– other causes of dark stools (for example, intake of iron, beets, berries, or greens)
– dietary recommendations, as ordered (for example, avoidance of caffeine).

3. Additional individualized interventions: _____

RATIONALES

1. The "Knowledge deficit" care plan contains detailed interventions related to patient and family teaching.

2. The patient's condition may limit teaching, but abbreviated teaching may lay the groundwork for more detailed education before discharge.
– Awareness of contributing factors over which the patient has control may decrease the likelihood of a recurrence.
– Early medical attention if bleeding recurs may avert the need for a prolonged hospital stay.

– Knowing other causes may avert undue alarm.

– Careful dietary management may be the primary preventive therapy for some conditions.

3. Rationales: _____

> **Suggested NIC Interventions**
> *Teaching: Individual; Teaching: Procedure/treatment*

> **Suggested NOC Outcomes**
> *Knowledge: Illness care*

Discharge planning
DISCHARGE CHECKLIST
Before discharge, the patient shows evidence of:
- ❏ stable vital signs within normal limits
- ❏ urine output of at least 60 ml/hour
- ❏ normal or decreasing BUN values
- ❏ normal serum electrolytes
- ❏ normal skin perfusion
- ❏ gastric pH of 4.0 or greater
- ❏ normal guaiac test of stools or vomitus
- ❏ stable LOC for more than 12 hours
- ❏ balanced fluid intake and output.

TEACHING CHECKLIST
Document evidence that the patient and his family demonstrate an understanding of:
- ❏ the cause and site of bleeding
- ❏ precipitating or contributing factors
- ❏ the signs and symptoms indicating possible recurrence of bleeding
- ❏ dietary recommendations, if any.

DOCUMENTATION CHECKLIST
Using outcome criteria as a guide, document:
- ❏ clinical status on admission
- ❏ significant changes in status
- ❏ pertinent diagnostic test findings

❒ bleeding episodes
❒ fluid and blood replacement measures
❒ fluid intake and output
❒ emotional response
❒ pharmacologic interventions
❒ procedures to stop bleeding
❒ patient and family teaching
❒ discharge planning.

Associated care plans

- Acute renal failure
- Disseminated intravascular coagulation
- Dying
- Hypovolemic shock
- Impaired physical mobility
- Ineffective individual coping
- Knowledge deficit
- Liver failure
- Nutritional deficit
- Pancreatitis

References

Brackman, M.R., et al. "Acute Lower Gastroenteric Bleeding Retrospective Analysis (The ALGEBRA Study): An Analysis of the Triage, Management and Outcomes of Patients with Acute Aower Gastrointestinal Bleeding," *The American Surgeon* 9(2):145-49, February 2003.

Foga, M.M., and Leslie, W.D. "Gastrointestinal Bleeding, Munchausen Style," *Clinical Nuclear Medicine* 28(4):330-331, April 2003.

Jordan, K. (ed). *Emergency Nursing Core Curriculum.* Emergency Nurses Association. Philadelphia: W.B. Saunders Co., 2000.

Lynn-McHale, D.J., and Carlson, K.K. American Association of Critical Care Nurses *AACN Procedure Manual for Critical Care,* 4th ed. Philadelphia: W.B. Saunders Co., 2001.

Shoemaker, W.C., et al. *Textbook of Critical Care* 4th ed. Philadelphia: W.B. Saunders Co., 2002.

Gastrointestinal disorders

Inflammatory bowel disease

DRG INFORMATION
DRG 179   Inflammatory Bowel Disease (IBD).
            Mean LOS = 6.0 days
DRG 182   Esophagitis, Gastroenteritis, and Miscellaneous Digestive Disorders; Age 17+ with Complications or Comorbidity (CC).
            Mean LOS = 4.3 days
DRG 183   Esophagitis, Gastroenteritis, and Miscellaneous Digestive Disorders; Age 17+ without CC.
            Mean LOS = 2.8 days
DRG 184   Esophagitis, Gastroenteritis, and Miscellaneous Digestive Disorders; Ages 0 to 17.
            Mean LOS = 2.9 days

Introduction
DEFINITION AND TIME FOCUS
IBD is a broad diagnostic category that includes ulcerative colitis, Crohn's disease (regional enteritis), appendicitis, diverticulitis, infectious diarrhea, functional bowel disorders, and humorally mediated diarrheal syndromes. Hospitalized IBD patients may be acutely ill and may demonstrate similar management problems. This care plan focuses on the problems associated with acute exacerbations of ulcerative colitis and regional enteritis.

Ulcerative colitis and regional enteritis involve local defects characterized by excavation of the bowel surface from sloughing of necrotic inflammatory tissue. The ulcerations in regional enteritis are transmural, involving all layers of the bowel; those of ulcerative colitis begin in the crypts of Lieberkühn and usually involve the mucosa and submucosa. The lesions in ulcerative colitis are usually confined to the descending large bowel and sigmoid colon and are continuous in nature; the defects in regional enteritis occur predominantly in, but aren't confined to, the terminal ileum and tend to alternate with areas of normal bowel surface. (See *Clinical snapshot: Inflammatory bowel disease,* page 500.)

ETIOLOGY AND PRECIPITATING FACTORS
- Exact cause unknown — infectious agents, genetic or familial tendencies, immunologic mechanisms, and stress-related psychological factors may be involved
- Stressful event, possibly preceding an acute attack by 4 to 6 months
- Bacterial infection, possibly occurring several weeks before an acute attack
- Age — attacks are more severe, with a higher mortality, after age 40 in regional enteritis and after age 60 with ulcerative colitis

Focused assessment guidelines
NURSING HISTORY
(FUNCTIONAL HEALTH PATTERN FINDINGS)
Health-perception–health-management pattern
- Gradual or acute onset of abdominal cramping, anorexia, and weight loss related to fear of intake of food and fluids that increase cramping; low-grade fever (may be high-grade if perforation present); change in bowel habits with increasing frequency of stools (in ulcerative colitis, stools may exceed 15 per day, be accompanied by urgency and tenesmus [the frequent, painful, unproductive urge to defecate], and contain blood, mucus, or pus)
- History of acute exacerbations
- Drug regimen that includes corticosteroids or immunosuppressants
- Family history of disorder
- Whites, typically, but an unexplained increase in regional enteritis among Blacks has been observed
- Growth retardation (seen in childhood onset of IBD)

Nutritional-metabolic pattern
- Anorexia with weight loss
- Signs and symptoms of chronic malnutrition
- Intake of fatty foods or other dietary indiscretions; if disease is chronic, may report being on a low-residue, low-fiber, bland diet

Elimination pattern
- Increasing frequency of bowel movements (may have been gradual or acute in onset)
- Abdominal pain and possible audible bowel sounds (borborygmi) before onset of discomfort
- Bright red rectal bleeding with fecal incontinence, particularly with ulcerative colitis
- Visible peristaltic waves over the abdomen

Activity-exercise pattern
- Malaise and fatigue
- Muscle weakness

Sleep-rest pattern
- Sleep disturbance related to abdominal discomfort and nocturnal defecation

Self-perception–self-concept pattern
- Low self-esteem, compensated for by ambitious, hard-driving lifestyle

Role-relationship pattern
- Use of dependent behavior to cope with feelings of anger, hostility, and anxiety

- may report family history of similar GI problems

Sexuality-reproductive pattern

- Altered ability to cope with human relationships (with chronic disease)
- Delayed development of secondary sex characteristics and sexual function if IBD begins before puberty
- Decreased fertility

Coping–stress tolerance pattern

- Feelings of hopelessness and despair
- Use of somatization (recurrent, multiple physical complaints with no organic cause), expressions of helplessness, crying, excessive demands on staff time, and excessive praise as mechanisms for individual coping

PHYSICAL FINDINGS

Cardiovascular

- Hypotension
- Tachycardia
- Arrhythmias

Renal

- Decreased output
- Fecal material in urine (if bladder fistula present)

Gastrointestinal

- Diarrhea
- Weight loss
- Hyperactive or hypoactive bowel sounds
- Abdominal tenderness and mass
- Abdominal distention and rigidity
- Rectal bleeding
- Liver tenderness

Neurologic

- Restlessness
- Irritability
- Blurred vision (uncommon)
- Iritis (uncommon)
- Conjunctivitis (uncommon)
- Uveitis (uncommon)

Integumentary

- Poor skin turgor
- Pallor
- Pustules (uncommon)
- Erythematous lesions (uncommon)
- Pyoderma gangrenosum (uncommon skin infection)
- Icterus (if hepatitis present)
- Draining fistulas (particularly around umbilicus or surgical scars)
- Ecchymoses

Musculoskeletal

- Muscle weakness
- Joint pain and tenderness
- Ankylosing spondylitis (uncommon)

DIAGNOSTIC STUDIES

- Complete blood count — may reveal moderate elevation in white blood cell (WBC) count, unless perforation is present (which causes a major elevation above normal); hemoglobin level and hematocrit are decreased with chronic blood loss; if blood loss is sudden and dramatic, hemoglobin level and hematocrit may not immediately reflect the change in blood volume; the red blood cell (RBC) count may reflect megaloblastic anemia if the part of the ileum responsible for vitamin B absorption is affected
- Electrolyte profile — sodium, potassium, and chloride may be deficient with persistent or acute loss of fluids from the GI tract with inadequate replacement
- Total protein levels — decreased because a significant amount of protein is lost in inflammatory exudate in the bowel and through bleeding of damaged tissues, which can deplete albumin and other plasma proteins
- Blood urea nitrogen (BUN) level — decreased because significant nutritional deficits cause the catabolism of body proteins; reflected in negative nitrogen balance
- Bleeding and clotting time — prolonged because vitamin K synthesis decreases as bowel surfaces are destroyed; liver involvement may disturb clotting factor synthesis, altering clotting mechanisms
- Stool studies — culture and sensitivity testing and examination for ova and parasites and fecal leukocyte count are usually ordered to rule out an infectious origin for the symptoms; a guaiac test is usually abnormal for occult blood; fat may also be found in stools (steatorrhea) if destruction of bowel surfaces impairs bile reabsorption
- Liver function tests — hepatitis is a complication of IBD; consequently, elevated bilirubin and liver enzyme levels may be observed
- Alkaline phosphatase levels — increased if arthritic skeletal involvement or hepatitis is present
- Urine studies — culture and sensitivity testing may be ordered if a fistula to the bladder is suspected; opportunistic infections may also occur in the genitourinary tract from overall immunosuppression
- Tuberculin skin test — tuberculosis of the cecum may mimic symptoms of IBD
- Antibody titers — anticolon antibodies are demonstrated commonly in patients with ulcerative colitis but not usually observed in other IBD patients
- Carcinoembryonic antigen — may be ordered for patients with ulcerative colitis because they tend to develop colon cancer after 10 years with the disorder. Carcinoembryonic antigen may become elevated by a variety of noncancerous conditions
- Barium enema — in ulcerative colitis, demonstrates the characteristic obliteration of haustral folds, blurring of bowel margins, and narrowing and stenosis of the large bowel; in regional enteritis, changes usually are found in the small bowel but may occur in the large bowel, so distinguishing between the two disorders on the basis of a barium enema is difficult; procedure may be omitted if abscess or fistula is suspected because the bowel preparation for the procedure, and the procedure itself, may aggravate the condition

- Carotene and Schilling tests — reflect the intestine's absorptive capacity; estimate degree of damaged bowel surface in regional enteritis
- Proctoscopy or colonoscopy — demonstrates hyperemic, edematous, friable bowel mucosa; if lesion is beyond the ileocecal valve, narrowing and stenosis of the valve may be evident; can't be used for small bowel involvement
- Rectal biopsy — inflammation and abscesses of the crypts are evident in ulcerative colitis; biopsy usually doesn't contribute to regional enteritis diagnosis
- Computed tomography scan — reveals abdominal masses that could be fistulas or abscesses
- Upper GI series — lesions in regional enteritis can occur at any point along the GI tract and tend to alternate with segments of normal tissue; upper GI series reveals the extent of involvement and indicates segments where scarring and stenosis may obstruct intestinal flow
- Skeletal X-rays — used to demonstrate the presence and extent of arthritic changes and ankylosing spondylitis, which can occur with IBD

- Magnetic resonance imaging (MRI) — imaging technologies including positron emission tomography scans are increasingly being used as noninvasive procedures to diagnose IBD and complications of the disorders (MRI at present is the preferred procedure because intraluminal bowel visualization can be performed using MRI.)

POTENTIAL COMPLICATIONS
- Malnutrition
- Bowel obstruction
- Arrhythmias
- Peritonitis
- Hepatitis
- Sepsis
- Toxic megacolon
- Malabsorption syndrome
- Gangrenous skin lesions
- Ankylosing spondylitis
- Exudative retinopathy
- Renal calculi
- Pericarditis
- Carcinoma of the colon

CLINICAL SNAPSHOT

Inflammatory bowel disease

Major nursing diagnoses and collaborative problems	Key patient outcomes
CP: Risk for cardiac arrhythmias	Show stable vital signs, typically: heart rate, 60 to 100 beats/minute; systolic blood pressure, 90 to 140 mm Hg; and diastolic blood pressure, 50 to 90 mm Hg.
ND: Excess fluid volume	Maintain fluid intake that equals output.
ND: Imbalanced nutrition: Less than body requirements	Tolerate diet without undue distress.
ND: Risk for infection	Show no signs of infection.
ND: Chronic pain	Rate pain as absent or mild on a pain rating scale.
ND: Distrubed sleep pattern	Experience adequate rest and sleep.
ND: Impaired skin integrity, perianal	Show no evidence of skin breakdown.
ND: Social isolation	Decrease use of ineffective coping behaviors.
ND: Ineffective sexuality patterns	Identify techniques for minimizing physical demands of sexual activity.

Collaborative problem
Risk for cardiac arrhythmias related to electrolyte depletion

NURSING PRIORITY
Maintain electrolyte levels within normal limits.

PATIENT OUTCOME CRITERIA
Within 24 hours of admission, the patient will:

■ show vital signs within normal limits, typically: heart rate, 60 to 100 beats/minute; systolic blood pressure, 90 to 140 mm Hg; and diastolic blood pressure, 50 to 90 mm Hg.
   Within 3 days of admission, the patient will:
■ have serum electrolyte levels within normal limits.

INTERVENTIONS	RATIONALES
1. *Monitor and record fluid losses.* * Evaluate serum electrolyte levels daily, as ordered. Monitor apical and radial pulses, changes in tendon reflexes, and muscle strength every 4 hours or more frequently, depending on the severity of the patient's condition.	**1.** Diarrhea and internal fluid sequestration can cause significant electrolyte loss. Frequent observations for signs of alterations in the cellular membrane potential are necessary. Reminders to the physician to order electrolyte determinations may also be necessary.
2. *Administer and document electrolyte replacement therapy.*	**2.** Normal saline or lactated Ringer's solution and potassium supplements usually are ordered during the acute stage, when oral replacement may be contraindicated. Total parenteral nutrition may be ordered in severely decompensated patients.
3. *Notify the physician immediately of any evidence of arrhythmias* (for example, pulse irregularity, syncopal episodes, or altered level of consciousness [LOC]). See appendix C, Fluid and electrolyte imbalances.	**3.** Cardiac arrest can occur without warning in severe hypokalemia or hyperkalemia. See appendix C, Fluid and electrolyte imbalances for details on specific imbalances.
4. *Notify physician of any evidence of worsening heart failure (HF)* (for example, sudden weight gain, edema, cough, shortness of breath)	**4.** Crohn's patients with previously diagnosed Type I or Type II HF may experience worsening of symptoms upon administration of Remicade (Infleximab).
5. Additional individualized interventions: _____	5. Rationales: _____

Nursing diagnosis

Excess fluid volume related to decreased fluid intake, increased fluid loss through diarrhea or internal sequestration of fluid, or hemorrhage

NURSING PRIORITY

Maintain fluid balance or replace fluid loss to improve cellular perfusion.

PATIENT OUTCOME CRITERIA

Within 24 hours of admission, the patient will:
■ show stable vital signs, typically: heart rate, 60 to 100 beats/minute; systolic blood pressure, 90 to 140 mm Hg; and diastolic blood pressure, 50 to 90 mm Hg
■ maintain urine output of at least 30 ml/hour
■ show good skin turgor.
   Within 3 days of admission, the patient will:
■ maintain urine output within normal limits.

INTERVENTIONS	RATIONALES
1. *Measure and document hourly urine output* with specific gravity determinations for the acutely ill patient. Report a urine output of less than 30 ml/hour. Weigh the patient daily.	**1.** Urine output and specific gravity determinations provide an immediate, objective indication of the need for volume replacement. Weight loss may indicate loss of fluid volume.

*Italics indicate key interventions.

2. *Maintain accurate records of the type and amount of fluid lost.*

2. The type and amount of fluid lost will guide replacement therapy.

3. *Monitor and record indicators of fluid balance,* such as skin color, turgor, and temperature; LOC; body temperature; and vital signs every 1 to 4 hours, depending on the severity of the patient's condition. Note trends.

3. A persistent or dramatic change in the parameters listed indicates either sequestration of fluid or blood volume loss. Hypovolemia is indicated by hypotension, tachycardia, and signs of decreased peripheral perfusion.

4. *Monitor abdominal status.* Auscultate and palpate the abdomen, and observe for increasing pain. Document evidence of distention and changes in bowel sounds.

4. Sudden, acute distention, increased pain, and loss of or diminished bowel sounds can be early indications of serious bowel injury. Increased bowel activity may also indicate early obstruction or increasing tissue damage and inflammation.

5. *Administer and document fluid replacement, as ordered.*

5. The preferred route for fluid replacement is by mouth. However, the patient with IBD may be too ill or oral replacement may increase distressing symptoms. I.V. fluids usually include volume expanders such as normal saline solution. Whole blood or packed RBCs may also be ordered if hypotension is related to blood loss.

6. Additional individualized interventions: _____

6. Rationales: _____

Suggested NIC Interventions
Acid-base management; Fluid and electrolyte management; Fluid monitoring; Hypovolemia management; Intravenous (I.V.) therapy

Suggested NOC Outcomes
Electrolyte and acid-base balance; Fluid balance; Hydration

Nursing diagnosis

Imbalanced nutrition: Less than body requirements related to decreased nutrient intake, increased nutrient loss, and possible decreased bowel absorption

NURSING PRIORITIES
- Maintain or increase body weight.
- Improve general nutritional status.

PATIENT OUTCOME CRITERIA
Within 2 days of admission, the patient will:
- comply with the agreed-upon treatment plan.
  By the time of discharge, the patient will:
- gain mutually agreed-upon weight
- perform activities of daily living (ADLs)
- tolerate diet without undue distress.

INTERVENTIONS

1. *Initiate consultation with a nutritional expert* to estimate and document the extent of the nutritional deficit based on body mass index (BMI); character, color, and texture of hair and skin; the presence or absence of corneal plaques, cracked and bleeding gums and mucous membranes, muscle wasting and weakness, and anemia; changes in visual acuity; and decreased BUN level.

RATIONALES

1. BMI has become the standard for estimating nutritional status. A BMI less than 25 suggests nutritional deficit. Rapidly reproducing cells, such as those of the hair, skin, mucous membranes, and retinas, tend to be the first to demonstrate the changes characteristic of nutritional deficit. Later manifestations of a severe deficit include muscle wasting, weakness, decreased BUN level, and anemia.

2. *Collaborate with the patient, family, and other health team members to set goals and plan for normal nutritional maintenance.*

2. The patient with IBD tends to ignore dietary recommendations and may eat irritating foods. The IBD patient also learns to associate food and fluid intake with unpleasant sensations and may voluntarily decrease intake to avoid distressing symptoms. The patient must have the support of both family and caregivers for the dietary plan to succeed.

3. *Administer medications, as ordered,* to control peristalsis before meals.

3. The presence of food in the gut stimulates peristalsis and causes increased discomfort and diarrhea. Diphenoxylate with atropine (Lomotil) or camphorated opium tincture (paregoric) are commonly used to control peristalsis.

4. *Serve small, frequent meals* rather than three large meals a day. Assess patient response.

4. Small, frequent meals tend to be better tolerated and cause fewer distressing symptoms.

5. *Administer I.V. nutritional supplements,* such as fat emulsions (Intralipid) and vitamins, or parenteral nutrition, as ordered. See the "Parenteral nutrition" care plan, page 510, for further details.

5. I.V. nutritional supplements or parenteral nutrition may be indicated for the IBD patient who can't take anything by mouth, to rest the gut and promote healing, and for the patient too malnourished to tolerate surgery. Vitamin B_{12} is useful in reversing anemia associated with decreased blood cell formation and for treating immunosuppression associated with chronic inflammation. The "Parenteral nutrition" care plan contains details about this therapy.

6. Additional individualized interventions: _____

6. Rationales: _____

Suggested NIC Interventions
Diet staging; Nutrition management; Weight gain assistance; Fluid monitoring; Nutritional monitoring

Suggested NOC Outcomes
Nutritional status; Nutritional status: Food and fluid intake; Nutritional status: Nutrient intake; Weight control

---

Nursing diagnosis
Risk for infection related to bowel perforation, immunosuppression, and general debilitation

NURSING PRIORITY
Prevent opportunistic infections.

PATIENT OUTCOME CRITERIA
By the time of discharge, the patient will:
- have a normal body temperature
- show no signs of infection.

INTERVENTIONS

1. *Monitor and record indicators of infection,* including: vital signs, body temperature, bowel sounds, breath sounds, urine character and odor, and the presence or absence of abdominal distention, joint pain, hepatic tenderness, icterus, increasing malaise, and exudative skin or eye lesions.

RATIONALES

1. The patient with IBD is susceptible to many opportunistic infections. Close observation is necessary because such infections may not produce the usual dramatic rise in body temperature and WBC count as a result of medication-related immunosuppression and the condition's chronicity.

Gastrointestinal disorders

2. *Administer antibiotics, as ordered.*

2. Typically, broad-spectrum antibiotics, such as sulfasalazine (Azulfidine), are ordered as a prophylactic measure.

3. *Obtain specimens for culture and sensitivity testing,* as ordered, before beginning antibiotic therapy.

3. Culture and sensitivity testing tend to be inaccurate when performed after initiation of antibiotic therapy.

4. *Practice careful aseptic technique for all nursing procedures.*

4. The patient with IBD tends to be immunosuppressed, as noted previously.

5. *Question orders for extensive bowel preparation* for the patient with abdominal tenderness or masses, decreased or absent bowel sounds, or abdominal distention or rigidity.

5. Enemas and purgatives are irritants that can cause or exacerbate detrimental changes in the patient with acute abdominal pathology.

6. *Administer Remicade (Infliximab) I.V., if ordered* for Crohn's patients. Monitor patients with previously diagnosed Type I or Type II HF for signs and symptoms of worsening HF. Also observe for development of tuberculosis, fungal infections, and other opportunistic infections. Also observe for increased fatigue, malaise, cough, night sweats, muscle weakness, and other new signs or symptoms.

6. Remicade is a chimeric monoclonal antibody, a new drug class that suppresses the tumor necrosing factor, one of the activators of acute Crohn's episodes. The biggest risks for this drug are worsening of HF and development of disseminated tuberculosis, fungal infections, and other opportunistic infections. Potentially, lethal infections may not present with fever or leukocytosis due to general debilitation.

7. Additional individualized interventions: _____

7. Rationales: _____

Suggested NIC Interventions
Infection control; Infection protection; Incision site care; Wound care

Suggested NOC Outcomes
Infection status; Wound healing: primary intention

Nursing diagnosis
Chronic pain related to abdominal distention and possible skeletal pathology

NURSING PRIORITY
Prevent or control pain.

PATIENT OUTCOME CRITERIA
Within 3 days of admission, the patient will:
- verbalize pain relief.
  By the time of discharge, the patient will:
- verbalize rationale for pain-control measures
- use nonpharmacologic pain-control methods, as appropriate
- rate pain as mild on a pain rating scale.

INTERVENTIONS

1. *Assess and document complaints of pain, using a pain rating scale.* Be especially alert for sudden and severe abdominal pain, guarding, rigidity, or distention, and for vomiting, and report their occurrence to the physician immediately.

RATIONALES

1. Changes in the character and severity of abdominal pain may indicate a life-threatening condition such as perforation of the GI tract.

2. *Administer appropriate analgesic medication, as ordered.* Teach the patient about nonpharmacologic pain control measures. See the "Chronic pain" care plan, page 63.

2. Narcotic analgesics are administered judiciously in IBD because they tend to mask potentially life-threatening conditions. Medications that inhibit GI motility and abdominal cramping, such as diphenoxylate with atropine or camphorated opium tincture, may be ordered. Skeletal discomfort related to arthritis is best handled with gentle exercise, warm soaks, and frequent repositioning because many of the oral anti-inflammatory medications used to control skeletal pain are GI irritants. The "Chronic pain" care plan contains general interventions for pain control.

3. *Administer anti-inflammatory medications, as ordered,* and document their therapeutic and adverse effects.

3. Control of IBD reduces distressing and painful symptoms. Common medications used to suppress inflammation include hydrocortisone sodium succinate (Solu-Cortef), methylprednisolone sodium succinate (Solu-Medrol), and dexamethasone (Decadron).

4. Additional individualized interventions: _____

4. Rationales: _____

Suggested NIC Interventions
Medication management; Pain management; Analgesic administration

Suggested NOC Outcomes
Comfort level; Pain control; Pain: Disruptive effects; Pain level

Gastrointestinal disorders

Nursing diagnosis
Disturbed sleep pattern related to uncomfortable sensations, possible anxiety related to hospitalization, nocturnal defecation, or change in usual sleep environment

NURSING PRIORITY
Promote adequate rest and sleep.

PATIENT OUTCOME CRITERIA
Within 2 days of admission, the patient will:
- verbalize feelings of being rested.
  Throughout the hospital stay, the patient will:
- experience adequate rest and sleep.

INTERVENTIONS

1. Ask the patient to describe the usual sleep environment; when possible, modify the patient's surroundings to match that environment.

2. *Avoid performing prolonged or painful procedures within the hour before bedtime.*

3. *Group all nursing procedures that must be done while the patient sleeps.*

4. Encourage the patient to express fears. Offer reassurance as appropriate.

RATIONALES

1. An unfamiliar environment may inhibit sleep.

2. Autonomic nervous system stimulation, with increased catecholamine secretion, may interfere with sleep.

3. The sleep cycle is 90 to 120 minutes long. Grouping nursing procedures allows the patient to complete sleep cycles.

4. Some patients may feel that if they fall asleep they won't wake up. They may need to be reassured that the staff will be available to meet their needs and watch over them.

5. Allow the patient to follow rituals that promote sleep at home.

5. At home, most individuals follow sleep rituals, such as reading, which help them fall asleep.

6. *Encourage relaxation.* Reposition the patient for comfort, and offer soothing back rubs.

6. If the patient is on bed rest, immobility can increase discomfort.

7. *Provide a bedside commode for night use.* Administer antidiarrheal medication at bedtime.

7. These measures help minimize sleep disturbance related to nocturnal defecation.

8. Additional individualized interventions: _____

8. Rationales:_____

Suggested NIC Interventions
Energy management; Sleep enhancement; Coping enhancement

Suggested NOC Outcomes
Rest; Sleep; Well-being

Nursing diagnosis
Impaired skin integrity, perianal related to frequent stools and altered nutritional status

NURSING PRIORITY
Prevent skin breakdown.

PATIENT OUTCOME CRITERION
By the time of discharge, the patient will show no evidence of skin breakdown.

INTERVENTIONS

1. *Provide and document perianal care* after each bowel movement.

RATIONALES

1. The acid secretions and digestive enzymes from diarrhea quickly excoriate the perianal area. A protective ointment, such as lanolin and petroleum jelly (A&D), is commonly used because the skin is vulnerable to breakdown.

2. *Institute and document a skin care routine,* based on the patient's general condition, to be performed every 2 to 4 hours.

2. Anticipating and preventing skin breakdown on other body surfaces is important because tissue damage heals slowly, if at all, in the critically ill patient with IBD.

3. *Promote and document food and fluid intake,* paying special attention to protein consumption.

3. Adequate intake of nutrients (especially protein) and fluids is necessary for tissue repair.

4. Additional individualized interventions: _____

4. Rationales:_____

Suggested NIC Interventions
Pressure management; Pressure ulcer care; Skin surveillance; Incision site care; Wound care

Suggested NOC Outcomes
Tissue integrity; Skin and mucous membranes; Wound healing: Primary intention; Wound healing: Secondary intention

Nursing diagnosis

Social isolation related to dependent behavior

NURSING PRIORITIES
- Decrease use of dependent behavior.
- Facilitate direct expression of feelings.

PATIENT OUTCOME CRITERIA
By the time of discharge, the patient will:
- decrease use of ineffective coping behaviors
- express anger, hostility, and anxiety appropriately.

INTERVENTIONS	RATIONALES
1. *Identify dependent behavior* for patient, self, staff, and family.	1. Dependent behavior may be manifested by crying, expressions of hopelessness, endless requests for staff attention, or excessive praise of staff. Although such behavior represents an attempt to control and manage underlying feelings of anger, hostility, and anxiety, it commonly provokes social isolation, reinforcing negative feelings.
2. *Collaborate with staff and family to set limits on unacceptable behavior.* Ensure that all staff members agree to maintain the limits and to share concerns with each other.	2. Limit setting and consistent enforcement allow the patient to know exactly what's expected and interrupts the cycle of dependency and isolation. The dependent patient may attempt to turn staff members against each other through manipulative behavior.
3. *Enforce limits without apology.* Avoid bargaining about or justifying limits.	3. Engaging in dialogue concerning limits creates doubt about their enforcement.
4. *Discuss the patient's feelings concerning limits.* Encourage expressions of feelings of anxiety, hostility, and anger.	4. The patient may have difficulty identifying feelings. A nonjudgmental atmosphere provides a way to recognize and discuss uncomfortable emotions.
5. *Investigate somatic complaints immediately and matter-of-factly.*	5. Somatization is an attention-getting behavior used by people with inadequate coping skills. The seriousness of the illness warrants investigation of complaints; avoid prolonged discussions of physical complaints, however, and focus instead on the patient's feelings.
6. *If behavioral problems persist, consult a psychiatric clinical nurse specialist or other mental health professional.*	6. A mental health professional can offer expertise for dealing with manipulative behavior and the staff's negative response to such behavior.
7. Additional individualized interventions: _____	7. Rationales: _____

> ### Suggested NIC Interventions
> *Family integrity promotion; Recreation therapy; Socialization enhancement; Support system enhancement; Mood management; Therapeutic play; Behavior modification: Social skills; Complex relationship building; Coping enhancement; Self-awareness enhancement*

> ### Suggested NOC Outcomes
> *Family environment: Internal; Leisure participation; Loneliness; Mood equilibrium; Play participation; Social interaction skills; Social involvement; Social support; Well-being*

Gastrointestinal disorders

Nursing diagnosis

Ineffective sexuality patterns related to diminished physical energy and persistence of uncomfortable physical symptoms

NURSING PRIORITY

Encourage the discussion and expression of sexual desires.

PATIENT OUTCOME CRITERIA

By the time of discharge, the patient will:
- discuss sexual feelings openly with partner, if desired
- identify techniques for minimizing physical demands of sexual activity.

INTERVENTIONS

1. Initiate discussion about values, beliefs, and feelings concerning sexuality. Assess for sexual dysfunction. Include the patient's spouse or partner in discussions, if possible.

2. Allow the patient to discuss feelings, values, and beliefs concerning sexuality in a nonjudgmental atmosphere. It's important to be aware of personal feelings about sexuality. If you're too uncomfortable to counsel the patient and spouse or partner effectively, make an appropriate referral.

3. To the extent possible, allow the patient and spouse or partner uninterrupted private time together.

4. Construct a teaching plan for sexual expression. Address energy-conserving positions for intercourse, timing activity to coincide with peak energy levels, alternatives to intercourse, specific patient concerns, and potential interactions between contraceptives and medications used to treat IBD. Patient teaching should also cover the potential interactions between various types of contraceptives and the medications used to treat chronic IBD.

5. Additional individualized interventions: _____

RATIONALES

1. Discussions concerning sexuality are difficult for many patients to initiate, although the topic may be of considerable importance. The nurse must anticipate that altered sexual function is common in patients who have chronic or debilitating illnesses and who have diminished energy and persistent, uncomfortable physical sensations. The patient with IBD may also be facing surgery for fecal diversion; thus, body-image changes and altered sexual function should be anticipated. The patient may or may not communicate openly with his spouse or partner. Both may welcome frank discussions of sexual matters.

2. The nurse's values and beliefs concerning sexual behavior may interfere with the ability to provide professional care. If this occurs, refer the patient to another professional who may provide acceptance and counsel to benefit the patient and partner.

3. Sexuality can be expressed in many forms besides sexual intercourse, such as cuddling and fondling. The patient with IBD may be hospitalized for prolonged periods and needs privacy to express intimate feelings.

4. The sexual intercourse guidelines for cardiac patients can be modified to meet the needs of the patient with chronic IBD who has diminished physical energy and uncomfortable physical sensations. Teaching the patient about potential interactions between contraceptives and medications helps to prevent unexpected contraceptive failure.

5. Rationales: _____

Suggested NIC Interventions
Body image enhancement; Role enhancement; Self-esteem enhancement; Sexual counseling

Suggested NOC Outcomes
Body image; Role performance; Self-esteem; Sexual identity: Acceptance

Discharge planning

DISCHARGE CHECKLIST

Before discharge, the patient shows evidence of:
- ❏ absence of fever
- ❏ absence of signs and symptoms of infection
- ❏ stable vital signs
- ❏ ability to tolerate oral nutritional intake
- ❏ I.V. lines discontinued for at least 24 hours before discharge
- ❏ stabilized weight
- ❏ ability to control pain using oral medications
- ❏ ability to perform perianal care
- ❏ controlled bowel movements
- ❏ absence of skin breakdown
- ❏ electrolyte levels within acceptable parameters
- ❏ ability to ambulate and perform ADLs
- ❏ adequate home support system, or referral to home care if indicated by inability to perform ADLs and perianal care independently, by inadequacy of the home support system, or by the need to reinforce teaching.

TEACHING CHECKLIST

Document evidence that the patient and his family demonstrate an understanding of:
- ❏ the extent of disease
- ❏ all discharge medications' purpose, dosage, administration schedule, and adverse effects requiring medical attention (usual discharge medications include steroids and immunosuppressants)
- ❏ recommended dietary modifications (usual diet is low-fiber, low-residue, and bland)
- ❏ community support groups and resources, including an ostomy club, when appropriate
- ❏ resumption of normal role activity
- ❏ the signs and symptoms indicating exacerbation of illness
- ❏ the dates, times, and locations of follow-up appointments
- ❏ how to contact the physician.

DOCUMENTATION CHECKLIST

Using outcome criteria as a guide, document:
- ❏ clinical status on admission
- ❏ changes in status
- ❏ pertinent laboratory and diagnostic findings
- ❏ pain-relief measures
- ❏ I.V. line patency
- ❏ fluid intake
- ❏ acute abdominal pain episodes
- ❏ use of emergency protocols
- ❏ nutritional intake
- ❏ other therapies
- ❏ patient and family teaching
- ❏ discharge planning.

Associated care plans

- ■ Chronic pain
- ■ Colostomy
- ■ Grieving
- ■ Ineffective individual coping
- ■ Parenteral nutrition

References

Berhman, R., and Kleigman, N. *Essentials of Pediatrics,* 4th ed. Philadelphia: W.B. Saunders Co., 2002.

Goroll, A., and Mulley, A. *Primary Care Medicine.* Philadelphia: Lippincott Williams & Wilkins, 2000.

Orth, R.M. "Remicade." *www.endo-world.com/newpage12. htm* (8-16-02).

"Remicade." *www.remicade-ra.com/indication2/Hp/index.jsp* (p-86-2002).

www.niddk.nih/.gov/health/digest/pubs/chrons/crohns.html, (8-13-02).

Gastrointestinal disorders

Parenteral nutrition

DRG INFORMATION

DRG 296 Nutritional and Miscellaneous Metabolic Disorders; Age 17+ with Complication or Comorbidity (CC).
Mean LOS = 5.2 days

DRG 297 Nutritional and Miscellaneous Metabolic Disorders; Age 17+ without CC.
Mean LOS = 3.4 days

DRG 298 Nutritional and Miscellaneous Metabolic Disorders; Ages 0 to 17.
Mean LOS = 2.9 days

Introduction

DEFINITION AND TIME FOCUS

Parenteral nutrition (PN) is the delivery of nutrients through a venous infusion of glucose, amino acids, fats, vitamins, and trace elements in sufficient quantities to promote growth, weight gain, anabolism, and wound healing. The patient requiring PN typically exhibits one of four problems:

■ can't eat — the patient may have an obstruction or ileus at any point along the GI tract or may be at risk for aspiration if fed orally

■ won't eat — the geriatric, cancer, or anorexic patient may be unwilling to ingest food

■ shouldn't eat — the patient may have a disease or condition aggravated by oral intake, such as intestinal fistula, severe pancreatitis, small-bowel obstruction, or inflammatory bowel disease

■ can't eat enough — the patient has such a severe disease or degree of injury that sufficient nutrients can't be provided enterally. Examples are short-bowel syndrome, multiple trauma, and major burns.

PN is indicated when:

■ the patient has a nonfunctioning GI tract

■ the patient is in a stressed state or preexisting state of malnutrition that precludes waiting until the GI tract is available

■ the patient has an irreversible condition that will preclude using the GI tract in the foreseeable future.

Safe delivery of PN depends on four basic principles of care:

■ sterile technique in catheter placement

■ sterile technique in catheter care

■ proper preparation and delivery of the PN solution

■ careful patient monitoring.

This care plan focuses on the patient who requires PN to maintain nutritional status during the hospital stay.

(See *Clinical snapshot: Parenteral nutrition,* page 511, and *Major elements monitored in PN,* page 512.)

Focused assessment guidelines

NURSING HISTORY
(FUNCTIONAL HEALTH PATTERN FINDINGS)

Health-perception–health-management pattern

■ Chronic illness or have an acute condition that increases nutritional needs

Activity-exercise pattern

■ Decreased energy level

■ Generalized weakness or weak extremities related to muscle wasting

Nutritional-metabolic pattern

■ Nausea, vomiting, diarrhea, or constipation

■ Lack of appetite

■ Recent weight loss

■ Lack of interest in food

■ Improperly fitting dentures

■ Chronically thirsty

■ Change in the taste of food

PHYSICAL FINDINGS

Clinical signs of malnutrition are rarely observed and may not be recognized as clinically significant.

Musculoskeletal

■ Generalized muscle wasting and weakness (muscle mass and major organs are spared unless the patient has moderate to severe malnutrition)

■ Edematous extremities

Integumentary

■ Skin — subcutaneous fat loss, scaly dermatitis (primarily on legs and feet), pellagrous dermatitis, seborrheic dermatitis of face, nasolabial seborrhea (greasy and scaly skin of the nasolabial folds of the nose, from riboflavin deficiency), thinning of the innermost layer of the epidermis (possibly from vitamin A deficiency), dilated veins, petechiae, purpura, poor skin turgor, dry mucous membranes

■ Hair — increased pluckability, lack of luster, alopecia, sparsity, decreased pigmentation

■ Nails — brittle, lined, increased rigidity, thin, flattened or spoon-shaped

Eye

■ Xerosis (dryness) of conjunctivae

■ Keratomalacia (a condition linked to vitamin A deficiency that causes softening of the cornea; early signs include xerotic spots on conjunctivae and xerotic, insensitive, and hazy cornea)

- Corneal vascularization
- Blepharitis (scaly inflammation of eyelid edges)
- Bitot's spots (gray, triangular conjunctival spots, linked to vitamin A deficiency)
- "Spectacle eye" (inflammation of the periorbital skin associated with a vitamin B [biotin] deficiency)

Neurologic
- Lethargy
- Hyporeflexia
- Decreased proprioception
- Disorientation
- Confabulation
- Paresthesia
- Weakness of legs
- Irritability
- Seizures
- Flaccid paralysis
- Confusion

Gastrointestinal
- Tongue — baldness, glossitis, edema
- Lips — cheilosis, angular stomatitis

Glandular
- Parotid enlargement
- Thyroid enlargement

DIAGNOSTIC STUDIES
See *Major elements monitored in PN,* page 512.

POTENTIAL COMPLICATIONS
- Sepsis
- Mechanical injury from catheter
- Pneumothorax, hemothorax
- Arterial puncture
- Air emboli
- Catheter emboli
- Catheter and venous thrombosis
- Metabolic disorders
- Hypoglycemia
- Fluid and electrolyte abnormalities
- Hyperglycemia
- Essential fatty acid deficiency

CLINICAL SNAPSHOT

Parenteral nutrition

Major nursing diagnoses	Key patient outcomes
Risk for injury	Show no signs of catheter-related injury.
Imbalanced nutrition: Less than body requirements	Exhibit increased weight, muscle strength, and energy level.
Excess fluid volume	Manifest no signs or symptoms of fluid imbalance.
Deficient knowledge (PN care)	List signs and symptoms of potential PN complications.
Risk for infection	Show no signs or symptoms of infection.

Nursing diagnosis
Risk for injury related to complications of PN catheter insertion, displacement, use, or removal

NURSING PRIORITY
Prevent or promptly treat complications that may result from PN catheter.

PATIENT OUTCOME CRITERIA
While the central venous catheter (CVC) is in place, the patient will:
- exhibit unrestricted, pain-free inhalation and exhalation
- exhibit symmetrical chest movement
- exhibit normal respirations
- present a normal chest X-ray
- have a patent catheter
- show no fluid infiltration
- show no evidence of catheter emboli.

Major elements monitored in PN

Glucose — serum levels may be elevated above 200 mg/dl when parenteral nutrition (PN) infusion is begun, decreasing to 150 to 200 mg/dl after 24 to 48 hours as the body adjusts to increased glucose load. (Serum glucose levels greater than 200 mg/dl indicate glucose intolerance or hyperglycemia. Levels less than 60 mg/dl indicate hypoglycemia, the more dangerous of the two states; without glucose, the brain can't function and death is imminent if hypoglycemia continues.)

Electrolytes — sodium, potassium, and chloride levels obtained for baseline and as guide for replacement therapy. (Fluid and electrolyte management is the most important aspect of PN because the patient requiring nutritional repletion typically has fluid and electrolyte abnormalities. Electrolytes are provided as needed to replace loss from fistulas, nasogastric [NG] drainage, diarrhea, or excessive output or—in an appropriate ratio—to promote lean muscle mass, nutritional repletion, and positive nitrogen balance.)

Magnesium — low serum levels may occur in intestinal malabsorption syndrome, bowel resection, intestinal fistula, or in patients with extended NG suction. (Magnesium requirements increase with nutritional repletion related to new tissue synthesis: 0.35 to 0.45 mEq/kg/day is sufficient to prevent magnesium depletion in patients receiving PN. Magnesium levels need to be monitored at least every week and twice per week for patients in renal failure. The normal range of magnesium is 1.4 to 2.2 mEq/L.)

Phosphorus — low serum levels occur in patients receiving PN because of increased use of phosphorus for glucose metabolism. (For each kilocalorie of PN administered, 2 mEq/dl of phosphorus is required. Serum levels should be measured weekly. Serum phosphorus levels below 1 mg/dl will produce clinical signs and symptoms of hypophosphatemia. The normal range is 2.5 to 4.5 mg/dl.)

INTERVENTIONS	RATIONALES
1. *Observe for signs and symptoms of respiratory distress and shock during insertion of the CVC,* * including tachypnea, tachycardia, dropping systolic blood pressure, dyspnea, use of accessory muscles for respiration, and decreased or absent breath sounds on side of insertion.	**1.** After using a local anesthetic, the physician inserts the catheter into the subclavian or internal jugular vein and positions the tip in the superior vena cava. He then sutures the catheter in place and applies an occlusive dressing. The lungs or an artery may be punctured during subclavian venous cannulation. The artery may bleed to the point of compressing the trachea, causing life-threatening respiratory distress. A puncture of the lung creates a pneumothorax, causing respiratory compromise from entry of air into the pleural space and collapse of all or part of the lung on the venipuncture side.
2. *Maintain the patient in Trendelenburg's position during CVC insertion.*	**2.** Trendelenburg's position increases venous pressure in the upper half of the body. This prevents air influx into the venous system through the insertion needle or I.V. catheters when their lumens are open to air.
3. *After CVC insertion, assess for bilateral breath sounds in all lung fields and ensure that a chest X-ray is obtained.* Monitor the patient's respiratory status and breath sounds at least every 8 hours thereafter.	**3.** Bilateral breath sounds and symmetrical pain-free chest movement indicate fully inflated lungs. Chest X-ray confirms placement of the catheter tip in the superior vena cava and rules out hemothorax, chylothorax (from puncture of a lymph vessel), and pneumothorax.
4. *Don't begin administering the PN solution until the position of the catheter tip is confirmed by chest X-ray.*	**4.** The hyperosmolar PN solution irritates veins smaller than the superior vena cava. Thrombophlebitis can result if the PN solution is infused into the jugular, subclavian, or innominate vein.
5. *Use locking (luer-lock) connections, or tape the connections securely.*	**5.** Secure connections are essential to prevent accidental tubing disconnection. Accidental disconnection may cause bleeding, loss of catheter patency from clot formation, air emboli, hub contamination, and sepsis.

---

*Italics indicate key interventions.

6. *Before opening the I.V. system to the air, instruct the patient to perform Valsalva's maneuver (hold the breath and bear down), or clamp the catheter.* If the patient is unable to perform Valsalva's maneuver, change the tubing only during exhalation.

7. *Observe for signs and symptoms of air emboli,* such as extreme anxiousness, sharp chest pain, cyanosis, or churning precordial murmur. If air emboli are suspected, position the patient in Trendelenburg's position on the left side, administer oxygen, and notify the physician immediately.

8. *During dressing changes, observe for a suture* at the insertion site of a temporary CVC, a suture at the exit site of a permanent CVC, or increased external catheter length.

9. *Observe for inability to withdraw blood; complaints of chest pain or burning; leaking fluid; and swelling around the insertion site, shoulder, clavicle, and upper extremity.*

10. *Observe for visible collateral circulation on the chest wall.*

11. *When the catheter is being removed, take appropriate safety measures.* Make sure that:
– the patient is in a supine position

– the patient performs Valsalva's maneuver before the catheter is removed

– a completely sealed airtight dressing is applied over the insertion site after the CVC is removed.

12. *When the catheter is removed, measure its length and observe for jagged edges.*

13. Additional individualized interventions: _____

_____

6. Valsalva's maneuver increases intrathoracic pressure, forcing blood through the area of least resistance (in this case, the catheter) and preventing inflow of air. Air will enter the catheter only as the patient inhales. (Negative intrathoracic pressure allows the lungs to fill with air. If the I.V. catheter is open to the air during inhalation, air can be pulled into the bloodstream as well.)

7. Small amounts of air may produce no symptoms. Large amounts, however, may cause an air lock in the heart, in which case no blood can pass through the heart. The patient may die from cardiac arrest related to blocked blood flow and resultant ischemia.

Trendelenburg's and the left lateral recumbent positions allow air to collect at the apex of the right ventricle. Small amounts of air may pass into the pulmonary circulation and be reabsorbed. Large amounts of air in the heart may need to be aspirated through a catheter passed into the right atrium.

8. A suture at the insertion or exit site stabilizes the catheter. Increased external catheter length indicates movement and possible catheter displacement.

9. These signs and symptoms may indicate catheter displacement and vein thrombosis.

10. Development of collateral circulation on the chest wall is a sign of vein thrombosis.

11. Conscientious attention to the details of catheter removal is important for several reasons:
– The supine position allows a clear view while removing stitches and the catheter and applying a sealed dressing.
– Air can be sucked in through the CVC sinus tract if the catheter is pulled out during inhalation, causing air emboli.
– The CVC sinus tract allows air to enter the venous system with each inhalation if an airtight dressing isn't applied.

12. To ensure that the entire catheter was removed, the catheter should be measured and inspected for breaks.

13. Rationales: _____

_____

> **Suggested NIC Interventions**
> *Surveillance: Safety*

> **Suggested NOC Outcomes**
> *Safety status: Physical injury*

Nursing diagnosis

Imbalanced nutrition: Less than body requirements related to inability to ingest nutrients orally or digest them satisfactorily, or to increased metabolic need

NURSING PRIORITY

Provide for adequate nutritional intake.

PATIENT OUTCOME CRITERIA

Within 24 hours of starting PN and throughout PN therapy, the patient will:

- maintain serum glucose level of 100 to 200 mg/dl
- show no signs or symptoms of hypoglycemia, hyperglycemia, hyperosmolar hyperglycemic nonketotic syndrome (HHNS), electrolyte imbalance, or vitamin or trace metal deficiencies.

  Within 7 days of starting PN, the patient will:

- exhibit weight gain of less than ½ lb (0.2 kg)/day
- exhibit increased muscle strength
- exhibit increased energy level
- verbalize increased sense of well-being.

INTERVENTIONS	RATIONALES
1. *Administer the appropriate PN solution via a peripheral or central venous route,* including tunneled catheters and peripherally inserted central catheter.	**1.** PN solution composition is based on the individual patient's calculated needs. Usual nutrient requirements for critically ill patients include calories, 1,500 to 2,000 cal/day; protein, 1.2 to 1.5 g/kg/day; fat, 30% of non-protein calories; trace elements; and vitamins. Peripheral PN contains a lesser concentration of the same ingredients found in central formula PN. Solutions containing higher concentrations of dextrose (greater than 10%) must be delivered via a central vein because chemical phlebitis may result if a peripheral vein is used.
2. *Infuse PN solution at a constant rate with an infusion pump.*	**2.** The infusion pump regulates the flow rate with greater accuracy than does a standard I.V. set, decreasing the likelihood of accidentally infusing a bag of PN solution too quickly.
– Check the volume of solution, flow rate, and patient tolerance every half hour.	– This prevents a hyperglycemic, hyperosmolar load. (The hyperosmolar state results in osmotic diuresis that can lead to dehydration, lethargy, and coma.)
– Don't interrupt the flow of PN solution.	– Turning PN on and off at intervals creates fluctuations in the serum glucose level. The pancreas responds to high or low serum glucose by altering the secretion of glucagon and insulin. This system keeps the serum glucose level within the normal range; if changes in flow rate are made too quickly, the body can't adjust and signs and symptoms of hypoglycemia or hyperglycemia may occur.
– Don't attempt to "catch up" if the PN infusion is behind schedule or "slow down" if it's ahead of schedule. Set the I.V. infusion to the ordered rate.	– If PN on gravity drip has fallen behind the ordered drip rate, there will be less glucose circulating in the blood and less insulin secreted to handle the glucose (insulin decreases serum glucose levels by transporting glucose into the cells to be converted to glycogen for storage). A rapid infusion of PN solution results in a rapid rise in serum glucose to above normal levels without a corresponding increase in insulin production. (The body takes 30 to 60 minutes to sense the high serum glucose level and respond by increasing insulin production.)

The physiologic effect of high serum glucose levels is dehydration. Water is drained out of the interstitial spaces into the vascular system in an attempt to equalize serum and interstitial glucose levels. This results in dehydrated interstitial spaces, causing excessive thirst and hunger. The kidneys sense the increased vascular volume and excrete the excess fluid and glucose. Dehydration, if not treated, will lead to lethargy, confusion, and coma.

– When discontinuing central formula PN, lower the rate to 50 ml/hour for 3 to 4 hours.

– Slowing the PN rate to 50 ml/hour for 3 to 4 hours allows the body to sense the lower serum glucose level and adjust to it. The pancreas responds by decreasing insulin production. These mechanisms prevent development of hypoglycemia, which can occur if PN is discontinued too rapidly.

3. *Ensure that the PN infusion doesn't stop suddenly, or take appropriate corrective action.*

3. If the PN infusion stops suddenly, another source of glucose must be supplied to prevent hypoglycemia. The high levels of insulin in the bloodstream will deplete the serum glucose level to less than 60 mg/dl within an hour.

– For a clotted catheter, hang dextrose 10% in water at another I.V. site to infuse at the ordered PN rate.

– Brain cells can't function without glucose as an energy source. Another source of I.V. glucose prevents a rapid drop in the serum glucose level.

– During cardiopulmonary arrest stop the PN infusion and provide one or more boluses of dextrose 50% in water, as ordered.

– This precaution prevents accidentally giving a bolus of PN solution during an emergency. One or more boluses of dextrose prevents hypoglycemia and allows more control. In an emergency situation, a rapidly decreasing serum glucose level may otherwise go unnoticed.

4. *Monitor fingerstick glucose levels and laboratory serum glucose levels* every 6 hours, as ordered. Maintain serum glucose level at 100 to 200 mg/dl.

4. Monitoring serum glucose levels evaluates the patient's tolerance of the glucose load being infused. Levels greater than 200 mg/dl may indicate that the body isn't using glucose, and additional insulin may be necessary to increase conversion of glucose to glycogen. Levels greater than 200 mg/dl may also indicate new stressors: Medications, surgery, and sepsis all can cause hyperglycemia. To handle the stress, the body increases the amount of glucose available for energy. Blood glucose checks may be less frequent if hyperglycemia doesn't exist.

5. *Observe for signs and symptoms of serious problems:*

5. The complex nature of PN therapy places the patient at risk for numerous complications:

– hypoglycemia — weakness; agitation; tremors; cold, clammy skin; serum glucose level less than 60 mg/dl

– The brain can't survive without glucose. Death may occur within 1 hour if glucose levels aren't restored to normal.

– hyperglycemia — thirst, acetone breath, diuresis, dehydration; serum glucose level above 200 mg/dl

– Monitoring for signs and symptoms of hyperglycemia promotes early identification of glucose intolerance and its cause. This may be related to a new stress such as sepsis. Unchecked, hyperglycemia leads to osmolar diuresis, causing dehydration, thirst, confusion, lethargy, seizures, and coma.

– protein overload — elevated blood urea nitrogen and creatinine levels

– Protein overload can cause osmotic diuresis.

– hyperosmolar overload — thirst, headache, lethargy, seizures, and urine positive for glucose and negative for acetone

– electrolyte imbalances (see appendix C, Fluid and electrolyte imbalances) — hypocalcemia (numbness and tingling), hypokalemia (muscle weakness, cramps, paresthesia, lethargy, confusion, ileus, and arrhythmias), hypomagnesemia (confusion, positive Chvostek's sign, and tetany), hyponatremia (lethargy and confusion), and hypophosphatemia (weakness, anorexia, dizziness, bone pain, signs of encephalopathy, poor resistance to infection, and severe congestive cardiomyopathy). Monitor serum electrolyte levels as ordered, typically daily until stable and then 2 to 3 times per week. Obtain 24-hour urine for urine urea nitrogen once per week for nutritional assessment.

– vitamin and trace mineral deficiencies (see *Signs and symptoms of vitamin and trace mineral deficiencies,* page 518).

6. *Infuse I.V. fat emulsion as ordered* through one of two infusion methods:

– through a Y-connector added between the PN catheter and the I.V. tubing

– as a 3-in-1 solution or total nutrient admixture.

– HHNS may occur if the PN solution is infused over too short a time. A serum osmolar level above 300 mOsm/kg water pulls fluid into the vascular bed to dilute the osmolar load. The excess vascular fluid results in osmotic diuresis. Also, HHNS may occur with simultaneous infusion of PN solution and tube feeding. To prevent this problem, decrease the PN rate as the tube feeding rate is increased.
– The Fluid and electrolyte imbalances appendix contains general information on these disorders; this section covers information specific to PN. Fluid and electrolyte status requires careful monitoring for several reasons:
  – Increased glucose metabolism and protein synthesis tend to deplete potassium and phosphate; if they aren't replaced appropriately with PN, a deficit may result.
  – The primary diagnosis may alter fluid and electrolyte balance. Fluid and electrolyte losses from fistulas, diarrhea, or nasogastric tubes can cause electrolyte and acid-base abnormalities.
  – To promote lean body mass repletion and positive nitrogen balance, electrolytes have to be supplied in a specific ratio: phosphorus 0.8 g, sodium 3.9 mg, potassium 3 mEq, chloride 2.5 mEq, and calcium 1.2 mEq for every gram of nitrogen infused.
– Vitamins and trace minerals are necessary for vital processes. Vitamins may function as hormones and as catalysts in enzyme systems. Minerals serve as coenzyme activators and as major factors in the regulation of acid-base and fluid and electrolyte balance.
  Deficiencies of vitamins and minerals result from inadequate intake, inability to digest and absorb, poor utilization of nutrients, excess losses, and increased requirements related to medication or severity of illness.

6. Fat emulsions are used as an adjunct to PN therapy to prevent essential fatty acid deficiency. Fats can also be used as a source of calories if calories from PN alone aren't sufficient. For example, if hyperglycemia is a consistent problem and insulin can't control the serum glucose level, the glucose infusion is decreased and the lost calories are supplied as fat.
– The Y-connector allows fats to infuse with minimal mixing with the PN solution, preventing breakdown of the fat emulsion and decreasing the risk of fat emboli. Fats appear to float on top of the PN solution when administered through a Y-connector.
– The pharmacy can mix carbohydrates, protein, and fat in one bag to hang over a 24-hour period. This method saves nursing time because there's no Y-connector to add and pharmacy time because only one bag must be mixed and dispensed. These solutions are also cost-effective because they use less I.V. tubing and fewer I.V. catheters. They also have the potential for decreased contamination because the catheter requires less manipulation. Most important, the patient is spared the pain of venipuncture for a fat emulsion I.V.

7. *If a 3-in-1 solution is used, ensure that it's mixed in a ratio of calcium, as appropriate,* less than or equal to 15 mEq/L; phosphorus, less than or equal to 30 mEq/L; and magnesium, less than or equal to 10 mEq/L.

7. The milky color of 3-in-1 solutions obscures particulate matter. The ratio listed prevents precipitate formation.

8. *Check that the infusion pump delivers the correct volume* of the 3-in-1 solution. Adjust the infusion rate as needed to ensure delivery of the desired volume.

8. When fats are added to a PN solution, the solution's increased viscosity may alter infusion pump delivery.

9. *Observe for fat separation in the 3-in-1 solution* as indicated by a yellow ring around the edges of the solution. Stop the infusion if this occurs, and replace the solution bag with a fresh one.

9. The 3-in-1 solution can separate if it isn't mixed properly or if it hangs for more than 24 hours. Separation may cause fat emboli.

10. *Culture the 3-in-1 solution if the patient develops sepsis.*

10. If it becomes contaminated, the 3-in-1 solution is more likely to support microbial growth than is a PN solution without fat.

11. *If a separate fat infusion is used, administer it slowly over the first 15 to 20 minutes* (1 ml/minute for a 10% fat infusion or 0.5 ml/minute for a 20% fat infusion). Observe for dyspnea, pain at the I.V. site, or chest or back pain. If any of these signs or symptoms occur, stop the infusion and notify the physician. Otherwise, increase the rate as ordered.

11. Allergic reactions to the fat emulsion may be local or systemic. Slow administration allows time to observe for an allergic reaction before a dangerous amount of antigen is administered.

12. *If the fat emulsion is to be infused separately, infuse it over 4 hours* (for a 10% fat emulsion) or 8 hours (for a 20% fat emulsion). Don't allow fat emulsions to hang more than 12 hours unless mixed in a 3-in-1 solution.

12. The patient with renal failure or heart failure may not tolerate an additional 500 ml of fluid 2 to 3 times per week. The slower infusion rate allows the body to assimilate the emulsion and prevents hyperlipidemia.

13. *Don't use I.V. filters with separate fat emulsion infusions.* When infusing fats on a long-term basis (longer than 3 months), ensure that thiosalicylate-free tubing is used.

13. The fat emulsion particle size exceeds the filter pore size, so the solution won't infuse through the filter. Fats leach thiosalicylate from ordinary tubing; it can accumulate in the body, with unknown effects.

14. *Encourage walking or mild exercise* to promote nitrogen retention and nutrient use. Consider a referral to physical therapy, occupational therapy, or both.

14. Exercise improves use of nutrients and promotes lean muscle mass development rather than the storage of fatty acids. Exercise also prevents muscle wasting, which occurs with inactivity.

15. *Weigh the patient daily,* at the same time, with the same amount of clothing, and using the same scale.

15. Weighing is necessary to determine if nutritional goals are being met. Weight is also used to assess the patient's fluid status. Weight gain of more than $1/2$ lb (0.2 kg) per day may indicate fluid retention.

16. *When oral intake resumes, initiate a daily calorie count and measure fat intake.* Observe for nausea, vomiting, or diarrhea.

16. Daily monitoring of fat intake and calories provides guidelines for therapy. If used for essential fatty acid deficiency only, I.V. fat emulsions can be discontinued when the patient is taking 10 g of fat per day orally. When the patient can consume 1,000 cal/day or half of the estimated caloric intake without nausea, vomiting, or diarrhea, PN can be discontinued.

17. *Observe for changes in muscle strength, wound healing, and energy level.*

17. Increased strength, energy level, sense of well-being, and tissue granulation indicate that PN is meeting the body's nutritional needs.

18. Additional individualized interventions: _____

18. Rationales:_____

Suggested NIC Interventions
Diet staging; Nutrition management; Fluid monitoring; Nutritional monitoring

Suggested NOC Outcomes
Nutritional status; Nutritional status: Food and fluid intake; Nutritional status: Nutrient intake; Weight control

Signs and symptoms of vitamin and trace mineral deficiencies

Vitamin deficiencies are avoided by adding 1 unit of a multivitamin preparation to the parenteral nutrition solution every day. Trace mineral deficiencies usually won't develop until 2 to 4 weeks after oral intake has stopped.

Water-soluble vitamins	Fat-soluble vitamins	Trace mineral deficiencies
Vitamin B complex Blepharitis, periorbital fissures, cheilosis, glossitis, weakness, paresthesia of legs, dermatoses	**Vitamin A** Night blindness, Bitot's spots	**Chromium** Glucose intolerance, mental confusion
	Vitamin D Bone tenderness	**Copper** Depigmentation of skin and hair within 2 to 4 weeks, kinky hair
Vitamin C (ascorbic acid) Bleeding gums, joint and muscle aching	**Vitamin E** Myopathy, creatinuria prolonged blood clotting	**Iodine** Enlarged thyroid, impaired memory, hoarseness, hearing loss
		Manganese Transient dermatitis
		Molybdenum Night blindness, irritability
		Selenium Muscle pain and tenderness
		Zinc Hypogeusia (abnormally diminished sense of taste); moist, excoriated rash in paranasal, anal, and groin areas

Nursing diagnosis
Excess fluid volume related to fluid retention, altered oral intake, or osmotic diuresis

NURSING PRIORITY
Maintain optimal fluid balance.

PATIENT OUTCOME CRITERIA
Throughout PN therapy, the patient will:
- maintain fluid intake that approximately equals output
- exhibit no signs or symptoms of fluid imbalance
- maintain urine output greater than 200 ml/8 hours
- exhibit weight gain less than $\frac{1}{2}$ lb (0.2 kg)/day.

INTERVENTIONS

1. *See appendix C, Fluid and electrolyte imbalances.*

RATIONALES

1. The Fluid and Electrolyte Imbalances appendix contains further details related to fluid and electrolyte disorders.

2. *Observe for edema, increased pulse rate, and increased blood pressure.* If any of these signs are present, consult with the physician about decreasing overall fluid administration.

2. Edema, increased pulse rate, and increased blood pressure may be signs of excess fluid volume. This may result from the body's inability to tolerate the increased cardiac and renal workload imposed by total parenteral nutrition or from the underlying disease itself (for example, heart failure or renal failure). Edema in the malnourished patient is also commonly related to protein depletion, in which circulating serum protein levels are lower than protein levels in the interstitial spaces. This inequality causes fluids to shift into the interstitial spaces to equalize protein-to-fluid ratios.

3. *Observe for thirst, dry mucous membranes, dry skin, decreased urine output, and increased urine specific gravity.*

3. These may be signs and symptoms of fluid deficit or dehydration.

4. *Assess breath sounds* each shift.

4. Crackles or gurgles may indicate fluid overload.

5. *Record fluid intake and output each shift.* Maintain approximate balance.

5. An intake consistently lower than output indicates a fluid deficit and the need for additional fluid to prevent dehydration and renal failure. An intake higher than output may reflect fluid overload and result in pulmonary complications.

6. *Weigh the patient daily.* For every liter lost or gained, weight should change approximately 2 lb (1 kg). Generally, maintain weight gain at less than $\frac{1}{2}$ lb (0.2 kg)/day.

6. Daily weight is another way to determine whether the patient is being given too much or too little fluid. Weight gain of more than $\frac{1}{2}$ lb/day is too rapid and reflects fluid retention.

7. Additional individualized interventions: _____

7. Rationales: _____

Suggested NIC Interventions
Fluid monitoring; Fluid and electrolyte management; Hypovolemia management

Suggested NOC Outcomes
Electrolyte and acid-base balance; Fluid balance; Hydration

Nursing diagnosis
Deficient knowledge (PN care) related to lack of experience with PN

NURSING PRIORITY
Teach the patient and family about PN.

PATIENT OUTCOME CRITERIA
Within 48 hours of starting PN, the patient or his family will on request:
- describe PN
- discuss medical reasons for PN
- discuss the role of the nutrition support service staff
- use appropriate problem-solving skills for hypothetical problems with PN
- list signs and symptoms of complications and what to do about them.

Gastrointestinal disorders

INTERVENTIONS	**RATIONALES**
1. *Briefly explain the purpose and method of PN therapy.*	**1.** A general understanding of PN provides a framework within which to understand the specific details of therapy.
– Explain that in PN calories and nutrients infuse directly into the bloodstream until the patient can resume oral intake.	– This defines PN in terms the patient can understand.
– Define the roles of the dietitian, nurse, pharmacist, physician, and other health care team members in PN.	– Describing the roles of the health care team members ensures patient awareness of resources.
– Explain that the PN solution contains carbohydrate, protein, fat, vitamins, and electrolytes and will provide all the calories and protein the patient needs.	– Describing the PN solution may reassure the patient and family.
– Describe the route and equipment used, the length of time PN may be infused, and the patient's responsibilities.	– A thorough understanding of PN administration, clear expectations, and acceptance of responsibility for self-monitoring promote optimum therapeutic benefit.
– Provide the patient and family with written material on PN therapy.	– Written material reinforces the nurse's explanation.
2. *If the patient is to receive PN at home, teach necessary management:*	**2.** PN is a complex therapy requiring substantial expertise on the patient's part for successful home management.
– Collaborate with the nutrition support service to determine appropriate teaching strategies.	– The nutrition support service can provide expert advice on adapting teaching to the home setting. The patient receiving PN at home will need to be followed by the service (or by a home care agency specializing in PN management).
– Teach the signs, symptoms, and necessary actions for managing complications, such as infection, abnormal serum glucose levels, air emboli, clotted catheter, and displaced catheter. Ask the patient to report any signs or symptoms to the nutrition support team.	– Knowledge of how to detect and manage complications may increase the patient's confidence about managing this therapy at home. Prompt reporting facilitates timely intervention.
–Review the information, and answer questions. Ask the patient "what if" questions.	– Reviewing, clarifying, and using practical "what if" examples promote understanding and boost problem-solving skills.
– Provide written instructions on home PN protocols.	– Written information reinforces teaching and provides a permanent reference.
3. See the "Knowledge deficit" care plan, page 129, for further details.	**3.** The "Knowledge deficit" care plan contains interventions related to patient teaching.
4. Additional individualized interventions: _____	**4.** Rationales: _____

Suggested NIC Interventions
Teaching: Disease process; Teaching: Individual; Teaching: Prescribed medication

Suggested NOC Outcomes
Knowledge: Disease process; Knowledge: Health behaviors; Knowledge: Treatment regimen

---

Nursing diagnosis
Risk for infection related to invasive CVC, leukopenia, or damp dressing

NURSING PRIORITY
Prevent or detect and promptly treat infection.

PATIENT OUTCOME CRITERIA

Throughout PN therapy, the patient will:

- be afebrile
- present urine negative for glucose
- show no infection or inflammation at the catheter site
- maintain serum glucose level between 100 and 200 g/dl.

INTERVENTIONS	RATIONALES
1. *Follow facility protocol for dressing changes.* Use sterile technique and standard precautions. Apply a clear, completely sealed dressing.	1. Good technique decreases the risk of infection. Dressing change frequency ranges from every day to once per week.
2. *Inspect the dressing* every 8 hours, and change it anytime it's unsealed or damp.	2. Moisture and exposure to air encourage microbial growth at the insertion site. Colonization may lead to sepsis.
3. *Observe the insertion site* every 8 hours for signs and symptoms of infection. Report any redness, swelling, pain, or purulent drainage.	3. These signs and symptoms may indicate infection of the insertion site.
4. *Follow facility protocol for tubing changes and antibacterial preparation* at all connections before changing I.V. tubing.	4. Using proper technique when changing and disconnecting tubing decreases the risk of PN line contamination. Tubing changes are usually performed every 24 hours.
5. *Use filter appropriate for type of solution.*	5. The reason for use of in-line filters centers on removal of microprecipitates rather than microorganisms. Using a 0.22 micron filter for dextrose–amino acid solution with lipids piggybacked below the filter will effectively retain bacteria, fungi, and particulate matter. The total nutrient admixture or 3:1 solution requires the use of a 1.2 micron filter.
6. *Infuse only PN solution through the PN catheter.* Don't use the PN line for injecting medications or drawing blood samples.	6. Using the PN catheter for other solutions provides another possible source of contamination and increases the risk of sepsis.
7. *Use only solutions prepared in the pharmacy under a laminar flow hood.* Don't make any additions on the unit. If additions are necessary, request that they be made in the pharmacy under a laminar flow hood.	7. Preparing the solution in a sterile area decreases the risk of contamination. The laminar flow hood minimizes contamination from airborne microorganisms.
8. *Return cloudy or precipitated solution* to the pharmacy.	8. Cloudy solution indicates possible bacterial contamination. Precipitate may occlude the catheter or cause thrombus formation.
9. *Allow each bag or bottle to hang no more than 24 hours.*	9. Infusing solutions over longer periods allows for rapid multiplication of microorganisms inadvertently introduced during mixing of the PN solution.
10. *Monitor for signs and symptoms of infection:* – increased pulse and respiratory rates – temperature above 101° F (38.3° C) – white blood cell (WBC) count over 10,000/μl – serum glucose level over 200 mg/dl – glycosuria – chills, diaphoresis, or lethargy.	10. A change in vital signs or WBC count, hyperglycemia, glycosuria, chills, or diaphoresis may indicate developing infection.

11. *Notify the physician if signs and symptoms of infection are present.*

11. Prompt notification allows the physician to identify source of infection and order appropriate therapy. Infection may require removal of venous catheter and culture of the tip and any other potential source of infection

12. Additional individualized interventions: _____

12. Rationales: _____

Suggested NIC Interventions
Infection control; Infection protection; Incision site care; Wound care

Suggested NOC Outcomes
Infection status; Wound healing: Primary intention

Discharge planning
DISCHARGE CHECKLIST
Before discharge, the patient shows evidence of:
❐ absence of fever
❐ stabilizing weight
❐ absence of pulmonary or cardiovascular complications
❐ electrolytes within acceptable parameters
❐ WBC counts within normal parameters
❐ absence of redness, swelling, pain, and drainage at catheter site
❐ absence of nausea and vomiting
❐ ability to perform activities of daily living (ADLs), transfer, and ambulate same as before hospitalization
❐ adequate home support system, or referral to home care or a nursing home if indicated by an inadequate home support system or the patient's inability to perform ADLs, transfers, and ambulation
❐ a plan for follow-up by nutrition support service or home care agency specializing in PN for the patient receiving PN at home.

TEACHING CHECKLIST
If the patient is to receive PN at home, document evidence that the patient and his family demonstrate an understanding of:
❐ preventing complications
❐ actions to take if complications do occur
❐ where and how to obtain supplies
❐ catheter site care
❐ procedure for PN administration
❐ community resources
❐ date, time, and location of follow-up appointments
❐ how to contact the physician.

DOCUMENTATION CHECKLIST
Using outcome criteria as a guide, document:
❐ nutritional status on admission
❐ any significant changes in status
❐ CVC insertion — difficulties or complications; length of catheter; position and any change in position; signs and symptoms of infection, thrombosis, emboli, or other postinsertion complication
❐ dressing and tubing changes
❐ PN solution and fat emulsion — for each bag or bottle, record date, time, and name of nurse hanging solution; all ingredients; rate of infusion
❐ patient and family teaching
❐ discharge planning.

Associated care plans
■ Knowledge deficit
■ Nutritional deficit

References
Adam, S. "Standardization of Nutrition Support: Are Protocols Useful?" *NursingTimes* 16(5):283-89, October 2000.

ASPEN Board of Directors and Clinical Guidelines for Use of Parenteral and Enteral Nutrition in Adults and Pediatric Patients. *Journal of Parenteral and Enteral Nutrition* 26(supp):15A-136SA, 2002.

Cahill, G. "Starvation in Man," *New England Journal of Medicine* 282(12):668-75, March 1970.

Cameron, J. *Current Surgical Therapy,* 7th ed. St. Louis: Mosby-Year Book, Inc., 2001.

Corson, J. *Surgery.* St. Louis: Mosby–Year Book, Inc., 2001.

Hankin, J. *Infusion Therapy in Clinical Practice,* 2nd ed. Philadelphia: W.B. Saunders Co., 2001.

"Infusion Nursing Standards of Practice," *Journal of Intravenous Nursing* (supp) 23(65):S1-S85, November-December 2000.

Mahan, L. *Krause's Food Nutrition and Diet Therapy,* 10th ed. Philadelphia: W.B. Saunders Co., 2000.

McCowen, K. "Hypocaloric Total Parenteral Nutrition: Effectiveness in Prevention of Hyperglycemia and Infectious Complications — A Randomized Clinical Trial," *Critical Care Medicine* 28(11):3606-11, November 2000.

Townsend, C. *Sabiston Textbook of Surgery,* 16th ed. Philadelphia: W.B. Saunders Co., 2001.

Weinstein, S. *Plummer's Principles and Practice of Infusion Therapy,* 7th ed. Philadelphia: Lippincott Williams & Wilkins, 2001.

Hepatobiliary and pancreatic disorders

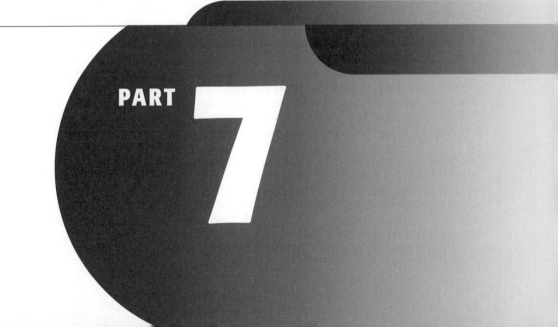

PART 7

Cholecystectomy

DRG INFORMATION

DRG 195   Cholecystectomy with Common Bile Duct Exploration with Complication or Comorbidity (CC).
Mean LOS = 8.2 days

DRG 196   Cholecystectomy with Common Bile Duct Exploration without CC.
Mean LOS = 5.5 days

DRG 197   Cholecystectomy Except by Laparoscope without Common Bile Duct Exploration with CC.
Mean LOS = 7.2 days

DRG 198   Cholecystectomy Except by Laparoscope without Common Bile Duct Exploration without CC.
Mean LOS = 4.7 days

DRG 493   Laparoscopic Cholecystectomy without Common Bile Duct Exploration with CC.
Mean LOS = 4.1 days

DRG 494   Laparoscopic Cholecystectomy without Common Bile Duct Exploration without CC.
Mean LOS = 1.8

Introduction

DEFINITION AND TIME FOCUS

Cholecystitis (inflammation of the gallbladder) is an extremely common disorder usually associated with cholelithiasis (gallstone formation). Cholelithiasis may be symptomatic or asymptomatic. Cholecystitis may be acute or chronic. Some patients who have asymptomatic cholelithiasis or short, infrequent periods of biliary colic may be treated with oral bile salts. Prophylactic cholecystectomy for asymptomatic persons isn't recommended.

Acute cholecystitis may be associated with transient gallstone impaction at the gallbladder–cystic duct junction, infections such as cytomegalovirus, ischemic changes after critical illness or major surgery, or rapid weight loss. Most gallstones are composed predominantly of cholesterol or calcium bilirubinate. Cholecystectomy is the treatment of choice for symptomatic cholecystitis.

Laparoscopic cholecystectomy is now more commonly performed than the traditional, or open, cholecystectomy. Although the only absolute contraindication to laparoscopic cholecystectomy is third trimester normal pregnancy, relative contraindications include bleeding or coagulopathy, abscess or fistula formation, peritonitis, multiple abdominal surgeries, or gallbladder malignancy.

Approximately 5% of laparoscopic cholecystectomies convert to open cholecystectomy due to technical problems or excessive bleeding encountered during surgery. Laparoscopic cholecystectomy may be performed in an outpatient surgery setting or as a short-stay procedure.

For laparoscopic cholecystectomy, several small incisions or punctures are made. Carbon dioxide is instilled through the umbilical incision to inflate the abdomen; then the laparoscope is inserted. Instruments, such as the cautery, laser, and operative instruments, are inserted through other small skin incisions in the upper right abdomen. After the procedure is completed, adhesive bandages are placed over the small incisions; sutures are usually unnecessary. The traditional, or open, cholecystectomy generally requires a 5″ to 8″ (12.5 to 20 cm) incision that's sutured after the procedure. Biliary drains are more commonly used in postoperative care of the open cholecystectomy patient. Bile leaks are a more common complication after laparoscopic cholecystectomy.

This care plan focuses on preoperative and postoperative care for the patient with acute cholecystitis who requires traditional, or open, cholecystectomy. (See *Clinical snapshot: Cholecystectomy*, page 526.)

ETIOLOGY AND PRECIPITATING FACTORS
Cholecystitis

■ Critically ill patients may develop cholecystitis without the formation of gallstones related to localized ischemic reactions.

■ Human immunodeficiency virus-positive patients may develop either calculus or acalculus cholecystitis. Gallbladder infections resistant to antibiotic therapy may develop.

■ Patients with sickle cell disease may develop cholecystitis related to hemolysis of the sickled cells.

■ Ninety percent of all cases of cholecystitis are related to impaction of gallstones in the cystic duct causing inflammation and obstruction. Gangrene may develop or perforation may occur. Repeated episodes of biliary colic may result in chronic cholecystitis and the development of a scarred, nonfunctional gallbladder.

Cholelithiasis

■ Diabetes (also contributes to higher complication and comorbidity rates postoperatively)
■ Obesity
■ Significant weight loss or extensive fasting
■ Oral contraceptive use
■ For women, more than one child
■ Recent childbirth

Focused assessment guidelines

NURSING HISTORY (FUNCTIONAL HEALTH PATTERN FINDINGS)

Health-perception–health-management pattern

- Pain, initially situated in midepigastrium, that becomes pronounced in the right upper quadrant (RUQ); pain is initially mild but persistent and intensifies as inflammation spreads; pain may be referred to the right scapula or right shoulder and is exacerbated by movement, coughing, and deep breathing
- History of diabetes, extensive bowel resections, or hemolytic anemia
- Increased risk if over age 50
- Ethnic background: Native American, Jewish, Asian, Italian

Nutritional-metabolic pattern

- Ingestion of heavy or fatty meal
- Intolerance of heavy meals or fatty foods
- Indigestion leading to anorexia
- Nausea, possibly with vomiting
- Recent weight loss

Elimination pattern

- Flatulence
- Change in color of urine or stool (indicates obstructed bile flow)
- Pruritus

Activity-exercise pattern

- Sedentary lifestyle; increases risk for gallstones and therefore cholecystitis

Sleep-rest pattern

- Pain that disturbs sleep

PHYSICAL FINDINGS

General

- Elevated temperature
- Obesity

Eyes

- Icteric sclera

Mouth

- Jaundiced mucous membranes

Cardiovascular

- Tachycardia
- Hypertension

Pulmonary

- Short and shallow respirations

Abdomen

- Pain in RUQ, referred to right scapula and intensified by deep breathing or percussion above right costal margin
- Localized rebound tenderness in RUQ
- Distention
- Light-colored stools
- Murphy's sign (tenderness in subcostal area with deep aspiration)

Urinary

- Dark, frothy urine

Integumentary

- Jaundice, especially on inner aspects of forearms
- Bruising
- Pruritis

DIAGNOSTIC STUDIES

- White blood cell count — typically 10,000 to 15,000/ml, although it may not be elevated
- Serum bilirubin level (direct and indirect) — may be elevated when gallstones obstruct the bile duct
- Prothrombin time/international normalized ratio (PT/INR) — may be prolonged because bile is necessary for vitamin K absorption (prothrombin synthesis depends on vitamin K)
- Alkaline phosphatase level — may be elevated because normal excretion through the biliary system may be impeded
- Oral cholecystogram — may not visualize gallbladder because of biliary duct obstruction or inability of the gallbladder to concentrate the dye; repetition may be ordered to rule out inadequate preparation
- Cholangiogram — may show gallstones or strictures in biliary tree
- Ultrasonography — may show gallstones, gallbladder wall thickness, or sludge

POTENTIAL COMPLICATIONS

- Perforation of the gallbladder
- Hemorrhage
- Empyema of the gallbladder
- Subphrenic or hepatic abscess
- Fistulas
- Pancreatitis
- Cholangitis
- Pneumonia
- Cancer of the gallbladder

Hepatobiliary and pancreatic disorders

Cholecystectomy

Major nursing diagnoses and collaborative problems	Key patient outcomes
CP: Risk for peritonitis	Show stable vital signs, typically: heart rate, 60 to 100 beats/minute; systolic blood pressure, 90 to 140 mm Hg; diastolic blood pressure, 50 to 90 mm Hg.
CP: Risk for hemorrhage	Show no evidence of bleeding.
ND: Acute pain	Have no abdominal pain or distention, nausea, vomiting, or anorexia.
ND: Risk for infection	Show no signs of infection.
ND: Ineffective breathing pattern	Display nonlabored, deep respirations.
ND: Imbalanced nutrition: Less than body requirements	Have a sufficient caloric intake by mouth.
ND: Impaired oral mucous membrane	Have an intact, moist mucous membrane.

Collaborative problem

Risk for peritonitis related to possible preoperative perforation of the gallbladder

NURSING PRIORITIES

- Detect perforation.
- Minimize possible complications.

PATIENT OUTCOME CRITERIA

Within 24 hours of admission, the patient will:

- display stable vital signs, typically: heart rate, 60 to 100 beats/minute; systolic blood pressure, 90 to 140 mm Hg; and diastolic blood pressure, 50 to 90 mm Hg
- verbalize reduction of pain
- show lessening of abnormal abdominal signs.

INTERVENTIONS

1. *Monitor vital signs* * every 2 hours for 12 hours, then every 4 hours if stable. *Document and report abnormalities,* especially fever, tachycardia, or dropping blood pressure.

2. *Assess the abdomen* during vital sign checks, particularly noting bowel sounds, distention, firmness, and presence or absence of a mass in the RUQ. Document and report any changes.

3. *During vital sign checks, note the location and character of pain.* Document and report any changes.

4. *Maintain antibiotic therapy* as ordered.

5. Additional individualized interventions: _____

RATIONALES

1. Early detection of changes in vital signs will alert caregivers to possible perforation and the need for emergency surgery. Temperature changes indicate further inflammation or a response to antibiotics.

2. Muscle rigidity and a palpable mass in the RUQ suggest peritonitis. In peritonitis, an initial period of hypermotility is followed by hypoactive or absent bowel sounds.

3. RUQ pain that becomes generalized may indicate perforation.

4. Antibiotics excreted through the biliary tree are given to prevent or treat infection and to decrease the risk of perforation from a friable or necrotic gallbladder wall.

5. Rationales: _____

*Italics indicate key interventions.

Collaborative problem

Risk for hemorrhage related to decreased vitamin K absorption and decreased prothrombin synthesis

NURSING PRIORITIES
- Prevent hemorrhage.
- Detect clotting abnormalities so that they can be corrected before surgery.

PATIENT OUTCOME CRITERIA
Within 48 hours of admission, the patient will:
- have PT/INR level approaching normal
- show no evidence of bleeding.

INTERVENTIONS	RATIONALES
1. *Monitor PT/INR, as ordered. Alert the physician to an abnormally prolonged PT/INR.*	**1.** Prothrombin is manufactured in the liver and depends on vitamin K for synthesis. Bile is necessary for vitamin K absorption; thus, PT may be prolonged and INR level may be elevated if an obstruction interferes with bile excretion.
2. *Administer vitamin K, as ordered.*	**2.** Administration of vitamin K will correct any deficiency and promote prothrombin synthesis.
3. *Observe for bleeding* from the gums, nose, or injection sites and for blood in the urine or stool. Document and report bleeding.	**3.** Observing for bleeding aids in detecting coagulation problems.
4. *Give injections using small-gauge needles.* If an increased bleeding tendency is noted, limit the number of injections or venipunctures as much as possible, and apply direct pressure for at least 5 minutes after such procedures.	**4.** Small-gauge needles reduce the risk of bleeding at injection sites. Minimizing the number of punctures reduces the risk of significant blood loss. Direct pressure controls bleeding and allows clot formation.
5. *Apply gentle pressure to injection sites* instead of massaging them.	**5.** Gentle pressure reduces the trauma at injection sites and controls bleeding.
6. Additional individualized interventions: _____	**6.** Rationales: _____

Nursing diagnosis
Acute pain related to gallbladder inflammation

NURSING PRIORITY
Relieve RUQ pain.

PATIENT OUTCOME CRITERIA
Within 1 hour of admission, and then continuously, the patient will:
- verbalize pain relief
- with pain medications, rate pain as less than 3 on a 0 to 10 pain rating scale.

INTERVENTIONS	RATIONALES
1. *See the "Acute pain" care plan,* page 32.	**1.** Generalized interventions regarding pain management are included in the "Acute pain" care plan.
2. *Maintain nothing by mouth (NPO) status.*	**2.** NPO status decreases stimulation of the gallbladder.

Hepatobiliary and pancreatic disorders

3. Administer medications, as ordered, and document their effectiveness. Meperidine (Demerol) is the analgesic of choice; papaverine (Pavabid) may be used.

4. Additional individualized interventions: _____

3. Specific medications are most appropriate for pain from cholecystitis. Meperidine is less likely than morphine to cause spasm of the sphincter of Oddi. Papaverine exerts a nonspecific spasmolytic effect on smooth muscle.

4. Rationales: _____

Suggested NIC Interventions
Medication management; Pain management; Patient-controlled analgesia (PCA) assistance; Analgesic administration; Conscious sedation

Suggested NOC Outcomes
Comfort level; Pain control; Pain: Disruptive effects; Pain level

---

Nursing diagnosis

Risk for infection (postoperative) related to obstruction or dislodgment of external biliary drainage tube

NURSING PRIORITIES

- Prevent or promptly detect complications.
- Maintain patency of the drainage system.

PATIENT OUTCOME CRITERIA

Throughout the period of external biliary drainage, the patient will:
- be afebrile
- show no signs of infection or peritonitis
- show no signs of tube obstruction
- show no signs of tube dislodgment.

INTERVENTIONS

1. *Monitor vital signs* every 4 hours. Document and report abnormalities.

2. *Assess the abdomen every shift,* noting any abdominal pain or rigidity. Document and report any changes.

3. *Assess for signs of infection at the T-tube insertion site.* Document and report any redness, swelling, warmth, or purulent drainage. Teach the patient and his family to recognize and report signs of infection.

4. *Assess for signs of T-tube obstruction.* Document and report pain in the RUQ, biliary drainage around the T-tube, nausea and vomiting, clay-colored stools, jaundice, or dark yellow urine.

5. *Assess for signs of tube dislodgment:* decreased drainage or a change in tube position.

6. *Maintain a drainage system,* using sterile technique. Connect the T-tube to a closed gravity drainage system, and attach sufficient tubing so it doesn't kink or pull as the patient moves.

RATIONALES

1. Elevated temperature may indicate infection.

2. Generalized abdominal pain and rigidity, combined with an elevated temperature, may indicate biliary peritonitis.

3. Early detection of infection facilitates prompt treatment.

4. These signs indicate the backup of bile into the common bile duct and liver.

5. Prompt detection and treatment of tube dislodgment reduces the risk of complications (such as peritonitis) from bile leakage.

6. After choledochostomy, a T-tube is inserted into the hepatic duct and the common bile duct to allow biliary drainage and maintain patency until edema subsides. A closed biliary drainage system ensures sterility. Providing enough tubing reduces the risk of obstructing or dislodging the T-tube.

7. *Monitor the amount and character of any drainage.* Measure and record the drainage every 4 hours for 12 hours, then once per shift and as needed.

7. Initially, all bile output (500 to 1,000 ml/day) may flow through the T-tube. Within 7 to 10 days, however, most of the bile should flow into the duodenum. Monitoring the amount of drainage permits early detection of an obstructed or dislodged tube.

8. *Monitor and record the patient's stool color.*

8. Stools will be light-colored initially, when most of the bile is flowing out through the T-tube. Stools should gradually become normal in color as bile passes into the duodenum. Persistence of light-colored stools for more than 7 days may indicate tube obstruction.

9. *Place the patient in low Fowler's position* upon return from surgery.

9. Low Fowler's position facilitates T-tube drainage.

10. *Teach the patient and his family how to care for the drainage system.* If the patient will be discharged with a T-tube in place, include the expected amount of drainage, frequency of bag emptying and dressing changes, techniques for site care and dressing changes, and signs to report to the physician (excessive drainage, leakage, and signs of obstruction).

10. To successfully manage the T-tube at home, the patient and his family need to know about routine care as well as what to do about potential complications.

11. Additional individualized interventions: _____

11. Rationales: _____

Suggested NIC Interventions
Infection control; Infection protection; Incision site care; Wound care

Suggested NOC Outcomes
Infection status; Wound healing: Primary intention

Nursing diagnosis
Ineffective breathing pattern related to high abdominal incision and pain

NURSING PRIORITIES
- Maintain optimal air exchange.
- Prevent atelectasis.

PATIENT OUTCOME CRITERIA
Throughout the postoperative period, the patient will:
- maintain a respiratory rate of 12 to 24 breaths/minute
- display nonlabored, deep respirations
- have clear breath sounds in all lobes.

INTERVENTIONS

1. *Monitor respiratory rate and character* every 4 hours. Note the depth of respirations. Document and report abnormalities. Measure oxygen saturation (Sao_2) and report Sao_2 less than 95%.

RATIONALES

1. After an open cholecystectomy, the patient may breathe shallowly to avoid pain associated with deep breathing. In a laparoscopic cholecystectomy, Sao_2 less than 95% may indicate the need for supplemental oxygen and more aggressive spirometry. Carbon dioxide (CO_2) is used for inflating the abdominal area. Afterwards the migration of the CO_2 up the thorax may cause pain associated with deep breathing.

2. *Auscultate for breath sounds once per shift.* Document and report changes.

2. Breath sounds may be diminished at the bases, especially on the right side.

3. *Instruct and coach the patient in diaphragmatic breathing.*

3. Diaphragmatic breathing increases lung expansion by allowing the diaphragm to descend fully.

4. *Assist the patient to use the incentive spirometer —* 10 breaths/hour during the day and every 2 hours at night.

4. Using the incentive spirometer promotes sustained maximal inspiration, which fully inflates alveoli.

5. *Turn the patient every 2 hours.*

5. Position changes promote ventilation of all lung lobes and drainage of secretions.

6. *Assess pain and administer pain medication,* as needed, before breathing exercises and ambulation.

6. The pain-free patient is better able to take deep breaths, therefore is likely to cooperate with prescribed pulmonary hygiene measures and activity level.

7. *Assist the patient to splint the incisions* with a pillow or bath blanket while coughing.

7. Splinting relieves stress and pulling on the incisions.

8. *Encourage the patient to increase ambulation progressively.*

8. Ambulation promotes adequate ventilation by increasing the depth of respirations.

9. After a laparoscopic cholecystectomy, apply a heating pad to the abdominal area and thorax for 20 minutes.

9. Heat may decrease pain from the CO_2 gas migration.

10. Additional individualized interventions: _____

10. Rationales: _____

Suggested NIC Interventions
Airway management; Airway suctioning; Respiratory monitoring; Ventilation assistance; Vital signs monitoring

Suggested NOC Outcomes
Respiratory status: Airway patency; Respiratory status; Ventilation; Vital signs status

---

Nursing diagnosis

Imbalanced nutrition: Less than body requirements related to preoperative nausea and vomiting, postoperative NPO status, nasogastric (NG) suction, altered lipid metabolism, and increased nutritional needs during healing

NURSING PRIORITIES

- Maintain optimal nutritional status.
- Teach the patient and his family about postoperative dietary recommendations.

PATIENT OUTCOME CRITERIA

Throughout the hospital stay, the patient will:
- have normal fluid and electrolyte status.
  By the time of discharge, the patient will:
- list three general dietary considerations
- identify specific foods that may need to be restricted.

INTERVENTIONS

1. *Maintain I.V. fluid replacement,* as ordered. (See appendix C, Fluid and electrolyte imbalances.)

RATIONALES

1. During the immediate postoperative period, the patient will receive nothing by mouth until peristalsis returns. The patient may also have an NG tube in place to reduce distention and minimize the pancreatic stimulation normally triggered by gastric juices. Gastric suction and NPO status increase the risk of fluid and electrolyte disorders.

2. *When peristalsis returns, remove the NG tube and encourage a progressive dietary intake,* as ordered.

3. *Clamp the T-tube during meals,* as ordered.

4. *Teach the patient and his family about a fat-restricted diet,* as ordered. Involve a dietitian in meal planning and home care teaching.

5. Suggest small, frequent meals.

6. Instruct the patient to minimize alcohol intake during recovery.

7. Flatulence is common after surgery. Typically, these patients have other GI disorders (such as hiatal hernia or ulcer) that may cause persistent symptoms, such as bloating and nausea. Dietary modifications and treatment of the underlying disorder may reduce symptoms.

8. Additional individualized interventions: _____
_____

2. Patients are usually able to take clear liquids 24 to 48 hours after surgery and gradually increase to a full diet, with fat restrictions as ordered.

3. Clamping the T-tube during meals may aid fat absorption by allowing additional bile to flow into the duodenum.

4. After cholecystectomy, the liver must store and release all bile for lipid digestion; thus, fat absorption may be altered, especially if postoperative edema limits hepatic bile excretion. Fat intake is usually limited for $1\frac{1}{2}$ to 6 months, depending on the physician's preference and the patient's response to gradual increases in fat intake. A dietitian can help ensure that the patient's diet compensates for the calories normally provided by fats.

5. Large meals may contribute to distention and increase discomfort.

6. Pancreatitis is a common complication after cholecystectomy. Alcohol intake commonly triggers acute pancreatic inflammation.

7. Prepare the patient for the possibility of persistent flatulence.

8. Rationales: _____
_____

Suggested NIC Interventions
Diet staging; Nutrition management; Weight gain assistance; Fluid monitoring; Nutritional monitoring

Suggested NOC Outcomes
Nutritional status; Nutritional status: Food and fluid intake; Nutritional status: Nutrient intake; Weight control

Nursing diagnosis
Impaired oral mucous membrane related to NPO status and possible NG suction

NURSING PRIORITY
Maintain integrity of the oral mucous membrane.

PATIENT OUTCOME CRITERIA
Throughout the period of NPO status, the patient will:
- have an intact, moist oral mucous membrane
- display no evidence of an inflamed oral mucosa.

INTERVENTIONS

1. *Assess the oral mucous membrane* once per shift for dryness, cracks, coating, or lesions.

RATIONALES

1. Early identification of potential problems facilitates prompt treatment.

2. *Assist the patient with gentle mouth care* at least twice daily or as needed. Make sure that water and oral hygiene materials are within the patient's reach.

3. Apply lubricant to the lips every 2 hours while the patient is awake or more frequently as needed.

4. Additional individualized interventions: _____
_____

2. NPO status and NG suction (as well as any previously existing nutritional deficits) may contribute to fragility of the oral mucosa and increase the risk of infection or injury. Frequent mouth care reduces accumulation of bacteria and decreases discomfort associated with NPO status.

3. Lubricant keeps lips smooth and moist.

4. Rationales: _____
_____

Suggested NIC Interventions
Oral health restoration

Suggested NOC Outcomes
Oral health; Tissue integrity: Skin and mucous membranes

Discharge planning

DISCHARGE CHECKLIST
Before discharge, the patient shows evidence of:
❏ absence of wound infection
❏ absence of fever
❏ stable vital signs
❏ absence of pulmonary and cardiovascular complications
❏ ability to tolerate diet as ordered
❏ same ability to ambulate as before surgery
❏ ability to perform activities of daily living (ADLs) independently
❏ adequate support system after discharge, or referral to home care if indicated by inadequate home support system or inability to perform ADLs.

TEACHING CHECKLIST
Document evidence that the patient and his family demonstrate an understanding of:
❏ signs and symptoms of wound infection
❏ dietary modifications (patient may be on a low-fat diet for up to 6 months; a normal diet is resumed as soon as tolerated)
❏ resumption of normal activities
❏ lifting restricted to less than 10 lb (4.5 kg) for 3 to 4 weeks with open cholecystectomy, for 1 week with a laparoscopic cholecystectomy
❏ resumption of normal activities
❏ resumption of sexual activity (when cleared by physician, usually after 2 weeks or when pain-free)
❏ all discharge medications' purpose, dosage, administration schedule, and adverse effects (postoperative patients may be discharged with oral analgesics)
❏ if discharged with a T-tube, routine care and signs to report to the physician
❏ date, time, and location of follow-up appointment
❏ how to contact the physician.

DOCUMENTATION CHECKLIST
Using outcome criteria as a guide, document:
❏ clinical status on admission
❏ significant changes in status
❏ pertinent laboratory and diagnostic test findings
❏ wound assessment
❏ amount and character of T-tube drainage
❏ pain-relief measures
❏ pulmonary hygiene measures
❏ observations of oral mucous membrane
❏ nutritional intake
❏ GI assessment
❏ patient and family teaching
❏ discharge planning.

Associated care plans
- Acute pain
- Knowledge deficit
- Pancreatitis
- Perioperative care

References
Ignatavicius, D., and Workman, L. *Medical-Surgical Nursing, Critical Thinking for Collaborative Care,* 4th ed. Philadelphia: W.B. Saunders Co., 2002.
Smeltzer, S., and Bare, B. *Brunner & Suddarth's Medical-Surgical Nursing.* Philadelphia: Lippincott Williams & Wilkins, 2002.

Liver failure

DRG INFORMATION

DRG 205   Disorders of Liver Except Malignancy, Cirrhosis, or Alcoholic Hepatitis with Complications or Comorbidity (CC).
         Mean LOS = 5.0 days

Principal diagnoses include:
- acute or chronic liver failure
- various types of hepatitis
- hepatomegaly
- jaundice, unspecified etiology
- hepatic infarction
- liver abscess.

DRG 206   Disorders of Liver Except Malignancy, Cirrhosis, or Alcoholic Hepatitis without CC.
         Mean LOS = 3.2 days

Principal diagnoses include selected principal diagnoses listed under DRG 205. The distinction is that a case assigned DRG 206 has no CC.

Introduction

DEFINITION AND TIME FOCUS

The liver is an organ essential for life, with metabolic, secretory, excretory, and vascular functions. Metabolic functions include glycogen formation, storage, and breakdown; glucose formation; fat storage, breakdown, and synthesis; amino acid deamination; ammonia conversion; and synthesis of plasma proteins, including clotting factors. Secretory functions include bile production and bilirubin conjugation. Excretory functions include detoxification of hormones and drugs. Vascular functions include blood storage and filtration.

In liver failure, which can result from almost all forms of liver disease, parenchymal cells are progressively destroyed and replaced with fibrotic tissue. Once chronically damaged, the liver will never regain normal structure. However, because liver cells retain an enormous regenerative capacity, functional compensation may be attained if precipitating factors are eliminated. This care plan focuses on the critically ill patient presenting with acute symptoms of liver failure. These symptoms include hepatic encephalopathy, fluid and electrolyte imbalance from ascites, and related complications of liver failure. (See *Clinical snapshot: Liver failure*, page 534.)

ETIOLOGY AND PRECIPITATING FACTORS

- Laënnec's (alcoholic) cirrhosis with an acute episode of alcohol ingestion, hypovolemia from rapid diuresis or shock, GI bleeding, or infection
- Acute hepatic failure caused by fulminant hepatitis, hepatotoxic chemicals, or biliary obstruction
- Primary biliary cirrhosis

Focused assessment guidelines

NURSING HISTORY (FUNCTIONAL HEALTH PATTERN FINDINGS)

Health-perception–health-management pattern
- Commonly complains about weakness and fatigue
- Treatment for chronic alcoholism, hepatitis, or biliary obstructive disease

Nutritional-metabolic pattern
- Diet history that includes excessive alcohol consumption and fat intolerance
- Anorexia and resulting weight loss
- Ingestion of certain drugs, such as large doses of acetaminophen (Tylenol), tetracycline (Tetracyn), or antituberculosis drugs such as isoniazid (Laniazid)

Elimination pattern
- Clay-colored stools or dark urine resulting from jaundice

Activity-exercise pattern
- Psychomotor defects

Sleep-rest pattern
- Increased drowsiness

Cognitive-perceptual pattern
- Intellectual deterioration and slurred speech in beginning stages of hepatic encephalopathy commonly reported by the patient's family
- Personality changes or altered moods reported by the patient's family

Sexuality-reproductive pattern
- Impotence in male patients because of endocrine changes
- Erratic menstruation among female patients

Role-relationship pattern
- Job involving hepatotoxic chemicals such as vinyl chloride

PHYSICAL FINDINGS

General appearance
- Fever unaffected by antibiotics; reason for fever is unknown

Cardiovascular
- Hyperkinetic circulation: flushed extremities, bounding pulse, and capillary pulsations that result primarily from liver cell failure but also may occur with the opening of many normal but functionally inactive arteriovenous anastomoses

Pulmonary
- Cyanosis

Neurologic
- Hyperactive reflexes, positive Babinski's reflex
- Various stages of encephalopathy with resultant altered level of consciousness (LOC)

Gastrointestinal
- Fetor hepaticus: sweetish, slightly fecal breath smell, presumably intestinal in origin
- Hepatomegaly, splenomegaly
- Ascites
- Distant bowel sounds and muffled percussion notes

Endocrine
- Male: hypogonadism, gynecomastia
- Female: gonadal atrophy

Integumentary
- Jaundiced skin, sclera, and mucous membranes from failure to metabolize bilirubin
- Vascular spiders: consist of central arteriole with radiating small vessels; usually in vascular territory of superior vena cava (above nipple line)
- Palmar erythema: hands warm, palms bright red from estrogen excess
- Easy bruising from inadequate clotting factors
- "Paper money skin": numerous small blood vessels that resemble silk threads in a dollar bill

DIAGNOSTIC STUDIES

- Complete blood count — may reveal decreased hematocrit and hemoglobin values, which reflect the liver's inability to store hematopoietic factors (such as iron, folic acid, and vitamin B_{12}); decreased white blood cell (WBC) count and thrombocyte levels, which appear with splenomegaly; and elevated WBC count, which may indicate infection
- Prolonged prothrombin time/international normalized ratio (PT/INR) — reflects decreased synthesis of prothrombin, impaired vitamin K absorption, or both

- Enzyme tests — may show elevated serum aspartate aminotransferase, serum alanine aminotransferase, alkaline phosphatase, and lactate dehydrogenase values, which reflect hepatocellular or biliary tissue dysfunction and necrosis
- Protein metabolite tests (serum albumin and total protein levels) — may reflect impaired protein synthesis
- Lipid and carbohydrate tests — may reveal decreased serum cholesterol levels, reflecting impaired hepatic synthesis, or increased levels, reflecting obstructive pathology; elevated serum ammonia values, reflecting impaired hepatic synthesis of urea; and decreased serum glucose levels, which accompany malnutrition
- Bilirubin levels — increased in liver disease
- Urine and stool tests — may reveal increased urine urobilinogen and reduced fecal urobilinogen values, which accompany jaundice
- Testosterone level — reduced
- Abdominal ultrasound — may be performed if biliary obstruction is suspected
- Abdominal X-rays — may reveal liver enlargement
- Angiography or superior mesenteric arteriography — important for evaluation of portal hypertension
- Liver scan — reveals abnormalities in hepatic structure
- Liver biopsy — indicates extent of hepatic tissue changes
- EEG — may show generalized slowing of frequency, which substantiates encephalopathy
- Endoscopy — helps locate GI bleeding site

POTENTIAL COMPLICATIONS

- Hepatorenal failure
- Disseminated intravascular coagulation
- Bleeding esophageal varices

CLINICAL SNAPSHOT ☀

Liver failure

Major nursing diagnoses and collaborative problems	Key patient outcomes
CP: Deteriorating neurologic status	Display improved neurologic status.
CP: Risk for fever	Have a temperature of 97.5° to 99.5°F (36.4° to 37.5° C).
CP: Fluid and electrolyte imbalance	Show reduced ascites and edema.
CP: Risk for GI hemorrhage	Show stable vital signs, typically: heart rate, 60 to 100 beats/minute; systolic blood pressure, 90 to 140 mm Hg; and diastolic blood pressure, 50 to 90 mm Hg.
ND: Imbalanced nutrition: Less than body requirements	Tolerate protein intake without encephalopathy recurring.
ND: Impaired skin integrity	Have no apparent skin breakdown.

Collaborative problem

Deteriorating neurologic status related to hepatic encephalopathy syndrome

NURSING PRIORITIES
■ Monitor changes in psychomotor skills, mental status, and speech.
■ Eliminate factors that decrease hepatocellular function.

PATIENT OUTCOME CRITERIA
Within 24 to 48 hours of admission, the patient will:
■ display improved neurologic status
■ display a decreased need for respiratory support.

INTERVENTIONS	RATIONALES
1. *Assess neurologic status hourly. Assess and implement safety measures.* * Describe the changes observed, typically: – Stage 1: confusion, altered mood or behavior, psychomotor deficits – Stage 2: drowsiness, inappropriate behavior – Stage 3: stupor, marked confusion, and inarticulate speech (although the patient may speak or obey simple commands) – Stage 4: coma, but response to painful stimuli still present – Stage 5: deep coma; no response to painful stimuli.	1. Symptoms vary; therefore, close monitoring and implementation of appropriate safety measures is important. The encephalopathy syndrome results from impaired nitrogen metabolism, passage of toxic substances of intestinal origin (ammonia, active amines, and short-chain fatty acids) to the brain, and numerous other metabolic abnormalities occurring in hepatocellular failure. The toxic substances are thought to interfere with glucose metabolism and cerebral blood flow. Chronic exposure of brain cells to these substances through repeated bouts of encephalopathy results in irreversible damage.
2. *Assess for asterixis* (flapping tremor of the wrist).	2. This sign, caused by impaired flow of proprioceptive information to the brain stem reticular formation, indicates that the patient is in the early stages of encephalopathy.
3. *Auscultate the chest and assess respiratory rate hourly.* Administer oxygen therapy using nasal prongs, as ordered. Monitor pulse oximetry continuously. Anticipate more aggressive measures, such as intubation, if the encephalopathy progresses to coma.	3. The patient with long-standing liver disease will have developed decreased oxygen saturation and decreased diffusing capacity before the onset of encephalopathy. Therefore, respiratory support measures are commonly required.
4. *Stop intake of dietary protein.* Also stop administration of all drugs containing nitrogen, such as ammonium chloride, urea (Ureaphil), and methionine, as ordered.	4. Intake of dietary protein and drugs containing nitrogen increase the accumulation of nitrogenous substances that the liver can't break down.
5. Administer neomycin (Mycifradin) by a nasogastric tube, if ordered. The usual dose is 1 g.	5. Neomycin decreases the intestinal bacteria that produce ammonia.
6. Administer lactulose (Cephulac) by an NG tube, if ordered. The usual dose is 10 to 30 ml. Expect frequent bowel movements due to lactulose. Keep patient clean and comfortable. Monitor closely for skin breakdown due to excessive bowel movements. Monitor for diarrhea; if it occurs, consult with the physician about reducing the dose.	6. Although lactulose's exact mechanism of action is unclear, it may be instrumental in chelating ammonia (NH_3), acting as an osmotic agent for inducing diarrhea, changing gut pH resulting in excretion of ammonium (NH_4^+), or changing gut flora to decrease the growth of NH_3-forming bacteria. Diarrhea is a sign of excessive dosage.
7. Stop any diuretic therapy, as ordered.	7. If the patient has hepatic cirrhosis, the most common cause of hepatic encephalopathy is excessive diuresis from diuretic therapy. The resulting hypovolemia further reduces hepatic perfusion, causing the encephalopathy.

*Italics indicate key interventions.

Hepatobiliary and
pancreatic disorders

8. Administer neutral, acid-free enema solutions, as ordered.

8. Purging the intestines reduces NH_4^+ absorption and may result in improvement of clinical symptoms and EEG readings.

9. *Avoid all sedatives metabolized primarily by the liver.* If the patient is uncontrollable, administer half the usual dose of barbiturate, as ordered. Morphine and paraldehyde (Paral) are contraindicated.

9. The patient in impending coma is extremely sensitive to sedatives. Drugs metabolized primarily by the liver are particularly dangerous because toxic accumulations can occur rapidly from impaired hepatic perfusion. Some sedation may be necessary, however, if the patient becomes agitated as hepatic failure worsens and toxic metabolic substances accumulate. Long-acting, short-chain barbiturates that are excreted largely by the kidney are preferred. Morphine and paraldehyde may cause coma.

10. *Teach the patient and his family about necessary interventions,* as appropriate. Emphasize causes of changes in neurologic status and rationales for methods to reduce encephalopathy.

10. Although patient teaching may be of limited success because of altered LOC, brief and repeated explanations may help the patient feel more secure psychologically. Teaching family members may help them understand mood swings and behavior changes.

11. Additional individualized interventions: _____

11. Rationales: _____

Collaborative problem

Risk for fever related to liver disease or infection

NURSING PRIORITY

Assist in determining the cause of the fever.

PATIENT OUTCOME CRITERION

Within 24 to 48 hours of admission, the patient will have a temperature less than 100.4° F (38° C).

INTERVENTIONS

1. *Assess temperature every 4 hours.* If elevated, assess more frequently. Consult with the physician about abnormal readings.

RATIONALES

1. Continuous, low-grade fever rarely exceeding 100.4° F is seen in about one-third of patients with liver disease. This fever is unaffected by antibiotics and attributable to liver disease alone, although the reason for it is unknown. However, the patient may have fever from infection. The liver normally is bacteriologically sterile and filters bacteria from the bloodstream. Cirrhosis allows bacteria to pass into the circulation. Differentiation of possible causes of fever is necessary for effective treatment.

2. *Observe for cloudy, concentrated urine and pain upon urination,* if a catheter isn't in place. Avoid catheterization, if possible.

2. These signs indicate urinary tract infection. Avoiding catheterization reduces the risk of infection. However, accurate measurement of input and output is crucial for the critically ill patient with liver disease. An indwelling urinary catheter may be necessary to monitor accurate hourly urine output. Remember, urine may be dark amber because of jaundice.

3. *Auscultate lung fields at least every 2 hours.* Also assess respiratory rate, skin color, and level of cyanosis.

3. Respiratory difficulties may indicate aspiration pneumonia. Pulmonary arteriovenous shunting from liver disease and the resultant decreased oxygen saturation place the patient at increased risk for pneumonia.

4. *Ausculate bowel sounds at least every 4 hours.* Observe for abdominal rigidity, increased abdominal girth, or vomiting.

5. If infection is diagnosed, assist with treatment, as ordered; for example, administer antibiotics. If the fever stems solely from liver disease, provide symptomatic care such as frequent linen changes.

6. Additional individualized interventions: _____
_____

4. Spontaneous peritonitis is known to occur in patients with liver disease.

5. Infection requires prompt, aggressive treatment because it promotes protein accumulation from tissue catabolism. Low-grade fever may remain if fever results solely from liver disease. Frequent linen changes reduce discomfort from diaphoresis.

6. Rationales: _____
_____

Collaborative problem
Fluid and electrolyte imbalance related to ascites

NURSING PRIORITY
Restore a normal fluid balance (as described in outcome criteria).

PATIENT OUTCOME CRITERIA
Within 4 days of admission, the patient will:
- manifest urine output of at least 60 ml/hour
- display urinary sodium excretion greater than 10 mEq/day
- show reduced ascites and edema, as evidenced by decreased weight and improved respiratory status.

INTERVENTIONS

1. *Closely monitor fluid and electrolyte status,* including strict intake and output measurements, hourly determination of urine specific gravity, daily weights, and assessment of lung fields at least every 2 hours for crackles or gurgles.

2. *Percuss and palpate the abdomen every 4 hours.* Don't rely solely on abdominal girth measurements.

3. *Maintain strict bed rest.*

RATIONALES

1. Close monitoring of fluid status is necessary to judge the degree of cardiovascular and pulmonary compromise imposed by ascites. In liver failure, ascites develops from lowered plasma oncotic pressure, portal venous hypertension, and sodium and water retention. The lowered plasma oncotic pressure results from the liver's failure to synthesize albumin. This lowered oncotic pressure, combined with increased hydrostatic pressure from portal hypertension, causes fluid to shift into interstitial spaces (third spacing) in the peritoneal cavity. The resulting depletion of effective intravascular volume causes the renal tubules to retain sodium and water through the aldosterone effect.

2. Percussion and palpation allow evaluation of changes in fluid shifting. Dullness on percussion in the flanks is the earliest sign of ascites and indicates approximately 2 L of fluid. The liver and spleen may be palpated if only moderate amounts of fluid are present; with tense ascites, it's difficult to palpate abdominal viscera. A fluid thrill indicates a large amount of free fluid. It's a very late sign of fluid under tension. Abdominal girth measurements are unreliable as gaseous distention is common.

3. Bed rest increases renal perfusion and the kidneys' ability to excrete excess fluid. Placing the patient with ascites in the semi-Fowler's or Fowler's position may impair ventilation due to excessive pressure on the diaphragm.

Hepatobiliary and pancreatic disorders

4. Implement therapy, as ordered:
– dietary restrictions, typically sodium intake of 0.5 g/day and fluid intake of 1 L/day
– diuretic administration, typically furosemide (Lasix) or spironolactone (Aldactone)
– postoperative care after peritoneovenous (LeVeen) shunt insertion.

5. *Teach the patient and his family about necessary interventions,* as appropriate.

6. Additional individualized interventions: _____
_____

4. The rate of ascitic fluid reabsorption is limited to 700 to 900 ml/day. Limiting sodium and water intake reduces ascitic fluid production, while diuretic administration increases fluid excretion. Shunt insertion controls ascites in less than 5% of patients with liver failure.

5. Understanding the effects of ascites and treatment methods improves the patient and his family's cooperation with the treatment plan, increasing the likelihood of its effectiveness.

6. Rationales: _____
_____

Collaborative problem
Risk for GI hemorrhage related to esophageal varices

NURSING PRIORITY
Monitor for, prevent, or promptly treat hemorrhage.

PATIENT OUTCOME CRITERIA
Within 24 hours of detection of bleeding, the patient will:
- show stable vital signs, typically: heart rate, 60 to 100 beats/minute; systolic blood pressure, 90 to 140 mm Hg; and diastolic blood pressure, 50 to 90 mm Hg
- have warm, dry skin.

INTERVENTIONS

1. *Observe for and report signs of esophageal bleeding* such as hematemesis. Anticipate drug treatment with vasopressin (Pitressin), propranolol (Inderal), or octreotide (Sandostatin), or insertion of a gastric compression tube. *See the "Gastrointestinal hemorrhage" care plan,* page 487, for specific nursing interventions.

2. Additional individualized interventions: _____
_____

RATIONALES

1. The mechanism of esophageal varices formation is unclear; they're thought to be caused by excessive portal venous backflow into the esophageal vasculature. Hematemesis of frank red blood indicates active bleeding. Vasopressin constricts blood vessels and smooth muscle in the GI tract. Octreotide suppresses secretion of serotonin and gastroenteropancreatic peptides, while propranolol lowers blood pressure. A compression tube may control bleeding varices temporarily. The "Gastrointestinal hemorrhage" care plan contains detailed information on detecting and treating bleeding varices.

2. Rationales: _____
_____

Nursing diagnosis
Imbalanced nutrition: Less than body requirements related to catabolism caused by liver disease

NURSING PRIORITY
Restore metabolism to an anabolic state.

PATIENT OUTCOME CRITERION
Within 96 hours of admission, the patient will tolerate protein intake without recurrence of encephalopathy.

INTERVENTIONS	RATIONALES
1. *Implement dietary restrictions,* as ordered. Maintain high caloric intake, usually 1,600 calories/day, by administering high carbohydrate I.V. infusions, as ordered. If jaundice is present, don't administer oral fat or fat infusions.	1. Dietary control of precursors to toxic metabolites plays an important role in the control of symptoms. High-caloric intake is necessary to meet energy needs. Jaundice indicates decreased bile salt levels, which impair fat absorption.
2. *If encephalopathy is present, stop protein intake,* as ordered. *Once encephalopathy has subsided, start protein* intake at 20-g/day increments. *Monitor closely for recurrence of encephalopathy.*	2. Inability to metabolize protein causes the blood ammonia level to rise, producing encephalopathy. Restricting protein intake helps eliminate symptoms. Gradual reintroduction of protein helps determine the amount the patient can metabolize safely. Recurrence of symptoms indicates the need for permanent protein restriction.
3. *Emphasize to the patient and his family the importance of dietary restrictions.*	3. The necessary restrictions may make the diet unpalatable and difficult to accept. Understanding the rationale increases the patient's motivation to follow recommendations and the likelihood of family support.
4. Additional individualized interventions: _____	4. Rationales: _____

> **Suggested NIC Interventions**
> *Diet staging; Nutrition management; Weight gain assistance; Fluid monitoring; Nutritional monitoring*

> **Suggested NOC Outcomes**
> *Nutritional status; Nutritional status: Food and fluid intake; Nutritional status: Nutrient intake; Weight control*

Nursing diagnosis
Impaired skin integrity related to jaundice, increased bleeding tendencies, malnutrition, and ascites

NURSING PRIORITY
Maintain or restore skin integrity.

PATIENT OUTCOME CRITERION
Within 48 hours of admission, and then continuously, the patient will have no apparent skin breakdown.

INTERVENTIONS	RATIONALES
1. *Monitor skin condition.* Particularly note the presence of vascular spiders.	1. Careful monitoring of skin status, commonly overlooked, allows early detection of skin problems to which liver failure patients are particularly susceptible. Vascular spiders can bleed profusely.
2. *Monitor PT/INR,* as ordered.	2. Liver failure impairs the synthesis of clotting factors. A prolonged PT increases the risk of skin bruising and breakdown.
3. Turn the patient and rub bony prominences every 2 hours. Implement additional measures found in the "Impaired physical mobility" care plan, page 111, as appropriate.	3. Malnutrition and ascites predispose the patient to pressure ulcer formation. The "Impaired physical mobility" care plan presents detailed information on potential skin problems.

Hepatobiliary and pancreatic disorders

4. Provide symptomatic treatment of pruritus, as necessary; for example, bathe the skin with cool water.

4. Pruritus, which results from jaundice, can cause extreme discomfort. Treatment may be limited because phenothiazides and antihistamines are contraindicated if the patient has encephalopathy.

5. Additional individualized interventions: _____

5. Rationales: _____

Suggested NIC Interventions
Pressure management; Pressure ulcer care; Skin surveillance; Incision site care; Wound care

Suggested NOC Outcomes
Tissue integrity: Skin and mucous membranes; Wound healing: Primary intention; Wound healing: Secondary intention

---

Discharge planning

DISCHARGE CHECKLIST
Before discharge, the patient shows evidence of:
- ❏ improved neurologic status
- ❏ absence of respiratory complications
- ❏ adequate urine output
- ❏ reduction of ascites and weight
- ❏ normal temperature or stable low-grade fever
- ❏ resumption of I.V. or oral protein and fat intake.

TEACHING CHECKLIST
Document evidence that the patient and his family demonstrate an understanding of:
- ❏ the relationship between alcohol consumption and exacerbation of liver disease
- ❏ the causes of changes in neurologic status and relationship to liver disease
- ❏ the effects of ascites and methods of treatment
- ❏ the importance of diet in liver disease.

DOCUMENTATION CHECKLIST
Using outcome criteria as a guide, document:
- ❏ clinical status on admission
- ❏ significant changes in status
- ❏ pertinent laboratory and diagnostic test findings
- ❏ weight
- ❏ fluid intake and output measurements
- ❏ fluctuations in fever and associated symptoms
- ❏ skin integrity
- ❏ signs of GI bleeding
- ❏ patient and family teaching
- ❏ discharge planning.

Associated care plans
- ■ Confusion
- ■ Gastrointestinal hemorrhage
- ■ Impaired physical mobility
- ■ Nutritional deficit

References
Jordan, K. (ed). *Emergency Nursing Core Curriculum.* Emergency Nurses Association. Philadelphia: W.B. Saunders Co., 2000.

Kjaergard L.L., et al. "Artificial and Bioartificial Support Systems for Acute and Acute-on-Chronic Liver Failure: A Systematic Review," *JAMA* 289(2):217-22, January 2003.

Lynn-McHale, D.J., and Carlson, K.K. American Association of Critical Care Nurses *AACN Procedure Manual for Critical Care,* 4th ed. Philadelphia: W.B. Saunders Co., 2001.

Sanyal, A.J., et al. "The North American Study for the Treatment of Refractory Ascites," *Gastroenterology* 124(3):634-41, March 2003.

Saseen, J.J. "Does Acetaminophen Affect Liver Function in Alcoholic Patients?" *Journal of Family Practice* 52(3): 187-88, January 2003.

Shoemaker, W.C., et al. *Textbook of Critical Care,* 4th ed. Philadelphia: W.B. Saunders Co., 2002.

Pancreatitis

DRG INFORMATION

DRG 204   Disorder of Pancreas Except Malignancy.
          Mean LOS = 4.9 days

Principal diagnoses include:

- pancreatitis
- benign neoplasm of pancreas, except islets of Langerhans
- injury to any portion of the pancreas.

Introduction
DEFINITION AND TIME FOCUS

Pancreatitis (inflammation of the pancreas) is an autodigestive disorder in which premature activation of pancreatic proteolytic enzymes damages the organ itself. The exact physiologic mechanism is unknown but, theoretically, duodenal reflux or spasm, or blockage of pancreatic ducts by gallstones or edema, may result in the backup of pancreatic secretions. Pancreatitis may be a complication of surgery for other biliary tract or GI disease; numerous other causative factors have also been implicated.

Depending on the nature and severity of the disorder, significant edema, tissue necrosis, and life-threatening hemorrhage may result. Pancreatitis may be either acute or chronic. Chronic pancreatitis causes progressive loss of pancreatic function and may be associated with repeated bouts of acute pancreatitis. This care plan focuses on the care of the patient who is admitted for diagnosis and management of an episode of acute pancreatitis. (See *Clinical snapshot: Pancreatitis,* page 542.)

ETIOLOGY AND PRECIPITATING FACTORS

- Alcohol abuse
- Cholecystitis or cholelithiasis
- Abdominal surgery
- Trauma
- Peptic or duodenal ulcer
- Hyperparathyroidism
- Viral hepatitis
- Mumps
- Hyperlipidemia
- Anorexia nervosa
- Ischemia related to shock
- Metabolic disorders
- Use of certain medications: thiazide diuretics, steroids, sulfonamides, hormonal contraceptives, tetracycline, acetaminophen (in excessive doses)

Focused assessment guidelines
NURSING HISTORY
(FUNCTIONAL HEALTH PATTERN FINDINGS)
Health-perception–health-management pattern

- Severe abdominal pain in epigastric or umbilical region that radiates into back or flank
- Pain that increases when the patient is supine or when food is taken and after administration of certain narcotics
- History of gallbladder disease or alcoholism with recent dietary indiscretion or drinking binge

Nutritional-metabolic pattern

- Nausea or vomiting
- Anorexia
- Recent weight loss

Elimination pattern

- Increased flatus
- Steatorrhea (associated with chronic disease)

Activity-exercise pattern

- Preference for a hunched sitting position because of pain
- Dizziness or faintness when standing

Cognitive-perceptual pattern

- Shoulder pain or frequent hiccups (if diaphragmatic irritation is present)
- Pleuritic-like pain that increases with deep inspiration

Coping–stress tolerance pattern

- Habitual use of unhealthy coping mechanisms (such as alcoholism)

PHYSICAL FINDINGS
General appearance

- Hunched posture
- Restlessness

Cardiovascular

- Fever
- Tachycardia
- Hypotension

Pulmonary

If pleural effusion is present:

- reduced chest excursion
- crackles
- tachypnea

Gastrointestinal

- Abdominal distention
- Guarding
- Reduced or absent bowel sounds
- Ascites

Neurologic

- Seizures

- Stupor
- Neuromuscular irritability

Integumentary
- Jaundice
- Pallor
- Diaphoresis
- Cullen's sign (ecchymosis around umbilicus)
- Turner's sign (ecchymosis in flank, retroperitoneal, and groin area)
- Cool extremities
- Cyanosis (if advanced shock)

Musculoskeletal
If hypocalcemia is present:
- tetany
- positive Chvostek's sign
- positive Trousseau's sign

Renal
- Oliguria (if prerenal azotemia or acute tubular necrosis present)

DIAGNOSTIC STUDIES

- Serum amylase level — elevated in acute pancreatitis; although not specific for pancreatitis, increased enzyme levels occur during pancreatic inflammation
- Amylase-creatinine-clearance ratio — indicates acute pancreatitis if greater than 5%
- Urine amylase level — elevated for the first 3 to 5 days of illness; it reflects pancreatic secretion better than serum value; in acute pancreatitis, renal clearance of amylase is markedly increased
- Serum calcium level — decreased, usually less than 8 mg/dl (unless hyperparathyroidism is present, in which instance value may be normal)
- Complete blood count — likely to reveal leukocytosis; hemoglobin and hematocrit values vary depending on fluid status, hemorrhage, or degree of compensation
- Serum and urine glucose levels — may be elevated because of altered insulin production
- Serum lipase level — elevated

- Serum and urine bilirubin levels — elevated
- Serum albumin value — usually less than 3.2 g/dl
- Serum triglyceride levels — may be elevated
- Serum electrolyte levels — may reveal hypokalemia or hyponatremia
- Computed tomography (CT) scan — visualizes tumors, dilated pancreatic ducts, calcification, or pseudocyst
- Abdominal ultrasound — may provide evidence of inflammation, edema, gallstones, calcified pancreatic ducts, abscess, organ enlargement, hematoma, or pseudocyst (cavities of exudate, blood, and pancreatic products that may expand and compress other organs)
- Abdominal X-rays — may reveal areas of calcification or adhesion, or identify indicators of reduced bowel motility
- Upper GI X-rays — may show enlarged pancreas or may reveal stomach displacement from pseudocyst formation
- Chest X-ray — may reveal diaphragmatic elevation if abscess formation or peritonitis is present; may identify areas of atelectasis or effusion
- I.V. cholangiography — used to rule out acute cholecystitis as cause of symptoms
- Paracentesis — may reveal elevated amylase levels or blood, both associated with acute pancreatitis

POTENTIAL COMPLICATIONS

- Hypovolemic shock
- Hemorrhage
- Acute respiratory distress syndrome
- Renal failure
- Pulmonary edema
- Myocardial infarction
- Peritonitis or sepsis
- Pleural effusion
- Abscess formation
- Hyperglycemia or diabetes mellitus
- Paralytic ileus
- Pseudocyst formation

CLINICAL SNAPSHOT

Pancreatitis

Major nursing diagnoses and collaborative problems	Key patient outcomes
CP: Risk for hypovolemic shock	Show stable vital signs, typically: heart rate, 60 to 100 beats/minute; systolic blood pressure, 90 to 140 mm Hg; and diastolic blood pressure, 50 to 90 mm Hg.
ND: Acute pain	Rate pain as less than 3 on a 0 to 10 pain rating scale.
ND: Risk for injury: Complications	Display no evidence of complications.
ND: Imbalanced nutrition: Less than body requirements	Maintain prescribed nutritional intake.

Collaborative problem

Risk for hypovolemic shock related to hemorrhage, fluid shifts, hyperglycemia, or vomiting

NURSING PRIORITY
Maintain fluid volume.

PATIENT OUTCOME CRITERIA
Within 24 hours of admission and then continuously, the patient will:
- have stable vital signs, typically: heart rate, 60 to 100 beats/minute; systolic blood pressure, 90 to 140 mm Hg; and diastolic blood pressure, 50 to 90 mm Hg
- display serum glucose, urine glucose, and ketone levels returning to normal
- have serum electrolyte levels returning to normal.

INTERVENTIONS	RATIONALES
1. *Monitor vital signs, fluid intake and output, hemodynamic pressures, and electrocardiography* findings according to appendix A, Monitoring standards, or unit protocol. Immediately report any findings indicating hypovolemia.	1. The damaged pancreas releases several substances that have systemic vasoactive effects. Kinins increase vascular permeability and cause vasodilation, increasing the likelihood of shock. Elastase and chymotrypsin cause necrosis and damage blood vessels, which may cause hemorrhage. In addition, pancreatic fluid and blood entering the peritoneum may cause chemical irritation of the bowel and bowel atony, resulting in fluid shift into interstitial spaces (third spacing) as fluid leaks out of the damaged intestine. Reduced renal blood flow may lead to acute tubular necrosis.
2. *Maintain I.V. access* through peripheral or central lines. Monitor I.V. fluid replacement, usually with lactated Ringer's solution, dextran, or albumin. If hemorrhage is suspected, anticipate and monitor transfusion, as ordered.	2. Rapid I.V. infusion of large volumes of fluid or blood is the primary immediate treatment indicated for hypovolemia. Untreated, hypovolemia quickly results in circulatory collapse and tissue death.
3. *Assess serum glucose* or fingerstick glucose and urine ketone levels every 4 to 6 hours or more frequently if severe hyperglycemia is present. Administer regular insulin, as ordered, and monitor and document effects.	3. Injury to the insulin-producing islet cells of the pancreas commonly decreases insulin production and causes at least transient hyperglycemia. If damage is severe, particularly if chronic pancreatitis is also present, overt diabetes mellitus may develop. Hyperglycemia may contribute further to functional hypovolemia as the body responds to the hyperosmolar state with further fluid shifts.
4. *Monitor serum electrolytes daily,* as ordered, including serum calcium. (See appendix C, Fluid and electrolyte imbalances.) Stay alert for characteristic signs of severe hypocalcemia: neuromuscular irritability and tetany.	4. Fluid shifts associated with acute pancreatitis may result in various electrolyte imbalances, including hypokalemia and hyponatremia. Hypocalcemia is a common finding, possibly caused by the bonding of calcium with fatty substances. Clinically significant hypocalcemia is associated with a poor prognosis.

*Italics indicate key interventions.

5. *Maintain continuous gastric drainage with low suction,* as ordered, preferably with a double-lumen tube. Administer anticholinergic medications, if ordered. Test gastric drainage for blood at least every 8 hours. Withhold food and fluids.

5. Draining gastric secretions removes a stimulus for pancreatic secretions, thus reducing the release of vasoactive substances and allowing the damaged pancreas to rest. A double-lumen tube is preferable for continuous suction because the air vent minimizes the risk of damage to the gastric mucosa. Anticholinergic use is controversial because such medication may contribute to ileus; some practitioners believe anticholinergics effectively reduce pancreatic secretions, but this is unproved. Withholding food and fluids prevents stimulation of gastric secretions.

6. *Administer I.V. dopamine (Intropin) or other vasopressor, as ordered,* if hypotension persists.

6. In acute pancreatitis, the release of myocardial depressant factor from the pancreas is thought to reduce cardiac output. Dopamine increases blood pressure and cardiac output by increasing heart rate and peripheral vasoconstriction. Low-dose dopamine (2 to 5 mcg/kg/minute) causes increased blood flow to renal arteries, thus increasing urinary output. The patient must be well hydrated prior to administration of any vasoactive agent.

7. Prepare the patient for surgery if hemodynamic parameters don't stabilize in response to therapeutic interventions.

7. Persistent shock indicates the need for surgical intervention to stop bleeding, relieve duct obstruction, drain an abscess or pseudocyst, or evaluate other possible intra-abdominal pathology

8. Additional individualized interventions: _____

8. Rationales: _____

Nursing diagnosis

Acute pain related to edema, necrosis, autodigestive processes, abdominal distention, abscess formation, ileus, or peritonitis

NURSING PRIORITY
Monitor, evaluate, and relieve pain and treat underlying cause.

PATIENT OUTCOME CRITERIA
Within 1 hour of the onset of pain, and then continuously, the patient will:
- rate pain as less than 3 on a 0 to 10 pain rating scale.
  Within 2 days, the patient will:
- upon request, state two recommended dietary or lifestyle changes.

INTERVENTIONS

1. *Assess pain,* noting location, character, severity, radiation, frequency, and any accompanying symptoms. Immediately report changes in pain quality or location, particularly if abdominal rigidity, reduced or absent bowel sounds, palpable abdominal mass, or other indications of generalized peritonitis or abscess occur. *See the "Acute pain" care plan,* page 32.

RATIONALES

1. Evaluating the nature of the patient's pain is essential for early detection of complications. Typically, the pain accompanying acute pancreatitis is severe, steady, and felt across the entire abdomen, and it commonly radiates to the back or flank. Tenderness on deep palpation may occur; however, the abdomen usually remains soft. Abdominal rigidity and reduced bowel sounds may indicate peritonitis; a mass may indicate abscess or pseudocyst. Prompt surgical intervention is warranted if these occur. The "Acute pain" care plan contains general interventions for any patient in pain.

2. Ensure that blood samples for serum amylase and lipase levels are obtained before administering analgesics.

2. Many analgesics, including meperidine (Demerol) and morphine, may elevate serum amylase and lipase levels, limiting the usefulness of these findings in diagnosis.

3. Medicate, as ordered, with narcotic analgesics, usually meperidine. Observe for increased pain after narcotic administration and collaborate with the physician to adjust pain control regimen, as indicated. Consider administering narcotic analgesics via patient controlled analgesia (PCA) pump.

3. The severity of pain associated with acute pancreatitis generally warrants narcotic analgesia. Morphine is thought to increase spasm of Oddi's sphincter and, thus, is usually avoided for these patients. However, other analgesics, including meperidine, may also have such effects to some degree. PCA maintains a steady level of narcotic analgesia in the blood stream.

4. Administer antacids, as ordered, clamping the gastric tube for 30 minutes after administration. When oral intake is resumed, avoid simultaneous administration of antacids with oral cimetidine (Tagamet).

4. Antacids reduce gastric acidity and associated discomfort; some products may also act to relieve flatulence and distention. Antacids may impair cimetidine absorption if given at the same time.

5. If the patient's condition permits, begin teaching dietary and lifestyle measures that reduce discomfort and help avert recurrence of acute attacks. Include family members in all teaching. Address the following considerations:
– need for lifelong avoidance of alcohol
– low-fat diet, depending on presence of gallbladder disease
– avoidance of caffeine or other substances linked to increased gastric secretions.

5. The patient's condition may limit teaching, but introductory material can lay the groundwork for more thorough discussion after the patient has stabilized. Alcohol is a common factor in the recurrence of acute pancreatitis, although the exact physiologic mechanism isn't known. Gallbladder disease may indicate the need for a low-fat diet to avoid exacerbating symptoms. Caffeine causes increased gastric acid secretion, thus increasing pancreatic activity.

6. Additional individualized interventions: _____

6. Rationales: _____

> ### *Suggested NIC Interventions*
> *Medication management; Pain management; Analgesic administration; Patient-controlled analgesia (PCA) assistance; Conscious sedation*

> ### *Suggested NOC Outcomes*
> *Comfort level; Pain control; Pain: Disruptive effects; Pain level*

Nursing diagnosis
Risk for injury: Complications related to pulmonary insults, hypovolemia, alcoholism, or other factors

NURSING PRIORITY
Prevent or detect and promptly treat complications.

PATIENT OUTCOME CRITERIA
Throughout the hospital stay, the patient will:
- perform pulmonary hygiene measures as instructed
- show no evidence of complications.

Hepatobiliary and pancreatic disorders

INTERVENTIONS

1. *Assess lung sounds, sputum production, skin color, and respiratory rate and effort frequently,* at least every 2 hours. Report decreased breath sounds, crackles, productive cough, increased respiratory rate or effort or other signs of respiratory complications immediately. Monitor arterial blood gas levels daily or as ordered and report abnormal results.

2. *Encourage deep breathing, coughing, incentive spirometer use, and position changes at least every 2 hours.*

3. *Assess for indicators of paralytic ileus, perforated viscus, or peritonitis,* such as reduced or absent bowel sounds, vomiting, increased abdominal distention, rigid or boardlike abdomen, and tympany.

4. *Monitor for signs and symptoms of pseudocyst development,* such as increasing tenderness, palpable mass, upper abdominal pain, diarrhea, and worsening of general condition despite interventions.

5. After surgical intervention, assess for and report indications of colonic, enteric, or pancreatic fistula. Observe for signs of a fistula opening to the skin: pinpoint openings at wound edges or within the wound, green or yellow wound drainage, and excoriated wound edges. If the fistula opens to the skin, collect drainage; provide frequent, meticulous skin care; measure drainage pH; and replace fluids and electrolytes as ordered. Also observe for signs of an internal fistula: electrolyte imbalance, hypovolemia, fever, and peritonitis. If the fistula is internal, anticipate surgery.

6. *Assess for and report indications of disseminated intravascular coagulation* (DIC), such as bleeding or oozing from wounds, drains, or puncture sites; purpura of the chest or abdomen; petechiae; hematuria; melena; or epistaxis. Guaiac test all drainage. See the "Disseminated intravascular coagulation" care plan, page 764, for details.

7. *Assess for early indications of renal impairment,* such as oliguria or anuria, increased urine osmolality, and elevated blood urea nitrogen level.

RATIONALES

1. The patient with acute pancreatitis is at increased risk for pulmonary complications from edema, fluid shifts, diaphragmatic irritation, and possible decreased myocardial contractility. Adult respiratory distress syndrome, pulmonary edema, pleural effusion, or pneumonia may occur. Endotracheal intubation and mechanical ventilation may be required for adequate oxygenation if respiratory impairment is a factor. Early intervention reduces the risk of significant hypoxic damage.

2. Abdominal distention, pain, and the use of narcotic medications may contribute to reduced chest expansion, predisposing the patient to pulmonary abnormalities. These measures help reexpand atelectatic areas and improve clearance of pulmonary secretions.

3. These conditions may arise as a result of chemical irritation of the bowel, necrosis, and abscess formation associated with acute pancreatitis. Without immediate surgical intervention, sepsis may develop.

4. Pseudocysts are pockets left in the pancreas after tissue necrosis, in which blood, tissue debris, and pancreatic secretions accumulate. They may resolve spontaneously, rupture and cause chemical peritonitis, or grow so large that they compress other organs. Intervention may include drainage with percutaneous aspiration guided by CT scan, or surgical resection.

5. Fistulas (abnormal openings from body cavities or hollow organs to other cavities or the skin surface) can result from impaired wound healing around surgical anastomosis sites or an anastamotic leak. Pancreatic fistulas are more common when necrosis of the head or midportion of the pancreas leaves behind a viable, pancreatic-juice-secreting tail. Because pancreatic secretions have a high enzyme content, drainage collection minimizes skin excoriation; it also helps predict fluid replacement needs. The pancreas produces bicarbonate, so an alkaline pH confirms pancreatic fistula drainage. Fluid and electrolyte loss from fistula drainage can cause dehydration, hypokalemia, and hyponatremia.

6. DIC is a major potential complication associated with acute pancreatitis, possibly from release of tissue fragments, toxins associated with shock, or other physiologic mechanisms. Early detection allows prompt treatment. The "Disseminated intravascular coagulation" care plan contains interventions for this disorder.

7. Hypovolemia may decrease renal perfusion and lead to acute renal failure. Renal impairment may also occur in acute pancreatitis when volume status is normal; the mechanism involved is unclear, but may involve DIC.

8. *Be alert for indications of alcohol withdrawal syndrome,* such as agitation, tremors, insomnia, hypertension, and anxiety. If alcoholism is a likely contributing factor to the patient's condition, consult with the physician regarding measures to prevent or minimize alcohol withdrawal syndrome.

9. Additional individualized interventions: _____

8. Because excessive alcohol intake is a common factor in acute pancreatitis, always consider the possibility of overt or hidden alcoholism. Untreated, the withdrawal syndrome may progress rapidly to seizures, hallucinations, hyperthermia, other severe complications, or death.

9. Rationales: _____

Suggested NIC Interventions
Surveillance: Safety

Suggested NOC Outcomes
Safety status: Physical injury

Nursing diagnosis

Imbalanced nutrition: Less than body requirements related to vomiting, pain, gastric suction, nothing by mouth (NPO) status, and impaired digestion

NURSING PRIORITY
Maintain or restore adequate nutritional intake.

PATIENT OUTCOME CRITERION
Throughout the hospital stay, the patient will maintain prescribed nutritional intake (see the "Nutritional deficit" care plan, page 138, for specific criteria).

INTERVENTIONS

1. *Assess nutritional status.* See the "Nutritional deficit" plan, for details.

2. Administer parenteral nutrition (PN), as ordered, and monitor the patient's response, including careful monitoring of glucose levels. Consult the "Parenteral nutrition" care plan, page 510, for details.

3. As the patient's condition permits, institute dietary teaching, as indicated, including:
– diabetic diet
– use of pancreatic enzymes, if recommended
– avoidance of alcohol and caffeine.

4. Additional individualized interventions: _____

RATIONALES

1. Baseline assessment of nutritional status is essential for planning appropriate maintenance or replacement therapy. The "Nutritional deficit" care plan provides details on evaluating nutritional status.

2. Oral nutrient intake during an acute pancreatitis episode tends to exacerbate pain and increase pancreatic activity. In the patient requiring prolonged NPO status, PN may be indicated to avert malnutrition. Increased protein and calories are necessary for healing and for maintenance of the body's immunologic defenses. In pancreatitis, glucose levels may be elevated because of damage to the insulin-producing islet cells in the pancreas; if hyperglycemia has been present, the additional glucose in the PN solution makes insulin dosage adjustment necessary. Enteral products may be contraindicated during the initial phases of pancreatitis.

3. Careful dietary teaching may help the patient avoid recurrences. A diabetic diet may be necessary because of reduced insulin production. Oral intake of pancreatic enzymes helps correct deficiencies. Alcohol and caffeine avoidance eliminates common triggers of acute pancreatitis.

4. Rationales: _____

Hepatobiliary and pancreatic disorders

> **Suggested NIC Interventions**
> *Diet staging; Nutrition management; Weight gain assistance; Fluid monitoring; Nutrition monitoring*

> **Suggested NOC Outcomes**
> *Nutritional status; Nutritional status: Food and fluid intake; Nutritional status: Nutrient intake; Weight control*

Discharge planning

DISCHARGE CHECKLIST

Before discharge, the patient shows evidence of:
❒ stable vital signs
❒ normal electrolyte values
❒ serum glucose controlled by medication, as needed
❒ pain controlled by medication
❒ absence of pulmonary or cardiovascular complications
❒ normal bowel sounds and elimination
❒ normal urine output
❒ adequate nutritional intake.

TEACHING CHECKLIST

Document evidence that the patient and his family demonstrate an understanding of:
❒ the disease, precipitating factors, and prognosis
❒ dietary considerations
❒ diabetic teaching, as required
❒ the signs and symptoms indicating recurrence or complications
❒ pain-relief measures.

DOCUMENTATION CHECKLIST

Using outcome criteria as a guide, document:
❒ clinical status on admission
❒ significant changes in status
❒ pertinent laboratory and diagnostic test findings
❒ fluid intake and output
❒ bowel function
❒ patient and family teaching
❒ discharge planning.

Associated care plans

- Acute pain
- Acute respiratory distress syndrome
- Diabetic ketoacidosis
- Disseminated intravascular coagulation
- Ineffective individual coping
- Knowledge deficit
- Nutritional deficit
- Parenteral nutrition
- Pulmonary embolism

References

Jordan, K. (ed). *Emergency Nursing Core Curriculum.* Emergency Nurses Association. Philadelphia: W.B. Saunders Co., 2000.

Lynn-McHale, D.J., and Carlson, K.K. American Association of Critical Care Nurses *AACN Procedure Manual for Critical Care,* 4th ed. Philadelphia: W.B. Saunders Co., 2001.

Mohan, V., et al. "Tropical Chronic Pancreatitis: An Update," *Journal of Clinical Gastroenterology* 36(4):337-46, April 2003.

Pezzilli, R., et al. "Early Activation of Peripheral Lymphocytes in Human Acute Pancreatitis," *Journal of Clinical Gastroenterology* 36(4):360-63, April 2003.

Shoemaker, W.C., et al. *Textbook of Critical Care* 4th ed. Philadelphia: W.B. Saunders Co., 2002.

Musculoskeletal and integumentary disorders

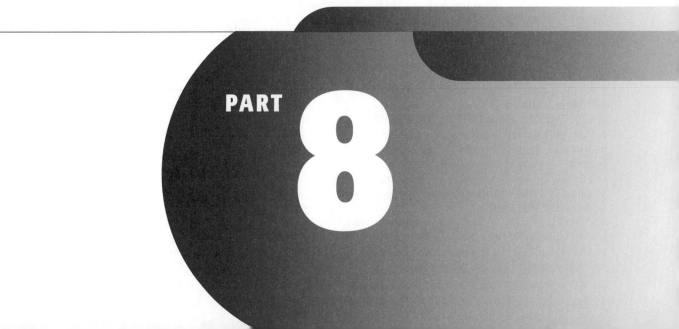

PART 8

Amputation

DRG INFORMATION

DRG 213   Amputation for Musculoskeletal System and Connective Tissue Disorders.

Mean LOS = 9.0 days

Additional DRG information: DRG 213 is only provided as a rough guideline. Determining the correct DRG for amputations depends on the underlying disease or type of trauma and the site and level of amputation.

Introduction

DEFINITION AND TIME FOCUS

Amputation is the surgical removal of an irreparably damaged or diseased limb. An amputation may be immediate because of the nature of an injury (from such factors as a motor vehicle crash or burn) or offered together with a prosthesis to improve function. The stump is closed with sutures or staples unless massive infection was present before surgery, in which case a guillotine-like surgery is performed and the wound is left unsutured. Traction may be applied to prevent skin retraction and to allow healing.

This care plan focuses on providing care after amputation of an upper or lower extremity. (See *Clinical snapshot: Amputation.*)

ETIOLOGY AND PRECIPITATING FACTORS

- Advanced peripheral vascular disease (especially when associated with diabetes mellitus, infection, or smoking)
- Trauma (such as that from crushing injuries, motor vehicle crashes, or industrial incidents)
- Thermal injury (such as that from frostbite, chemical exposure, or burns)
- Tumor
- Congenital anomaly

Focused assessment guidelines

NURSING HISTORY (FUNCTIONAL HEALTH PATTERN FINDINGS)

Health-perception–health-management pattern
- Treatment for diabetes mellitus, atherosclerotic arterial occlusive disease, or osteomyelitis
- The likelihood of amputation is significantly increased if patient is a smoker with peripheral vascular disease

Activity-exercise pattern
- Difficulty in ambulation if lower limb is involved, leading to an altered exercise pattern
- Severe pain associated with exercise in lower limbs if peripheral vascular disease is present

Sleep-rest pattern
- Interrupted sleep pattern associated with discomfort

Cognitive-perceptual pattern
- Tingling or burning sensation or paresthesia

Self-perception–self-concept pattern
- Difficulty accepting body image change
- Verbalized concern about returning to work

Role-relationship pattern
- Concern about relationships and rejection by others
- Verbalized fear of role change

Coping–stress tolerance pattern
- Failure to seek or follow medical treatment for problem, necessitating amputation
- Failure to deal with current experience

PHYSICAL FINDINGS

Integumentary
(in affected extremity)
- Shiny skin
- Skin atrophy
- Skin cool to touch
- Cyanosis or redness of extremities when in dependent position
- Thickened nails
- Stasis ulcer
- Edema
- Nonhealing wound
- Palpable mass

Cardiovascular
- Capillary refill time greater than 3 seconds
- Severe, cramping pain with exercise, usually relieved by rest
- Decreased pulse amplitude
- Diminished or absent peripheral pulses

Musculoskeletal
- Limited limb movement
- Limited ambulation
- Pain
- Contractures
- Protective holding of affected extremity

DIAGNOSTIC STUDIES

- Wound culture and sensitivity — if infection is present, may identify causative microorganism and identify appropriate antibiotics
- Complete blood count — elevated white blood cell count indicates infection
- Erythrocyte sedimentation rate — elevation indicates an inflammatory response
- X-rays — may reveal skeletal trauma, anomalies, or a mass

- Computed tomography scan — may reveal primary and metastatic tumors, infection, or trauma
- Arteriography and Doppler flow studies — may confirm circulatory inadequacy in major arteries or veins
- Biopsy — confirms presence of a malignant or benign mass
- Physical and occupational therapy evaluation — extent of gross and fine motor function determines ability to use assistive devices (such as prosthesis, crutches, and walker)

POTENTIAL COMPLICATIONS
- Hemorrhage
- Infection
- Flexion contracture
- Psychopathologic adaptation to limb loss

CLINICAL SNAPSHOT ✷

Amputation

Major nursing diagnoses and collaborative problems	Key patient outcomes
CP: Risk for hemorrhage	Have stable vital signs, typically: heart rate, 60 to 100 beats/minute; systolic blood pressure, 90 to 140 mm Hg; and diastolic blood pressure, 50 to 90 mm Hg.
ND: Acute pain	Rate pain as absent or mild on a 0 to 10 pain rating scale.
ND: Risk for infection	Show no signs or symptoms of infection.
ND: Risk for disuse syndrome (loss of joint function)	Demonstrate independent use of transfer techniques.
ND: Disturbed body image	Verbalize feelings and concerns regarding amputation.

Collaborative problem
Risk for hemorrhage related to amputation

NURSING PRIORITY
Maintain circulatory volume.

PATIENT OUTCOME CRITERIA
Within 1 day after surgery and then continuously, the patient will:
- have stable vital signs, typically: heart rate, 60 to 100 beats/minute; systolic blood pressure, 90 to 140 mm Hg; and diastolic blood pressure, 50 to 90 mm Hg.

Within 3 days after surgery, the patient will:
- have decreased wound drainage.

INTERVENTIONS

1. *Assess the surgical site** immediately upon the patient's arrival on the unit after surgery. Document your findings, including the type of dressing and a description of any drainage and closed drainage system.

2. *Observe and document signs of oozing on the dressing.* Reinforce the dressing as required. Don't remove the dressing until ordered. Document the amount of supplies used and the frequency of reinforcement.

RATIONALES

1. Baseline assessment permits comparison of data, which assists in the ongoing status evaluation. A drain or portable wound suction device may be in place to remove fluid or blood that might interfere with granulation. Observed drainage will be minimal and serosanguineous. Increased amounts of bright red drainage may indicate hemorrhage.

2. A small amount of oozing from the incision is normal. Documenting the supplies used and drainage characteristics helps other caregivers assess status changes. Initially, most postamputation dressings are pressure or pressure-cast dressings; premature removal may result in undesirable edema and bleeding.

---

*Italics indicate key interventions.

3. *Maintain an I.V. line.* Document its site, appearance, and patency.

4. *Keep a tourniquet at the bedside.* Apply it to the limb or apply direct pressure to the artery if significant bleeding occurs. Notify the physician immediately, remain with the patient until the physician arrives, and document the events.

5. Additional individualized interventions: _____
_____

3. Loss of circulating blood volume results in vessel constriction, increasing the difficulty of venipuncture. An established I.V. line provides a route for rapid fluid replacement, if necessary.

4. If hemorrhage occurs, immediate tourniquet application prevents significant blood loss and shock. If bleeding is severe, direct arterial pressure may be necessary. The patient may be frightened by the amount of blood lost; the nurse's presence can be reassuring.

5. Rationales: _____
_____

Nursing diagnosis

Acute pain related to postoperative tissue, nerve, and bone trauma

NURSING PRIORITIES

Relieve pain, provide reassurance, and teach about phantom limb phenomena.

PATIENT OUTCOME CRITERIA

Within 4 hours after surgery, the patient will:
- show no associated pain behaviors
- rate pain (with pain medication) as less than 3 on a 0 to 10 pain rating scale.
  Within 1 day after surgery, the patient will:
- verbalize understanding of phantom limb pain and sensation.
  Within 3 days after surgery, the patient will:
- decrease requests for pain medication.

INTERVENTIONS

1. *Provide standard nursing care related to acute pain.* See the "Acute pain" care plan, page 32.

2. *Monitor for pain continually.* Listen to complaints of discomfort and observe for tense posture, tightening fists, diaphoresis, and increased pulse rate. Have patient rate pain level using a pain rating scale.

3. *Document pain episodes,* noting location, characteristics, radiation, frequency, severity, and associated findings.

4. *When pain occurs, administer medication promptly* as ordered. Evaluate and document the patient's response. Taper the frequency of intramuscular medication administration after the 3rd or 4th postoperative day as ordered; substitute oral medication as ordered and as needed.

5. *Evaluate the dressing or cast for tightness* each time the patient complains of pain and every 3 to 4 hours. Document the findings. If circulation, sensation, or movement is impaired, notify the physician and reapply the dressing more loosely.

6. *Reposition the patient or the affected limb* every 2 to 3 hours. Document repositionings.

RATIONALES

1. The "Acute pain" care plan provides general guidelines and interventions for pain.

2. Pain is what the patient states it is; early detection and intervention promote patient comfort. Pain stimulates the sympathetic nervous system, resulting in physical symptoms.

3. Documentation provides a baseline to help others interpret pain-related behaviors.

4. Early administration of pain medication is more effective in controlling pain than is medication administered after pain becomes severe. Pain normally begins to diminish in intensity 3 or 4 days after surgery.

5. Decreased circulation causes tissue hypoxia and increases the pain response.

6. Pain increases with external pressure or fatigue. Changing position relieves pressure and the risk of complications from immobility.

7. *Gently massage the stump* every 4 hours after the surgeon removes the dressing. Avoid using emollients. Evaluate and document the patient's response.

7. Massage increases circulation to the traumatized area. Emollients can cause skin maceration.

8. *Explain the cause of phantom limb sensation and pain.* Inform the patient that this may last as long as 6 months (rarely longer), although phantom limb pain may arise again even years later.

8. Phantom limb sensation is the feeling or perception of the amputated limb's presence. Phantom limb pain, a separate phenomenon, is the awareness of pain in the amputated body part. Unfortunately, treatment methods for persistent phantom limb pain are of limited value. The cause of these relatively uncommon phenomena is unknown. Knowing that phantom limb sensation and pain are normal responses to amputation may reassure the patient.

9. *Use nonpharmacologic pain relief measures* between doses of pain medication and when the patient doesn't experience pain relief. Consider diversion, activity, back rubs, relaxation techniques, imagery, or cutaneous stimulation (such as counterirritation with oil of wintergreen). Consider consulting the physician about a transcutaneous electrical nerve stimulation device.

9. These methods decrease awareness of painful stimuli.

10. Additional individualized interventions:_____

10. Rationales:_____

Suggested NIC Interventions
Medication management; Pain management; Analgesic administration; Patient-controlled analgesia (PCA) assistance

Suggested NOC Outcomes
Comfort level; Pain control; Pain: Disruptive effects; Pain level.

Nursing diagnosis
Risk for infection related to impaired tissue integrity

NURSING PRIORITY
Promote wound healing.

PATIENT OUTCOME CRITERIA
By the time of discharge, the patient will:
- show no signs or symptoms of infection
- list signs of stump breakdown
- demonstrate stump-toughening exercises.

INTERVENTIONS

1. *Observe the incision line for redness, edema, or exudate* during each dressing change. Document all findings. If a plaster cast is in place, check for signs of tissue necrosis: "hot" spots, drainage on the cast, unrelieved pain, or foul odor.

2. *Protect the stump from contamination and trauma.* If the patient is incontinent, protect the limb with a plastic covering. Always use sterile technique during dressing changes.

RATIONALES

1. Assessment of the incision line during the first dressing change provides baseline data for future comparison. Histamine release causes the classic signs of inflammation. Diminished tissue perfusion, resulting from decreased circulation secondary to external pressure, causes cell death. Tissue necrosis results in pain, a sensation of local heat, drainage, and odor.

2. Exposing the stump to microorganisms increases the risk of infection. Trauma causes tissue death and slows healing.

3. *Always rewrap dressings securely but not tightly.* Don't apply tape to skin.

4. Encourage the patient to follow the prescribed diet. Document the patient's likes and dislikes, and assist with menu selection. Promote intake of foods high in protein, vitamins, calories, and minerals.

5. *After a dressing is no longer necessary, bathe the stump daily* with mild soap and water. Dry it thoroughly and leave it exposed to air twice daily for at least 20 minutes.

6. *Teach the signs and symptoms of stump breakdown.* Examine the stump daily for edema, redness, and skin breaks. Teach the patient to examine the stump regularly after discharge, such as during exercise or bathing.

7. *Teach stump-toughening exercises.* Have the patient push the stump against a soft pillow four to six times daily. Increase resistance gradually. Document progress.

8. Additional individualized interventions:_____
_____

3. Tight dressings may inhibit blood flow to the healing wound, reducing the availability of oxygen and essential nutrients. Tape can cause tissue trauma during removal.

4. Preexisting diseases, such as diabetes, may require that the patient follow a specific diet. Additional amounts of protein, calories, vitamins, and minerals are needed for wound healing.

5. Hygiene is essential to maintaining healthy skin that can tolerate a prosthesis. Moist skin allows maceration to occur.

6. Early detection of stump breakdown allows prompt treatment. Undetected complications jeopardize the patient's rehabilitation program and may make further amputation necessary.

7. Fragile, delicate skin won't withstand the pressure a prosthesis will apply. Toughening the skin prepares the patient to wear a prosthesis and reduces the chance of infection related to skin breakdown.

8. Rationales: _____
_____

Suggested NIC Interventions
Infection control; Infection protection; Incision site care; Wound care

Suggested NOC Outcomes
Infection status; Wound healing: Primary intention

Nursing diagnosis

Risk for disuse syndrome (loss of joint function) related to impaired physical mobility

NURSING PRIORITY

Maintain range of motion (ROM) in affected joint.

PATIENT OUTCOME CRITERIA

By the time of discharge, the patient will:
- display no signs of joint contracture
- demonstrate independent use of transfer techniques
- use assistive devices independently
- demonstrate muscle-strengthening exercises
- initiate discussion of follow-up plans.

INTERVENTIONS

1. *Promote joint extension.* Don't use pillows under a lower-extremity stump; raise the foot of the bed instead. Use slings and pillows under an upper-extremity stump.

2. *Place the patient in the prone position* for 30 minutes four times daily and for sleep (for lower-limb amputation), if not contraindicated.

RATIONALES

1. Proper positioning promotes venous return and decreases edema without causing flexion contracture.

2. The prone position facilitates normal joint alignment in extension.

3. *Don't allow the knee to bend over the edge of the chair or bed* if the patient had a below-the-knee amputation.

4. *Institute ROM exercises for the affected limb* two to three times daily, beginning on the 1st day after surgery. Gradually increase the frequency on subsequent days. Evaluate and document the patient's response.

5. *Provide a trapeze bar over the patient's bed.*

6. *Plan activities around the time of peak pain medication effect.* Be alert for medication effects that can decrease alertness or increase the patient's potential for injury.

7. Position items within the patient's reach at all times, particularly if an arm was amputated. (Include personal belongings, water, the telephone, and the call light.)

8. *Instruct a patient with a lower-extremity amputation to call for assistance when getting out of bed.* Keep the bed in the low position at all times.

9. *Teach transfer techniques* appropriate to the patient's amputation (for example, repositioning in bed, or bed-to-chair or bed-to-wheelchair transfer). Document the teaching and the patient's use of the techniques.

10. *Teach muscle-strengthening exercises* specific to the limb amputated. Gluteal-setting exercises for above-the-knee amputation, hamstring-setting exercises for below-the-knee amputation, and straightening the flexed proximal joint against resistance are examples of valuable exercises. Include exercises for increasing triceps strength, such as pushing against the bed with the fists and raising the buttocks off the bed. Tell the patient to exercise twice daily, gradually increasing frequency as muscle strength increases.

11. *Explain that stance will be altered.* Teach abdominal and gluteal muscle–tightening exercises to perform while standing. Have the patient practice balancing on the toes. Teach him to bend the knee and hop while holding onto a chair. Remain with the patient during these exercises.

12. Consult with the physician concerning physical therapy or occupational therapy referrals.

13. *After a lower-extremity amputation, reinforce ambulation skills* (unassisted ambulation, crutch walking, or use of assistive devices) learned during physical therapy. Encourage the patient to use these techniques whenever ambulating.

3. Allowing the stump to hang in a dependent position decreases venous return and increases edema. Flexion contracture may occur if the stump remains bent.

4. ROM exercises are directed toward maintaining normal joint mobility. Disuse can cause permanent shortening of the muscles, resulting in contractures.

5. A trapeze increases mobility in bed, allows the patient to be more independent, and prevents exclusive use of the heel or elbow for pushing when the patient moves (which may contribute to skin breakdown).

6. Pain prevents full participation in activities. Narcotics may cause orthostatic hypotension and fainting from vascular dilation.

7. Being able to reach needed items promotes independence and increases self-confidence in a patient with an altered self-concept.

8. Muscle weakness and impaired balance after a lower-limb amputation may result in an injury.

9. Learning transfer techniques reestablishes the patient's independence and promotes a feeling of security when moving in and out of bed.

10. Optimal muscle strength is required to maintain balance while using assistive devices, such as crutches, a walker, and a prosthesis.

11. An altered center of gravity requires increased muscle strength, balance, and coordination to compensate for the amputated extremity. Remaining with the patient during practice provides reassurance and helps prevent injury related to loss of balance.

12. Early intervention by physical and occupational therapy specialists increases the patient's rehabilitation potential.

13. Consistent use of learned methods increases the patient's skill, self-confidence, and awareness of their importance.

14. *Ensure appropriate referral for home care* if self-care ability or motivation is a problem. Emphasize the importance of ongoing rehabilitative follow-up.

14. Inadequate follow-up may lead to functional limitations or further limb compromise. Ongoing follow-up allows early detection of problems.

15. Additional individualized interventions: _____

15. Rationales:_____

Suggested NIC Interventions
Activity therapy; Energy management; Cognitive stimulation; Environmental management; Exercise therapy: Ambulation; Exercise therapy: Balance; Exercise therapy: Joint mobility; Exercise therapy: Muscle control

Suggested NOC Outcomes
Endurance; Immobility consequences: Physiological; Immobility consequences: Psycho-cognitive; Mobility level

---

Nursing diagnosis
Disturbed body image related to loss of a body part

NURSING PRIORITY
Promote acceptance of the loss of a body part.

PATIENT OUTCOME CRITERIA
By the time of discharge, the patient will:
- verbalize feelings and concerns regarding amputation
- participate in stump care
- express knowledge about the availability of a prosthesis (if appropriate).

INTERVENTIONS

1. Show an accepting attitude toward the patient. Anticipate a period of mourning for the lost limb. See the "Grieving" care plan, page 105.

2. Spend time with the patient each shift. Encourage verbalization of feelings about the amputation. Clarify areas of misunderstanding and reassure the patient that feelings are normal.

3. *Encourage family and friends to interact with the patient.* Explain the patient's response, if necessary. Refer family members to a counselor as needed.

4. Encourage the patient to look at the stump and to help in its care during the early postoperative period. Don't force this, however, if the patient is hesitant.

5. *Introduce the patient to others with similar amputations who have adapted successfully.*

RATIONALES

1. Acceptance helps the patient feel valued as an individual. The patient may experience various manifestations of the grieving process, such as directing anger and frustration toward staff and family members. The "Grieving" care plan contains detailed information on assisting with the grieving process.

2. Clarifying knowledge and encouraging expression of feelings helps the patient pass through the stages of grief.

3. The demonstration of acceptance and love by family and friends is essential to completing the grieving process.

4. Acknowledging the stump helps the patient recognize reality and promotes acceptance of an altered body image. Acceptance is a highly individualized process; forcing the patient to look at the stump may provoke undue distress.

5. Seeing someone who has adapted successfully demonstrates that the amputation doesn't have to interfere with a normal lifestyle. Peers may provide realistic encouragement and practical help in adapting to the change.

6. *Provide information about an appropriate prosthesis and its use,* reinforcing the teaching of the prosthetist or physical therapist.

6. Replacement of the amputated body part with a prosthesis gives the body a more normal appearance and increases the patient's participation in daily activities. Knowing that a prosthesis is available provides the patient with a goal to work toward.

A prosthesis may be applied immediately after surgery. This reduces residual limb edema, loss of muscle strength, and complications of immobility and also promotes healing through increased tissue perfusion at the operative site as a result of early ambulation. More important, immediate application of a prosthesis improves the patient's psychological outlook.

A prosthesis may also be applied 1 to 6 months after surgery. This occurs when wound healing is delayed because of infection, peripheral vascular disease, or the patient's debilitated status.

7. *Consult a counseling professional if the patient can't progress through the grieving process.* Consider a member of the clergy, psychiatric clinician, or social worker. See the "Ineffective individual coping" care plan, page 124.

7. Special assistance may be necessary to help the patient accept the amputation. Maladaptation to amputation may result in severe depression or suicidal behavior.

8. Additional individualized interventions:_____
_____

8. Rationales: _____
_____

Suggested NIC Interventions
Body image enhancement; Grief work facilitation; Anticipatory guidance; Coping enhancement; Self-esteem enhancement

Suggested NOC Outcomes
Body image; Grief resolution; Self-esteem

Discharge planning

DISCHARGE CHECKLIST
Before discharge, the patient shows evidence of:
- ❏ stable vital signs
- ❏ absence of pulmonary or cardiovascular complications
- ❏ a healing incision with no signs of swelling, redness, inflammation, or drainage
- ❏ absence of fever
- ❏ absence of contractures
- ❏ pain controlled by oral medication
- ❏ ability to tolerate diet
- ❏ ability to perform stump care independently or with minimal assistance
- ❏ ability to perform activities of daily living (ADLs) independently or with minimal assistance
- ❏ completion of initial physical therapy program with appropriate assistive devices
- ❏ ability to transfer and ambulate independently or with minimal assistance (with a lower-extremity amputation)
- ❏ adequate home support or referral for home care or to a rehabilitation setting if indicated by lack of home support system; inability to perform ADLs, stump care, and safe transfers; or continued need for physical therapy.

TEACHING CHECKLIST
Document evidence that the patient and family demonstrate an understanding of:
- ❏ underlying disease and implications
- ❏ all discharge medications' purposes, dosages, administration schedules, and adverse effects requiring medical attention (discharge medications are prescribed only if the patient has an infection or a preexisting condition such as diabetes mellitus; patient may be prescribed pain medication to be taken as needed)
- ❏ prescribed diet
- ❏ necessary equipment and supplies
- ❏ care of stump and prosthesis
- ❏ phantom limb sensation and pain
- ❏ signs of wound inflammation and infection that require medical attention
- ❏ prescribed exercises for the residual limb
- ❏ need for smoking cessation program (if appropriate)

Musculoskeletal and integumentary disorders

❏ name and telephone number of contact person for additional information or answers to questions
❏ date, time, and location of follow-up appointments
❏ how to contact the physician
❏ available community resources.

DOCUMENTATION CHECKLIST

Using outcome criteria as a guide, document:
❏ clinical status on return from surgery
❏ significant changes in status
❏ pertinent laboratory and diagnostic test findings
❏ pain at surgical site
❏ phantom limb pain
❏ phantom limb sensation
❏ pain-relief measures
❏ mobility and positioning
❏ dressing changes
❏ appearance of wound
❏ drainage devices
❏ I.V. line patency
❏ oxygen therapy
❏ nutritional intake
❏ psychological status
❏ physical therapy, occupational therapy, or both
❏ assistive devices, such as a walker, crutches, and prosthesis
❏ patient and family teaching
❏ discharge planning.

Associated care plans

- Acute pain
- Diabetes mellitus
- Grieving
- Ineffective individual coping
- Knowledge deficit
- Perioperative care

References

Hansen, S.T. "Salvage or Amputation after Complex Foot and Ankle Trauma," *Orthopedic Clinics of North America* 32(1):181-86, January 2001.

Hoover, T.J., and Siefert, J.A. "Soft Tissue Complications of Orthopedic Emergencies," *Emergency Medical Clinics of North America* 18(1):115-39, February 2000.

MacKenzie, E.J., et al. "Factors Influencing the Decision to Amputate or Reconstruct after High-Energy Lower Extremity Trauma," *The Journal of Trauma* 52(4):641-49, April 2002.

Mattox, K., et al. *Trauma*, 4th ed. New York: McGraw-Hill Book Co., 2000.

Peitzman, A.B., et al. *The Trauma Manual*, 2nd ed. Philadelphia: Lippincott Williams & Wilkins, 2002.

Pezzin, E.E. "Rehabilitation and the Long-Term Outcomes of Persons with Trauma-Related Amputations," *Archives of Physical Medicine and Rehabilitation* 81(3):292-300, March 2000.

Smeltzer, S.C., and Bare, B.G., eds. *Brunner and Suddarth's Textbook of Medical-Surgical Nursing,* 9th ed. Philadelphia: Lippincott Williams & Wilkins, March 2000.

Treat-Jacobson, D., et al. "A Patient-Derived Perspective of Health-Related Quality of Life with Peripheral Arterial Disease," *Journal of Nursing Scholarship* 34(1):55-60, 2002.

Walton, J. "Helping High-Risk Surgical Patients Beat the Odds," *Nursing* 31(3):54-59, March 2001.

Fractured femur

DRG INFORMATION

DRG 210   Hip and Femur Procedures, Except Major
Joint; Age 17 + with Complication or Comor-
bidity (CC).
Mean LOS = 6.8 days

DRG 211   Hip and Femur Procedures, Except Major
Joint; Age 17 + without CC.
Mean LOS = 4.9 days

DRG 212   Hip and Femur Procedures, Except Major
Joint; Ages 0 to 17.
Mean LOS = Not available

Introduction

DEFINITION AND TIME FOCUS

The femur, which connects the hip and knee joints, is
the longest and strongest bone in the body. Because of
its strength, most fractures of the femur are the result of
traumatic events involving considerable force.

The two primary classifications of femur fractures are:
- proximal end fractures, involving the portion of the femur that engages with the acetabulum (These fractures
may be further classified into two subtypes: intracapsu-
lar, involving the head and neck of the femur within the
hip joint, and extracapsular, involving the area from the
femoral neck distally to about 20″ [5 cm] below the lesser trochanter.)
- femoral shaft fractures, involving the distal portion of
the femur.

This care plan focuses on preoperative and postoperative care of the patient admitted to the hospital for treatment of a femur fracture. See the "Total joint replacement in a lower extremity" care plan, page 612, for more
information on fractures involving the hip joint. (See
Clinical snapshot: Fractured femur, page 560.)

ETIOLOGY AND PRECIPITATING FACTORS

- Proximal end fractures — fall injuries most common,
with osteoporosis a significant contributing factor in older patients
- Femoral shaft fractures — high-impact traumatic
events, most often in younger patients
- Related fractures of sacrum or lumbar spine

Focused assessment guidelines

NURSING HISTORY (FUNCTIONAL HEALTH PATTERN FINDINGS)

Health-perception–health-management pattern
- If older, history of coexisting medical conditions (such
as heart disease, diabetes, and hypertension) that caused
or contributed to the fall
- If younger, may be the first contact with an inpatient
setting

Activity-exercise pattern
- Ability to walk (in proximal end fractures) but more
typically, can't bear weight
- Inability to bear weight (in femoral shaft fractures)

Cognitive-perceptual pattern
- Severe, localized pain in the affected limb
- Numbness or tingling in the affected limb

Value-belief pattern
- Disbelief that injury is severe (in proximal end fractures); an older patient may insist that only pain relief is
necessary; may deny need for surgical intervention

PHYSICAL FINDINGS

Cardiovascular
- Edema at injury site or distally
- Tachycardia
- Hypotension
- If severe vascular involvement: absent pulse, reduced
pulse rate, or reduced or absent pulse amplitude in the
affected limb

Pulmonary
- Hyperventilation, tachypnea

Musculoskeletal
- Deformity at injury site (for example, external rotation
or shortening)
- Severe pain with movement of affected limb
- Ecchymosis
- Crepitus

Integumentary
- Diaphoresis
- Pallor (if significant blood is lost)

DIAGNOSTIC STUDIES

Diagnostic studies may reveal no significant abnormalities initially, unless related to a coexisting condition.
- Complete blood count — performed before surgery to
establish baseline; may reveal extent of blood loss associated with the injury (loss of up to 1.5 L may occur);
decreased hemoglobin and hematocrit values result from
dilution by crystalloid fluid replacement during resusci-

tation; white blood cell count may be elevated in response to injury

■ Blood typing and crossmatching — performed in preparation for blood replacement if significant blood loss is present or incurred during surgery

■ Chemistry panel — obtained before surgery to establish baseline and assess for underlying imbalances that may have contributed to the injury or that may affect intraoperative care (for example, potassium imbalances, which can cause increased cardiac irritability during anesthesia); blood urea nitrogen and creatinine levels evaluate renal function

■ Prothrombin time, international normalized ratio, and partial thromboplastin time — performed before surgery to establish baseline; usually are normal unless an underlying bleeding disorder is present or the patient is taking anticoagulant medication; older patients may be started on anticoagulant therapy after surgery to minimize the risk of thromboembolism

■ Urinalysis — performed for baseline evaluation of renal function

■ Serum drug levels — performed if medication overdose or noncompliance is suspected as contributing factor to injury

■ Femur X-ray — identifies location and type of fracture

■ Chest X-ray — routinely obtained before surgery to rule out associated injuries or preexisting conditions affecting surgical care (such as cardiomegaly and heart failure)

■ 12-lead electrocardiography (ECG) — obtained before surgery to establish baseline and to identify preexisting cardiac abnormalities, if any; may be especially significant in older patients or in those with blunt trauma to the chest (possible blunt cardiac injury) in addition to the leg injury

POTENTIAL COMPLICATIONS

■ Shock
■ Hemorrhage
■ Pulmonary embolism
■ Fat embolism
■ Thrombophlebitis
■ Aseptic necrosis of the femoral head
■ Nonunion of the affected portions
■ Osteomyelitis
■ Pneumonia
■ Arthritic deformities
■ Hemoglobin depletion related to iron depletion or deprivation

---

CLINICAL SNAPSHOT ☀

Fractured femur

Major nursing diagnoses and collaborative problems	Key patient outcomes
CP: Risk for preoperative complications	Have stable vital signs, typically: heart rate, 60 to 100 beats/minute; systolic blood pressure, 90 to 140 mm Hg; and diastolic blood pressure, 50 to 90 mm Hg.
ND: Risk for injury	Have no signs of excessive bleeding, neurovascular impairment, or infection.
ND: Deficient knowledge (home care)	Identify signs and symptoms of complications.

Collaborative problem

Risk for preoperative complications related to nature of traumatic injury

NURSING PRIORITIES

■ Prepare the patient to undergo surgery in optimal physical condition.
■ Prevent or identify and promptly treat preoperative complications.

PATIENT OUTCOME CRITERIA

Before surgery, the patient will:

■ have normal respirations or, if abnormal, receive treatment for respiratory problems
■ achieve stable vital signs, typically: heart rate, 60 to 100 beats/minute; systolic blood pressure, 90 to 140 mm Hg; and diastolic blood pressure, 50 to 90 mm Hg
■ have no uncontrolled bleeding
■ have neurovascular findings within expected limits
■ rate pain (with pain medications) as absent or mild on a pain rating scale
■ have received initial tetanus and infection prophylaxis, if indicated.

INTERVENTIONS

1. *Ensure adequacy of respirations.** Auscultate the lungs and note any evidence of unequal chest excursion, unequal or diminished breath sounds, pain on respiration, cyanosis, restlessness, or dyspnea. Report any respiratory difficulty to the physician immediately, and prepare to support ventilation or assist with insertion of chest tubes, if indicated.

2. *Assess for signs of bleeding and maintain circulatory volume.* Report increasing pulse rate, decreasing blood pressure, pallor, diaphoresis, or decreasing alertness. Establish and maintain an I.V. line as ordered, usually with 0.9 normal saline solution or lactated Ringer's solution initially. If an open fracture is bleeding, apply direct, continuous pressure to the area and notify the physician.

3. *Assess the limb's neurovascular status.* Note weakened or absent pulses, mottling, cyanosis, paresthesia, or loss of sensation. Compare pulse rates bilaterally. Avoid moving the limb unnecessarily. Report deficits to the physician immediately.

4. *Control pain.* Assess level of pain using a pain rating scale. Administer analgesics as ordered during the preoperative period, making sure all medications are noted on the surgical checklist. Apply cold packs to the fracture area. Maintain traction or splinting as ordered.

5. *If an open fracture is present, make sure tetanus and infection prophylaxis is considered before surgery.* Cover the wound with a sterile dressing.

6. *Prepare the patient for surgery, if indicated.* See the "Perioperative care" care plan, page 146, for details.

7. Additional individualized interventions:_____
_____

RATIONALES

1. High-impact events or forces, such as those that cause femoral fractures, have a high incidence of multisystem injuries, including chest trauma. Pulmonary or chest abnormalities may indicate tracheal injury, pneumothorax, rib fractures, or other complications. In older patients, preexisting medical conditions may involve cardiac or central nervous system functions, affecting respiratory capability and adequacy.

2. Femoral fractures are associated with significant blood loss because of the vascularity of long bones and the proximity of large vessels. The parameters noted are signs of shock and require immediate intervention. Intravenous infusions help replace fluids lost from bleeding; 0.9 normal saline solution or lactated Ringer's solution expands blood volume and replaces electrolyte losses. Active bleeding is controlled by direct pressure controls until it can be stopped surgically.

3. Blood vessels and nerves in the fracture area may be displaced or severed by bone fragments or by edema and deformity. Movement may cause further injury. Inadequate perfusion of the limb may result in permanent functional impairment or loss of the affected portion.

4. Pain contributes to increasing anxiety, stresses the cardiovascular system, and may contribute to increased muscle tension and associated displacement at the injury site. Noting medications on the checklist ensures that their effects are considered in the administration of anesthetics. Cold packs help minimize edema by causing local vasoconstriction. Traction and splints may help reduce muscle spasms and pain.

5. Tetanus immunization, if not current, should be updated because open wounds associated with trauma are considered tetanus-prone. Any break in skin integrity predisposes the patient to infection. Covering the wound minimizes further contamination from airborne bacteria.

6. Depending on the location and type of fracture, a femoral fracture may be treated with traction or a cast; however, surgery is usually the treatment of choice. Various surgical procedures are used to repair these fractures, including placement of a prosthesis, pins, intramedullary rods, or nails and bone grafts. Proper preoperative preparation helps minimize postoperative problems. General interventions for the surgical patient are included in the "Perioperative care" care plan.

7. Rationales: _____
_____

Musculoskeletal and integumentary disorders

*Italics indicate key interventions.

Nursing diagnosis

Risk for injury: Postoperative complications related to the initial trauma injury, surgical intervention, or immobility

NURSING PRIORITIES

Prevent, or identify and promptly treat, postoperative complications and promote healing.

PATIENT OUTCOME CRITERIA

Within 2 hours of arrival on the unit after surgery, the patient will:
- maintain vital signs within normal limits, typically: heart rate, 60 to 100 beats/minute; systolic blood pressure, 90 to 140 mm Hg; and diastolic blood pressure, 50 to 90 mm Hg
- have no signs of excessive bleeding, neurovascular impairment, or infection
- rate pain (with pain medication) as less than 3 on a 0 to 10 pain rating scale
- manage coughing and deep breathing well
- maintain proper positioning.
   Within 24 hours after surgery, the patient will:
- perform exercises as permitted
- show no signs of skin breakdown
- show no signs of embolism
- verbalize awareness of positioning restrictions
- take adequate food and fluids by mouth, if permitted.

INTERVENTIONS	RATIONALES
1. *Provide standard nursing care related to acute pain.* See the "Acute pain" care plan, page 32, and the "Perioperative care" care plan, page 146.	**1.** General guidelines for care of the surgical patient and for pain management are included in the "Perioperative care" and "Acute pain" care plans.
2. *Assess vital signs* according to postoperative protocol or more often if unstable. Check dressings and drains for bleeding. Report abnormalities in vital signs; excessive bleeding from the wound, surgical sites, drains, or graft sites; increasing edema; or ecchymosis. Assess for associated injuries if a high-impact trauma was involved.	**2.** As noted previously, femoral fractures may cause massive bleeding. Tachycardia and hypotension may indicate inadequate fluid replacement, excessive blood loss related to injury and repair, or other undetected injuries.
3. *Assess neurovascular status* at least once every hour and more often if compromised. Note weakened or absent pulses, mottling, cyanosis, paresthesia, loss of sensation, or a significant increase in edema after surgery. Be especially alert for signs and symptoms of compartment syndrome: increasing pain exacerbated by stretching, sensory deficits, paralysis, tense or hard swelling, or decreasing distal pulses. Notify the physician immediately if neurovascular status becomes impaired.	**3.** Careful assessment ensures prompt intervention should the limb's neurovascular status be compromised after surgery. Increasing edema may put pressure on surrounding vascular structures, impairing oxygenation of tissue. Immediate intervention is needed to restore circulation. Compartment syndrome is a complication caused by muscle swelling by which increased tissue pressure causes circulatory impairment and ischemia. This condition may occur immediately after injury or may develop over several days. Immediate treatment (fasciotomy) may prevent permanent damage.
4. *Maintain a patent I.V. line and administer fluids* as ordered, usually for at least 24 hours after surgery.	**4.** I.V. infusions replace fluid losses related to bleeding, restricted oral intake, preexisting dehydration, or tissue loss during surgery. Also, maintaining venous access allows administration of I.V. medication.

5. *Administer antibiotics,* if ordered. Observe the wound carefully and report increases in erythema or swelling, fever, purulent drainage, and other signs and symptoms of infection.

5. I.V. antibiotics are usually ordered during the initial postoperative period, particularly for the patient with an open fracture or increased susceptibility to infection. Infected bone wounds can be particularly serious; untreated, they may lead to osteomyelitis and bone disintegration. If the patient is already on antibiotic therapy when the infection develops, a different antibiotic may be indicated because the causative organism may be resistant to current therapy.

6. *Prevent complications associated with immobility.*

6. Immobility predisposes the patient to serious complications.

– Encourage the patient to perform gentle range-of-motion exercises for unaffected extremities; encourage alternate flexion and extension or quadriceps-setting exercises for the affected limb, as permitted. Increase activity level as permitted and as tolerated.
– Apply antiembolism stockings or sequential compression devices as prescribed.

– Exercise, as allowed, decreases venous stasis and helps maintain muscle tone.

– Antiembolism stockings or sequential compression devices increase venous return and may help prevent thrombus formation.

– Provide a trapeze to assist movement.

– A trapeze allows the patient to assist with repositioning.

– Encourage coughing and deep breathing hourly while the patient is awake.

– Pulmonary hygiene measures help prevent postoperative lung infections related to immobility, anesthesia, decreased respiratory effort, and accumulation of secretions.

– Urge adequate fluid intake, when allowed, forcing fluids unless contraindicated. Document intake and output.

– Forcing fluids helps maintain hydration, liquefy secretions, maintain renal function, and minimize risk of urinary infection from stasis. Documenting intake and output identifies fluid imbalances.

– Provide clean, dry bedding and a special bed or mattress as needed; reposition the patient at least every 2 hours, and provide frequent skin care, with special attention to bony prominences.
– Encourage verbalization of feelings. Provide diversionary activities.

– The immobilized patient is at increased risk for skin breakdown from constant pressure. A warm, moist environment encourages bacterial growth. Special beds and careful skin care prevent pressure ulcers.
– Prolonged immobilization contributes to depression, anxiety, and frustration. Verbalizing feelings to an accepting caregiver may help decrease stress. Diversionary activities decrease boredom and give the patient some sense of self-control.

– Consult the "Impaired physical mobility" care plan, page 111.

– The "Impaired physical mobility" care plan provides further information about this condition.

7. *Observe for signs and symptoms of embolism,* as follows:
– fat embolism — tachycardia, dyspnea, pleuritic pain, pallor and cyanosis, petechiae, crackles, wheezing, nausea, syncope, weakness, altered mentation, ECG changes, or fever; in the affected limb, pallor, numbness, and coldness to touch
– pulmonary embolism — sudden chest pain, dyspnea, tachycardia, cough, hemoptysis, anxiety, syncope, ECG changes, hypotension, and fever

7. The nature of the injury and the period of postoperative immobility predispose the patient to embolism.
– Fat embolism occurs most commonly with long-bone fractures, usually within the first 3 days after injury. The exact physiologic mechanism is unknown. Fat emboli may lodge in the lungs, heart, brain, or extremities and associated lipase release may cause tissue irritation.
– Pulmonary embolism is usually a later complication, occurring 10 to 24 days after injury. Signs may be related to obstruction from a blood clot that travels to the lungs and from reflex vasoconstriction.

Musculoskeletal and integumentary disorders

– thrombophlebitis — positive Homans' sign, pain in calf, swelling, and local redness in the limb. Report any signs to the physician immediately, and initiate treatment as ordered.

8. *Maintain proper immobilization of the affected limb,* depending on the fracture site and the type of repair. Usually, adduction, external rotation, and acute hip flexion should be avoided in a patient with a proximal end fracture; lateral pressure or overpulling with traction must be avoided in a patient with a femoral shaft fracture. Verify specific positioning orders with the physician.

9. *Observe for and immediately report any indicators of dislocation or necrosis:* sudden, sharp pain, shortening or rotation of the affected limb, or persistent muscle spasm.

10. Encourage adequate nutritional intake, especially of protein-rich foods and foods high in vitamins and minerals.

11. Additional individualized interventions: _____
_____

– Thrombophlebitis usually occurs in the lower extremities as the result of clot formation and obstruction of superficial veins, although thrombi can occlude major vessels as well. Immediate intervention is required because these complications may be life-threatening. Treatment may include ventilatory support, anticoagulants, or thrombolytic agents.

8. Movement at the fracture site may displace bone fragments and interfere with healing. Positioning of the affected limb depends on the fracture location and the surgical approach; common rules don't hold true for all patients. Verifying positioning recommendations and careful positioning prevent dislocation during turning.

9. Signs and symptoms indicating dislocation of the joint or necrosis of the femoral head in a patient with a proximal end fracture need immediate intervention to prevent permanent damage.

10. Healing requires additional calories and protein. Deficits in vitamins and minerals (particularly vitamins B and C and calcium) retard healing and can contribute to long-term bone disorders such as osteomalacia. Careful dietary assessment and monitoring may be required for the patient with impaired renal, hepatic, or pulmonary function.

11. Rationales: _____
_____

Suggested NIC Interventions
Infection control: Intraoperative; Surgical precautions; Teaching: Preoperative

Suggested NOC Outcomes
Risk control; Risk detection; Safety behavior: Fall prevention; Knowledge: Infection control

Nursing diagnosis

Deficient knowledge (home care) related to lack of exposure to information and ongoing care of injury after discharge

NURSING PRIORITIES
- Reinforce the physician's recommendations for home care.
- Identify potential problems related to home care and intervene as appropriate.

PATIENT OUTCOME CRITERIA
By the time of discharge, the patient and family will:
- verbalize and demonstrate understanding of positioning, activity restrictions, and care of the injury
- verbalize understanding of the recommended diet and medication regimen
- identify signs and symptoms of complications.

INTERVENTIONS

1. *Provide standard nursing care related to knowledge deficit.* See the "Knowledge deficit" care plan, page 129.

2. *Provide patient and family teaching related to specifics of fractured femur:* positioning, activity restrictions, cast care, crutch walking, use of a cane or walker, diet, complications, and medications. Verify recommendations with the physician, and incorporate teaching throughout the hospital stay.

3. *Assess available resources for home care and make appropriate referrals.*

4. Additional individualized interventions:_____
_____

RATIONALES

1. General interventions for patient and family teaching are included in the "Knowledge deficit" care plan.

2. Home care recommendations vary widely depending on the nature of the fracture and repair, the patient's age and condition, and any associated or preexisting conditions. The patient may be more responsive to continual, repetitive instruction during inpatient care routines than to a large amount of information just before discharge.

3. Depending on the factors mentioned above and on the family support structure, the patient may require home medical or nursing assistance or other follow-up care to ensure an uncomplicated recovery.

4. Rationales: _____
_____

> **Suggested NIC Interventions**
> Teaching: Procedure/treatment

> **Suggested NOC Outcomes**
> Knowledge: Treatment regimen

Discharge planning

DISCHARGE CHECKLIST

Before discharge, the patient shows evidence of:
- ❐ stable vital signs
- ❐ absence of pulmonary or cardiovascular complications
- ❐ healing incision with no signs of swelling, redness, inflammation, or drainage
- ❐ ability to control pain using oral medication
- ❐ absence of fever
- ❐ hemoglobin levels within expected parameters
- ❐ ability to perform activities of daily living (ADLs) independently or with minimal assistance
- ❐ ability to transfer independently or with minimal assistance
- ❐ ability to demonstrate weight-bearing restrictions when transferring
- ❐ ability to verbalize activity restrictions
- ❐ completion of initial ambulation training with the appropriate assistive device
- ❐ ability to tolerate diet
- ❐ normal voiding and bowel movements
- ❐ referral to home care if indicated by inability to perform ADLs or safe transfer technique or by continued need for physical therapy
- ❐ adequate home support or, if home support isn't adequate, ability to verbalize agreement with temporary placement in a nursing home to convalesce and continue physical therapy.

TEACHING CHECKLIST

Document evidence that the patient and family demonstrate an understanding of:
- ❐ site and nature of injury and repair
- ❐ implications of injury
- ❐ all discharge medications' purposes, dosages, administration schedules, and adverse effects requiring medical attention (discharge medications may include antibiotics, analgesics, anticoagulants, and antispasmodics)
- ❐ signs and symptoms of complications
- ❐ activity and positioning recommendations
- ❐ care of cast, if present
- ❐ dietary recommendations
- ❐ when and how to access the emergency medical system
- ❐ home care and follow-up referrals
- ❐ date, time, and location of follow-up appointments, and availability of transportation, if indicated
- ❐ how to contact the physician
- ❐ injury prevention strategies.

DOCUMENTATION CHECKLIST

Using outcome criteria as a guide, document:
- ❐ clinical status on admission
- ❐ preoperative assessment and treatment
- ❐ postoperative assessment and treatment
- ❐ significant changes in status
- ❐ pertinent laboratory and diagnostic findings
- ❐ pain-relief measures

Musculoskeletal and integumentary disorders

❏ recommendations for and tolerance of activity and positioning
❏ nutritional intake
❏ fluid intake and output
❏ bowel status
❏ patient and family teaching
❏ discharge planning.

Associated care plans

- Acute pain
- Geriatric
- Impaired physical mobility
- Knowledge deficit
- Perioperative care
- Pulmonary embolism
- Thrombophlebitis
- Total joint replacement in a lower extremity

References

Hoover, T.H., and Siefert, J.A. "Soft Tissue Complications of Orthopedic Emergencies," *Emergency Medicine Clinics of North America* 18(1):115-39, February 2000.

Mattox, K., et al. *Trauma,* 4th ed. New York: McGraw-Hill Book Co., 2000.

Norris, B.L., et al. "Pulmonary Dysfunction in Patients with Femoral Shaft Fracture Treated with Intramedullary Nailing" *Journal of Bone and Joint Surgery* 83-A(8):1162-68, August 2001.

Peitzman, A.B., et al. *The Trauma Manual,* 2nd ed. Philadelphia: Lippincott Williams & Wilkins, 2002.

Santy, J., and Mackintosh, C. "A Phenomenological Study of Pain Following Fractured Shaft of Femur," *Journal of Clinical Nursing* 10(4):521-27, July 2001.

Smeltzer, S.C., and Bare, B.G., eds. *Brunner and Suddarth's Textbook of Medical-Surgical Nursing,* 9th ed. Philadelphia: Lippincott Williams & Wilkins, 2000.

Trauma Nursing Care Course, 5th ed. Park Ridge, Ill.: Emergency Nurses Association, 2000.

Wolinsky, P., et al. "Controversies in Intramedullary Nailing of Femoral Shaft Fractures," *Instructional Course Lectures* 51:291-303, 2002.

Major burns

DRG INFORMATION
DRGs involving burns may be assigned based on degree of burn, extent of body surface burned, and presence of significant trauma, inhalation injury, or skin graft. The following are examples of some DRG classifications for burns.

DRG 504 Extensive Third-Degree Burn with Skin Graft.
Mean LOS = 29.6 days

DRG 505 Extensive Third-Degree Burn without Skin Graft.
Mean LOS = 4 days

DRG 506 Full-Thickness Burn with Skin Graft or Inhalation Injury with CC or Significant Trauma.
Mean LOS = 17.4 days

DRG 507 Full-Thickness Burn with Skin Graft or Inhalation Injury without CC or Significant Trauma.
Mean LOS = 8.6 days

DRG 508 Full-Thickness Burn without Skin Graft or Inhalation Injury with CC or Significant Trauma.
Mean LOS = 7.9 days

DRG 509 Full-Thickness Burn without Skin Graft or Inhalation Injury without CC or Significant Trauma.
Mean LOS = 4.6 days

DRG 510 Nonextensive Burns with CC or Significant Trauma.
Mean LOS = 7.5 days

DRG 511 Nonextensive Burns without CC or Significant Trauma.
Mean LOS = 5.0 days

Introduction
DEFINITION AND TIME FOCUS
A burn is a traumatic skin injury caused by exposure to heat, chemicals, or electricity. A burn's severity depends on its depth and the body surface area (BSA) affected. Partial-thickness burns can be superficial (first-degree), involving only the epidermis, or deep (second-degree), involving the epidermal and dermal layers of the skin. Because some epithelial tissue, such as hair follicles, is uninjured, the skin can regenerate. Full-thickness burns (third- and fourth-degree) involve the epidermis, dermis, subcutaneous tissues and, sometimes, underlying muscle, tendon, and bone. Full-thickness burns require skin grafting to heal.

The total BSA burned is estimated using the Rule of Nines or the Lund-Browder classification system. The burn's depth and area are used to determine the initial treatment and if admission to a burn unit is necessary. Treatment in a burn unit is indicated for patients with a partial-thickness burn involving more than 25% of BSA; a full-thickness burn involving more than 10% of BSA; burns complicated by trauma, chronic illness, or inhalation or electrical injuries; or burns affecting such special areas as the face, eyes, ears, hands, feet, or perineum. Treatment in a burn unit is also indicated for children younger than age 2 and adults older than age 60.

Minor burns can be treated in the emergency department or in the physician's office. Patients with moderate burns without complications can be treated in a general critical care setting. This care plan focuses on the patient admitted for treatment of superficial and deep partial-thickness burns involving more than 25% of total BSA. (See *Clinical snapshot: Major burns,* page 569.)

ETIOLOGY AND PRECIPITATING FACTORS
■ Occupational exposure to such elements as fuels, chemicals, electricity, or hot substances
■ Home exposure to such elements as stoves, hot water, electricity, heaters, chemicals, matches, or cigarettes
■ Outdoor exposure to such elements as ultraviolet light, lightning, barbecues, or flammable liquids
■ High-risk populations, such as young children, older adults, drug or alcohol abusers, chronically ill or debilitated patients, or those working in high-risk jobs

Focused assessment guidelines
NURSING HISTORY (FUNCTIONAL HEALTH PATTERN FINDINGS)
Health-perception–health-management pattern
■ High occupational risk for burns
■ High-risk activity that caused the burn
■ Chronic illness or debilitation
Nutritional-metabolic pattern
■ Thirst
■ Nausea, vomiting, and loss of appetite
■ Feelings of abdominal fullness
Elimination pattern
■ Decreased or absent urination
Activity-exercise pattern
■ Pain and stiffness when moving involved area
■ Difficulty breathing at rest and during movement
Cognitive-perceptual pattern
■ Pain
■ Repeated discussion of the circumstances of the burn, or confusion and loss of memory about burn incident

Self-perception–self-concept pattern
- Fear of disfigurement or loss of body part
- Fear of dying

Role-relationship pattern
- Concern about whereabouts and condition of others involved in the burn incident
- Fear about maintaining role in family and in relationships
- Concern over effects of injury on family
- Fear about not being able to work again

Sexuality-reproductive pattern
- Fear about future sexual performance
- Fear about lack of sexual attractiveness because of injury

Coping–stress tolerance pattern
- Initial lack of concern about burn
- Fear and anxiety
- Expressed feelings of being overwhelmed by burn

Value-belief pattern
- Expressed need to see member of clergy

PHYSICAL FINDINGS
Physical findings may vary depending on the burn's type, depth, surface area, and location.

Pulmonary
- Tachypnea, dyspnea, shortness of breath on exertion
- Soot in nostrils or sputum, with an inhalation injury
- Stridor
- Wheezing
- Hoarse voice
- Diminished lung sounds
- Mucosal edema, vesicles, redness

Cardiovascular
- Tachycardia
- Hypotension
- Arrhythmias
- Pale, clammy, diaphoretic, or cool skin
- Cardiac arrest (from an electrical injury) with ventricular fibrillation, chest pain, or cardiac irritability

Neurologic
- Agitation
- Memory loss
- Confusion
- Headache
- Mentation changes

Gastrointestinal
- Decreased or absent bowel sounds
- Distention
- Vomiting
- Dry mouth and mucous membranes

Genitourinary
- Oliguria or anuria
- Cloudy or tea-colored urine

Musculoskeletal
- Pain and stiffness on movement of affected areas
- Tetany (from an electrical injury) and bone fractures caused by tetany or fall

Integumentary
- Bright red to pink color, glistening blisters, blanching on pressure, and pain (with a superficial partial-thickness burn)
- Pink to white color, blanching, pain, sensitivity to pressure, and blisters (with a deep partial-thickness burn)
- White, gray, brown, or black skin color (with a full-thickness burn); eschar (coagulated and necrotic tissue) formation; no pain or pressure sensations; no blanching; dry, easily pulled out hair
- Massive edema
- Hypothermia
- Shivering

DIAGNOSTIC STUDIES
- Complete blood count — determines red blood cell count, hemoglobin level, and hematocrit, reflecting any blood loss or destruction and indicating the blood's oxygen-carrying ability; the white blood cell (WBC) count reflects the ability of the WBCs to respond to the inflammatory process; baseline data and serial evaluations may reflect the seriousness of the fluid shifts and cell destruction accompanying major burns
- Serum electrolyte level — monitors fluid, electrolyte, and acid-base status; hyperkalemia initially occurs because of the release of potassium into the serum during cell destruction and the hemoconcentration caused by fluid shifts into the interstitium; hypokalemia may occur during the 2nd day after injury as electrolytes are excreted into the urine; levels of other electrolytes may be low during the initial period after injury because of the massive shifts of fluid and electrolytes into the interstitium
- Blood glucose level — monitors the effect of the catabolic burn state on sugar metabolism and insulin production
- Blood urea nitrogen and creatinine levels — monitor the adequacy of kidney function; acute tubular necrosis is a common complication after major tissue destruction
- Clotting time (prothrombin time/international normalized ratio and partial thromboplastin time) — prolonged clotting time may reflect coagulation problems associated with major tissue destruction
- Serum proteins (albumin and globulin) and serum osmolality — may reflect movement of intravascular colloids in and out of the interstitium
- Arterial blood gas (ABG) values — monitor oxygenation, ventilation, and acid-base status, especially with a suspected inhalation injury; initially, ABG values may reveal respiratory alkalosis, reflecting hyperventilation; later, metabolic acidosis, reflecting hypoxemia and shock
- Carboxyhemoglobin level — may be elevated, confirming carbon monoxide poisoning and smoke inhalation

- Urinalysis, specific gravity, urine electrolytes, and urine myoglobin levels — monitor kidney status; total urine output monitors hydration status
- Blood and tissue cultures — provide baseline data and monitor infections
- Chest X-ray — usually normal at first; in 1 to 2 days, may reveal atelectasis or pulmonary edema
- Electrocardiogram — may reveal arrhythmias
- Ventilation-perfusion pulmonary scan — may reveal areas of nonventilation and nonperfusion
- Bronchoscopy — may reveal abnormalities of the bronchial tree such as redness, blistering, edema, or the presence of soot
- Tissue biopsies and repeat cultures — may reveal excessive wound contamination

POTENTIAL COMPLICATIONS

- Hypovolemic shock
- Cardiac arrhythmias
- Cardiac arrest
- Respiratory arrest
- Atelectasis, pneumonia
- Pulmonary edema
- Infection, sepsis, septic shock
- Acute tubular necrosis
- Acute renal failure
- Conversion of partial-thickness burns to full-thickness burns
- Contractures
- Loss of mobility and function
- Scarring
- Social and emotional isolation
- Hematologic disorders

CLINICAL SNAPSHOT ✳

Major burns

Major nursing diagnoses	Key patient outcomes
Risk for injury	Display minimal or no continuing tissue damage.
Impaired gas exchange	Maintain a patent airway and show no signs of respiratory distress.
Deficient fluid volume	Have stable vital signs, typically: heart rate, 60 to 100 beats/minute; systolic blood pressure, 90 to 140 mm Hg; and diastolic blood pressure, 50 to 90 mm Hg.
Ineffective tissue perfusion (peripheral)	Display signs of adequate tissue perfusion such as warm, dry skin.
Risk for infection	Have no signs of infection.
Acute pain	Rate pain as absent or mild on a 0 to 10 pain rating scale.
Risk for impaired skin integrity	Display an intact and healing graft.
Imbalanced nutrition: More than body requirements	Manifest minimal or no signs of imbalanced nutrition.
Impaired physical mobility	Display active ROM of affected extremity.
Disturbed body image	Express fears and concerns openly.

Nursing diagnosis
Risk for injury related to continued exposure to heat or chemicals

NURSING PRIORITY
Stop the burn from expanding.

PATIENT OUTCOME CRITERIA
Within the 1st hour after admission, the patient will:
- display minimal or no continuing tissue damage, such as additional areas of redness, blistering, or sensation loss
- manifest no signs of chemical residue on skin.

INTERVENTIONS

1. *Remove any jewelry, belts, coins, or other metal objects from the patient and then immediately flush the burn with cool water for 10 to 15 minutes.* * Document your actions.

2. *For a chemical burn, quickly remove the patient's clothes, brush off dry chemicals, and flush the burns with large amounts of water.* Observe the site for chemical residues. After flushing, use a neutralizer, if appropriate, on any remaining chemicals; consult a burn center or poison control center for the appropriate agent. Assess the site hourly and as needed for continuing damage, such as spreading redness, blistering, or loss of sensation. Document your findings.

3. *Temporarily cover the flushed burn with a clean or sterile dressing or sheet* while other interventions continue.

4. Additional individualized interventions:_____

_____

RATIONALES

1. Metal items retain heat and permit continued thermal burning. Immediate flushing with cool water will cool the tissue and may limit the damage. Prolonged flushing or using ice water may cause such complications as arrhythmias, hypothermia, or shock.

2. Clothes may contain chemical residues and should be removed to prevent further injury. Thorough flushing with water will remove most chemicals. Neutralization may be helpful, but flushing is a higher initial priority than is finding an appropriate neutralizer. Some chemicals, such as alkali, may continue to cause damage even when neutralized, making ongoing assessments necessary.

3. Covering the burn may limit contamination and decrease pain from air exposure. Further burn care, such as debridement and application of topical antibiotics, has a low priority compared with stabilization of airway, breathing, and circulation.

4. Rationales: _____

_____

Suggested NIC Interventions
Surveillance: Safety

Suggested NOC Outcomes
Safety status: Physical injury

Nursing diagnosis

Impaired gas exchange related to airway burns and carbon monoxide inhalation

NURSING PRIORITY

Promote ventilation and gas exchange.

PATIENT OUTCOME CRITERIA

Within 24 hours of admission, the patient will:
- maintain a patent airway
- display no signs of respiratory distress
- display improving breath sounds
- remain alert and oriented.

INTERVENTIONS

1. *Maintain a patent airway.* Anticipate the possible need for endotracheal intubation and mechanical ventilation.

RATIONALES

1. Airway burns or inhalation of hot air can cause laryngospasm, progressive edema, and rapid airway occlusion up to 8 hours after the burn. Intubation is usually performed before progressive edema occludes the airway.

---

*Italics indicate key interventions.

2. *Assess the patient's respiratory status* on admission, then every 15 minutes until stable, then every 1 to 2 hours. Monitor respiratory rate; chest movements; use of accessory muscles; signs of anxiety or restlessness; color; breath sounds; adventitious sounds, such as crackles, gurgles, or wheezes; hoarseness when speaking; and soot around the nostrils. Notify the physician and document findings. Be prepared to assist with chest wall escharotomy, if necessary.

2. Abnormal findings, including hoarseness, crackles, wheezes, gurgles, signs of hypoxemia, restlessness, and soot around the nostrils, may indicate an inhalation injury and impending respiratory failure. Circumferential chest burns can restrict chest wall expansion and require escharotomy to allow ventilation.

3. *Monitor oxygenation closely.* Monitor pulse oximetry oxygen saturation levels continuously for 24 hours and then every 2 hours or as needed. Monitor ABG values initially and then every shift and as needed for changes in respiratory status. Monitor initial and serial carboxyhemoglobin levels. Document and notify physician of abnormalities.

3. Pulse oximetry monitors oxygen saturation noninvasively. ABG values reflect general oxygenation and acid-base levels. Low oxygen and high carbon dioxide levels may indicate a need for oxygen therapy or mechanical ventilation. Carbon monoxide interferes with oxygen transport because of its strong affinity for hemoglobin. Carboxyhemoglobin levels reflect the amount of abnormal hemoglobin present.

4. *Provide 100% humidified oxygen therapy,* as needed and ordered, especially for smoke inhalation or respiratory distress. Document oxygen administration.

4. Oxygen therapy may be required during the initial postinjury period to maintain desirable ABG levels, help eliminate carbon monoxide, and assist burn healing.

5. *Obtain initial and serial chest X-rays* as ordered.

5. Pulmonary involvement may not appear on X-ray for up to 24 hours.

6. *Encourage deep-breathing and coughing exercises* every hour and as needed. Assist with incentive spirometer use. Document pulmonary hygiene measures.

6. Regular deep-breathing and coughing exercises promote lung expansion, mobilize secretions, and prevent atelectasis. Incentive spirometry encourages deep inspiratory efforts that expand the alveoli more effectively than forceful expiratory efforts.

7. *Administer bronchodilators* every 4 to 8 hours, if ordered. Document their use.

7. Bronchodilators may interrupt bronchospasms and counteract the narrowing effect of airway edema.

8. *Monitor sputum characteristics.* Assess the amount, color, and consistency of sputum, including the presence of soot, every shift. Notify the physician and document your findings.

8. Soot in the sputum may confirm an inhalation injury. Excessive sputum may indicate an infection.

9. *Assist with bronchoscopy,* if ordered.

9. Bronchoscopy is used diagnostically to locate soot in smaller airways, airway burns, and pulmonary inflammation. It's also used therapeutically to remove soot and secretions, minimizing the risk of later infection and atelectasis.

10. *After stabilization, assist with intermittent positive-pressure breathing* (IPPB) therapy every 4 hours, if ordered. Document all treatments.

10. IPPB therapy promotes lung expansion by the deep delivery of bronchodilators and positive pressure breaths.

11. Additional individualized interventions: _____

11. Rationales: _____

Suggested NIC Interventions
Acid-base management; Electrolyte management; Laboratory data interpretation; Oxygen therapy; Ventilation assistance; Airway management; Respiratory monitoring; Embolus care: Pulmonary; Hemodynamic regulation; Vital signs monitoring

Suggested NOC Outcomes
Electrolyte and acid-base balance; Respiratory status: Gas exchange; Respiratory status: Ventilation; Tissue perfusion: Pulmonary; Vital signs status

Musculoskeletal and integumentary disorders

Nursing diagnosis

Deficient fluid volume related to movement of vascular fluids to the interstitium and water evaporation from burns

NURSING PRIORITY
Maintain vascular fluid volume.

PATIENT OUTCOME CRITERIA
Within 24 hours of admission, the patient will:
- maintain stable vital signs, typically: heart rate, 60 to 100 beats/minute; systolic blood pressure, 90 to 140 mm Hg; and diastolic blood pressure, 50 to 90 mm Hg
- have a urine output of 50 to 100 ml/hour
- stay within normal ranges for urine specific gravity, serum electrolyte levels, serum osmolality, and hematocrit
- have no observable changes in mentation.
  Within 48 to 72 hours of admission, the patient will:
- manifest a weight loss of no more than 2% per day.

INTERVENTIONS

1. *On admission, place one or two large-bore I.V. lines* in large veins in the arms, as ordered, using sterile technique. Document your actions.

2. *Collaborate with the physician on fluid replacement therapy.* Administer fluids, as ordered, and document their use.
– On admission, assess the patient's fluid needs. Use the Rule of Nines or the Lund-Browder classification system to determine the total BSA burned; use a fluid replacement formula, preferably the Parkland formula (4 ml lactated Ringer's solution × kg body weight × % total BSA), to determine the volume of fluid needed in the first 24 hours after injury.
– Give crystalloid fluid replacements during the first 24 hours after injury. According to the Parkland formula, administer half the volume in the first 8 hours, a quarter in the next 8 hours, and a quarter in the last 8 hours.
– After 24 to 48 hours, administer colloids and dextrose in water solutions.

3. *Assess adequacy of fluid replacement* every 1 to 2 hours and as needed, including vital signs, urine output, urine specific gravity, mentation, weight, serum electrolytes and osmolality, and hematocrit. Document your findings.

4. *Assess serum electrolyte levels and administer replacements* as ordered. Document your actions. See appendix C, Fluid and electrolyte imbalances, for general assessments and interventions.

RATIONALES

1. Large I.V. access lines are needed to give the large amount of fluids required during the fluid resuscitation period.

2. Appropriate fluid therapy is critical to the patient's survival.

– Fluid replacement formulas, in conjunction with the total BSA burned, estimate the fluid replacement needed every 24 hours. Numerous fluid replacement formulas are available. The American College of Surgeons and the American Burn Association recommend the Parkland formula.

– Large amounts of crystalloid fluids are needed to replace the massive amounts of vascular fluids that leak into the interstitium during the first 24 hours, a result of inflammation and increased capillary permeability.
– After the capillary membranes stabilize, colloids such as plasma can be administered to replace colloid losses. Dextrose in water solutions is also given to replace evaporative fluid loss and as a maintenance solution.

3. Stable vital signs, urine output (50 to 100 ml/hour), specific gravity and osmolality, mental status, serum electrolyte levels, and hematocrit all reflect adequate fluid replacement. Diuresis commonly begins on the 3rd day after injury. A weight loss of less than 2% per day during this time reflects adequate fluid replacement.

4. During the first 24 to 48 hours, electrolytes follow the fluid shifts into the interstitium, reducing the amounts available in the intravascular areas. Electrolyte replacement may be necessary except for potassium, whose serum levels increase because of cell destruction during the immediate postburn period. Careful monitoring guides electrolyte replacement. The Fluid and electrolyte imbalances appendix includes general assessments and interventions for electrolyte imbalances.

5. *After fluid replacement is complete and the patient's GI function returns, begin enteral feedings and remove the I.V. lines* as ordered. Document your actions.

6. Additional individualized interventions:_____
_____

5. Enteral feedings should begin as soon as possible to decrease the risk of infection at the I.V. insertion sites.

6. Rationales: _____
_____

Suggested NIC Interventions
Acid-base management; Fluid and electrolyte management; Fluid monitoring; Hypovolemia management; Intravenous (I.V.) therapy

Suggested NOC Outcomes
Electrolyte and acid-base balance; Fluid balance; Hydration

Nursing diagnosis

Ineffective tissue perfusion (peripheral) related to circumferential eschar formation on arms and legs, compartment syndrome, or vascular disruption

NURSING PRIORITY
Maintain adequate tissue perfusion.

PATIENT OUTCOME CRITERIA
Within 1 to 2 days of admission, the patient will:
- display signs of adequate tissue perfusion distal to the burned area, such as pink color, capillary refill less than 3 seconds, normal sensation, adequate function, minimal pain, and warm, dry skin
- display minimal bleeding or other complications at eschar site.

INTERVENTIONS

1. *When possible, elevate burned areas* but not above the level of the heart.

2. *Assess tissue perfusion distal to the burn site* every 1 to 2 hours, noting color, temperature, capillary refill, pulses, sensation, function, and pain. Notify the physician of and document any abnormalities.

3. *Assist the physician in performing an escharotomy,* if necessary. Assess the escharotomy site for bleeding and circulation return. Apply dressings to the site. Document your actions.

4. *If ordered, apply proteolytic enzymes to eschar.* Assess and document their effect.

5. Additional individualized interventions:_____
_____

RATIONALES

1. Elevation may decrease edema by using gravity to optimize venous return.

2. As eschar hardens, it may constrict circulation, particularly if it's circumferential. The patient with arm or leg burns is also at great risk for compartment syndrome, in which edema increases pressure in a fascial compartment and compresses nerves, blood vessels, and muscle. Early recognition of impaired circulation allows early intervention and minimizes the risk of permanent damage.

3. Incisions across areas of eschar formation release tissue tension and allow circulation to return to constricted areas. Assessment provides for early identification and correction of complications.

4. Proteolytic enzymes selectively digest necrotic tissue. By softening the eschar, they decrease its constricting effects.

5. Rationales: _____
_____

Musculoskeletal and integumentary disorders

Nursing diagnosis

Risk for infection related to loss of protective integument, exposure to contamination, decreased perfusion, and impaired immunologic response

NURSING PRIORITIES

- Protect the burn.
- Prevent or minimize infection.

PATIENT OUTCOME CRITERIA

Within 7 days of admission, the patient will:

- display clean and healing superficial burns, including scab formation
- display development of red granulation tissue over deeper partial-thickness wounds that are also free from odor, purulent drainage, and elevations or depressions
- display no complications of topical antibiotic use, such as pain, leukopenia, tissue damage, electrolyte or fluid loss, and secondary infections
- display intact wound covers
- manifest vital signs, WBC count, urine output, and mentation within normal ranges.

INTERVENTIONS	RATIONALES
1. *Explain the purpose and methods of burn care* to the patient and family.	**1.** Understanding the purpose of wound care may help the patient cope with the inevitable pain such care causes, while understanding the general methods may decrease fear of the unknown. Involving family members in teaching and care, when appropriate, acknowledges their learning needs and the importance of their emotional support to the patient.
2. *Use strict sterile technique,* including the wearing of cap, mask, gown, and sterile gloves, during all burn care. Wash the burn once or twice daily with a mild soap or normal saline solution. A hydrotherapy tub, shower stretcher, or basins at the bedside may be used. Use a gentle circular scrubbing motion. Debride with scissors, if necessary. Shave hair over involved areas, except for the eyebrows. Rinse with water. Document your actions.	**2.** To reduce the risk of infection, strict sterile technique must be used when the burn is uncovered. Regular washing and debridement removes dead tissue and stimulates the development of granulation tissue, which serves as the base for skin grafts. Shaving excess hair removes a medium for bacterial growth. Eyebrows aren't shaved because they may not grow back, leaving the patient with an odd facial appearance.
3. *During washing and debridement, assess the burn* for color, drainage, size, odor, elevations or depressions, and pain. Document your findings.	**3.** Regular assessment may identify early signs of infection and allow timely treatment.

4. *Apply topical antibiotics,* if ordered, after washing and debridement, typically silver nitrate, mafenide acetate solution, Sulfamylon solution, silver sulfadiazine (Silvadene), or povidone-iodine (Betadine). Use sterile technique including the wearing of mask, cap, gown, and sterile gloves. Cover the burn with gauze or stretch bandages after applying antibiotics. Monitor for medication-related complications, such as pain, leukopenia, tissue damage, or electrolyte depletion. If signs of medication-related complications occur, notify the physician and document your findings.

4. Topical antibiotics are commonly used to prevent massive bacterial colonization of burns from the patient's skin flora or contaminants. Strict sterile technique reduces the risk of infection. Monitoring for adverse effects or complications of antibiotic therapy helps avoid further compromise of the patient's status.

5. *Leave partial-thickness burns exposed to air,* if ordered. Document scab formation and condition of the burn.

5. Partial-thickness burns may heal in a week without complications when left exposed to air.

6. *Monitor temporary wound covers,* such as biologic, biosynthetic, or synthetic dressings, if used. Change as needed, observing for infection and excessive exudate. Remove excess liquid as necessary. Document your actions.

6. Temporary wound covers used early in treatment prevent infection and evaporative losses and promote granulation tissue development. The dressings are left in place for varying amounts of time. Usually, excessive exudate should be removed to enhance the dressing's adherence.

7. *Maintain patient warmth* during washing, debridement, and dressing changes. Limit procedures to 30 minutes or less. Document the procedure and the patient's tolerance.

7. Evaporative water loss during procedures may increase the risks of volume deficit, electrolyte loss, and shock.

8. *Assist in obtaining needle biopsy cultures* from burns as ordered. Document the procedure.

8. Needle biopsy cultures are more accurate monitors of wound infection than are surface cultures. Early detection of wound infection allows timely treatment and may prevent sepsis.

9. *Assess for signs of sepsis,* including increased pulse rate, respiratory rate and temperature, decreased blood pressure, decreased urine output, and mentation changes, every 2 to 4 hours and as needed. Document and notify the physician of abnormal findings.

9. Loss of the skin barrier, frequent manipulation of burn wounds, and the general catabolic state place the patient at high risk for sepsis. Early recognition and treatment may prevent irreversible sepsis and septic shock, a major cause of death in burn patients.

10. *Administer tetanus toxoid* on admission as ordered. Administer tetanus immunoglobulin in another site, if tetanus toxoid hasn't been given during the preceding 10 years. Document their administrations.

10. Burns are at high risk for anaerobic infections, including tetanus. Tetanus toxoid stimulates antibody production. Tetanus immunoglobulin provides protection until tetanus antibodies develop. Using different sites prevents inactivation of the immunoglobulin.

11. *Give I.V. antibiotics,* as ordered, if major wound sepsis occurs. Observe for secondary infections of the mouth, GI tract, and the genitalia. Monitor for resistance to topical and systemic antibiotics. Document your findings.

11. I.V. antibiotics usually are given only for major wound sepsis because areas of eschar have poor circulation and are better treated with topical antibiotics. Secondary infections may result from overgrowth of normally suppressed pathogens. Development of resistant strains of microorganisms is a common result of long-term topical antibiotic use.

12. Additional individualized interventions: _____

12. Rationales:_____

Suggested NIC Interventions
Infection control; Infection protection; Incision site care; Wound care

Suggested NOC Outcomes
Infection status; Wound healing; Primary intention

Musculoskeletal and integumentary disorders

Nursing diagnosis

Acute pain related to tissue destruction and exposure of nerves in partially destroyed tissue

NURSING PRIORITY

Relieve pain.

PATIENT OUTCOME CRITERIA

Within 24 to 48 hours of admission, the patient will:
- rate pain (with pain medications) as less than 3 on a 0 to 10 pain rating scale
- verbalize pain relief from pain medication.

INTERVENTIONS	RATIONALES
1. *Provide standard nursing care related to pain.* See the "Acute pain" care plan, page 32.	1. The "Acute pain" care plan includes general assessments and interventions for a patient with pain. This plan contains additional information specific to the burn patient.
2. *Administer I.V. analgesics 10 to 20 minutes before burn cleaning, debridement, and dressing changes.* Medicate frequently and liberally within the ordered parameters. Document administration and degree of pain relief achieved.	2. Burn care is excruciatingly painful and may need to be repeated several times daily. Anticipation increases the patient's perceived pain. Frequent and liberal analgesic administration may prevent the pain from reaching intolerable levels. Addiction to pain medication is rare in burn patients. The I.V. route is preferred because massive edema and inflammation reduce medication absorption through the subcutaneous and intramuscular routes.
3. *Decrease anxiety and fear* by explaining procedures and treatments thoroughly. Document teaching. See the "Knowledge deficit" care plan, page 129, and the "Ineffective individual coping" care plan, page 124.	3. Fear of the unknown, helplessness, and powerlessness may increase pain. Burn care is complex and long term. Thorough teaching and emotional support may allay fear of the unknown and provide the patient some sense of control over treatment, which may lessen the pain experience. The "Knowledge deficit" and "Ineffective individual coping" care plans contain general assessments and interventions applicable to any patient.
4. Additional individualized interventions:_____	4. Rationales: _____

Suggested NIC Interventions

Medication management: Pain management; Analgesic administration

Suggested NOC Outcomes

Comfort level; Pain control; Pain: Disruptive effects; Pain level

---

Nursing diagnosis

Risk for impaired skin integrity related to nonadherence of graft and impaired donor site healing

NURSING PRIORITY

Optimize burn healing.

PATIENT OUTCOME CRITERIA

Within 2 to 5 days after grafting, the patient will:
- display an intact and healing graft without redness, swelling, exudate formation, bleeding, or foul odor

- display a dry and healed donor site
- maintain stable vital signs, typically: heart rate, 60 to 100 beats/minute; systolic blood pressure, 90 to 140 mm Hg; and diastolic blood pressure, 50 to 90 mm Hg
- display no signs of wound sepsis
- maintain activity limitations.

INTERVENTIONS

1. *Apply homografts or heterografts* in single sheets to freshly cleaned burns, as ordered, using sterile technique. Trim to prevent overlapping. Smooth the graft, removing wrinkles and air. Apply thin gauze (with or without antibiotic ointment) over the graft as ordered. Apply a dressing over the gauze. Protect the site from movement or trauma. Document your actions.

2. *After surgery for autografting, immobilize the graft and protect it from injury* for at least 48 hours. Keep the large, bulky dressings in place. Use a bed cradle. Prevent prolonged pressure over the graft. Elevate the graft site to the highest position possible. Use splints and elastic bandages over graft sites, particularly when the patient walks. Discontinue activities, such as hydrotherapy or active physical therapy, for several days after grafting. Document your actions.

3. *Protect the donor site from infection or trauma.* If outer dressings are used, keep them in place by using splints and limiting exercise for several days. Leave the inner gauze dressing in place until it falls off, usually in 2 to 3 weeks. Use a heat lamp or hair dryer to dry the site for 15 to 20 minutes four times daily or as ordered. Leave the site exposed to air as ordered. Document treatments and the condition of the site every shift.

4. *Observe the homograft, heterograft, or autograft for signs of rejection.* Monitor all grafts and donor sites for signs of infection. Report immediately any redness, exudate, blood under the graft, swelling, separation, drainage, foul odor, or increased temperature, pulse rate, or respirations. Document your findings.

5. *Apply moist, warm compresses to the donor site,* if ordered, for 20 to 30 minutes four times per day. Document your actions.

6. *Apply topical antibiotics to the burn and donor site and administer systemic antibiotics I.V.,* if ordered. Document your actions.

7. Additional individualized interventions:_____

RATIONALES

1. Homografts and heterografts are temporary biological dressings that protect burns and stimulate formation of granulation tissue until autografts can be applied. Removing wrinkles and air pockets promotes adherence. Gauze and dressings protect the graft. Freshly grafted sites must be protected from accidental dislodgment until circulation has been established with underlying tissue.

2. The graft must be immobilized and protected from trauma and movement for several days to prevent dislodgment and promote circulation until it adheres. Large dressings provide protective padding. A bed cradle prevents pressure from bed linens. Elevation limits edema. Splints and elastic bandages provide support, maintain dressing placement, prevent excessive movement of the graft site, and allow some activity. Excessive moisture or exercise may dislodge the graft in the 1st days after grafting.

3. The donor site must be protected to prevent its conversion from a partial-thickness wound to a deeper-thickness wound. Using dressings and splints and limiting exercise may protect the site and promote tissue regeneration. The inner gauze is left in place to stabilize and cover the site during tissue regeneration; early removal could traumatize the new tissue. Heat increases circulation and promotes healing. Air exposure promotes drying and scab formation.

4. Regular assessment may permit early detection of graft rejection or wound sepsis.

5. Warmth and moisture may increase circulation and promote epithelialization.

6. As previously described, topical antibiotics are commonly used to prevent wound sepsis from the patient's skin flora. Systemic antibiotics are used when major wound sepsis occurs.

7. Rationales: _____

Musculoskeletal and integumentary disorders

Nursing diagnosis

Imbalanced nutrition: More than body requirements related to increased metabolic needs of burn healing

NURSING PRIORITY

Provide adequate nutrition to promote burn healing.

PATIENT OUTCOME CRITERIA

Within 7 days of admission, the patient will:
- display minimal or no signs of imbalanced nutrition
- manifest expected wound healing
- display no more than a 10% weight loss.

INTERVENTIONS

1. *Provide standard nursing care related to deficient nutrition.* See the "Nutritional deficit" care plan, page 138.

2. *Upon admission, insert a nasogastric tube and withhold food and fluids until bowel sounds return.* Provide I.V. fluids and parenteral nutrition continuously as ordered. Assess patient tolerance, including weights, intake and output, edema, and blood glucose, electrolyte, and protein levels. Document your findings.

3. *After bowel function returns, collaborate with the dietitian or nutritional support nurse to provide a high-calorie, high-protein diet with vitamin supplements,* as ordered. Provide high-calorie liquids, such as milk shakes or prepared liquid diet supplements, instead of water. Take the patient's food preferences into consideration whenever possible. Document daily intake.

4. Additional individualized interventions:_____
_____

RATIONALES

1. The "Nutritional deficit" care plan contains general assessments and interventions for a patient with a nutritional deficit. This section provides additional information pertinent to the burn patient.

2. A burn commonly causes paralytic ileus, which prevents oral intake for 2 to 4 days. Nutritional requirements are met through I.V. administration during this time. Regular assessments monitor the adequacy of fluid and nutrient intake.

3. A high-calorie, high-protein diet (between 5,000 and 6,000 calories daily) may be required to meet the increased metabolic needs for tissue healing. All intake must help meet these increased needs, so milk shakes are preferable to water. Because the burn patient commonly experiences loss of appetite, offering favorite foods may improve intake. Extra vitamins are needed to meet tissue-healing needs.

4. Rationales: _____
_____

Nursing diagnosis

Impaired physical mobility related to prescribed position and movement limitations

NURSING PRIORITY

Maintain mobility within the range of limitations.

PATIENT OUTCOME CRITERIA

Within 14 days of admission, the patient will:
- have no contractures
- maintain proper anatomic and functional positions of arms and legs
- perform range-of-motion (ROM) and other exercises
- experience minimal pain during activities.

INTERVENTIONS	RATIONALES
1. *Provide standard nursing care related to impaired mobility.* Implement measures in the "Impaired physical mobility" care plan, page 111, as appropriate.	**1.** The "Impaired physical mobility" care plan covers general information about this problem. This section provides additional information pertinent to burn patients.
2. *Provide active and passive ROM exercises to arms and legs with a healing graft* every 2 hours and as needed, as ordered. Document patient tolerance.	**2.** ROM exercises prevent contractures and promote circulation, healing, and a sense of well-being.
3. *Promote self-care* within the patient's limitations.	**3.** Self-care increases the patient's activity level and promotes a sense of well-being and control over the environment.
4. *Provide protective devices, such as splints and dressings, during exercise* as ordered. Document their use.	**4.** Protective devices allow mobility while maintaining the integrity of the graft site.
5. *Position body parts in anatomic and functional alignment.* Document your actions.	**5.** Anatomic and functional alignment prevents contracture formation and promotes eventual return to normal activities.
6. Provide pain medication as needed and ordered. Document its administration.	**6.** Pain relief encourages movement and activity.
7. Additional individualized interventions:_____	**7.** Rationales: _____

> ### Suggested NIC Interventions
> *Exercise therapy: Ambulation; Exercise therapy: Balance; Exercise therapy: Joint mobility; Exercise therapy: Muscle control; Exercise promotion: Strength training*

> ### Suggested NOC Outcomes
> *Ambulation: Walking; Ambulation: Wheelchair; Joint movement: Active; Mobility level*

Nursing diagnosis

Disturbed body image related to extensive burns and potential scarring

NURSING PRIORITY

Promote adjustment to body changes.

Musculoskeletal and integumentary disorders

PATIENT OUTCOME CRITERIA

Throughout the recovery period, the patient will:

■ express fears and concerns openly
■ set small, realistic goals for recovery
■ participate in recovery.

INTERVENTIONS	RATIONALES
1. *Provide standard nursing care related to ineffective coping and anticipatory grieving.* See the "Ineffective individual coping" care plan, page 124, and the "Grieving" care plan, page 105.	**1.** The extensive emotional adjustments necessary to recover from the burn may severely tax the patient's and family's coping abilities. Grieving for lost appearance or the function of body parts is a necessary first step in emotional recovery. "Ineffective individual coping" and "Grieving" care plans provide multiple interventions helpful to recovery.
2. *Encourage verbalization of feelings* about the burn, potential scarring, and loss of function. Document concerns.	**2.** Verbalization of concerns decreases anxiety and fear and encourages self-appraisal to determine realistic goals.
3. *Provide information about procedures and expected results.* Document teaching and the patient's response.	**3.** Knowledge of procedures and expected results decreases fear of the unknown and encourages patient participation and cooperation during recovery.
4. *Encourage realistic goals.*	**4.** Focusing on realistic goals, such as small, obtainable daily goals, may prevent disappointment and despair during recovery
5. Additional individualized interventions:_____	**5.** Rationales: _____

> **Suggested NIC Interventions**
> *Body image enhancement; Grief work facilitation; Anticipatory guidance; Coping enhancement; Self-esteem enhancement*

> **Suggested NOC Outcomes**
> *Body image; Grief resolution; Self-esteem*

Discharge planning

DISCHARGE CHECKLIST

Before discharge, the patient shows evidence of:

❐ stable vital signs and monitoring parameters
❐ healing graft and donor sites
❐ absence of wound or systemic sepsis
❐ stable fluid and electrolyte status
❐ renal status within normal limits
❐ adequate nutrition and fluid intake
❐ ability to perform ROM and other exercises
❐ ability to maintain proper anatomic and functional positions of arms and legs
❐ absence of such complications as shock, cardiac arrhythmias, renal failure, contractures, or bleeding
❐ minimal edema
❐ ability to take medication as prescribed.

TEACHING CHECKLIST

Document evidence that the patient and family demonstrate an understanding of:

❐ grafting and wound care procedures, including expected course of healing
❐ signs and symptoms of such complications as shock, bleeding, infection, and graft rejection and who to contact if these occur
❐ importance of ROM exercises and proper anatomic and functional positioning of affected arms and legs
❐ nutritional needs
❐ comfort measures for pain
❐ protective measures, such as splints and dressings, for wounds
❐ long-term recovery goals
❐ medication, dose, time, and so on.

DOCUMENTATION CHECKLIST

If there's a home health referral, document when to expect a call or visit and who to notify if the visit isn't received. Using outcome criteria as a guide, document:
- ❐ clinical status on admission
- ❐ significant changes in status
- ❐ pertinent diagnostic test findings
- ❐ status of graft and donor sites
- ❐ complications, such as shock, arrhythmias, sepsis, renal failure, or contractures
- ❐ oxygen therapy
- ❐ ROM and other exercises
- ❐ tolerance of tube insertions, debridement, and wound care
- ❐ pain and effect of medication
- ❐ mental and emotional status
- ❐ patient and family teaching
- ❐ discharge planning.

Associated care plans

- Acute pain
- Grieving
- Impaired physical mobility
- Ineffective individual coping
- Knowledge deficit
- Nutritional deficit

References

Graham, J.S., et al. "Efficacy of Laser Debridement with Autologous Split-thickness Skin Grafting in Promoting Improved Healing of Deep Cutaneous Sulfur Mustard Burns," *Burns* 28(8):719-30, December 2002.

Jordan, K. (ed). *Emergency Nursing Core Curriculum.* Emergency Nurses Association. Philadelphia: W.B. Saunders Co., 2000.

Lynn-McHale, D.J., and Carlson, K.K. American Association of Critical Care Nurses *AACN Procedure Manual for Critical Care,* 4th ed. Philadelphia: W.B. Saunders Co., 2001.

Mordjikian, E. "Severe Microstomia Due to Burn by Caustic Soda," *Burns* 28(8):802-805, December 2002.

Saetti, R., et al. "Endoscopic Treatment of Upper Airway and Digestive Tract Lesions Caused by Caustic Agents," *The Annals of Otology, Rhinology, and Laryngology* 112(1): 29-36, January 2003.

Santucci, S.G., et al. "Infections in a Burn Intensive Care Unit: Experience of Seven Years," *The Journal of Hospital Infection* 53(1):6-13, January 2003.

Schrage, N.F., et al. "Use of an Amphoteric Lavage Solution for Emergency Treatment of Eye Burns. First Animal Type Experimental Clinical Considerations," *Burns* 28(8):782-86, December 2002.

Shoemaker, W.C., et al. *Textbook of Critical Care,* 4th ed. Philadelphia: W.B. Saunders Co., 2002.

Musculoskeletal and integumentary disorders

Multiple trauma

DRG INFORMATION
DRG 484 Craniotomy for Multiple Significant Trauma.
Mean LOS = 12.9 days
DRG 485 Limb Reattachment, Hip and Femur Procedures for Multiple Significant Trauma.
Mean LOS = 9.8 days
DRG 486 Other Operating Room Procedures for Multiple Significant Trauma.
Mean LOS = 12.4 days
DRG 487 Other Multiple Significant Trauma.
Mean LOS = 7.6 days

To attain the correct DRG for a multiple trauma patient, the injuries must include significant trauma to different significant trauma body site categories as outlined by DRG guidelines. It's important to document all injuries sustained and procedures (surgical and nonsurgical) performed because, for instance, a bedside excisional debridement could enhance the DRG; similarly, an injury to a separate body site that seems minor might be the injury that prompts the multiple injury DRGs.

Introduction
DEFINITION AND TIME FOCUS
Multiple trauma results from accidental or intentional injury to more than one body part, organ, or system. Trauma usually can be described as blunt or penetrating, depending on whether the skin is broken.

    This care plan focuses on the first days after trauma — the critical care phase. It assumes that the patient has been moved from the field to the emergency department for stabilization, to surgery where essential repairs have been accomplished, and then to the unit. If the patient isn't already stable, plan and implement appropriate cardiopulmonary support and cervical spine protection, and provide preoperative care based on your facility's policies. Although every possible complication can't be included, this plan reviews major complications in detail and refers to other plans where appropriate. Long-term rehabilitation isn't covered here, but prevention of long-term disability — the focus of nursing care — is discussed. The care plan refers to special equipment used to care for the trauma patient, but no endorsement of a specific product or manufacturer is implied. (See *Clinical snapshot: Multiple trauma*, page 584.)

ETIOLOGY AND PRECIPITATING FACTORS
- Chemical impairment of mentation and judgment by such drugs as alcohol, narcotics, cocaine, or other street drugs
- Suicide attempts
- Assaults
- Falls, especially in the elderly
- Industrial incidents
- Motor vehicle crashes
- Pedestrian-vehicle collisions
- Sports injuries
- Underlying physical problems, such as acute myocardial infarction (AMI) and stroke
- Major psychiatric disorders
- Recent personal stress

Focused assessment guidelines
NURSING HISTORY
(FUNCTIONAL HEALTH PATTERN FINDINGS)
Health-perception–health-management pattern
- Male (likely) ages 15 to 35; about 75% of trauma patients are male

Nutritional-metabolic pattern
- Well-nourished

Activity-exercise pattern
- History of athletic competition

Cognitive-perceptual pattern
- Complaints of pain, if conscious
- Reported or displayed confusion, anxiety, or amnesia, if conscious

Coping–stress tolerance pattern
- Situational or maturational life crisis
- History of psychiatric problems

PHYSICAL FINDINGS
Alcohol, drugs, anxiety, restlessness, decreased level of consciousness (LOC), or altered sensory function commonly interfere with accurate assessment. Serial observations and analysis of trends in findings are critical. Physical findings vary with the particular trauma present.

Cardiovascular
- Hypotension and tachycardia (if shock is present)
- Hypertension and tachycardia (if shock is absent)
- Diminished or absent pulse (if trauma is to an extremity or if blood circulation is impaired)
- Arrhythmias

- Jugular vein distention (if cardiac tamponade or tension pneumothorax is present)
- Muffled heart sounds (if cardiac tamponade or tension pneumothorax is present)
- Capillary refill time greater than 3 seconds (if shock or vascular disruption is present)

Pulmonary
- Tachypnea
- Shallow respirations
- Paradoxical chest movement (if flail chest is present)
- Crepitus and ecchymoses (if chest trauma is present)

Gastrointestinal
- Cullen's sign (ecchymoses around umbilicus) and Turner's sign (ecchymoses in flanks) if intra-abdominal or retroperitoneal bleeding present (a late sign)

Neurologic
- Decreased LOC
- Rhinorrhea or otorrhea (if cerebrospinal fluid [CSF] leak is present)
- Pupillary changes
- Sensory or motor impairment (if trauma is to the head, the spinal cord, or an extremity)

Integumentary
- Abrasions
- Lacerations
- Ecchymoses
- Road burns
- Battle's sign (ecchymoses over mastoid area) and raccoon eyes (periorbital ecchymoses) if basilar skull fracture or facial fracture is present
- Pallor, mottling, or cyanosis
- Cool, cold, or clammy skin

Musculoskeletal
- Fractures
- Amputations

DIAGNOSTIC STUDIES

- Complete blood count — commonly reveals decreased hemoglobin level and hematocrit secondary to hemorrhage; white blood cell count may be elevated
- Serum electrolyte levels — monitor fluid and electrolyte status
- Blood urea nitrogen and serum creatinine levels — may be elevated secondary to decreased renal perfusion in shock and in renal failure
- Lactate levels — may be elevated, reflecting anaerobic metabolism in shock; high initial levels are associated with low probability of survival
- Serum bilirubin levels — assess hepatic damage
- Cardiac isoenzyme levels — determine AMI, a common cause of trauma, or cardiac injury
- Arterial blood gas (ABG) levels — vary, depending on cardiopulmonary status; generally, respiratory alkalosis occurs if tachypnea is present; respiratory acidosis occurs if respiratory depression is present; metabolic acidosis occurs if shock is present

- Coagulation panel — monitors for disseminated intravascular coagulation (DIC) and coagulopathy
- Serum aspartate aminotransferase, alanine aminotransferase, and lactic dehydrogenase levels — monitor for liver damage
- Anteroposterior, odontoid, and lateral cervical spine radiography — an essential procedure to visualize cervical vertebrae C1 to C7; can detect spinal injury
- 12-lead electrocardiography (ECG) — can help evaluate AMI or ischemia, arrhythmias, electrolyte imbalance, or antiarrhythmic agent effects
- Chest X-ray — can detect fractured ribs, widened mediastinum, pneumothorax, hemothorax, or other life-threatening chest injuries; a chest X-ray can also confirm placement of an endotracheal tube and central lines and monitor for acute respiratory distress syndrome (ARDS), pneumonia, and other complications
- Anteroposterior pelvic X-ray, including both hips — can detect pelvic ring disruption or hip dislocation
- Diagnostic peritoneal lavage — may reveal blood, feces, bile, or amylase, indicating abdominal injury
- Excretory urogram, cystogram, or ureterogram — used to identify the size, location, and filling of the renal pelvis, ureters, and urethra
- Computed tomography (CT) scan — can visualize injuries to the head, neck, spine, abdomen, and kidneys
- Arteriography — determines vessel integrity
- Radionuclide scanning and sonography — assists in the identification of organ structure and function; especially useful in suspected chest, abdominal, or pelvic injuries

POTENTIAL COMPLICATIONS

- Infection or sepsis
- Pulmonary embolism
- Atelectasis or pneumonia
- ARDS
- DIC
- Renal failure
- Cardiac failure
- Liver failure
- Increased intracranial pressure (ICP)
- Paralysis
- Fat embolism
- Compartment syndrome
- Malnutrition
- Multisystem organ failure
- Posttraumatic stress disorder

Musculoskeletal and integumentary disorders

Multiple trauma

Major nursing diagnoses and collaborative problems	Key patient outcomes
ND: Impaired gas exchange	Achieve ABGs within normal limits (pH, 7.35 to 7.45; $Paco_2$, 35 to 45 mm Hg; HCO_3^-, 23 to 28 mEq/L) and pulse oximetry levels 93% or higher.
CP: Risk for shock	Have stable vital signs, typically: heart rate, 60 to 100 beats/minute; systolic blood pressure, 90 to 140 mm Hg; and diastolic blood pressure, 50 to 90 mm Hg.
ND: Risk for injury	Have no signs or symptoms of previously unapparent injury.
ND: Impaired physical mobility	Have no new evidence of skin breakdown or other hazards of immobility.
ND: Risk for posttrauma syndrome	Discuss feelings about the traumatic incident.
ND: Risk for injury (complications)	Show no signs or symptoms of complications.

Nursing diagnosis

Impaired gas exchange related to pulmonary injury, head injury, shock, or other factors

NURSING PRIORITY
Maintain optimal airway, ventilation, and oxygenation.

PATIENT OUTCOME CRITERIA
According to individual readiness, the patient will:
- display ABGs within normal limits (pH, 7.35 to 7.45; $Paco_2$, 35 to 45 mm Hg; HCO_3^-, 23 to 28 mEq/L) and pulse oximetry levels 93% or higher
- have clear breath sounds bilaterally
- have clear lung fields on chest X-ray.

INTERVENTIONS

1. *Maintain a patent airway.** Maintain cervical spine precautions until clinical, radiologic, or tomographic findings have ruled out ligamentous injury or fracture.

2. *Monitor ventilatory status.* Observe respiratory rate, rhythm, effort of breathing, and tidal volume. Monitor trends in pulse oximetry and ABG values. Consult physician about acceptable limits. Prepare for intubation and mechanical ventilation, as ordered, particularly if the patient has flail chest, pulmonary contusion, or shock. See the "Mechanical ventilation" care plan, page 281.

RATIONALES

1. Although airway patency will have been evaluated before unit admission, trauma to the head, face, neck, or torso can compromise a previously patent airway at any time. Although cervical spine clearance is usually done before unit admission, general precautions may still be required while awaiting the official radiologic reading. The C6 and C7 vertebrae may be difficult to clear in a patient with large shoulders, and CT scan may be required.

2. If the patient's condition deteriorates, ventilatory status may change abruptly. Deterioration also may be insidious (for example, if the patient tires), so close monitoring is essential. The "Mechanical ventilation" care plan presents comprehensive information on indications for mechanical ventilation, types of ventilators, and associated nursing care.

---

*Italics indicate key interventions.

3. *Provide supplemental oxygen,* as ordered.	**3.** All multiple-trauma patients need supplemental oxygenation. Hypoxemia involves many factors and may result from pulmonary injury, depressed LOC, decreased cardiac output, ischemia, acidosis, and other factors. Supplemental oxygen elevates arterial oxygen tension, ensuring that the blood reaching the tissues provides the maximum amount of oxygen possible.
4. *Obtain serial chest X-rays at least daily,* as ordered.	**4.** Serial chest X-rays can detect complications in time for corrective action.
5. Additional individualized interventions:_____ _____	**5.** Rationales: _____ _____

> **Suggested NIC Interventions**
> *Acid-base management: Electrolyte management; Laboratory data interpretation; Oxygen therapy; Ventilation assistance; Airway management; Respiratory monitoring; Embolus care: Pulmonary; Hemodynamic regulation; Vital signs monitoring*

> **Suggested NOC Outcomes**
> *Electrolyte and acid-base balance: Respiratory status: Gas exchange; Respiratory status: Ventilation; Tissue perfusion: Pulmonary; Vital signs status*

Collaborative problem
Risk for shock related to hypovolemia, cardiac injury, spinal cord injury, or sepsis

NURSING PRIORITIES
Monitor for shock, and restore circulating blood volume and tissue perfusion if shock occurs.

PATIENT OUTCOME CRITERIA
Within 24 hours of the onset of therapy, the patient will:
■ achieve stable vital signs, typically: heart rate, 60 to 100 beats/minute; systolic blood pressure, 90 to 140 mm Hg; and diastolic blood pressure, 50 to 90 mm Hg
■ have an adequate circulating volume, as manifested by warm, dry skin; urine output within normal limits; and strong, bilaterally equal peripheral pulses
■ have a core temperature within normal limits.

INTERVENTIONS	**RATIONALES**
1. *Provide standard nursing care related to hypovolemic shock.* Implement measures in the "Hypovolemic shock" care plan, page 424, as appropriate, such as monitoring LOC, vital signs, urine output, ECG pattern, hemodynamic measurements, and laboratory values; maintaining patency of two large-bore I.V. lines; and administering fluids and positive inotropic agents, as ordered.	**1.** The "Hypovolemic shock" care plan covers assessment and interventions for this potential problem in detail. This plan provides additional information specific to the trauma patient.
2. *Implement autotransfusion, when possible.* Follow the manufacturer's directions for acid-citrate-dextrose (ACD) anticoagulant, if used, and reinfusion.	**2.** The patient's blood, when captured in drainage, is an ideal source of blood replacement because it decreases the possibility of transfusion reactions and infection. ACD anticoagulant may be used to prevent the retrieved blood from coagulating in the autotransfusor.
3. *Monitor continually for new or ongoing bleeding.*	**3.** Commonly, restoration of adequate blood pressure reverses peripheral vasoconstriction and dislodges fragile clots, so additional bleeding becomes apparent.

4. *Collaborate with the physician to adjust blood replacement* according to the sites of suspected or obvious bleeding and estimated amount lost.

4. Rough guidelines exist for the amount of blood loss to expect with particular injuries, such as for the following closed orthopedic injuries: humerus, 1 to 2 units; ulna-radius, $\frac{1}{2}$ to 1 unit; pelvis, 2 to 12 units or greater; tibia-fibula, $\frac{1}{2}$ to 4 units; and ankle, $\frac{1}{2}$ to 2 units. With open injuries, an estimated 1 to 3 additional units may be lost per site. Such guidelines, when used with clinical findings, help determine appropriate blood replacement.

5. Warm I.V. fluids before administration.

5. The volume of fluid required in a major trauma resuscitation is so massive that infusing room temperature solutions and cold blood products may cause hypothermia and shivering. Shivering requires an extraordinary energy expenditure the patient can ill afford.

6. Additional individualized interventions:_____
_____

6. Rationales: _____
_____

Nursing diagnosis
Risk for injury related to mechanism of injury

NURSING PRIORITIES
- Correlate the mechanism of injury with the patient's clinical presentation.
- Remain alert for new signs of injury.

PATIENT OUTCOME CRITERION
Throughout the unit stay, the patient will have no signs or symptoms of previously unapparent injury.

INTERVENTIONS

Blunt head trauma

1. *Provide standard nursing care related to increased intracranial pressure.* Implement measures in the "Increased intracranial pressure" care plan, page 190, as appropriate.

2. *Monitor for neurologic deterioration.* Observe LOC, pupillary reactions, motor function, and sensory function. Alert the physician immediately to any signs of neurologic deterioration.

RATIONALES

1. Brain damage may not reflect velocity and duration of the injuring force because a contrecoup injury (which is opposite the site of injury) may be worse than the coup injury (the injury at point of contact) to the head. Preadmission health status, the specific injury, and immediate detection and treatment of increased ICP are critical to survival. The "Increased intracranial pressure" care plan discusses these problems in detail.

2. Brain damage may not be apparent until days or weeks after injury. An epidural hematoma, usually from arterial bleeding secondary to blows to the temple that tear the middle meningeal artery, is life-threatening and requires immediate surgical evacuation. Signs of acute subdural hematoma usually appear within 24 hours of injury. Signs of concussion usually reverse within 24 hours, while those from contusion may persist for several days or longer. Failure to recover within the expected time may indicate ongoing pathology or previously undetected injury and requires medical evaluation.

Blunt chest trauma

1. *Observe for signs and symptoms of tracheoesophageal injury.* Notify the physician promptly of the onset of subcutaneous emphysema in the chest or neck, gastric contents in tracheal secretions, severe chest pain, deteriorating ABG values, or dyspnea.

1. Signs and symptoms of tracheoesophageal injury may indicate tracheal disruption or esophageal or bronchial tears. The trachea, esophagus, and bronchi are attached to other body structures by stalks that are prone to tearing from direct impact, deceleration, and shearing or rotary forces associated with blunt trauma.

2. *Monitor for indicators of cardiac tamponade,* such as rising central venous pressure, falling blood pressure, jugular vein distention, or muffled heart sounds. Notify the physician immediately and prepare for pericardiocentesis or thoracotomy.

2. When the chest strikes the steering wheel in a motor vehicle crash, for instance, the heart is compressed between the sternum and vertebrae. The abrupt increase in intracardiac pressure may cause cardiac rupture. Damage may also occur to great vessels, especially to the venae cavae and pulmonary veins, which are thought to have different deceleration rates than the atria.

3. *Monitor for signs of blunt cardiac injury,* including tachycardia, chest pain, arrhythmias, elevated pulmonary artery wedge pressure, and indicators of heart failure. Obtain serial ECGs and an echocardiogram during the diagnostic phase as ordered. Provide care, as ordered, depending on the injury's effect on the patient.

3. Blunt cardiac injury may result from horizontal or vertical deceleration, compression, or shock wave damage in a gunshot wound to the chest or abdomen. Some controversy exists over management of blunt cardiac injury. Recent studies show little risk for most patients. If an ECG and echocardiogram don't reveal electrical or mechanical dysfunction, this disorder may not be critical. If function is impaired or arrhythmias threaten cardiac output, however, treatment should be similar to that for AMI.

4. *Monitor for signs of pulmonary contusion,* such as dyspnea, increasing pulmonary secretions (usually bloody), increasing inspiratory pressure while on a ventilator, and hypoxemia. Follow pulse oximetry, serial ABG measurements and chest X-ray results.

4. Pulmonary insufficiency from contusions increases within the first hours after injury. Contusion creates swelling, a natural inflammatory process, and a capillary leak, which is worsened by the aggressive fluid resuscitation necessary for the multiple-trauma patient.

5. Additional individualized interventions:_____

5. Rationales: _____

Blunt abdominal trauma

1. *Observe for abdominal bleeding.* Report changes in abdominal pain, tenderness, rebound tenderness, absent bowel sounds, and increased abdominal distention.

1. Lap belt restraints may produce intraperitoneal, retroperitoneal, or pelvic disruption, resulting in life-threatening hemorrhage. These acceleration-deceleration injuries may not appear immediately after injury but hours or even days later.

2. *Maintain placement and patency of gastric and urinary catheters* as ordered. Avoid nasogastric (NG) tube placement if facial fractures or cribriform plate injury is suspected. Insert an orogastric tube instead. Avoid urinary catheter insertion if blood is present at the urinary meatus; notify the physician.

2. A gastric catheter decompresses the stomach and helps detect gastric bleeding; a urinary catheter does the same for the bladder. Attempts to insert an NG tube when facial fractures or cribriform plate injury is present may result in catheter placement into the brain. Bleeding at the urinary meatus may indicate urethral transection and requires medical evaluation.

3. Additional individualized interventions:_____

3. Rationales: _____

Blunt spinal cord injury

1. *Perform and document a motor and sensory examination every shift.*

1. Mechanisms of spinal cord injury include horizontal loading, vertical loading, and acceleration or deceleration. Horizontal loading causes lateral cord motion, for instance, when the patient hits the ground after being ejected from an automobile. Vertical loading results in cord compression, for instance, with a vertical fall or diving injury. Acceleration or deceleration injuries are common in falls.

2. Additional individualized interventions:_____

2. Rationales: _____

Penetrating wounds

1. *With bullet wounds, observe the wound edge for necrosis and distal tissue for perfusion.* Also inspect carefully for other wounds.

1. Bullet wounds usually are explored surgically because of the erratic path the bullet may take as it moves through tissue and because the bullet's kinetic energy (which depends on its mass and velocity) creates a much larger internal wound than the surface may indicate.

2. *With stab wounds, observe distal vascular supply and tissue integrity, and assess signs of underlying organ function.* Assume underlying vessel, tissue, and organ damage until proven otherwise.

2. Depending on the length of the weapon and the direction of penetration, body areas other than that of the surface wound may be injured. For example, an abdominal stab wound may penetrate the diaphragm and involve the chest cavity, or a buttock stab wound may enter the abdomen. Maintain suspicion regarding the extent of the wound.

3. Additional individualized interventions:_____

3. Rationales: _____

All injuries

1. *Assess and report to the physician if the apparent mechanism of injury and observed injuries don't match.*

1. Inconsistencies between the apparent mechanism of injury and pattern of observed injuries may indicate previously undetected mechanisms of injury or abuse.

2. Additional individualized interventions:_____

2. Rationales: _____

Suggested NIC Interventions
Surveillance: Safety

Suggested NOC Outcomes
Safety status: Physical injury

Nursing diagnosis
Impaired physical mobility related to orthopedic injury

NURSING PRIORITIES
- Restore maximum mobility.
- Strengthen muscle groups involved in weight bearing and range of motion (ROM).
- Prevent orthopedic complications.

PATIENT OUTCOME CRITERION
By the 3rd day after traumatic injury, the patient will have no new evidence of skin breakdown or other hazards of immobility.

INTERVENTIONS

1. *Provide standard nursing care related to impaired mobility.* Implement measures in the "Impaired physical mobility" care plan, page 111, as appropriate.

2. *Elevate casted extremities.* Check neurovascular function every 1 to 2 hours. Report to the physician altered sensation, increased pain, decreased ability to move fingers or toes, and capillary refill time greater than 3 seconds.

3. *Observe uncasted extremities* for crepitus, deformity, swelling, discoloration, pain, paralysis, pulse loss, and muscle spasms. If present, splint the extremity and notify the physician.

4. *If reimplantation is planned for a severed body part, maintain the viability of the body part.* Wrap the part in sterile gauze slightly moistened with sterile normal saline. Place it in a sealed plastic bag and immerse it in a slurry of iced normal saline. Don't allow the part to soak in liquid or freeze. Don't use dry ice. Prepare the patient for reimplantation surgery.

5. *Maintain traction and immobilization of all cervical spine injuries and all other unstable spinal fractures.* Besides halo traction, methods include using Gardner-Wells or Crutchfield tongs.

6. *Prevent skin breakdown and other hazards of immobility* by obtaining turning orders and restrictions, as appropriate, instituting a program of diligent side-to-side turning, at least every 2 hours as ordered, or using trauma beds. Trauma beds include:
– Roto kinetic bed

– air bag beds (avoid these for the patient in spinal traction)

– Stryker frame

7. *Apply, monitor, and maintain sequential compression devices,* if ordered.

8. Additional individualized interventions: _____
_____

RATIONALES

1. The "Impaired physical mobility" care plan presents comprehensive information on the hazards of immobility and their prevention. This care plan provides additional information pertinent to the trauma patient.

2. Extremities in casts commonly swell from tissue edema; elevation decreases the amount of swelling. Altered sensation, increased pain, limited movement, and prolonged capillary refill time indicate that the swelling is causing neurovascular compromise. Unrecognized damage can threaten limb survival or function.

3. Occasionally, injuries may be missed during resuscitation, especially if other life-threatening injuries require immediate surgery.

4. Several hours may elapse before reimplantation. Maintaining the body part as described preserves viability. Dry ice isn't recommended because it may freeze the body part and possibly cause tissue damage.

5. Maintaining traction prevents further injury to the spinal cord. Although cervical spine injuries require immediate treatment along with other life-threatening injuries, treatment of thoracolumbar injuries can be deferred until the patient is stable.

6. Skin breakdown, thromboembolism, and other complications of immobility may threaten life or markedly prolong recovery. Preventive methods depend on the injury and degree of activity allowed.

– A Roto kinetic bed cycles automatically and continuously to 90-degree positions and has been used with various injuries, including cervical spine fractures. A patient on a ventilator can be cared for easily on this bed.
– Various air bag beds are available. Benefits include side-to-side turning, bacterial filtration, and prevention of skin breakdown. Because of the potential for deflation with air bag beds, they're contraindicated for the patient with an unstable spine. A Roto kinetic bed is better suited for the patient in spinal traction.
– Although a Stryker frame bed facilitates turning, it doesn't automatically change the patient's position and thus the patient requires more nursing supervision.

7. These devices are designed to prevent deep vein stasis and thromboembolism.

8. Rationales: _____
_____

Musculoskeletal and integumentary disorders

<table>
<tr><td>

Suggested NIC Interventions

Exercise therapy: Ambulation; Exercise therapy: Balance; Exercise therapy: Joint mobility; Exercise therapy: Muscle control; Exercise promotion: Strength training

</td><td>

Suggested NOC Outcomes

Ambulation: Walking; Ambulation: Wheelchair; Joint movement: Active; Mobility level

</td></tr>
</table>

Nursing diagnosis

Risk for posttrauma syndrome related to overwhelming psychological assault from sudden, unexpected injury

NURSING PRIORITY

Facilitate effective coping.

PATIENT OUTCOME CRITERIA

According to individual readiness, the patient will:
- discuss feelings about the traumatic incident
- learn to cope with flashbacks and other signs of the posttraumatic response.

INTERVENTIONS	RATIONALES
1. *Provide standard nursing care related to ineffective coping, grieving, and dying.* Refer to the "Ineffective individual coping" care plan, page 124, the "Grieving" care plan, page 129, and the "Dying" care plan, page 78.	**1.** The "Ineffective individual coping," "Grieving," and "Dying" care plans contain helpful interventions for the trauma patient and his family. These care plans provide additional specific information.
2. *Observe for indications that the patient is reexperiencing the traumatic incident,* such as flashbacks, intrusive thoughts, nightmares, guilt over survival, and excessive talking about the event. Also observe for indications of psychic numbing, such as confusion, amnesia, limited affect, misinterpretation of reality, and poor impulse control.	**2.** Identifying these signs and symptoms that characterize the posttraumatic response may help you to assist the patient in identifying triggers to the episodes.
3. *Encourage the patient to discuss feelings and reach out to others for help in coping with them.* Explicitly acknowledge the intense feelings involved and the difficulty in coping with them.	**3.** Retelling the incident and verbalizing feelings are important steps toward psychic integration of the experience. Reaching out to others provides comfort and reestablishes psychological security. By recognizing the powerful feelings involved and acknowledging the patient's difficulty in coping with the experience, the nurse conveys respect and establishes rapport and trust.
4. *Reassure the patient about being safe now.* Praise behaviors contributing to survival, if appropriate.	**4.** The posttrauma syndrome can be so intense that the patient becomes absorbed in reexperiencing the terrifying incident. Reassurance helps reorient the patient to reality and brings closure to the terrifying incident. Praise for survival behaviors helps restore a sense of control.
5. *Support the family members and help them understand the patient's response.*	**5.** Distress at seeing the patient upset may cause the family to shut off verbalizations, crying, and other expressions of emotion. Although well intentioned, such blocking may ultimately interfere with the patient's ability to integrate the experience.
6. *With the consent of the patient and family, call in counseling professionals,* such as a spiritual advisor, social worker, or trauma stress specialist. Refer the patient and family to a trauma support group, if available.	**6.** Counseling professionals offer special skills that may facilitate coping. Calling them in without consent, however, may reinforce the powerless feeling the patient experienced during the traumatic incident.

7. Additional individualized interventions:_____

7. Rationales: _____

Suggested NIC Interventions
Coping enhancement; Counseling; Security enhancement

Suggested NOC Outcomes
Coping; Fear control

Nursing diagnosis

Risk for injury (complications) related to impaired immunologic defenses, hypermetabolic state, stress, and other factors

NURSING PRIORITY
Prevent or minimize complications.

PATIENT OUTCOME CRITERION
Throughout the hospital stay, the patient will show no signs or symptoms of complications.

INTERVENTIONS

1. *Identify and minimize potential sources of infection.* For example, use strict sterile technique when opening invasive lines; provide care at the insertion site of skeletal pins, wires, and tongs as ordered; and administer antibiotics as ordered. If a CSF leak is present, avoid suctioning and packing the nose or ears, and tell the patient to avoid nose blowing. Ideally, remove and replace I.V. lines and urinary catheters within 24 hours of insertion in the field or emergency department.

2. *Verify that tetanus prophylaxis was administered,* if needed.

3. *Provide adequate nutrition* within 24 hours of admission as ordered. See the "Nutritional deficit" care plan, page 138, for details.

4. *Prevent stress ulcers* by administering antacids, titrated to gastric pH, and histamine antagonists or anticholinergic agents as ordered. Monitor gastric drainage for occult blood.

RATIONALES

1. Breach of the skin barrier, ischemia and necrotic tissue, inadequate inflammatory response, chronic disease, many invasive procedures, malnutrition, and pharmacologic agents contribute to the high risk of infection for the trauma patient. The measures listed prevent or treat infection. Lines and catheters placed hurriedly tend to become contaminated and serve as a wick for infection. Early replacement minimizes the infection risk.

2. Although tetanus prophylaxis is usually accomplished in the emergency department, it may have been overlooked if life-threatening injuries required immediate surgery.

3. Adequate nutrition is critically important to recovery because trauma induces a hypermetabolic response. Commonly, paralytic ileus or facial, airway, esophageal, chest, or abdominal injuries preclude oral nutrition. If these injuries are substantial, a jejunostomy tube is placed during the initial chest or abdominal surgery. If the enteral route is unavailable, parenteral nutrition should be started. Nutritional goals include achieving positive nitrogen balance and preventing complications from inadequate nutrition, such as sepsis, delayed wound healing, and multiple organ failure. The "Nutritional deficit" care plan discusses this potential complication in detail.

4. The trauma patient is at increased risk for stress ulcers. Prevention is the best therapy. The medications indicated reduce the secretion and acidity of gastric fluids, and gastric drainage monitoring can detect incipient stress ulcers.

Musculoskeletal and integumentary disorders

5. *Monitor for signs and symptoms of compartment syndrome,* such as unrelievable pain, muscle tension, and neurovascular compromise. If any of these signs and symptoms is present, alert the physician and assist with measurement of compartmental pressure or transfer to surgery for fasciotomy.

5. Compartment syndrome results from excessive pressure within a fascial compartment caused by swollen tissue or blood confined within the compartment. Soft-tissue injury, burns, pneumatic antishock garment use, and tight casts or dressings increase the risk of compartment syndrome. Neurovascular compromise results and, if the pressure isn't relieved by fasciotomy, the end result may be nerve damage or paralysis or necrosis.

6. *Monitor for signs and symptoms of myoglobinuric renal failure,* such as decreased urine output and elevated specific gravity. Notify the physician and obtain plasma creatine kinase (CK) and urine myoglobin levels as ordered. If myoglobinuria is present, administer fluids and mannitol as ordered.

6. Myoglobinuria reflects myoglobin release from muscle damage associated with crush injury or compartment syndrome. When circulation is restored to the damaged tissue, a flood of myoglobin enters the central circulation. Myoglobinuria peaks about 3 hours after circulation is restored and may persist for as long as 12 hours after the ischemic event. If myoglobin precipitates in the renal tubules, it may cause acute renal failure. Elevated plasma CK and urine myoglobin levels confirm the diagnosis. Fluid administration and osmotic diuresis maintain renal tubular flow and lessen the risk of myoglobin clogging the renal tubules.

7. *If musculoskeletal, soft tissue, burn, arterial, or multisystem trauma is present, observe for signs of fat embolism,* such as sudden onset of respiratory distress, tachypnea, tachycardia, decreased LOC, and personality changes. If any of these signs or symptoms is present, alert the physician.

7. Fat embolism results from mobilization of fat globules (for example, fat escaping from a fractured bone) or altered fat metabolism. The signs and symptoms from fat globules lodging in the lungs, brain, and kidneys usually occur 24 to 48 hours after injury. The early signs listed may be followed by petechiae (which appear 2 to 4 days after injury), retinal changes, and hematuria. Untreated, fat embolism may result in ARDS. Treatment is controversial but usually includes mechanical ventilation with positive end-expiratory pressure and possibly corticosteroids.

8. *If death is imminent, consider possible organ donation.* Consult with the physician, family, and organ transplant team per hospital policy.

8. Because trauma commonly involves young, previously healthy people, the trauma patient may be a suitable organ donor. Although contemplating the end of a loved one's life is naturally distressing, donating the patient's organs may bring meaning and comfort to his family.

9. Additional individualized interventions:_____

9. Rationales: _____

Suggested NIC Interventions
Surveillance: Safety

Suggested NOC Outcomes
Safety status: Physical injury

Discharge planning

DISCHARGE CHECKLIST
Upon discharge, the patient shows evidence of:
- stable vital signs
- stable laboratory values
- absence of major complications, such as sepsis, renal failure, and increased ICP.

TEACHING CHECKLIST
Document evidence that the patient and family demonstrate an understanding of:
- extent of injuries
- prognosis
- treatments
- pain management
- posttrauma syndrome

❏ coping resources
❏ organ donation process, if appropriate.

DOCUMENTATION CHECKLIST
Using outcome criteria as a guide, document:
❏ clinical status on admission
❏ significant changes in status
❏ pertinent laboratory and diagnostic test findings
❏ airway and ventilation support
❏ fluid administration
❏ medication administration
❏ nutritional support
❏ emotional support
❏ measures to prevent or treat complications
❏ patient and family teaching
❏ discharge planning.

Associated care plans

■ Acute pain
■ Acute renal failure
■ Acute respiratory distress syndrome
■ Disseminated intravascular coagulation
■ Dying
■ Grieving
■ Hypovolemic shock
■ Impaired physical mobility
■ Increased intracranial pressure
■ Ineffective individual coping
■ Knowledge deficit
■ Mechanical ventilation
■ Nutritional deficit
■ Septic shock

References

Buduhan G., and McRitchie, D.I. "Missed Injuries in Patients with Multiple Trauma," *The Journal of Trauma* 49(4):600-605, October 2000.

Dewar, A. "Protecting Strategies Used by Sufferers of Catastrophic Illnesses and Injuries," *Journal of Clinical Nursing* 10(5):600-608, September 2001.

Fritsch, D.E., and Steinmann, R.A. "Managing Trauma Patients with Abdominal Compartment Syndrome," *Critical Care Nurse* 20(6):48-58, December 2000.

Harrahill, M. "Tracheobronchial injuries," *Journal of Emergency Nursing* 28(3):265-66, June 2002.

Hoover, T.J., and Siefert, J.A. "Soft Tissue Complications of Orthopedic Emergencies," *Emergency Medical Clinics of North America* 18(1):115-39, February 2000.

Laskowski-Jones, L. "Managing Spleen Trauma Without Surgery," *Nursing* 32(1):36-41, January 2002.

Mattox, K., et al. *Trauma,* 4th ed. New York: McGraw-Hill Book Co., 2000.

Miller, C.A. "The Connection Between Drugs and Falls in Elders," *Geriatric Nursing* 23(2):109-10, March-April 2002.

Peitzman, A.B., et al. *The Trauma Manual,* 2nd ed. Philadelphia: Lippincott Williams & Wilkins, 2002.

Smeltzer, S.C., and Bare, B.G., eds. *Brunner and Suddarth's Textbook of Medical-Surgical Nursing,* 9th ed. Philadelphia: Lippincott Williams & Wilkins, 2000.

Trauma Nursing Care Course, 5th ed. Park Ridge, Ill.: Emergency Nurses Association, 2000.

Musculoskeletal and integumentary disorders

Osteomyelitis

DRG INFORMATION
DRG 238   Osteomyelitis.
> Mean LOS = 8.6 days

Principal diagnoses include:
- acute osteomyelitis
- chronic osteomyelitis
- unspecified osteomyelitis.

Introduction
DEFINITION AND TIME FOCUS
Osteomyelitis is a bone infection that may be classified as primary, secondary, or chronic. *Primary osteomyelitis* occurs from compound fractures, penetrating wounds, or surgery. *Secondary osteomyelitis* may be hematogenous (blood-borne) or may represent extension of nearby infections (especially pressure ulcers). *Chronic osteomyelitis*, a persistent bone infection manifested by draining sinus tracts, is rare.

This care plan focuses on the patient receiving nonsurgical treatment of osteomyelitis for which postdischarge antibiotic therapy is anticipated. (See *Clinical snapshot: Osteomyelitis*.)

ETIOLOGY AND PRECIPITATING FACTORS
- Bone infection (either blood-borne or from an open wound) with sufficient numbers of pathogenic bacteria, most commonly *Staphylococcus aureus*
- Sufficient bone and soft-tissue trauma and hematoma to provide growth media for the infecting agent
- Implantation of foreign material (joint replacements or metallic internal fixation devices) that may impair the body's ability to control bacterial growth
- Infection near bone or joints
- I.V. drug abuse

Focused assessment guidelines
NURSING HISTORY
(FUNCTIONAL HEALTH PATTERN FINDINGS)
Health-perception–health-management pattern
- Deficient knowledge about basic health care practices, especially hand washing and signs and symptoms of infection
- History of unreported local infection
- Unreported systemic indicators of infection, such as fever, malaise, weakness, irritability, anorexia, and generalized sepsis (rare)
- Recent upper respiratory tract infection, urinary tract infection, otitis media, impetigo, tonsillitis, or dental procedure
- History of disinterest in learning about care of an immobilization device or devices (for example, cast, splint, external fixator, or brace) needed previously

Activity-exercise pattern
- Weakness and fatigue

Cognitive-perceptual pattern
- Pain in affected limb, increasing with movement

Sleep-rest pattern
- Night sweats
- Pain affecting sleep

PHYSICAL FINDINGS
General
- Emotional irritability

Cardiovascular
- Tachycardia

Integumentary
- Localized edema and erythema in infection area
- Localized tenderness in infection area
- Draining wound, with either serous or gross purulent drainage (may not be present in all patients)
- Diaphoresis and flushing with fever
- Chronically draining sinus tracts (rare)

Musculoskeletal
- Pseudoparalysis (inability to move joints adjacent to area of osteomyelitis because of anticipated pain)
- Muscle spasm in infected extremity

DIAGNOSTIC STUDIES
- Wound aspirate or bone biopsy of sequestrum (involved bone) — demonstrates the infecting organism
- Complete blood count — reveals leukocytosis and, after prolonged infection, anemia related to associated decrease in erythropoietin production and reduced red blood cell life span
- Erythrocyte sedimentation rate — elevated; degree of elevation relates to extent of infection
- Blood cultures — may reveal infecting organism when shaking chills and temperature spikes are associated with osteomyelitis
- X-rays of involved bones — may eventually show evidence of osteonecrosis and new bone formation
- Radioisotope scanning — may reveal areas of increased vascularity, indicating infection
- Sinography of draining sinus tract — may outline involved areas of chronic osteomyelitis

- Computed tomography scan — may reveal changes indicating osteonecrosis
- Magnetic resonance imaging — may reveal soft-tissue inflammation
- Myelogram — may be required for vertebral infections

POTENTIAL COMPLICATIONS
- Chronic osteomyelitis
- Sepsis
- Dysfunctional limb
- Refractory, life-threatening infection requiring amputation
- Pathologic fractures
- Nonunion of existing fractures

CLINICAL SNAPSHOT

Osteomyelitis

Major nursing diagnoses and collaborative problems	Key patient outcomes
ND: Acute pain	Rate pain a less than 3 on a 0 to 10 pain rating scale.
CP: Risk for repeat infection	List, on request, local and systemic signs and symptoms of infection.
ND: Risk for injury	Monitor responses as needed for specific antibiotics.
ND: Risk for disuse syndrome	Independently perform prescribed exercises; show no signs or symptoms of complications.

Nursing diagnosis
Acute pain related to inflammation

NURSING PRIORITY
Relieve pain.

PATIENT OUTCOME CRITERIA
Within 1 day of admission, the patient will:
- show no indications of uncontrolled pain, such as facial grimacing, tachycardia, increased blood pressure, or groaning
- verbalize pain control
- rate pain severity as less than 3 on a 0 to 10 pain rating scale while using pain medications.
  Within 2 days of admission, the patient will:
- verbalize or demonstrate an understanding of at least two personally effective nonpharmacologic methods of pain control
- verbalize an understanding of the need to report increasing or uncontrolled pain.

INTERVENTIONS	RATIONALES
1. *Provide standard nursing care related to acute pain.** See the "Acute pain" care plan, page 32.	1. General interventions for pain are detailed in the "Acute pain" care plan.
2. *Clearly identify and document the source and degree of pain.* Aid the patient in rating pain, using a scale.	2. Continuing or increasing severe pain may indicate increasing inflammation.
3. *Medicate the patient with narcotics and nonsteroidal anti-inflammatory drugs (NSAIDs),* as ordered, and carefully document their effectiveness. Monitor for adverse reactions.	3. Bone pain is usually severe.

*Italics indicate key interventions.

4. *Instruct the patient in nonpharmacologic pain control methods,* including relaxation, enhanced relaxation, guided imagery, distraction (verbal, auditory, visual, or tactile), rhythmic breathing, massage, transcutaneous electrical nerve stimulation, use of heat and cold, and biofeedback. Document methods that the patient finds helpful.

4. Nonpharmacologic pain control allows self-control of pain without possible adverse drug reactions to medications. Ice, for example, acts as a tactile distraction, stimulates large-diameter cutaneous sensory neurons, which decreases deeper pain sensation (the gate control theory), and causes vasoconstriction, which reduces edema that contributes to pain.

5. *Elevate and support the affected extremity.*

5. Elevation enhances venous return to reduce inflammatory edema; supportive positioning protects against muscle strain and spasm.

6. *Schedule necessary activity of the involved extremity to coincide with the peak effectiveness of analgesics or NSAIDs.*

6. Scheduling activity to coincide with the peak of medication action decreases discomfort while allowing necessary mobility.

7. *Instruct the patient to report increasing or uncontrolled pain.*

7. Increasing or uncontrolled pain may indicate worsening osteomyelitis, ineffective therapy, or both.

8. *Use adjunctive devices* (such as a bed cradle, antirotation boots, or a mechanical bed) to aid in pain control.

8. Reducing direct pressure, rotational force, and discomfort from turning may help control pain in some circumstances.

9. *Maintain traction and support devices* (such as a cast, a splint, or internal fixators), as ordered.

9. Immobilization and external support devices aid fracture healing, protect the infected bone from excessive stress, and decrease pain.

10. Additional individualized interventions:_____

10. Rationales:_____

> **Suggested NIC Interventions**
> *Medication management; Pain management; Patient controlled analgesia (PCA) assistance; Analgesic administration; Conscious sedation*

> **Suggested NOC Outcomes**
> *Comfort level; Pain control; Pain: Disruptive effects; Pain level*

Collaborative problem
Risk for repeat infection related to deficient knowledge of infection control

NURSING PRIORITY
Teach the patient to recognize local and systemic indicators of infection.

PATIENT OUTCOME CRITERIA
Within 2 days of admission, the patient will:
- list, on request, local and systemic signs and symptoms of infection
- verbalize an understanding of the need to alert health care providers promptly if infection occurs.

INTERVENTIONS

1. *Instruct about signs and symptoms of local infection* (erythema, edema, localized tenderness, serous or purulent discharge, and local warmth) *and systemic infection* (fever, chills, malaise, weakness, and irritability). Teach the need to report limited range of motion (ROM) as a possible indication of spreading infection. Stress the need to report these findings promptly; provide a phone number for postdischarge contact.

RATIONALES

1. Prompt reporting of signs and symptoms of local and systemic infections ensures early identification and treatment of infection.

2. *Evaluate learning* by having the patient list the signs and symptoms of infection, preferably in writing. Document learning. See the "Knowledge deficit" care plan, page 129.

3. *Provide the patient with a written list of local and systemic signs and symptoms of infection* for periodic review. Document the material provided.

4. When necessary, establish continuity for continued education or evaluation of learning through community health nurse referrals.

5. Additional individualized interventions:_____
_____

2. Having the patient list signs and symptoms provides feedback about learning and an opportunity to identify omissions and correct misconceptions. The "Knowledge deficit" care plan contains further details related to patient teaching.

3. Readily accessible review materials help the patient retain new knowledge.

4. Some patients won't benefit from the patient education provided and will require continued instruction or appropriate follow-up care.

5. Rationales: _____
_____

Nursing diagnosis
Risk for injury related to use of antibiotics with high potential for toxic effects

NURSING PRIORITY
Prevent or minimize toxic effects of antibiotic therapy.

PATIENT OUTCOME CRITERIA
Within 2 days after initiation of therapy, the patient will:
- (with aminoglycoside therapy) list signs and symptoms of ototoxicity, nephrotoxicity, and superimposed infections
- (with penicillin therapy) list signs and symptoms of anemia, hypersensitivity reaction, and opportunistic infections
- (with cephalosporin therapy) list signs and symptoms of photosensitivity, hepatotoxicity, nephrotoxicity, and opportunistic infections
- (with sulfonamide therapy) list signs and symptoms of nephrotoxicity, agranulocytosis, crystalluria, and hemorrhagic tendencies
- (with fluoroquinolone therapy) list the signs and symptoms of nephrotoxicity and potential drug interactions
- with vancomycin therapy) list the signs and symptoms of ototoxicity, nephrotoxicity, hypersensitivity reactions and "red man" syndrome
- verbalize the importance of rapidly reporting signs and symptoms of untoward effects.
  By the time of discharge, the patient will:
- monitor responses as needed for specific antibiotics.

INTERVENTIONS

1. *Teach the patient about antibiotic administration,* especially monitoring for significant antibiotic adverse effects. See *Minimizing adverse effects of antibiotic therapy,* pages 599 and 600.

2. *Instruct the patient to report any adverse effects promptly.*

3. Additional individualized interventions:_____
_____

RATIONALES

1. A patient's knowledgeable participation in self-care while in the hospital improves the quality of care, allows for rapid identification of complications, and prepares the patient for self-care after discharge.

2. Prompt identification and notification reduce the potential for long-term complications.

3. Rationales:_____
_____

Nursing diagnosis

Risk for disuse syndrome with risk factors of prolonged infection, pain, and immobilization

NURSING PRIORITY

Help the patient regain or exceed usual activity level.

PATIENT OUTCOME CRITERIA

Within 2 days of admission, the patient will:
- verbalize an understanding of the need for exercise when mobility is restricted
- list exercise goals
- demonstrate the exercise regimen.
  By the time of discharge, the patient will:
- independently perform prescribed exercises
- show no signs or symptoms of complications due to immobilization.

INTERVENTIONS

1. *Assess and document the patient's baseline activity level,* including muscle strength and ability to perform activities of daily living (ADLs).

2. *Document activity goals* set in collaboration with the patient.

3. *Teach the patient about the need to maintain muscle strength and endurance while immobilized.* Provide instruction in isotonic and isometric exercises that can be accomplished within the patient's activity limitations.

4. *Have the patient demonstrate the exercises,* and evaluate and document the patient's learning. Establish and monitor an exercise regimen throughout the hospital stay. Help the patient establish a home exercise program as well, and ensure community health care follow-up after discharge, when needed.

5. Provide abundant positive reinforcement. Develop goals of increasing strength (increasing increments of resistance or weight) and endurance (increasing numbers or repetitions or longer exercise periods), when feasible.

6. *Provide written materials on exercises* for review as needed. Document the materials provided.

7. Additional individualized interventions:_____

RATIONALES

1. Adequate baseline information allows determination of individualized goals.

2. Involving the patient in planning increases the potential for success. Goals provide focus.

3. Maintenance exercise programs decrease loss of muscle strength and endurance during immobilization by maintaining adequate blood flow to muscle and by stressing bone to ensure continued balance in bone remodeling.

4. Return demonstration of exercises allows effective evaluation of patient learning. Monitoring the exercise regimen ensures that the patient will maintain strength and endurance.

5. Positive reinforcement helps establish health-promoting behaviors. Isometric and isotonic exercises performed within activity restrictions may increase strength and endurance in unaffected body areas.

6. Written materials increase understanding of exercises and the potential for doing exercises as required.

7. Rationales: _____

Minimizing adverse effects of antibiotic therapy

The following chart lists common antibiotics and appropriate interventions.

Drugs	Nursing interventions
Aminoglycosides (gentamicin, neomycin, streptomycin, and tobramycin)	• Teach the potential for ototoxicity (as shown by high-frequency hearing loss [for example, decreased ability to hear a ticking wristwatch], tinnitus, vertigo, and dizziness); superimposed infections (especially fungal infections of mucous membranes or at the site of indwelling vascular access catheters); and nephrotoxicity (as shown by oliguria, polyuria, abnormal specific gravity, and rapid weight gain). • Explain the rationale for baseline and weekly audiograms and serum creatinine and blood urea nitrogen (BUN) studies. • Explain the need for laboratory assessment of serum peak and trough levels (respectively the highest and lowest drug levels). These specimens are collected to ensure the lowest effective dose to maintain bactericidal levels while reducing the potential for adverse effects. • Monitor and document fluid intake and output and urine specific gravity while the patient is hospitalized. Report oliguria, polyuria, and specific gravity extremes (less than 1.010 and greater than 1.030). When appropriate, instruct the patient about continuing this monitoring after discharge. • Weigh the patient twice weekly and document. Teach him about twice weekly weight measurement after discharge. Report weight gain exceeding 3 lb (1.4 kg). • Teach the patient to closely monitor mucous membranes for indications of fungal infection (redness, tenderness, cheesy white discharge, black or furry tongue, fever, nausea, and diarrhea) and the need to report any that occur.
Penicillins (ampicillin, carbenicillin, dicloxacillin, nafcillin, and oxacillin)	• Teach the potential for anemia (as shown by weakness, paleness, and malaise), hypersensitivity reactions (as shown by asthmatic reactions, erythematous-maculopapular rash, urticaria, and anaphylaxis), and overgrowth of nonsusceptible organisms leading to opportunistic infection (as shown by fever, chills, and continuing or increasing indications of infection or inflammation).
Cephalosporins (cefamandole, cefazolin, cefepime, cefoxitin, cephapirin, and cephradine)	• Teach the potential for opportunistic infections (as shown by fever, chills, and continuing or increasing indications of infection or inflammation), photosensitivity and, in the patient with suspected renal or hepatic disease, nephrotoxicity (as shown by oliguria, polyuria, abnormal specific gravity, and rapid weight gain) and hepatotoxicity (as shown by jaundice, icteric sclera, dark brown urine, and pale, pasty stools). • Explain the rationale for baseline and weekly measurement of serum creatinine, BUN, lactic dehydrogenase, serum aspartate aminotransferase, and serum alanine aminotransferase levels. • Monitor and instruct the patient about nephrotoxicity and weight gain, as discussed under "Aminoglycosides" above. • When oral medications are used, teach the patient to avoid concurrent intake of iron products or dairy foods because they decrease cephalosporin absorption. • Instruct the patient to avoid direct sunlight and to use sunblocking agents when sun exposure is unavoidable.
Sulfonamides (sulfadiazine, sulfamethoxazole, and sulfisoxazole)	• Teach the potential for nephrotoxicity (as shown by polyuria, oliguria, abnormal specific gravity, and rapid weight gain), agranulocytosis (as shown by fever and lesions of the mucous membranes, GI tract, and skin), crystalluria (as shown by evidence of renal calculi — hematuria, pyuria, frequency, urgency, retention, and pain in the flank, lower back, perineum, thighs, groin, labia, or scrotum), and hemorrhagic tendencies (as shown by epistaxis, bleeding gums, prolonged bleeding from wounds, ecchymoses, melena, hematuria, hemoptysis, and hematemesis from disruption of intestinal flora and synthesis of vitamin K). • Explain the rationale for baseline and weekly measurement of serum creatinine, BUN, and granulocyte levels. • Monitor and instruct the patient about nephrotoxicity and weight gain, as discussed under "Aminoglycosides" above. • Instruct the patient taking oral sulfonamides to drink 8 oz (237 ml) of fluid with each dose. Encourage total fluid intake of at least eight 8-oz glasses daily.

(continued)

Minimizing adverse effects of antibiotic therapy *(continued)*

Drugs	Nursing interventions
Fluoroquinolones (ciprofloxacin, enoxacin)	• Teach the potential for adverse reactions (such as nausea, vomiting, diarrhea, abdominal discomfort, dizziness, headaches, insomnia, slit lamp eye changes, and skin disorders). Nausea associated with enoxacin may be decreased by taking the medication within 1 hour of a meal. • Teach the potential for drug interactions, especially when taking theophylline, because all these agents slow the clearance of theophylline and increase its potential for toxicity. Under the physician's supervision, the theophylline dosage may need to be decreased. Similarly, concurrent use of antacids may decrease absorption of fluoroquinolones. • Explain the need to take ciprofloxacin 2 hours after meals and to drink plenty of fluids while taking this agent. • Monitor for and instruct the patient about nephrotoxicity and weight gain, as discussed under "Aminoglycosides" above.
Vancomycin (Vancocin, Vancoled)	• Teach the potential for ototoxicity (high-frequency hearing loss [for example decreased ability to hear a ticking wristwatch], tinnitus, vertigo, or dizziness), nephrotoxicity (as shown by oliguria, polyuria, abnormal specific gravity, and rapid weight gain), hypersensitivity reactions (urticaria, chills, fever, skin rash, and anaphylactoid reaction with accompanying vascular collapse) and, following too-rapid I.V. infusion, "red man" syndrome (flushing and erythematous rash on the upper thorax and face accompanied by hypotension). • Explain the need for laboratory assessment of serum peak and trough levels (respectively the highest and lowest drug levels). These specimens are collected to ensure the lowest effective dose to maintain bactericidal levels while reducing the potential for adverse effects. • Monitor for nephrotoxicity and weight gain, as discussed under "Aminoglycosides" above.
I.V. antibiotics	• When indwelling vascular access catheters are used for antibiotic administration, closely monitor the insertion sites for inflammation or irritation that doesn't respond to treatment with topical antibiotics. Teach the patient to monitor for this complication and promptly report it to the health care provider. • Teach close monitoring of wounds for indications of unresolving or increasing inflammation or infection (which are evidence of opportunistic infection).
Any oral antibiotic	• Instruct the patient about the need to take medication, as ordered. Although some antibiotic therapy (such as with fluoroquinolones) may be administered orally, this doesn't decrease the need to ensure that medications are administered on schedule to provide adequate serum drug levels.

Suggested NIC Interventions

Activity therapy; Energy management; Cognitive stimulation; Environmental management; Exercise therapy: Ambulation; Exercise therapy: Balance; Exercise therapy: Joint mobility; Exercise therapy: Muscle control

Suggested NOC Outcomes

Endurance; Immobility consequences: Physiological; Immobility consequences: Psycho-cognitive; Mobility level

---

Discharge planning

DISCHARGE CHECKLIST

Before discharge, the patient shows evidence of:

❏ wound drainage within expected parameters, with little or no purulent or bloody drainage

❏ stable vital signs

❏ absence of fever

❏ absence of pulmonary or cardiovascular complications

❏ absence of erythema, edema, or tenderness at wound site

- absence of loss of ROM in joints adjacent to the infection
- ability to control pain using oral medications
- stabilizing weight and adequate nutritional intake
- ability to perform ADLs at usual level
- ability to transfer, ambulate, and perform prescribed exercise regimen at usual level or with minimal assistance
- ability to perform wound care and dressing changes as prescribed, with minimal assistance
- hemoglobin level and blood cultures within normal parameters
- white blood cell count within expected parameters
- normal bowel and bladder function
- adequate home support system, or referral to home care if indicated by inadequate home support system or inability to perform self-care.

If the patient is discharged with an indwelling vascular access catheter, documentation also shows:
- evidence of automatic referral to home care or arrangements for short-term stay in a nursing home (depending on the patient's home support system and ability to care for catheter and administer medications independently)
- knowledge of where to obtain additional supplies
- knowledge of signs and symptoms indicating catheter dysfunction or infection
- ability to follow prescribed medication regimen and I.V. administration technique
- ability to monitor weight and follow instructions for oral intake as directed
- knowledge of signs and symptoms indicating fungal or other systemic infection.

TEACHING CHECKLIST

Document evidence that the patient and family demonstrate an understanding of:
- disease and implications
- hand-washing techniques
- dressing changes, pin site care, cast care, or care of braces or splints as appropriate
- nonpharmacologic pain-control interventions
- use of elevation and supportive positioning
- ROM exercise of the affected extremity as appropriate
- dietary requirements
- all discharge medications' purposes, dosages, administration schedules, precautions, and adverse effects requiring medical attention (usual discharge medications include antibiotics, analgesics, and NSAIDs)
- need to report increasing or uncontrolled pain
- care of indwelling vascular access catheters
- self-administration of I.V. antibiotics
- vascular access complications
- patient exercise regimen
- how to obtain clarification of instructions or further information

- date, time, and place of follow-up appointments
- referral agencies and medical supply resources
- how to contact the physician.

DOCUMENTATION CHECKLIST

Using outcome criteria as a guide, document:
- clinical status on admission
- significant changes in status
- pertinent laboratory and diagnostic test findings
- baseline information on muscle strength, ADLs performed, endurance, and collaborative goals established with the patient
- source and degree of pain, especially if persistent or increasing
- effective pain-relief measures
- daily or biweekly measurement of weight, intake, output, and urine specific gravity, when appropriate
- appearance of indwelling vascular access catheter site and catheter care
- patient and family teaching
- discharge planning.

Associated care plans

- Acute pain
- Chronic renal failure
- Ineffective individual coping
- Knowledge deficit
- Perioperative care
- Urolithiasis

References

Bibbo, C., et al. "Neutropenic Enterocolitis in a Trauma Patient During Antibiotic Therapy for Osteomyelitis," *The Journal of Trauma* 49(4):760-63, October 2000.

DiPasquale, D. "Chronic Osteomyelitis in Adults: Aggressive Management Required," *Journal of Musculoskeletal Medicine* 17(5):250-53, 2000.

Hoover, T.J., and Siefert, J.A. "Soft Tissue Complications Orthopedic Emergencies," *Emergency Medicine Clinics of North America* 18(1):115-39, February 2000.

Mattox, K., et al. *Trauma,* 4th ed. New York: McGraw-Hill Book Co., 2000.

Nursing2004 Drug Handbook, 24nd ed. Philadelphia: Lippincott Williams & Wilkins, 2003.

Smeltzer, S.C., and Bare, B.G., eds. *Brunner and Suddarth's Textbook of Medical-Surgical Nursing,* 9th ed. Philadelphia: Lippincott Williams & Wilkins, 2000.

Musculoskeletal and integumentary disorders

Skin grafts

DRG INFORMATION
DRG 263   Skin Grafts or Debridement for Skin Ulcer or Cellulitis with Complication or Comorbidity (CC).
Mean LOS = 11.7 days
DRG 264   Skin Grafts or Debridement for Skin Ulcer or Cellulitis without CC.
Mean LOS = 7.0 days
DRG 439   Skin Grafts for Injuries.
Mean LOS = 8.4 days

Introduction
DEFINITION AND TIME FOCUS
Skin grafting is the process of covering damaged tissue, such as burns or pressure ulcers, with healthy skin transplants. The skin transplants may be autografts from the patient's body, allografts or homografts from another person, or heterografts from a different species (such as porcine grafts). Grafts vary in thickness, depending on the extent of the wound, the availability of donor sites, the mobility and vascularity of the area to be covered, and the desired cosmetic results. The usual types are:
■ split-thickness grafts — epidermis and part of the dermis, varying from thin to thick, meshed or nonmeshed; thinner grafts are used for large, hidden areas; thicker grafts, large, visible areas
■ full-thickness grafts — epidermis and dermis, used for visible, mobile areas, such as the eyelids and hands
■ flap grafts — autografts of skin and subcutaneous tissue where part of the flap is left attached to the donor site; used for large areas with a poor blood supply
■ allogenic or autologous cultured epithelial sheets — healthy skin cell biopsies minced and cultured into thin sheets over 3 to 4 weeks; sheets can cover large body surface areas.

This care plan focuses on the patient with any large, open skin wound who is admitted for preoperative wound preparation and skin grafting with a split-thickness autograft. (See *Clinical snapshot: Skin grafts,* page 604.)

ETIOLOGY AND PRECIPITATING FACTORS
■ Burns of sufficient extent or depth to require grafting for protection and healing
■ Large pressure or vascular ulcers, particularly over bony, avascular areas, that can't heal effectively through normal epithelialization and granulation from the wound edges inward

■ Major trauma, such as avulsion of an extremity, that may require grafting for protection and to preserve function

Focused assessment guidelines
NURSING HISTORY (FUNCTIONAL HEALTH PATTERN FINDINGS)
Because skin grafts are performed for different reasons, such as burns, wounds, and trauma, a typical presenting picture doesn't exist. However, the nurse must assess all patients undergoing skin grafting for preoperative preparedness to ensure optimal outcomes; therefore, this section presents preoperative assessment guidelines.
Health-perception–health-management pattern
■ Determine the purpose for grafting, including the cause and extent of the injury; the grafting procedure; expectations for successful graft adherence; and the potential for return of function as the basis for care, patient teaching, and discharge planning.
■ Determine the patient's perceptions regarding potential disfigurement and its impact on health status and lifestyle.
Nutritional-metabolic pattern
■ Assess typical nutritional intake for adequate fluids, calories, proteins, and vitamins.
■ Assess nutritional status for signs of nutritional deficiency, such as weight loss, poor skin and hair condition, and low albumin levels, that may increase the risk of graft loss and infection.
■ Assess for general conditions that may contribute to poor healing, such as general debilitation, immobility, age, prolonged bed rest, skin and circulatory problems, steroid use, hyperglycemia, and inability to perform activities of daily living (ADLs).
■ Assess the graft site for the presence of healthy granulation tissue and the absence of necrotic areas, drainage, and odor. Grafts will adhere only to healthy granulated tissue.
Elimination pattern
■ Assess for elimination problems, such as frequent bowel and bladder incontinence, that may contribute to skin breakdown and poor healing.
Activity-exercise pattern
■ Assess normal activity and exercise habits to determine the patient's potential for adjusting to position and activity limitations.

■ Establish a baseline assessment of present musculoskeletal and neurologic functions for comparison to potential postoperative changes in function and sensation.

Sleep-rest pattern
■ Assess normal sleep patterns to guide postoperative management of pain and rest.

Cognitive-perceptual pattern
■ Determine the patient's readiness for treatment by assessing understanding of the injury's extent, the prognosis for return of function, the surgical procedure, and rehabilitation phases during the hospital stay and home care.

Self-perception–self-concept pattern
■ Assess the patient's usual self-perception–self-concept pattern to determine ability to adapt positively during the hospital stay and recovery at home.
■ Assess the impact of body changes on the patient's feelings of self-worth.

Role-relationship pattern
■ Assess the patient's concerns regarding the impact of current or potential disfigurement on relationships with family and others.
■ Assess family members' and friends' ability to support the patient.

Sexuality-reproductive pattern
■ Assess the patient's concerns regarding alterations in physical attractiveness, ability to feel sensations, and ability to perform sexually. (*Note:* Grafted tissue may have a decreased touch sensation.)

Coping–stress tolerance pattern
■ Assess for anxiety, anger, and depression related to changes in body image and potentially permanent disfigurement. (*Note:* Regression is a common coping pattern for the patient with large wounds needing grafting.)

Value-belief pattern
■ Assess the effect of cultural and value-belief systems on the patient's response to illness.

PHYSICAL FINDINGS
Cardiovascular
■ Poor capillary refill

Neurologic
■ Diminished sensation, including pain response, over wound
■ Increased pain response around wound edges

Integumentary
■ Fragile skin
■ Poor skin turgor
■ Ulcerated area (damage may extend to subcutaneous tissue, underlying fat, and muscle; tissue may be reddened, draining, and necrotic)
■ Bleeding and clot formation from early excision of eschar and necrotic tissue

Musculoskeletal
■ Limited mobility
■ Limited range of motion (ROM)

DIAGNOSTIC STUDIES
■ Culture and sensitivity testing of wound drainage — may indicate infecting organism and help determine the most desirable antibiotic treatment
■ White blood cell (WBC) count — may be elevated in presence of inflammation and infection
■ Complete blood count — may show a low hematocrit, which may affect tissue healing
■ Clotting time — may be prolonged, affecting tissue healing
■ Serum protein (albumin and globulin) and fat (cholesterol and triglyceride) levels — may be depressed in poor nutritional status
■ Postoperative tissue biopsy — may show infection or indicate degree of graft success
■ Ultrasound — may determine size of wound, particularly if deep

POTENTIAL COMPLICATIONS
■ Nonadherence of graft
■ Infection
■ Contractures
■ Hypertrophic scar formation at donor or recipient site

Musculoskeletal and integumentary disorders

CLINICAL SNAPSHOT ✴

Skin grafts

Major nursing diagnoses and collaborative problems	Key patient outcomes
CP: Risk for nonadherence of graft related to inadequate wound preparation	Exhibit signs of wound healing.
CP: Risk for nonadherance of graft related to postoperative exudate or blood accumulation, movement, or infection	Have a healing graft free from infection, swelling, and accumulation of blood or exudates.
ND: Risk for infection	Exhibit a dry, infection-free donor site.
ND: Impaired physical mobility	Perform ADLs, position changes, ROM exercises, and other activities as allowed.
ND: Imbalanced nutrition: More than body requirements	Exhibit no signs or symptoms of inadequate nutritional intake.
ND: Disturbed body image	Verbalize feelings about the wound and healing on request.
ND: Deficient knowledge (home care of donor and graft sites)	Describe appropriate graft and donor site appearance and care.

Collaborative problem

Risk for nonadherence of graft related to inadequate wound preparation

NURSING PRIORITY

Prepare the wound properly for grafting.

PATIENT OUTCOME CRITERIA

Within 2 days of admission, the patient will:
- exhibit signs of wound healing
- exhibit no redness over pressure points.

INTERVENTIONS	RATIONALES
1. *Assess and document wound condition and surrounding skin** on admission and at least every shift. Indicate the wound's size, color, and depth and the presence or absence of odor, drainage, necrotic tissue, and swelling.	1. Initial documentation provides baseline data concerning wound condition. Regular assessment and documentation provide data on the pattern of healing.
2. *Change dressings* as ordered, using good hand-washing and sterile techniques. Use dressings that are nonadherent, absorptive, immobilizing, and protective.	2. Conscientious attention to technique helps prevent infection. The dressing needs to keep the wound moist, to protect it from infection, and be absorbent, to protect the area.
3. *Clean the wound and surrounding skin* with soap and water, as ordered, every shift. Apply topical agents as ordered.	3. Cleaning the skin prevents bacterial colonization and spread. Topical microbicidal agents such as povidone-iodine may help prevent infections, if indicated.
4. *Irrigate the wound with normal saline solution* as ordered.	4. Wound irrigation with large amounts of normal saline solution removes drainage, debriding agents, and contaminants.
5. *Apply hydrophilic agents* as ordered.	5. Hydrophilic agents such as dextranomer (Debrisan) absorb drainage and aid in wound debridement.

*Italics indicate key interventions.

6. *Apply enzymes to the wound* every shift as ordered. Examples are fibrinolysin and desoxyribonuclease (Elase). Apply only to the wound, protecting healthy tissue with an ointment such as zinc oxide.

6. Enzymes soften necrotic tissue by fibrinolytic action, breaking up clots and exudates. Although enzymes act primarily on necrotic tissue, healthy tissue may be irritated unless protected.

7. *Assist the physician, as needed, with surgical debridement of necrotic tissue.*

7. Removal of necrotic tissue speeds healing and granulation tissue development.

8. *Apply barrier dressings,* if ordered, every 3 to 4 days or as needed for leakage.

8. Barrier dressings maintain a moist environment, which promotes granulation tissue formation.

9. *Change the patient's position* every $1\frac{1}{2}$ to 2 hours, protecting the affected area from pressure by using rubber rings, extra padding, or special positioning.

9. Position changes promote circulation and prevent tissue damage from prolonged pressure.

10. Additional individualized interventions:_____

10. Rationales:_____

Collaborative problem

Risk for nonadherence of graft related to postoperative exudate or blood accumulation, movement, or infection

NURSING PRIORITIES
Maintain graft integrity and promote graft healing.

PATIENT OUTCOME CRITERIA
Within 2 days after surgery, the patient will:
- exhibit an intact graft
- exhibit a graft free from injury
- keep the dressing intact.
  Within 2 weeks after surgery, the patient will:
- exhibit a graft free from infection, swelling, and exudate or blood accumulation
- exhibit graft adherence and blood supply formation.

INTERVENTIONS

1. *Maintain movement restrictions* for 3 days or as ordered. Use splints, restraints, pillows, or other devices to maintain the desired position. Teach the patient about position and activity limitations.

2. *Elevate the grafted area,* if possible, for 1 week after surgery.

3. *Continuously protect the graft from injury,* using splints or bed cradles.

4. *Assist the physician during initial removal of inner dressings and graft inspection,* usually 1 to 2 days after surgery. Document findings. Thereafter, carefully assess the graft every 8 hours and document its appearance. Report immediately any swelling, redness, and exudate or blood under the graft.

RATIONALES

1. Movement of the tissue under the graft may dislodge it. Adherence will be evident several days after surgery, although 2 to 3 weeks are needed for vascularization.

2. Elevation prevents swelling, which could cause graft separation.

3. Jarring or pressure may dislodge the graft.

4. Initial dressing removal must be done with utmost care to prevent separating the graft from the underlying tissue. Regular inspections allow prompt treatment of complications. Any substance, such as exudate or blood, coming between the graft and underlying tissue may cause separation. Swelling or redness may indicate infection, which can dislodge the graft. The physician must carefully remove any drainage by aspiration or by rolling an applicator toward a nicked area.

5. *Apply dressings and maintain continuously,* as ordered. Report unusual drainage or dislodged dressings.

5. Various dressings — including petroleum gauze, nonadhesive gauze, coarse mesh gauze, and moist saline-soaked gauze — may be used to maintain gentle pressure on the graft. Newer dressings, semipermeable films, semiocclusive hydrogels and occlusive hydrocolloids are designed to provide a microenvironment conducive to the healing process. Drainage or dislodged dressings may prevent adherence.

6. *Administer topical or systemic antibiotics, or both,* as ordered.

6. Antibiotics may be used to prevent or treat graft infection.

7. Additional individualized interventions:_____

7. Rationales:_____

Nursing diagnosis

Risk for infection of donor site related to surgical excision of half of the skin layer

NURSING PRIORITY
Promote healing of the donor site.

PATIENT OUTCOME CRITERIA
Within 2 days after surgery, the patient will:
- exhibit a dry, infection-free donor site.
  Within 2 weeks after surgery, the patient will:
- exhibit a reepithelialized donor site
- exhibit soft and unscarred skin.

INTERVENTIONS

1. *Maintain dressings over the donor site* for 1 to 2 days. Document your actions. Then lightly dress or leave the site open to air, leaving the fine mesh gauze intact.

2. *Promote air circulation to the donor site* by using a cradle to keep bedding and clothing away from the site.

3. *If infection occurs, notify provider immediately,* apply wet antiseptic dressings such as acetic acid or topical agents, as ordered.

4. *After healing (usually in 2 to 3 weeks), apply lotion to the site* four times daily or as ordered.

5. Additional individualized interventions:_____

RATIONALES

1. Dressings are left over the site until serum dries. The inner dressing is either a nonadherent dressing or fine mesh gauze; it's left in place until it falls off (usually 2 to 3 weeks).

2. Air circulation aids drying and healing.

3. Antiseptic dressings decrease microorganism growth and aid healing.

4. Lotions keep the skin soft and help prevent scarring.

5. Rationales: _____

Suggested NIC Interventions
Infection control; Infection protection; Incision site care; Wound care

Suggested NOC Outcomes
Infection status; Wound healing: Primary intention

Nursing diagnosis

Impaired physical mobility related to position and movement limitations

NURSING PRIORITY
Promote maintenance of muscle tone and skin integrity.

PATIENT OUTCOME CRITERIA
Within 8 hours after surgery, the patient will:
- have no uncontrolled pain or discomfort
- exhibit an intact graft
- perform ADLs, position changes, ROM exercises, and other activities as allowed.

INTERVENTIONS	RATIONALES
1. *Provide active and passive ROM exercises to unaffected areas* every 2 hours as ordered.	**1.** ROM exercises promote muscle tone, circulation, and a feeling of well-being; they also help prevent contractures.
2. *Promote self-care* according to the patient's tolerance and the physician's orders.	**2.** Self-care enhances feelings of independence and control over the course of recovery.
3. *Apply splints and other devices,* as ordered, either continuously or as needed during activities or ambulation.	**3.** Protective devices allow some mobility while protecting the graft site.
4. *Provide relief as needed for discomfort or pain.* See the "Acute pain" care plan, page 32.	**4.** The patient will experience pain from the graft and donor sites and discomfort from immobility. Relief from pain or discomfort encourages movement, as allowed, and aids healing by promoting a sense of well-being. The "Acute pain" care plan contains general interventions for pain management.
5. Additional individualized interventions:_____	**5.** Rationales: _____

> **Suggested NIC Interventions**
> *Exercise therapy: Ambulation; Exercise therapy: Balance; Exercise therapy: Joint mobility; Exercise therapy: Muscle control; Exercise promotion: Strength training*

> **Suggested NOC Outcomes**
> *Ambulation: Walking; Ambulation: Wheelchair; Joint movement: Active; Mobility level*

Nursing diagnosis
Imbalanced nutrition: More than body requirements related to increased metabolic needs secondary to tissue healing

NURSING PRIORITY
Provide adequate calories and protein to promote tissue healing.

PATIENT OUTCOME CRITERIA
Within 1 week after surgery, the patient will:
- exhibit no signs or symptoms of inadequate nutritional intake
- exhibit a healing wound.

INTERVENTIONS	RATIONALES
1. *Assess and document nutritional status* daily, including weight, wound healing, and condition of skin, hair, and mucous membranes. Note baseline serum total protein findings.	**1.** Baseline and ongoing assessment data help guide dietary intake.
2. *Provide a high-calorie, high-protein diet* along with vitamin supplements. Document calorie intake and fluid intake and output daily.	**2.** A diet high in calories, protein, and vitamins aids tissue healing. Maintaining fluid balance is necessary for supple skin.
3. Additional individualized interventions: _____	**3.** Rationales: _____

> **Suggested NIC Interventions**
> *Diet staging: Nutrition management; Weight gain assistance; Fluid monitoring; Nutritional monitoring*

> **Suggested NOC Outcomes**
> *Nutritional status; Nutritional status: Food and fluid intake; Nutritional status: Nutrient intake; Weight control*

Nursing diagnosis
Disturbed body image related to wound and potential scarring

NURSING PRIORITY
Optimize adjustment to body changes.

PATIENT OUTCOME CRITERIA
Within 8 hours after surgery, the patient will:
- verbalize feelings about the wound and healing, on request
- express appropriate expectations regarding healing.

INTERVENTIONS	RATIONALES
1. *Allow expression of fears and concerns related to wounds and scarring.* Document patient concerns. Encourage continuity of discussion by all health team members on all shifts by documenting the patient's current psychological status on the care plan.	**1.** Sharing concerns releases tension and opens discussion, which may lead to more realistic self-appraisal of body changes.
2. *Provide information about the expected stages of graft healing* during nursing care and as needed.	**2.** Knowing what to expect decreases fear of the unknown and allows the patient to participate in assessment of healing. Initially, the area will be reddened, swollen, and different in appearance from surrounding tissue. After 6 months, the area will be more normal in appearance as swelling decreases and color matches other tissue.
3. Additional individualized interventions: _____	**3.** Rationales: _____

> **Suggested NIC Interventions**
> *Body image enhancement; Grief work facilitation; Anticipatory guidance; Coping enhancement; Self-esteem enhancement*

> **Suggested NOC Outcomes**
> *Body image; Grief resolution; Self-esteem*

Nursing diagnosis

Deficient knowledge (home care of donor and graft sites) related to lack of exposure to information

NURSING PRIORITY
Provide information to optimize long-term healing of donor and graft sites.

PATIENT OUTCOME CRITERIA
By the time of discharge, the patient will:
- demonstrate ointment and dressing application
- describe specific activity and position limitations
- explain skin protection methods
- identify diet requirements
- describe appropriate graft and donor site appearance and care
- list two risk factors for poor healing
- list four signs of complications and what to do about them.

INTERVENTIONS

1. *Provide standard nursing care related to deficient knowledge.* See the "Knowledge deficit" care plan, page 129.

2. *Teach the patient and family skin graft care measures:*

– Apply topical ointments, and skin softeners (lanolin and mineral oil), to the donor and graft sites.

– Maintain pressure and protective dressings as ordered.

– Avoid sun exposure by wearing protective clothing and using sunscreen lotions until the graft heals completely (usually in 6 to 12 months).
– Maintain activity and position limitations as ordered.
– Perform ROM exercises and maintain a positioning program, as ordered, until the tissue heals and matures in 6 to 12 months.
– Maintain a diet high in calories, protein, and vitamins.

– Avoid smoking. Attend a smoking-cessation program, if needed.
– Assess the donor and graft sites daily for healing progress and absence of such complications as redness or other discolorations, swelling, drainage, bad odor, pain, and excessive warmth. Promptly report signs of complications to the physician.

3. Additional individualized interventions:_____
_____

RATIONALES

1. The "Knowledge deficit" care plan contains general interventions related to patient teaching.

2. Skin graft care measures provide the following benefits:
– Grafted tissue may lack lubricating glands and may dry more readily. Topical ointments and skin softeners may help eliminate dryness.
– Pressure dressings inhibit excessive scar formation. Protective dressings may be necessary because new tissue is sensitive and easily injured.
– New tissue lacks melanin-producing cells and is more susceptible to sunburn. Melanin-producing cells may regenerate in 6 to 12 months.
– Premature or excessive activity may dislodge the graft.
– ROM exercises and positioning extend the affected area and prevent contractures.

– Additional calories, protein, and vitamins are necessary for tissue healing because the stresses of an open wound, surgery, and hospitalization create a catabolic state.
– Smoking decreases blood flow and oxygen supply to peripheral tissues, thus inhibiting healing.
– Healing tissue should be warm, flat, only slightly more reddened than the surrounding tissue, and flexible, and it should have a capillary refill time of less than 3 seconds. Such signs and symptoms as redness, swelling, and pain may indicate an infection, which could prevent permanent graft adherence. Prompt reporting of complications allows early intervention and preservation of the graft.

3. Rationales: _____
_____

Discharge planning

DISCHARGE CHECKLIST
Before discharge, the patient shows evidence of:
❏ healing and intact donor and graft sites with no evidence of abnormal drainage or swelling
❏ ability to control pain using oral medications
❏ stable vital signs
❏ absence of fever
❏ absence of pulmonary or cardiovascular complications
❏ hemoglobin level and WBC count within normal parameters
❏ ability to perform proper graft and donor-site care independently or with minimal assistance
❏ ability to tolerate adequate nutritional intake
❏ absence of hospital-acquired contractures
❏ ability to verbalize and demonstrate activity and position limitations
❏ absence of bowel and bladder dysfunction
❏ ability to perform ADLs, transfers, and ambulation at usual level with minimal assistance
❏ an adequate home support system or referral to home care or a nursing home if indicated by an inadequate home support system, inability to perform ADLs, or inability to care for graft and donor sites independently.

Additional information: The patient undergoing skin grafts for pressure ulcers is commonly disabled, not independently mobile, and dependent on others for care. Because of this, the patient is considered a "vulnerable adult." Any patient with pressure ulcers should automatically be referred to the social services department so that the ulcers' cause can be investigated. Most states have an automatic reporting mechanism for vulnerable adults, and nurses should be aware of this.

The patient with this diagnosis commonly lives in a nursing home, in which case the nursing home staff should be contacted to ascertain their ability to care for the patient during convalescence. Important questions to consider include: Does the nursing home have adequate staff to care for the patient? Does the nursing home have access to a special mattress or bed that promotes healing? What's the charge for such equipment? Where can the patient be discharged if the nursing home can't provide adequate care or supply needed equipment?

Under Medicare, the cost of special equipment — such as a Clinitron bed — is covered in an acute care setting but isn't covered in a nursing home at the daily rate. This creates a problem if the patient is discharged to a nursing home that can't supply the necessary equipment. Another issue to consider is whether the patient meets Medicare's criteria for extended care benefits. Many patients who undergo skin grafting are eligible for care in extended care facilities upon discharge. If the patient lives at home with a capable, willing caregiver, obtaining and paying for equipment and supplies must be addressed. All of these issues must be considered early in the hospital stay to prevent a delay in discharge. Although these are all nursing considerations, the social services department will probably address them, which is why a social services referral should be automatic.

TEACHING CHECKLIST
Document evidence that the patient and family demonstrate an understanding of:
❏ care of the graft and donor sites
❏ signs and symptoms of complications
❏ activity and position limitations
❏ all discharge medications' purposes, dosages, administration schedules, and adverse effects requiring medical attention (usual discharge medications include topical ointments, such as corticosteroids, and skin softeners, such as lanolin or mineral oil)
❏ recommended dietary modifications
❏ date, time, and location of follow-up appointments
❏ how to contact the physician.

DOCUMENTATION CHECKLIST
Using outcome criteria as a guide, document:
❏ clinical status on admission
❏ significant changes in status
❏ pertinent laboratory and diagnostic test findings
❏ wound condition (donor and graft sites)
❏ pain episodes
❏ pain-relief measures
❏ activity and position limitations
❏ resumption of ADLs
❏ nutritional intake
❏ psychological adjustment
❏ patient and family teaching
❏ discharge planning.

Associated care plans
- Acute pain
- Compromised family coping
- Grieving
- Ineffective individual coping

- Knowledge deficit
- Perioperative care

References

Deunk, J., et al. "Long-term Results of Syndactyly Correction: Full-thickness versus Split-thickness Skin Grafts," *Journal of Hand Surgery* [Br] 28(2):125-30, April 2003.

Jordan, K. (ed). *Emergency Nursing Core Curriculum.* Emergency Nurses Association. Philadelphia: W.B. Saunders Co., 2000.

Lynn-McHale, D.J., and Carlson, K.K. American Association of Critical Care Nurses *AACN Procedure Manual for Critical Care,* 4th ed. Philadelphia: W.B. Saunders Co., 2001.

Shoemaker, W.C., et al. *Textbook of Critical Care,* 4th ed. Philadelphia: W.B. Saunders Co., 2002.

Thourani, V.H., et al. "Factors Affecting Success of Split-thickness Skin Grafts in the Modern Burn Unit," *The Journal of Trauma* 54(3):562-68, March 2003.

Wang C., et al. "Hyperbaric Oxygen for Treating Wounds: A Systematic Review of the Literature," *Archives of Surgery* 138(3):272-79, March 2003.

Musculoskeletal and integumentary disorders

Total joint replacement in a lower extremity

DRG INFORMATION

DRG 209   Major Joint and Limb Reattachment Procedure.
          Mean LOS = 5.1 days
DRG 471   Bilateral or Multiple Major Joint Procedures of the Lower Extremity.
          Mean LOS = 5.6 days

Additional DRG information: These DRGs have been significant money losers because of the cost of surgical components and the rehabilitation time. Although the surgeon may inform the patient before surgery about transfer to a nursing home or extended care facility (ECF), most patients want to stay in the hospital until they feel ready to go home. Nurses can help prepare the patient for an early discharge and transfer.

Introduction

DEFINITION AND TIME FOCUS

Total joint replacement involves the surgical implantation of a prosthesis, which replaces the damaged articulating surfaces of the joint. Joint damage may result from debilitating arthritis or from traumatic degenerative bone disease. In the lower extremity, total joint replacement entails removing the damaged tissues, including bone, synovium, and cartilage. An acrylic cement may be used to attach a metallic prosthesis, which replaces the femoral head or the femoral condyle, or a polyethylene prosthesis, which replaces the acetabulum or tibial plateau. Porous, coated metal implants have been developed that allow bone to grow into the joint area; this method may be used instead of the acrylic cement.

This care plan focuses on preoperative and postoperative care of the patient admitted for total hip or knee replacement. (See *Clinical snapshot: Total joint replacement in a lower extremity.*)

ETIOLOGY AND PRECIPITATING FACTORS

- Factors contributing to joint debilitation, including arthritis, infection, trauma, and obesity
- Causes of degenerative joint incongruity, including hormonal imbalance, instability related to dysplasia, calcium deficiency from menopause, and physiologic changes from aging
- Femoral head irregularities from Legg-Calvé-Perthes disease or avascular necrosis

Focused assessment guidelines

NURSING HISTORY (FUNCTIONAL HEALTH PATTERN FINDINGS)

Health-perception–health-management pattern
- Decreased motivation to carry out a previously prescribed rehabilitation program for an injured or painful joint
- History of misconceptions about care of injured or painful joint — for example, may report exercise during acute pain episodes or inappropriate use of mobility aids
- Accompanying problems, such as obesity, excessive involvement in sports, neurologic deficits, arthritis, or evidence of osteoporosis
- History of problems with or surgical procedures involving this or other joints
- Need for specific aids (such as a knee immobilizer) to prevent falls or further damage
- Short- or long-term use of prescribed corticosteroids

Nutritional-metabolic pattern
- Inadequate nutrient intake before admission, indicating poor tissue state for wound healing

Elimination pattern
- Constipation (related to decreased mobility)

Activity-exercise pattern
- Inability to ambulate, sit up, change position, move extremities, or get in and out of bed
- Inability to tolerate an exercise program because of unusual fatigue and weakness before or after exercise
- Some soreness over bony prominences
- History of unusual swelling around affected joint
- Decreased ability to perform activities of daily living (ADLs)
- Decreased leisure activity related to joint problems

Sleep-rest pattern
- Ineffective rest and sleep patterns, with frequent waking because of pain or stiffness
- Stiffness after sleep or periods of rest

Cognitive-perceptual pattern
- Pain, stiffness, or both, usually chronic and associated with movement or weight bearing
- Lack of knowledge about the specific joint condition, causes of the condition, aggravating factors, ways this procedure will change the condition, stages of recovery and rehabilitation, and personal responsibility during recovery and rehabilitation
- Displayed inability to recognize needs related to healing of affected joint, especially concerning nutrition

needed for healing and limitations on ADLs and planned exercise
Role-relationship pattern
■ Inadequate support system during planned rehabilitation program
Coping–stress tolerance pattern
■ Concern about recovery of full function in affected joint

PHYSICAL FINDINGS

Physical findings vary, depending on the joint involved and the nature and extent of the injury or disease.
Cardiovascular
■ Normal peripheral pulses in affected extremity
Neurologic
■ Decreased bilateral patellar and Achilles reflexes
Musculoskeletal
■ Pain on active or passive range-of-motion (ROM) exercise of affected joint
■ Limited ROM or contracture of affected joint
■ Varus, valgus, or flexion deformity of knees
■ Decreased leg strength
■ Shortening of affected limb
■ Impaired gait
■ Joint enlargement, inflammation, or tenderness
■ Distorted posture from pain or effort to maintain balance

■ Crepitation on movement
Integumentary
■ Ischemic blanching or redness over bony prominences

DIAGNOSTIC STUDIES
■ Serum electrolyte levels — may show hypokalemia from corticosteroid use
■ Fasting blood glucose levels — may show hyperglycemia from corticosteroid use
■ Bilateral X-ray of hip or knee joints — demonstrates extent of degenerative changes
■ Chest X-ray — may demonstrate presence of lung disease, indicating that the patient is a poor surgical risk during anesthesia and the first 3 to 5 postoperative days

POTENTIAL COMPLICATIONS
■ Hemorrhage
■ Thrombophlebitis
■ Infection (systemic, wound, or joint)
■ Disarticulation of prosthesis
■ Pulmonary embolus
■ Atelectasis
■ Pneumonia
■ Neurovascular damage in the extremity
■ Fat embolism
■ Osteomyelitis

CLINICAL SNAPSHOT ✳

Total joint replacement in a lower extremity

Major nursing diagnoses and collaborative problems	Key patient outcomes
CP: Risk for postoperative complications (hypovolemic shock, neurovascular damage, or thromboembolic phenomena)	Have stable vital signs, typically: heart rate, 60 to 100 beats/minute; systolic blood pressure, 90 to 140 mm Hg; and diastolic blood pressure, 50 to 90 mm Hg.
ND: Impaired physical mobility	Perform self-care activities independently and ambulate 50′ (15.2 m) with a walker and prescribed amount of weight bearing.
ND: Impaired skin integrity	Exhibit a clean healing wound well-approximated edges.

Collaborative problem

Risk for postoperative complications (hypovolemic shock, neurovascular damage, or thromboembolic phenomena) related to surgical trauma, bleeding, edema, improper positioning, or immobility

NURSING PRIORITY

Prevent or promptly detect complications.

PATIENT OUTCOME CRITERIA

Within 2 hours after surgery and then continuously, the patient will exhibit stable vital signs, typically: heart rate, 60 to 100 beats/minute; systolic blood pressure, 90 to 140 mm Hg; and diastolic blood pressure, 50 to 90 mm Hg.
For hypovolemic shock
Within 2 hours after surgery, the patient will:

- exhibit drainage changing from frank bleeding to serosanguineous drainage.
  Within 1 day after surgery, the patient will:
- exhibit drainage less than 300 ml/day
- exhibit serosanguineous drainage.
  Within 2 days after surgery, the patient will:
- exhibit drainage less than 100 ml/day.

For neurovascular damage

Throughout the hospital stay, the patient will:
- exhibit bilaterally equal pedal pulses and toe temperature
- exhibit capillary refill time less than 3 seconds
- have no foot numbness or tingling
- be able to move the toes spontaneously and dorsiflex the ankle.

For thromboembolic phenomena

Within 3 days after surgery, the patient will:
- exhibit no signs or symptoms of fat embolism
- be alert and oriented
- experience no respiratory distress
- exhibit no petechiae
- have a partial pressure of arterial oxygen level of 80 to 100 mm Hg.
  Throughout the hospital stay, the patient will:
- exhibit no signs or symptoms of thromboembolism
- present bilaterally clear breath sounds
- exhibit vital signs within normal limits
- experience no calf pain on foot dorsiflexion (negative Homans' sign).

INTERVENTIONS

1. *Implement standard care related to hypovolemic shock:* *

– See the "Perioperative care" care plan, page 146, and the "Hypovolemic shock" care plan, page 147.

– Maintain patency of the wound drainage device (such as a Hemovac). Assess, measure, and record the amount of drainage every 8 hours or as needed to maintain continuous suction. Monitor the amount of bleeding, and report unusual increases. Monitor results of hematocrit studies.

2. *Provide nursing care related to neurovascular damage.* Implement these measures:

– Perform neurovascular checks every hour for the first 4 hours after the patient's return from surgery, then every 2 hours for 12 hours, and then every 4 hours until ambulatory. Assess pedal pulses, capillary refill time, toe temperature, skin color, foot sensation, and ability to move the toes and dorsiflex the ankle. Compare findings with the other extremity as well as with earlier findings. Once the patient is ambulatory, reassess at least daily.

RATIONALES

1. Usual postoperative factors and the unique nature of joint replacement place the patient at risk for hypovolemic shock.
– The "Perioperative care" and "Hypovolemic shock" care plans contain general interventions related to postoperative shock. These care plans present information pertinent to the patient undergoing hip or knee replacement.
– The hip area is highly vascular. Also, the patient may be taking an anticoagulant to prevent thromboembolism. Initial drainage may be frankly bloody but should become serosanguineous within a few hours. A typical amount is 200 to 300 ml in the first 24 hours after surgery, decreasing to less than 100 ml within 48 hours. The drainage device usually is removed by the 2nd postoperative day.

2. Altered neurovascular status may be associated with trauma to the nerves or blood vessels as a result of surgery, joint dislocation, edema, improper positioning, or excessive tightness of abduction pillow straps.
– Early detection of neurovascular damage facilitates prompt intervention to correct the underlying cause and minimize the chance of permanent damage.

---

*Italics indicate key interventions.

– Notify the physician immediately if pedal pulses are absent or unequal bilaterally; if capillary refill time is greater than 3 seconds; if the patient has cold toes, pale skin, foot numbness, tingling, or pain; or if the patient can't move his toes.

– Maintain positioning as recommended. See "Impaired physical mobility" below for further details.

– Apply ice packs to the affected joint for 24 to 48 hours after surgery, if ordered.

– Maintain patency of the drainage device as previously described.

3. *Provide astute nursing care related to thromboembolic phenomena.* Implement these measures:

– Instruct and coach preoperative exercises for calves, quadriceps, gluteals, and ankles. After surgery, supervise performance of exercises 5 to 10 times hourly while the patient is awake.

– Monitor for signs of thromboembolism, assessing daily for calf pain, a positive Homans' sign, redness, and swelling. See the "Perioperative care" care plan, page 146, and the "Thrombophlebitis" care plan, page 459, for details.

– Apply elastic stockings to both legs (to the affected extremity only after the dressing is removed). Remove daily for 1 hour every 8 hours. Check the skin for signs of pressure. Use pneumatic compression devices as ordered.

– Monitor for signs of fat embolism daily. Immediately report sudden onset of dyspnea, tachycardia, pallor or cyanosis, or pleuritic pain. See the "Perioperative care" care plan, page 146, for details.

– Administer prophylactic anticoagulants (aspirin, heparin, or warfarin [Coumadin]) as ordered. Monitor clotting studies and report findings outside the recommended therapeutic range. Observe for (and advise the patient and family to report) melena, petechiae, epistaxis, hematuria, ecchymoses, or other unusual bleeding. (See *Clinical pathway: Managing joint replacement [elective]*, pages 616 and 617.)

4. Additional individualized interventions:_____

_____

– Early medical intervention can prevent permanent damage in the affected extremity.

– Proper positioning is critical to prevent prosthesis dislocation, which can trap and irreparably damage nerves or blood vessels.

– Ice packs promote vasoconstriction, thereby decreasing inflammation, edema, and bleeding.

– Drainage must be maintained because fluid accumulation could exert pressure on nearby nerves and vessels.

3. The patient undergoing total joint replacement is at particular risk for thrombophlebitis, embolism, and fat embolism because of immobility-induced venous stasis and possible surgical trauma to veins.

– Practice before surgery enhances the patient's ability to perform exercises later. These exercises are designed to promote venous return, minimizing the risk of thromboembolic phenomena.

– Calf pain, redness, or swelling may indicate thrombus formation. The "Perioperative care" care plan contains general interventions related to various thrombotic and embolic phenomena. The "Thrombophlebitis" care plan provides additional details on assessing for this complication.

– Elastic support stockings and pneumatic compression devices may promote venous return by redirecting flow from superficial veins to deeper veins.

– The patient undergoing total joint replacement is at particular risk for fat embolism because of bone marrow release from surgical disruption of flat (pelvic) or long bones.

– Prophylactic anticoagulants may reduce the risk of thrombophlebitis or thromboembolism. However, the patient must be monitored carefully because anticoagulant use may cause uncontrolled bleeding.

4. Rationales:_____

_____

Nursing diagnosis
Impaired physical mobility related to hip or knee surgery

NURSING PRIORITIES
- Maintain proper alignment of the affected extremity to prevent dislocation of the prosthesis.
- Increase mobility in the extremity through implementation of the rehabilitation plan.
- Educate the patient concerning rehabilitation needs.

(Text continues on page 618.)

CLINICAL PATHWAY

Managing joint replacement (elective)

Plan	Before surgery	Day 1	Day 2
Laboratory studies	• CBC • CXR, ECG as indicated per anesthesia protocol requirements		• PT/INR, if on warfarin • Chem 7 profile • CBC
Tests	• Medical comanagement, if ordered	• VS, neurologic and circulatory checks per policy • Pain scale q 2 h while awake	• VS q shift, if stable • Check pain scale q 2 h while awake
Consults		• PT • OT • Respiratory care • Pharmacist consult for warfarin teaching • Case management social work • Medical comanagement, if ordered	• Diet consult if < 80% ideal body weight or > 120% ideal body weight (Use HAMWI formula: 106 lb for 5' plus 6 lb for q inch; 100 lb for 5' plus 5 lb for q inch) • ET nurse regarding skin care
Medication/I.V.	• Bring all medications to hospital	• PCA • Epidural • Pain controlled (< 4 on pain scale) • Enoxaparin • Warfarin • Home medications • Nausea controlled with antiemetics	• Maintenance I.V. – PCA/Epidural • Pain controlled (< 4 on pain scale) • Enoxaparin • Warfarin
Treatments	• SCDs	• Drain • THR: abductor pillow • Granulex/ET mix • Spenco boots	• Drain • Nurse to check heels, sacrum, and elbows q shift
Nutrition	• NPO after midnight	• Tolerating diet without N/V	• Diet consistent with Dx and condition
Elimination		• Indwelling urinary catheter • u.l. > 60 ml/2° x 16 hr • Voiding without difficulty	• D/C indwelling urinary catheter in morning or when D/C epidural and patient is out of bed
Activity		• Hips: reposition q 2 h to unaffected side with abductor pillow between legs • Knee: immobilizer, if ordered • Knee: CPM, if ordered	• Exercise program per rehabilitation • Activity wall chart posted • Dangle • THR: transfer to chair, if tolerated • TKR: transfer to chair, if tolerated
Patient teaching	• Pain management • Pain scale • Cough and deep breathe • Incentive spirometry	• Preadmission: video, class, tour • Exercise sheets • Hip or knee folder during class • Pain management (0 to 10 pain scale) • PCA, if receiving PCA • Incentive spirometry	• Joint precautions • Demonstrate adaptive equipment • Review: – Incentive spirometry – Pain management – PCA review, if indicated
Discharge planning	• High-risk cases referred to case management through office	• Interdisciplinary consultation with case management, if high-risk case	• Interdisciplinary consultation with case management, if high-risk case

Day 3	Day 4	Outcome goals met
• PT/INR, if on warfarin	• PT/INR, if on warfarin • CBC • If discharged on warfarin, F/U PT/INR planned	• Lab results WNL • PT/INR therapeutic, if on warfarin
• Check pain scale q 2 h while awake • Rehabilitation: performs FIM scores		• Temp < 101° F (38.3° C)
• D/C PCA/epidural • Pain controlled (< 4 on pain scale) with P.O. analgesics • D/C I.V. • Saline well • Warfarin • Enoxaparin	• Warfarin dose before discharge • Enoxaparin, continue for ___ days	• Adequate pain control and anti-coagulation
• Drain D/C • Nurse to check heels, sacrum, and elbows q shift • No skin breakdown	• D/C SCDs when fully ambulatory • 1st dressing change/physician within 72 hr • Independent with wound care • Nurse to check heels, sacrum, and elbows q shift	• Wounds without infection • No skin breakdown
• Diet consistent with Dx and condition	• Diet consistent with Dx and condition	• Tolerating food
• If no BM, give laxative	• Last BM date:	• Normal elimination
• Initiate gait training • Progressive exercise • OT instruction on use of adaptive equipment and home recommendations • Up in chair for meals/t.i.d.: breakfast, lunch, dinner, other	• Transfers to commode, bed, chair with standby assist • Ind. with exercise program • Bathing, dressing, tub with SBA • Transfer with assistive device • Functional gait • Ind. with usage/knowledge of adaptive equipment	• > 70° flexion (knee) • Independent ADLs, transfer, functional gait with equipment • Independent with home exercises • Demonstrates safety precautions

• Pharmacist to teach about warfarin
• Nurse to instruct on:
   – S.C. injection of enoxaparin, if ordered
   – Rehabilitation to dispense hip/knee booklet
	• Drug/nutrient interaction sheet (if applicable)
	• Incision care
	• Anticoagulant therapy
	• Medications
	• Patient/family provide wound care with supervision
	• Home care precautions with pain medications
	• Car transfers
		• Patient and family verbalize:
		   – Signs and symptoms of complications
		   – Name, dose, adverse effects, purpose, schedule, food/drug interactions of medications
		   – Wound care

• Case management assessment and planning for discharge needs	• Appropriate follow-up scheduled • Durable medical equipment needs met • Interventions on home health, outpatient therapy, rehabilitation unit, or ECF	• Discharge disposition/plan is appropriate and meets patient's needs • Discharge information completed: discharge date, length of stay

Musculoskeletal and integumentary disorders

PATIENT OUTCOME CRITERIA

By the time of discharge, the patient will:

- maintain mobility of unaffected joints equal to or greater than preoperative level
- perform self-care activities independently
- verbalize an understanding of the rehabilitation plan.
  By the time of discharge, the patient with a hip replacement will:
- ambulate 50′ (15.2 m) with a walker and partial weight bearing on the affected side as tolerated
- observe ROM restrictions — flexion of the affected joint limited to 90 degrees during the rehabilitation phase.
  By the time of discharge, the patient with a knee replacement will:
- ambulate with an assistive device and lightweight bearing as tolerated
- flex the knee up to 90 degrees of flexion
- not extend the knee (0-degree extension).

INTERVENTIONS	RATIONALES
1. *Before surgery, instruct the patient about the correct postoperative positioning of the affected extremity:* – hip — maintain flexion of the hip joint at a 45-degree angle or less. Don't rotate the hip joint externally. Don't adduct the hip joint (don't cross the legs). – knee — don't flex or hyperextend the leg. Maintain the leg slightly elevated from the hip, using a pillow or continuous passive motion machine as ordered, typically for 48 to 72 hours.	**1.** Preoperative teaching provides information that helps the patient maintain proper positioning of the joint after surgery. The positions described help prevent prosthesis dislocation.
2. *Before surgery, teach the patient how to use the appropriate walking device* (walker or crutches). Provide practice with the device, if possible.	**2.** Preoperative instruction and practice, if possible, allow the patient to feel more secure when using a walking device.
3. *After surgery, maintain the patient on bed rest* as ordered, usually for 12 to 24 hours. Place the affected joint in the prescribed position (usually in the neutral position), using rolls, splints, pillows, or abduction pillows, as ordered and appropriate. Observe position and activity precautions as noted above.	**3.** The affected joint must be stabilized to prevent dislocation. Excessive flexion, internal rotation, or adduction will cause postoperative hip dislocation. Knee elevation helps reduce swelling and pain.
4. *Observe for signs of prosthesis dislocation,* shortening of the extremity, a sudden increase in pain, a bulge over the femoral head on the affected side (in hip replacement), and decreased neurovascular status of the affected extremity. Report any such findings to the physician immediately.	**4.** Signs of prosthesis dislocation, a common occurrence in hip replacement, indicate need for immediate attention.
5. *Supervise position changes* at least every 2 hours. Have the patient use a trapeze and either shift weight in bed or turn to the unaffected side. Assist only as necessary.	**5.** Self-propelled movement helps the patient maintain muscle tone and reduces the risk of skin breakdown.
6. *Implement a planned and progressive daily ambulation schedule,* as ordered, 1 to 3 days after surgery. Use either crutches or a walker to allow weight bearing as recommended. Coordinate this activity with the physical therapy program.	**6.** Progressive daily ambulation promotes the patient's return to increased physical activity and self-care.
7. *Ensure that unaffected joints are put through at least ten repetitions of full ROM exercises,* at least 10 repetitions three to four times daily.	**7.** ROM exercises of unaffected joints must be maintained during periods of decreased activity. Arthritic joints lose function more rapidly when activity is restricted.

8. *Help the patient maintain preferred rest and sleep routines.* Use back rubs, other skin care measures, positioning, and ordered medications as necessary.

9. *Collaborate with the health care team to design an appropriate rehabilitation plan* that includes:
– muscle-strengthening activities until maximum potential strength is reached
– increasing ROM of the affected joint until full ROM is attained
– return to occupational and leisure activities.

10. Identify, with the patient, the specific methods that will be used to implement the plan.

11. Additional individualized interventions: _____
_____

8. Uninterrupted periods of full relaxation and deep sleep help maintain the energy needed for remobilization of the affected joint.

9. An effective rehabilitation plan requires input from the physician, physical therapist, occupational therapist, and professionals from other appropriate disciplines to maximize the patient's rehabilitation potential.

10. For a rehabilitation program to be successful, the patient must agree to the plan and be able to describe its implementation.

11. Rationales: _____
_____

Suggested NIC Interventions
Exercise therapy: Ambulation; Exercise therapy: Balance; Exercise therapy: Joint mobility; Exercise therapy: Muscle control; Exercise promotion: Strength training

Suggested NOC Outcomes
Ambulation: Walking; Ambulation: Wheelchair; Joint movement: Active; Mobility level

---

Nursing diagnosis
Impaired skin integrity related to surgery

NURSING PRIORITIES
■ Promote wound healing.
■ Prevent infection.

PATIENT OUTCOME CRITERIA
By the time of discharge, the patient will:
■ exhibit clean wound healing with well-approximated edges
■ be afebrile
■ exhibit warm and dry skin
■ exhibit no bleeding
■ exhibit no signs or symptoms of infection
■ list signs and symptoms to report.

INTERVENTIONS

1. *Maintain the patency of the drainage device,* as previously described. Avoid contaminating the drainage port when emptying the device.

2. *Don't administer injections in the affected extremity.* Teach the patient to take precautions to minimize the risk of injury.

RATIONALES

1. Adequate suction with a self-controlled vacuum must be maintained to prevent blood collection in the joint — an excellent medium for bacterial growth. Contamination of the device may lead to wound infection.

2. Any break in the skin may predispose the patient to infection.

3. *Assess daily for signs and symptoms of infection:* fever, chills, purulent drainage, incisional swelling, redness, and increasing tenderness. Teach the patient which signs and symptoms to report.

4. Additional individualized interventions:_____
_____

3. Infection is devastating to a patient with total joint replacement because the joint can't be saved once infection and prosthetic loss occur.

4. Rationales: _____
_____

Suggested NIC Interventions
Pressure management; Pressure ulcer care; Skin surveillance; Incision site care; Wound care

Suggested NOC Outcomes
Tissue integrity: Skin and mucous membranes; Wound healing: Primary intention; Wound healing: Secondary intention

---

Discharge planning
DISCHARGE CHECKLIST
Before discharge, the patient shows evidence of:
❒ absence of fever
❒ vital signs within acceptable limits
❒ absence of signs and symptoms of infection at the incision
❒ absence of contractures or skin breakdown
❒ administration of oral anticoagulant medication for at least the previous 48 to 72 hours and partial thromboplastin time within acceptable parameters
❒ ability to control pain using oral medications
❒ absence of bowel or bladder dysfunction
❒ absence of pulmonary or cardiovascular complications
❒ ability to perform ADLs independently or with minimal assistance
❒ adherence to hip flexion and adduction restrictions when transferring and ambulating
❒ adherence to weight-bearing restrictions when transferring or ambulating
❒ ability to transfer and ambulate independently or with minimal assistance, using appropriate assistive devices
❒ ability to tolerate adequate nutritional intake
❒ absence of signs and symptoms of prosthesis dislocation
❒ adequate home support system or referral to home care or nursing home if indicated by an inadequate home support system; inability to perform ADLs, transfers, and ambulation independently; or inability to adhere to flexion or weight-bearing restrictions
❒ demonstration of maximum hospital rehabilitation benefit.

One of the peer review organization criteria used when reviewing total joint replacement is whether the patient received maximum hospital benefit. The major criteria are whether the patient had a physical therapy evaluation and whether discharge planning was appropriate. The discharge would be deemed premature if a rehabilitation program had not been designed and if the patient showed evidence of medical instability.

Discharge planning for a patient who undergoes total hip or knee replacement should include automatic referral to the social services department. Most patients can't function at their usual level after this procedure, especially if it's bilateral. Documentation should indicate plans for long-term rehabilitation. The nurse isn't necessarily responsible for this documentation; the physical therapist, occupational therapist, or discharge planner–social worker may provide it.

After discharge, many patients are eligible for care in a nursing home or ECF until they can ambulate 50' to 80' (15 to 24 m) independently or with minimal assistance. Because the discharge plan commonly includes early discharge with transfer to an ECF, timely referral to the social services department is essential to allow adequate time to find an opening at an appropriate facility.

TEACHING CHECKLIST
Document evidence that the patient and family demonstrate an understanding of:
❒ implications of joint replacement
❒ rationale for continued use of antiembolism stockings
❒ all discharge medications' purposes, dosages, administration schedules, and adverse effects requiring medical attention (discharge medications typically include analgesics, antibiotics, anti-inflammatories, and anticoagulants)
❒ need for laboratory and medical follow-up if discharged on warfarin
❒ schedule for progressive ambulation and weight bearing
❒ additional activity restrictions
❒ signs and symptoms of infection, bleeding, and dislocation
❒ use of self-help devices, such as a raised toilet seat
❒ appropriate resources for posthospitalization care
❒ diet to promote healing

❏ wound care
❏ date, time, and location of follow-up appointments
❏ how to contact the physician
❏ need for antibiotic prophylaxis prior to dental and GI or genitourinary procedures.

DOCUMENTATION CHECKLIST
Using outcome criteria as a guide, document:
❏ clinical status on admission
❏ significant changes in status
❏ preoperative and postoperative teaching
❏ position of affected extremity
❏ exercises and ROM achieved
❏ neurovascular checks
❏ calf pain
❏ wound drainage
❏ progressive ambulation
❏ pain-relief measures
❏ presence or absence of disabling fatigue
❏ nutritional intake
❏ patient and family teaching
❏ discharge planning and referrals.

Associated care plans

- Acute pain
- Hypovolemic shock
- Ineffective individual coping
- Knowledge deficit
- Perioperative care
- Thrombophlebitis

References

Chan, Y.K., et al. "Full Weight Bearing after Non-cemented Total Hip Replacement is Compatible with Satisfactory Results," *International Orthopedics* 27(2):94-97, 2003.

Jordan, K. (ed). *Emergency Nursing Core Curriculum.* Emergency Nurses Association. Philadelphia: W.B. Saunders Co., 2000.

Loft, M., et al. "Patient Empowerment after Total Hip and Knee Replacement," *Orthopedic Nursing* 22(1):42-47, January-February 2003.

Lynn-Mchale, D.J., and Carlson, K.K. American Association of Critical Care Nurses *AACN Procedure Manual for Critical Care,* 4th ed. Philadelphia: W.B. Saunders Co., 2001.

Shoemaker, W.C., et al. *Textbook of Critical Care,* 4th ed. Philadelphia: W.B. Saunders Co., 2002.

Weil, Y., et al. "Brucella Prosthetic Joint Infection: A Report of 3 cases and a Review of the Literature," *Clinical Journal of Infectious Diseases* 36(7):81-86, April 2003.

Endocrine disorders

PART

9

Diabetes mellitus

DRG INFORMATION
DRG 294   Diabetes; Age 35+.
          Mean LOS = 4.6 days
DRG 295   Diabetes; Ages 0 to 35.
          Mean LOS = 3.8 days

Introduction
DEFINITION AND TIME FOCUS
Diabetes mellitus (DM) is a chronic metabolic disorder in which an absolute or relative lack of endogenous insulin causes abnormal metabolism of carbohydrates, proteins, and fats. The clinical hallmark of diabetes is hyperglycemia. Altered glucose metabolism provokes a pattern of associated acute and chronic complications. The chronic hyperglycemia of diabetes is associated with long-term damage to various organs, especially the eyes, kidneys, nerves, heart, and blood vessels. Landmark studies have demonstrated that in the two most common types of diabetes, type 1 and type 2, this damage can be slowed and reduced by strict control of blood glucose levels. This plan focuses on both types of diabetes, their diagnosis, and initiation of a treatment and management regimen.

Note: Although type 2 was previously called non-insulin-dependent DM, patients with type 2 DM may require insulin as part of their management plans, either initially or later in the course of the disease. Classification of diabetes is now based on disease etiology and not the pharmacological approach to treatment. The terms insulin-dependent diabetes mellitus and non-insulin dependent diabetes mellitus have been eliminated. (See *Clinical snapshot: Diabetes mellitus,* page 626.)

ETIOLOGY AND PRECIPITATING FACTORS
Type 1 (5% to 10% of cases): primary defect is inadequate or absent insulin production secondary to destruction of beta (insulin-producing) cells in the pancreas. There are two forms of type 1 DM. In the most common form, immune-mediated diabetes, an autoimmune process attacks the beta cells and produces islet-cell and insulin antibodies that can be measured. While this form usually occurs prior to adulthood, it can occur at any age.
- Genetic predisposition, related to genes of human leukocyte antigen (HLA) affecting immune system for autoimmune type 1
- Viral infections

The second form, idiopathic type 1, is rare, has no known cause, and has a strong genetic predisposition not related to HLA.

Type 2 (approximately 90% to 95% of cases): primary defect is insulin resistance by skeletal muscle, fat, and liver receptors for insulin; hyperglycemia leads to increased insulin production and eventual beta cell secretory exhaustion
- Strong genetic predisposition, not yet as clearly defined as in type 1
- Obesity (in 80% to 90% of patients at diagnosis)
- Sedentary lifestyle
- Age (most patients develop type 2 after age 45)
- Higher incidence in Native Americans, Latinos, and Blacks than in Whites
- Hypertension and dyslipidemia

Focused assessment guidelines
NURSING HISTORY
(FUNCTIONAL HEALTH PATTERN FINDINGS)
Type 1 DM is commonly diagnosed when the patient presents in diabetic ketoacidosis (DKA); type 2 is commonly diagnosed when the patient seeks treatment for one of the many associated symptoms, but may go undiagnosed for years. Many medications may be associated with impaired glucose tolerance, including steroids, some diuretics, hormonal contraceptives, anticonvulsants, and psychoactive medications. The physician who suspects DM should ensure that medication-related factors are identified and ruled out before making a diagnosis.

Health-perception–health-management pattern
Type 1
- Family history of diabetes
- Patient usually under age 30
- Acute onset of symptoms (flulike syndrome)

Type 2
- Family history of diabetes
- Patient usually over age 45
- Gradual onset of symptoms
- Patient may report multiple minor symptoms

Nutritional-metabolic pattern
Type 1
- Increased thirst (polydipsia)
- Increased appetite (polyphagia)
- Weight loss
- Ketosis
- Nausea (occasionally)

Type 2
- Polydipsia and polyphagia
- History of diet high in refined carbohydrates and calories
- Usually overweight (possibly recent weight gain)

Elimination pattern
Type 1
- Polyuria
- Constipation or diarrhea
Type 2
- Nocturia
- Polyuria
- Constipation or diarrhea
- Diuretics taken for another condition
- Recurrent urinary tract infections (UTIs)

Activity-exercise pattern
Type 1
- Sudden weakness
- Increased fatigue or sleepiness
Type 2
- Gradually increasing weakness and fatigability
- History of lack of regular exercise

Sleep-rest pattern
Type 1
- Sleep disturbance related to nocturia
Type 2
- Nocturia
- Drowsiness after meals

Cognitive-perceptual pattern
Type 1
- Dizziness or orthostatic hypotension
- Abdominal pain
Type 2
- Pruritus, acute or recurrent UTIs, recurrent vaginitis, or vaginal infection
- Poorly healing skin infections
- Myopia or blurred vision
- Muscle cramping
- Abdominal pain
- Numbness, pain, or tingling in extremities
- Irritability

Sexuality pattern
Type 2
- Loss of sex drive or erectile dysfunction
- Recurrent vaginal infections

PHYSICAL FINDINGS
Cardiovascular
- Tachycardia
- Postural hypotension
- Hypertension
- Cool extremities and decreased pulses

Pulmonary
- Deep, rapid (Kussmaul's) respirations; fruity breath odor (in DKA)

Gastrointestinal
- Abdominal distention
- Decreased bowel sounds
- Abdominal tenderness

Integumentary
- Poorly healing skin wounds, especially on feet
- Skin infections
- Warm, flushed, dry skin (in DKA)

Neurologic
- Drowsiness
- Confusion
- Coma (in DKA)
- Altered reflexes

Genitourinary
- Vaginal discharge
- Perineal irritation

DIAGNOSTIC STUDIES
- Random serum glucose test — a level greater than or equal to 200 mg/dl plus classic signs and symptoms confirms DM
- Fasting serum glucose test — elevation greater than or equal to 126 mg/dl confirms DM
- Urinalysis — reveals glycosuria and (in type 1) ketonuria (Urine microalbumin is the earliest indication of diabetic renal disease.)
- Glucose tolerance test — confirms DM if levels are greater than or equal to 200 mg/dl in the 2-hour sample (This test should be performed after a glucose load dose of 75 g anhydrous glucose.)
- Blood insulin level — type 1, absent or minimal; type 2, low, normal, or high
- Glycosylated hemoglobin (HbA_{1C} or A_{IC}) — evaluates overall glucose control over previous 120 days (life of red blood cell) by detecting elevations or wide fluctuations in blood glucose over time; greater than 8% indicates poor glucose control in either type 1 or type 2
- Arterial blood gas levels — may reveal metabolic acidosis, particularly common in type 1, with compensatory respiratory alkalosis
- Electrolyte panel — may be normal or may reveal hyponatremia or hyperkalemia associated with dehydration or DKA (type 1); needed to establish baseline
- Blood urea nitrogen (BUN) and creatinine levels — BUN may be normal or elevated in DKA or hyperosmolar hyperglycemic nonketotic syndrome (HHNS); both may be normal or elevated in presence of renal involvement; needed to establish baseline
- Thyroid function studies — may be ordered to rule out coexisting thyroid dysfunction, which could increase the need for insulin and contribute to hyperglycemia (thyroid disorders more common in type 1)
- Electrocardiography — commonly ordered to establish baseline and to rule out underlying cardiac disorders
- Lipid profile — needed to establish baseline and monitor levels every 1 to 2 years

- Dilated eye examination and vision testing by an ophthalmologist — needed to establish baseline and monitor for early indication of retinopathy

POTENTIAL COMPLICATIONS
- Coma related to DKA, hypoglycemia, or HHNS
- Renal failure (nephropathy)

- Conditions related to degenerative vascular disease: accelerated atherosclerosis, myocardial infarction, thrombophlebitis, peripheral vascular disease, and stroke
  - Retinopathy, blindness, or cataracts
  - Neuropathies, autonomic and especially peripheral
  - Microangiopathies

CLINICAL SNAPSHOT ✸

Diabetes mellitus

Major nursing diagnoses and collaborative problems	Key patient outcomes
CP: Hyperglycemia	Maintain blood glucose levels between 80 and 120 mg/dl.
ND: Deficient knowledge (self-care)	Discuss disease management in relation to medication, diet, exercise, and stress.
ND: Ineffective therapeutic regimen management	Have resource deficits resolved or appropriate referrals completed.

Collaborative problem

Hyperglycemia related to inadequate endogenous insulin (type 1 DM) or inadequate endogenous insulin and insulin resistance (type 2 DM)

NURSING PRIORITY
Prevent or minimize complications when establishing treatment regimen to control altered glucose metabolism.

PATIENT OUTCOME CRITERIA
Within 2 hours of admission, the patient will:
- have an improved blood glucose level
- be awake and alert
- maintain vital signs within normal limits, typically: heart rate, 60 to 100 beats/minute; systolic blood pressure, 90 to 140 mm Hg; and diastolic blood pressure, 50 to 90 mm Hg.
  Within 24 to 48 hours of admission, the patient will:
- show no signs of dehydration
- maintain preprandial blood glucose levels between 80 and 120 mg/dl and bedtime blood glucose between 100 and 140 mg/dl
- have no hypoglycemia, or have promptly treated hypoglycemic episodes with no associated complications.

INTERVENTIONS

1. *Administer insulin or oral hypoglycemics,* * as ordered.

– Monitor fingerstick blood glucose levels according to facility protocol, typically every 6 hours or before meals and at bedtime. Always check the blood glucose level before giving hypoglycemic medications. Follow established protocol for withholding the dose based on normal values.

– Be aware of differences in peak action and duration of action for various hypoglycemic medications: Rapid-acting insulins (lispro, insulin aspart) peak between 1 and 2 hours; short-acting insulins (regular, Humulin R), peak within 2 and 4 hours; intermediate-acting insulins (NPH, Lente) peak between 6 and 12 hours; and long-acting insulins (Ultralente, insulin glargine) peak between 10 and 30 hours. Oral hypoglycemics with a 24-hour duration peak on the average between 3 and 4 hours.

RATIONALES

1. Insulin increases cellular glucose uptake and decreases gluconeogenesis. Exogenous insulin is essential for controlling type 1 DM and may also be used in type 2 DM. In initial treatment of type 1 or 2, especially if DKA is present, I.V. infusion of regular insulin may be ordered concurrently with aggressive fluid replacement. The I.V. route is preferred because it offers the fastest absorption rate, but too-rapid lowering of blood glucose without adequate fluid replacement may cause vascular collapse or cerebral edema. Circulatory insufficiency can make insulin uptake from subcutaneous sites unpredictable; however, it's the route of choice for ongoing therapy. Oral hypoglycemics are indicated only in type 2 DM. Oral agents include several types of drugs, which have four different actions to lower blood glucose. Sulfonylureas (such as glyburide [Micronase] and glimepiride [Amaryl]) stimulate beta cells to secrete insulin. Meglitinides (repaglinide [Prandin]) and D-phenylalanines (nateglinide [Starlix]), also stimulate insulin release but have a much shorter duration of action. Alpha-glucosidase inhibitors, such as acarbose (Precose), block glucose absorption in the small intestine, slowing its absorption after meals. The drug class, thiazolidinediones, also known as the glitazones (such as rosiglitazone [Avandia]), increase insulin sensitivity in peripheral tissue, partially reversing insulin resistance. The biguanide drug metformin (Glucophage) reduces glucose production in the liver; secondarily, it increases insulin sensitivity in muscle and fat cells. The drugs that stimulate insulin secretion can be used in combination with oral hypoglycemic agents, which have other mechanisms to lower blood glucose levels. Combination products are becoming available.

– In the initial diagnosis and treatment of DM, frequent assessment of glucose levels is essential for monitoring the patient's response. Checking the glucose level and withholding the dose if the level is acceptable prevents medication-induced hypoglycemia. Protocols for withholding doses vary depending on the hypoglycemic ordered and patient status.

– Awareness of these characteristics helps the nurse correlate onset and duration of signs and symptoms with peaks and troughs in serum drug levels.

---

*Italics indicate key interventions.

– Insulins differ according to onset, peak, and duration of action. The type of insulin, timing of injections, and individual response influence when a reaction is most likely to occur. With insulins given in the morning, a reaction from a short-acting insulin is most likely between breakfast and lunch; an intermediate-acting insulin, between midafternoon and dinner; and a long-acting insulin, between 2 a.m. and 7 a.m.

– Because duration of action is more prolonged with oral agents, a single daily or divided dose is usually sufficient for control. Reactions are most likely to coincide with peak action.

2. *Establish and maintain an I.V. fluid infusion* (usually normal saline solution), as ordered. Monitor for dry mucous membranes, poor skin turgor, cracked lips, abdominal pain, elevated urine specific gravity, elevated hematocrit, and other signs or symptoms of dehydration. *Keep an accurate intake and output record. Document daily weight.*

2. Hyperglycemia causes dehydration through hyperosmolality. Water is drawn from the cells into the vascular system and then into the urine in an attempt to maintain homeostasis. Normal saline is the preferred solution to prevent further elevation of blood glucose (and to replace sodium in DKA). Accurate intake and output documentation and daily weights are essential for assessing fluid status and for early detection of inadequate renal function. Daily weight is a gross indicator of general fluid and nutritional status.

3. *Observe for signs and symptoms of medication-induced hypoglycemia,* including pallor, confusion, diaphoresis, headache, weakness, shallow respirations, irritability, and restlessness or stupor. Reactions are most likely to coincide with peak insulin effect or late or missed meals, depending on the type of insulin and the patient's response. *If a reaction occurs, notify the physician, measure blood glucose level, and treat immediately with oral glucose, I.V. glucose, or glucagon, depending on protocol and the patient's responsiveness.* Recheck blood glucose in 10 minutes. Feed a small snack of carbohydrate and protein if the patient's next meal is more than 1 hour away. Once the patient is stable, use the episode as an example for teaching. *See the "Hypoglycemia" care plan,* page 651, for details.

3. Insulin reactions can occur with relative suddenness. Oral glucose is used for mild to moderate hypoglycemia when the patient can swallow; parenteral glucagon or glucose is used when the person is unconscious or unable to swallow. If the patient with newly diagnosed diabetes is unaware of the symptoms' significance and doesn't seek treatment, a hypoglycemic reaction may be life-threatening.

4. *Make sure the patient is served the prescribed therapeutic diet at consistent times.*

4. The patient with DM — especially type 1 DM — needs diet guidelines tailored to meet his specific needs. Generally, concentrated sweets and alcohol are avoided for patients with either type of DM. Increased dietary fiber is recommended. Consistent carbohydrate intake distributed over the day is fundamental to all types of medical nutrition therapy for DM because it helps stabilize blood glucose level. The "ADA diet" (calorie levels with percentages of carbohydrate, fat, and protein) and "no added sugar" diet are no longer recommended.

– The patient with type 1 DM adjusts insulin to dietary intake and exercise and distributes carbohydrate consumption equally throughout the day. If necessary, the patient's diet may include bedtime snacks, depending on insulin use. (If the patient needs intensive therapy, frequent blood glucose monitoring and multiple daily injections of insulin or an insulin pump allow adjustment of insulin to compensate for the patient's diet.)

– Clear or full liquid diets should provide 200 g of carbohydrates distributed over the day

– After surgery, encourage progression to solid foods as soon as tolerated.

5. *Observe for signs of DKA* (in type 1 DM only):
– early — nausea; fatigue; polyuria; dry, flushed skin; dry mucous membranes; thirst; and tachycardia
– late — vomiting, poor skin turgor, lethargy, Kussmaul's respirations, acetone breath, hypotension, and abdominal pain.

If the patient's condition suggests DKA, notify the physician immediately. Obtain a blood glucose level (usually 300 to 800 mg/dl), and check urine ketones (typically positive). Treat according to protocol (usually rapid hypotonic or isotonic I.V. fluid replacement, I.V. insulin, and — as hyperglycemia and dehydration resolve — potassium replacement; ensure that the patient has had some urine output before adding potassium to I.V. fluids). Once the patient is stable, use the episode as an example for teaching. *See the "Diabetic ketoacidosis" care plan,* page 635, for details.

6. *Observe for signs and symptoms of HHNS (in type 2 DM),* including lethargy or stupor, fatigue, drowsiness, confusion, coma, seizures, intense thirst, and very dry mucous membranes. *If the patient's condition suggests HHNS, notify the physician immediately.* Obtain a blood glucose level (typically over 800 mg/dl), check urine ketones (usually negative), and obtain a serum osmolality level, as ordered (characteristically over 350 mOsm/kg). Treat according to protocol, typically vigorous hypotonic fluid replacement, low-dose insulin, and potassium repletion. Once the patient is stable, use the episode as an example for teaching. *Refer to the "Hyperosmolar hyperglycemic nonketotic syndrome" care plan,* page 645, for further details.

7. Additional individualized interventions: _____
_____

– The patient with type 2 DM restricts calories to achieve moderate weight loss (usually necessary), lowers fat intake, spaces meals, and avoids snacks. Insulin and oral hypoglycemics are prescribed to fit the normal diet schedule; a missed or delayed meal can lead to hypoglycemia.

5. Inadequate pharmacologic control, increased dietary intake, infection, stress, or the interaction of other factors may cause DKA in type 1 DM. Hyperglycemia causes osmotic diuresis, which provokes compensatory mechanisms to maintain blood volume and pressure. In DKA, incomplete breakdown of fatty acids leads to accumulation of ketones in the bloodstream in addition to high (unusable) glucose levels. This leads to a state of metabolic acidosis, usually with a compensatory respiratory alkalosis. I.V. fluids correct dehydration and insulin facilitates glucose metabolism. As hyperglycemia and dehydration resolve, potassium shifting from the plasma back into the cells may unmask hypokalemia related to urinary potassium loss. The "Diabetic ketoacidosis" care plan contains comprehensive information on managing this complication.

6. HHNS, a complication that occurs over days to weeks, develops most commonly in the older and infirm patient with type 2 DM who doesn't recognize (or doesn't react to) fluid loss. It's usually caused by infection or massive fluid loss. The pathophysiology includes severe hyperglycemia and profound dehydration in the absence of ketosis. Perhaps because of pancreatic exhaustion, not enough insulin is produced to metabolize glucose, so glucose accumulates. However, enough insulin is produced to prevent adipose tissue breakdown, so ketosis doesn't occur. Blood glucose and osmolality levels are much more elevated in HHNS than in DKA.

Hypotonic fluids help reverse high serum osmolality; vigorous replacement is necessary because of the extent of dehydration. The patient with HHNS may be more sensitive to insulin than the patient with DKA. Urinary potassium loss may require earlier replacement in HHNS than in DKA. The "Hyperosmolar hyperglycemic nonketotic syndrome" care plan contains detailed guidance on managing this complication.

7. Rationales: _____
_____

Nursing diagnosis
Deficient knowledge (self-care) related to newly diagnosed complex chronic disease

NURSING PRIORITY
Establish a diabetes control regimen, emphasizing self-care.

PATIENT OUTCOME CRITERIA

Within 48 hours of diagnosis, the patient will:

- initiate diet planning with dietitian
- observe and practice injection technique (if insulin is ordered)
- practice blood glucose testing.

By the time of discharge, the patient will:

- demonstrate proficiency in injection technique
- produce evidence of site rotation documentation
- discuss disease management in relation to medication, diet, exercise, and stress
- demonstrate proper foot care
- discuss hypoglycemia and appropriate treatment
- discuss hyperglycemia and appropriate treatment
- plan adequate diet for 3-day period
- perform and interpret blood glucose tests accurately.

INTERVENTIONS

1. *See the "Knowledge deficit" care plan,* page 129.

2. *Emphasize that DM control involves coordinating many aspects of daily living with prescribed interventions.* Teach the significance of insulin or oral hypoglycemics for disease control. Demonstrate injection techniques, and observe patient performance. Rotate sites for subcutaneous injections every 7 to 10 days (abdominal sites are preferred over arms or legs). Document site rotation. Link medication needs to other factors, such as diet and exercise. Ensure that the patient and his family are aware of signs and treatment of hypoglycemia as well as the protocol for managing persistent hyperglycemia, DKA (for type 1 DM), and HHNS (for type 2 DM). Involve family members in all teaching. Use the patient's symptomatic episodes as teaching tools. Where possible, link changes in habits to the prevention of complications.

3. *Involve the patient, his family, and dietitian in planning a therapeutic diet.* Reinforce nutritional guidelines. Encourage supervised weight loss if the patient is overweight. Ensure that the patient has been given written diet guidelines before discharge. Provide referral for further questions and special situations (such as "sick day" management, pregnancy, dining out, exercise, use of alcohol, or complications).

RATIONALES

1. The "Knowledge deficit" care plan provides general guidelines for patient teaching. This care plan provides additional information pertinent to diabetes.

2. Patient understanding is essential for home management of DM. A patient may mistakenly believe that attention to a single factor (for example, medication) will control the disorder. Compliance may increase if the patient links control with personal preventive efforts. Observing the patient's injection technique and providing opportunities for supervised practice help ensure accuracy. Rotating injection sites (after using same site for 7 to 10 days) minimizes lipodystrophy and helps prevent scar tissue formation; documentation serves as a reminder. Insulin absorption is fastest from abdominal sites (followed by arm sites, then leg sites) and abdominal sites are minimally affected by exercise. The need for medication increases with stress, infection, and higher caloric intake but may decrease with excessive activity, decreased caloric intake, or vomiting. Awareness of hyperglycemia and hypoglycemia (signs and symptoms, possible causes, treatment, and prevention) decreases patient anxiety and increases self-control; using the patient's personal experiences as teaching tools helps the patient identify and recognize personal responses to the disease.

3. Involving the patient and his family with dietary planning helps ensure compliance at home. Diet is specific for each patient. For the patient with type 2 DM, diet alone or diet with weight loss may be sufficient to control hyperglycemia. Written materials help minimize misunderstanding. Referral ensures an ongoing source of dietary information. The registered dietitian is an important member of the health care team and the best professional to provide nutrition planning and counseling. The nurse's role is typically to provide reinforcement and support.

4. *For type 1 and most type 2 DM, teach blood glucose testing methods for home use.* If possible, use a Certified Diabetes Educator to help select the specific blood glucose monitor best suited to the individual patient. Observe patient demonstrations for accuracy of testing, interpretation of results, calibration, and documentation. Provide target glucose ranges. Be aware that the patient may think "the lower the better" regarding blood glucose; ensure that the patient understands the body's need for glucose in regulated amounts. Encourage the patient to keep a daily record of glucose monitoring. At least annually, evaluate the patient's technique and provide revised target glucose ranges, if necessary.

5. *Emphasize the importance of regular activity and exercise and of maintaining the same level of activity from day to day.* Teach the importance of warm-up, stretching, and cool-down periods. Teach the patient to check his blood glucose level before exercise and consume a carbohydrate snack if blood glucose is lower than 100 mg/dl. Emphasize the need to use protective footwear, and teach foot care. (See #8).

6. *Teach or review "sick day" management techniques:* testing blood glucose more often, increasing fluids, continuing to take diabetes medication, contacting the physician early in illness, and postponing exercise. Explain the importance of contacting the physician if fever, nausea, or vomiting lasts for more than 24 hours or if blood glucose levels rise above 250 mg/dl.

7. *Tell the patient to be aware of increased susceptibility to infections;* discuss ways to avoid exposure. Review signs of infection, such as redness, swelling, exudate, and fever. Emphasize the importance of prompt, appropriate treatment of even minor injuries to avoid serious complications.

8. *Discuss ways to prevent the vascular complications of DM:*

– Discuss leg and foot care. Teach the patient how to perform foot care, skin care, leg exercises, and to assess circulatory status; observe return demonstration of all techniques. If the patient smokes, emphasize the importance of quitting and provide a referral to a smoking-cessation program. Ensure that the patient and his family receive a written plan of foot care.

4. Successful home management of DM requires that the patient perform self-monitoring to ensure that the prescribed regimen of medication, diet, and exercise remains appropriate to needs. Blood glucose testing for type 1 DM patients is usually 3 or more times per day; type 2 DM patients on medication will test blood glucose at least once per day. Type 2 DM patients on diet alone may not test blood glucose at home. Glucose monitors differ in complexity of operation, size of screen (some are voice activated for the blind), and sample size needed. Newer monitors allow use of body sites, such as forearm or abdomen. Stressors (or disease progression) may change body requirements; blood and urine testing alerts the patient to such changes and helps avert complications. Misconceptions about the disease may have disastrous consequences. Keeping a record of glucose levels helps identify trends. Periodic evaluation helps detect errors in the testing methods and ensures that target glucose ranges reflect the patient's current needs.

5. Regular, consistent exercise is an essential part of DM management. Exercise stimulates carbohydrate metabolism, lowers blood pressure, aids in weight control, and may help avert or minimize circulatory complications by increasing levels of high-density lipoproteins. Increases or decreases in activity may require dietary or medication changes. Exercise induces blood glucose fluctuations. Checking blood glucose before exercising and eating a carbohydrate snack minimize hypoglycemia.

6. Unless managed carefully, even minor illnesses can quickly lead to such diabetic emergencies as hyperglycemia, hypoglycemia, DKA, or HHNS. During illness, patients with type 2 DM, who usually treat with oral agents or diet alone, may temporarily need insulin to control blood glucose.

7. A compromised state of health may make the patient with DM more susceptible to some infections; also, healing may be impaired or prolonged due to associated vascular insufficiency. Awareness of signs of infection may help ensure prompt treatment. Because of impaired healing from DM, even minor cuts or scratches may develop into gangrenous lesions. Infection also affects medication and dietary needs.

8. DM is characterized by degenerative vascular changes that predispose the patient to infections, ulcerations, and gangrene, particularly of the legs and feet.
– Careful skin care may help avert serious problems. Leg exercises may help develop collateral circulation and promote venous return. Nicotine causes vasoconstriction and contributes to circulatory impairment; additionally, smoking greatly increases the risk of significant heart disease. Written instructions help ensure full compliance.

– Discuss potential eye complications of DM. Help the patient understand the significance of careful disease control (especially glucose and blood pressure) in preventing or slowing diabetic retinopathy. Emphasize the importance of early reporting of vision changes and annual ophthalmologic evaluation.

– Teach the symptoms of UTI and renal impairment — flank pain, fever, dysuria, pyuria, frequency, urgency, and oliguria — and emphasize the importance of prompt treatment. Emphasize the importance of an annual kidney function evaluation (microalbumin, urea, and 24-hour urine collection for protein and creatinine). Help the patient understand the importance of glucose and blood pressure control in preventing nephropathy.

9. *Discuss the implications of diabetic neuropathy (autonomic and peripheral).* Explain peripheral symptoms, such as paresthesia, pain, and sensory loss. Emphasize the importance of foot care. Instruct the patient and his family to report urine retention or incontinence, orthostatic hypotension, decreased perspiration, diarrhea, or impotence.

10. Additional individualized interventions: _____
_____

– The retina consumes oxygen at a higher rate than other body tissues; thus, it's sensitive to the effects of vascular degeneration (microangiopathy) associated with DM. These effects may eventually lead to retinopathy, retinal detachment, and blindness. Although some treatment is available, the most effective deterrent to blindness is careful disease control. Early reporting of vision changes may permit palliative treatment.
– Glycosuria predisposes the patient to UTIs; recurrent severe UTIs or pyelonephritis may increase the likelihood of renal failure. Nephropathy is a long-term complication related to vascular changes in the small vessels of the glomerulus. Proteinuria is the hallmark of changes in renal function.

9. Gradual degeneration of peripheral nerves may cause paresthesia and pain, followed by loss of sensation, particularly in the legs and feet; the patient may thus be unaware of injuries. The signs listed may indicate autonomic nerve dysfunction; if so, the patient may not exhibit the usual signs of hypoglycemia.

10. Rationales:_____

Suggested NIC Interventions
Teaching: Disease process; Teaching: Individual; Teaching: Prescribed medication

Suggested NOC Outcomes
Knowledge: Disease process; Knowledge: Health behaviors; Knowledge: Treatment regimen

Nursing diagnosis
Ineffective therapeutic regimen management related to lack of material resources, lack of support, or ineffective coping

NURSING PRIORITY
Optimize management of personal therapeutic regimen.

PATIENT OUTCOME CRITERIA
By the time of discharge, the patient will:
- verbalize understanding of need for lifestyle changes
- ask appropriate questions
- verbalize feelings about diagnosis
- participate actively in disease control planning
- have resource deficits resolved or appropriate referrals completed
- have a home visit or outpatient follow-up appointments scheduled.

INTERVENTIONS
1. *Assess the patient's resources,* including financial management capabilities and family support system.

RATIONALES
1. Independent home management of DM requires the ability to organize activities in a relatively stable setting. Patients are commonly admitted to the hospital "out of control" because of poor financial management and lack of a support system.

2. *Involve the patient's family in all teaching and planning.*

3. *Arrange appropriate follow-up home health visits.*

4. *Link the patient and his family with community resources and mutual support groups.*

5. *Encourage verbalization of feelings, and support healthy coping behaviors.* See the "Ineffective individual coping" care plan, page 124.

6. Additional individualized interventions:_____
_____

2. Family members may help reinforce teaching and encourage compliance.

3. Transferring new knowledge and skills for disease management from the hospital to the home may be difficult. Home visits allow assessment of environmental factors that may contribute to noncompliance.

4. Diagnosis of DM commonly involves major patient reeducation and lifestyle changes. Community or mutual support groups can offer ongoing education and support. Because hospitalization for DM is less frequent than in the past, or of short duration, outpatient diabetes education programs are essential. Many local and state health departments are participating in the National Diabetes Education Program, which provides increased educational programs and materials in many areas. Educational materials are also available online at *www.ndep/nih.gov/materials.*

5. As with the diagnosis of any serious chronic disease, the patient with DM may experience denial, anger, grief, and other emotions as part of a normal response. Expression of feelings is a necessary prelude to acceptance of the disease and active, responsible management. Supporting healthy coping behaviors helps maintain the patient's independence and sense of self-control — both essential for compliance. The "Ineffective individual coping" care plan contains detailed interventions related to this problem.

6. Rationales:_____
_____

Suggested NIC Interventions
Behavior modification; Mutual goal setting; Patient contracting; Self-modification assistance; Teaching: Procedure/treatment; Decision-making support; Health system guidance; Self-responsibility facilitation; Teaching: Disease process

Suggested NOC Outcomes
Compliance behavior; Knowledge: Treatment regimen; Participation: Health care decisions; Treatment behavior: Illness or injury

---

Discharge planning
DISCHARGE CHECKLIST
Before discharge, the patient shows evidence of:
- ❏ blood glucose level less than 200 mg/dl
- ❏ ability to manage medication administration
- ❏ ability to understand and follow dietary guidelines
- ❏ ability to follow and perform exercise regimen
- ❏ ability to perform foot and skin care
- ❏ ability to perform and interpret results of blood glucose testing (type 1 DM [usually], type 2)
- ❏ adequate home support system
- ❏ referral to home care or outpatient services for reinforcement of teaching or if home support is unavailable (because patients with DM are rarely admitted to the hospital unless the disease is out of control or is causing complications, always consider a referral to home care or an outpatient or community diabetes program to reinforce hospital teaching and to allow further observation)
- ❏ no signs of infection
- ❏ stable vital signs
- ❏ ability to describe emergency measures for managing hyperglycemia and hypoglycemia.

TEACHING CHECKLIST
Document evidence that the patient and his family demonstrate an understanding of:

❏ the disease and its repercussions
❏ for all medications: purpose, dosage, administration schedule, and adverse effects requiring medical attention (usual discharge medications include insulin or oral hypoglycemics)
❏ blood glucose testing (type 1 DM [usually], type 2)
❏ interrelationship of diet, exercise, and other factors in disease management
❏ hypoglycemia (signs and symptoms, possible causes, treatment, and prevention)
❏ hyperglycemia (signs and symptoms, possible causes, treatment, and prevention)
❏ diet management and exercise regimen
❏ foot care
❏ signs and symptoms of infection, the need to report them, and appropriate treatment
❏ signs and symptoms of neuropathy, the need to report them, and appropriate treatment
❏ signs and symptoms of retinopathy, the need to report them, and appropriate treatment
❏ signs and symptoms of urinary and renal complications, the need to report them, and appropriate treatment
❏ community resources
❏ when and how to access emergency medical treatment
❏ date, time, and location of follow-up appointments
❏ how to contact the physician
❏ written materials, insulin, and syringes, as provided.

DOCUMENTATION CHECKLIST
Using outcome criteria as a guide, document:
❏ clinical status on admission
❏ significant changes in status
❏ pertinent laboratory and diagnostic test findings
❏ episodes of hyperglycemia and hypoglycemia
❏ dietary intake and planning
❏ activity and exercise regimen
❏ medication therapy
❏ I.V. line patency
❏ patient and family teaching
❏ discharge planning and availability of community resources.

Associated care plans
- Chronic renal failure
- Diabetic ketoacidosis
- Grieving
- Hyperosmolar hyperglycemic nonketotic syndrome
- Hypoglycemia
- Ineffective individual coping
- Knowledge deficit
- Thrombophlebitis

References

American Diabetes Association: *www.diabetes.org.*

American Diabetes Association. "Evidence-based Nutrition Principles and Recommendations for the Treatment and Prevention of Diabetes and Related Complications," *Diabetes Care* 25(Suppl 1):S50-61, January 2002.

American Diabetes Association. "Insulin Administration," *Diabetes Care* 25(Suppl 1):S112-115, January 2002.

American Diabetes Association. "Report of the Expert Committee on the Diagnosis and Classification of Diabetes Mellitus," *Diabetes Care* 25(Suppl 1):S5-20, January 2002.

American Diabetes Association. "Screening for Diabetes," *Diabetes Care 25* (Suppl 1):S21-25, January 2002.

American Diabetes Association. "Standards of Medical Care for Patients with Diabetes," Diabetes Care 25 (Suppl 1):S33-49, January 2002.

American Diabetes Association. "Tests of Glycemia in Diabetes," *Diabetes Care* 25(Suppl 1):S97-99, January 2002.

Cameron, B.L. "Making Diabetes Management Routine," *AJN* 102(92):26-33, February 2002.

Centers for Disease Control and Prevention: *www.cdc.gov/diabetes/.*

Cincinnati, R., and Veliko, J. "Diabetes Update: Oral Medications," *RN* 64(8):30-36, August 2001.

Guthrie, D.W., and Guthrie, R. *Nursing Management of Diabetes Mellitus: A Guide to Pattern Approach.* 5th ed. New York: Springer Publishing Co., 2002.

Passanza C.E. "Diabetes Update: Monitor Options," *RN* 64(6):36-43, June 2001.

Diabetic ketoacidosis

DRG INFORMATION
DRG 294   Diabetes; Age 35+.
             Mean LOS = 4.6 days
DRG 295   Diabetes; Ages 0 to 35.
             Mean LOS = 3.8 days

Introduction
DEFINITION AND TIME FOCUS
Diabetic ketoacidosis (DKA) is a life-threatening endocrine emergency in which an acute or absolute insulin
deficiency produces metabolic acidosis. Clinical hallmarks include hyperglycemia, dehydration, ketosis, and
electrolyte imbalance. DKA is most commonly seen in
type 1 diabetes mellitus (DM) and may be present at the
time of diagnosis.

DM, the disease of insulin deficiency, alters the metabolism of carbohydrates, fats, and proteins, resulting in
various physiologic derangements that may become
life-threatening. Insulin, an anabolic hormone secreted
by pancreatic islet cells, facilitates glucose transport
across cell membranes. It thus promotes glucose uptake,
metabolism, and storage (as glycogen). Insulin also promotes fatty acid synthesis and amino acid transport
while inhibiting excessive breakdown of fats and proteins. In type 1 DM, the basic defect is thought to be inadequate or absent insulin secretion, whereas in type 2
DM, inadequate insulin secretion or insulin resistance or
both are thought to be responsible.

This care plan focuses on the critically ill diabetic patient admitted with ketoacidosis. (See *Clinical snapshot:
Diabetic ketoacidosis*, page 636.)

ETIOLOGY AND PRECIPITATING FACTORS
- Most commonly occurs in type 1 DM
- Mortality reported as less than 5%
- Most common causes include newly diagnosed type 1
DM; incorrect exogenous insulin dosage (omitted or de-
creased); and stressful states (such as infection, acute ill-
ness, myocardial infarction, or trauma), which stimulate
the release of counterregulatory hormones, such as epi-
nephrine, cortisol, and glucagon
- Occasionally, cause isn't identified

Focused assessment guidelines
NURSING HISTORY
(FUNCTIONAL HEALTH PATTERN FINDINGS)
Health-perception–health-management pattern
- New diagnosis or known history of type 1 DM

- Recent onset of infection
- Insulin, diet, and exercise to control blood glucose level in patient with known type 1 DM
- Insulin secretion level can't prevent ketosis in patient
with known type 2 M and severe illness or stress
- Onset of symptoms usually occurring over hours to
days

Nutritional-metabolic pattern
- Anorexia, nausea, abdominal pain, and vomiting
- Increased thirst (polydipsia) reported or displayed
- Increased hunger (polyphagia) reported or displayed
- Weight loss

Elimination pattern
- Excessive urination (polyuria) and nighttime urination
(nocturia) common
- Diarrhea or constipation

Activity-exercise pattern
- Weakness, fatigue, or lethargy

Sleep-rest pattern
- Disturbed sleep (from nocturia)

Cognitive-perceptual pattern
- Dizziness or confusion
- Blurred vision

PHYSICAL FINDINGS
Cardiovascular
- Postural (orthostatic) hypotension
- Weak, rapid pulse
- Low to normal blood pressure
- Hyperthermia possible
- Capillary refill time greater than 3 seconds

Pulmonary
- Deep, rapid (Kussmaul's) respirations
- Ketotic, acetone breath odor
- Dyspnea, tachypnea

Gastrointestinal
- Abdominal distention
- Decreased bowel sounds
- Abdominal tenderness or pain
- Dry mucous membranes

Integumentary
- Dry skin and mucous membranes
- Warm, flushed skin, especially on face
- Poor or decreased skin turgor
- Sunken eyes
- Skin infections or poorly healing skin wounds

Neurologic
- Lethargy, stupor, or coma
- Fatigue, drowsiness, disorientation, or confusion
- Normal, decreased, or absent reflexes

Genitourinary
- Polyuria initially; oliguria and anuria may follow
- Underlying renal involvement

Musculoskeletal
- Weakness

DIAGNOSTIC STUDIES

- Serum glucose level — elevated (300 to 800 mg/dl or higher)
- Arterial blood gas (ABG) levels — may reveal mild to severe metabolic acidosis with respiratory compensation (pH less than 7.35 and bicarbonate less than 10 mEq/L)
- Electrolyte panel levels — may be low, normal, or elevated depending on severity of dehydration and DKA; sodium and potassium imbalances common; acidosis causes potassium shifts in and out of cells, but a total body potassium deficit exists no matter what the current serum level
- Blood urea nitrogen and creatinine levels — may be normal or elevated depending on severity of dehydration and DKA and presence of underlying renal disease
- Osmolality — usually less than 350 mOsm/kg

- Complete blood count and white blood cell count — may be elevated in presence of infection; hemoglobin levels and hematocrit may be elevated secondary to dehydration
- Ketones — positive in urine and serum
- Electrocardiography — used to rule out myocardial infarction and evaluate potassium abnormalities
- Chest X-ray — rules out infection
- Cardiac enzymes — rule out myocardial infarction
- Blood, urine, sputum cultures — detect infection's source

POTENTIAL COMPLICATIONS

- Long-term complications of DM (retinopathy, neuropathy, nephropathy, cardiovascular disease, and peripheral vascular disease) that will influence nursing interventions and treatment strategies
- Coma and death if DKA untreated
- Fluid overload
- Hypoglycemia if DKA overtreated
- Hypovolemic shock

CLINICAL SNAPSHOT

Diabetic ketoacidosis

Major nursing diagnoses and collaborative problems	Key patient outcomes
CP: Hypovolemia	Maintain vital signs within normal limits, typically: pulse rate, 60 to 100 beats/minute; systolic blood pressure, 90 to 140 mm Hg; and diastolic blood pressure, 50 to 90 mm Hg.
CP: Hyperglycemia	Display a blood glucose level of less than 200 mg/dl or within therapeutic limits as specified by the physician.
ND: Risk for injury	Return to baseline LOC.
CP: Acidosis	Maintain ABG levels within normal limits: pH, 7.35 to 7.45; $Paco_2$, 35 to 45 mm Hg; and HCO_3^-, 23 to 28 mEq/L.
ND: Deficient knowledge (self-care)	On request, state care plan for "sick day" management.

Collaborative problem

Hypovolemia related to osmotic diuresis or vomiting, or both

NURSING PRIORITY

Restore fluid volume rapidly.

PATIENT OUTCOME CRITERIA

Within 12 hours after the onset of therapy, the patient will:
- maintain vital signs within normal limits, typically: heart rate, 60 to 100 beats/minute; systolic blood pressure, 90 to 140 mm Hg; and diastolic blood pressure, 50 to 90 mm Hg
- display adequate peripheral perfusion, as manifested by strong peripheral pulses and capillary refill time less than 3 seconds.

Within 24 hours after the onset of therapy, the patient will:
- have urine output of 60 to 100 ml/hour
- have a balanced intake and output
- have normal skin turgor, mucous membrane moisture, and other clinical signs of adequate hydration
- show no signs or symptoms of electrolyte imbalances.

INTERVENTIONS	RATIONALES
1. *Monitor for signs and symptoms of dehydration and shock,** such as tachycardia; hypotension; weak peripheral pulses; capillary refill time greater than 3 seconds; warm, dry, flushed skin and mucus membranes; poor skin turgor; and polyuria or oliguria. Continuously monitor blood pressure and cardiac rate and rhythm.	**1.** In DKA, the blood glucose level is elevated because of decreased cellular uptake and use of glucose. The resulting hyperglycemia increases serum osmolality and triggers a fluid shift from the intracellular to the extracellular space, producing intracellular dehydration. Compensatory renal glucose spillage, a powerful control mechanism to prevent excessive hyperglycemia, produces intense, obligatory osmotic diuresis resulting in extracellular dehydration. Eventually, severe dehydration decreases glomerular filtration. The resulting oliguria aggravates hyperglycemia and hyperosmolality. Signs and symptoms indicate the severity of the deficit and the adequacy of fluid replacement. As volume is restored, signs and symptoms should gradually resolve; failure to do so indicates inadequate fluid replacement or continuing fluid losses.
2. *Observe for signs and symptoms of electrolyte imbalances* (see appendix C, Fluid and electrolyte imbalances, for details): – hyperkalemia in the first 1 to 4 hours of treatment – hypokalemia after 1 to 4 hours of treatment – hyponatremia early in treatment – hypernatremia later in treatment	**2.** Electrolyte status may change rapidly, so monitor closely to identify any imbalances. – Buffering of excess hydrogen ions released in acidosis displaces intracellular potassium into the serum. – Renal excretion of potassium accelerates because of hyperkalemia, and the high serum level masks the resulting total body potassium deficit. As therapy reduces acidosis, potassium ions move into the cells from the serum, unmasking the underlying deficit. – Diuresis and ketone excretion cause hyponatremia from urinary sodium losses. – As metabolic control is restored, the kidneys begin to conserve sodium. This sodium retention, added to sodium administration in I.V. fluids, may produce hypernatremia.
3. *Monitor serum osmolality and electrolyte values,* as ordered. Report abnormal values to the physician.	**3.** Laboratory values provide objective data on the type and degree of physiologic derangements present. In addition, serum osmolality values guide fluid replacement, while electrolyte values guide electrolyte repletion.
4. *On admission, establish and maintain one or more I.V. lines* in large peripheral veins, as ordered.	**4.** Dehydration is the most immediately life-threatening aspect of DKA. In addition, the body must be adequately hydrated for insulin to be effective. Large veins permit rapid administration of the large amounts of fluid necessary to reverse severe dehydration.

*Italics indicate key interventions.

5. *Monitor intake and output meticulously. Report urine output below 30 ml/hour.* Weigh the patient daily, and document findings. Insert an indwelling urinary catheter, as ordered.

5. Intake and output and weight records reflect the degree of fluid imbalance and effectiveness of therapy. Renal function, as reflected by hourly urine output, must be assured before I.V. potassium replacement is begun or continued. Initially, output greatly exceeds intake, unless severe dehydration and oliguria are present. As the patient is rehydrated, fluid losses continue for the first several hours until glycosuria and osmotic diuresis are controlled. An indwelling catheter facilitates accurate measurement of urinary fluid loss. An indwelling catheter is rarely used in a conscious patient.

6. *Administer I.V. solutions,* as ordered. Replacement may include 4 to 9 L in the first 24 hours, typically:

– normal saline solution, 1 to 2 L in the first 2 hours

– half normal saline, after the first few hours, or half normal saline with 5% dextrose in water at 150 to 250 ml/hour when blood glucose level reaches 250 mg/dl

– plasma volume expanders, such as albumin, if dehydration is severe (administer only after normal saline solution administration is underway).

6. The selection of I.V. fluid depends on the patient's blood glucose and electrolyte levels, whereas the amount depends on the existing fluid deficit and ongoing fluid losses. The average fluid deficit on admission ranges from 4 to 9 L. Volume repletion is essential in reversing hypovolemia and allowing continued renal glucose excretion, an important compensatory mechanism in restoring glucose levels to normal.
– Normal saline solution replaces lost volume and sodium without increasing the blood glucose level.
– As the serum sodium level returns to normal, the saline concentration of I.V. solutions is reduced to prevent sodium overload. As the blood glucose level returns to normal, a solution containing glucose may be used to prevent hypoglycemia.
– Usually, normal saline administration is sufficient to reverse volume depletion. Although rarely used, plasma volume expanders may be necessary in severe dehydration. If they're administered before normal saline solution, however, their hypertonicity increases cellular dehydration.

7. *Administer therapy for electrolyte imbalances,* as ordered.

7. Hyperkalemia, hyponatremia, and hypernatremia usually resolve with appropriate fluid administration and control of hyperglycemia. Hypokalemia usually requires I.V. administration of supplemental potassium. Don't add potassium until urine output is established. Potassium replacement usually includes $^2/_3$ potassium chloride with $^1/_3$ potassium phosphate.

8. *For at least 24 hours after rapid fluid repletion, observe for signs and symptoms of pulmonary edema,* such as crackles, dyspnea, cough, or frothy sputum. If any are present, alert the physician immediately.

8. Rapid fluid repletion causes hemodilution. Lowered plasma oncotic pressure may allow fluid to leak into the pulmonary interstitial space, producing pulmonary edema. Pulmonary edema requires prompt aggressive medical intervention.

9. Additional individualized interventions: _____

_____

9. Rationales:_____

_____

Collaborative problem

Hyperglycemia related to decreased cellular glucose uptake and use

NURSING PRIORITY
Restore glucose control gradually.

PATIENT OUTCOME CRITERIA

Within 2 hours of the onset of therapy, the patient's blood glucose level will:
- be decreasing toward normal at a rate of approximately 50 to 75 mg/dl/hour.

Within 24 to 48 hours of the onset of therapy, the patient will:
- display a blood glucose level between 80 and 120 mg/dl
- have a small or negative urine ketone level.

INTERVENTIONS

1. *Assess blood glucose levels according to facility protocol.* Typically, obtain blood and fingerstick glucose levels on admission; correlate values, then fingerstick monitoring every hour until normal, then every 6 hours, then before meals and at bedtime, or as ordered.

2. *Administer insulin as ordered.* The I.V. route is preferred. Typically, an I.V. bolus of regular insulin at 0.15 unit/kg body weight is followed by a continuous infusion of regular insulin at 0.1 unit/kg/hour. Before starting the infusion, flush the I.V. line with 100 ml of the insulin solution. Occasionally, boluses of regular insulin may be given by I.V., I.M., or subcutaneous (S.C.) injection in conjunction with the I.V. infusion. Monitor blood glucose levels hourly, and adjust insulin I.V. infusion rates accordingly.

3. *Take steps to prevent hypoglycemia.* Alert the physician when the blood glucose level reaches 50 mg/ml. Change the normal saline solution to a glucose solution, or decrease the insulin dose, as ordered. Alert the physician again. Switch to S.C. insulin; continue I.V. insulin infusion for 1 to 2 hours, more, as ordered.

4. *If ordered, assess blood ketone level on admission and as ordered.* Perform bedside urine monitoring, every void, until ketone level is low, then every 6 hours or before meals and at bedtime.

RATIONALES

1. Blood glucose levels are the most direct indicators of deranged glucose metabolism and are used to determine therapy. As glomerular filtration of glucose exceeds the transport maximum, glucose spills into the urine. Because blood glucose levels are much more accurate than urine glucose levels, bedside fingersticks are the favored monitoring method. The goal is to reduce the glucose level approximately 50 to 75 mg/dl an hour.

2. Exogenous insulin controls gluconeogenesis and ketogenesis and increases cellular glucose uptake. In profound dehydration, medication absorption may be erratic, so the I.V. route is most reliable. A small amount of insulin may bind to I.V. tubing and bottles; flushing the line first limits the amount of insulin absorbed by the tubing during administration. Periodic boluses may allow swings in blood glucose level; the goal is to lower the glucose level 50 to 75 mg/dl/hour. Gradual lowering of the blood glucose levels reduces the possibility of cerebral edema or cerebral hypoglycemia due to fluid shifts from a brain-blood glucose gradient. Continuous infusion allows delivery of low dosage. Remember, I.V. absorption is greater than I.M. absorption, which in turn is greater than S.C. absorption. I.M. and S.C. absorption may be erratic; I.V. administration is preferred.

3. As metabolic control is reestablished, the blood glucose level may drop precipitously from the combined effects of therapy and continuing glycosuria. The measures listed help avoid hypoglycemia. Continuing I.V. insulin infusion for 1 to 2 hours after S.C. insulin is begun ensures adequate plasma insulin levels.

4. When carbohydrate metabolism is impaired, the body uses fat as a fuel source. Lipolysis produces free fatty aids, which when oxidized produce ketone bodies. Blood ketone levels directly reflect the degree of ketogenesis. The body initially compensates by buffering ketoacids with bicarbonate. When ketoacid production exceeds buffering, ketoacids accumulate in the blood, producing acidosis. Direct measurement of beta-hydroxybutyric acid is the preferred method to monitor ketoacidosis. Some of the excess ketoacids are excreted in the urine (largely as sodium salts). Urine ketone levels measure ketone excretion. Urine ketones may be positive for 24 to 48 hours after DKA resolves.

5. *Observe for signs and symptoms of medication-induced hypoglycemia,* such as headache, confusion, irritability, restlessness, trembling, pallor, diaphoresis, and stupor. If these signs and symptoms are present, notify the physician, obtain a bedside fingerstick blood glucose level without delay, and treat immediately with food, oral glucose gel, or I.V. glucose or glucagon, depending upon unit protocol and the patient's level of consciousness (LOC).

6. Additional individualized interventions: _____
_____

5. The brain depends on glucose almost exclusively for energy. Hypoglycemia produces dramatic cerebral dysfunction and a profound stress response. The longer hypoglycemia persists, the greater the chance of transient or permanent neurologic damage. Hypoglycemic reactions may be fatal if left untreated. Mild reactions should be treated with protein and carbohydrates (such as milk and crackers). Simple sugars should be reserved for severe reactions.

6. Rationales: _____
_____

Nursing diagnosis

Risk for injury related to cerebral dehydration, decreased perfusion, hypoxemia, or acidosis

NURSING PRIORITIES
- Ensure patient safety.
- Monitor return to the patient's usual LOC.

PATIENT OUTCOME CRITERION
Within 24 hours of the onset of therapy, the patient's LOC will return to baseline.

INTERVENTIONS

1. *Implement standard safety precautions* such as keeping side rails up for the critically ill patient.

2. *Monitor LOC constantly.* Alert the physician if LOC doesn't improve within 2 hours of the onset of therapy.

3. Additional individualized interventions: _____
_____

RATIONALES

1. A decreased LOC makes the patient unable to guard against accidental injury.

2. Decreased LOC in early DKA may result from hyperosmolality, marked cellular dehydration from osmotic diuresis, altered cellular function from anaerobic metabolism, or acidotic cerebrospinal fluid. Persistently decreased or worsening LOC may result from cerebral edema caused by a precipitous lowering of the blood glucose level. A substantial difference between blood glucose concentration and the concentration of glucose metabolites in the brain creates an osmotic gradient, drawing water into the brain and producing cerebral edema. LOC should return to normal with therapy; failure to do so suggests another disorder and requires further medical evaluation.

3. Rationales: _____
_____

Suggested NIC Interventions
Fall prevention; Surveillance: Safety

Suggested NOC Outcomes
Safety status: Physical injury

Collaborative problem

Acidosis related to altered LOC, ketosis, and decreased tissue perfusion

NURSING PRIORITIES

- Maintain optimal ventilation and oxygenation.
- Restore normal acid-base balance.

PATIENT OUTCOME CRITERIA

Within 24 hours of the onset of therapy, the patient will:
- breathe at a rate of 12 to 24 respirations/minute
- display eupnea.
  Within 36 hours of the onset of therapy, the patient will:
- have ABG levels within normal limits: pH, 7.35 to 7.45; $Paco_2$, 35 to 45 mm Hg; and HCO_3^-, 23 to 28 mEq/L
- have normal bowel sounds
- be able to take oral food and fluids safely.

INTERVENTIONS	RATIONALES
1. *Maintain a patent airway.*	1. Decreased LOC increases risk of aspiration.
2. *Every hour, monitor ease, rate, and depth of respiration continuously.* Document respiratory status: – respiratory rate and depth	2. Serial assessments allow timely detection of respiratory abnormalities. – The body responds to ketoacidosis, a form of metabolic acidosis, by increasing the rate and depth of ventilation to blow off carbon dioxide and induce a compensatory respiratory alkalosis. The presence of Kussmaul's respirations indicates severe acidosis.
– breath odor	– Acetone breath indicates respiratory excretion of ketones.
– breath sounds.	– Breath sounds indicate the adequacy of ventilation. Abnormal sounds may suggest pneumonia (an infection that can cause DKA) or fluid overload.
3. *Anticipate intubation and mechanical ventilation if respiratory distress increases.*	3. Although rarely needed, these measures may be necessary to maintain airway patency and ventilatory adequacy.
4. *Administer oxygen,* as ordered.	4. Acidosis impairs oxygen delivery to tissues. Hypoxia provokes anaerobic metabolism, which produces lactic acid and further worsens the metabolic acidosis. Supplemental oxygen elevates arterial oxygen tension, reducing the need for anaerobic metabolism.
5. *Monitor ABG levels or venous pH and anion gap,* as ordered.	5. ABG levels document the type and degree of acid-base imbalances present and the effectiveness of therapy for DKA. After initial ABG measurement, venous pH (which is 0.03 units lower than arterial pH) and anion gap can be used to monitor acidosis. These measures can be included with electrolyte and other metabolic measures in venous blood samples. Abnormalities normally resolve with fluid and electrolyte replacement and insulin therapy.
6. *Administer I.V. sodium bicarbonate,* as ordered, if pH is 7.0 or less	6. These parameters indicate severe acidosis. Bicarbonate administration replenishes bicarbonate ions, which buffer excess hydrogen ions, thus returning pH to normal. Use of I.V. sodium bicarbonate is uncommon.

7. *While the patient is acutely ill, withhold food and fluids, even if the patient is extremely thirsty.* Auscultate bowel sounds every 8 hours. Insert a gastric tube, as ordered, and connect to suction. Remove the gastric tube and allow oral intake of food and fluids only after LOC and bowel sounds return to normal.

7. Intense thirst is a compensatory mechanism for dehydration, but oral fluid intake can be dangerous. Because hyperglycemia decreases bowel motility, abdominal pain, nausea, and vomiting are common. Vomiting increases the risk of aspiration. Bowel sounds reflect GI motility. Allowing oral intake only after bowel sounds and LOC are normal reduces the risk of aspiration. Use of gastric tubes is rare, unless the patient is unconscious.

8. Additional individualized interventions: _____

_____

8. Rationales: _____

_____

Nursing diagnosis

Deficient knowledge (self-care) related to lack of exposure to complex disease and therapy

NURSING PRIORITY

Identify and meet immediate learning needs.

PATIENT OUTCOME CRITERIA

By the time of discharge, the patient and his family will:
- identify learning needs
- show beginning involvement in learning, if appropriate
- on request, state plan of care for "sick day" management.

INTERVENTIONS

1. *Refer to the "Knowledge deficit" care plan,* page 129.

2. *When the patient's condition allows, determine learning needs.* Ascertain whether DM is a new or previously identified diagnosis. If the patient is a known diabetic, assess for possible causes of DKA, for example, a missed insulin dose or undetected infection.

3. *When the patient's condition allows, begin a teaching program* that emphasizes principles of "sick day" management:
– continue to take insulin or oral hypoglycemic agents
– change diet to frequent small meals of soft or liquid foods containing carbohydrate content of usual meals.
– contact the physician early in the illness
– check blood glucose level at least every 4 hours
– check blood or urine ketones if blood glucose is greater than 300 mg/dl
– increase sugar-free fluids to more than 8 oz (240 ml) per hour
– postpone exercise
  Notify the health care provider if:
– blood glucose level is greater than 250 mg/dl
– unable to take food or fluids
– illness persists for more than 1 day
– ketonuria is moderate or present for more than 24 hours.

RATIONALES

1. The "Knowledge deficit" care plan provides general guidelines for patient teaching.

2. Learning needs vary depending on whether the patient is a new or known diabetic. If the patient is newly diagnosed, extensive teaching is necessary. With a known diabetic, DKA episodes are usually preventable, and instruction may focus on unmet learning needs or areas needing reinforcement.

3. Although teaching is crucial to successful management of DM, physiologic needs take precedence in the critically ill patient. Extensive teaching may need to be deferred until after the patient's condition stabilizes. Understanding principles of "sick day" management may avert future crises.

4. *Use the patient's symptomatic episode as a teaching tool.* Involve the patient's family in all teaching sessions.

5. *As appropriate, initiate teaching about DM.* Include, for example, the cause of DM, signs and symptoms, significance of insulin, injection techniques, factors affecting medication needs (such as food intake and exercise), therapeutic diet, blood and urine testing, importance of consistent level of daily exercise, increased susceptibility to infections, recognition and management of hyperglycemic and hypoglycemic episodes, and long-range complications, such as neuropathy and retinopathy. *Refer to the "Diabetes mellitus" care plan,* page 624.

6. *Document learning needs and make appropriate referrals.* When the patient is discharged, communicate learning needs and arrange for teaching to continue on an outpatient basis.

7. Additional individualized interventions: _____
_____

4. The immediacy of the DKA episode makes it a powerful teaching tool for actively involving the patient and his family.

5. Although the patient's and family's knowledge of all these topics is essential for ongoing home management of DM, only initial teaching is feasible for the critically ill patient. The "Diabetes mellitus" care plan contains detailed information on these topics.

6. The patient's condition, extensiveness of learning needs, and the hectic unit atmosphere means that the patient will be discharged before learning is complete. Documentation and communication enhance continuity of care.

7. Rationales:_____
_____

Suggested NIC Interventions
Teaching: Disease process; Teaching: Individual; Teaching: Prescribed medication

Suggested NOC Outcomes
Knowledge: Disease process; Knowledge: Health behaviors; Knowledge: Treatment regimen

---

Discharge planning

DISCHARGE CHECKLIST
Before discharge, the patient shows evidence of:
- ❑ stable vital signs within normal limits
- ❑ blood glucose level within normal limits without I.V. insulin
- ❑ return to premorbid LOC — ideally, alert and oriented
- ❑ ABG levels within normal limits
- ❑ patient's active participation in self-care.

TEACHING CHECKLIST
Document evidence that the patient and his family demonstrate an understanding of initial teaching related to:
- ❑ "sick day" management
- ❑ cause and consequences of DM
- ❑ causes of DKA, including signs and symptoms and appropriate responses
- ❑ significance of insulin
- ❑ signs, symptoms, and interventions for hyperglycemia and hypoglycemia
- ❑ dietary management
- ❑ exercise plan
- ❑ blood glucose and urine ketone testing

- ❑ plan for completing unmet learning needs, including use of community and outpatient resources.

DOCUMENTATION CHECKLIST
Using outcome criteria as a guide, document:
- ❑ clinical status on admission
- ❑ significant changes in status
- ❑ pertinent diagnostic test findings
- ❑ I.V. fluid therapy
- ❑ pharmacologic intervention
- ❑ oxygen administration
- ❑ patient and family teaching
- ❑ discharge planning.

Associated care plans
- Acute renal failure
- Diabetes mellitus
- Hyperosmolar hyperglycemic nonketotic syndrome
- Hypoglycemia
- Hypovolemic shock
- Knowledge deficit

References

Bryden, K.S., et al. "Poor Prognosis of Young Adults With Type 1 Diabetes: A Longitudinal Study," *Diabetes Care* 26(4):1052-57, April 2003.

Freire, A.X., et al. "Predictors of Intensive Care Unit and Hospital Length of Stay in Diabetic Ketoacidosis," *Journal of Critical Care* 17(4):207-11, December 2002.

Habib, G.S., et al. "Diabetic Ketoacidosis Associated with Oral Salbutamol Overdose," *American Journal of Medicine* 113(8):701-702, December 2002.

Jordan, K. (ed). *Emergency Nursing Core Curriculum.* Emergency Nurses Association. Philadelphia: W.B. Saunders Co., 2000.

Lynn-McHale, D.J., and Carlson, K.K. American Association of Critical Care Nurses *AACN Procedure Manual for Critical Care,* 4th ed. Philadelphia: W.B. Saunders Co., 2001.

Shoemaker, W.C., et al. *Textbook of Critical Care,* 4th ed. Philadelphia: W.B. Saunders Co., 2002.

Weissberg-Benchell, J., et al. "Insulin Pump Therapy: A Meta-analysis," *Diabetes Care* 26(4):1079-87, April 2003.

Hyperosmolar hyperglycemic nonketotic syndrome

DRG INFORMATION

DRG 294 Diabetes; Age 35+.
Mean LOS = 4.6 days
DRG 295 Diabetes; Ages 0 to 35.
Mean LOS = 3.8 days

Introduction
DEFINITION AND TIME FOCUS

Hyperosmolar hyperglycemic nonketotic syndrome (HHNS) is an endocrine emergency with a mortality greater than 15% in the general population and as high as 70% in the elderly, if left untreated. Like diabetic ketoacidosis (DKA), it produces profound hyperglycemia and dehydration, but unlike DKA, ketosis and acidosis are absent. It presents a diagnostic puzzle because its clinical picture is similar to both DKA and stroke. It may occur in type 1 or type 2 diabetes mellitus (DM) but is more common in type 2 and may be present at the time of diagnosis.

The basic defect in HHNS is a relative insulin deficiency in which enough insulin is secreted to prevent ketoacidosis but not enough to prevent hyperglycemia. Failure to recognize or respond to the thirst mechanism, which signals developing dehydration, exacerbates the problem. A precipitating factor (such as infection, new diagnosis of DM, stroke, or myocardial infarction) is also common. Clinical hallmarks include hyperglycemia, dehydration, hyperosmolality, and electrolyte imbalance without ketosis. This care plan focuses on the critically ill patient admitted with HHNS. (See *Clinical snapshot: Hyperosmolar hyperglycemic nonketotic syndrome,* page 646.)

ETIOLOGY AND PRECIPITATING FACTORS

- Usually only occurs in type 2 DM, but up to 50% of episodes occur in persons with no previous history of DM
- Infection (such as pneumonia or urinary tract infection)
- Acute illness (such as myocardial infarction or stroke)
- Loss of thirst mechanism or poor fluid intake
- Mortality reported at 15% with treatment
- Treatments (such as dialysis or total parenteral nutrition)
- Surgery
- Newly diagnosed DM
- Drugs (such as steroids, thiazides, or beta-adrenergic blockers)
- Pancreatitis

Focused assessment guidelines
NURSING HISTORY
(FUNCTIONAL HEALTH PATTERN FINDINGS)
Health-perception–health-management pattern
History is typically obtained from a family member or friend because the patient's level of consciousness is decreased.

- Patient newly diagnosed or has known history of type 2 DM
- Family history of DM common
- More common in older patients (over age 50)
- Slow onset of symptoms, typically over days to weeks

Nutritional-metabolic pattern
- Increased thirst (polydipsia) or loss of thirst mechanism
- Anorexia
- Weight loss

Elimination pattern
- Polyuria, nocturia, and incontinence (possible)
- Diarrhea or constipation (possible)

Activity-exercise pattern
- Weakness, fatigue, or lethargy (possible)

Sleep-rest pattern
- Sleep disturbance related to nocturia

Cognitive-perceptual pattern
- Dizziness or orthostatic hypotension (possible)
- Confusion
- Blurred vision (possible)
- Decreased or altered sensorium

PHYSICAL FINDINGS
Neurologic
- Lethargy or stupor
- Fatigue, drowsiness, disorientation, or confusion
- Seizures
- Normal, decreased, or absent reflexes

Pulmonary
- Tachypnea or dyspnea
- Absence of Kussmaul's respirations (differential finding from DKA)
- Absence of acetone breath (differential finding from DKA)

645

Cardiovascular
- Tachycardia
- Postural hypotension
- Other cardiovascular disease (such as hypertension or heart failure)
- Hyperthermia possible
- Capillary refill time greater than 3 seconds

Renal
- Polyuria (early stage)
- Oliguria (late stage)
- Nocturia
- Incontinence

Integumentary
- Dry skin and mucous membranes
- Poor skin turgor
- Warm, flushed skin
- Sunken or soft eyes
- Skin infections or poorly healing wounds

Gastrointestinal
- Abdominal distention
- Decreased bowel sounds

DIAGNOSTIC STUDIES

- Serum glucose levels — usually greater than 800 mg/dl, may be as high as 3,000 mg/dl
- Arterial blood gas (ABG) levels — usually normal
- Electrolyte panel levels — may be low, normal, or elevated depending on severity of dehydration and HHNS (Extreme hyperglycemia produces profound diuresis with resulting potassium loss. A total body potassium deficit exists no matter what current serum level.)
- Blood urea nitrogen (BUN) and creatinine levels — BUN levels may be normal to elevated depending on severity of dehydration and HHNS; both may be normal to elevated in presence of underlying renal disease
- Urine ketones — usually negative
- Serum osmolality — usually greater than 350 mOsm/kg
- Complete blood count and white blood cell count — may be elevated in presence of infection
- Hemoglobin levels and hematocrit — may be elevated secondary to dehydration
- Electrocardiography — may reveal underlying cardiac disorder or arrhythmias
- Chest X-ray — needed to establish baseline and rule out infection
- Blood, urine, and sputum cultures — used to detect infection's source
- Serum amylase — rules out pancreatitis

POTENTIAL COMPLICATIONS

- Diabetes-related complications (retinopathy, neuropathy, nephropathy, cardiovascular disease, and peripheral vascular disease) that will influence nursing interventions and treatment strategies
- Fluid overload, heart failure, or pulmonary edema
- Disseminated intravascular coagulation
- Hypoglycemia (if HHNS overtreated)
- Hypovolemic shock
- Cerebral edema
- Coma and death if untreated

CLINICAL SNAPSHOT ✸

Hyperosmolar hyperglycemic nonketotic syndrome

Major nursing diagnoses and collaborative problems	Key patient outcomes
CP: Hypovolemia	Maintain stable vital signs, typically: heart rate, 60 to 100 beats/minute; systolic blood pressure, 90 to 140 mm Hg; and diastolic blood pressure, 50 to 90 mm Hg.
CP: Hyperglycemia	Display a blood glucose level of less than 200 mg/dl or within therapeutic limits as specified by the physician.
ND: Risk for injury	Return to baseline LOC.
ND: Deficient knowledge (self-care)	On request, state care plan for "sick day" management.

Collaborative problem
Hypovolemia related to osmotic diuresis

NURSING PRIORITY
Restore fluid volume.

PATIENT OUTCOME CRITERIA

Within 36 to 48 hours of the onset of therapy, the patient will:
- maintain vital signs within normal limits, typically: heart rate, 60 to 100 beats/minute; systolic blood pressure, 90 to 140 mm Hg; and diastolic blood pressure, 50 to 90 mm Hg
- peripheral perfusion within normal limits, as evidenced by warm, dry skin and bilaterally equal pedal pulses
- maintain a urine output of 60 to 100 ml/hour
- manifest serum osmolality levels within normal limits
- display normal skin turgor, mucous membrane moisture, and other clinical signs of adequate hydration
- exhibit serum electrolyte levels within normal limits.

INTERVENTIONS

1. *Monitor for signs and symptoms of dehydration and shock,** such as tachycardia; hypotension; weak peripheral pulses; capillary refill time greater than 3 seconds; warm, dry, flushed skin; poor skin turgor; polyuria or oliguria; increased hematocrit; increased urine specific gravity; and increased serum osmolality. Monitor blood pressure and cardiac rate and rhythm continuously.

2. *Observe for signs and symptoms of electrolyte imbalances,* particularly hypernatremia and hypokalemia (see appendix C, Fluid and electrolyte imbalances, for details). Monitor serum electrolyte levels, as ordered, and report abnormal values to the physician. Administer electrolyte replacements, as ordered. Typically, administer I.V. potassium replacement ($^2/_3$ potassium chloride and $^1/_3$ potassium phosphate at 20 to 40 mEq/L to keep potassium level between 4 and 5 mEq/L.

3. *Monitor serum osmolality,* as ordered. Report levels greater than 295 mOsm/kg.

4. *Implement standard measures for hypovolemia,* as ordered. Maintain patency of one or more I.V. lines, insert an indwelling urinary catheter, and monitor intake and output and daily weights. Refer to the "Diabetic ketoacidosis" care plan, page 635, for details.

5. *Administer I.V. solutions,* as ordered, typically 6 to 8 L in the first 12 hours:
– normal saline solution if serum sodium level is less than 130 mEq/L

RATIONALES

1. Impaired insulin release or peripheral insulin resistance causes hyperglycemia, which in turn causes hyperosmolality. To compensate for the hyperosmolality, fluid shifts from the intracellular to the extracellular space, dehydrating cells. Renal glucose spillage, an important compensatory mechanism for hyperglycemia, triggers an intense osmotic diuresis. This diuresis causes obligatory fluid and electrolyte losses, reflected in an elevated hematocrit and increased serum osmolality. Severe hypovolemia decreases glomerular filtration, aggravating the hyperglycemia and hyperosmolality and eventually producing oliguria and increased specific gravity. Fluid loss is usually greater in HHNS than in DKA, so signs of dehydration may be severe. As volume is restored, signs and symptoms should resolve gradually; failure to do so indicates inadequate fluid replacement or continuing losses.

2. Electrolyte status may change rapidly in response to fluid shifts, so close observation for signs and symptoms of imbalances is essential. Hypernatremia results from the large water deficit. In contrast to DKA, where acidosis causes hyperkalemia that commonly masks a low total body potassium, urinary losses in HHNS result in hypokalemia. Hypernatremia usually resolves with fluid administration, while hypokalemia usually requires earlier potassium replacement than with DKA. Potassium doses depend on serum potassium levels.

3. Laboratory values document the extent of hyperosmolality, which usually is more marked than in DKA because of the failure of the thirst mechanism and the intense osmotic diuresis. Values greater than 320 mOsm/kg indicate severe hyperosmolality.

4. These measures are the same as with DKA. The "Diabetic ketoacidosis" care plan describes these interventions and associated rationales in detail. Because HHNS is seen more commonly in older patients, an indwelling urinary catheter is useful; it's necessary in the unconscious patient.

5. Aggressive fluid repletion is necessary due to the severity of dehydration in HHNS.
– A very low serum sodium level reflects large urinary sodium losses. Isotonic saline solution replaces sodium and replenishes volume.

*Italics indicate key interventions.

– half-normal saline solution if serum sodium level is greater than 145 mEq/L

– 5% dextrose in 0.45% saline when blood glucose levels reach 300 mg/dl

6. *During fluid replacement, monitor closely for signs and symptoms of fluid overload,* including crackles, S_3 heart sound, jugular vein distention, dyspnea, or persistently depressed LOC. If any indicators are present, notify the physician.

7. Additional individualized interventions: _____

– An elevated serum sodium level reflects decreased glomerular filtration and sodium retention in severe hypovolemia. Hypotonic fluid provides free water to reverse hyperosmolality.
– As blood glucose or serum osmolality approaches normal, changing to a glucose-containing solution prevents hypoglycemia.

6. Because the patient with HHNS is usually older and has significant preexisting disease, the risk for heart failure, pulmonary edema, or cerebral edema is higher than in DKA. These signs and symptoms require prompt nursing intervention and medical evaluation.

7. Rationales: _____

Collaborative problem

Hyperglycemia related to inadequate insulin secretion or peripheral insulin resistance, or both

NURSING PRIORITY

Lower blood glucose level.

PATIENT OUTCOME CRITERION

Within 24 to 48 hours of the onset of therapy, the patient will display a blood glucose level between 80 and 120 mg/dl.

INTERVENTIONS	RATIONALES
1. *Adapt measures for this problem contained in the "Diabetic ketoacidosis" care plan,* page 635. Implement the following modifications: – Judiciously administer low-dose insulin I.V., as ordered. Discontinue the infusion if the blood glucose level drops more than 70 mg/dl in 1 hour and alert the physician. – Notify the physician when blood glucose reaches 300 mg/dl. Reduce insulin infusion to maintain blood glucose between 250 and 300 mg/dl, until plasma osmolality is less than 315 mOsm/kg and the patient is mentally alert.	**1.** Care for hyperglycemia is similar in both HHNS and DKA, but with different emphasis on two points. – Because some endogenous insulin is produced, the patient with HHNS is more sensitive to exogenous insulin than a patient with DKA, and lower insulin doses are usually needed. – Risk of cerebral edema is greater with the more profound dehydration of HHNS.
– Monitor closely for medication-induced hypoglycemia.	– Because the patient with HHNS retains some control of glucose metabolism, the risk for developing hypoglycemia in response to measures that lower blood glucose is high.
2. *If the patient developed HHNS while on high-carbohydrate enteral nutrition or hyperosmolar dialysis, consult with the physician about revising orders for these therapies.*	**2.** Modifying or discontinuing these causes of HHNS removes an unnecessary glucose load for the patient.
3. Additional individualized interventions: _____	**3.** Rationales: _____

Nursing diagnosis

Risk for injury related to cerebral dehydration, decreased perfusion, hypoxemia, glucose deprivation, or cerebral edema during rapid rehydration

NURSING PRIORITIES
- Restore the patient's baseline level of consciousness (LOC).
- Protect the patient from injury.

PATIENT OUTCOME CRITERIA
Within 24 hours, the patient will:
- display baseline LOC
- (ideally) be alert, oriented, and able to move all extremities.

INTERVENTIONS	RATIONALES
1. *Evaluate neurologic status* according to facility protocol or at least every 1 to 4 hours, as indicated by the rapidity of other changes in the patient's condition. *Alert the physician to deepening coma or other indications of deteriorating neurologic functioning.*	1. Neurologic changes, which are characteristic of this disorder, correlate closely with the degree of hyperosmolality. Deteriorating neurologic function may indicate serious pathophysiologic derangements, other previously undetected disorders, or inadequate therapy, and it requires medical evaluation.
2. *Institute seizure precautions. Promptly report seizures to the physician.*	2. Seizures occur commonly with HHNS, as a result of cerebral dehydration, cerebral edema (during rehydration), or glucose deprivation (if hypoglycemia occurs).
3. Additional individualized interventions: _____	3. Rationales:_____

> **Suggested NIC Interventions**
> *Fall prevention; Surveillance: Safety*

> **Suggested NOC Outcomes**
> *Safety status: Physical injury*

Nursing diagnosis

Deficient knowledge (self-care) related to lack of exposure to complex disease and management

NURSING PRIORITY
Teach the patient and his family to avoid recurrence of HHNS, if appropriate.

PATIENT OUTCOME CRITERIA
By the time of discharge, the patient and his family will:
- identify learning needs, if appropriate, as manifested by curiosity, asking questions, and attentiveness to teaching
- show beginning involvement in learning, if appropriate
- state plan of care for "sick day" management on request.

INTERVENTIONS	RATIONALES
1. *Collaborate with the physician to identify cause of HHNS. If it's DM, implement measures in the "Diabetic ketoacidosis" care plan (with the exception of ketone testing), page 635, and the "Diabetes Mellitus" care plan, page 624, as appropriate.*	1. These care plans detail measures that also apply to teaching some HHNS patients. It's pertinent to patients with uncontrolled DM in whom HHNS may recur. It's inappropriate when HHNS results from high-carbohydrate nutrition or hyperosmolar dialysis; in those instances, HHNS shouldn't recur once the cause has been removed.

2. Additional individualized interventions: _____

2. Rationales: _____

Suggested NIC Interventions
Teaching: Disease process; Teaching: Individual; Teaching: Prescribed medication

Suggested NOC Outcomes
Knowledge: Disease process; Knowledge: Health behaviors; Knowledge: Treatment regimen

---

Discharge planning

DISCHARGE CHECKLIST
Before discharge, the patient shows evidence of:
❒ stable vital signs within normal limits
❒ blood glucose level within normal limits without I.V. insulin
❒ return to baseline LOC
❒ ABG levels within normal limits
❒ electrolyte levels within normal limits.

TEACHING CHECKLIST
Document evidence that the patient and his family demonstrate an understanding of:
❒ cause and significance of HHNS
❒ methods to decrease risk, if appropriate.
  If the patient has DM, also document understanding of the following items:
❒ oral hypoglycemic agents and insulin, if appropriate
❒ hyperglycemia and hypoglycemia (signs and symptoms, possible causes, treatment, and prevention)
❒ "sick day" management plan
❒ dietary plan
❒ exercise and activity plan
❒ blood glucose testing
❒ learning needs at time of discharge
❒ community resources.

DOCUMENTATION CHECKLIST
Using outcome criteria as a guide, document:
❒ clinical status on admission
❒ significant changes in status
❒ pertinent laboratory and diagnostic test findings
❒ I.V. fluid therapy
❒ pharmacologic intervention
❒ patient and family teaching
❒ discharge planning.

Associated care plans

■ Acute renal failure
■ Diabetic ketoacidosis
■ Disseminated intravascular coagulation
■ Hypovolemic shock
■ Knowledge deficit

References

American Diabetes Association. "Hyperglycemic Crises in Patients with *Diabetes Mellitus*," *Diabetes Care 25* (Suppl 1): S100-108, January 2002.

Fain, J.A. "Lowering the Boom on Hyperglycemia," *Nursing31* (8):48-50, August 2001.

Guthrie, D.W., and Guthrie R. *Nursing Management of Diabetes Mellitus: A Guide to Pattern Approach*, 5th ed. New York: Springer Publishing Co., 2002.

McLeod, M.E. "Interventions for Clients with Diabetes Mellitus," in *Medical-Surgical Nursing: Critical Thinking for Collaborative Care*, 4th ed. Edited by Ignatavicius, D.D., and Workman, M.L. Philadelphia: W.B. Saunders Co., 2002.

Quinn, L. "Diabetes Emergencies in the Patient with Type 2 Diabetes," *Nursing Clinics of North America* 36(2):341-60, June 2001.

Umipierrez, G.E., et al. "Diabetic Ketoacidosis and Hyperglycemic Hyperosmolar Syndrome," *Diabetes Spectrum* 15(1):28-36, January 2002.

Hypoglycemia

DRG INFORMATION
DRG 296   Nutritional and Miscellaneous Metabolic Disorders with Complication or Comorbidity (CC); Age 17+.
Mean LOS = 5.2 days
DRG 297   Nutritional and Miscellaneous Metabolic Disorders without CC; Ages 0 to 17.
Mean LOS = 3.4 days
DRG 298   Nutritional and Miscellaneous Metabolic Disorders; Ages 0 to 17.
Mean LOS = 2.9 days

Introduction

DEFINITION AND TIME FOCUS
Diabetes mellitus (DM) is a chronic metabolic condition involving an absolute (as in type 1 DM) or relative (as in type 2 DM) lack of endogenous insulin. A delicate balance of diet, medicine (insulin or oral hypoglycemics), and exercise is needed to achieve glucose homeostasis. However, alterations in glucose metabolism can provoke acute complications. This care plan focuses on one of the most common acute complications of DM: hypoglycemia. Also called low blood sugar, insulin reaction, and insulin shock, it usually occurs when the serum glucose level falls below 50 mg/dl (normal is 80 to 120 mg/dl). Symptoms can also occur in many patients with DM when the blood glucose levels are above 50 mg/dl, or when a high blood glucose level is lowered rapidly to 180 mg/dl.

Hypoglycemia can be life-threatening if left untreated. Usually, it's an acute complication of type 1 DM, with a prevalence ranging from 4% to 26%, and is seen more commonly with attempts to establish normoglycemia to diminish chronic complications of DM. It also can occur in type 2 DM with the use of oral agents that stimulate the release of endogenous insulin.

Many patients with long-standing type 1 DM (and some type 2 DM) don't experience the warning symptoms of hypoglycemia, a problem called hypoglycemia unawareness. The blood glucose may fall as low as 40 mg/dl while the person feels normal. (See *Clinical snapshot: Hypoglycemia,* page 652.)

ETIOLOGY AND PRECIPITATING FACTORS
- Excessive or unplanned exercise
- Delayed or missed meal
- Tight serum glucose control
- Inappropriate insulin regimen
- Too much insulin or oral hypoglycemic medicine
- Renal failure
- Alcohol use
- Underlying renal disease (nephropathy)
- Pancreatic tumor (rare)

Focused assessment guidelines

NURSING HISTORY (FUNCTIONAL HEALTH PATTERN FINDINGS)

Health-perception–health-management pattern
- History of diabetes
- Use of oral hypoglycemics or insulin

Nutritional-metabolic pattern
- Feeling of hunger
- Nausea

Elimination pattern
- Increased perspiration

Activity-exercise pattern
- Weakness, lethargy
- Feeling of faintness or dizziness

Sleep-rest pattern
- Bizarre dreams or nightmares
- Restless sleep
- Difficulty waking in the morning

Cognitive-perceptual pattern
- Headache or lack of concentration
- Blurred vision

PHYSICAL FINDINGS

Cardiovascular
- Tachycardia
- Palpitations
- Syncope

Integumentary
- Pallor
- Flushing
- Sweating (diaphoresis)

Neurologic
- Irritability and mood swings
- Confusion or uncontrollable behavior
- Seizures
- Decreased level of consciousness (LOC) or coma

Musculoskeletal
- Weakness

DIAGNOSTIC STUDIES
- Random serum glucose level — less than 50 mg/dl

POTENTIAL COMPLICATIONS

- Chronic complications of DM (retinopathy, neuropathy, nephropathy, cardiovascular disease, or peripheral vascular disease)

- Rebound hyperglycemia (if hypoglycemia overtreated)
- Coma, brain damage, or death, if untreated

CLINICAL SNAPSHOT ☀

Hypoglycemia

Major nursing diagnoses	Key patient outcomes
Risk for injury	Have a serum blood glucose level above 80 mg/dl.
Deficient knowledge (self-care)	On request, state the signs and symptoms, possible causes, treatment, and preventive strategies related to hypoglycemia.

Nursing diagnosis

Risk for injury related to inappropriate exogenous insulin use, lack of food, or excessive exercise

NURSING PRIORITY

Restore serum glucose level to normal.

PATIENT OUTCOME CRITERIA

Within 15 minutes of the onset of treatment, the patient will:
- have a serum glucose level above 80 mg/dl
- be alert, oriented, and able to communicate.

INTERVENTIONS	RATIONALES
1. *Observe for signs and symptoms of hypoglycemia constantly:* * – autonomic signs and symptoms (anxiety, tremor, nervousness, and flushing, numbness, weakness, hunger, nausea, pallor, irritability, sweating, and palpitations) – neuroglycopenic signs and symptoms (moderate: headache, mental dullness, confusion, and fatigue; or severe: glazed stare, bizarre dreams, difficulty waking, nightmares, coma, and seizures). Document findings.	**1.** With hypoglycemia, autonomic signs and symptoms occur first because low blood glucose triggers the sympathetic nervous system to stimulate the release of counter-regulatory hormones: epinephrine, cortisol, and glucagon. These hormones increase glucose production from the liver, raising the blood glucose level. In mild hypoglycemia, these may be the only signs and symptoms that occur. If hypoglycemia remains untreated, neuroglycopenic symptoms emerge because of starvation of cerebral neurons, which are only able to use glucose for energy. Symptoms may be moderate or severe. In long-standing type 1 DM, especially with intensive insulin therapy, many patients have "hypoglycemia unawareness," which causes them to experience none of the usual symptoms of hypoglycemia until they suddenly lose consciousness. This is a dangerous and life-threatening situation.
2. *Document suspected hypoglycemia with bedside glucose fingerstick or serum glucose,* following facility protocol.	**2.** If the fingerstick glucose is less than 50 mg/dl, most facilities obtain a serum glucose level if the fingerstick glucose is less than 50 mg/dl before treatment. A patient may complain of symptoms of hypoglycemia when the glucose level is normal or elevated. Symptoms may occur with a normal glucose level if the glucose level is quickly lowered or if the patient has had a high glucose level recently brought under control.

---

*Italics indicate key interventions.

3. *Treat hypoglycemia promptly:*
– If the patient is alert and the glucose level is less than 60 mg/dl (or below normal level specified by your facility), give a simple carbohydrate, such as glucose gel, by mouth. For mild symptoms, give 10 to 20 g; for moderate symptoms, 20 to 30 g. Follow with a complex carbohydrate and protein snack, such as one-half glass of milk with two graham crackers or four soda crackers (unless a meal will be eaten within 1 hour).

– If the patient is alert and the glucose level is greater than 80 mg/dl, don't treat. Check on the patient and reassure him frequently.

– If the patient is unconscious with a glucose level less than 60 mg/dl, ensure airway patency, check pulse rate, and administer 50% dextrose (25 g by I.V. push) or glucagon (1 mg I.M. or subcutaneously), according to protocol.

4. *Recheck the glucose level 10 to 15 minutes after treatment.* Repeat treatment if glucose level remains low. If the patient was unconscious, give a protein and carbohydrate snack when fully awake.

5. *If hypoglycemia occurs frequently, consult the physician.*

6. Additional individualized interventions: _____

_____

3. Prompt treatment reduces the risk of injury.
– Glucose gel or liquids containing simple sugars provide a measured amount of simple, rapidly acting glucose. Using fruit juice is no longer recommended because it provides a variable amount of fructose, a concentrated form of glucose that's absorbed very rapidly and may cause rebound hyperglycemia. However, 4 to 6 oz (118 to 177 ml) of orange juice can be used if glucose gel isn't available. Other concentrated forms of glucose, such as sugared soda or candy, also cause an unreliable rise in blood glucose and may cause rebound hyperglycemia. Carbohydrates and protein cause a gradual rise in the glucose level to prevent recurrence of hypoglycemia.
– This is a normal glucose level. The goal of diabetes management is to keep the glucose level as near to normal as possible to prevent, reverse, or delay DM-related complications.
– The patient with DM may also have cardiac disease, so it's important to recognize that unconsciousness may not be related to hypoglycemia. The patient's airway and pulse should be assessed immediately to detect emergency cardiac conditions. The unconscious hypoglycemic patient usually suffers from severe hypoglycemia. Because of the effect of glucose deprivation on cerebral neurons, immediate measures must be taken to reverse the hypoglycemic state. I.V. dextrose supplies glucose most rapidly. Glucagon administration stimulates glycogenolysis, the release of glucose from liver glycogen stores. Never give an unconscious patient liquids by mouth because of the risk of aspiration.

4. Blood glucose may drop again rapidly. Rechecking may indicate the need for further treatment. Carbohydrates and protein will cause a sustained rise in blood glucose.

5. The patient's medication, diet, and activity regimens may need adjustment.

6. Rationales: _____

_____

Suggested NIC Interventions
Fall prevention; Surveillance: Safety

Suggested NOC Outcomes
Safety status: Physical injury

Nursing diagnosis
Deficient knowledge (self-care) related to complexity of disease and therapeutic regimen

NURSING PRIORITY
Teach the patient and his family how to avoid and appropriately manage hypoglycemia.

PATIENT OUTCOME CRITERIA

By the time of discharge, the patient and his family will be able to:
- recognize the risk of hypoglycemia
- state signs and symptoms, possible causes, treatment, and preventive strategies related to hypoglycemia.

INTERVENTIONS	RATIONALES
1. *Use the hypoglycemic episode as a learning experience. Involve family members in all teaching sessions.* Help them to identify the causes of hypoglycemia, if possible.	1. The patient needs to realize that occasional episodes of hypoglycemia can and will happen. By being prepared, the patient and his family will be able to alleviate symptoms quickly. Common causes of hypoglycemia usually involve too much insulin or oral hypoglycemic, missed or delayed meals and snacks, or excessive exercise. In the hospital, the patient who can take nothing by mouth because of tests, procedures, surgery, or nausea and vomiting is also at risk for hypoglycemia. Identifying causes may help the patient avoid future episodes.
2. *Review the signs and symptoms of hypoglycemia.* If possible, have the patient identify personal signs and symptoms. Stress the importance of early recognition and treatment.	2. Each patient responds individually to hypoglycemia. Symptoms may be mild to severe. Some patients have no symptoms. Early identification of symptoms promotes prompt treatment and possibly a less severe hypoglycemic episode. Repeated severe episodes can lead to memory loss and learning impairment.
3. *Discuss appropriate treatment strategies for hypoglycemia:* – If symptoms are mild and the blood glucose level is less than 60 mg/dl, eat a carbohydrate and protein snack. – If symptoms are severe, eat a simple sugar. – If the patient is unconscious, a family member should administer glucagon and call for emergency medical assistance.	3. A protein and carbohydrate snack causes a gradual rise in the glucose level. Because the goal of management is a normal glucose level, rebound hyperglycemia can occur if the patient eats too much food or uses simple sugars. If the episode occurs close to a meal, the patient may elect to eat a little earlier as treatment. Family members may need one-on-one teaching before administering glucagon.
4. *Review strategies to prevent hypoglycemia.* Encourage the patient to: – wear a medical identification bracelet and carry a medical identification card – have a source of food available at all times at home, in the car, at work, and any other place the patient frequents – monitor glucose level regularly and record results – work closely with the physician and health care team if a pattern of hypoglycemia develops.	4. Carrying and wearing medical identification will alert others to the potential for hypoglycemia if the patient can't speak. Having food available ensures quick treatment of hypoglycemia. Regularly monitoring glucose level and recording the results helps identify patterns of hypoglycemia. These records should be reviewed at each outpatient visit. Correct insulin administration is essential for optimal effectiveness.
5. Additional individualized interventions: _____	5. Rationales: _____

> **Suggested NIC Interventions**
> *Teaching: Disease process; Teaching: Individual; Teaching: Prescribed medicine*

> **Suggested NOC Outcomes**
> *Knowledge: Disease process; Knowledge: Health behaviors; Knowledge: Treatment regimen*

Discharge planning

DISCHARGE CHECKLIST

Before discharge, the patient shows evidence of:
❏ stable vital signs within normal limits
❏ blood glucose level within normal limits without I.V. glucose
❏ return to usual LOC.

TEACHING CHECKLIST

Document evidence that the patient and his family demonstrate an understanding of:
❏ cause and significance of hypoglycemia
❏ signs and symptoms
❏ preventive measures
❏ treatment strategies
❏ proper use of insulin or oral agents
❏ dietary management
❏ exercise and activity plan
❏ blood glucose monitoring
❏ chronic complications related to DM
❏ learning needs at time of discharge
❏ community resources.

DOCUMENTATION CHECKLIST

Using outcome criteria as a guide, document:
❏ clinical status on admission
❏ significant changes in status
❏ pertinent laboratory and diagnostic test findings
❏ I.V. fluid therapy
❏ pharmacologic intervention
❏ patient and family teaching
❏ discharge planning.

Associated care plans

- Diabetic ketoacidosis
- Hyperosmolar hyperglycemic nonketotic syndrome
- Hypovolemic shock
- Knowledge deficit

References

Bloomgarden, J.T. "Treatment Issues in Type 1 Diabetes," *Diabetes Care* 25(1):230-236, January 2002.

Guthrie, D.W., and Guthrie, R. *Nursing Management of Diabetes Mellitus: A guide to Pattern Approach,* 5th ed. New York: Springer Publishing Co., 2002.

McLeod, M.E. "Interventions for Clients with Diabetes Mellitus," in *Medical-Surgical Nursing: Critical Thinking for Collaborative Care,* 4th ed. Edited by Ignatavicius D.D., and Workman M.L. Philadelphia: W.B. Saunders Co., 2002.

Tkacs, N.C. "Hypoglycemia Unawareness," *AJN* 102(2):34-41, February 2002.

Obesity

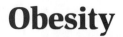

DRG INFORMATION

DRG 292 Other Endocrine, Nutritional, and Metabolic Disorders or Procedures with Complication or Comorbidity (CC).
Mean LOS = 10.2

DRG 293 Other Endocrine, Nutritional, and Metabolic Disorders or Procedures without CC.
Mean LOS = 5.3

DRG 296 Nutritional and Miscellaneous Metabolic Disorders with CC; Age 17+.
Mean LOS = 5.2

DRG 297 Nutritional and Miscellaneous Metabolic Disorders without CC; Age 17+.
Mean LOS = 3.4

DRG 298 Nutritional and Miscellaneous Metabolic Disorders; Age 0 to 17.
Mean LOS = 2.9

DRG 299 Inborn Errors of Metabolism.
Mean LOS = 5.3

DRG 300 Endocrine Disorders with CC.
Mean LOS = 6.1

DRG 301 Endocrine Disorders without CC.
Mean LOS = 3.6

DRG 170 Other Digestive System Disorders or Procedures with CC.
Mean LOS = 11.2

DRG 171 Other Digestive System Disorders or Procedures without CC.
Mean LOS = 4.6

Introduction

DEFINITION AND TIME FOCUS

Obesity is defined as a chronic disease manifested by an excess of body fat. Associated with serious medical complications, impaired quality of life, and premature mortality, obesity has become an epidemic in the United States. As of 2002, the *Annals of Internal Medicine* indicated that 100 million Americans are overweight or obese. In fact, the *British Medical Journal* (in that same year) reported that more than 300,000 people die annually from obesity in the United States.

Obesity can be diagnosed using the body mass index (BMI) formula — the most widely accepted classification of weight status. To calculate BMI, you divide body weight in kilograms by height in meters squared. A BMI over 25 is categorized as overweight; 30 to 34.9, Class I obesity; 35 to 39.9, Class II obesity; and over 40, Class III obesity. Because morbidity and mortality increase proportionately to BMI, this measurement is used to estimate health risk. Body shape or distribution of adipose tissue also correlates with risk. For example, an individual with an "apple" shape is at higher risk for hypertension, coronary artery disease, stroke, or diabetes; whereas, an individual with a "pear" shape is at increased risk for hernia, osteoarthritis, and venous stasis disease.

The obese individual is also at risk for additional health problems such as those secondary to physiologic factors, including cardiovascular system changes; increased intra-abdominal pressure; hypertension; respiratory compromise; endocrine system changes; degenerative joint disease; and poor wound healing. Those who suffer from obesity may be more vulnerable to psychosocial complications because of prejudice and discrimination, impaired mobility, and alterations in quality of life due to diminished social interactions.

Obesity complicates the care and prolongs the length of stay in a significant proportion of hospitalized patients. This care plan focuses on care needs specific to the obese patient admitted to the hospital with either a medical or surgical condition. (See *Clinical snapshot: Obesity*, page 658.)

ETIOLOGY AND PRECIPITATING FACTORS

■ Environmental factors including nutrition, physical inactivity, trauma (physical, psychological), use of medications, socioeconomic factors, and level of education

■ Physiological factors including the number and size of an individual's fat cells, regulatory systems affecting satiety, fat storing enzymes, and taste for fat

Focused assessment guidelines

NURSING HISTORY
(FUNCTIONAL HEALTH PATTERN FINDINGS)

Health-perception–health-management pattern

■ Various presenting problems, depending on the comorbid conditions

■ Restricted mobility, limited transportation options, and embarrassment contribute to a resistance in seeking health care and participating in health maintenance activities (Commonly, the obese patient will defer seeking health care until the need is urgent.)

■ Commonly perceive general health as poor

Nutritional-metabolic pattern

■ BMI over 25

■ Percentage of body fat greater than 20% for females; 19% for males

- Food intake — energy expenditure imbalance
- Binge eating behaviors common, concentrates food intake at end of day
- Pairs food with other activities
- Dieting history, common use of over-the-counter aides, fad diets
- "Yo-yo" weight loss and gain pattern common; recurrent weight loss with regain
- Eats in response to external and or internal cues

Elimination pattern
- Heartburn (common)
- Constipation
- Diarrhea
- Incontinence with coughing, sneezing, or any activity increasing intra-abdominal pressure
- Urinary urgency and frequency
- Odor problems due to excessive perspiration and fungal rash

Activity-exercise pattern
- Inability or lack of desire to be active or engage in regular exercise
- Fatigue common, doesn't have sufficient energy for desired or required activities
- Decreased muscle strength and endurance
- Dyspnea on exertion
- Respirations shallow and rapid
- Dizziness during activity
- May require assistance with bathing, hygiene, dressing, or toileting due to decreased mobility

Sleep-rest pattern
- Daytime somnolence
- Awakens with headache
- Frequent nighttime awakenings
- Snoring
- Observed apneic episodes during sleep

Cognitive-perceptual pattern
- Inadequate knowledge regarding nutrition and exercise (less common)

Self-perception–self-concept pattern
- Lack of self confidence
- Low self esteem (common)
- Negative body image (common)
- Verbalizes fear of rejection by others
- Depression (common)

Role-relationship pattern
- Social isolation

Sexuality-reproductive pattern
- Infertility (common)
- Menstrual irregularities; amenorrhea

Coping–stress tolerance pattern
- Coping mechanisms (commonly ineffective)
- Emotional eating (common)

PHYSICAL FINDINGS
Examination will be limited based on body characteristics; body size may render standard assessment methods ineffective.

Vital signs and anthropometrics
- A false high blood pressure reading will be obtained if the cuff is too small. The width of the bladder should be 40% to 50% of the arm circumference and the length 80%.
- Height and weight should be measured precisely. Special equipment may be necessary.
- Observe body shape and distribution of body fat.

Integumentary
- Chronic dermatitis especially under breasts, abdominal folds, back skin folds, and perineal area
- Fungal rash in skin folds
- Bilateral lower extremity edema or edema of the abdominal wall — may be brawny, non pitting, or indurated
- Hirsutism or excess body hair in females in a male pattern (upper lip, face, chest, abdomen, arms, and legs)
- Acanthosis nigrans — dark, hypertrophic velvety skin areas on lateral aspect of neck and axilla; may signal endocrine disorder or insulin resistance (less common)
- Acne
- Striae
- Skin tags
- Pressure ulcer

Endocrine
- Moon facies — plethoric, rounded with prominent jowls and red cheeks; associated with hirsutism
- Thyromegaly (less common)

Cardiovascular
- Heart tones distant — heart tones best heard over the left lateral chest wall with the patient turned to the left side, or over the aortic or pulmonic areas to the left or right of the sternal border at the second intercostal space
- Lower extremities: swelling may be present; skin changes consistent with venous stasis — dusky rubor when extremity dependent, brownish discoloration secondary to hemosiderin deposits; ulcers present at the medial malleolus
- Varicose veins
- Clubbing of distal phalanx (less common)

Pulmonary
- Respirations rapid and shallow
- Breath sounds distant — displace all skin folds over the areas and place diaphragm of stethoscope firmly over the exposed area; may best be heard over dependent areas where lung tissue is closest to chest wall and fluid is likely to accumulate
- Gynecomastia
- "Buffalo hump" (rare)

Abdomen
- On inspection will be uniformly round; umbilicus may be sunken; bowel sounds are normal, but may take longer to distinguish; on percussion — tympany with scattered dullness over adipose tissue
- Purple striae on abdominal wall
- Hernias

Neurologic
■ Meralgia paresthetica — numbness and tingling over the anterior thigh
■ Sciatica

Musculoskeletal
■ Limited motion
■ Pain with motion
■ Gait changes

DIAGNOSTIC STUDIES
■ Bioimpedance analysis — estimates percentage of body fat: lean mass

Laboratory data
A combination of biochemical values should be obtained to assess nutritional status, the underlying etiology for the obesity, and common metabolic abnormalities.
■ Markers for nutritional status
– Albumin
   Normal values: 3.5 to 5.0 g/dl
   Low value may reflect protein malnutrition
– Transferrin
   Normal values: 202 to 336 mg/dl
   Low value may reflect protein malnutrition
– Metabolic abnormalities
– Glucose
   Normal values: 70 to 110 mg/dl
   Elevation may reflect diabetes mellitus
– Total cholesterol, triglycerides, high-density lipoprotein (HDL)
   Normal values:
   Cholesterol — < 200 mg/dl
   Triglycerides — < 200 mg/dl

Elevation may reflect hyperlipidemias
   HDL — 45 to 85 mg/dl
■ Etiologic factors
– Thyroid-stimulating hormone
   Normal values: 0.49 to 4.67 μIU/ml
   Elevation may reflect hypothyroidism

POTENTIAL COMPLICATIONS
■ Osteoarthritis of the weight bearing joints
■ Hypertension
■ Gastroesophageal reflux disease
■ Urinary stress incontinence
■ Pancreatic insufficiency
■ Gallbladder disease
■ Depression
■ Dyslipidemia
■ Hypertriglyceridemia
■ Low HDL cholesterol
■ Hypercholesterolemia
■ Diabetes mellitus
■ Hyperinsulinemia and insulin resistance
■ Asthma
■ Sleep apnea
■ Heart failure
■ Cancer — uterine, breast, or colon
■ Stroke
■ Hypoventilation syndrome
■ Myocardial infarction
■ Nonalcoholic steatohepatitis with or without cirrhosis
■ Respiratory failure
■ Thrombophlebitis; deep venous thrombosis

CLINICAL SNAPSHOT ✳

Obesity

Major nursing diagnoses	Key patient outcomes
Impaired gas exchange	Maintain a clear airway.
Imbalanced nutrition: More than body requirements	Maintain consistent weight loss.
Risk for impaired skin integrity	Improved or maintained skin integrity.
Impaired physical mobility	Maintain functional alignment.
Activity intolerance	Progress to the highest level of activity possible.
Social isolation	Identify new behaviors to promote effective socialization.
Disturbed body image	Verbalize a more realistic self-image.

Nursing diagnosis

Impaired gas exchange related to ventilation-perfusion imbalance

NURSING PRIORITY
Improve gas exchange and oxygenation.

PATIENT OUTCOME CRITERIA
Throughout the hospital stay the patient will exhibit:
- partial pressure of arterial oxygen (Pao_2) $\geq$ 90% or baseline
- absence of cyanosis, restlessness, confusion, irritability, and dizziness
- a clear airway.

INTERVENTIONS	RATIONALES
1. *Assess respiratory function.* ∗ – Assess respiratory rate, depth, and use of accessory muscles, vital signs, and cardiac rhythm. – Assess color of skin and mucous membranes. – Auscultate breath sounds. – Monitor for mental status changes. – Evaluate level of activity tolerance.	1. Baseline and ongoing assessment provides for early recognition of problems with oxygenation and airway clearance. Change in vital signs and mental function, such as altered LOC and anxiety, may indicate hypoxia and are key guides to determining the seriousness of the problem. Activity levels are monitored; lack of rest and excessive activity will increase oxygen needs.
2. *Eliminate, or reduce causative factors affecting respiratory function*: – Assess patient for presence and level of pain. – Assess patient's level of consciousness (LOC). – Investigate the patient's medication history and present regime.	2. Pain may limit maximal thoracic expansion. Relief of pain will improve respiratory function by maximizing thoracic expansion. Altered LOC may precede respiratory collapse. Medications, such as narcotics, anxiolytics, and sedatives, may depress respirations.
3. *Monitor pulse oximetry and arterial blood gas levels.*	3. Pao_2 reflects oxygen levels in the blood. An oxygen saturation less than 90% will compromise oxygen transport.
4. *Provide supplemental humidification.*	4. Humidification prevents drying of the mucous membranes and reduces viscosity of secretions.
5. *Administer oxygen as prescribed.*	5. Oxygen may need to be administered to improve gas exchange.
6. *Assist with respiratory treatments:* incentive spirometry, turn, cough and deep-breathing exercises, or continuous positive airway pressure (CPAP).	6. CPAP causes alveolar hyperinflation, increasing the surface area available for gas exchange. Obesity affects ventilation by limiting chest wall expansion. Alveolar ventilation is promoted by change in position, incentive spirometry, and turning, coughing and deep-breathing exercises. Deep-breathing exercises also help to reinflate collapsed alveoli.
7. *Tracheal suctioning as needed.*	7. Suctioning removes secretions from the main airways.
8. Additional individualized interventions: _____	8. Rationales: _____

∗Italics indicate key interventions.

> **Suggested NIC Interventions**
> Acid-base management; Electrolyte management; Laboratory data interpretation; Oxygen therapy; Ventilation assistance; Airway management; Respiratory monitoring; Embolus care: Pulmonary; Hemodynamic regulation; Vital signs monitoring

> **Suggested NOC Outcomes**
> Electrolyte and acid-base balance; Respiratory status: Gas exchange; Respiratory status: Ventilation; Tissue perfusion: Pulmonary; Vital signs status

Nursing diagnosis

Imbalanced nutrition: More than body requirements related to food intake, energy expenditure imbalance, dysfunctional eating patterns, sedentary activity level, or inherited disposition

NURSING PRIORITIES

- Assist the patient to identify desirable method of weight control.
- Promote optimal nutrition intake and lifestyle changes for lifelong weight control.

PATIENT OUTCOME CRITERIA

By the time of discharge, the patient will:

- express the need to maintain or stabilize weight within 5 to 10 lb (2 to 4.5 kg) of goal weight
- develop a plan to reduce body weight by 10% at a rate of 1 to 2 lb (0.5 to 1 kg) per week
- plan to monitor weight and sustain target weight
- identify internal and external cues that lead to increased food consumption.

INTERVENTIONS	RATIONALES
1. *Weigh patient weekly or as prescribed.*	**1.** Weighing the patient weekly or as prescribed will monitor the effectiveness of the weight reduction program.
2. *Work with the patient to establish realistic goals.* Instruct the patient on how to record his weight.	**2.** Working with the patient to set realistic goals helps to make the goals more attainable and helps the patient comply with the program. Involving the patient in his plan of care improves compliance.
3. *Instruct the patient to keep a food diary.*	**3.** Keeping a food diary helps the patient confront his actual intake, break through denial, and achieve a more objective view of his eating habits.
4. *Monitor fluid intake and output.*	**4.** Fluid retention may increase body weight.
5. *Encourage the patient to express his feelings about his dietary restrictions.* Help him to identify emotions associated with food and situations that trigger eating episodes.	**5.** Helping the patient to express his feelings helps him assess his perception of the problem. Permanent weight maintenance requires an understanding of risk factors that contribute to weight gain.
6. *Have the patient meet with a dietitian to discuss meal planning.* Encourage consumption of foods that are low in calories and fat and high in complex carbohydrates and fiber.	**6.** Education and counseling will help the patient plan nutritious, well-balanced meals.
7. *Refer the patient to appropriate resources for behavior modification and cognitive therapy.*	**7.** Behavior modification and cognitive therapy help to prevent the patient from relapsing into high-risk eating behaviors.
8. *Give the patient emotional support and positive feedback* when he adheres to the prescribed diet.	**8.** Support and positive feedback foster compliance and help ensure adherence to the program.

9. *Discuss the importance of incorporating exercise into his lifestyle.* Help the patient select an exercise program with a variety of activities (such as swimming, walking, aerobics, and biking) appropriate for his age and physical ability.

10. Additional individualized interventions:_____
_____

9. Exercise burns calories, offers an alternative to eating to alleviate stress, and builds a sense of accomplishment.

10. Rationales:_____
_____

Suggested NIC Interventions
Diet staging; Nutrition management; Fluid monitoring; Nutritional monitoring

Suggested NOC Outcomes
Nutritional status; Nutritional status: Food and fluid intake; Nutritional status: Nutrient intake; Weight control

Nursing diagnosis
Risk for impaired skin integrity related to nutritional deficit and altered circulation (edema) and decreased mobility

NURSING PRIORITIES
- Promote optimal skin care.
- Prevent break in skin integrity.

PATIENT OUTCOME CRITERIA
Within 24 hours of admission the patient will:
- display maintained or improved skin integrity
- show no signs of infection.

INTERVENTIONS

1. *Assess skin daily for color, turgor, circulation, sensation, and moistness or dryness.* Observe for erythema, blanching, and edema. Palpate for warmth or tissue sponginess. Monitor for rashes or abrasions. Using a formal scale to assess the risk for impaired skin integrity will facilitate a thorough skin assessment.

2. *Consult the dietitian for evaluation and maintenance of nutrition status.*
– Maintain hydration; 2500 ml per day unless contraindicated.

3. *Maintain and instruct in skin hygiene measures;* wash the patient thoroughly with soap that doesn't alter pH, pat dry, and gently massage with lotion or appropriate cream.
– Use drying powders in deep skin folds.
– Clean the perineal area of stool and urine with water and mineral oil or a commercial product.
– Apply protective creams, such as A&D or zinc oxide.

RATIONALES

1. Skin assessment provides baseline for comparison and permits identification of patients at risk for skin disturbance so that the appropriate preventive interventions can be instituted. Frequency of reevaluation of the skin will depend on the patient's level of risk and mobility. Several scales to help assess risk of have been researched. The Norton and the Braden scales have been studied most extensively.

2. Maintaining nutrition and hydration of skin will help promote skin integrity.

3. Clean, dry, intact skin is a barrier to infection. Patting dry decreases dermal damage. Massage improves circulation and prevents maceration. Maceration causes tissues to become waterlogged, weakens cells, and the epidermis is easily damaged as a result. Maceration will decrease the tensile strength of a tissue.

4. *Turn and reposition or shift weight every 30 minutes to 2 hours depending on skin condition.* Small shifts in body weight should be encouraged. Relieve vulnerable areas more often. Increase frequency of repositioning if reddened areas appear and don't disappear in 2 hours.
– Protect bony prominences; suspend the patient's heels off the bed surface.
– Maintain dry, clean, wrinkle free linen.
– Alternate pressure mattress or bed to relieve pressure; surface must not be fully compressed by the patient's body, must redistribute body weight across a surface.
– Keep bed as flat as possible. Provide a support surface, such as foam, gel, or alternating pressure surface.
– Provide support to edematous areas.
– Use the appropriate number of personal and assist devices when repositioning the patient to decrease the risk to the patient and personnel.
– Encourage ambulation.

5. Additional individualized interventions: _____
_____

4. Pressure reduction is the single most important initial intervention and is achieved by repositioning or by altering the physical properties of the support surface. The primary objective is to maintain capillary blood flow because pressure against tissue greater than intra-capillary pressure may occlude capillaries. Friction will alter the ability of a tissue to tolerate pressure. Shear or parallel forces occur as one layer of tissue moves in a direction opposite to another tissue layer; subepidermal capillaries may occlude. Both pressure and shear forces cause tissue damage as a result of hypoxia. Pressure relief will also allow occult tissue injury to heal, preventing repetitive insults, which may lead to perceptible skin damage and breakdown.

5. Rationales: _____
_____

Suggested NIC Interventions
Pressure management; Pressure ulcer care; Skin surveillance; Wound care

Suggested NOC Outcomes
Tissue integrity: Skin and mucous membranes; Wound healing: Primary intention; Wound healing: Secondary intention

---

Nursing diagnosis
Impaired physical mobility related to intolerance to activity and uncompensated musculoskeletal impairment

NURSING PRIORITY
Promote improved mobility in a safe environment.

PATIENT OUTCOME CRITERIA
Throughout the hospital stay, the patient will:
- maintain functional alignment
- perform as much self-care as possible.

INTERVENTIONS

1. *Implement measures described in the "Impaired physical mobility" care plan,* page 111.

2. Additional individualized interventions: _____
_____

RATIONALES

1. The "Impaired physical mobility" care plan contains multiple interventions to address the patient's physical mobility.

2. Rationales: _____
_____

Suggested NIC Interventions
Exercise therapy: Ambulation; Exercise therapy: Balance; Exercise therapy: Joint mobility; Exercise therapy: Muscle control; Exercise promotion: Strength training

Suggested NOC Outcomes
Ambulation: Walking; Ambulation: Wheelchair; Joint movement: Active; Mobility level

Nursing diagnosis

Activity intolerance related to deconditioned status and excessive energy demands secondary to obesity

NURSING PRIORITY

Promote participation in activities to achieve a desired or required level of tolerance.

PATIENT OUTCOME CRITERIA

Throughout the hospital stay the patient will:
- identify factors that reduce activity tolerance
- progress to the highest level of activity possible
- exhibit an improved physiologic response to activity as evidenced by a decrease in pulse, blood pressure, and respirations
- report reduced symptoms of activity intolerance.

INTERVENTIONS

1. *Assess response to activity.* Note resting heart rate, blood pressure, and respirations. Repeat assessment at the end of activity and after 3 minutes of rest.

2. *Increase activity gradually.*
– Mutually set goals for activity schedule.
– Identify and obtain resources: collaborate with physical therapy, occupational therapy, and exercise physiologist.
– Allow for rest periods.
– Allow patient to set pace.
– Perform activity slowly with frequent rest periods.
– Increase tolerance by increasing time out of bed by 15 minutes a day, three times per day.

3. *Promote energy conservation.*
– Schedule rest periods during activity and at intervals throughout the day.
– Rest 3 minutes for every 5 minutes of activity.
– Stop for perceived increase in heart rate, dyspnea, or chest pain.

4. Additional individualized interventions:_____

RATIONALES

1. Resting heart rate is normally 60 to 90 beats/minute, blood pressure less than 140/90 mm Hg, respirations less than 20 breaths/minute. Immediately after activity, the heart rate, blood pressure, and respirations should increase. A decrease in these parameters is abnormal. Within 3 minutes of activity ending, the heart rate should be within 6 beats of the resting pulse. Response to an activity can be evaluated by comparing preactivity vital signs with postactivity and recovery parameters.

2. Activity should be planned based on the patient's knowledge of activity demands, values, beliefs, and perceived ability. Tolerance develops by adjusting frequency, duration, and intensity until the desired activity level is achieved. Frequency is increased first followed by duration and intensity.

3. Interventions should be directed at delaying the onset of fatigue and optimizing muscle efficiency. Work simplification delays the onset of fatigue. Symptoms of activity intolerance are alleviated with rest.

4. Rationales: _____

Suggested NIC Interventions
Activity therapy; Energy management; Exercise promotion: Strength training; Nutrition management; Self-care assistance; Home maintenance assistance

Suggested NOC Outcomes
Activity intolerance; Endurance; Energy conservation; Self-care: Activities of daily living (ADL); Self-care: Instrumental activities of daily living (IADL)

Nursing diagnosis

Social isolation related to impaired mobility and body image disturbance

NURSING PRIORITY
Promote effective social interaction.

PATIENT OUTCOME CRITERIA
Throughout the hospital stay the patient will:
- verbalize problems with socialization
- identify new behaviors to promote effective socialization.

INTERVENTIONS

1. *Provide an individual, supportive relationship.*
– Help the patient increase awareness of his strengths and limits in communicating with others and identify family patterns for social behaviors.
– Encourage the patient to express feelings and perceptions about the problem.
– Confront the patient about impaired judgment when appropriate. Request and expect verbal communication. Provide positive feedback when patient reaches out to others.
– Assess the patient's coping strategies and defense mechanisms.
– Support healthy defenses. Encourage involvement in already established relationships.

2. *Provide the opportunity for the development of social skills.*
– Identify with the patient environments in which social interaction is impaired.
– Collaborate with speech, occupational and physical therapy personnel to develop an individualized social skill program (grooming, posture and gait training, and conversational skills)
– Help to identify alternative courses of action and appropriate support. Use a wide variety of agencies and services.

3. Additional individualized interventions: _____
_____

RATIONALES

1. Social interaction is learned within the family. Interpersonal relationships are important to assist a person through both positive and negative life experiences. Identifying inadequate patterns of communication help to heighten awareness of the underlying cause of ineffective interactions with others. Effective social interactions depend on positive self-esteem. Satisfactory interaction is also dependent on acknowledging and accepting limitations. Social competence relies on the ability to problem-solve as well as the use of a variety of coping mechanisms.

2. To interact effectively one must have social competence. Positive self-concept, social skills, and social sensitivity contribute to the development of positive relationships with others. Ineffective interactions with others if extreme or prolonged contribute to social isolation. An individual who is socially competent will interact effectively with people in his environment. Group activities will encourage the sharing of common problems and solutions with others.

3. Rationales: _____
_____

Suggested NIC Interventions	Suggested NOC Outcomes
Socialization enhancement	*Social interaction skills; Social involvement; Social support*

Nursing diagnosis

Disturbed body image related to obesity

NURSING PRIORITY
Encourage positive body image.

PATIENT OUTCOME CRITERIA

Throughout the hospital stay the patient will:
- verbalize and demonstrate acceptance of appearance
- verbalize a more realistic self-image
- establish or strengthen support systems.

INTERVENTIONS	RATIONALES
1. *Determine patient's body image expectations* (view of being overweight).	1. Personal beliefs about the ideal body shape or size can sabotage efforts directed at weight loss.
2. Encourage expression of feelings about patient's view of self. *Assist the patient to separate physical appearance from feelings of personal worth. Monitor frequency of self-criticizing statements and those addressing body shape and weight.*	2. To facilitate actions for change, the nurse should determine the patient's feelings about himself.
3. *Identify the influence of culture, religion, race, sex, and age on body image.*	3. Self-concept is influenced by others and by our perceptions of how others view us. It's influenced by interactions with others and by societal and cultural mores.
4. *Determine if body image perception has contributed to social isolation.*	4. A disturbance in body image may contribute to feelings of isolation.
5. *Identify support groups to provide opportunity for sharing with others* facing similar experiences. Teach about available community resources for weight loss.	5. Support groups can provide companionship, enhance motivation for weight loss, and decrease loneliness. Sharing may provide solutions to common problems.
6. Refer the patient to a psychologist or psychotherapist.	6. Compulsive eating behaviors may have deep rooted psychological implications. Group or individual therapy can be helpful in addressing psychological concerns.
7. Work with staff to identify and deal with their own feelings when caring for an obese patient.	7. The nurse needs to be aware of her feelings and attitudes in order to deal more effectively with others. Judgmental attitudes, anger, and negative feelings will interfere with patient care and may reinforce patient's negative self-image.
8. Additional individualized interventions: _____	8. Rationales: _____

> **Suggested NIC Interventions**
> *Body image enhancement; Grief work facilitation; Anticipatory guidance; Coping enhancement; Self-esteem enhancement*

> **Suggested NOC Outcomes**
> *Body image; Grief resolution; Self-esteem*

Discharge planning

The inpatient setting isn't the ideal environment in which to focus on initiating and implementing a weight loss program. It's the time to gauge the patient's interest in such a program and initiate appropriate referrals. Treatment of obesity should be based on a multimodality approach including education on nutrition, exercise, behavior modification, and strategies for maintenance. Referrals to a dietitian, exercise physiologist, and psycholo-gist may be indicated. A variety of community and governmental resources are also available.

DISCHARGE CHECKLIST

Before discharge, the patient shows evidence of:
- ❏ improved gas exchange and oxygenation
- ❏ knowledge of desirable method of weight control
- ❏ optimal nutrition intake and lifestyle changes for life-long weight control
- ❏ maintained or improved skin integrity

❏ ability to identify internal and external cues that lead to increased food consumption
❏ being free from infection
❏ functional alignment
❏ ability to perform self-care
❏ progression in activity to the highest level possible
❏ improved physical response to activity
❏ improved socialization
❏ established or strengthened supports systems
❏ acceptance of appearance.

TEACHING CHECKLIST

Document evidence that the patient and his family demonstrate an understanding of:
❏ internal and external cues that lead to increased food consumption
❏ plan to monitor weight and regime to sustain weight loss
❏ optimal skin care
❏ hygiene measures
❏ measures to improve physical mobility
❏ factors that reduce activity intolerance
❏ taking pulse, blood pressure and respiration
❏ signs and symptoms of activity intolerance
❏ ways to improve socialization
❏ awareness of present and initiation of new coping skills.

DOCUMENTATION CHECKLIST

Using outcome criteria, document:
❏ clinical status on admission
❏ significant changes in status
❏ pertinent laboratory and diagnostic test findings
❏ I.V. therapy
❏ pharmacologic interventions
❏ patient and family teaching
❏ discharge planning.

Associated care plans

■ Impaired physical mobility
■ Ineffective individual coping
■ Knowledge deficit
■ Nutritional deficit

References

Braden, B.J., and Bergstrom, N. "Clinical Utility of the Braden Scale for Predicting Pressure Sore Risk," *Decubitus* 2(3):44-46, 50-51, August 1989.

Goldstone, L., and Goldstone, J. "The Norton score: An Early Warning of Pressure sores?" *Journal of Advanced Nursing* 7(5):419-26, September 1982.

Hahler, B. "Morbid Obesity: A Nursing Care Challenge," *Medsurg Nursing* 11(2):85-90, April 2002.

National Institutes of Health, National Heart, Lung, and Blood Institute, National Institute of Diabetes and Digestive and Kidney Diseases. *The Practice Guideline identification, Evaluation, and Treatment of Overweight and Obesity in Adults: The Evidence Report.* Bethesda, Md.: NIH Publication 98-4083, 1998.

National Institutes of Health, National Heart, Lung, and Blood Institute, and the North American Association for the Study of Obesity. *The Practice Guideline Identification, Evaluation, and Treatment of Overweight and Obesity in Adults.* Washington, D.C.: Department of Health and Human Services, Public Health Services, 2000

Renal disorders

## PART 10

Acute renal failure

DRG INFORMATION

DRG 316   Renal Failure.
           Mean LOS = 6.6 days
  Principal diagnoses include:
- chronic or unspecified renal failure
- acute renal failure (unspecified, with renal cortical necrosis, renal medullary necrosis, or tubular necrosis, or with other specified pathologic lesion in kidney)
- oliguria or anuria.

Renal failure accompanied by any operative procedure won't be classified under DRG 316.

DRG 317   Admit for Renal Dialysis.
           Mean LOS = 2.9 days
  Principal diagnoses include aftercare involving intermittent dialysis.

Renal failure without intermittent dialysis is coded differently from renal failure with intermittent dialysis. For the latter, the principal diagnosis is actually admission for dialysis; renal failure becomes a secondary diagnosis.

Introduction

DEFINITION AND TIME FOCUS

Acute renal failure (ARF) is a sudden cessation or decrease in renal function. In ARF, the kidneys can't maintain fluid and electrolyte balance or filter metabolic waste products. ARF disrupts all body systems and may cause problems in cardiac, respiratory, GI, neurologic, musculoskeletal, integumentary, genitourinary, and endocrine-metabolic functions. Mortality can be high depending on the cause, the patient's age, and related physical problems.

Most patients with ARF who recover, progress through three stages: oliguria, diuresis, and recovery. The oliguric stage lasts about 2 weeks (a shorter period represents a better prognosis). The diuretic stage may last several weeks. The recovery stage may last up to 1 year, with initial rapid improvement and a continuing slow return to near-normal function. In some cases, patients have nonoliguric ARF with increasing azotemia and urine volumes for 12 days and a return to normal in another 12 days. If the patient doesn't recover, long-term hemodialysis, peritoneal dialysis, continuous renal replacement therapy, or kidney transplantation is necessary.

This care plan focuses on the patient admitted for treatment of ARF, including identification of its cause and support of body systems until the kidneys begin to recover, or evaluation for dialysis or transplantation. (See *Clinical snapshot: Acute renal failure,* page 670.)

ETIOLOGY AND PRECIPITATING FACTORS

- Prerenal problems leading to decreased renal perfusion, such as hemorrhage, all forms of shock, excessive vomiting or diarrhea, heart failure or other causes of decreased cardiac output, burns, excessive diuresis, third-spacing of fluids, hypotension, vasodilation, or obstruction of the aorta or renal arteries
- Renal (parenchymal) problems leading to destruction of kidney tissue, such as acute tubular necrosis from ischemia or nephrotoxins, glomerulonephritis, emboli, allergic inflammation, or infections
- Postrenal problems leading to obstruction of urine flow, such as calculi, prostate enlargement, tumors, or retroperitoneal fibrosis
- Preexisting multisystem problems increase risk of ARF, especially in an older patient

Focused assessment guidelines

NURSING HISTORY
(FUNCTIONAL HEALTH PATTERN FINDINGS)

Health-perception–health-management pattern
- Decreased amount and frequency of urination
- Headaches, swelling of feet and ankles, and palpitations
- Recent high-risk episode such as infection; cardiac, aortic, or biliary surgery; trauma; ingestion of aspirin, antibiotics, or other drugs; exposure to toxins; or an allergic response to food, drugs, or blood transfusions
- History of urinary tract infections, diabetes mellitus, hypertension, kidney disease, or cardiac or liver problems
- Pain around the flank or costal margin areas

Nutritional-metabolic pattern
- Loss of appetite, nausea
- Weight gain or loss
- Odd taste in mouth
- Increased saliva or a dry mouth
- GI bleeding

Elimination pattern
- Decreased or absent urination
- Change in urine color and smell
- Abdominal cramps, a feeling of fullness, diarrhea, or constipation
- Pruritus

Activity-exercise pattern
- Difficulty in breathing at rest and during exercise
- Weakness and fatigue
- Muscle cramps

Sleep-rest pattern
- Fatigue
- Longer than usual sleep periods

Cognitive-perceptual pattern
- Periods of dizziness
- Memory loss and inability to concentrate
- Confusion

Role-relationship pattern
- Job-related exposure to nephrotoxic chemicals, such as carbon tetrachloride, dyes, fungicides, pesticides, or heavy metals

Sexuality-reproductive pattern
- Loss of sexual drive, impotence, or cessation of menstruation

Coping–stress tolerance pattern
- Increased irritability and decreased ability to handle stress

PHYSICAL FINDINGS
Physical findings may vary, depending on the cause, type, and stage of ARF.

Genitourinary
- Oliguria (less than 400 ml/day)
- Less commonly, anuria (less than 50 ml/day) or high urine output (1 to 2 L/day in nonoliguric ARF)
- Abnormal urine color, clarity, or smell (such as red or brown color, cloudiness, or foul smell)

Neurologic
- Lethargy, apathy
- Tremors, seizures
- Memory loss, confusion
- Coma

Cardiovascular
- Arrhythmias
- Bounding, rapid pulse; normal or high blood pressure; and distended jugular veins (with hypervolemia)
- Tachycardia, low blood pressure, or orthostatic hypotension (with hypovolemia)
- Pericardial-type chest pain (mild to severe pain that may increase with movement or decrease with leaning forward)
- Anemia

Pulmonary
- Rapid respirations, dyspnea, or crackles (with hypervolemia)
- Tachypnea (with hypovolemia)
- Kussmaul's respirations (with acidosis)

Gastrointestinal
- Moist tongue and increased saliva (with hypervolemia)
- Dry tongue and mucous membranes (with hypovolemia)
- Vomiting
- Diarrhea
- Stomatitis

Musculoskeletal
- Muscle spasms (tetany)
- Weakness
- Asterixis

Integumentary
- Moist, warm skin and pitting edema over bony areas (with hypervolemia)
- Decreased skin turgor and dry skin (with hypovolemia)
- Bruises
- Thin, brittle hair and nails
- Pallor

DIAGNOSTIC STUDIES
- 24-hour urine output and serum creatinine and blood urea nitrogen (BUN) levels — monitor the kidneys' ability to excrete fluid and waste products. Oliguric ARF is characterized by oliguria and rising BUN and creatinine levels. Patients with nonoliguric ARF exhibit a urine output of 1 to 2 L/day and rising BUN and creatinine levels. The diuretic stage is characterized by increasing urine output (2 to 3 L/day), indicating returning glomerular filtration. BUN and creatinine levels remain high during this stage because the kidneys can't concentrate the urine effectively. As the kidneys regain concentrating ability during the recovery stage, the BUN and creatinine levels begin to fall and stabilize at normal or near normal levels depending upon the residual damage to the kidneys.
- Serum electrolyte panel — monitors fluid, electrolyte, and acid-base status. Elevated potassium, sodium, and phosphate levels; decreased calcium level; and a decreased pH level indicate poor renal function.
- Urinalysis — monitors renal excretion and concentration abilities. Sodium and potassium concentrations may vary, depending on the cause and type of ARF. Casts, crystals, hematuria, and proteinuria may be present. White blood cells (WBCs) may indicate infection. With prerenal conditions, specific gravity and osmolality may be high; with renal conditions, they may be constant at 1.010 and approximately 300 mOsm/kg respectively.
- Creatinine clearance — reflects glomerular filtration rate (GFR) and is an accurate indication of renal function. A decrease indicates a poor GFR. A value of 50 to 84 ml/minute indicates mild failure; 10 to 49 ml/minute, moderate failure; and less than 10 ml/minute, severe failure.
- Fractional sodium excretion or renal failure index — compares the clearance of sodium to the clearance of creatinine; indexes greater than 1 may indicate nonfunctioning tubules.
- Urine-plasma creatinine concentration ratios and urine-plasma urea concentration ratios — reflect the kidneys' ability to save water and excrete wastes. Values vary depending upon the cause and type of ARF. In prerenal failure, ratios are high, reflecting kidney conserva-

tion of sodium and water; in acute tubular insufficiency, the kidneys' inability to perform these functions results in low urine-plasma ratios.

■ BUN-creatinine ratio — reflects GFR and tubular function. In prerenal failure, the ratio is high (usually greater than 20:1), reflecting increased tubular reabsorption of urea. In acute tubular insufficiency, the ratio remains approximately 10:1, reflecting increased reabsorption of both urea and creatinine by the damaged tubules.

■ Complete blood count (CBC) — may reveal low red blood cell (RBC) count, hemoglobin, and hematocrit, reflecting anemia. An elevated WBC count may reflect infection.

■ Coagulation studies — may be abnormal if disseminated intravascular coagulation causes ARF

■ Renal concentration tests — may show the kidneys' inability to concentrate solutes in urine

■ Electrocardiography (ECG) — may show arrhythmias or high peaked T waves, flattened P waves, and widened QRS complexes associated with high potassium levels

■ Kidney-ureter-bladder X-rays — show size, structure, and position of kidneys, ureters, and bladder. The kidneys may be normal or enlarged in ARF. Changes in bladder or ureters suggest postrenal ARF.

■ Computed tomography scan — shows cross-sectional views of renal structures

■ Magnetic resonance imaging — differentiates normal from abnormal cells

■ Ultrasound scan — may show internal and external abnormalities in kidney size and shape

■ Excretory urography (I.V. or retrograde pyelogram) — may show obstruction, constriction, or masses

■ Renal biopsy — may help differentiate among parenchymal kidney diseases

■ Renal angiography — may show renal artery abnormalities, cysts, or tumors

■ Radionuclide tests (renal scan and renogram) — may show abnormal distributions of radioactive compounds, indicating structural abnormalities or impaired perfusion or uptake

■ Cystoscopy — may show urethra and bladder abnormalities

POTENTIAL COMPLICATIONS

Most complications result from the uremic syndrome — the accumulation of waste products in the blood. Some complications result from the kidneys' inability to maintain the normal hormonal functions of stimulating RBC production, regulating calcium absorption, and controlling the renin-angiotensin-aldosterone system.

■ Infection (sepsis is the most dangerous complication of ARF)
■ Stress ulcer
■ Heart failure
■ Pericarditis
■ Pneumonitis
■ Encephalopathy
■ Peripheral neuropathy
■ Coagulation defects
■ Pathologic fractures from bone demineralization
■ GI bleeding

CLINICAL SNAPSHOT ✷

Acute renal failure

Major nursing diagnoses and collaborative problems	Key patient outcomes
CP: Electrolyte imbalance	Maintain serum electrolyte levels within acceptable limits for the patient.
ND: Excess fluid volume	Maintain vital signs and hemodynamic readings within acceptable limits for the patient.
ND: Risk for injury	Display no signs or symptoms of uremia such as mentation changes.
ND: Risk for infection	Have clean, dry access sites for lines and catheters.
ND: Imbalanced nutrition: Less than body requirements	Have only limited weight loss, muscle wasting, or edema.
ND: Deficient knowledge (ARF and dialysis)	Express commitment to comply with treatments, including dialysis, dietary modifications, and activity restrictions.

Collaborative problem

Electrolyte imbalance related to decreased electrolyte excretion, excessive electrolyte intake, or metabolic acidosis

NURSING PRIORITY
Prevent complications of electrolyte imbalance.

PATIENT OUTCOME CRITERIA
Within 8 hours after treatment for hyperkalemia, the patient will:
- have a serum potassium level within normal limits (3.5 to 5.5 mEq/L)
- show no tented T waves or other signs of hyperkalemia on ECG
- display arterial blood gas (ABG) levels within normal limits: pH, 7.35 to 7.45; $Paco_2$, 35 to 45 mm Hg; HCO_3^-, 23 to 28 mEq/L.
    Within 24 hours of admission and then continuously, the patient will:
- maintain serum electrolyte levels within acceptable limits
- have normal sinus rhythm.

INTERVENTIONS	RATIONALES
1. *Monitor and document electrolyte levels every 8 to 12 hours,* * as ordered, particularly potassium, phosphate, calcium, and magnesium. See appendix C, Fluid and electrolyte imbalances, for general assessment parameters and interventions for abnormal electrolyte levels. Consult the nephrologist about acceptable electrolyte levels for the patient.	**1.** The kidneys' inability to regulate electrolyte excretion and reabsorption may result in high potassium and phosphate levels, a low calcium level, and a high or low magnesium level. These levels can change quickly and result in such complications as cardiac arrhythmias, muscle response changes, mentation changes, skin irritation, and even death. General assessment parameters and interventions are included in the Fluid and electrolyte imbalances appendix. The nephrologist can help determine appropriate electrolyte levels for each patient.
2. *Continuously monitor the ECG* and document your findings. See appendix A, Monitoring standards. Note and promptly report peaked, high ("tented") T waves; prolonged PR interval; or a widened QRS complex.	**2.** Electrolyte abnormalities can trigger arrhythmias and cardiac arrest. The Monitoring standards appendix contains general assessments for arrhythmias. The signs listed indicate hyperkalemia severe enough to cause a cardiac emergency.
3. *If hyperkalemia is present, administer* and document the following, as ordered:	**3.** The kidneys' inability to excrete the potassium released into the serum by normal cellular metabolism results in dangerously high potassium levels.
– I.V. glucose (50%) and insulin solution	– Glucose and insulin may transport potassium into cells temporarily, thus lowering serum potassium in an emergency.
– I.V. calcium chloride or calcium gluconate	– Calcium competes with potassium for entry into heart cells, thus decreasing the dangerous effect of hyperkalemia on cardiac rhythm.
– Cation-exchange resins such as sodium polystyrene sulfonate (Kayexalate) with sorbitol, orally or rectally (don't give oral doses with fruit juices); never give if patient has hypoactive bowel sounds	– Sodium polystyrene sulfonate removes potassium at the rate of 1 mEq/g of drug by exchanging it for sodium in the bowel. Sorbitol helps remove the exchanged and bound potassium from the bowel by acting as an osmotic diarrheic. Fruit juices may bind with sodium polystyrene sulfonate and decrease its effectiveness.
– Fluid (water) and sodium retention	– Hypoactive bowel sounds could be an indication of potential fluid shifts that could lead to necrosis.

---

*Italics indicate key interventions.

– I.V. sodium bicarbonate solution

– ARF causes metabolic acidosis, which may increase the release of potassium from cells in exchange for hydrogen ions. Sodium bicarbonate corrects acidosis by combining with hydrogen ions, allowing potassium to move back into the cells.

4. *Limit dietary and drug intake of potassium;* for example, avoid juices high in potassium and drugs such as potassium penicillin (Penicillin VK) or potassium-containing antacids.

4. When the kidneys can't excrete potassium, excess intake can push serum potassium to dangerously high levels.

5. Give aluminum hydroxide antacid (Amphojel) with meals and every 4 hours, as ordered. Document administration.

5. The kidneys can't excrete the phosphates released from normal cellular metabolism or from dietary phosphate intake. Aluminum hydroxide binds with phosphate in the bowels and prevents absorption into the bloodstream, thus decreasing hyperphosphatemia.

6. Give calcium and vitamin supplements as needed and ordered. Document their administration.

6. The kidneys' inability to stimulate the absorption of calcium in the bowel results in hypocalcemia and bone demineralization. High phosphate levels also cause hypocalcemia. Calcium and vitamin D supplements increase the serum calcium levels, helping to prevent bone demineralization and other adverse effects of hypocalcemia.

7. *Limit intake of magnesium,* as from magnesium-containing antacids.

7. The kidneys can't excrete magnesium.

8. *Give sodium chloride I.V.,* as needed and ordered. Document its administration.

8. Usually, sodium intake is restricted to prevent fluid overload. However, major losses through vomiting, diarrhea, and wound drainage may create a need for sodium replacement.

9. Additional individualized interventions: _____
_____

9. Rationales: _____
_____

Nursing diagnosis

Excess fluid volume related to sodium and water retention

NURSING PRIORITIES
- Maintain adequate hydration.
- Prevent fluid overload.

PATIENT OUTCOME CRITERIA
By the time of discharge, the patient will:
- maintain vital signs and hemodynamic readings within acceptable parameters
- have clear lungs
- display minimal or absent peripheral edema
- manifest normal skin turgor
- have moist and clean mucous membranes
- experience weight loss of no more than 1 lb (0.5 kg) per day.

INTERVENTIONS

1. See appendix C, Fluid and electrolyte imbalances.

RATIONALES

1. The Fluid and electrolyte imbalances appendix contains general information on fluid and electrolyte imbalances. This care plan presents additional information specific to ARF.

2. *Assess for signs of fluid overload* and document findings.

– Assess vital signs, breath sounds, and peripheral edema every 4 hours, or more frequently if appropriate. Assess weight and CBC, especially hematocrit, daily. If the patient has an invasive hemodynamic monitoring line, measure right atrial pressure, pulmonary artery pressures, pulmonary artery wedge pressure, mean arterial pressure, and cardiac output according to facility protocol.
– Report the following promptly: high blood pressure, rapid pulse, rapid respirations, high hemodynamic parameters, crackles or gurgles, peripheral edema, increasing daily weight, or low hematocrit.
– Also promptly report: low hemodynamic monitoring parameters, rapid pulse, low blood pressure, dry skin and mucous membranes, poor skin turgor, decreased weight, or high hematocrit.

3. *Measure and document intake and output* every 8 hours.

4. *Restrict fluid intake to measured losses plus 400 ml/day, unless fluid or weight losses are excessive.* Correlate the intake and output record with daily weights. Consult the physician about increasing fluid replacement if excessive fluid losses are present or if weight loss exceeds 1 lb (0.5 kg) per day. Document fluid administration.

5. *Give I.V. infusions continuously through an infusion pump,* as ordered.

6. Provide hard candies, ice chips, and mouth care every 2 hours as needed and ordered. Document your actions.

7. *Give diuretics,* such as mannitol, furosemide (Lasix), or ethacrynic acid (Edecrin), as needed and ordered. Document administration and results. Administer vasodilators, as ordered, such as low-dose dopamine (Intropin).

8. Additional individualized interventions: _____

2. Inability to maintain normal fluid homeostasis results in fluid overload during the oliguric stage and potential dehydration during the diuretic stage.
– Regular assessment of indicated parameters provides for early detection of imbalances.

– Prompt medical intervention is necessary to resolve imbalances. These signs indicate fluid overload. A low hematocrit may reflect hemodilution from overhydration.

– These signs reflect a low circulating fluid volume. High hematocrit may reflect hemoconcentration.

3. A careful comparison of intake and output is necessary to prevent fluid overload or dehydration.

4. Because the kidneys can't eliminate excess fluids, intake must be restricted to replacement of lost fluids. The additional 400 ml represents insensible fluid losses (through lungs, skin, and stool). Although such losses are estimated at 400 ml/day, excess losses from high temperatures, wound drainage, diarrhea, or vomiting may require increasing this amount. Daily weight may help guide fluid replacement because the ARF patient usually loses ³/₄ lb (0.3 kg) to 1 lb/day from catabolism. A loss of more than 1 lb/day may indicate a need for additional fluids.

5. The patient with ARF is susceptible to fluid overload. An infusion pump prevents accidental administration of fluid boluses.

6. Fluid restrictions cause dry mouth and thirst. These measures aid mouth comfort by stimulating salivation and removing debris during fluid restriction.

7. Diuretics may be given initially in prerenal conditions to increase fluid volume through the kidneys in an attempt to prevent ARF. However, diuretics may cause ARF in marginally functioning kidneys and are not effective in nonfunctioning kidneys. Vasodilators expand the vascular bed, lessening vascular congestion and the risk of pulmonary edema. Low-dose dopamine causes dopaminergic stimulation of renal blood vessels, thus increasing renal perfusion.

8. Rationales: _____

Suggested NIC Interventions
Fluid and electrolyte management; Fluid management; Fluid monitoring; Fluid resuscitation

Suggested NOC Outcomes
Urinary elimination; Electrolyte and acid base balance; Fluid balance; Hydration

Renal disorders

Nursing diagnosis

Risk for injury related to uremic syndrome

NURSING PRIORITIES

- Assess for signs and symptoms of uremia.
- Monitor for complications.
- Prevent injuries.

PATIENT OUTCOME CRITERIA

Immediately at the start of dialysis, the patient will:

- have a patent dialysis shunt or catheter
- display no signs of infection
- manifest no signs of hemorrhage.
  Within 3 days of admission, the patient will:
- have an acceptable blood pressure
- display strong, regular peripheral pulses
- show a level of consciousness (LOC) within normal limits
- manifest a normal temperature.
  Within 7 days of admission, the patient will:
- have BUN, creatinine, uric acid, and pH values within expected limits
- display ABG levels within normal limits
- manifest no signs or symptoms of uremia
- maintain therapeutic drug levels
- have a hemoglobin level and hematocrit within expected limits
- display no signs of pericarditis, such as pericardial friction rub and chest pain.

INTERVENTIONS

1. See appendix B, Acid-base imbalances.

2. *Monitor BUN, creatinine, uric acid, and pH levels* once daily or as needed and ordered. *Monitor ABG levels* once daily or as needed and ordered. Document your findings.

3. *Assess for and document signs and symptoms of uremia* every 2 to 4 hours and as needed. Note headache, mentation changes, fatigue, confusion, lethargy, pruritus, uremic frost, stomatitis, nausea and vomiting, ammonia breath odor, weight loss, muscle wasting, Kussmaul's respirations, seizures, or coma. Report significant findings to the physician.

4. *Give sodium bicarbonate I.V. as needed and ordered,* typically if the plasma bicarbonate level is 10 to 15 mEq/L or less. Document administration.

5. *Assess the hemodialysis access site,* if present, every 2 hours for patency, warmth, color, thrill, and bruit. Check circulation above and below the access site. Don't use the access site for I.V. infusions or to draw blood. Don't take blood pressures on an arm or leg with an access site. Inject heparinized normal saline solution into the catheter every 12 hours to maintain patency, as ordered. Document access site status and promptly report abnormalities to the physician.

RATIONALES

1. The Acid-base imbalances appendix contains general information on acid-base imbalances. This plan presents additional information specific to ARF.

2. Accumulation of the metabolic waste products in the blood and increasing acidosis reflect worsening failure and may indicate the need for dialysis.

3. Uremia affects every system and may cause subtle changes as the condition worsens. Careful assessments are valuable in determining the need for dialysis and gauging its frequency.

4. Acidosis is commonly treated by dialysis, but severe cases may be treated with sodium bicarbonate.

5. The access site must remain patent because of the limited number of large vessels available for dialysis. Early discovery of a clotted catheter may allow clot removal and salvaging of the site. Using the site for purposes other than dialysis increases the risk of infection and loss of the site. Regular heparinization prevents clotting.

6. *Assess the peritoneal dialysis access catheter site,* if present, every 24 hours and as needed for signs and symptoms of infection, including redness, swelling, excess warmth, and drainage. Also assess for general signs and symptoms of infection, including fever, malaise, abdominal pain, and cloudy drainage. Maintain surgical aseptic technique when manipulating the site, changing dressings, or adding medication to the dialysate.

6. The patient undergoing peritoneal dialysis is at high risk for peritonitis, a life-threatening complication. Early detection of infection permits aggressive intervention and increases the likelihood of its success.

7. Prepare the patient for dialysis, as needed and ordered, when potassium, BUN, and creatinine levels, and other parameters indicate worsening uremia, usually every 1 to 3 days.

7. Both hemodialysis and peritoneal dialysis remove serum waste products and excess fluids and electrolytes, allowing a more homeostatic metabolic state.

8. Monitor drug administration and blood levels, as ordered. Assess potential nephrotoxicity, electrolyte content, dosage, and timing with dialysis.

8. Renal dysfunction may decrease drug excretion, resulting in excessive blood levels and varying durations of drug effects. Certain drugs, including antibiotics, may be nephrotoxic and may worsen kidney damage. Drugs containing electrolytes should be limited to prevent undesirable effects. Dialysis may remove some drugs from the blood, so drug administration should be timed with dialysis treatments. Monitoring blood levels provides accurate guidelines for drug therapy.

9. *Monitor hematocrit and hemoglobin level* daily for signs of anemia. Give packed RBCs, folic acid, and iron supplements as needed and ordered. Document your findings and actions.

9. Erythropoietin, a hormone manufactured by the kidneys, normally stimulates RBC production. Diminished erythropoietin production in ARF results in anemia. Folic acid and iron supplements stimulate RBC production and may correct the anemia. Administering packed cells instead of whole blood provides oxygen-carrying RBCs without exacerbating fluid overload.

10. *Assess continually for signs and symptoms of hemorrhage,* including changes in vital signs, CBC, and coagulation panel. If present, alert the physician immediately. Give vitamin K, packed RBCs, and other blood components as needed and ordered, and document their use. See the "Gastrointestinal hemorrhage" care plan, page 487.

10. Uremic syndrome places the patient at high risk for stress ulcers and coagulation problems. General interventions for the patient with GI bleeding are included in the "Gastrointestinal hemorrhage" care plan.

11. *Assess daily for signs and symptoms of pericarditis,* including tachycardia, fever, friction rub, and pleuritic pain that is relieved by sitting forward. If these indicators are present:
– Notify the physician. Administer steroids or nonsteroidal anti-inflammatory agents, as ordered. Document their use.
– Monitor every 4 hours for indicators of pericardial effusion and a small cardiac tamponade: weak peripheral pulses, paradoxical pulse greater than 10 mm Hg, or a decreased LOC. If present, alert the physician immediately.
– Monitor continually for indicators of a large cardiac tamponade: distended jugular veins, profound hypotension, and rapid loss of consciousness. Summon immediate medical assistance and prepare for emergency pericardial aspiration.

11. About 20% of patients with ARF develop pericarditis (inflammation of the pericardial sac).

– Untreated, pericarditis can lead to pericardial effusion and cardiac tamponade. The medications listed relieve inflammation.
– Pericardial effusion can range from mild to major. Mild effusion produces a small cardiac tamponade and mildly decreased cardiac output. Increased dialysis may be used to remove the uremic toxins causing mild effusion.
– A large cardiac tamponade — a medical emergency — compromises cardiac output severely. Immediate removal of pericardial fluid is necessary to allow ventricular filling and prevent cardiac arrest.

12. Additional individualized interventions: _____

12. Rationales:_____

Nursing diagnosis

Risk for infection related to decreased immune response and skin changes secondary to uremia

NURSING PRIORITY

Assess for and prevent infection.

PATIENT OUTCOME CRITERIA

Within 72 hours of admission and then continuously, the patient will:
- have a normal temperature
- have clean, dry access sites for I.V. lines and catheters
- have negative cultures
- have a therapeutic blood level, if taking antibiotics.

INTERVENTIONS	RATIONALES
1. *Assess continually for signs of infection,* such as increased temperature, redness, swelling, warmth, and drainage. Document findings and report them to the physician.	1. Uremic syndrome suppresses normal cell metabolism and immune response, resulting in an increased risk for infection, a major cause of death for ARF patients. Continuous assessment is necessary to identify infection and to begin early treatment, reducing the risk of life-threatening sepsis and septicemia.
2. *Continually protect the patient from cross-contamination by practicing strict medical and surgical asepsis.*	2. Carefully washing hands and using aseptic technique during procedures and when handling equipment may prevent infection.
3. *Give antibiotics every 4 to 12 hours, as ordered,* and document their use. Follow the guidelines for drug administration in "Risk for injury," page 674.	3. Antibiotics are a potent weapon against infection; however, many are nephrotoxic. Because the kidneys may be unable to excrete antibiotics normally, lower-than-normal doses may be needed. Coordination with dialysis is important to minimize drug removal and maintain therapeutic blood levels.
4. Provide site care and dressing changes for central and peripheral I.V. lines, catheters, and dialysis access every 12 to 48 hours, according to policy. Assess and document condition of skin and puncture sites; document date and care given.	4. Site care may prevent the accumulation of secretions that could serve as growth media for infective organisms, while regular assessment may allow the early identification of infection. Careful documentation of site care promotes continuity of care.
5. Provide skin care at frequent intervals. Use preventive measures, such as position changes, range-of-motion exercises, massage, wrinkle-free linens, and protective pads and mattresses. Document skin condition and nursing care given. See the "Impaired physical mobility" care plan, page 111.	5. Skin integrity is compromised in the patient with ARF and uremia because of altered metabolism and the accumulation of fluid and waste products in the tissues. Frequent skin care may counteract the increased risk of skin breakdown and infection. The "Impaired physical mobility" care plan provides further detail on preventing skin breakdown.
6. *Avoid continuous invasive procedures* such as indwelling urinary catheterization. Catheterize intermittently, as needed and as ordered.	6. Continuous invasive procedures provide reservoirs for infective organisms in a patient already at high risk for infection.

7. Collect urine, blood, and secretion specimens for culture and sensitivity laboratory tests, as needed and ordered. Document your actions.

8. Additional individualized interventions: _____
_____

7. Careful monitoring of body secretions for infection may allow timely and appropriate treatment if needed.

8. Rationales: _____
_____

> **Suggested NIC Interventions**
> *Infection control; Infection protection; Risk identification*

> **Suggested NOC Outcomes**
> *Infection status; Wound healing: Primary intention*

Nursing diagnosis
Imbalanced nutrition: Less than body requirements related to anorexia, nausea and vomiting, and restricted dietary intake

NURSING PRIORITIES
- Maintain nutritional status.
- Minimize protein catabolism.

PATIENT OUTCOME CRITERIA
Upon discharge, the patient will:
- be free from nausea and vomiting
- have only limited weight loss, muscle wasting, or edema
- display a pattern of regular and adequate meal intake
- verbalize having enough energy for activities of daily living.

INTERVENTIONS

1. *See the "Nutritional deficit" care plan,* page 138.

2. *Administer medication to control nausea and vomiting,* as needed and as ordered. Document administration and patient response. Provide small, frequent meals. Document dietary intake.

3. Collaborate with the physician and nutritionist to design a high-carbohydrate diet that provides small quantities of high-quality proteins (containing essential amino acids); limits fluids, potassium, and sodium; and includes vitamin supplements.

4. Additional individualized interventions: _____
_____

RATIONALES

1. General assessments and interventions are included in the "Nutritional deficit" care plan. This nursing diagnosis focuses on information specific to ARF.

2. The patient with ARF commonly experiences nausea and vomiting because of uremia's effects on the GI system. Medication and smaller servings enhance tolerance to the diet.

3. A high-carbohydrate diet provides calories for energy while sparing proteins and preventing protein catabolism. Because the kidneys can't excrete the waste products of protein metabolism, proteins are limited to easily used, high-quality proteins. The kidneys can't regulate water balance, so fluids are limited. Electrolytes, such as potassium, are limited because the kidneys can't excrete them. Sodium is limited to prevent volume overload. Dialysis may remove vitamins, requiring administration of supplements.

4. Rationales: _____
_____

> **Suggested NIC Interventions**
> *Nutrition therapy; Nutrition management; Nutritional monitoring*

> **Suggested NOC Outcomes**
> *Nutritional status: Body mass; Nutritional status: Energy; Nutritional status: Food and fluid intake; Nutritional status: Nutrient intake*

Nursing diagnosis

Deficient knowledge (ARF and dialysis) related to lack of exposure to information on complex disease and its management

NURSING PRIORITY
Provide information on ARF and dialysis, as appropriate.

PATIENT OUTCOME CRITERIA
According to individual readiness, the patient will be able to relate on request:
- signs and symptoms, such as headache, nausea, and vomiting, to be reported to the nurse
- commitment to comply with treatments, including dialysis, dietary modifications, and activity restrictions.

INTERVENTIONS	RATIONALES
1. *See the "Knowledge deficit" care plan,* page 129.	**1.** General interventions appropriate for any patient are included in the "Knowledge deficit" care plan. This nursing diagnosis focuses on information specific to ARF.
2. *Provide, as appropriate, information about the complexity and life-threatening nature of ARF and dialysis,* including: – the common stages of ARF – medications – signs and symptoms that should be reported to the nurse, such as dizziness and nausea – procedures, including hemodialysis or peritoneal dialysis – dietary modifications – activity restrictions.	**2.** The acutely ill patient may not be receptive to extensive teaching. However, if appropriate, teaching may decrease anxiety and enhance recovery.
3. Additional individualized interventions: _____	**3.** Rationales: _____

> **Suggested NIC Interventions**
> *Teaching: Disease process; Teaching: Individual; Teaching: Prescribed medication*

> **Suggested NOC Outcomes**
> *Knowledge: Disease process; Knowledge: Health behaviors; Knowledge: Treatment regimen*

Discharge planning

DISCHARGE CHECKLIST
Before discharge, the patient shows evidence of:
- ❏ stable vital signs and monitoring parameters
- ❏ absence of infection, hemorrhage, and major complications in all systems
- ❏ stabilized fluid and electrolyte status, including limited edema and appropriate potassium, calcium, sodium, phosphate, and magnesium levels
- ❏ stabilized BUN, creatinine, uric acid, and pH levels
- ❏ intact and healing dialysis access site
- ❏ stable nutritional status including a positive nitrogen balance and minimal weight loss
- ❏ therapeutic drug levels.

TEACHING CHECKLIST

Document evidence that the patient and his family demonstrate an understanding of:

❑ common stages of ARF and the patient's current stage
❑ fluid and diet regimen, including limitations of proteins, electrolytes, and fluids
❑ rest and activity schedule
❑ medications, including action and adverse effects
❑ dialysis treatment if appropriate, including schedule and adverse effects
❑ signs and symptoms, including fever, pain, nausea, vomiting, and dizziness, to report to the nurse
❑ changes in neurologic status.

DOCUMENTATION CHECKLIST

Using outcome criteria as a guide, document:

❑ clinical status on admission
❑ significant changes in status
❑ pertinent laboratory and diagnostic test findings, including serum drug levels
❑ dialysis access site condition and care
❑ urine characteristics and quantity, if appropriate
❑ intake and output
❑ daily weights
❑ diet tolerance
❑ activity tolerance
❑ mentation status
❑ skin status
❑ pertinent procedures including dialysis.

Associated care plans

- Gastrointestinal hemorrhage
- Knowledge deficit
- Nutritional deficit

References

Jordan, K. (ed). *Emergency Nursing Core Curriculum.* Emergency Nurses Association. Philadelphia: W.B. Saunders Co. 2000.

Lewis, S.M., et al. *Medical-Surgical Nursing: Assessment and Management of Clinical Problems.* St. Louis: Mosby–Year Book, Inc., 2000.

Lynn-McHale, D.J., and Carlson, K.K. American Association of Critical Care Nurses *AACN Procedure Manual for Critical Care,* 4th ed. Philadelphia: W.B. Saunders Co., 2001.

Shoemaker, W.C., et al. *Textbook of Critical Care,* 4th ed. Philadelphia: W.B. Saunders Co., 2002.

Chronic renal failure

DRG INFORMATION

DRG 316   Renal Failure.
          Mean LOS = 6.6 days
   Principal diagnoses include chronic renal failure.
DRG 317   Admit for Renal Dialysis.
          Mean LOS = 2.9 days
DRG 315   Other Kidney and Urinary Tract Operating
          Room Procedures.
          Mean LOS = 7.0 days
   Principal diagnoses include arteriovenostomy for renal
dialysis.

Introduction

DEFINITION AND TIME FOCUS

Chronic renal failure (CRF) is a progressive, irreversible
decrease in kidney function to the point where homeostasis can no longer be maintained. Usually slow and
insidious, CRF eventually has consequences in all organ
systems and physiologic processes. The final stage of
CRF, when more than 90% of kidney function is perma-
nently lost, is called end-stage renal disease (ESRD).
During ESRD, chronic abnormalities occur, and patient
survival depends on maintenance dialysis or kidney
transplantation. This care plan focuses on the ESRD patient receiving maintenance hemodialysis or peritoneal
dialysis, who has been admitted for evaluation of the
systemic consequences of CRF and the effectiveness of
therapy. (See *Clinical snapshot: Chronic renal failure,*
page 683.)

ETIOLOGY AND PRECIPITATING FACTORS

- Untreated acute renal failure or poor response to treat-
ment (for example, acute tubular necrosis)
- Diabetes mellitus (DM) leading to diabetic nephropa-
thy
- Severe hypertension leading to hypertensive
nephropathy
- Lupus erythematosus leading to lupus nephritis
- Recurrent glomerulonephritis, typically related to
chronic streptococcal infection
- Pyelonephritis
- Polycystic kidney disease
- Chronic use of nephrotoxic drugs
- Frequent lower urinary tract infections (UTIs) with
eventual kidney involvement
- Neoplasms (metastatic or primary)
- Developmental and congenital disorders

- Complications of pregnancy (for example, eclampsia,
UTI, hemorrhage, or abruptio placenta)
- Sarcoidosis
- Amyloidosis
- Goodpasture's syndrome (autoimmune disease involv-
ing basement membrane of glomerular capillaries)

Focused assessment guidelines

NURSING HISTORY
(FUNCTIONAL HEALTH PATTERN FINDINGS)

Health-perception–health-management pattern

- Signs and symptoms that cause the patient to seek
health care vary widely and may include decreased urine
output, edema, extreme fatigue, depression, loss of interest in environment, impotence, and flank pain
- Commonly has a history of acute or chronic renal
problems and may be receiving treatment for acute renal
failure, chronic renal insufficiency, hypertension, DM,
generalized arteriosclerosis and atherosclerosis, lupus
erythematosus, or other systemic diseases involving the
kidneys

Nutritional-metabolic pattern

- Anorexia, nausea, and vomiting
- Weight loss related to decreased intake of nutrients or
weight gain related to fluid retention
- Unpleasant taste in mouth

Elimination pattern

- Polyuria and nocturia if patient is in an early stage of
CRF
- Oliguria (with polycystic kidney disease, urine output
may be normal, or polyuria may occur), if patient is in
advanced stage of CRF
- Diarrhea alternating with constipation

Activity-exercise pattern

- Fatigue, malaise, and decreased energy level

Sleep-rest pattern

- Extreme somnolence or insomnia and restlessness
- Sleep often interrupted by muscle cramps and leg pain

Cognitive-perceptual pattern

- Shortened attention span
- Memory loss
- Decreased ability to perform abstract reasoning or
mathematical calculations
- Loss of interest in environment

Self-perception–self-concept pattern

- Depression or frequent mood swings
- Altered self-concept and body image
- Decreased self-esteem

- Reduced level of independence and self-care
- Sense of powerlessness and hopelessness

Role-relationship pattern
- Inability to work
- Inability to maintain spousal and parental roles
- Decrease in social contacts and activities

Sexuality-reproductive pattern
- Amenorrhea, infertility, decreased libido, and decreased or absent sexual expression in female patient
- Impotence, decreased libido, and decreased or absent sexual expression in male patient

Coping–stress tolerance pattern
- Ineffective individual and family coping patterns in response to changes caused by chronic catastrophic disease and its treatment
- Defense mechanisms (for example, denial, projection, displacement, or rationalization)

Value-belief pattern
- Loss of confidence in health care providers
- Questioning or reaffirming lifelong religious and philosophical values and beliefs

PHYSICAL FINDINGS
Integumentary
- Rough, dry skin
- Bronze-gray, pallid skin color
- Pruritus
- Ecchymoses
- Poor skin mobility and turgor (skin mobility is the ease with which the skin can be lifted between the fingers; turgor is the speed with which it resumes position)
- Excoriation
- Signs and symptoms of inflammation
- Thin, brittle nails
- Coarse and thinning hair

Cardiovascular
- Hypertension, or hypotension (uncommon)
- Orthostatic hypotension
- Pitting edema of feet, legs, fingers, and hands
- Periorbital edema
- Sacral edema
- Engorged jugular veins
- Arrhythmias
- Pericardial friction rub (with pericarditis)
- Paradoxical pulse (with pericardial effusion or tamponade)
- Palpitations

Pulmonary
- Crackles
- Shortness of breath
- Coughing
- Thick, tenacious sputum
- Deep, rapid respirations (with acidosis)

Gastrointestinal
- Smell of urine and ammonia on the breath
- Gum ulcerations and bleeding

- Dry, cracked, bleeding mucous membranes and tongue
- Vomiting
- Bleeding from GI tract
- Constipation or diarrhea
- Weight loss related to decreased intake of nutrients masked by fluid retention (peripheral edema), leading to increase in overall body weight; after the patient receives appropriate treatment (fluid restriction and dialysis), excess fluid is decreased and weight loss is especially evident
- Liver enlargement
- Ascites

Neurologic
- Malaise, weakness, and fatigue
- Confusion and disorientation
- Memory loss
- Slowing of thought processes
- Changes in sensorium (somnolence, stupor, or coma)
- Seizures
- Changes in behavior (irritability, withdrawal, depression, psychosis, or delusions)
- Numbness and burning of soles
- Decreased sensory perception
- Muscle cramps
- Restlessness of legs
- Diminished deep tendon reflexes
- Positive Chvostek's and Trousseau's signs (rare)

Musculoskeletal
- Muscle cramps (especially in the legs)
- Loss of muscle strength
- Limited range of motion (ROM) in joints
- Bone fractures
- Lumps (calcium-phosphate deposits) in skin, soft tissues, and joints
- Footdrop with motor nerve involvement

Reproductive
- Amenorrhea (in females)
- Atrophy of testicles (in males)
- Gynecomastia

DIAGNOSTIC STUDIES
- Blood urea nitrogen (BUN) levels — elevated
- Serum creatinine levels — elevated (see *Creatinine ranges in renal failure*, page 682)
- Creatinine clearance — decreased by more than 90% in ESRD (see *Creatinine ranges in renal failure*, page 682)
- Serum electrolyte levels — hypernatremia (common), hyperkalemia, hyperphosphatemia, hypocalcemia, elevated calcium-phosphate product, hypermagnesemia
- Venous carbon dioxide (comparable to arterial bicarbonate) levels — decreased
- Arterial blood gas levels — acid-base imbalance, typically metabolic acidosis

Creatinine ranges in renal failure

Renal function	Serum creatinine (approximate mg/100 ml)	Creatinine clearance (ml/minute)
Normal	1.0 to 1.4	85 to 150
Mild failure	1.5 to 2.0	50 to 84
Moderate failure	2.1 to 6.5	10 to 49
Severe failure	> 6.5	< 10
End-stage failure	> 12	0

- Hemoglobin levels and hematocrit — decreased (hemoglobin usually 6 to 8 mg, hematocrit usually 20% to 25%)
- Red blood cell (RBC) count — decreased
- Serum albumin and total protein levels — commonly decreased
- Alkaline phosphatase levels — may be elevated
- White blood cell count — may be elevated
- Electrocardiogram (ECG) — may show abnormal rhythms or altered waveform appearance
- Urinalysis — of minimal diagnostic value in ESRD
- Renal biopsy — indicates the nature and extent of renal disease; necessary to diagnose cause of CRF
- Radionuclide tests (renal scan and renogram) — may show abnormal renal structure and function
- Renal arteriogram — may identify narrowed, stenosed, missing, or misplaced blood vessels
- Plain X-ray of kidneys, ureters, and bladder — may indicate gross structural abnormalities
- Ultrasonography — may indicate gross structural abnormalities
- Computed tomography scan — may show renal masses, abnormal filling of the collecting system, or vascular disorders

Note: Because CRF commonly coexists with other systemic diseases and because it affects all organ systems and physiologic processes, numerous additional laboratory tests and diagnostic procedures are commonly required to assess the other diseases and systemic consequences of CRF.

POTENTIAL COMPLICATIONS
- Uncontrollable hypertension
- Hyperkalemia and related cardiac electrical conduction deficits
- Pericarditis, pericardial effusion, or cardiac tamponade
- Pulmonary edema
- Heart failure
- Osteodystrophy
- Metastatic calcium-phosphate calcifications
- Aluminum intoxication
- Profound neurologic impairment
- Profound psychosocial disequilibrium
- Abnormal protein, lipid, and carbohydrate metabolism
- Accelerated atherosclerosis
- Anemia
- Fluid and electrolyte imbalance
- GI bleeding
- Hyperparathyroidism
- Infections
- Fluid overload
- Medication toxicity
- Metabolic acidosis
- Pleural effusion
- Uremia

CLINICAL SNAPSHOT ✸

Chronic renal failure

Major nursing diagnoses and collaborative problems	Key patient outcomes
CP: Risk for hyperkalemia	Maintain serum potassium levels within acceptable limits as specified by the physician, ideally 3.5 to 5.5 mEq/L.
CP: Risk for pericarditis, pericardial effusion, and cardiac tamponade	Display no signs of pericarditis, such as fever, chest pain, and pericardial friction rub.
CP: Hypertension	Maintain blood pressure within acceptable limits as specified by the physician.
CP: Anemia	Maintain a stable hematocrit within a defined range, usually 20% to 25%.
CP: Risk for osteodystrophy and metastatic calcifications	Exhibit serum calcium, phosphorus, alkaline phosphatase, aluminum, and calcium-phosphate product levels within an acceptable range.
ND: Imbalanced nutrition: Less than body requirements	Demonstrate ability to weigh self and to maintain weight and intake and output records.
ND: Impaired oral mucous membrane	Maintain clean, moist oral mucous membrane without ulcers, bleeding, or signs of infection.
CP: Risk for peripheral neuropathy	Ambulate and carry out ADLs safely and comfortably.
ND: Risk for impaired skin integrity	Maintain clean, intact, infection-free skin.
ND: Disturbed thought processes	Show no neurologic complications, such as seizures and encephalopathy.
ND: Noncompliance (treatment regimen)	Express commitment to comply with therapeutic regimen.
ND: Sexual dysfunction	Express concerns about sexual and reproductive functioning with spouse or partner.
ND: Deficient knowledge (vascular access care)	Describe all protective measures appropriate to the vascular access.

Renal disorders

Collaborative problem

Risk for hyperkalemia related to decreased renal excretion, metabolic acidosis, excessive dietary intake, blood transfusion, catabolism, and noncompliance with therapeutic regimen

NURSING PRIORITIES

- Implement measures to prevent or treat hyperkalemia.
- Monitor their effectiveness.

PATIENT OUTCOME CRITERIA

Within 2 hours after treatment is initiated, the patient will:
- maintain serum potassium levels within acceptable limits as specified by the physician, ideally 3.5 to 5.5 mEq/L
- exhibit no signs of hyperkalemia on ECG
- have an arterial pH of 7.35 to 7.45 and a venous carbon dioxide of 22 to 25 mEq/L (or as defined as acceptable for the patient).
    By the time of discharge, the patient will:
- demonstrate an ability to plan a 3-day diet incorporating potassium restrictions and other dietary requirements.

INTERVENTIONS	RATIONALES
1. *Monitor serum potassium** daily, and notify the physician if the level exceeds 5.5 mEq/L.	1. Hyperkalemia causes adverse and even lethal physiologic effects.
2. *Assess and report signs and symptoms of hyperkalemia* — slow, irregular pulse; muscle weakness and flaccidity; diarrhea; and ECG changes (tall, tented T wave; ST-segment depression; prolonged PR interval; wide QRS complex; or cardiac standstill, indicating extreme hyperkalemia).	2. Cardiovascular signs and symptoms are the most important physiologic indicators of the effects of hyperkalemia.
3. *Implement measures to prevent or treat metabolic acidosis,* as ordered, such as administering alkaline medications (for example, sodium bicarbonate) and maintenance dialysis.	3. In the acidotic state, hydrogen ions move into the cell to compensate for the acidosis to maintain electrochemical neutrality; potassium ions move out of the cell and into the plasma, producing hyperkalemia.
4. If blood transfusions are necessary, *administer fresh packed RBCs during dialysis,* as ordered.	4. In fresh blood, fewer RBCs have hemolyzed and released potassium as compared with stored blood. Dialysis removes excess potassium.
5. *Decrease catabolism by encouraging the patient to consume prescribed amounts of dietary protein and carbohydrates, by treating infections, and by decreasing fever.*	5. Catabolism causes release of intracellular potassium into the plasma. Appropriate intake of dietary protein reduces breakdown of the body's cells. Infections and fever increase the metabolic rate and can lead to a catabolic state.
6. Encourage compliance with the therapeutic regimen.	6. Dietary noncompliance can result in excessive potassium intake; noncompliance with the dialysis regimen causes hyperkalemia from decreased removal of potassium.
7. *Implement and evaluate therapy for hyperkalemia, as ordered:* – sodium bicarbonate I.V. – hypertonic glucose and insulin I.V. – calcium lactate or calcium gluconate I.V. – cation-exchange resin (such as Kayexalate) – dialysis.	7. Rationales for hyperkalemia therapy include the following: – Sodium bicarbonate helps correct acidosis and causes potassium to shift from the plasma back into the cells. – Hypertonic glucose and insulin cause potassium to move from the extracellular to the intracellular space. – Calcium antagonizes potassium and reduces its potentially deleterious effects on the cardiac conduction system. – This medication exchanges sodium for potassium and increases potassium excretion through the intestines. – Hemodialysis rapidly and efficiently removes potassium from the blood; peritoneal dialysis removes potassium at a much slower rate.
8. *Monitor serial serum potassium levels and ECG readings* for signs of hypokalemia during treatment.	8. Overtreatment of hyperkalemia may result in hypokalemia.
9. Additional individualized interventions: _____	9. Rationales: _____

Collaborative problem
Risk for pericarditis, pericardial effusion, and cardiac tamponade related to uremia or inadequate dialysis

NURSING PRIORITY
Detect complications and intervene promptly to maintain hemodynamic status.

---

*Italics indicate key interventions.

PATIENT OUTCOME CRITERIA

With adequate treatment, the patient will exhibit relief of pericarditis (if present), maintenance of hemodynamic status, and prevention of complications as evidenced by:

- blood pressure within defined parameters
- strong, regular peripheral pulses
- normal heart sounds (strong, readily audible apical impulse without friction rub)
- normal temperature
- maintenance of alert and oriented (or usual) mental status
- maintenance of usual respiratory status
- absent or decreased peripheral edema
- ECG without evidence of pericarditis
- maintenance of usual energy level.

INTERVENTIONS	RATIONALES
1. *Assess for signs and symptoms of pericarditis* daily: fever, chest pain, and pericardial friction rub. Report their occurrence to the physician.	**1.** Of patients with CRF on dialysis, 30% to 50% develop uremic pericarditis; the classic triad of fever, chest pain, and pericardial friction rub is the hallmark of this condition.
2. If signs and symptoms of pericarditis are present, collaborate with the nephrology team to *assess the adequacy of dialysis* and increase frequency as necessary and as ordered.	**2.** Inadequate dialysis, with subsequent uremic toxin accumulation, is one cause of pericarditis; intense dialysis therapy is the usual treatment.
3. If signs and symptoms of pericarditis are present, *assess for signs and symptoms of pericardial effusion and tamponade* every 4 hours, as follows: – Palpate peripheral pulses for rate, quality, waxing, and waning. – Assess for paradoxical pulse greater than 10 mm Hg. – Assess for peripheral edema. – Assess for decrease in sensorium. – Assess for profound hypotension, narrow pulse pressure, weak or absent peripheral pulses, cold and poorly perfused extremities, rapid decrease in sensorium, and bulging jugular veins (signs of rapidly occurring large tamponade).	**3.** Pericardial effusion is a common complication that can lead to tamponade, a life-threatening condition. Signs and symptoms vary from mild compromise of cardiac output with small effusion to severely compromised hemodynamic status in tamponade. To assess paradoxical pulse, place a blood pressure cuff on the patient's arm and instruct him to breathe normally. Inflate the cuff above the systolic level. Slowly deflate the cuff and note the systolic pressure on expiration. Wait, reinflate the cuff, and deflate it again, this time noting the systolic pressure on inspiration. The difference between the two readings is the paradoxical pulse. A paradoxical pulse of 10 mm Hg or less indicates a normal blood pressure response to inspiration. A value greater than 10 mm Hg indicates an exaggerated response to inspiration typical of cardiac tamponade.
4. *If tamponade develops, prepare the patient for emergency pericardial aspiration.*	**4.** The mortality rate in tamponade is 95%. Immediate aspiration of fluid from the pericardial cavity is essential to restore cardiac function and hemodynamic status.
5. Encourage compliance with the therapeutic regimen.	**5.** Dialysis removes uremic toxins that can cause pericarditis. Dialysis combined with fluid restriction reduces the risk of effusion.
6. Additional individualized interventions: _____	**6.** Rationales: _____

Collaborative problem

Hypertension related to sodium and water retention and malfunction of the renin-angiotensin-aldosterone system

NURSING PRIORITY

Implement the therapeutic regimen and patient teaching to control hypertension.

Renal disorders

PATIENT OUTCOME CRITERIA

Throughout the hospital stay, the patient will:
- maintain blood pressure within acceptable limits
- show no hypertensive complications.

By the time of discharge, the patient will:
- demonstrate ability to measure blood pressure and pulse rate.

INTERVENTIONS	RATIONALES
1. *Administer antihypertensive medications,* as ordered, and assess for desired and adverse effects. Reassure the patient that some adverse effects may decrease once the body adjusts to the medication.	**1.** Antihypertensive medications are an essential part of treatment of CRF. Antihypertensives act by vasodilation, beta-adrenergic blocking, angiotensin blocking, alpha$_1$-adrenergic receptor blocking, or calcium channel blocking. Reassurance helps prevent noncompliance because of initial adverse effects.
2. With the physician, determine an acceptable range for the patient's blood pressure. Measure blood pressure at various times of the day with the patient in a supine position, sitting, and standing. Record blood pressure readings on a flow sheet to correlate the influence of time of day, positioning, medications, diet, and weight. Teach the patient to measure blood pressure and pulse rate.	**2.** Blood pressure measurements commonly vary throughout the day and in relation to medication administration, diet, weight, and positioning. Excessive doses of antihypertensives or dehydration can cause orthostatic hypotension.
3. *Teach the patient how to avoid orthostatic hypotension* by changing position slowly such as sitting for 5 minutes when changing from a supine to a standing position.	**3.** Orthostatic hypotension may cause falls and injuries. Medication noncompliance may result if the patient can't prevent orthostatic hypotension.
4. Encourage compliance with therapy.	**4.** Dialysis removes sodium and water and controls vascular volume; diet restrictions prevent excessive sodium and fluid intake.
5. *Instruct the patient to report any changes that may indicate fluid overload, hypertensive encephalopathy, or vision disturbances.* These include periorbital, sacral, or peripheral edema; headaches; seizures; and blurred vision.	**5.** These signs and symptoms may indicate poor control of hypertension and the need to alter therapy.
6. Recognize the significance of funduscopic changes reported on medical or nursing examination: arteriovenous nicking, exudates, hemorrhages, and papilledema.	**6.** These conditions suggest uncontrolled hypertension and the need to reevaluate the therapeutic regimen.
7. Additional individualized interventions: _____	**7.** Rationales: _____

Collaborative problem

Anemia related to decreased life span of RBCs in CRF, bleeding, decreased production of erythropoietin and RBCs, and blood loss during hemodialysis

NURSING PRIORITIES
- Stabilize the RBC count.
- Maximize tissue perfusion.

PATIENT OUTCOME CRITERIA

Throughout the hospital stay, the patient will:
- maintain a stable hematocrit within a defined range, usually 20% to 25%
- exhibit symptomatic relief of the effects of anemia
- verbalize ways to protect self from trauma
- perform activities of daily living (ADLs) without undue fatigue.

INTERVENTIONS	RATIONALES
1. *Assess daily the degree of anemia* (as reflected by hemoglobin level, hematocrit, and RBC count) and its physiologic effects, such as fatigue, pallor, dyspnea, palpitations, ecchymoses, and tachycardia.	1. The severity of anemia and its physiologic effects vary. The therapeutic plan is based on anemia's effects on the individual patient.
2. *Administer vitamins and minerals,* as ordered, and assess for desired and adverse effects: iron and folic acid supplements, vitamin B complex, vitamin C, and epoetin alfa (Epogen). Don't administer folic acid and vitamins during dialysis or iron with phosphate binders.	2. Iron, folic acid, and vitamins are required for RBC production, but are commonly deficient in the CRF patient's diet. Like endogenous erythropoietin, epoetin alfa (erythropoietin produced through recombinant DNA techniques) stimulates RBC production. However, the patient's iron stores must be adequate for epoetin alfa to be effective. Dialysis removes folic acid and vitamins. Phosphate binders decrease iron absorption.
3. Assist the patient to develop an activity and exercise schedule, with regular rest periods, to avoid undue fatigue.	3. Decreased hemoglobin decreases tissue oxygenation and increases fatigue. A carefully developed plan of activity and exercise can lessen fatigue and allow the patient to perform ADLs.
4. *Avoid taking unnecessary blood specimens.*	4. Frequent collection of blood specimens worsens anemia.
5. *Instruct the patient how to prevent bleeding:* using a soft toothbrush, avoiding vigorous nose blowing, preventing constipation, and avoiding contact sports.	5. Bleeding from any site worsens anemia.
6. *Administer blood transfusions,* as indicated and ordered.	6. Blood transfusions are administered only when the patient becomes symptomatic with low hematocrit; frequent blood transfusions suppress RBC production even further. Fresh packed RBCs are administered during dialysis, as noted previously.
7. Additional individualized interventions: _____	7. Rationales: _____

Collaborative problem
Risk for osteodystrophy and metastatic calcifications related to hyperphosphatemia, hypocalcemia, abnormal vitamin D metabolism, hyperparathyroidism, and elevated aluminum levels

NURSING PRIORITY
Minimize bone demineralization and metastatic calcifications.

PATIENT OUTCOME CRITERIA
Throughout the hospital stay, the patient will:
- exhibit serum calcium, phosphorus, alkaline phosphatase, aluminum, and calcium-phosphate product levels within an acceptable range
- exhibit minimal bone demineralization on bone scan
- exhibit minimal calcium-phosphate deposits
- show no signs or symptoms of hypocalcemia, such as numbness or tingling fingertips and toes
- maintain a safe, painless level of activity.

INTERVENTIONS	RATIONALES
1. *Administer phosphate binders, calcium supplements, and vitamin D supplements,* as ordered, and assess their effects: – Weekly, monitor serum levels of calcium, phosphate, alkaline phosphatase, aluminum, and calcium-phosphate product; report abnormal findings to the physician. – Monitor X-rays for bone fractures and joint deposits. – Weekly, palpate joints for enlargement, swelling, and tenderness. – Weekly, inspect the patient's gait, ROM in joints, and muscle strength.	**1.** In renal failure, the decreased glomerular filtration rate causes phosphate retention and hyperphosphatemia; plasma calcium levels decrease to compensate. Decreased vitamin D metabolism by the kidneys decreases calcium absorption from the GI tract. The decrease in plasma calcium levels stimulates production of parathyroid hormone, which causes reabsorption of calcium and phosphate from the bones and eventual bone demineralization. As plasma calcium and phosphate levels rise, the plasma calcium phosphate product level also rises; the excess calcium phosphate is deposited as metastatic calcifications in joints, soft tissue, eyes, heart, and brain. These metastatic calcifications decrease function of the involved organs. Administering phosphate binders, such as aluminum hydroxide (Amphojel), aluminum carbonate (Basaljel), calcium carbonate (BioCal), or calcium acetate (Phos-Lo), with meals binds phosphate in the GI tract and decreases its absorption. Calcium and vitamin D supplements help support normal plasma calcium levels. Excess aluminum (absorbed from phosphate binders and from high levels of aluminum in water used to prepare dialysate) is deposited into the bones and exacerbates osteodystrophy.
2. With the patient, develop an activity and exercise schedule to avoid immobilization.	**2.** Immobilization increases bone demineralization.
3. *Question the patient daily about signs and symptoms of hypocalcemia:* numbness, tingling, and twitching of fingertips and toes; carpopedal spasms; seizures; and confusion.	**3.** Hypocalcemia causes central nervous system (CNS) irritability and alters nerve conduction. The signs and symptoms listed indicate tetany, hypocalcemia's most obvious manifestation.
4. *Monitor each ECG* (or ECG report) for prolonged QT interval, irritable arrhythmias, and atrioventricular conduction defects.	**4.** Hypocalcemia can alter normal cardiac electrical conduction.
5. *Assess for positive Chvostek's and Trousseau's signs,* daily. See appendix C, Fluid and electrolyte imbalances, for details.	**5.** Positive Chvostek's and Trousseau's signs indicate hypocalcemia.
6. Encourage the patient to comply with therapy.	**6.** Dialysis, medications, and diet work together to maintain acceptable calcium-phosphate balance.
7. Additional individualized interventions: _____	**7.** Rationales: _____

Nursing diagnosis

Imbalanced nutrition: Less than body requirements related to anorexia, nausea, vomiting, diarrhea, restricted dietary intake, GI inflammation with poor absorption, and altered metabolism of proteins, lipids, and carbohydrates

NURSING PRIORITY

Maintain acceptable nutritional status.

PATIENT OUTCOME CRITERIA

During the hospital stay, the patient will:
- maintain weight within 2 lb (1 kg) of ideal body weight

- exhibit BUN, serum sodium, potassium, albumin, and total protein levels within acceptable limits
- maintain preillness pattern of elimination.
  By the time of discharge, the patient will:
- plan a 3-day dietary intake (including fluid)
- demonstrate ability to weigh himself and to maintain weight and intake and output records.

INTERVENTIONS	RATIONALES
1. *Assess nutritional status on admission* by determining weight in relation to height and body build; serum albumin, protein, cholesterol, and transferrin values; triceps skinfold thickness; degree of weakness and fatigue; dietary intake; and history of anorexia, nausea, vomiting, and diarrhea.	**1.** A baseline assessment is necessary to monitor progress and the need to modify the patient's diet.
2. *Weigh the patient daily,* comparing actual and ideal body weights. Be sure to consider the effect of excess fluid on actual weight by comparing the current weight with nonedematous weight (500 ml fluid = 1 lb body weight). Teach the patient to measure weight under consistent conditions, to maintain a weight record, and to maintain an intake and output record.	**2.** Achieving ideal body weight is the goal. If the patient weighs less than the ideal body weight, additional calories may be added to the diet; if more, calorie restriction may be necessary.
3. Encourage the patient to eat the maximum amount of nutrients allowed. Encourage compliance with the dialysis regimen.	**3.** Diet and dialysis must complement each other to minimize toxin accumulation and maintain fluid and electrolyte and acid-base balance.
4. Encourage intake of foods high in calories from carbohydrates and low in protein, potassium, sodium, and water. Provide related teaching, including planning of food and fluid intake.	**4.** High-carbohydrate foods provide calories for energy and allow storage of dietary proteins. Restriction of potassium, sodium, and water is necessary to prevent electrolyte imbalances and volume overload. Protein is restricted to control the degree of uremia.
5. As necessary, consult with a dietitian to find ways to include the patient's preferences in the prescribed diet.	**5.** Including preferred foods makes the diet more palatable and increases dietary compliance.
6. Implement interventions to reduce nausea and vomiting, diarrhea or constipation, and stomatitis.	**6.** These conditions commonly result in anorexia or decreased GI absorption of nutrients.
7. *Monitor BUN, serum creatinine, sodium, potassium, albumin, and total protein* levels as indicators of dietary adequacy and compliance with dietary restrictions. (Consult with the physician regarding appropriate laboratory values for the patient.)	**7.** BUN levels may be elevated from excessive dietary protein; serum creatinine levels may be elevated from inadequate dietary protein and subsequent muscle breakdown; serum albumin levels are decreased in the malnourished patient; serum sodium and potassium levels are elevated by excessive intake. Appropriate laboratory values vary depending on the type of dialysis and other therapeutic measures, and so must be determined for the individual patient.
8. Additional individualized interventions: _____	**8.** Rationales: _____

> **Suggested NIC Interventions**
> *Diet staging; Nutrition management; Weight-gain assistance; Fluid monitoring; Nutritional monitoring*

> **Suggested NOC Outcomes**
> *Nutritional status: Food and fluid intake; Nutritional status: Nutrient intake; Weight control*

Renal disorders

Nursing diagnosis

Impaired oral mucous membrane related to accumulation of urea and ammonia

NURSING PRIORITY

Maintain intact oral mucous membrane.

PATIENT OUTCOME CRITERION

Throughout the hospital stay, the patient will maintain clean, moist oral mucous membrane without ulcers, bleeding, or signs of infection

INTERVENTIONS	RATIONALES
1. *On admission, inspect oral mucous membrane for ulcers and bleeding.*	**1.** Early detection and treatment can lessen consequences of severe stomatitis. (Excessive uremic toxins cause stomatitis.)
2. *Teach the patient an appropriate mouth care regimen* that includes rinsing with a dilute vinegar mouthwash as needed, using a soft toothbrush to clean teeth at least twice daily, sucking sour candies or lemon wedges as needed, and drinking cool liquids (within fluid restrictions).	**2.** Vinegar achieves the same results by neutralizing ammonia. A soft toothbrush reduces the risk of bleeding, and frequent mouth care decreases bacterial growth and the chance of infection. Sour candies or lemon wedges improve taste in the mouth while decreasing thirst.
3. Encourage the patient to comply with therapy.	**3.** Dialysis removes uremic toxins, which are partly responsible for stomatitis.
4. Additional individualized interventions: _____	**4.** Rationales: _____

> *Suggested NIC Interventions*
> Skin surveillance

> *Suggested NOC Outcomes*
> Tissue integrity: Skin and mucous membranes

Collaborative problem

Risk for peripheral neuropathy related to effects of uremia, fluid and electrolyte imbalances, and acid-base imbalances on the peripheral nervous system

NURSING PRIORITY

Ameliorate effects of peripheral neuropathy.

PATIENT OUTCOME CRITERION

Throughout the hospital stay, the patient will ambulate and carry out ADLs safely and comfortably.

INTERVENTIONS	RATIONALES
1. On admission, have a physical therapist *assess muscle strength, gait, and degree of neuromuscular impairment.*	**1.** A baseline assessment is essential for devising an individualized activity and exercise schedule.
2. In collaboration with a physical therapist, help the patient develop an activity and exercise regimen.	**2.** Regular activity and exercise prevent the hazards of immobility.
3. *Guard against leg and foot trauma.*	**3.** With decreased peripheral sensation, the patient may be unaware of impending trauma.

4. Administer analgesics as ordered and indicated; observe for desired effects.

5. Encourage the patient to comply with therapy.

6. Additional individualized interventions: _____
_____

4. Analgesics may be necessary for severe pain; if the medication ordered is excreted by the kidneys, observe for toxic effects.

5. Dialysis removes uremic toxins and improves fluid and electrolyte and acid-base balance.

6. Rationales: _____
_____

Nursing diagnosis

Risk for impaired skin integrity related to decreased activity of oil and sweat glands, scratching, capillary fragility, abnormal blood clotting, anemia, retention of pigments, and calcium phosphate deposits on the skin

NURSING PRIORITIES
- Maintain intact skin.
- Relieve dryness and itching.

PATIENT OUTCOME CRITERIA
Throughout the hospital stay, the patient will:
- maintain intact, clean, infection-free skin
- exhibit relief from dryness and itching.

INTERVENTIONS	**RATIONALES**
1. On admission and twice daily, *assess skin for color, turgor, ecchymoses, texture, and edema.*	**1.** A baseline assessment is essential for developing an individualized plan of skin care. Regular follow-up assessments allow modification as necessary.
2. Keep the skin clean while relieving dryness and itching using superfatted soap, oatmeal baths, and bath oils; apply lotion daily and as needed, especially while the skin is still moist after bathing.	**2.** These measures help relieve dry skin. Applying lotion immediately after bathing helps the skin retain moisture. Itching decreases when the skin is kept moist; decreased itching prevents scratching and subsequent skin excoriation.
3. Keep the patient's nails trimmed.	**3.** Trimming the patient's nails prevents excoriation from scratching.
4. *Monitor serum calcium and phosphorus levels weekly.*	**4.** Excess calcium phosphate deposited in the skin causes dryness and itching.
5. *Administer phosphate binders,* as ordered.	**5.** These medications decrease serum phosphate levels and thus lessen irritating deposits in the skin.
6. *Administer antipruritic medications,* as indicated and ordered; assess effects.	**6.** These medications are indicated in severe pruritus when other measures aren't effective.
7. Encourage the patient to comply with therapy.	**7.** Dialysis removes uremic toxins that dry and irritate the skin and helps normalize serum calcium and phosphorus levels.
8. Additional individualized interventions: _____	**8.** Rationales: _____

> ### *Suggested NIC Interventions*
> *Pressure management; Pressure ulcer care; Skin surveillance; Incision site care; Wound care*

> ### *Suggested NOC Outcomes*
> *Tissue integrity: Skin and mucous membranes; Wound healing: Primary intention; Wound healing: Secondary intention*

Nursing diagnosis

Disturbed thought processes related to the effects of uremic toxins, acidosis, fluid and electrolyte imbalances, and hypoxia on the CNS

NURSING PRIORITY
Protect the patient from neurologic complications.

PATIENT OUTCOME CRITERIA
By the time of discharge, the patient will:
- show improved memory and reasoning ability
- show an increased interest in ADLs
- show no neurologic complications, such as seizures and encephalopathy.

INTERVENTIONS	RATIONALES
1. On admission and daily, *assess the patient's thought processes.* With assistance from his family, compare current findings with premorbid intellectual status.	**1.** The premorbid status provides guidelines for establishing realistic goals. Ongoing assessment allows prompt detection of any changes and modification of treatment as needed.
2. Alter communication methods, as needed.	**2.** The patient will typically require short periods of simple communication, responding best to direct questions.
3. *Minimize environmental stimuli.* Alter the environment as needed to ensure the patient's safety.	**3.** Excessive environmental stimuli may cause sensory overload and disorientation. The patient usually functions best in a consistently quiet, organized environment that's free from hazards.
4. *Don't administer opiates or barbiturates.*	**4.** Opiates and barbiturates have an increased half-life in renal failure. Mental status worsens as a result.
5. Encourage the patient to comply with therapy, including following dietary restrictions, undergoing dialysis, and taking epoetin alfa as directed.	**5.** Dietary restrictions and dialysis are essential to control uremic toxin buildup and fluid and electrolyte and acid-base balance, and to reduce the risk of adverse effects on the CNS. Epoetin alfa enhances RBC production, increasing oxygen delivery to the brain.
6. Additional individualized interventions: _____	**6.** Rationales: _____

> **Suggested NIC Interventions**
> *Health education; Learning facilitation; Learning readiness; Enhancement; Teaching: Individual*

> **Suggested NOC Outcomes**
> *Adherence behavior; Compliance behavior; Treatment behavior: Illness or injury*

Nursing diagnosis

Noncompliance (treatment regimen) related to knowledge deficit; lack of resources; adverse effects of diet, dialysis, and medications; denial; and lack of social support systems

NURSING PRIORITY
Help the patient make informed choices about compliance and noncompliance.

PATIENT OUTCOME CRITERIA
Throughout the hospital stay, the patient will:
- state knowledge of the therapeutic regimen
- express commitment to comply with therapeutic regimen or a realistic treatment alternative more in keeping with personal beliefs and lifestyle.

By the time of discharge, the patient will:
- explain the cause and implications of the disease
- name each medication and its dosage, interval, desired effects, and adverse effects
- describe associated problems, how to manage them, and when to report them
- explain the plan for follow-up care.

INTERVENTIONS	RATIONALES
1. *Clarify the patient's understanding of the therapeutic regimen and the consequences of noncompliance.*	**1.** In many cases, noncompliance results from the patient's lack of understanding about the nature of the disease and the objectives of therapy.
2. Assess for physiologic, psychological, social, and cultural factors that could contribute to noncompliance. Explore ways to alter treatment to fit the patient's social and cultural beliefs.	**2.** Many patients deny that they have a chronic, irreversible illness. Compliance is more likely if treatment is congruent with the patient's beliefs.
3. *Teach the patient about the therapeutic regimen,* including medications, common problems related to CRF and their management, and plans for follow-up care. Clarify areas of misunderstanding in relation to the disease and therapeutic regimen. Allow the patient to make as many informed decisions and choices from as many alternatives as possible.	**3.** The patient is more likely to comply if encouraged to participate in decision making and allowed maximum independence. Thus, each patient requires an individualized care plan that considers physiologic, psychosocial, and cultural factors and the patient's desires.
4. Additional individualized interventions: _____	**4.** Rationales: _____

> **Suggested NIC Interventions**
> *Health education; Self-modification assistance; Self-responsibility facilitation; Health system guidance; Mutual goal setting; Energy management; Nutrition management; Teaching: Disease process; Teaching: Individual*

> **Suggested NOC Outcomes**
> *Adherance behavior; Compliance behavior; Symptom control; Treatment behavior: Illness or injury*

Nursing diagnosis
Sexual dysfunction related to the effects of uremia on the endocrine system and CNS and to the psychosocial impact of CRF and its treatment

NURSING PRIORITY
Help the patient and spouse (or partner) achieve satisfying sexual expression.

PATIENT OUTCOME CRITERIA
Throughout the hospital stay, the patient will:
- express concerns about sexual and reproductive functioning with spouse or partner
- express satisfaction with sexual relationship with spouse or partner.

INTERVENTIONS	RATIONALES
1. Discuss with the patient and spouse (or partner) the meaning of sexuality and reproduction to them, how changes in sexual functioning affect masculine and feminine roles, and mutual goals for their sexual functioning.	**1.** Sexuality and reproduction assume different levels of significance at various stages of maturity and at various times during CRF. Sex drive varies from person to person; therefore, sexuality and reproduction are personal experiences. Sexual dysfunction affects sex role in many ways, based on experiences and expectations. Thus, the nurse must explore sexuality with the couple to establish baseline data and to determine their mutual goals.
2. *Evaluate the couple's receptiveness to learning,* and discuss alternative methods of sexual expression.	**2.** If impotence or decreased libido is present or if intercourse causes fatigue, and if the couple is receptive to experimentation, then fellatio, cunnilingus, or mutual masturbation may provide sexual gratification.
3. Emphasize the importance of giving and receiving love and affection as alternatives to intercourse.	**3.** Sexual intercourse and orgasm aren't necessarily the goal of all meaningful intimate interactions: Love and affection are also important in strengthening a relationship.
4. Consult with the physician about the appropriateness of a penile prosthesis for a male patient, if indicated.	**4.** If a male patient can't achieve or maintain an erection, a penile prosthesis may provide a means for successful intercourse.
5. Additional individualized interventions: _____	**5.** Rationales: _____

Suggested NIC Interventions
Sexual counseling

Suggested NOC Outcomes
Sexual functioning

Nursing diagnosis
Deficient knowledge (vascular access care) related to lack of exposure to information

NURSING PRIORITY
Teach the patient about care and precautions related to vascular access. (If the patient is receiving peritoneal dialysis, consult the "Renal dialysis" care plan, page 713.)

PATIENT OUTCOME CRITERIA
Throughout the hospital stay, the patient will:
- describe all protective measures appropriate to the vascular access
- correctly demonstrate the procedure for checking fistula patency
- describe specific measures to control bleeding
- state how to contact a nephrology professional.

INTERVENTIONS	RATIONALES
1. *Emphasize the patient's crucial role in protecting the vascular access.*	**1.** The vascular access is essential for hemodialysis. Loss of access may disrupt the dialysis schedule and require surgery. Various vascular access methods may be used. The most common is the internal arteriovenous fistula, an internal surgical anastomosis of an artery and vein. It's usually placed in the nondominant forearm and requires 2 to 3 months for the venous wall to thicken and the fistula to distend. The major complications are occlusion and postdialysis bleeding.

2. *Explain these activity restrictions for the affected extremity:*
– Don't wear constrictive clothing or jewelry.
– Don't carry heavy objects.
– Don't allow blood pressure measurements.
– Don't allow venipunctures for I.V. fluids or laboratory blood specimens.
– Don't lie on the access.

3. *Teach these additional measures to maintain fistula patency:*
– Assess patency daily by feeling for pulsation at the anastomosis site.

– If pulsation is absent, contact a nephrology professional immediately.
– If a pressure dressing is applied after dialysis, remove it after 4 hours.

– Check needle insertion sites for bleeding for 4 hours after dialysis, or longer if bleeding occurs.

4. Additional individualized interventions: _____
_____

2. These activities threaten the integrity of the vascular access and may cause occlusion, dislodgment, or infection.

3. These interventions protect the patency of the internal fistula:
– Because the fistula is internal, patency can't be determined visually. Pulsation is caused by the surge of arterial blood into the vein to which the artery has been anastomosed.
– Loss of pulsation implies impending loss of patency. A clotted fistula may require surgery.
– Direct pressure on the venipuncture sites is necessary to control bleeding. Usually 10 minutes of firm finger pressure is sufficient, but at times a pressure dressing may be applied. If left on too long, a pressure dressing may cause occlusion.
– Because the patient is heparinized during hemodialysis, bleeding may occur after dialysis.

4. Rationales: _____
_____

> **Suggested NIC Interventions**
> *Teaching: Disease process; Teaching: Individual; Teaching: Prescribed medication*

> **Suggested NOC Outcomes**
> *Knowledge: Disease process; Knowledge: Health behaviors; Knowledge: Treatment regimen*

Discharge planning

DISCHARGE CHECKLIST
Before discharge, the patient shows evidence of:
❏ ability to perform care of the fistula
❏ vital signs within expected parameters
❏ stable nutritional status
❏ intact skin
❏ ability to control pain using oral medications
❏ acceptable hemoglobin levels
❏ absence of pulmonary complications
❏ absence of cardiovascular complications
❏ ability to comply with and tolerate diet and fluid restrictions
❏ weight within expected parameters
❏ home support adequate to ensure compliance with therapy or appropriate referrals made for follow-up care
❏ appropriate activity tolerance
❏ absence of fever and other signs of infection
❏ ability to manage ADLs.

TEACHING CHECKLIST
Document evidence that the patient and his family demonstrate an understanding of:
❏ cause and implications of renal failure
❏ purpose of dialysis
❏ all discharge medications' purpose, dosage, administration schedule, desired effects, and adverse effects (usual discharge medications include antihypertensives, phosphate binders, calcium, vitamin D, folic acid, iron, vitamins B and C, and others, depending on patient's response to the disease)
❏ recommended diet and fluid modifications
❏ common problems related to CRF and their management
❏ care of the fistula (if receiving hemodialysis)
❏ how to obtain and record weights
❏ how to measure and record blood pressure and pulse rate
❏ how to maintain an intake and output record
❏ problems to report to health care provider
❏ financial and community resources to assist with treatment of CRF

❑ dialysis schedule, location of dialysis facility, and day and time of appointments
❑ resources for counseling
❑ how to contact the physician or nephrology nurse.

DOCUMENTATION CHECKLIST
Using outcome criteria as a guide, document:
❑ clinical status on admission
❑ significant changes in status
❑ pertinent laboratory and diagnostic test findings
❑ response to medication
❑ physical and psychological response to dialysis
❑ nutritional intake
❑ activity and exercise tolerance
❑ ability to perform self-care
❑ compliance with therapy
❑ patient and family teaching
❑ discharge planning (postdischarge referrals and plans for long-term and follow-up care).

Associated care plans

▪ Acute pain
▪ Anemia
▪ Dying
▪ Grieving
▪ Ineffective individual coping
▪ Knowledge deficit
▪ Renal dialysis

References

Alfaro-Lefevre, R. *Applying Nursing Process: Promoting Collaborative Care.* 5th ed. Philadelphia: Lippincott Williams & Wilkins, 2002.

Greenberg, A. (ed). *Primer on Kidney Diseases.* 2nd ed. San Diego: Academic Press, 1998.

Nursing Procedures, 3rd ed. Springhouse, Pa.: Springhouse Corp., 2000.

Parker, J. (ed). *Contemporary Nephrology Nursing.* American Nephrology Nurses, 1997. (Classic)

Schrier, R. (ed). *Manual of Nephrology,* 5th ed. Philadelphia: Lippincott Williams & Wilkins, 2000.

Ileal conduit urinary diversion

DRG INFORMATION

DRG 303   Kidney, Ureter, and Major Bladder Procedure for Neoplasm.
Mean LOS = 8.4 days

DRG 304   Kidney, Ureter, and Major Bladder Procedure for Nonneoplasm with Complication or Comorbidity (CC).
Mean LOS = 8.8 days

DRG 305   Kidney, Ureter, and Major Bladder Procedure for Nonneoplasm without CC.
Mean LOS = 3.7 days

Introduction

DEFINITION AND TIME FOCUS

An ileal conduit urinary diversion, also known as a *urostomy* or *Bricker procedure,* is the most common urinary diversion procedure for adults. It's usually performed with a cystectomy and involves isolating a 6½" to 8½" (15 to 20.5 cm) segment of the terminal ileum, with its mesentery intact, then reanastomosing the GI tract. The proximal end of the isolated ileal segment is sutured closed, and the distal end of the ileal segment is brought out through the right lower abdominal quadrant and everted to form a stoma. The ureters are implanted into the body of the ileal segment, which then becomes a conduit for urine. Other segments of the small or large intestine can be used as conduits for urinary diversion, especially if the ileum has been damaged by radiation.

Ileal conduit urinary diversion is most commonly performed for transitional cell cancer of the bladder; however, in rare instances, it may also be done for other conditions requiring total cystectomy, such as severe trauma to the bladder or persistent, severe urinary tract infections (UTIs). This care plan focuses on the immediate preoperative and postoperative care of a patient undergoing ileal conduit diversion for transitional cell cancer of the bladder. (See *Clinical snapshot: Ileal conduit urinary diversion,* page 698.)

ETIOLOGY AND PRECIPITATING FACTORS

■ Transitional cell carcinoma, accounting for 90% of bladder cancers that require cystectomy — that is, lesions unresponsive to conservative treatment, lesions found at or near the bladder neck in the female, or deep infiltrating tumors that may involve the lymphatic system

Focused assessment guidelines

NURSING HISTORY (FUNCTIONAL HEALTH PATTERN FINDINGS)

Health-perception–health-management pattern

■ Sudden onset of gross painless hematuria, which may be intermittent

■ Treatment for transitional cell carcinoma of the bladder (being followed by cystoscopy every 3 to 6 months)

■ History of intravesical instillations of chemotherapeutic agents, such as thiotepa (Thioplex), mitomycin-C (Mutamycin), or doxorubicin (Adriamycin), after transurethral resection of a bladder tumor, or may have received intravesical bacillus Calmette-Guérin (BCG; TheraCys) as prophylactic treatment against tumor recurrence (BCG is most effective when combined with the others.)

■ Preoperative radiation therapy to shrink the tumor and reduce spread at the time of surgery. (10% to 15% of patients will develop bladder, bowel, or rectal complications.)

■ Fluorouracil (5-FU) use for recurrent or progressive invasive bladder cancer

■ Photodynamic techniques, which cause cancer cells to retain toxic chemicals

■ Limited information received from physician about upcoming urinary diversion surgery and its effects on activities of daily living (ADLs)

■ Increased risk if patient is between ages 50 and 70

■ Cigarette smoker (increases risk of bladder cancer)

Elimination pattern

■ History of urinary urgency or frequency for 3 to 8 months before diagnosis of transitional cell carcinoma of bladder

■ Cystitis as an adverse effect of intravesical chemotherapy

Sleep-rest pattern

■ Sleep disturbances from nocturia

Self-perception–self-concept pattern

■ Expressed negative feelings about self, along with anger; disappointment; fear of pain, mutilation, and loss of control; and distaste for altered bodily functions

Role-relationship pattern

■ Occupational exposure to dust and fumes from dyes, rubber, leather, leather products, paint, or organic chemicals (increases risk of bladder cancer)

■ Concern about spouse's or partner's adjustment to ostomy and possibility that ostomy may change that person's feelings toward the patient

■ Concerns about sexual dysfunction following cystectomy

Coping–stress tolerance pattern

■ With recent diagnosis of bladder cancer, concern about cancer treatment rather than the creation of an ostomy

Value-belief pattern

■ Delay in seeking medical attention because of fear combined with embarrassment over the intimate nature of problem

PHYSICAL FINDINGS

Transitional cell carcinoma may be asymptomatic except for the following symptoms.

Genitourinary

■ Gross hematuria
■ Urgency, frequency, and dysuria unrelieved by antibiotics

DIAGNOSTIC STUDIES

■ Complete blood count — drop in hematocrit and hemoglobin level may indicate internal bleeding; elevated white blood cell count may signify beginning of infection or abscess
■ Electrolyte panel — monitors fluid status and acid-base balance
■ Serum creatinine and blood urea nitrogen levels — used to monitor renal function

■ Preoperative excretory urography — helpful in evaluating upper urinary tract functioning; size and location of kidneys, filling of the renal pelvis, and outline of ureters
■ Postoperative conduitogram or loopogram — assesses length and emptying ability of the conduit along with the presence or absence of stricture, reflux, angulation, or obstruction
■ X-ray of kidneys, ureter, and bladder — indicates structural changes in the urinary tract along with presence or absence of stool or gas in GI tract

POTENTIAL COMPLICATIONS

■ Peritonitis
■ Leakage at point of GI anastomosis
■ Leakage at proximal end of the conduit
■ Ureteral-ileum anastomotic leakage
■ Abscess formation
■ Thrombophlebitis
■ Stoma necrosis
■ Ureteral obstruction from edema or mucus
■ Wound dehiscence
■ Small-bowel obstruction
■ Pneumonia
■ Ileus
■ Atelectasis
■ Wound infection
■ Mucocutaneous separation around stoma

CLINICAL SNAPSHOT ✳

Ileal conduit urinary diversion

Major nursing diagnoses and collaborative problems	Key patient outcomes
ND: Deficient knowledge (care of an ileal conduit)	On request, express understanding of upcoming surgery and its expected effects.
CP: Risk for postoperative peritonitis	Show no signs of peritonitis.
CP: Risk for stoma ischemia and necrosis	Have a viable stoma with red, moist mucosa.
CP: Risk for stoma retraction and mucocutaneous separation	Have a healed mucocutaneous border around a budded stoma.
ND: Impaired urinary elimination	Describe normal stoma and urine characteristics after creation of an ileal conduit.
ND: Disturbed body image	Express feelings about the ostomy.
ND: Deficient knowledge (care of the ileal conduit)	Change the pouch two to three times with minimal assistance from the nurse.
ND: Sexual dysfunction	Ask questions about impact on sexual function or agree to appropriate referrals.

Nursing diagnosis

Deficient knowledge (care of an ileal conduit) related to lack of exposure to information

NURSING PRIORITY
Prepare the patient physically and emotionally for upcoming urinary tract alterations.

PATIENT OUTCOME CRITERION
Before surgery, the patient will express understanding of upcoming surgery and its expected effects.

INTERVENTIONS

1. *Assess what the patient already knows about the upcoming cystectomy and creation of an ileal conduit** from information the physician has provided or from someone who has had an ostomy.

2. *Assess the patient's ability to learn.* Check occupation, level of education, and hobbies, and note if the patient may have difficulty learning.

3. *Assess the patient's manual dexterity and visual acuity, and determine if any sensory deficits are present.* Enlist the help of a family member, if possible and appropriate. Allow the patient to see and handle a pouch at eye level before surgery.

4. *Inquire about the patient's past and recent fluid intake habits,* especially quantity and preferred types of fluids.

5. *Describe construction of the conduit,* bowel preparation, and normal stoma characteristics.

6. *Anticipate problems with pouch use.* Assess the patient for allergies or sensitivity to tape or adhesives.

7. Request a physician's order for an enterostomal nurse to mark the stoma site before surgery. This mark should place the stoma away from old scars, dimples, the umbilicus, belt line, fat folds, and skin creases, and within the rectus muscle in a spot the patient can see. The stoma may be placed above the umbilicus in an obese patient or one who uses a wheelchair.

8. *If the patient is male, discuss what effect the cystectomy may have on sexual functioning.* Explain that a urologist or sex therapist can give him more information in the future.

9. Additional individualized interventions: _____

_____

RATIONALES

1. The patient may have received limited or confusing information from the physician. If the patient knows anyone with an ostomy, impressions gained from that person will strongly influence personal expectations of surgery and adaptation to the ostomy.

2. Learning difficulties, especially reduced reading ability, will affect the strategy and choice of literature used to teach ostomy care.

3. Degree of dexterity will affect the patient's ability to care for the stoma and apply a pouch effectively. If the patient can't care for the stoma, a family member is the best substitute. Handling the pouch before surgery increases later adaptation.

4. Inadequate fluid intake may cause odor problems from urine concentration and peristomal skin problems from dehydration.

5. The patient should know that an ileal conduit isn't a substitute bladder. Bowel preparation usually consists of 1 to 2 days of a clear liquid diet, a bowel-cleaning oral liquid such as polyethylene glycol and electrolyte solution the day before surgery, and then nothing by mouth after midnight the night before surgery.

6. Any allergy to these products suggests a need to patch-test the patient for sensitivity before selecting ostomy equipment.

7. The stoma should be marked where the pouch will have an optimal seal, giving the patient some sense of control. Placing the stoma within the rectus muscle reduces the risk of hernia or prolapse. To achieve independence, the patient must be able to see the stoma.

8. Informed consent includes the male patient's understanding that erectile dysfunction can be expected along with ejaculatory incompetence. It's important to give the patient "permission" to discuss sexual concerns.

9. Rationales: _____

_____

---

*Italics indicate key interventions.

Collaborative problem

Risk for postoperative peritonitis related to GI or genitourinary anastomosis breakdown or leakage

NURSING PRIORITY
Prevent and assess for signs of peritonitis.

PATIENT OUTCOME CRITERIA
Within 2 to 3 days after surgery, the patient will:
- have stabilized urine output
- have no gross hematuria.
  Within 4 to 5 days after surgery, the patient will:
- pass flatus
- have normal bowel sounds
- be afebrile
- show no signs of peritonitis.

INTERVENTIONS

1. *Monitor and document nasogastric (NG) tube patency, NG output, abdominal pain and distention, bowel sounds, and appearance of and drainage from the abdominal incision.*

2. *Evaluate for signs of GI anastomosis leakage and peritonitis,* such as paralytic ileus and abdominal pain with muscle rigidity, vomiting, and leukocytosis.

3. *Monitor for signs of urine leakage.* Assess carefully for pouch leakage to allow for accurate output measurement. Document characteristics of urine output, and presence of ureteral stents or catheters. When changing pouch (if necessary because of leakage), observe that urine is dropping from each stent. Also, note abdominal wound drainage, abdominal tenderness or distention, bowel sounds, and temperature.

4. Additional individualized interventions: _____
_____

RATIONALES

1. A dynamic ileus usually resolves within 72 hours after surgery. Changes in NG output, rapid abdominal distention, and crampy pain with hyperactive and tinkling bowel sounds may indicate small-bowel obstruction. Obstruction increases pressure on newly anastomosed sites.

2. A GI anastomosis is weakest until the 4th day after surgery. Leakage of intestinal secretions may result in peritonitis. I.V. fluids, electrolyte replacement, intestinal decompression, and appropriate I.V. antibiotic therapy are indicated if peritonitis is present.

3. Urine should be blood-tinged for only 1 to 2 days after surgery. Improper pouch fit or application can cause ongoing stomal bleeding. Ureteral stents prevent ureteral obstruction from edema or mucus; it's normal for urine to flow out around the stents. Signs of urine leakage may include a sudden decrease in urine output with a corresponding increase in drainage from the wound or a drain. Abdominal distention, an increase in abdominal pain, prolonged ileus, and fever may also indicate urine leakage. Small leaks may seal themselves within 8 to 12 hours; otherwise, surgery is needed.

4. Rationales: _____
_____

Collaborative problem
Risk for stoma ischemia and necrosis related to vascular compromise of conduit

NURSING PRIORITY
Monitor stoma viability.

PATIENT OUTCOME CRITERION
Immediately postoperatively and then continuously, the patient will have a viable stoma with red, moist mucosa.

INTERVENTIONS	RATIONALES
1. *Apply a disposable transparent urinary pouch,* as ordered, and attach the pouch to a bedside drainage bag.	**1.** A transparent pouch with continual bedside drainage allows visualization of the stoma.
2. *Observe the stoma for color changes* every 4 hours and as needed.	**2.** Color changes reflect adequacy of perfusion. Stoma should stay red or pink.
3. *Report color change of stoma* (to purple, brown, or black) immediately to the physician.	**3.** Color changes may imply ischemia leading to a necrotic, nonviable stoma. A necrotic stoma can develop from tension on the mesentery, possibly from abdominal distention; from twisting of the conduit during surgery; or from arterial or venous insufficiency. A necrotic stoma requires surgery.
4. To differentiate superficial ischemia from necrosis, insert a small, lubricated test tube about ½ (1.5 cm) into the stoma, then shine a flashlight into the lumen of the test tube. Observe for red, moist mucosa indicating that the body of conduit is viable.	**4.** If the inner lumen of conduit is viable, the stoma may be showing only minimal ischemia from edema; the stoma may then change color and appear viable. A dusky stoma may slough its outer layer during the next 5 to 7 days.
5. Additional individualized interventions: _____	**5.** Rationales: _____

Collaborative problem
Risk for stoma retraction and mucocutaneous separation related to peristomal trauma or tension on the intestinal mesentery

NURSING PRIORITIES
- Monitor the mucocutaneous border.
- Minimize the risk of separation.
- Encourage healing.

PATIENT OUTCOME CRITERION
By 5 to 7 days after surgery, the patient will have a healed mucocutaneous border around a budded stoma.

INTERVENTIONS	RATIONALES
1. *Apply a pouch with an antireflux valve,* as ordered. Make sure the opening of the adhesive barrier is ⅛″ (3 mm) larger than the diameter of the stoma.	**1.** An antireflux valve promotes healing by preventing urine from pooling on the stoma and mucocutaneous border. An opening that's too small can compromise circulation to the stoma at the mucocutaneous junction or lacerate the stoma.

Renal disorders

2. *If compatible with the pouch barrier, use a skin sealant under the pouch to protect and waterproof peristomal skin.*

3. If mucocutaneous separation occurs, protect the separated area and take measures to encourage granulation. Fill the mucocutaneous separation with desiccated hydrocolloid starch powder; then apply stoma adhesive paste and a properly sized skin barrier and pouch. Notify the surgeon of the separation.

4. Additional individualized interventions: _____
_____

2. Protecting and waterproofing the peristomal skin by routinely applying a skin sealant encourages healing of the mucocutaneous border and minimizes trauma when removing the pouch.

3. Mucocutaneous separation doesn't usually require surgery. The measures described increase the rate of healing and provide additional support for the stoma. If, however, the stoma retracts through the fascia into the peritoneum, peritonitis may develop and surgery is essential.

4. Rationales: _____
_____

Nursing diagnosis

Impaired urinary elimination related to creation of an ileal conduit

NURSING PRIORITIES
- Protect peristomal skin and contain urine.
- Teach the patient the conduit's function and purpose.

PATIENT OUTCOME CRITERIA

Within 3 days after surgery, the patient will:
- have intact skin around the stoma
- describe normal stoma and urine characteristics after creation of an ileal conduit.

INTERVENTIONS

1. *Maintain a good pouch seal, and protect peristomal skin with sealants.*

2. *Review the construction and function of the conduit,* assuring the patient of GI tract continuity. Use diagrams and pictures.

3. *Describe and show normal urine and stoma characteristics.* Explain the following: The conduit and stoma are made from the GI tract, so they have the same red, moist lining as the mouth. The stoma has no sensory nerve endings, so it's insensitive to pain. Without a sphincter, voluntary control of urination is gone. The stoma is vascular and may bleed when cleaned. The GI tract makes mucus, so mucus in the urine is to be expected.

4. Additional individualized interventions: _____
_____

RATIONALES

1. Urine can irritate and macerate the skin after prolonged contact.

2. Reviewing preoperative teaching after surgery reinforces information the patient may have forgotten or misunderstood. The patient should understand the nature of the surgery and its anatomical effects. The patient may mistakenly expect the ileal conduit to act as a substitute bladder.

3. The patient needs to know what is now normal. Blood in the urine can result from stomal bleeding. Urine will flow continuously from the stoma. There will be a greater amount of mucus in the urine during the early postoperative period, when oral intake is low, or when a urinary infection is present. The patient may mistake mucus for pus.

4. Rationales: _____
_____

Suggested NIC Interventions
Urinary elimination

Suggested NOC Outcomes
Tube care: Urinary; Urinary elimination

Nursing diagnosis

Disturbed body image related to urinary diversion

NURSING PRIORITIES
- Minimize damage to self-concept.
- Promote a healthy body image.

PATIENT OUTCOME CRITERIA
Within 2 to 4 days after surgery, the patient will:
- express feelings about the ostomy
- demonstrate ability to empty pouch in bathroom
- express confidence about ability to care for himself.

INTERVENTIONS	RATIONALES
1. Encourage the patient to express feelings and beliefs about the diagnosis, surgery, and stoma.	**1.** The patient may feel fear or isolation or may harbor misconceptions. Expression of feelings is the first step in the coping process.
2. *Allow for privacy when teaching ostomy care.*	**2.** Privacy encourages the patient to ask questions and facilitates learning.
3. Have the patient empty the pouch in the bathroom.	**3.** Mimicking normal bathroom behavior minimizes feelings of being disabled or different.
4. Suggest a visit from a United Ostomy Association (UOA) member (may also be helpful before surgery). The local chapter will be listed in the telephone directory's white pages.	**4.** The UOA provides the patient with fellowship, information, and support from others with ostomies. Seeing a well-adjusted person with an ostomy can encourage hope and provide a positive role model for the patient.
5. Show an accepting, tolerant attitude when performing or teaching ostomy care. Explain that wearing gloves is necessary to comply with standard precautions.	**5.** The nurse's acceptance and tolerance reassure the patient and facilitate advancement to complete self-care. The patient may perceive the nurse's gloves as a sign of unacceptance of or disgust for the new stoma.
6. Additional individualized interventions: _____	**6.** Rationales: _____

> **Suggested NIC Interventions**
> *Body image enhancement; Self-esteem enhancement*

> **Suggested NOC Outcomes**
> *Body image*

Nursing diagnosis

Deficient knowledge (care of the ileal conduit) related to lack of exposure to information

NURSING PRIORITY
Encourage independence in caring for the ileal conduit.

PATIENT OUTCOME CRITERIA
Within 5 days after surgery, the patient will:
- display learning readiness, such as looking at the stoma or holding wicks (rolled-up gauze or tampons) during pouch changes.

By the time of discharge, the patient will:
- change the pouch two or three times with minimal assistance from the nurse.

INTERVENTIONS	RATIONALES

INTERVENTIONS

1. *Instruct the patient how to empty the pouch when it's one-third to one-half full.* Demonstrate the emptying procedure using a pouch the patient isn't wearing. (A female can sit on the toilet to empty; a male can stand.)

2. *Demonstrate the use and care of the nighttime bedside drainage bag.* Run tubing from the drainage bag down the patient's pajama leg, or attach it to the leg with a Velcro strap. Attach the pouch, with urine in it, to the drainage bag. Explain that the drainage bag is easily cleaned with white vinegar and water or a commercial cleaner.

3. *Encourage the patient to change the pouch in the morning and provide step-by-step written instructions,* teaching the use of wicks, having the patient practice on a stoma model, explaining that he should clean urine and mucus from stoma and skin with warm water only, using a mirror if necessary to help him see the underside of the stoma, and having him apply the pouch while standing.

4. *Teach the patient how to treat minor peristomal skin irritations* using karaya powder and a skin sealant. Explain that momentary stinging may result if desiccated hydrocolloid starch powder or sealant is applied to denuded skin, but they should be used to prevent more serious peristomal skin complications.

5. *Explain fluid intake requirements.* Demonstrate pH testing of urine. Check pH routinely on the first few drops of urine in a freshly changed pouch. Warn against touching nitrazine paper to the skin or stoma. Explain why the patient shouldn't drink more than 3 or 4 glasses of citrus juice or milk per day.

6. List recommended ways to control urine odor through diet. Explain that pouches are odor-proof except during emptying and changing.

7. Define routine follow-up care, and explain the rationale for it.

RATIONALES

1. Emptying is usually taught first because it's done most often. A too-full pouch may pull away and have to be changed. Opening and closing the spout is easier to practice on a pouch the patient can hold out and see. Mimicking normal toileting behavior facilitates the patient's adjustment.

2. A bedside drainage bag prevents pouch overfilling and leakage at night. Attaching a partially filled pouch prevents suction vacuum, which can lead to overfilling and leakage. Cleaning keeps the drainage bag free from odor and urine sediment or crystals.

3. Written instructions promote continuity of care. Changing the pouch in the morning before consuming liquids will allow for less output during the procedure and an improved seal. Wicks are placed on the stoma to absorb urine and keep the peristomal skin dry so the pouch can seal. Practicing on a stoma model decreases fear and allows for repetition. Water is used for cleaning because soap can leave a film on the skin and disrupt the pouch seal. The patient needs to monitor the condition of the peristomal skin during each pouch change. Standing minimizes abdominal creases, which predispose the pouch to leakage.

4. Routinely applying a skin sealant before pouch application protects skin from adhesives and urine. Treating minor skin irritations with karaya powder and sealant minimizes the risk of serious complications. Intact, healthy skin increases a pouch's wearing time and prevents unexpected leaks.

5. Normal urine is acidic in a well-hydrated adult. Touching nitrazine paper to the skin or stoma will yield inaccurate results. The patient may need to drink 10 to 12 glasses of fluid daily to keep urine acidic; drinking large amounts of citrus juice or milk will negate this effect and make urine alkaline. Alkaline urine predisposes the patient to foul-smelling urine, urinary infections, peristomal skin irritations, stomal stenosis, increased mucus production from the conduit, urine crystals and calculi, and pyelonephritis.

6. Increased urine odor is associated with eating fish, eggs, asparagus, onions, and spicy foods.

7. The patient will see the urologist routinely every 6 to 12 months. Routine follow-up includes urine culture and sensitivity testing to rule out or detect infection, plus excretory urography or a renal scan to check upper urinary tract function and evaluate for recurrent tumor. The stoma and skin should be checked and pouch problems evaluated.

8. Address any special concerns the patient has about living with an ostomy. Consult an enterostomal nurse for specialized ostomy care.

9. Additional individualized interventions: _____
_____

8. Enterostomal nurses are specially trained to teach, counsel, and help rehabilitate the ostomy patient. They are knowledgeable about the newest pouch supplies and can assist the patient in coping with problems of daily living.

9. Rationales: _____
_____

Suggested NIC Interventions
Teaching: Disease process; Teaching: Individual; Teaching: Prescribed medication

Suggested NOC Outcomes
Knowledge: Disease process; Knowledge: Health behaviors; Knowledge: Treatment regimen

---

Nursing diagnosis

Sexual dysfunction: Male erectile dysfunction related to cystectomy and possible ejaculatory incompetence with prostatectomy

NURSING PRIORITIES
- Help the patient maximize remaining sexual function.
- Provide information or referrals as needed.

PATIENT OUTCOME CRITERION
During the postoperative teaching phase, the patient will ask questions about impact on sexual function or agree to appropriate referrals.

INTERVENTIONS

1. Assess the patient's readiness to discuss sexual matters. If the patient isn't ready, arrange for outpatient follow-up.

2. Describe the separate nerve pathways for sexual excitement, erection, ejaculation, and orgasm. Explain which ones may be affected by surgery and why.

3. If indicated, mention alternatives, such as a penile prosthesis or external devices that aid erection. Refer the patient to the urologist or enterostomal nurse for details.

4. Additional individualized interventions: _____
_____

RATIONALES

1. The patient may deny interest in resumption of sexual activity at first, while learning to cope with the ostomy and the diagnosis of cancer.

2. Cystectomy may only affect the patient's ability to experience erection or ejaculation, or it may affect both.

3. The patient may need specific suggestions for resumption of fulfilling sexual activity. A urologist may surgically implant a penile prosthesis or prescribe medications to facilitate erections. The enterostomal nurse can counsel the patient on alternatives, help obtain information on external devices, and suggest ways to minimize the ostomy's presence during sex.

4. Rationales: _____
_____

Suggested NIC Interventions
Sexual counseling

Suggested NOC Outcomes
Sexual identity: Acceptance

Renal disorders

Discharge planning
DISCHARGE CHECKLIST
Before discharge, the patient shows evidence of:
- ❏ a viable stoma
- ❏ stable vital signs
- ❏ stable nutritional status
- ❏ absence of pulmonary or cardiovascular complications
- ❏ adequate support system for postdischarge assistance and ability to perform stoma care
- ❏ referral to home care if indicated by lack of a home support system or inability to perform ADLs and stoma care
- ❏ absence of fever
- ❏ ability to control pain using oral analgesics
- ❏ no need for I.V. support (discontinued for at least 24 hours before discharge)
- ❏ bowel sounds
- ❏ healing incision with no redness or other sign of infection
- ❏ ability to ambulate at preoperative level.

TEACHING CHECKLIST
Document evidence that the patient and his family demonstrate an understanding of:
- ❏ extent of tumor and resection
- ❏ nature of urinary diversion and its construction
- ❏ incision care (if not healed)
- ❏ procedure for emptying and changing pouch
- ❏ use and cleaning of bedside drainage system
- ❏ treatment of minor peristomal skin irritations
- ❏ written list of supplies and suppliers, with physician's prescription to facilitate insurance payment
- ❏ chemotherapy (if needed) and its expected adverse effects
- ❏ availability of support groups, such as UOA and the American Cancer Society (list their telephone numbers)
- ❏ amount and types of fluids preferred, along with any dietary considerations such as avoiding odor-causing foods
- ❏ signs and symptoms to report to the physician, such as fever, flank pain, or hematuria
- ❏ concerns to report to the enterostomal nurse, such as pouch problems and skin or stoma problems
- ❏ signs and symptoms of UTI
- ❏ considerations in resuming sexual activity
- ❏ date and time of follow-up appointments
- ❏ how to contact the physician
- ❏ how to contact the enterostomal nurse.

DOCUMENTATION CHECKLIST
Using outcome criteria as a guide, document:
- ❏ clinical status on admission
- ❏ significant changes in status

- ❏ pertinent laboratory and diagnostic test findings
- ❏ preoperative marking of stoma site
- ❏ preoperative teaching
- ❏ bowel preparation
- ❏ UOA visitor recommendation (if appropriate)
- ❏ stoma viability
- ❏ mucocutaneous border and sutures
- ❏ urine characteristics
- ❏ patient's response to ostomy
- ❏ fluid intake and output
- ❏ presence of stents
- ❏ GI status
- ❏ incision status
- ❏ patient's progress in learning ostomy care
- ❏ patient and family teaching
- ❏ discharge planning.

Associated care plans
- ■ Compromised family coping
- ■ Grieving
- ■ Ineffective individual coping
- ■ Knowledge deficit
- ■ Perioperative care

References
Current Medical Diagnosis & Treatment 2002, 41st Ed. Edited by Lawrence Tierney, et al. Stamford, Conn.: Appleton & Lange, 2002.

Jordan, K. (ed). *Emergency Nursing Core Curriculum.* Emergency Nurses Association. Philadelphia: W.B. Saunders Co., 2000.

Lynn-McHale, D.J., and Carlson, K.K. American Association of Critical Care Nurses *AACN Procedure Manual for Critical Care,* 4th ed. Philadelphia: W.B. Saunders Co., 2001.

Nursing Procedures & Protocols. Springhouse, Pa.: Lippincott Williams & Wilkins, 2003.

Shoemaker, W.C., et al. *Textbook of Critical Care,* 4th ed. Philadelphia: W.B. Saunders Co., 2002.

Nephrectomy

DRG INFORMATION
DRG 303   Kidney, Ureter, and Major Bladder Procedures for Neoplasm.
Mean LOS = 8.4 days

DRG 304   Kidney, Ureter, and Major Bladder Procedures for Nonneoplasms with Complication or Co-morbidity (CC).
Mean LOS = 8.8 days

DRG 305   Kidney, Ureter, and Major Bladder Procedures for Nonneoplasms without CC.
Mean LOS = 3.7 days

Introduction
DEFINITION AND TIME FOCUS
Kidney removal may be necessary for various reasons. The reason for the excision dictates the surgical approach. The flank or lumbar approach, the traditional approach through the retroperitoneum, is indicated in inflammatory renal disease, calculi, perinephric abscess, hydronephrosis, and renal cystic disease. The transabdominal approach allows easy access to the renal vessels, as is required in renal tumors, trauma, or renal vascular disease. Either approach may be used to remove a kidney for transplantation.

This care plan focuses on the immediate preoperative and postoperative care for the patient undergoing nephrectomy. Refer to the "Perioperative care" care plan, page 146, for more detailed information on preoperative and postoperative care. (See *Clinical snapshot: Nephrectomy*, page 708.)

ETIOLOGY AND PRECIPITATING FACTORS
- Renal tumors (benign or malignant)
- Obstructive uropathy (intrinsic or extrinsic), including renal calculi, vascular lesions (such as abdominal aortic aneurysm), pelvic disorders (such as endometriosis), GI disorders (such as Crohn's disease), retroperitoneal disorders (such as tumor or abscess), or effects of radiation therapy
- Blunt or penetrating trauma
- Kidney donation

Focused assessment guidelines
NURSING HISTORY (FUNCTIONAL HEALTH PATTERN FINDINGS)
Health-perception–health-management pattern
- History of concomitant health problems if the patient is older (such as diabetes mellitus, hypertension, hyper-parathyroidism, or vascular disease) that contributed to need for nephrectomy
- Concerns or fears about maintaining normal kidney function after surgery
- Concerns about diet and activity restrictions and need for adjuvant therapies after surgery
- History of contact with nephrotoxic substances

Activity-exercise pattern
- Fatigue

Nutritional-metabolic pattern
- Anorexia, nausea or vomiting, or weight loss

Self-perception–self-concept pattern
- Anxiety or depression

PHYSICAL FINDINGS
Cardiovascular
- Hypertension
- Tachycardia
- Edema
- Ecchymosis at injury site (with trauma)
- Hypotension (primarily with trauma)
- Signs of fluid overload (such as peripheral edema and distended neck veins)

Pulmonary
- Tachypnea
- Crackles

Genitourinary
- Dysuria
- Hematuria
- Oliguria
- Polyuria

Musculoskeletal
- Pain with movement
- Ecchymosis
- Muscle spasm (rarely)

Integumentary
- Diaphoresis
- Pallor

DIAGNOSTIC STUDIES
Diagnostic studies, performed before surgery, may reveal no significant abnormalities initially, unless related to a coexisting condition.
- Complete blood count — establishes baseline; may reveal preexisting disorder (such as anemia) or extent of blood loss from injury; white blood cell count may be elevated in response to injury
- Blood typing and crossmatching — allows blood replacement during surgery

- Chemistry panel — establishes baseline and reveals imbalances that may be related to renal dysfunction or that may affect care during surgery (such as potassium, calcium, or phosphate imbalances that may cause cardiac irritability during anesthesia); blood urea nitrogen and creatinine levels evaluate renal function
- Prothrombin time/international normalized ratio and partial thromboplastin time — establish baseline; some patients (older, obese, or with prosthetic valves) may receive anticoagulant therapy after surgery to minimize the risk of thromboembolism complications
- Urinalysis — establishes baseline and evaluates for presence of infection
- Chest X-ray — rules out preexisting conditions that may affect care during surgery

- 12-lead electrocardiography — establishes baseline and identifies preexisting cardiac abnormalities or pericardial effusion

POTENTIAL COMPLICATIONS
- Shock
- Hemorrhage
- Pulmonary embolism
- Pulmonary edema
- Atelectasis
- Pneumonia
- Wound infection, dehiscence, and evisceration
- Thrombophlebitis
- Paralytic ileus
- Acute renal failure

CLINICAL SNAPSHOT ✳

Nephrectomy

Major nursing diagnoses and collaborative problems	Key patient outcomes
ND: Deficient knowledge (perioperative procedures)	Verbalize understanding of perioperative procedures.
ND: Acute pain	Rate pain (while using pain medication) as less than 3 on a 0 to 10 pain rating scale.
CP: Risk for fluid and electrolyte imbalance	Have a urine output of 60 ml/hour or better.
CP: Risk for atelectasis	Display ABG levels within normal limits: pH, 7.35 to 7.45; $Paco_2$, 35 to 45 mm Hg; HCO_3^-, 23 to 28 mEq/L; and Sao_2, greater than 90%.
CP: Risk for postoperative paralytic ileus or intestinal obstruction	Have regular bowel movements.

Nursing diagnosis
Deficient knowledge (perioperative procedures) related to lack of exposure to information

NURSING PRIORITY
Prepare the patient for perioperative procedures.

PATIENT OUTCOME CRITERIA
Before surgery, the patient will:
- verbalize understanding of perioperative procedures
- demonstrate ability to perform coughing and deep-breathing exercises, use the incentive spirometer, splint the incision, and perform leg exercises.

INTERVENTIONS	**RATIONALES**
1. *See the "Knowledge deficit" care plan,** page 129.	1. General interventions related to patient teaching are included in the "Knowledge deficit" care plan. This care plan presents additional information about the nephrectomy patient's learning needs.

---

*Italics indicate key interventions.

2. See the "Perioperative care " care plan, page 146.

3. *Tell the patient where the incision will be made* (flank or abdomen), *whether to expect a chest tube* (for a flank incision) *or a drain* (for an abdominal incision), *and the potential effects of positioning during surgery.*

4. Additional individualized interventions: _____

2. General interventions related to perioperative procedures are included in the "Perioperative care" care plan.

3. Knowing what to expect decreases the patient's anxiety and increases the likelihood of compliance after surgery.

4. Rationales: _____

> **Suggested NIC Interventions**
> *Teaching: Disease process; Teaching: Individual; Teaching: Prescribed medication*

> **Suggested NOC Outcomes**
> *Knowledge: Disease process; Knowledge: Health behaviors; Knowledge: Treatment regimen*

Nursing diagnosis
Acute pain related to tissue injury, edema, or spasm after surgery

NURSING PRIORITY
Prevent or reduce pain.

PATIENT OUTCOME CRITERIA
Within 1 hour of pain onset, the patient will:
- rate pain (while using pain medication) as less than 3 on a 0 to 10 pain rating scale
- maintain vital signs within normal limits, typically: heart rate, 60 to 100 beats/minute; systolic blood pressure, 90 to 140 mm Hg; and diastolic blood pressure, 50 to 90 mm Hg.

INTERVENTIONS

1. See the "Acute pain" care plan, page 32.

2. Teach the patient about postoperative analgesia administration (injection, patient-controlled analgesia pump, or epidural infusion), potential adverse effects, and the importance of requesting medication before pain becomes severe.

3. Additional individualized interventions: _____

RATIONALES

1. The "Acute pain" care plan contains general interventions regarding pain management.

2. The patient is more likely to comply with postoperative care if pain is controlled.

3. Rationales: _____

> **Suggested NIC Interventions**
> *Pain management*

> **Suggested NOC Outcomes**
> *Pain control; Pain: Psychological response*

Collaborative problem
Risk for fluid and electrolyte imbalance related to decreased renal reserve and third-space fluid shifting immediately after surgery

NURSING PRIORITY
Prevent fluid and electrolyte imbalance.

PATIENT OUTCOME CRITERIA
Within 1 day after surgery, the patient will:
- have urine output of 30 ml/hour or greater
- have adequate I.V. or oral fluid intake
- exhibit normal electrolyte levels.
  By the time of discharge, the patient will:
- have urine output of 60 ml/hour or greater.

INTERVENTIONS	RATIONALES
1. See appendix C, Fluid and electrolyte imbalances.	1. The Fluid and electrolyte imbalances appendix contains detailed information on these imbalances.
2. *Preserve and protect the remaining kidney.*	2. Removal of one kidney makes preservation of remaining renal function imperative.
– Maintain adequate hydration. Monitor urine output, color, and specific gravity, as ordered. – Avoid or minimize use of nephrotoxic agents, such as aminoglycoside antibiotics and chemotherapeutic agents.	– Appropriate hydration preserves renal function and promotes efficient removal of metabolic wastes. – Nephrotoxic agents can damage the remaining kidney.
3. Additional individualized interventions: _____	3. Rationales: _____

Collaborative problem
Risk for atelectasis related to anesthesia, immobility, pain, presence of chest tube, and location of incision

NURSING PRIORITIES
- Maintain adequate oxygenation.
- Prevent pulmonary complications.

PATIENT OUTCOME CRITERIA
After surgery, the patient will:
- display ABG levels within normal limits: pH, 7.35 to 7.45; $Paco_2$, 35 to 45 mm Hg; HCO_3^-, 23 to 28 mEq/L; and Sao_2, greater than 90%
- have deep, unlabored respirations
- manifest audible, clear breath sounds in all lobes.

INTERVENTIONS	RATIONALES
1. Implement interventions listed under "Impaired gas exchange," page 149, in the "Perioperative care" care plan. As needed, *check pulmonary status frequently, help the patient to perform incentive spirometry, encourage frequent position changes, and promote early and progressive ambulation.*	1. In addition to the risk of atelectasis inherent to general anesthesia, the patient with a lumbar or flank incision is at increased risk because the intercostal muscles must be spread and the 12th rib may be removed. The resulting pain limits deep inspiration. If not detected and treated aggressively, atelectasis can lead to pneumonia. The "Perioperative care" care plan contains measures to prevent this complication.
2. Additional individualized interventions: _____	2. Rationales: _____

Collaborative problem

Risk for postoperative paralytic ileus or intestinal obstruction related to surgical manipulation, anesthesia, and immobility

NURSING PRIORITY

Promptly detect abnormal GI function.

PATIENT OUTCOME CRITERIA

By the time of discharge, the patient will:
- have normal, active bowel sounds
- tolerate a regular diet
- have regular bowel movements.

INTERVENTIONS	RATIONALES
1. Implement measures listed under "Risk for postoperative paralytic ileus," page 155, in the "Perioperative care" care plan. As appropriate, *assess the abdomen frequently, monitor nasogastric tube drainage, administer fluids, provide a diet appropriate to peristaltic activity, and encourage early and frequent ambulation.*	**1.** Bowel manipulation during nephrectomy increases the risk of paralytic ileus, the most common GI complication. Significant manipulation increases the risk of intestinal obstruction. The "Perioperative care" care plan details related interventions and their rationales.
2. Additional individualized interventions: _____	**2.** Rationales: _____

Discharge planning

DISCHARGE CHECKLIST

Before discharge, the patient shows evidence of:
- ❒ stable vital signs
- ❒ absence of cardiovascular or pulmonary complications
- ❒ absence of fever
- ❒ healing wound without signs or symptoms of infection (swelling, inflammation, tenderness, or drainage)
- ❒ ability to tolerate oral intake
- ❒ ability to ambulate and perform activities of daily living same as before surgery
- ❒ ability to void and have bowel movements same as before surgery
- ❒ ability to control pain using oral medications
- ❒ adequate home support system or referral to home health agency or nursing home, if indicated.

TEACHING CHECKLIST

Document evidence that the patient and his family demonstrate an understanding of:
- ❒ plan for resuming normal activity, with restrictions
- ❒ dietary recommendations
- ❒ wound care
- ❒ signs of wound infection or other complications

- ❒ all discharge medications' purpose, dosage, administration, and adverse effects requiring medical attention (discharge medications may include analgesics and antibiotics)
- ❒ necessary home care and referrals for follow-up care
- ❒ when and how to contact the physician
- ❒ date, time, and place of follow-up appointments.

DOCUMENTATION CHECKLIST

Using outcome criteria as a guide, document:
- ❒ clinical status on admission
- ❒ preoperative assessment and treatment
- ❒ preoperative teaching and its effectiveness
- ❒ preoperative checklist (usually includes documentation of operative consent, pertinent laboratory test results, skin preparation, voiding on call from the operating room, and removal of nail polish, jewelry, dentures, glasses, hearing aids, and prostheses — check hospital's specific requirements)
- ❒ postoperative assessment and treatment
- ❒ amount and character of drainage on dressing and through drains
- ❒ patency of I.V. lines, nasogastric tube, indwelling urinary catheter, and drains
- ❒ pulmonary hygiene
- ❒ pain-relief measures

❏ activity tolerance
❏ nutritional intake and tolerance
❏ fluid intake and output
❏ bladder and bowel function
❏ pertinent laboratory findings
❏ patient and family teaching
❏ discharge planning.

Associated care plans

■ Acute pain
■ Acute renal failure
■ Hypovolemic shock
■ Knowledge deficit
■ Perioperative care

References

Jordan, K. (ed). *Emergency Nursing Core Curriculum.* Emergency Nurses Association. Philadelphia: W.B. Saunders Co., 2000.

Lynn-McHale, D.J., and Carlson, K.K. American Association of Critical Care Nurses. *AACN Procedure Manual for Critical Care,* 4th ed. Philadelphia: W.B. Saunders Co., 2001.

Professional Guide to Diseases, 7th ed. Springhouse, Pa.: Springhouse Corp., 2001.

Shoemaker, W.C., et al. *Textbook of Critical Care,* 4th ed. Philadelphia: W.B. Saunders Co., 2002.

Smeltzer, S.C., and Bare, B.G. *Brunner and Suddarth's Textbook of Medical-Surgical Nursing,* 9th ed. Philadelphia: Lippincott Williams & Wilkins, 2000.

Tanago, E., and McAninch, J. *Smith's General Urology,* 15th ed. New York: McGraw-Hill Professional Publisher, 2000.

Renal dialysis

DRG INFORMATION
DRG 316   Renal Failure.
          Mean LOS = 6.6 days
DRG 449   Poisoning and Toxic Effects of Drugs; Age 17+.
          Mean LOS = 3.8 days
DRG 450   Poisoning and Toxic Effects of Drugs without Complication or Comorbidity (CC); Age 17 +.
          Mean LOS = 2.1 days
DRG 451   Poisoning and Toxic Effects of Drugs; Age 0 to 17.
          Mean LOS = 0 days
DRG 205   Disorders of the Liver except Malignancy, Cirrhosis, and Alcoholic Hepatitis with CC.
          Mean LOS = 6.2 days
DRG 206   Disorders of the Liver except Malignancy, Cirrhosis, and Alcoholic Hepatitis without CC.
          Mean LOS = 3.9 days

Renal dialysis is used to treat numerous disorders. Therefore, the diagnosis necessitating its use determines the DRG assigned. Examples of diagnoses for peritoneal dialysis are listed above.

Introduction
DEFINITION AND TIME FOCUS
Renal dialysis (RD) is a treatment process used to manage renal failure. RD is considered successful if two key outcomes are met: maintenance of the chemical balance of the blood and removal of excess water, solutes, and toxins from the body.

There are two main types of dialysis treatments: hemodialysis and peritoneal dialysis. *Hemodialysis* is a direct process that requires a vascular access and an artificial kidney machine. The patient's blood is pumped from the body into the machine, which removes excess water and impurities. The blood is then pumped back into the body. Usually, three treatments are required each week, each treatment lasting from 2 to 5 hours. *Peritoneal dialysis* (PD) is an indirect process that uses the peritoneal membrane as a dialyzing membrane. The dialysis solution is instilled through a catheter into the peritoneal cavity where it remains for a prescribed period of time (dwell time). The solution is then allowed to flow out (drain time) to remove excess water and waste products. The patient awaiting the creation of a vascular access for hemodialysis may receive PD until the vascular access is healed and functional. The number of treatments per week and length of treatments vary depending on the type of PD used and the need of the patient. This care plan focuses on the patient receiving PD or hemodialysis for the first time and then several times per week, as ordered and as necessary. (See *Clinical snapshot: Renal dialysis,* page 715.)

ETIOLOGY AND PRECIPITATING FACTORS
PD is indicated to treat chronic renal failure (CRF), acute renal failure (ARF), drug overdose, and hepatic coma. The patient awaiting hemodialysis whose vascular access device isn't yet operable may receive PD temporarily. Because RD isn't a diagnosis but a procedure, this care plan doesn't address specific illnesses. Refer to care plans for specific disorders for more information.

Focused assessment guidelines
NURSING HISTORY (FUNCTIONAL HEALTH PATTERN FINDINGS)
Health-perception–health-management pattern
- History of CRF or ARF
- Treatment for diabetes mellitus
- History of drug overdose or drug intolerance
- History of a clotting disorder or cardiovascular disease

Nutritional-metabolic pattern
- Anorexia, nausea, or vomiting
- Weight loss or diet intolerance

Elimination pattern
- Diminished urine output
- Constipation

Role-relationship pattern
- Inability to work or maintain usual roles because of chronic, disabling illness, treatment regimen, or both

Self-perception–self-concept pattern
- Verbalized decreased sense of self-worth

Coping–stress tolerance pattern
- Denial, anger, or depression over condition and needed treatment

Activity-exercise pattern
- Fatigue
- Shortness of breath or other signs of exercise intolerance

Value-belief pattern
- Religious or personal beliefs that don't allow blood transfusions

PHYSICAL FINDINGS
Cardiovascular
- Hypertension

- Periorbital, ankle, or sacral edema

Pulmonary
- Crackles
- Dyspnea

Gastrointestinal
- Nausea
- Anorexia
- Hiccoughs
- Constipation
- Stomatitis

Neurologic
- Lethargy
- Confusion
- Shortened attention span
- Restlessness

Integumentary
- Fragile skin
- Dry, flaky skin
- Yellow-gray skin hue
- Ecchymoses or purpura
- Poor skin turgor

Musculoskeletal
- Impaired mobility
- Bone deformities

DIAGNOSTIC STUDIES

- Creatinine clearance — determines glomerular filtration rate, which directly reflects renal function
  – normal, 85 to 150 ml/minute
  – mild renal failure, 50 to 84 ml/minute
  – moderate renal failure, 10 to 49 ml/minute
  – severe renal failure, less than 10 ml/minute
  – end-stage renal failure, 0 ml/minute
- Serum creatinine levels — determine renal function (normal is 1.0 to 1.4 mg/dl; elevation indicates renal impairment; see the "Chronic renal failure" care plan, page 680)
- Arterial blood gas (ABG) levels — determine acid-base abnormalities (normal pH is 7.35 to 7.45; the patient in renal failure is usually acidotic)
- serum electrolyte levels — usually show hyperkalemia (greater than 5 mEq/L)
- Sodium level — may be low (less than 120 mEq/L) because of kidney's inability to conserve sodium
- Phosphate and calcium levels — commonly show hypocalcemia and hyperphosphatemia
- Blood urea nitrogen levels — elevated in renal failure, reduced in severe liver damage
- Complete blood count — hemoglobin level may be reduced from decreased erythropoietin production
- Erythrocyte sedimentation rate — increased if infection present
- Serum drug levels — determine degree of overdose
- Culture and sensitivity of PD drainage — identifies causative organism and appropriate antibiotic for peritoneal infection

- Chest X-ray — rules out heart failure
- Electrocardiogram — determines cardiac status

POTENTIAL COMPLICATIONS
- Peritonitis (in patients receiving PD)
- Respiratory distress
- Cardiac arrhythmias
- Hypovolemia or hypervolemia
- Hyperglycemia
- Electrolyte imbalance
- Bowel or bladder perforation (in patients receiving PD)
- Thrombosis of vascular access (in patients receiving PD)
- Infection of vascular access (in patients receiving PD)

Renal dialysis

Major nursing diagnoses and collaborative problems	Key patient outcomes
CP: Risk for air embolism	Won't experience air embolism.
CP: Risk for confusion	Remain oriented to time, place, and person.
CP: Risk for transfusion reaction	Won't experience a blood transfusion reaction.
ND: Risk for injury related to bleeding from area around vascular access device	Have minimal bleeding from vascular access.
ND: Acute pain related to hemodialysis treatment	Rate pain as less than 3 on a 0 to 10 pain rating scale.
ND: Impaired physical mobility	Maintain normal function and mobility.
ND: Risk for injury: Perforation or ileus	Be free from trauma, injury, or bleeding.
ND: Ineffective breathing pattern	Show no dyspnea.
CP: Risk for fluid imbalance	Have a dialysate deficit less than 500 ml.
ND: Risk for infection	Be afebrile, have no exudate, edema, redness, or leakage at the catheter site or vascular access site.
ND: Acute pain related to diasylate temperature or rapid in-flow	Rate pain as less than 3 on a 0 to 10 pain rating scale.
ND: Imbalanced nutrition: Less than body requirements	Tolerate oral intake of at least 0.5 g/kg of ideal weight daily and 45 to 50 kcal/kg/day.

Collaborative problem

Risk for air embolism during and after dialysis treatment

NURSING PRIORITY
Maintain airtight system and monitor for signs of air embolism.

PATIENT OUTCOME CRITERION
During treatment the patient won't experience air embolism.

INTERVENTIONS	RATIONALES
1. *Ensure that all tubing connections are secure to prevent introduction of air into the system. Monitor fluid levels and tubing during treatment.**	1. The introduction of air into the tubing or system may cause an air embolism.
2. *Monitor skin color and rate, rhythm, depth, and effort of respirations. Auscultate breath sounds.*	2. Monitoring skin color and rate, rhythm, depth, and effort of respirations as well as auscultating breath sounds ensure airway patency and adequate gas exchange.
3. Additional individualized interventions: _____	3. Rationales: _____

*Italics indicate key interventions.

Collaborative problem

Risk for confusion related to consequences of long-term dialysis treatment

NURSING PRIORITY

Provide for security and safety.

PATIENT OUTCOME CRITERION

During treatment, the patient will remain oriented to time, place, and person.

INTERVENTIONS	RATIONALES
1. *Assess the patient's level of cognition at each treatment.*	**1.** Dialysis dementia is caused by the accumulation of aluminum in the brain as a result of long-term dialysis
2. *Monitor for signs of depression.*	**2.** Depression may result when long-term treatment regimens, such as hemodialysis, are implemented
3. Additional individualized interventions: _____ _____	**3.** Rationales: _____ _____

Collaborative problem

Risk for transfusion reaction related to multiple (repeat) transfusions

NURSING PRIORITY

Ensure the patient's safety.

PATIENT OUTCOME CRITERIA

During treatment, the patient won't experience a blood transfusion reaction.

INTERVENTIONS	RATIONALES
1. *Strictly follow your facility's policy and procedures regarding blood typing and transfusion administration.* *	**1.** Following facility policy helps to maintain patient safety during the procedure.
2. *Monitor the patient closely for signs of blood transfusion reaction, such as* chills, fever, back pain, chest tightness, or difficulty breathing.	**2.** Transfusion reaction is a medical emergency.
3. Stop the blood transfusion and flush the catheter with saline if reaction is suspected.	**3.** Stopping the transfusion and flushing the catheter with saline maintains an open venous access.
4. Additional individualized interventions: _____ _____	**4.** Rationales: _____ _____

Nursing diagnosis

Risk for injury related to bleeding from the area around the vascular access device; potential for thrombosis, stenosis or hematoma of vascular access

NURSING PRIORITY

Prevent or promptly detect and report injuries related to dialysis.

PATIENT OUTCOME CRITERION

During treatment, the patient will have minimal bleeding from vascular access (venous access is patent and free from thrombosis, stenosis or hematoma).

INTERVENTIONS	RATIONALES
1. *Observe for and report any unusual bleeding from the site.*	1. Anemia, decreased production of erythropoietin and loss of blood during dialysis may precipitate bleeding.
2. *Assess the patency of fistula prior to beginning each treatment. Assess for the bruit and thrill every shift.*	2. Patency of the vascular access device is vital for the success of dialysis treatment. If the vascular access device isn't patent, surgical intervention may be required to modify access.
3. Additional individualized interventions: _____	3. Rationales: _____

> **Suggested NIC Interventions**
> *Wound care; Skin surveillance; Incision site care*

> **Suggested NOC Outcomes**
> *Risk control*

Nursing diagnosis
Acute pain related to hemodialysis treatment

NURSING PRIORITY
Minimize discomfort during hemodialysis treatment.

PATIENT OUTCOME CRITERION
During treatment, the patient will rate pain or discomfort as less than 3 on a 0 to 10 pain rating scale.

INTERVENTIONS	RATIONALES
1. *Assess for pain at least every 2 hours during treatments. Assess pain level using a 0 to 10 pain rating scale.*	1. Acute pain may be an indication that the vascular access device isn't patent. Pain may indicate cardiac and or neurologic complications.
2. *Notify the physician if pain persists.*	2. Persistent pain may indicate infection.
3. *See the "Acute pain" care plan,* page 32.	3. The "Acute pain" care plan contains further details related to pain management.
4. Additional individualized interventions: _____	4. Rationales: _____

> **Suggested NIC Interventions**
> *Medication management; Pain management; Analgesic administration; Patient-controlled analgesia (PCA) assistance; Conscious sedation*

> **Suggested NOC Outcomes**
> *Comfort level; Pain control; Pain: Disruptive effects; Pain level*

Nursing diagnosis
Impaired physical mobility related to lengthy treatment regimen

NURSING PRIORITY
Promote comfort and prevent complications related to immobility.

PATIENT OUTCOME CRITERION
During treatment, the patient will maintain normal function and optimal mobility (as much as possible).

INTERVENTIONS	RATIONALES
1. *Assess for restriction of mobility and activity.*	1. Assessing the patient's activity and mobility restrictions helps with determining the patient's exercise and mobility needs.
2. Encourage and assist with active and passive exercise program.	2. A passive or active exercise program prevents skin breakdown, improves blood flow to extremities, and decreases discomfort.
3. *See the "Impaired physical mobility" care plan,* page 111.	3. The "Impaired physical mobility" care plan provides general information about this problem.
4. Additional individualized interventions: _____	4. Rationales: _____

> **Suggested NIC Interventions**
> *Positioning; Exercise promotion: Stretching*

> **Suggested NOC Outcomes**
> *Immobility consequences: Physiological; Joint movement: Active; Mobility level*

Nursing diagnosis

Risk for injury: Perforation or ileus related to catheter insertion or irritation from dialysate

NURSING PRIORITY

Prevent or promptly detect and report injuries related to PD.

PATIENT OUTCOME CRITERIA

After catheter insertion, the patient will:
- have no unusual urge to void or defecate
- produce his usual amount of urine and stool
- have dialysate returns free from fecal material or blood.
  Throughout the hospital stay, the patient will:
- have normal bowel sounds
- maintain a normal bowel elimination pattern
- show no abdominal distention and tenderness.

INTERVENTIONS	RATIONALES
1. *Have the patient void before catheter insertion.*	1. The catheter is inserted with a trocar near the bladder. Bladder distention increases the risk of perforation.
2. *During dialysate infusion, observe for indications of bladder or bowel perforation,* such as an extreme urge to urinate or defecate; large urine output; fecal color, odor, or material in returned dialysate; and liquid or watery stools. If any occur, stop the infusion and notify the physician immediately.	2. Bowel or bladder perforation may lead to severe peritonitis unless detected. Surgical repair and prompt antibiotic therapy are indicated. The signs listed appear when dialysate leaks into the bladder or bowel.
3. *Report persistently blood-tinged dialysate.*	3. Slight bleeding may be normal after catheter insertion, but the fluid should clear rapidly. Persistent bleeding or gross blood in the return flow requires prompt evaluation.

4. *Auscultate bowel sounds every 4 hours.*

4. Diminished or absent bowel sounds may suggest ileus or bowel obstruction from bowel injury or irritation from catheter placement or dialysate.

5. *Inspect and palpate the abdomen every 8 hours between dialysate infusions.*

5. Abdominal distention and tenderness may indicate ileus.

6. Monitor the patient's appetite and sense of well-being.

6. Anorexia, nausea, vomiting, and malaise can be signs and symptoms of ileus.

7. Encourage ambulation.

7. Ambulation stimulates peristalsis.

8. Apply warm compresses to the abdomen.

8. Heat increases peristalsis.

9. Additional individualized interventions: _____

9. Rationales: _____

Suggested NIC Interventions
Wound care; Skin surveillance; Incision site care

Suggested NOC Outcomes
Risk control

Nursing diagnosis

Ineffective breathing pattern related to elevation of diaphragm during PD exchanges and reduced mobility

NURSING PRIORITY

Prevent respiratory distress and pulmonary complications during PD exchanges.

PATIENT OUTCOME CRITERIA

During treatment, the patient will:
- show no dyspnea
- have minimal or no crackles
- perform pulmonary hygiene measures effectively.

INTERVENTIONS

1. *Elevate the head of the bed during exchanges.*

2. Administer oxygen, as ordered.

3. *Assess for possible causes of pain or discomfort.* Administer analgesics, as ordered.

4. Encourage deep-breathing and coughing exercises during PD exchanges, hourly while awake. Teach and promote hourly incentive spirometer use, as ordered.

5. *Auscultate the patient's lungs every hour,* assessing for and reporting crackles or other abnormal findings.

6. Turn and reposition the patient at least every hour.

7. Perform chest percussion every 2 hours.

RATIONALES

1. Elevating the head of the bed minimizes pressure on the diaphragm and allows fuller chest expansion.

2. Hypoventilation related to pressure on the diaphragm reduces partial pressure of arterial oxygen.

3. Pain may prevent effective breathing. Rapid inflow of dialysate, patient position, and air in the system can all cause discomfort; possible causes should be investigated before analgesics are given.

4. Good pulmonary hygiene helps prevent fluid accumulation in the lungs and air passages by promoting full chest expansion and preventing collapse of alveoli.

5. Crackles suggest pulmonary complications related to fluid retention.

6. Changing position promotes full chest expansion and optimal drainage of dialysate.

7. Percussion helps loosen secretions.

8. Additional individualized interventions:_____

8. Rationales: _____

Suggested NIC Interventions	**Suggested NOC Outcomes**
Airway management; Respiratory monitoring	*Respiratory status: Airway patency; Respiratory status: Ventilation; Respiratory status: Gas exchange*

Collaborative problem

Risk for fluid imbalance related to dialysis and underlying disease or disorder

NURSING PRIORITY

Maintain normal fluid balance.

PATIENT OUTCOME CRITERIA

During PD exchanges, the patient will:
- show no distended jugular veins
- have a decrease in peripheral edema
- have blood pressure within the normal range, typically: systolic blood pressure, 90 to 140 mm Hg and diastolic blood pressure, 50 to 90 mm Hg
- have a dialysate deficit less than 500 ml.

INTERVENTIONS	**RATIONALES**
1. See appendix C, Fluid and electrolyte imbalances. *Closely monitor vital signs,* observing for tachycardia or orthostatic changes.	**1.** The Fluid and electrolyte imbalances appendix provides detailed information on the fluid and electrolyte disturbances seen in the patient receiving PD.
2. *Monitor serum potassium levels,* as ordered, to help determine appropriate additions to the dialysate.	**2.** Dialysate normally contains no potassium. This is desirable for the hyperkalemic patient, but it may cause hypokalemia in others.
3. *Maintain accurate fluid intake and output records.* Notify the physician if the fluid return deficit exceeds 500 ml.	**3.** Normally, return should be equal to or slightly greater than the amount infused. A persistent deficit that isn't corrected by position changes may indicate fluid retention.
4. Additional individualized interventions: _____	**4.** Rationales: _____

Nursing diagnosis

Risk for infection related to invasive procedure

NURSING PRIORITY

Prevent infection.

PATIENT OUTCOME CRITERIA

By the time of discharge, the patient will:
- be afebrile for 24 hours
- have no exudate, edema, redness, or leakage at the catheter site
- show no signs or symptoms of peritonitis, such as abdominal pain or rebound tenderness
- have clear return drainage.

INTERVENTIONS	**RATIONALES**
1. *Use strict aseptic technique for all aspects of PD,* including daily dressing changes.	**1.** Introduction of pathogens through the catheter may cause peritonitis.
2. *Maintain a sterile, closed system during exchanges.*	**2.** Airborne bacteria can cause infection if introduced into the peritoneal cavity.
3. *Observe for and report leakage around the catheter.*	**3.** Further securing the catheter at the entry site and reducing the amount or rapidity of the infusion may control leakage. Moisture around the catheter provides a pathway for microorganisms and increases the risk of infection.
4. *Observe the catheter site for redness, exudate, and edema.*	**4.** These are signs of infection.
5. Observe the outflow for cloudiness, sediment, and odor. *Observe the patient for signs or symptoms of peritonitis,* such as abdominal pain, guarding, rigidity, and rebound tenderness.	**5.** Fluid appearance and odor may indicate peritonitis. Physical signs result from peritoneal inflammation.
6. Take and record the patient's temperature at least every 8 hours.	**6.** Temperature elevation is a sign of infection.
7. Administer systemic or local antibiotics, as ordered. Add antibiotics to the dialysate using the two-needle technique (one needle used to draw up the medication, another to inject it into the dialysate).	**7.** Antibiotics prevent the growth and reproduction of bacteria. The two-needle technique reduces the risk of contamination.
8. Additional individualized interventions: _____	**8.** Rationales:_____

> **Suggested NIC Interventions**
> *Infection status; Wound healing; Primary intention*

> **Suggested NOC Outcomes**
> *Infection control; Infection protection; Incision site and care; Wound care*

Nursing diagnosis

Acute pain related to dialysate temperature or rapid inflow

NURSING PRIORITY

Minimize discomfort during fluid exchanges.

PATIENT OUTCOME CRITERION

During treatment, the patient will rate pain as less than 3 on a 0 to 10 pain rating scale.

INTERVENTIONS	**RATIONALES**
1. *Warm the dialysate to body temperature before beginning the infusion.*	**1.** Cold dialysate causes vasoconstriction (which interferes with circulation to the peritoneal membrane) and discomfort.
2. Change the patient's position every 1 to 2 hours.	**2.** Frequent position changes improve dialysate drainage.
3. Slow the infusion rate by lowering the bottle and by clamping the tubing as needed.	**3.** Reducing bottle height decreases the infusion rate and reduces pressure during fill time.

4. *Prevent air from entering the catheter.*

4. Air introduced into the abdominal cavity causes distention and pain, sometimes referred to the shoulder area. Air in the tubing may also create an air lock, preventing adequate dialysate flow.

5. Assess pain level using a 0 to 10 pain rating scale. Notify the physician if pain persists.

5. Persistent pain may indicate peritonitis.

6. *See the "Acute pain" care plan,* page 32.

6. The "Acute pain" care plan contains further details related to pain management.

7. Additional individualized interventions: _____

7. Rationales: _____

Suggested NIC Interventions
Medication management; Pain management; Analgesic administration; Patient-controlled analgesia (PCA) assistance; Conscious sedation

Suggested NOC Outcomes
Comfort level; Pain control; Pain: Disruptive effects; Pain level

---

Nursing diagnosis

Imbalanced nutrition: Less than body requirements related to anorexia, abdominal distention, stomatitis, or nausea

NURSING PRIORITY
Promote adequate nutritional intake.

PATIENT OUTCOME CRITERIA
During treatment, the patient will:
- participate in dietary planning
- perform oral hygiene before and after meals
- eat adequate amounts of protein-rich foods.
  By the time of discharge, the patient will:
- retain food for at least 12 hours
- tolerate oral intake of at least 0.5 g/kg of ideal weight daily and 45 to 50 kcal/kg/day.

INTERVENTIONS

1. With the dietitian and patient, plan a menu that incorporates personal preferences, increased nutrient needs, and any restrictions related to the underlying disorder.

2. Offer snacks and supplements between meals, providing plenty of high-protein foods unless contraindicated. Avoid foods high in potassium if hyperkalemia is a problem. See the "Chronic renal failure" care plan, page 680, for more information.

3. Encourage frequent oral hygiene.

4. Offer small, frequent meals.

5. Avoid manipulating equipment or emptying drainage bags at mealtime.

RATIONALES

1. The dietitian's expertise may be helpful in selecting food for optimal nutritional value. When the patient's appetite is decreased, considering individual preferences is essential to promote adequate intake.

2. PD can cause weekly protein losses of 30 to 70 g. The adult dialysis patient requires 45 to 50 kcal/kg daily. Hyperkalemia is common in renal failure. The "Chronic renal failure" care plan contains specific interventions related to diet planning.

3. Good oral hygiene decreases unpleasant odors and tastes in the mouth that can decrease appetite.

4. Large amounts of food may seem overwhelming and unappetizing. The patient may complain of being too full to eat because of pressure from peritoneal fluid.

5. Unpleasant sights and odors may cause nausea and vomiting.

6. *Drain the peritoneal cavity before meals.* If possible, allow 1 to 2 hours between a meal and the next dialysate infusion.

7. If the patient can't tolerate adequate oral intake, discuss enteral or parenteral feedings with both the patient and physician.

8. Additional individualized interventions:_____
_____

6. Draining peritoneal fluid decreases intra-abdominal pressure and may enable the patient to eat and retain food more easily.

7. During acute illness, enteral or parenteral nutrition may be indicated.

8. Rationales:_____
_____

Suggested NIC Interventions
Diet staging; Nutrition management; Weight gain assistance; Fluid monitoring; Nutritional monitoring

Suggested NOC Outcomes
Nutritional status; Nutritional status:Food and fluid intake; Nutritional status: Nutrient intake

---

Discharge planning

DISCHARGE CHECKLIST
Before discharge, the patient shows evidence of:
- ❏ vital signs stable and within expected parameters
- ❏ electrolyte, ABG, and hemoglobin levels within acceptable parameters
- ❏ absence of drainage, redness, and edema at catheter site
- ❏ absence of cardiovascular and pulmonary complications
- ❏ absent or minimal peripheral edema
- ❏ ability to tolerate adequate nutritional intake, as ordered
- ❏ absence of abdominal distention and tenderness
- ❏ absence of nausea and vomiting
- ❏ normal bowel and bladder function
- ❏ stabilizing weight
- ❏ ability to control pain using oral medications
- ❏ ability to ambulate and perform activities of daily living independently or with minimal assistance
- ❏ adequate home support system or referral to home care or a nursing home as indicated by inadequate home support system, frequency of and tolerance to PD, and inability to care for self.

TEACHING CHECKLIST
Document evidence that the patient and his family demonstrate an understanding of:
- ❏ renal failure (pathophysiology, signs and symptoms, and implications)
- ❏ concepts of PD treatment
- ❏ importance of aseptic technique during treatment
- ❏ dietary modifications (sodium restrictions and high protein intake)
- ❏ all discharge medications' purpose, dosage, administration schedule, and adverse effects requiring medical attention (discharge medications vary, depending on underlying disorder)
- ❏ catheter care between treatments

- ❏ activity restrictions (usually only contact sports and swimming are prohibited)
- ❏ importance of a daily weight record
- ❏ changes in condition to report to the physician
- ❏ date, time, and location of next treatment
- ❏ community resources
- ❏ how to get help in an emergency.

DOCUMENTATION CHECKLIST
Using outcome criteria as a guide, document:
- ❏ clinical status at beginning of treatment, including vital signs and weight
- ❏ significant changes in clinical status
- ❏ appearance of catheter site
- ❏ time each exchange begins and ends
- ❏ fluid intake and output
- ❏ color, odor, and character of dialysate return
- ❏ care of catheter site
- ❏ weight at end of treatment
- ❏ nutritional intake
- ❏ pertinent laboratory and diagnostic test findings
- ❏ bowel status
- ❏ patient and family teaching
- ❏ discharge planning.

Associated care plans
- Acute pain
- Acute renal failure
- Chronic renal failure
- Knowledge deficit
- Liver failure
- Parenteral nutrition

References
Alfaro, R. *Applying Nursing Diagnosis and Nursing Process,* 5th ed. Philadelphia: Lippincott Williams & Wilkins, 2002.

Nettina, S. *The Lippincott Manual of Nursing Practice,* 7th ed. Philadelphia: Lippincott Williams & Wilkins, 2000.

Nursing Procedures, 3rd ed. Springhouse, Pa.: Springhouse Corp., 2002.

Renal disorders

Urolithiasis

DRG INFORMATION
DRG 323 Urinary Stones with Complication or Comorbidity (CC) or Treatment with Extracorporeal Shock-wave Lithotripsy.
Mean LOS = 3.2 days

DRG 324 Urinary Stones without CC.
Mean LOS = 1.9 days

DRG 304 Kidney, Ureter, and Bladder Procedures for Nonneoplasm with CC.
Mean LOS = 8.8 days

DRG 305 Kidney, Ureter, and Bladder Procedures for Nonneoplasm without CC.
Mean LOS = 3.7 days

DRG 310 Transurethral Procedures with CC.
Mean LOS = 4.4 days

Introduction
DEFINITION AND TIME FOCUS
Urolithiasis is the formation of mineral crystals (renal calculi or stones) around organic matter in the urinary tract. Calcium oxalate and calcium phosphate calculi are the most common. Calculi in the renal pelvis usually cause no symptoms until they pass into a ureter, where they commonly obstruct urine flow and cause severe pain, bleeding, and infection. This care plan focuses on the patient admitted for treatment of upper urinary tract calculi by percutaneous nephrolithotomy with ultrasonic lithotripsy. In this procedure, a nephroscope is passed through a small incision into the kidney. The calculi are then fragmented with ultrasonic waves, flushed, and aspirated by suction or grasped and removed with forceps or special baskets. (See *Clinical snapshot: Urolithiasis.*)

ETIOLOGY AND PRECIPITATING FACTORS
- Urinary tract infection (UTI), which increases the alkalinity of the urine and causes calcium and other substances to precipitate and form renal calculi
- Immobility, dehydration, and urinary obstruction or stasis, increasing likelihood that calculus-forming substances will precipitate
- Metabolic or dietary changes, such as hyperthyroidism; hyperparathyroidism; bone disease; corticosteroid use; excessive vitamin A and D intake; diet high in calcium or purine; or other factors increasing calcium, phosphorus, uric acid, and other calculus-forming substances in the blood or urine
- More common in males ages 30 to 50

Focused assessment guidelines
NURSING HISTORY
(FUNCTIONAL HEALTH PATTERN FINDINGS)
Health-perception–health-management pattern
- Severe pain is typical: If calculi are in the pelvis, patient reports dull constant pain, usually over costovertebral angle; if in a ureter, patient reports intermittent, excruciating pain radiating anteriorly down to vulva (female) or testes (male); in some cases, patient may not report pain or may report abdominal pain
- History of UTI or previous calculus formation and treatment (a history of calculi increases the risk of recurrence)

Nutritional-metabolic pattern
- Nausea, vomiting, diarrhea, and abdominal discomfort
- Diet high in calcium (milk, cheese, beans, nuts, and cocoa), purine (fish, fowl, meat, and organ meat), oxalate (spinach, parsley, rhubarb, cocoa, instant coffee, and tea), or vitamins A and D
- Decreased fluid intake

Elimination pattern
- History of UTI or urinary tract obstruction
- Blood in urine (hematuria)
- Cloudy, odorous urine (indicates infection); painful, urgent, and frequent urination; and decreasing urine output

Activity-exercise pattern
- Sedentary occupation or recent increased need for bed rest

Cognitive-perceptual pattern
- Difficulty understanding metabolic influences on calculus formation and the new treatment options available (percutaneous ultrasonic lithotripsy, extracorporeal shock-wave lithotripsy, electrohydraulic lithotripsy, and laser lithotripsy)

Role-relationship pattern
- Family history of renal calculi, gout, or other renal problems

Sexuality-reproductive pattern
- Sexual dysfunction related to UTI and pain

Coping–stress tolerance pattern
- Anxious appearance and obvious distress

PHYSICAL FINDINGS
Genitourinary
- Calculi in urine
- Costovertebral tenderness
- Hematuria

- Pyuria
- Oliguria
- Urinary frequency

Gastrointestinal
- Vomiting
- Abdominal tenderness or distention
- Diarrhea
- Absent bowel sounds

Integumentary
- Warm, flushed skin or chills and fever
- Pallor
- Diaphoresis

DIAGNOSTIC STUDIES

- Urinalysis — commonly shows red blood cells, white blood cells (WBCs), crystals, casts, minerals, and pH changes
- Urine culture — commonly shows presence of bacteria
- 24-hour urine study — commonly shows high levels of calcium, phosphorus, uric acid, creatinine, oxalate, or cystine
- Renal calculus analysis — shows mineral composition of stones
- Blood studies — may show high serum levels of calcium, protein, electrolytes, uric acid, phosphates, blood urea nitrogen, creatinine, or WBCs

- Serum and urine creatinine tests — may show renal dysfunction (creatinine levels high in serum, low in urine)
- Kidney-ureter-bladder radiography — commonly shows calcium calculi and gross anatomical changes, such as distortions or enlargement (uric acid calculi can't be visualized)
- Excretory urography (I.V. pyelography or retrograde pyelogram) — commonly shows anatomical abnormalities, obstruction, and outlines of radiopaque calculi
- Computed tomography scan, with or without dye — commonly shows calculi, masses, or other abnormalities
- Ultrasound (kidney sonogram) — shows size, density, and perfusion
- Cystoscopy — commonly shows obstruction or other problems

POTENTIAL COMPLICATIONS

- Bleeding (may be acute or delayed for 1 to 2 weeks)
- Sepsis
- Renal pelvis perforation and loss of irrigating fluid into retroperitoneal area
- Nonremovable calculi
- Loss of calculus fragments into retroperitoneum

CLINICAL SNAPSHOT ✳

Urolithiasis

Major nursing diagnoses	Key patient outcomes
Acute pain	Rate pain as less than 3 on a 0 to 10 pain rating scale.
Impaired urinary elimination	Void more than 200 ml of clear amber urine per attempt.
Deficient knowledge (potential causes of calculus formation)	On request, express understanding of dietary restrictions, the need for increased fluid intake, the recommended activity level, the need to monitor such metabolic problems as gout, and the signs and symptoms of a recurrence.

Nursing diagnosis

Acute pain related to procedural manipulation, incision, and passage of calculus fragments

NURSING PRIORITY

Relieve pain.

PATIENT OUTCOME CRITERION

Within 24 hours of the procedure, the patient will rate pain (with pain medication) as less than 3 on a 0 to 10 pain rating scale.

Renal disorders

INTERVENTIONS	RATIONALES
1. *See the "Acute pain" care plan,* * page 32.	**1.** General interventions for pain are included in the "Acute pain" care plan.
2. *Assess and document pain episodes,* asking the patient to rate pain on a scale of 0 to 10.	**2.** Pain may indicate calculus movement. Persistent pain may indicate obstruction or perforation. Sudden absence of pain may indicate calculus passage. Increased ureteral pressure may cause abdominal pain from extravasation of urine into perirenal spaces.
3. *Medicate with analgesics and antispasmodics, as ordered.* Narcotic analgesics are usually necessary.	**3.** These medications reduce pain, relax tense muscles, and reduce reflex spasms. Narcotic analgesics are warranted because of the pain's severity.
4. Apply heat to painful areas, as ordered, for 15 to 20 minutes every 2 hours as needed.	**4.** Heat relaxes tense muscles and diminishes reflex spasms.
5. Administer antiemetics, as ordered and needed.	**5.** Nausea and vomiting are commonly associated with renal pain from shared nerve pathways.
6. Encourage activity, as allowed. (The patient with an indwelling ureteral catheter may be on bed rest to prevent dislodgment.)	**6.** Activity prevents urine stasis, helps retard calculi formation, aids passage of calculus fragments, and promotes return of urinary tract function.
7. Additional individualized interventions: _____	**7.** Rationales: _____

> **Suggested NIC Interventions**
> *Pain management*

> **Suggested NOC Outcomes**
> *Pain control; Pain: Psychological response*

Nursing diagnosis

Impaired urinary elimination: Dysuria, oliguria, pyuria, or frequency related to calculus fragment passage, obstruction, hematuria, or infection

NURSING PRIORITIES
- Prevent urinary tract complications.
- Promote return of normal urinary function.

PATIENT OUTCOME CRITERIA
Within 3 days of surgery, the patient will:
- void more than 200 ml of clear amber urine per attempt
- have no infection
- have no hematuria
- show a reduced amount of calculus fragments in the urine
- have catheters removed without problems
- show adequate hydration
- maintain vital signs within normal limits, typically: heart rate, 60 to 100 beats/minute; systolic blood pressure, 90 to 140 mm Hg; and diastolic blood pressure, 50 to 90 mm Hg.

---

*Italics indicate key interventions.

INTERVENTIONS

1. *Measure each voiding and note urine characteristics. Monitor fluid intake and output every 4 to 8 hours,* more frequently if the patient is oliguric. Alert the physician if urine output is less than 30 ml/hour.

2. *Monitor the patency of an indwelling ureteral catheter or indwelling urinary catheter* every hour.

3. *Strain all urine for calculi and calculus fragments.* Send any calculi for laboratory analysis. Notify the physician of calculi passage and document your observations.

4. *Observe for signs or symptoms of ureteral obstruction* (increased flank pain and oliguria) or urethral obstruction (bladder distention and suprapubic pain), and report any that occur.

5. *Observe for signs of dehydration,* such as dry skin and mucous membranes, thirst, poor skin turgor, low urine output, decreased blood pressure, tachycardia, and weight loss.

6. Encourage intake of twelve to seventeen 8-oz (237-ml) glasses of fluid daily. Document intake.

7. Give antibiotics every 4 to 8 hours, as ordered.

8. Monitor and document vital signs every 2 to 4 hours, as ordered.

9. As ordered, irrigate the catheter with acid or alkaline solutions, depending on calculus composition.

10. Additional individualized interventions:_____

RATIONALES

1. Urine characteristics may indicate such complications as infection (cloudy, odorous urine) and hemorrhage. Some hematuria is expected for 1 to 2 days after surgery, but bright-red blood may indicate hemorrhage. Adequate fluid intake is necessary to flush calculi through the kidneys, prevent further calculus formation, and prevent tissue damage. Adequate urine output indicates proper kidney function. Calculi may increase the frequency and urgency of urination as they near the ureterovesical junction.

2. If present, a ureteral catheter aids passage of calculus fragments and prevents obstruction of urine flow. A patent urinary catheter aids in monitoring urine output and assessing calculus passage. Calculus fragments can easily obstruct catheters.

3. The type and amount of calculi passed may influence the treatment used to prevent recurrence.

4. Calculi are most likely to lodge in a ureter or the urethra.

5. Dehydration concentrates urine, increasing the risk of calculus formation and infection.

6. Fluids enhance passage of calculus fragments and help prevent obstruction and infection.

7. UTI is a major predisposing factor for urolithiasis. UTI provides organic material and alkalizes urine, precipitating minerals and causing calculi formation. Antibiotics are commonly given to prevent infection and recurrence.

8. Changes in vital signs may indicate infection or other complications. Fever is common.

9. Catheter irrigations with acid or alkaline solutions promote acidification or alkalinization of the urine and help prevent further calculus formation.

10. Rationales:_____

> ### *Suggested NIC Interventions*
> Urinary bladder training; Urinary elimination management

> ### *Suggested NOC Outcomes*
> Urinary incontinence; Urinary elimination

Nursing diagnosis

Deficient knowledge (potential causes of calculus formation) related to lack of exposure to information

NURSING PRIORITY

Promote understanding of the medical regimen to prevent calculi recurrence.

PATIENT OUTCOME CRITERIA

By the time of discharge, the patient will:
- on request, express understanding of the need for increased fluid intake, the recommended activity level, the need to monitor such metabolic problems as gout, and the signs and symptoms of recurrence
- demonstrate accurate testing and interpretation of urine pH.

INTERVENTIONS	RATIONALES
1. *See the "Knowledge deficit" care plan*, page 129.	1. The "Knowledge deficit" care plan contains general information on patient teaching. This care plan contains additional information specific to urolithiasis.
2. Provide information, reinforcing as necessary, and document teaching regarding: – dietary limitations for calcium calculi (dairy products and green leafy vegetables), uric acid calculi (meats, legumes, and whole grains), and oxalate calculi (chocolate, caffeinated beverages, beets, and spinach) – need for regular activity – need for adequate fluid intake – need to maintain desired urine pH with medications and regular urine pH testing, according to the physician's recommendations – need to monitor and treat metabolic and other conditions (such as gout) that predispose the patient to calculus formation – signs and symptoms of recurrence, such as pain, hematuria, oliguria.	2. The patient needs accurate information to comply with the preventive regimen. – Limiting foods rich in calculus-forming substances may inhibit recurrence. (A dietitian can provide details about specific diets, which vary considerably.) – Activity decreases urine stasis and the risk of calculus formation. – Fluids flush calculus fragments and help prevent recurrence. – Depending on their composition, calculi may form in either acid or alkaline urine. The goal of treatment is to prevent calculus formation by maintaining the urine at the desired pH using appropriate medications. – Treating underlying conditions such as gout (uric acid accumulation) is necessary to prevent calculus formation. – The incidence of recurrence is high.
3. Additional individualized interventions: _____	3. Rationales: _____

> **Suggested NIC Interventions**
> *Teaching: Disease process; Teaching: Individual; Teaching: Prescribed medication*

> **Suggested NOC Outcomes**
> *Knowledge: Disease process; Knowledge: Health behaviors; Knowledge: Treatment regimen*

Discharge planning

DISCHARGE CHECKLIST

Before discharge, the patient shows evidence of:
- ❏ absence of gross hematuria
- ❏ absence of fever
- ❏ healing incision with no redness or other signs of infection
- ❏ absence of pulmonary or cardiovascular complications
- ❏ ability to tolerate and follow dietary and fluid regimen
- ❏ ability to perform activities of daily living independently
- ❏ ability to ambulate same as before hospitalization
- ❏ ability to perform pH monitoring

- ❏ ability to control pain using oral medications
- ❏ absence of infection or appropriate antibiotic prescribed
- ❏ stable vital signs
- ❏ absence of indwelling ureteral or urinary catheter or, if urinary catheter is present, ability to perform appropriate catheter care
- ❏ referral to home care if catheter is in place or if the patient's home support system is inadequate.

TEACHING CHECKLIST

Document evidence that the patient and his family demonstrate an understanding of:
- ❏ care of incisions, drains, or catheters
- ❏ activity precautions
- ❏ dietary modifications
- ❏ desired fluid intake
- ❏ all discharge medications' purpose, dosage, administration schedule, and adverse effects requiring medical attention; usual medications include ascorbic acid (to increase urine acidity), ammonium chloride (for phosphate calculi), sodium or potassium phosphate (to decrease urine calcium for calcium calculi), sodium bicarbonate, acetazolamide (Diamox) and allopurinol (Lopurin) (for uric acid calculi), and antibiotics
- ❏ signs and symptoms of recurring calculi
- ❏ urine pH testing
- ❏ need for follow-up laboratory tests
- ❏ need for follow-up visits with the physician
- ❏ need for follow-up diagnostic tests
- ❏ date, time, and location of next appointment
- ❏ how to contact the physician.

DOCUMENTATION CHECKLIST

Using outcome criteria as a guide, document:
- ❏ clinical status on admission
- ❏ significant changes in status
- ❏ pertinent laboratory and diagnostic test findings
- ❏ renal pain episodes
- ❏ pain-relief measures
- ❏ passage of renal calculi fragments
- ❏ fluid intake
- ❏ urine output and characteristics
- ❏ other therapies
- ❏ nutritional intake
- ❏ patient and family teaching
- ❏ discharge planning.

Associated care plans

- ■ Acute pain
- ■ Chronic pain
- ■ Knowledge deficit
- ■ Perioperative care

References

Lewis, S.M., et al. *Medical-Surgical Nursing: Assessment and Management of Clinical Problems.* St. Louis: Mosby–Year Book, Inc., 2000.

Jordan, K. (ed). *Emergency Nursing Core Curriculum.* Emergency Nurses Association. Philadelphia: W.B. Saunders Co., 2000.

Lynn-McHale, D.J., and Carlson, K.K. American Association of Critical Care Nurses *AACN Procedure Manual for Critical Care,* 4th ed., Philadelphia: W.B. Saunders Co., 2001.

Shoemaker, W.C., et al. *Textbook of Critical Care,* 4th ed., Philadelphia: W.B. Saunders Co., 2002.

Renal disorders

Hematologic and immunologic disorders

## PART 11

Acquired immunodeficiency syndrome

DRG INFORMATION

DRG 488   Human immunodeficiency virus (HIV) with Extensive Operating Room Procedure.
Mean LOS = 17.3 days

DRG 489   HIV with Major Related Condition.
Mean LOS = 8.5 days

DRG 490   HIV with or without Other Related Condition.
Mean LOS = 5.5 days

Additional DRG information: To ensure maximum reimbursement, document all complications of acquired immunodeficiency syndrome (AIDS).

Introduction

DEFINITION AND TIME FOCUS

AIDS is a progressive, chronic disorder of cell-mediated and humoral immunity caused by HIV, a retrovirus previously referred to as the human T-lymphotropic virus type III or the lymphadenopathy-associated virus. HIV is a ribonucleic acid (RNA) virus that selectively infects human cells marked with a CD4+ surface antigen and, when stimulated, rapidly produces additional HIV, destroying and killing the human cell. Although T4 lymphocytes are most commonly infected, any cell with the CD4+ surface antigen is vulnerable to infection, including monocytes, macrophages, bone marrow progenitors, and glial, gut, and epithelial cells. HIV infection renders the patient immunodeficient and susceptible to opportunistic infections, unusual cancers, and other characteristic abnormalities.

The Centers for Disease Control and Prevention (CDC) first described AIDS in 1981. The 1993 modification of its case surveillance definition includes HIV-infected youths and adults with CD4+ counts of less than 200 cells/μl or total lymphocytes of less than 14%. HIV infection is seen as a continuum of disease, ranging from being asymptomatic to causing multiple opportunistic infections.

The current definition of AIDS includes three categories for CD4+ counts and three clinical categories, allowing the patient with HIV to be placed into one of nine mutually exclusive categories. See *CD4+ lymphocyte categories* for an illustration of the three CD4+ categories. The three clinical categories (A, B, and C) range from least to most severe. A patient in category A is an adolescent or adult with documented HIV infection who doesn't have any of the conditions included in categories B or C but has one or more of the following:

- asymptomatic HIV infection

- persistent generalized lymphadenopathy
- acute (primary) HIV infection with accompanying illness or history of acute HIV infection.

A patient in category B is an HIV-infected adolescent or adult with one or more of the following symptomatic conditions (the patient may also have other symptomatic conditions not listed below):

- bacillary angiomatosis
- candidiasis (thrush), oropharyngeal
- candidiasis, vulvovaginal; persistent, frequent, or poorly responsive to therapy
- cervical dysplasia, cervical carcinoma in situ
- hairy leukoplakia, oral
- herpes zoster (shingles), involving at least two distinct episodes or more than one dermatome
- idiopathic thrombocytopenic purpura
- listeriosis
- pelvic inflammatory disease, particularly if complicated by tubo-ovarian abscess
- peripheral neuropathy.

A category B patient also doesn't have any condition listed in category C, and his conditions (1) are attributed to HIV infection or indicate a defect in cell-mediated immunity or (2) are considered by the physician to have a clinical course or to require management that is complicated by HIV infection. For classification purposes, category B conditions take precedence over category A conditions. An HIV-positive patient who has been treated and hasn't developed a category C condition and is asymptomatic is classified as category B.

A patient in category C has one or more of the conditions listed in *Diagnostic criteria for AIDS,* page 735. After the patient has developed one of these conditions, he remains classified as category C. These guidelines may change with further study and developments in clinical practice.

Two disorders commonly linked with AIDS are *Pneumocystis carinii* pneumonia (PCP) and Kaposi's sarcoma. PCP, the most common opportunistic infection present at diagnosis, is a protozoal pneumonia. Kaposi's sarcoma is a malignant neoplasm that begins as reddish or purplish skin lesions with variable distribution that may gradually spread, involving internal organs, mucous membranes, and lymph nodes. Various other conditions may present with AIDS, including infections related to cytomegalovirus (CMV), *Mycobacterium avium* complex (MAC) — that's also known as *Mycobacterium avium-intracellulare*, *Mycobacterium intracellulare*, *Cryptococcus*, *Candida*, or herpesvirus.

CD4⁺ lymphocyte categories

Below are CD4⁺ lymphocyte categories

CD4⁺ T-cell category	CD4⁺ cells/µl	CD4⁺ percentage
1	500	≥ 29
2	200 to 499	14 to 28
3	< 200	< 14

AIDS currently has no cure, and the prognosis for long-term survival is unknown. The introduction in 1996 of protease inhibitors has greatly improved the projected life expectancy for patients with HIV. The so-called AIDS cocktail typically is made up of three drugs, one of which is a protease inhibitor. To keep the virus suppressed, the patient may take 20 pills or more daily on a strict dosing schedule that must continue indefinitely; the individual immune response seems to play a role in survival. Some patients can't comply with this strict regimen, and others can't tolerate the adverse effects of treatment. The cost of the treatment is prohibitively expensive for many developing nations as well as for those who are poor or uninsured in developed nations. The number of inpatient hospitalizations has decreased since the advent of this treatment. This care plan focuses on the patient admitted for diagnosis and treatment of one or more HIV-related conditions. (See *Clinical snapshot: Acquired immunodeficiency syndrome,* page 736.)

ETIOLOGY AND PRECIPITATING FACTORS

■ Sexual transmission (via semen, seminal fluid, or vaginal secretions) or artificial insemination
■ Blood-borne transmission from I.V. drug use, multiple blood transfusions (especially before 1985), blood product transfusions (including clotting factors), organ transplants, or cuts or punctures from needles or other sharp instruments that may be contaminated
■ High-risk groups include homosexual and bisexual men, I.V. drug users, recipients of contaminated blood or blood products, sexual partners of those considered at high risk, and neonates born to mothers who were HIV-positive during pregnancy

Focused assessment guidelines
NURSING HISTORY
(FUNCTIONAL HEALTH PATTERN FINDINGS)
Health-perception–health-management pattern
■ Asymptomatic or mononucleosis-like symptoms reported by the patient for 3 to 6 weeks after initial exposure
■ Weeks to months of fatigue, malaise, low-grade fever, drenching night sweats, anorexia, sore throat, upper respiratory disorder that lingers, cough, or shortness of breath
■ History of recurrent infections (including sexually transmitted diseases [STDs]), amebiasis, or herpes simplex infections
■ Known exposure to HIV
■ Self-identification for high risk, such as a male homosexual or bisexual, I.V. drug user, or recipient of blood products
■ History of multiple blood transfusions
■ Sexual partner of someone at high risk
Nutritional-metabolic pattern
■ Anorexia or dysphagia
■ Episodic oral candidiasis (thrush), which may interfere with eating and taste
■ Weight loss greater than 10 lb (4.5 kg) in 1 month
Elimination pattern
■ Persistent diarrhea, even with treatment
■ Incontinence (from myopathy)
Activity-exercise pattern
■ Severe exertional shortness of breath (with pulmonary involvement)
■ Dry mouth
■ Displayed lack of energy and malaise
■ Leg weakness (from myopathy) or pain and numbness (from neuropathy)
Sleep-rest pattern
■ Drenching night sweats
■ Erratic sleep patterns because of other symptoms
Cognitive-perceptual pattern
■ Forgetfulness, depression, mental dullness or lability, difficulty concentrating, or other changes in mental status
■ Headache
■ Pain from tumor invasion, fever, or neurogenic causes
Role-relationship pattern
■ Close friends or sexual partners who have died of AIDS
■ Expressed anxiety over the potential loss of social contact if the diagnosis becomes known to others or expressed distress over actual losses
Sexuality-reproductive pattern
■ Sexual activity with multiple partners

Hematologic and immunologic disorders

- Previous infection with other STDs

Coping–stress tolerance pattern
- Young to old age, previously healthy person who reports little experience with illness or death
- Delayed pursuit of medical attention until symptoms became severe because of fear, denial, lack of information, or low self-esteem
- Extreme anxiety and uncertainty expressed regarding diagnosis, current status, and prognosis
- Denial as initial coping behavior
- Signs of depression
- Suicidal thoughts expressed
- Fear expressed regarding lifetime antiretroviral and prophylaxis treatment regimen

Value-belief pattern
- Belief that illness is punishment for previous behavior
- Survivor guilt experienced by patient

PHYSICAL FINDINGS
Pulmonary
- Shortness of breath
- Dry cough
- Crackles

Gastrointestinal
- Diarrhea
- Hepatomegaly
- Splenomegaly
- Diffuse abdominal tenderness
- Thrush
- Mucosal lesions
- Oral hairy leukoplakia

Neurologic
- Anxiety
- Decreased mental acuity (as shown by slowed speech or impaired memory)
- Tendency to not initiate conversation
- Impaired sense of position or vibration
- Weakness
- Paresthesia or paralysis
- Hyperreflexia
- Retinal abnormalities
- Diffuse retinal hemorrhage or exudates
- Positive Babinski's sign

Integumentary
- Drenching night sweats
- In Kaposi's sarcoma, reddish or purplish lesions varying in size from a few millimeters to a few centimeters across; may be macules or papules, usually appearing first on the head and neck or mucous membranes
- Dermatitis
- Lymphadenopathy
- Herpes zoster or simplex
- Anal warts
- Diffuse dry skin
- Butterfly rash on nose or cheeks
- Tinea
- Edema (with advanced Kaposi's sarcoma)

- Hypersensitivity to light touch
- Molluscum contagiosum

Musculoskeletal
- Weakness
- Pain
- Stiff neck

DIAGNOSTIC STUDIES
The following are HIV antibody tests:

- Enzyme-linked immunosorbent assay (ELISA) — identifies HIV antibody (In the asymptomatic person, the ELISA isn't diagnostic for AIDS: An individual may have a positive test without subsequently developing signs or symptoms. In addition, the ELISA may be falsely negative if performed too soon after exposure to the virus or falsely negative or falsely positive if the person has had influenza or another viral illness recently. A positive ELISA in a patient who exhibits one or more indicator diseases, such as PCP, Kaposi's sarcoma, emaciation, or dementia, can be considered diagnostic. A positive result is usually followed by a Western blot assay for a more definitive diagnosis. Consult current CDC guidelines.)
- Western blot assay — uses electrophoretically marked proteins to distinguish and differentiate antibodies; used with ELISA to confirm diagnosis
- Radioimmunoprecipitation assay — more costly, time-consuming, and labor-intensive than the Western blot assay; generally used in cases that are hard to diagnose
- Anonymous home testing kit — manufactured by Home Access and approved by the Food and Drug Administration (FDA) in 1996, this test provides results in 3 to 7 days along with pretest and posttest counseling (1-800-HIV-TEST)
- Oral antibody testing (OraSure) — approved by the FDA in 1994, looks for antibodies, if present, in the blood vessels of the mucous membranes of the cheek and gum
- Urine testing for HIV antibodies — approved by the FDA in August of 1996, this test is usually followed by the Western blot assay for a more definitive diagnosis.

Viral load tests detect changes in viral load, referred to in "logs." A significant change is more than 0.5 log. These tests are used to decide when to initiate or change treatment in an attempt to keep the viral load below detectable levels. However, these tests are limited because they can't reveal viral levels in reservoirs where the virus may be hiding such as the brain. Such tests include the following:

- Polymerase chain reaction technique — amplifies target deoxyribonucleic acid (DNA) to estimate the virion population to levels as low as 20 copies/ml, considered "undetectable"
- Branched-chain DNA amplification technique — provides an estimate of HIV RNA levels and can measure levels as low as 500 copies/ml
- Nucleic acid sequence-based assay — quantifies HIV RNA in blood plasma; more commonly used in Europe

Diagnostic criteria for AIDS

According to the Centers for Disease Control and Prevention (1993), a patient who tests positive for human immunodeficiency virus and who has a CD4$^+$ count less than 200 cells/μl or who has one or more of the following diseases is diagnosed as having acquired immunodeficiency syndrome (AIDS).

Viruses
- Herpes simplex virus that causes a mucocutaneous infection of more than 1 month; or bronchitis, pneumonitis, or esophagitis
- Cytomegalovirus in an organ other than the liver, spleen, or lymph nodes
- Papovavirus such as progressive multifocal leukoencephalopathy

Bacteria
- Mycobacterium that causes disease outside of the lungs, skin, or cervical or hilar lymph nodes
- *Salmonella* infection that causes recurrent, nontyphoidal septicemia
- *Mycobacterium tuberculosis* at any site
- Recurrent bacterial pneumonia

Fungi
- Candidal infection that causes disease in the esophagus, trachea, bronchi, or lungs
- Cryptococcosis that causes extrapulmonary disease
- Histoplasmosis or coccidioidomycosis that causes disease outside of the lungs and cervical and hilar lymph nodes
- Disseminated coccidioidomycosis

Protozoa
- *Pneumocystis carinii* pneumonia
- Toxoplasmosis of the brain
- Cryptosporidiosis or isosporiasis that causes diarrhea for more than 1 month

Cancer
- Kaposi's sarcoma
- Primary lymphoma of the brain
- Other malignant lymphomas, such as B cell or unknown immunologic phenotype, small noncleaved lymphoma, and immunoblastic lymphoma
- Invasive cervical cancer

Other
- Wasting syndrome that causes unexplained weight loss of more than 10% of body weight and diarrhea or fever that lasts for more than 1 month
- Dementia that causes cognitive or motor dysfunction and interferes with work or activities of daily living
- HIV-related encephalopathy

■ Genotypic antiretroviral resistance testing — used to detect mutations in reverse transcriptase and protease genes associated with resistance to antiretroviral agents; used to determine which medication is likely to be most effective.

The following laboratory findings represent characteristic values in patients with AIDS but aren't specific to or diagnostic of AIDS:

■ Complete blood count (CBC) — reveals leukocytopenia and anemia

■ Total T-cell count — reduced; CD4$^+$ cell count commonly less than 400 cells/μl

■ CD4$^+$ to CD8$^+$ cell ratio — low; decrease depends on patient's status, usually less than 1.0 (CD4$^+$ cells are also known as helper or inducer T cells; CD8$^+$ cells are also known as cytotoxic or suppressor T cells)

■ Immunoglobulin (Ig) levels — usually elevated, especially IgG and IgA

■ Platelet count — shows thrombocytopenia

■ Absolute neutrophil count — may be low because of a reaction to a drug, underlying opportunistic infection, or disease progression; calculated by adding the percentage of bands and neutrophils and then multiplying by the total number of white blood cells (WBCs)

■ Skin test antigen studies — reveal anergy

■ Aspartate aminotransferase level — may be elevated (associated with hepatitis)

■ Lactate dehydrogenase level — may be elevated in PCP

■ Serum cholesterol level — may be low

■ Serum iron level — may be low

■ Hepatitis screen — may demonstrate carrier state or active disease (hepatitis A, B, C, and others)

■ Stool culture and examination — may reveal parasites or infection (such as cryptosporidiosis, salmonellosis, acid-fast bacilli, microsporidiosis, *Clostridium difficile*, MAC, *Isospora belli*, or *Giardia lamblia*)

■ Serum albumin and protein levels — may be low in emaciation

■ Blood urea nitrogen (BUN) level — may be elevated in emaciation.

The following diagnostic procedures may be ordered for patients with AIDS:

■ Bronchoscopy — to diagnose PCP or other disorders by transbronchial lung biopsy (to examine tissue) or by bronchoalveolar lavage to obtain a specimen containing PCP cysts, fungus, CMV, or Kaposi's sarcoma

Hematologic and immunologic disorders

■ Chest X-ray — may reveal diffuse interstitial infiltrates (associated with PCP); however, may not be diagnostic even in active PCP

■ Colonoscopy and endoscopy — used to visualize and biopsy a site for the diagnosis of Kaposi's sarcoma and other tumors

■ Culture of lesions — may demonstrate *Candida*, toxoplasmosis, or other organisms

■ Biopsy of lesions — may demonstrate Kaposi's sarcoma or other cancers

■ Gallium scan — may show radio-labeled gallium accumulation in WBCs of infected areas; used to help establish early diagnosis of PCP, although test is nonspecific

■ Blood cultures — may identify pathogen if bacteremia is present

■ Lumbar puncture — results vary; may reveal cryptococcal meningitis; culture of spinal fluid may reveal HIV; results may be inconclusive for CMV infection

■ Sputum test for acid-fast bacillus — may indicate *Mycobacterium*

■ Computed tomography scan or magnetic resonance imaging (MRI) — may identify lesions for later biopsy; MRI may be the only means to detect progressive multifocal leukoencephalopathy

■ Bone marrow aspiration — may reveal hypoplasia.

POTENTIAL COMPLICATIONS

For a list of potential complications, see *Diagnostic criteria for AIDS,* page 735.

CLINICAL SNAPSHOT ☀

Acquired immunodeficiency syndrome

Major nursing diagnoses and collaborative problems	Key patient outcomes
CP: Risk for infection	Maintain antiretroviral regimen.
ND: Ineffective coping	Identify specific personal stressors.
CP: Risk for hypoxemia	Exhibit oximeter or ABG measurements improved from baseline.
ND: Chronic confusion	Take appropriate precautions to prevent injury.
ND: Social isolation	Contact support and resource persons, as appropriate.
ND: Impaired physical mobility	Engage in physical activity as tolerated.
ND: Imbalanced nutrition: Less than body requirements	Take food orally without excessive nausea or vomiting *or* state and demonstrate understanding of outpatient or home parenteral nutrition therapy, if appropriate.
ND: Deficient fluid volume	Maintain normal fluid and electrolyte balance.
ND: Impaired oral mucous membrane	Perform or receive oral care at least four times daily.
ND: Risk for impaired skin integrity	Maintain clean, dry, intact skin.
ND: Sexual dysfunction	Share sexual concerns with partner, friends, or staff members.
ND: Deficient knowledge (symptoms of disease progression, risk factors, transmission of disease, home care, and treatment options)	List precautionary measures to avoid infections.

Collaborative problem

Risk for infection related to immunosuppression (low CD4$^+$ lymphocyte count, low CD4$^+$-CD8$^+$ ratio, or neutropenia)

NURSING PRIORITIES

■ Prevent or promptly treat new infections.
■ Minimize effects of associated hyperthermia.

PATIENT OUTCOME CRITERIA

Throughout the hospital stay, the patient will:

- maintain antiretroviral regimen
- display no unanticipated medication adverse effects
- exhibit no signs or symptoms of dehydration.

INTERVENTIONS

1. *Provide continuous protection against infection. Implement CDC and institution precautions for the immunosuppressed patient,* * including meticulous hand washing before entering and after leaving the patient's room, providing only cooked or well-washed foods, prohibiting standing water in the room (such as in flower vases), protecting the patient from visitors with infections, and preventing the patient from handling live flowers or plants.

2. *Monitor vital signs, including temperature, at least every 4 hours.* Report fever onset or temperature spikes immediately.

3. *Monitor CBC daily and report increasing leukopenia or neutropenia.*

4. *Monitor potential sites of infection daily.* Check I.V. and injection sites, mucous membranes (including the rectum and vagina), and any wounds or skin breaks for changes in color, texture, or sensation; swelling; pain; induration; purulent drainage; or other abnormalities. If the patient is alert, discuss the importance of ongoing monitoring and early reporting of signs and symptoms of infection to medical personnel.

5. *Be alert for signs and symptoms of neurologic infection,* including stiff neck, headache, visual or motor abnormalities, memory impairment, and altered level of consciousness (LOC). Compare new findings with baseline neurologic or mental status findings, and report abnormalities to the physician immediately. Consult with the physician about the need for a lumbar puncture or MRI series.

_____
*Italics indicate key interventions.

RATIONALES

1. The immunosuppressed patient is at risk for infection from any source, even those considered benign to a healthy person, such as raw fruits and vegetables. Such precautions minimize the patient's exposure to infectious organisms. Hand washing is the primary infection-control measure for any patient. Gloves are recommended along with protective gowns and eyewear, as indicated, to guard against exposure to HIV-contaminated blood or secretions. (See *Protecting yourself from HIV infection,* page 738, for more information on infection control.) Raw produce may harbor gram-negative bacilli; standing water provides a medium for microorganisms, particularly *Pseudomonas.* Visitors may transmit organisms through direct contact or airborne bacteria. Plants and soil may harbor fungi.

2. Fever is the body's response to pyrogens released from invading microorganisms. The increase in metabolic rate is accompanied by a corresponding increase in the heart and respiratory rates. In the severely immunocompromised patient, however, the usual response mechanisms may fail, and sepsis may occur in the absence of fever. For this reason, careful, frequent observation to detect subtle changes in the patient's condition is essential.

3. These changes indicate further compromise of the body's ability to resist or fight infection.

4. The skin is one of the body's most important barriers against infection, and any break in the skin provides an entry point for microorganisms. Classic signs and symptoms of infection may be masked or delayed in the immunocompromised patient; therefore, regular, careful observation for any changes is essential. For example, dysphagia may indicate esophagitis, while white patches in the mouth may signal candidiasis (both are common in AIDS). Any suspicious area warrants prompt investigation because even benign microorganisms can cause life-threatening illness in a patient with AIDS.

5. Neurologic abnormalities are common in AIDS. Encephalitis, a common neurologic complication, may be caused by various microorganisms, including CMV, *Toxoplasma gondii,* or HIV. Progressive multifocal leukoencephalopathy, another common finding, is usually detectable only by MRI. Early detection and treatment of neurologic infection is crucial; after such involvement is advanced, the patient's prognosis is poor.

Hematologic and immunologic disorders

Protecting yourself from HIV infection

When caring for patients with human immunodeficiency virus (HIV), health care providers are themselves at risk for infection because of exposure to infected waste, blood, body fluids, and needle-stick injury. Prevention of exposure to HIV and other infectious diseases should be the goal of all health care providers.

Take preventive measures
The Centers for Disease Control and Prevention (CDC) recommends that health care providers participate in in-service programs on current standard blood and body fluid precautions and body substance isolation. These techniques should be implemented to prevent the spread of HIV, hepatitis, and other contagious diseases.

Respond to exposure
If a needle-stick injury or exposure to infected waste, blood, or body fluid occurs, the health care worker will receive appropriate counseling with the options of testing and treatment. If an accidental injury or exposure occurs, follow your facility's policies and procedures, such as:

- wash the wound thoroughly and report the incident to the nursing supervisor
- seek counseling, including updated information on confidential testing and treatment.

The risk of seroconversion from a needle stick is 0.3%; the CDC recommends testing for HIV infection after the exposure and then at 6 weeks, 12 weeks, and 6 months.

Seek medication
Research shows that zidovudine may help prevent seroconversion if treatment starts within 1 hour after exposure. If the blood exposure came from a person known to have been using protease inhibitors, current clinical practice guidelines recommend the use of multiple antiretroviral agents within 1 hour or no more than 3 days after exposure to help prevent seroconversion.

---

6. *Monitor for evidence of new pulmonary infections,* checking breath sounds at least every 8 hours. Report crackles, decreased breath sounds, or other abnormal findings promptly.

7. *Obtain cultures, as ordered,* from blood, stool, urine, sputum, or wound drainage. Evaluate sensitivity results and verify appropriateness of antibiotic therapy.

8. *Watch closely for signs and symptoms of systemic, skin, mucocutaneous, hematologic, ophthalmologic, oral cavity, esophageal, GI, pulmonary, and central nervous system opportunistic infections.* Administer antibiotics and anti-infectives, as ordered. After treatment begins, look for indications of adverse effects and report your findings. Consult current guidelines because recommendations may change with further research and clinical practice:
– MAC: ethambutol (Myambutol), clarithromycin (Biaxin), azithromycin (Zithromax), clofazimine (Lamprene), and ciprofloxacin (Cipro). Potential adverse effects include nausea, uveitis, neutropenia, thrombocytopenia, anemia, flulike syndrome, and hepatitis.
– TB: Active TB is treated with isoniazid, rifampin, pyrazinamide (PZA), ethambutol, and streptomycin. Potential adverse effects include aminotransferase elevations and hepatitis, peripheral neuropathy, and drug interactions.

6. The most common AIDS-related pulmonary infection is PCP, but others — including tuberculosis (TB) and fungal infections — may occur. Although the effectiveness of current pharmacologic treatment for PCP is related to individual response, prompt treatment of other pulmonary infections may be lifesaving for the immunocompromised patient.

7. If a new infection is suspected, immediate cultures will identify causative organisms. Sensitivity results guide antibiotic therapy.

8. Depending on the organism, therapy may involve several drugs simultaneously. Antibiotics may also be ordered prophylactically. Specific acute and prophylactic drug treatment may vary with the patient, depending on the effectiveness of the medication and the patient's tolerance. Prophylactic treatment reduces the risk of developing an opportunistic infection and helps prevent a recurrence of an infection. More than any other intervention, this approach can improve the quality of life for an AIDS patient and increase his life span. Effectiveness varies, particularly in a second episode of PCP, which has a mortality rate of approximately 60%. If CMV is also involved, the mortality rate is higher.

– PCP: co-trimoxazole (SMZ-TMP septra), pentamidine isethionate (Pentam), clindamycin (Cleocin), primaquine, dapsone, and trimetrexate. Potential adverse effects include anaphylaxis, severe rashes, Stevens-Johnson syndrome, fever, pancreatitis, and renal, hematologic, and GI reactions.

– CMV: ganciclovir, foscarnet, and cidofovir (Vistide) given indefinitely to prevent the recurrence of retinitis. Potential adverse effects include anemia, leukopenia, nephrotoxicity, neuropathy, fever, rash, proteinuria, tremors, headaches, granulocytopenia, and penile ulceration.

– Histoplasmosis and coccidioidomycosis: amphotericin B (Fungizone) and itraconazole (Sporanox). Potential adverse effects include nausea, vomiting, adrenal insufficiency, and drug interactions.

9. If the patient is on a prophylactic antiretroviral regimen (as most patients are), keep up-to-date with the specific drugs the patient is taking. Maintain the strict schedule of every 8 hours for protease inhibitors. Consult current guidelines for treatment. Have the pharmacy run a drug interaction chart to help prevent interactions and to optimize the timing and use of medications.

9. Specific medications the patient takes may change while the patient is hospitalized. If protease inhibitors aren't taken on a strict schedule, resistance and mutations may occur rapidly. Treatment guidelines change with advances in research and clinical practice. Drug interactions are common with anti-HIV medications and other drugs the patient may need during hospitalization.

It's rare for any of these agents to be used alone, with the exception of zidovudine, didanosine, and stavudine. Combination therapy affects the virus at the integration and budding stages, decreasing the number of mutations and keeping the virus at undetectable levels. The patient needs close monitoring for drug interactions.

– Nucleoside reverse transcriptase inhibitors (NRTIs): zidovudine (Retrovir, AZT), didanosine (Videx, ddI), zalcitabine (HIVID, ddC), stavudine (Zerit, d4T), and lamivudine (Epivir, 3TC); lamivudine and zidovudine (Combivir); abacavir (Ziagen); and abacavir, lamivudine and zidovudine combined (Trizivir). Adverse effects of zidovudine include anemia, granulocytopenia, myositis, and myopathy; didanosine can cause pancreatitis, hepatotoxicity, and peripheral neuropathy; zalcitabine can cause peripheral neuropathy, pancreatitis, esophageal or mouth ulcers, cardiomyopathy, and anaphylaxis; stavudine can cause anemia, hepatotoxicity, neutropenia, and peripheral neuropathy; and lamivudine can cause headache, myalgia, pancreatitis, and peripheral neuropathy.

– NRTIs inhibit reverse transcriptase action. They impede binding and entry of the virus into the host CD4+ cell, resulting in DNA chain termination.

– Non-nucleoside reverse transcriptase inhibitors (NNRTIs): nevirapine (Viramune) and delavirdine (Rescriptor).

– NNRTIs also inhibit reverse transcriptase action. These drugs are still under study and are used only in combination with NRTIs and protease inhibitors.

– Protease inhibitors: indinavir (Crixivan), ritonavir (Norvir), saquinavir (Invirase, Fortovase), and nelfinavir (Viracept); lopinavir and ritonavir (Kaletra); and amprenavir (Agenerase); ritonavir (Norvir). Adverse effects of saquinavir include abdominal discomfort, diarrhea, nausea, and photosensitivity; ritonavir can cause nausea and diarrhea; indinavir can cause kidney stone formation and hyperbilirubinemia; and nelfinavir can cause abdominal discomfort and diarrhea.

– Protease inhibitors are active in the late stages of HIV replication. Protease is needed for budding, and protease inhibitors render the virions ineffective.

Hematologic and immunologic disorders

– Nucleotide reverse transcriptase inhibitor: tenofovir disoproxil fumarate (Viread). Adverse effects include nausea, vomiting, flatulence, diarrhea, headache and asthenia.

– Tenofovir inhibits HIV replication.

10. If fever is present, administer acetaminophen, as ordered. Consult the physician about alternating doses of acetaminophen with aspirin, naproxen (Naprosyn), or ibuprofen (Motrin) for persistent fever. Check platelet count and bleeding time before giving aspirin or ibuprofen, and withhold medication if clotting is prolonged.

10. Acetaminophen, aspirin, and ibuprofen inhibit the effects of pyrogens on the thermoregulatory center, thereby reducing fever. Aspirin and acetaminophen may impair zidovudine metabolism, resulting in toxicity; alternating antipyretics may avoid this effect. Aspirin and ibuprofen may decrease platelet adhesion, prolonging clotting time.

11. Institute the following measures for fever, as ordered and appropriate: administering antipyretics, using a hypothermia blanket, monitoring for signs of dehydration, and replacing fluids as needed. See appendix C, Fluid and electrolyte imbalances.

11. A hypothermia blanket may be necessary to reduce body temperature if aspirin and acetaminophen are ineffective or contraindicated. Prolonged fever increases the metabolic rate and promotes diaphoresis, contributing to dehydration and electrolyte imbalances. The Fluid and electrolyte imbalances appendix contains detailed information on these imbalances.

12. Additional individualized interventions: _____
_____

12. Rationales:_____
_____

Nursing diagnosis

Ineffective coping related to potentially life-threatening illness, decisions regarding treatment, or potentially uncertain prognosis for long-term survival

NURSING PRIORITY
Promote positive coping behaviors.

PATIENT OUTCOME CRITERIA
Throughout the hospital stay, the patient will:
- use positive coping behaviors, such as relaxation and verbalization of feelings
- display awareness of legal rights and available support, if appropriate to condition
- have opportunities to address issues of grieving and dying
- identify specific personal stressors
- identify resources and begin mobilizing them.

INTERVENTIONS

1. *Assess for excessive anxiety.* Note signs and symptoms, such as poor eye contact, agitation, or restlessness.

RATIONALES

1. Prolonged or excessive anxiety may have negative psychological and physiologic effects. Anxiety interferes with the ability to learn, make decisions, and mobilize resources. Anxiety also increases sympathetic nervous system activity, increasing metabolic and cardiac demands and placing further stress on the body.

2. Introduce yourself and other staff members. Provide continuity of caregivers; minimize use of unfamiliar staff whenever possible. Demonstrate acceptance by touching, making eye contact, and listening actively.

2. Consistency in staffing facilitates the development of trust. Unfamiliar staff members may increase the patient's anxiety. Demonstrating acceptance promotes a therapeutic relationship. Patients with AIDS commonly report "feeling like lepers"; touch reduces this sense of isolation.

3. Implement measures to promote physical relaxation, as indicated, including progressive relaxation or controlled breathing techniques, therapeutic use of heat or massage, environmental modifications (such as reducing noise, heat, light, and other stimuli), physical therapy, and providing familiar articles brought from home.

3. The patient may be unaware of physical tension and its contribution to anxiety. Physical relaxation promotes restoration of psychological equilibrium.

4. *Encourage verbalization of feelings.* Anticipate fear, guilt, and anger, and accept such expressions as normal. If uncomfortable discussing explicit issues, arrange for another nurse to care for the patient. Whenever possible, refer the patient at the time of diagnosis to a mental health professional who can provide ongoing counseling.

4. Some patients receive their HIV diagnosis at the same time as their first inpatient hospitalization. The diagnosis of AIDS carries an enormous psychosocial impact that may overwhelm the patient initially. The patient is typically unable to utilize his usual defenses and resources; for example, denial may be impossible because of the media's coverage of AIDS, and friends or family may abandon the patient when the diagnosis is confirmed. If the disease was contracted through sexual contact, the patient may experience guilt over unresolved issues, anxiety or anger toward previous partners, or ambivalence about past or future desires or behaviors. The diagnosis requires that the patient immediately rethink relationships and commonly involves a loss of intimacy at a time when the patient needs support. Multiple referrals may lead to fragmented care; consistency in follow-up promotes optimal use of resources.

5. *Identify and discuss unhealthy coping behaviors.* Teach the patient about the effects of alcohol or drug abuse on immune function.

5. The patient may use alcohol or illegal drugs to avoid painful realities. If the disease was contracted through I.V. drug use, the underlying dependency must be addressed when planning care. Alcohol and drug abuse can compromise immune activity. The harm-reduction model can lead to safer behaviors. Include referral to a counseling or rehabilitation program in discharge.

6. *Help the patient identify and list specific fears and concerns contributing to anxiety.* Focus on modifiable factors.

6. Anxiety increases when fears seem overwhelming and all-encompassing. Identifying specific concerns helps quantify feelings and allows the patient to begin planning a coping strategy. Focusing on modifiable factors may increase the patient's sense of control.

7. *Help the patient identify and activate resources,* considering inner strengths, coping ability, and such external supports as friends, family, and a spiritual advisor. See the "Ineffective individual coping" care plan, page 124.

7. Initial anxiety may be so overwhelming that the patient is unable to mobilize usual coping methods. The "Ineffective individual coping" care plan provides specific interventions for the patient experiencing anxiety.

8. *Assess the patient's knowledge about HIV, and teach him about anti-HIV medications.* Explain the use of the mediset (daily or weekly medication box) and timer.

8. The regimen for taking medications is complex and the patient may take 20 pills or more daily, some with food and some fasting, on a strict schedule. If the patient must also take prophylactic drugs, he'll need careful teaching to understand his schedule and the rationale behind treatment, including a written schedule, mediset, and timer.

Hematologic and immunologic disorders

9. Acknowledge the unknowns of AIDS. Answer questions honestly and accurately. Accept the patient's response to losses. See the "Dying" care plan, page 78, and the "Grieving" care plan, page 105.

9. Acknowledging unknowns reassures the patient that the caregiver understands and is sensitive to the profound changes AIDS implies. Reminding the patient that emotional reactions are a normal response to a realistic threat may reduce anxiety and facilitate coping. The "Grieving" and "Dying" care plans provide further interventions related to psychosocial adjustment to illness and the losses illness entails.

10. Additional individualized interventions:_____

10. Rationales:_____

Suggested NIC Interventions
Coping enhancement; Family involvement promotion

Suggested NOC Outcomes
Coping; Social support

Collaborative problem

Risk for hypoxemia related to pneumonia, respiratory failure, or ventilation-perfusion imbalance

NURSING PRIORITY

Promote oxygenation.

PATIENT OUTCOME CRITERIA

Within 2 days of admission, the patient will:
- exhibit decreased dyspnea
- exhibit oximeter or arterial blood gas (ABG) measurements improved from baseline
- cough and deep-breathe effectively
- initiate a plan for energy conservation.

INTERVENTIONS

1. *Assess continuously for signs of hypoxemia,* such as tachycardia, restlessness, anxiety, tachypnea, irritability, and pallor or cyanosis. Monitor oxygenation with an oximeter or take ABG measurements, as ordered and needed for increasing dyspnea or inadequate respiratory effort. Report abnormal findings immediately, and prepare the patient for ventilatory support, as his condition indicates. Administer corticosteroids, colloids, and crystalloids, as ordered.

2. *Administer oxygen therapy* via nasal cannula, face mask, nonrebreather mask, or continuous positive airway pressure mask according to unit protocol or as ordered.

RATIONALES

1. PCP causes hard cysts to form in the interstitial spaces of the lungs, displacing surfactant and decreasing diffusion across the alveolar-capillary membrane. As partial pressure of arterial oxygen (Pao_2) levels decrease, the sympathetic nervous system attempts to compensate by increasing the heart rate. Progressive deterioration in ventilatory status in moderate to severe PCP may lead to respiratory failure — a common cause of death in AIDS-related illness. Ventilatory support may be required to maintain oxygenation. Routine use of corticosteroids, which may blunt the inflammatory reaction resulting from antipneumocystis treatment, has significantly decreased the need for mechanical ventilation. Corticosteroids also protect the pulmonary parenchyma from accelerated injury. Colloids and crystalloids may reduce the risk of overhydration and alveolar flooding.

2. Supplemental oxygen elevates arterial oxygen content and decreases hypoxia.

3. *Perform airway clearance measures,* as needed:
– If the patient is cooperative, teach coughing and deep-breathing exercises, and encourage hourly use of the incentive spirometer, as ordered.
– If the patient is uncooperative, perform artificial sighing and coughing with a handheld resuscitation bag hourly. Suction as needed if the patient is unable to cough effectively, as indicated by noisy respirations or gurgles auscultated over the large airways. Use supplemental oxygen before, during, and after airway clearance procedures.

4. *Observe for complications of bronchoscopy;* report any bleeding, anxiety, or unusual findings.

5. Evaluate and document the following every 8 hours and as needed: presence or absence of an effective cough, sputum character and color, respiratory effort, skin color, breath sounds, and activity tolerance. Be alert for changes in LOC, and report promptly any that occur.

6. If narcotic analgesics are used to control pain, *be alert for signs of respiratory depression after analgesic administration.* Report an excessively slowed respiratory rate, frequent sighing, decreased alertness, or any other indications of inadequate respiratory effort.

7. Assist with self-care activities as needed. (See "Impaired physical mobility," page 111.) Teach energy conservation measures, such as using a shower chair, organizing activities and grouping procedures, using large muscles, avoiding activities that involve raising the arms over the head, and scheduling rest periods between activities.

8. Additional individualized interventions: _____
_____

3. The patient may be unable to clear his airway effectively because of general debilitation and weakness. Deep breathing helps expand the lungs fully and prevents areas of atelectasis associated with pneumonia and bed rest. Incentive spirometry and coughing also promote lung expansion; however, exercise caution because coughing and positive-pressure breathing may cause alveolar rupture secondary to decreased surfactant in PCP. All airway clearance procedures may reduce Pao_2 levels. Supplemental oxygen may be provided through nasal prongs during suctioning.

4. Irritation from the bronchoscope may cause bleeding, further decreasing oxygenation and threatening airway patency.

5. Careful serial observations of respiratory status are essential to detect subtle changes that may indicate the need to reevaluate therapy. The patient with PCP may require multiple antibiotics if other infections occur simultaneously. Changes in LOC may signal impending respiratory failure.

6. Narcotics cause central nervous system depression and may impair respiratory center function.

7. Because activity increases oxygen demand, hypoxemia may worsen with exertion. Sitting requires less energy than standing. Organizing and grouping procedures reduce unnecessary exertion. Large-muscle groups are more efficient. Raising the arms over the head rapidly causes fatigue.

8. Rationales: _____
_____

Nursing diagnosis
Chronic confusion related to neurologic involvement

NURSING PRIORITY
Minimize effects of neurologic changes.

PATIENT OUTCOME CRITERIA
Throughout the hospital stay, the patient will:
- use cues for reorientation
- take appropriate precautions to prevent injury
- acknowledge limitations appropriate to neurologic deficits.

INTERVENTIONS	**RATIONALES**
1. *Assess the patient's mental and neurologic status* on admission and at least daily thereafter, including LOC, orientation, long-term and recent memory, ability to follow directions and think abstractly, speech, pupillary responses, and strength and sensation in arms and legs.	**1.** Baseline and ongoing mental and neurologic assessments allow early detection of neurologic involvement, a common and usually ominous finding in the patient with AIDS. Such disorders range from encephalopathies and neuropathies, occurring in 8% of patients, to less specific manifestations such as headache, occurring in up to 45% of patients. Delirium and seizures may also occur, impairing cognitive function.
2. *Evaluate the patient's emotional state,* considering the effects of depression, anxiety, grief, or other emotions on mental status findings. Also be alert to the possibility that medications may cause confusion, memory impairment, or other unusual findings.	**2.** Emotional responses and medication adverse effects may contribute to reduced alertness, confusion, withdrawal, hyperactivity, anxiety, or other mental status changes.
3. *Assess for possible visual impairment by* using an eye chart, if possible. If the patient has significant visual impairment, prevent injury by placing items within easy reach and ensuring that side rails are always up.	**3.** CMV infection of the optic nerve can cause blindness. Vision changes may be particularly frightening and difficult for the patient to accept. Precautionary interventions, particularly if confusion is also a factor, reduce the risk of injury.
4. If confusion is present, *provide cues for reorientation,* such as identifying yourself when entering the room, putting identifying signs on doors and objects, providing a large calendar and clock, discussing the day's events, and encouraging frequent visits, if possible, from family and friends.	**4.** Reorientation may help decrease anxiety, reduce the risk of injury, and facilitate coping.
5. Explain neurologic symptoms to the patient and his family and friends. Emphasize supportive behaviors, such as using humor, changing the subject if repetitive or irrational behaviors are present, providing gentle reminders of appropriate behavior, and listening actively.	**5.** Explanations may help the patient feel less isolated and anxious about mentation changes. Family members and friends may be more supportive if they understand that mentation changes may be related to disease progression.
6. *Provide a safe and supportive environment,* instituting safety measures appropriate to the patient's deficits.	**6.** Confusion, disorientation, and loss of function are emotionally devastating. Because the disoriented patient is at increased risk for injury, safety measures must be instituted.
7. *Observe for involuntary movements, paresthesia, numbness, pain, weakness, and atrophy of extremities.* Consult the physician regarding treatment, if needed, and institute measures to protect the extremities if sensation is impaired.	**7.** Distal symmetrical sensorimotor neuropathy is a common peripheral nerve complication in AIDS. The cause is unknown. Although a relatively benign condition, it may cause significant discomfort. Treatment may include heat, range-of-motion exercises, and electrical stimulation.
8. Additional individualized interventions: _____	**8.** Rationales: _____

> ### *Suggested NIC Interventions*
> *Cognitive stimulation; Mood management; Dementia management; Reality orientation; Anxiety reduction; Decision-making support; Family involvement promotion; Delusional management; Cognitive restructuring; Memory training; Cerebral perfusion promotion; Neurologic monitoring*

> ### *Suggested NOC Outcomes*
> *Cognitive ability; Cognitive orientation; Concentration; Decision making; Distorted thought control; Identity; Information processing; Memory; Neurological status: Consciousness*

Nursing diagnosis

Social isolation related to communicable disease, associated social stigma, and fear of infection from social contact

NURSING PRIORITY
Minimize feelings of social isolation.

PATIENT OUTCOME CRITERIA
Throughout the hospital stay, the patient will:
- express feelings related to social losses
- express and receive affection
- contact support and resource persons, as appropriate.

INTERVENTIONS

1. *Assess the patient's support system,* such as his family, partner, and friends. Ask the patient and others in his support system about recent losses in their lives, recent changes in the patient's living situation, and attitudes of family and friends toward the disease.

2. *Provide opportunities for the patient and his family to express their feelings.*

3. *Provide an atmosphere of acceptance.* Encourage staff, family, and friends to touch and hug the patient.

4. Teach the patient's family and friends about ways the AIDS virus is *not* transmitted, including the following: toilet seats and bathroom fixtures, swimming pools, dishes, furniture, handshakes, hugging, social (dry) kissing and other nonsexual physical gestures of affection, pets (although pets may carry microorganisms threatening to the patient), doorknobs, or casual social contact. Saliva, tears, and coughing aren't considered sources of transmission. If an opportunistic infection is present, family members should observe the usual precautions, including hand washing, good health habits, and avoiding contact with contaminated secretions. Provide audio or written materials to reinforce these points.

5. Provide the patient and his family with telephone numbers of available resources for counseling, support, and information. Check with the local public health department for resources in your area. See *AIDS resource phone numbers and Web sites,* page 746, for more information. Refer the patient to the social services department for help with financial concerns.

6. Additional individualized interventions: _____
_____

RATIONALES

1. The patient's and others' lack of accurate knowledge as well as the social stigma associated with AIDS may diminish the patient's social contacts. In addition, the patient may isolate himself for fear of contracting infections from others. Assessing the patient's social support system helps identify resources and may allow the nurse to correct misconceptions about the disease.

2. Expressing feelings helps decrease the sense of isolation.

3. Physical contact decreases feelings of isolation and demonstrates caring. Family and friends may need gentle reminders that such contact doesn't transmit the virus. The nurse can be a good role model for family and friends.

4. The "worried well" (those who are healthy, but worried about contracting AIDS) may be torn between their desire to support the patient and their concern for personal health. Education may help reduce their conflicts and encourage normal interaction with the patient. The AIDS virus doesn't survive on inanimate objects and is killed by soap and hot water. Opportunistic infections can be transmitted to others, but healthy individuals aren't at greater risk than usual. Audio or written materials reinforce oral teaching and provide a source for future reference.

5. Ongoing support is essential for the AIDS patient and his family throughout the illness. Support groups offer understanding, practical advice, and the latest information on new developments, which may surpass the support clinicians can provide. In addition, such groups may provide enriching relationships that enhance the patient's ability to cope with the disease. Referral to a social services department is essential because treatment is expensive and the patient may have special housing needs.

6. Rationales:_____
_____

Hematologic and immunologic disorders

Suggested NIC Interventions
Counseling; Recreation therapy; Coping enhancement; Therapeutic play

Suggested NOC Outcomes
Loneliness; Self-esteem; Psychosocial Adjustment: Life change; Social interaction skills; Social involvement; Social support

AIDS resource phone numbers and Web sites

Centers for Disease Control and Prevention (CDC)
1-800-342-AIDS
www.cdc.gov

CDC in Spanish
1-800-344-7432

CDC National AIDS Clearinghouse
1-800-458-5231 or
www.cdcnpin.org

AIDS Foundation
(415) 487-3000

National AIDS Clinical Trials
1-800-874-2572

Office of AIDS Research
www.nih.gov/od/oar

HIV Insite from the University of California, San Francisco
www.hivinsite.ucsf.edu

AIDS Education Global Information System (AEGIS)
www.aegis.com

Nursing diagnosis

Impaired physical mobility related to fatigue, weakness, hypoxemia, depression, altered sleep patterns, medication adverse effects, and orthostatic hypotension

NURSING PRIORITIES
- Promote maximum physical mobility.
- Prevent complications associated with decreased mobility.

PATIENT OUTCOME CRITERIA
Throughout the hospital stay, the patient will:
- appear rested
- verbalize adequacy of rest
- call for assistance as appropriate
- experience no falls or other injuries related to weakness
- engage in physical activity as tolerated
- develop no complications from impaired mobility.

INTERVENTIONS	RATIONALES
1. *Provide standard nursing care for decreased mobility.* Refer to the "Impaired physical mobility" care plan, page 111.	**1.** The "Impaired physical mobility" care plan provides general nursing interventions for this condition. This care plan supplies additional information specific to the AIDS patient.
2. Assist with activities of daily living (ADLs), as necessary. Anticipate the patient's needs. Assess the patient's neurologic status. (See "Chronic confusion," page 743.)	**2.** The patient may never have been sick or hospitalized before and may feel uncomfortable asking for help. "Chronic confusion" provides interventions and rationales for this diagnosis.
3. *Assess the need for sedatives,* administer medications, as ordered, and monitor their effects.	**3.** Anxiety and worry commonly interrupt sleep in the patient with AIDS. Rest is essential for healing.

4. Encourage the patient experiencing weakness or orthostatic hypotension to use the call light, ask for assistance when standing and walking, and leave belongings within reach.

5. Additional individualized interventions: _____

4. The patient may have never been this weak or dizzy before and may need reminders to ask for assistance.

5. Rationales: _____

> ### *Suggested NIC Interventions*
> *Exercise therapy: Ambulation; Exercise therapy: Balance; Exercise therapy: Joint mobility; Exercise therapy: Muscle control; Exercise promotion: Strength training*

> ### *Suggested NOC Outcomes*
> *Ambulation: Walking; Ambulation: Wheelchair; Joint movement: Active; Mobility level*

Nursing diagnosis

Imbalanced nutrition: Less than body requirements related to nausea, vomiting, diarrhea, anorexia, medication adverse reactions, or decreased nutrient absorption secondary to the disease

NURSING PRIORITY

Promote adequate nutritional intake.

PATIENT OUTCOME CRITERIA

Throughout the hospital stay, the patient will:
- maintain adequate oral intake of food or tolerate enteral or parenteral feedings without complications.
  By the time of discharge, the patient will:
- exhibit BUN values that have decreased since admission
- take food orally without excessive nausea or vomiting or state and demonstrate an understanding of outpatient or home parenteral nutrition (PN) therapy, if appropriate.

INTERVENTIONS

1. Provide typical assessments and interventions for nutritional status. Refer to the "Nutritional deficit" care plan, page 138, for information.

2. *Administer appetite stimulants* (such as megestrol [Megace] and dronabinol [Marinol]), as ordered, to help stimulate the patient's appetite. Thalidomide, oxandrolone, nandrolone, and human growth hormone are being used to combat HIV wasting; watch for adverse effects, including neutropenia. Keep in mind that the goal of therapy is to increase lean body mass. Consult current guidelines for use of appetite stimulants to combat HIV wasting. Refer to "Impaired oral mucous membrane," page 749, for information on fungal infections.

3. *Administer antiemetics,* as ordered, if nausea and vomiting are present.

RATIONALES

1. The "Nutritional deficit" care plan discusses general interventions for this condition. This care plan contains additional information pertinent to AIDS.

2. First used in pregnant women to stimulate appetite, megestrol works well for some HIV patients. Dronabinol can stimulate appetite and decrease nausea. Thalidomide is thought to decrease the tumor necrosis factor, making it easier for the patient to gain weight. Human growth hormone and anabolic drugs (oxandrolone, nandrolone) promote muscle development and may prevent wasting. Long-term use of hormone stimulation is uncertain at this time. A weight gain from water retention or an increase in fat doesn't improve the patient's well-being. Guidelines for the use of appetite stimulants may change with advances in research and clinical practice. "Impaired oral mucous membrane" provides interventions for fungal infections.

3. Chemotherapeutic agents administered for infections commonly cause nausea and vomiting. Antiemetics block stimulation of the vomiting center.

4. Consult the physician about nasogastric (NG) tube feedings or PN if the patient is unable to tolerate adequate oral intake or has severe chronic diarrhea. See the "Parenteral nutrition" care plan, page 510, for further information.

5. Additional individualized interventions: _____
_____

4. NG tube feedings provide nutrients without as many associated complications as parenteral nutrition. However, severe diarrhea from cryptosporidiosis, salmonellosis, or intestinal Kaposi's sarcoma lesions may reduce GI absorption, making parenteral nutrition necessary.

5. Rationales:_____
_____

Suggested NIC Interventions
Diet staging; Nutrition management; Weight gain assistance; Fluid monitoring; Nutritional monitoring

Suggested NOC Outcomes
Nutritional status: Food and fluid intake; Nutritional status: Nutrient intake; Weight control

---

Nursing diagnosis

Deficient fluid volume related to chronic, persistent diarrhea associated with opportunistic infection

NURSING PRIORITY
Maintain optimal fluid status.

PATIENT OUTCOME CRITERION
Throughout the hospital stay, the patient will maintain normal fluid and electrolyte balance.

INTERVENTIONS

1. To rehydrate the patient, *encourage fluids by mouth or administer parenteral fluids,* as ordered. Monitor intake and output. See appendix C, Fluid and electrolyte imbalances.

2. As ordered, administer antidiarrheal agents, such as loperamide (Imodium), diphenoxylate (Lomotil), or opium tincture.

3. Additional individualized interventions: _____
_____

RATIONALES

1. Diarrhea is one of the most problematic signs for the AIDS patient. Various microorganisms contribute to the problem and rectal mucosal lesions, hemorrhoids, and nutritional deficits exacerbate it further. Fever increases the potential for dehydration. The Fluid and electrolyte imbalances appendix provides further guidelines for monitoring fluid and electrolyte status and intervening to maintain optimal hydration and metabolic balance.

2. Many anti-HIV drugs and opportunistic infections can cause diarrhea, although many patients adjust to the diarrheal effects of drugs over time. Because a patient can have up to 20 stools per day, antidiarrheal medications are important to prevent dehydration.

3. Rationales:_____
_____

Suggested NIC Interventions
Acid-base management; Fluid and electrolyte management; Fluid monitoring; Hypovolemia management; Intravenous (I.V.) therapy

Suggested NOC Outcomes
Electrolyte and acid-base balance; Fluid balance; Hydration

Nursing diagnosis

Impaired oral mucous membrane related to infections or masses

NURSING PRIORITY

Reduce discomfort and prevent further damage to the mucous membrane.

PATIENT OUTCOME CRITERIA

Throughout the hospital stay, the patient will:
- perform or receive oral care at least four times daily
- have oral mucous membrane lesions (if present) treated promptly.

INTERVENTIONS

1. *Assess the patient's mouth at least twice daily for signs and symptoms of thrush, lesions, or bleeding.*

2. *Ensure that the patient receives or completes mouth care after meals and at bedtime.* Provide the following instructions:
– Use a soft toothbrush or swabs.
– Use dilute hydrogen peroxide or toothpaste.

3. *Apply lubricant to the* lips as needed.

4. *Obtain cultures from suspicious oral lesions,* as ordered.

5. Administer medications to treat the underlying diseases that can cause oral lesions as well as antifungal medications. Thalidomide is used for aphthous ulcers. Protease inhibitors cause mouth lesions associated with Kaposi's sarcoma to recede, although some lesions only recede with the use of chemotherapeutic agents or radiotherapy. Antifungal agents used to treat thrush include clotrimazole (Mycelex), fluconazole, and itraconazole. Watch for adverse effects from treatments. No known treatment exists for hairy leukoplakia. Consult current treatment guidelines for oral lesions.

6. *Avoid using alcohol, lemon-glycerin swabs, and commercial mouthwashes.*

7. *Assess for and report inflammation or ulceration of the oral mucosa, leukoplakia, pain, dysphagia, or voice changes.*

8. Additional individualized interventions: _____
_____

RATIONALES

1. Candidiasis is extremely common in AIDS and has even been considered a harbinger of the disease. Lesions may occur as a medication adverse effect or from changes in normal oral flora.

2. Mouth care helps reduce the risk of infection by maintaining circulation to the mucous membrane and by decreasing bacteria in the mouth. Vigorous brushing is discouraged because it may cause bleeding and injure the mucous membrane, providing a place of entry for pathogens.

3. Lubricant helps prevent dry and cracked lips.

4. Culture results guide therapy.

5. Treatments that decrease oral lesions lessen discomfort and irritation, improving the patient's ability to swallow. Treatment guidelines may change with advances in research and clinical practice.

6. These products contain alcohol, which may dry and irritate mucous membranes.

7. Stomatitis, pharyngitis, and esophagitis are common AIDS-related infections. Initial signs and symptoms include inflammation of the mucous membranes, voice changes, and difficulty swallowing (if the inflammation involves the esophagus or larynx).

8. Rationales:_____
_____

Hematologic and immunologic disorders

Nursing diagnosis

Risk for impaired skin integrity related to effects of immobility, disease, medications, or poor nutritional status

NURSING PRIORITY
Prevent skin breakdown.

PATIENT OUTCOME CRITERION
Throughout the hospital stay, the patient will maintain clean, dry, intact skin.

INTERVENTIONS	RATIONALES
1. Implement usual measures to detect and prevent skin breakdown, such as inspection, frequent turning, and skin care.	1. Immunosuppression makes effective treatment of pressure ulcers difficult. Preventive care is essential.
2. If a pressure ulcer develops, institute therapeutic treatment, as ordered. This may include: – cleaning or debriding agents (according to facility protocol or the physician's recommendations) – topical antibiotics – blow-drying after bathing or treatments (follow facility policy) – positioning to avoid pressure on the lesion, using foam or other padding as needed.	2. Prompt treatment is essential to prevent further complications. – Agent selection depends on the patient's status and the physician's preference. Half-strength povidone-iodine solution (Betadine) is commonly used. – The choice of prophylactic antibiotic (which varies) should be reevaluated if infection develops. – A blow-dryer may be useful for certain areas such as the anus. – Additional pressure leads to further tissue breakdown.
3. *Observe for urticaria, maculopapular rash, pruritus, or other allergic reactions.*	3. Medications commonly used to treat opportunistic infections may cause skin irritation. Additionally, HIV infection itself may result in skin abnormalities.
4. Provide appropriate patient teaching related to the above measures.	4. For the able patient, such knowledge promotes self-care and a sense of increased control and self-esteem. For the patient unable to perform self-care, such knowledge promotes understanding of frequent interventions.
5. Additional individualized interventions:_____	5. Rationales:_____

Nursing diagnosis

Sexual dysfunction related to fatigue, depression, fear of rejection, and fear of disease transmission

NURSING PRIORITIES
■ Promote a positive sexual self-concept.
■ Teach safer sex practices.

PATIENT OUTCOME CRITERIA
By the time of discharge, the patient will:
■ list safer sex measures
■ exchange affection with loved ones
■ share sexual concerns with partner, friends, or staff members.

INTERVENTIONS

1. Determine if the patient is currently involved in a sexual relationship by asking direct questions in a nonjudgmental manner. If you're uncomfortable discussing sexuality, refer the patient to another professional or an AIDS counselor.

2. *Encourage open discussion and sharing of feelings between the patient and his partner.* Provide accurate information.

3. Encourage the expression of affection and nonsexual touching, such as hugging, massaging, and holding hands.

4. *Discuss safer sex practices.* Refer to current CDC guidelines for detailed, up-to-date recommendations. Teach the patient and his spouse or partner to observe the following guidelines:

– Abstain from sex or engage in a mutually monogamous relationship.
– Avoid the exchange of blood or body fluids, including swallowing semen.
– Use sexual techniques that don't involve the exchange of body fluids, such as mutual masturbation and fantasy.
– Avoid sex practices classified as "unsafe," such as intercourse without a condom, oral sex without a condom, and inserting objects into the rectum.
– Maintain safer sexual practices throughout life.

5. Additional individualized interventions: _____

RATIONALES

1. Because the disease may be transmitted through sexual contact, assessing sexual relationships is essential. Many patients with AIDS are abandoned by their partners after diagnosis. If the patient is a homosexual, the high incidence of AIDS among homosexual males may add to the anxiety of the patient and his partner. This is especially true if the patient's sexual orientation isn't known or accepted by his family or friends.

2. Sharing of feelings may help the couple maintain closeness and offer mutual support. Accurate information helps to dispel fears based on misunderstandings about AIDS.

3. Liberal use of touch reduces feelings of shame and abandonment.

4. Safer sex guidelines may help reduce the likelihood of disease transmission. CDC guidelines are revised frequently, so nurses should consult current information before providing specific teaching. The harm-reduction model encourages less risky sexual activities, decreasing the risk of sexual transmission.
– Multiple sexual contacts are associated with an increased risk of HIV transmission.
– The virus is transmitted through such exchanges.

– Alternative techniques may provide sexual satisfaction without the risk of disease transmission.
– Unsafe practices are associated with disease transmission.

– Even after AIDS education and years of safer sexual practices, the patient may relapse to unsafe behaviors.

5. Rationales: _____

Suggested NIC Interventions
Sexual counseling

Suggested NOC Outcomes
Sexual functioning

Nursing diagnosis

Deficient knowledge (symptoms of disease progression, risk factors, transmission of disease, home care, and treatment options) related to lack of exposure to information

NURSING PRIORITY

Provide the patient and his family with complete and accurate information.

PATIENT OUTCOME CRITERIA

By the time of discharge, the patient will:
- list precautionary measures to avoid infections
- list symptoms that may indicate infections or other complications
- discuss appropriate home care and waste disposal guidelines
- list precautions to prevent disease transmission
- verbalize awareness of legal rights.

INTERVENTIONS

1. See the "Knowledge deficit" care plan, page 129.

2. *Teach the patient and his loved ones about infection prevention measures,* including:
– regular cleaning of bathrooms and kitchen

– avoiding crowds and persons with known or suspected infections; using good hand-washing techniques
– avoiding touching fish tanks, animal waste, or bird-cages
– consulting the physician before obtaining pets
– thoroughly washing all raw fruits and vegetables and avoiding raw and undercooked meat, seafood, and eggs and unpasteurized milk
– smoking cessation, as indicated

– consulting the physician about vaccines

– following dietary recommendations, including high-protein, high-calorie intake
– eliminating sources of standing water

– practicing good health habits, such as getting adequate rest and regular exercise, and avoiding steroids or recreational drugs that may further decrease immune function

3. *Discuss the signs and symptoms that may indicate AIDS-related complications.* These include night sweats, chest pain, shortness of breath, swollen glands, persistent fever, weight loss, diarrhea, weakness, purplish blotches on the skin, white patches or ulcerations in the mouth, difficulty swallowing, dry cough, headache, confusion, easy bruising, and skin lesions. Emphasize the importance of promptly reporting signs and symptoms to health care providers.

RATIONALES

1. The "Knowledge deficit" care plan contains detailed interventions for patient and family teaching. This care plan contains additional information pertinent to AIDS.

2. Infection control is essential to minimize the risk of further complications.
– Moisture in bathrooms and kitchen may facilitate fungal growth.
– Immunosuppression renders the patient extremely susceptible to infections.
– Animal waste harbors microorganisms.

– Pets may carry intestinal protozoa.
– These may be sources of microorganisms.

– Smoking increases the incidence of respiratory infections.
– The immunosuppressed patient may not be able to manufacture appropriate antibodies and may develop the disease that the vaccine would normally protect against.
– Malnutrition predisposes the patient to infection.

– Standing water provides a medium for microbial growth.
– Overall health maintenance maximizes immune response.

3. Early reporting of new signs and symptoms and prompt treatment of complications, may prolong an active life.

4. *Review with the family the recommendations for home care and waste disposal:*
– Wash hands thoroughly before touching the patient and after contact with blood or secretions.
– Use 1:10 bleach-in-water solution for cleaning blood spills and washing soiled bedding, medical equipment, bedpans or commodes, and soiled surfaces.
– Dispose of contaminated waste carefully. Flush body fluids, blood, and used tissues down the toilet. Place needles in a puncture-proof container; when full, seal and dispose of it in the trash. Double-bag nonflushable items soiled with secretions in plastic bags, tie them closed, and dispose of them in the trash.
– Use masks only when suctioning or performing other measures that may allow direct contact with secretions or to protect the patient from the caregiver's infection.
– Wear gloves when handling body fluids or blood.
– Wash dishes and utensils in hot, soapy water.

4. Thorough, specific teaching reduces anxiety for family members and promotes safe and effective care. Current evidence doesn't suggest any danger of HIV transmission from casual contact. The CDC recommends that caregivers use blood and body fluid precautions.

5. *Teach the patient and his loved ones how the AIDS virus may be spread:* by sexual activity or by direct contact of an infected person's blood or body fluids with the broken skin or mucous membrane of an uninfected person. Discuss such precautionary measures as:
– avoiding sharing personal toiletry items (such as razors and toothbrushes) and needles (including piercing and tattoo needles)
– not donating blood or organs

– obtaining pregnancy counseling

5. Awareness of transmission factors may help the patient avoid spreading the disease to others.

– Sharing these items may permit transmission of the virus.

– The virus has been transmitted through blood transfusions and transplanted organs.
– The AIDS Clinical Trial Group study number 076 has demonstrated that when mothers are treated with AZT, the transmission rate from mother to child is 8.3%, compared to 25.5% in the group receiving placebos. The worldwide transmission rate varies from 8.3% to 45%. Increasingly, the use of AZT and other antiretrovirals is becoming the standard of care to decrease HIV transmission from mother to child.
– Sexual activity is a major method of HIV transmission.

– using safer sex practices (see "Sexual dysfunction," page 751, for details).

6. Provide information regarding the patient's legal rights, including privacy and confidentiality of medical records, laws protecting against discrimination in housing and employment, and the right to choose treatment and participate in research studies, as appropriate. If unable to provide such information yourself, refer the patient to an AIDS support group or AIDS hotline as appropriate.

6. Because of the widespread fear of AIDS, the patient may encounter discrimination. Knowledge of legal rights and options may help prevent further losses.

7. Encourage the patient to explore treatment options with the physician, including new or experimental medications and alternatives to traditional medicine (such as acupuncture, visualization, nutritional therapy, and stress control).

7. At this time, no cure for AIDS exists; however, new or alternative therapies may offer as-yet-undocumented benefits. In addition, such therapies may offer the patient hope, energy, and an increased sense of wellness.

8. Additional individualized interventions:_____

8. Rationales:_____

Hematologic and immunologic disorders

> **Suggested NIC Interventions**
> Teaching: Procedure/treatment; Teaching: Disease process; Teaching: Prescribed medication

> **Suggested NOC Outcomes**
> Knowledge: Treatment regimen; Knowledge: Disease process; Knowledge: Health behaviors; Knowledge: Health promotion

Discharge planning

DISCHARGE CHECKLIST

Before discharge, the patient shows evidence of:
- ❑ stable vital signs
- ❑ absence of cardiovascular and pulmonary symptoms
- ❑ absence of skin breakdown
- ❑ stabilizing weight
- ❑ ability to tolerate adequate nutritional intake
- ❑ ability to control pain and nausea using oral medications
- ❑ ability to transfer, ambulate, and perform ADLs independently or with minimal assistance
- ❑ absence of bowel or bladder dysfunction
- ❑ mentation indicating an ability for continued independent self-care
- ❑ adequate home support system or referral to home care or hospice if indicated by disease stage, inadequate home support system, or inability to manage ADLs and care independently.

TEACHING CHECKLIST

Document evidence that the patient and his family demonstrate an understanding of:
- ❑ disease and its implications
- ❑ the purpose, dosage, administration schedule, and adverse effects requiring medical attention for discharge medications
- ❑ community resources available for emotional support, financial counseling, grief counseling, and individual and family counseling
- ❑ treatment options, including investigational studies and compassionate-use medications
- ❑ resources for long-term care or terminal care, such as hospice or home care
- ❑ signs and symptoms of opportunistic infection or complications
- ❑ ways to prevent HIV transmission
- ❑ ways to decrease the risk of new infection
- ❑ symptoms to report to the health care provider
- ❑ importance of keeping follow-up appointments
- ❑ how to contact the physician
- ❑ legal rights and resources.

DOCUMENTATION CHECKLIST

Using outcome criteria as a guide, document:
- ❑ clinical status on admission
- ❑ significant changes in mental and physical status
- ❑ pertinent laboratory and diagnostic test findings

- ❑ occurrence of opportunistic infections
- ❑ treatment decisions
- ❑ nutritional program and support
- ❑ breathing patterns
- ❑ sleep patterns
- ❑ emotional coping
- ❑ support from family and friends
- ❑ patient and family teaching
- ❑ discharge planning.

Associated care plans

- Acute pain
- Compromised family coping
- Dying
- Grieving
- Impaired physical mobility
- Ineffective individual coping
- Knowledge deficit
- Lymphoma
- Nutritional deficit
- Parenteral nutrition
- Pneumonia

References

Board K.F., et al. "Experimental *Pneumocystis carinii* Pneumonia in Simian Immunodeficiency Virus-Infected Rhesus Macaques," *Journal of Infectious Disease* 187(4):576-88, February 2003.

Cozzolino, M., et al. "HIV-protease Inhibitors Impair Vitamin D Bioactivation to 1,25-dihydroxyvitamin D," *AIDS* 17(4): 513-20, March 2003.

Fauci, A.S., et al., eds. *Harrison's Principles of Internal Medicine*, 15th ed. New York: McGraw-Hill Book Co., 2001.

Hu, D.J., et al. "Key Issues for a Potential Human Immunodeficiency Virus Vaccine," *Clinical Infectious Diseases* 36(5): 638-44, March 2003.

Saurya, S., et al. "Characterization of Gag Gene of Plasma HIV Type 1 in Combination Therapy-treated AIDS Patients with High Viral Load and Stable CD4+ T Cell Counts," *AIDS Research and Human Retroviruses* 19(1):73-76, January 2003.

Twitchell, K.T. "Bloodborne Pathogens. What You Need to Know — Part I," *AAOHN Journal* 51(1):38-45, January 2003.

Anemia

DRG INFORMATION

DRG 395   Red Blood Cell Disorder; Age 17+.
      Mean LOS = 4.4 days
  Principal diagnoses include:
- acquired hemolytic anemia
- iron deficiency anemia
- aplastic anemia
- other.

DRG 396   Red Blood Cell Disorder; Ages 0 to 17.
      Mean LOS = 4.6 days

Introduction

DEFINITION AND TIME FOCUS

Anemia isn't a disease but a laboratory diagnosis comprising a constellation of physiologic symptoms. These symptoms result from an inadequate number of circulating red blood cells (RBCs) or from a decreased hemoglobin level. The primary function of the RBC is to carry oxygen from the lungs to the tissues; anemia reduces the blood's oxygen-carrying capacity and produces signs and symptoms of tissue hypoxia.

Anemia occurs in three situations:
- Life-threatening conditions, such as massive hemorrhage or bone marrow depression
- Life-threatening complications, such as arrhythmias, angina, or pulmonary edema
- As a complication of another disease such as lymphoma

Anemia may be classified by cause or by RBC morphology; both classifications are discussed in the appropriate sections. This care plan focuses on the newly diagnosed anemic patient with hemorrhagic or dietary deficiency anemia, the most common types. The principles of care can be generalized to other types of anemia but would be supplemented with condition-specific care, such as discontinuing medication (in toxic hemolytic reactions) or offering genetic counseling (in sickle cell disease). (See *Clinical snapshot: Anemia*, page 757.)

ETIOLOGY AND PRECIPITATING FACTORS

- Excessive bleeding (acute or chronic)
- Decreased RBC production, caused by:
– dietary deficiencies of iron, folic acid, or vitamin B_{12} (cobalamin)
– damaged bone marrow (aplastic anemia) from medications, such as chloramphenicol (Chloromycetin) or sulfonamides; from chemotherapy with alkylating and antimetabolite agents; or from radiation
– impaired production of erythropoietin (in kidney disease)
– defective hemoglobin synthesis (as in sickle cell disease and thalassemia)
– decreased metabolic oxygen demand (as in hypothyroidism).
- Increased RBC destruction (hemolytic anemia), caused by:
– hereditary disorders (such as sprue, sickle cell disease, or thalassemia)
– autoimmune hemolytic reactions (such as from transfusions or lupus erythematosus)
– toxic drug reactions (such as from penicillin, methyldopa [Aldomet], quinine [Quinine Sulfate], quinidine [Quinora], or sulfonamides)
– trauma (such as burns and crush injuries)
– systemic diseases (such as Hodgkin's disease and lymphomas).

Focused assessment guidelines

NURSING HISTORY (FUNCTIONAL HEALTH PATTERN FINDINGS)

The following signs and symptoms aren't present in all anemias. Because of the many types of anemias, symptoms vary widely. The symptoms also vary with the anemia's severity. The patient with mild anemia (hemoglobin level greater than 10 g/dl) is usually asymptomatic at rest but is symptomatic with exertion. The patient with moderate anemia (hemoglobin level 6 to 10 g/dl) is chronically fatigued as well as symptomatic on exertion. The patient with severe anemia (hemoglobin level less than 6 g/dl) is exhausted, cold, and symptomatic even at rest.

Health-perception–health-management pattern

- Fatigue, headaches, dizziness, irritability, sensation of being cold, or palpitations at rest
- History of bleeding (such as from ulcers or hemorrhoids), renal disease, liver disease, cancer, chronic infections, angina (especially in older patients), or inflammation
- Current or recent use of medications (see list above) that affect RBC production (rare)
- Recent exposure to a chemical or myelotoxic substance (such as benzene or a benzene derivative) or to large doses of radiation (rare)
- Family history of a disease such as sickle cell anemia, thalassemia major, or hereditary spherocytosis (all rare)

Activity-exercise pattern

- Fatigue, decreasing activity tolerance, weakness, shortness of breath, palpitations, or claudication

Cognitive-perceptual pattern

- Dizziness, headache, numbness, tingling of fingers and toes, or difficulty concentrating

Nutritional-metabolic pattern
- Weight loss, anorexia, nausea, indigestion, pruritus, or soreness of mouth, esophagus, or tongue (all rare)

Elimination pattern
- Tarry stools, constipation, diarrhea, or flatulence (all rare)
- Brown, hazy urine (rare)
- Gross blood in excretions (rare)

Sexuality-reproductive pattern
- Loss of libido, irregular menstruation or amenorrhea (if female), or impotence (if male)

PHYSICAL FINDINGS
Cardiovascular
- Tachycardia
- Cardiac enlargement (less common than other signs)
- Murmurs (less common than other signs)
- Dependent edema (less common than other signs)
- Vascular bruits (less common than other signs)
- Bounding arterial pulses (less common than other signs)

Pulmonary
- Dyspnea on exertion
- Tachypnea
- Orthopnea (less common than other signs)

Integumentary
- Pallor of skin and mucous membranes
- Diaphoresis
- Delayed wound healing
- Purpura (less common than other signs)
- Jaundice (less common than other signs)
- Spider angiomas (less common than other signs)
- Koilonychia (spoon nails) — late sign of iron deficiency
- Cool skin

DIAGNOSTIC STUDIES
- Hemoglobin level — may be decreased with iron deficiency, pernicious, hemolytic, and hemorrhagic anemias
- Hematocrit — may be low
- RBC count — may be below normal
- Microscopic evaluation of peripheral blood (performed by a hematologist) — reveals size, shape, color, and number of RBCs; useful in diagnosing the specific type of anemia

Note: The morphologic classification of anemias is based on structural changes seen in RBCs, which are classified by size and hemoglobin content:
– Normocytic (normal size) and normochromic (normal color) RBCs are associated with anemias of sudden blood loss; pregnancy; chronic disease such as cancer, kidney disease, or chronic infection; and some hemolytic anemias.
– Macrocytic (abnormally large) and normochromic RBCs are associated with pernicious anemia, folic acid anemia, vitamin B_{12} deficiency, and some hemolytic anemias.
– Microcytic (abnormally small) and normochromic RBCs are associated with anemias of chronic disease.
– Microcytic and hypochromic (pale-colored) RBCs are associated with iron-deficiency anemia and thalassemia.
- Erythrocyte indices — use the RBC count, hemoglobin level, and hematocrit to define the size, hemoglobin weight, and hemoglobin concentration of a typical RBC; mean corpuscular volume (MCV) gives the average cell size; mean corpuscular hemoglobin gives the average hemoglobin weight; and mean corpuscular hemoglobin concentration (MCHC) identifies the average hemoglobin volume. Low MCV and MCHC indicate microcytic, hypochromic anemia (such as iron-deficiency anemia and thalassemia); a high MCV suggests macrocytic anemia (such as folic acid anemia or vitamin B_{12} deficiency)
- Reticulocyte count — if low, may indicate hypoplastic or pernicious anemia; if high, may indicate bone marrow response to anemia resulting from blood loss or hemolysis
- Erythrocyte fragility test — if low, may indicate thalassemia, iron-deficiency anemia, or sickle cell disease; if high, may indicate spherocytosis (hereditary disorder associated with autoimmune hemolytic anemia)
- Direct Coombs' test — positive response may indicate autoimmune hemolytic anemia (idiopathic, drug-induced, or caused by an underlying disease such as cancer or lupus erythematosus)
- Hemoglobin electrophoresis — identifies hemoglobin types by measuring the degree of negative charge
- Sickle cell test — identifies sickle cell disease and trait (hemoglobin electrophoresis is then needed to differentiate the two disorders)
- Serum iron level and total iron-binding capacity (TIBC) — serum iron level decrease and TIBC increase indicate iron-deficiency anemia
- Serum folic acid levels — low levels may indicate megaloblastic anemia
- Serum vitamin B_{12} levels — low levels could indicate inadequate dietary intake of vitamin B_{12} or a malabsorption disorder
- Bone marrow aspiration and biopsy — histologic examination and differential count with erythroid-myeloid ratio useful for differential diagnosis of aplastic, hypoplastic, or pernicious anemia
- Liver-spleen scan — can detect splenomegaly associated with hereditary spherocytosis
- Chest X-ray — may show cardiac enlargement

POTENTIAL COMPLICATIONS
- Hemorrhagic shock
- Angina pectoris
- Heart failure
- Pulmonary edema
- Renal damage
- Arrhythmias

CLINICAL SNAPSHOT ✳

Anemia

Major nursing diagnoses and collaborative problems	Key patient outcomes
CP: Hypoxemia	Maintain stable vital signs, typically: heart rate, 60 to 100 beats/minute; systolic blood pressure, 90 to 140 mm Hg; and diastolic blood pressure, 50 to 90 mm Hg.
ND: Imbalanced nutrition: Less than body requirements	Follow the recommended diet.
ND: Risk for impaired skin integrity	Maintain dry, intact skin.
ND: Activity intolerance	Perform simple ADLs independently without reporting fatigue.
ND: Hopelessness	Identify pertinent community resources.

Collaborative problem

Hypoxemia related to decreased oxygen-carrying capacity of RBCs

NURSING PRIORITY

Prevent or promptly relieve hypoxemia.

PATIENT OUTCOME CRITERIA

Throughout the hospital stay, the patient will:
■ maintain vital signs within normal limits, typically: heart rate, 60 to 100 beats/minute; systolic blood pressure, 90 to 140 mm Hg; and diastolic blood pressure, 50 to 90 mm Hg
■ have no palpitations or chest pain
■ maintain usual mental status, ideally alert and oriented
■ display arterial blood gas (ABG) levels within normal limits: pH, 7.35 to 7.45; partial pressure of arterial carbon dioxide, 35 to 45 mm Hg; and HCO_3^-, 23 to 28 mEq/L
■ show normal skin color
■ have clear breath sounds
■ maintain acceptable hemoglobin level and hematocrit (as determined by the physician)
■ have no complaints of feeling cold.
   Note: The expected outcomes for a patient with newly diagnosed anemia vary, depending on the type of anemia, its severity, its chronicity, the treatment selected, and the underlying disease. Therefore, these outcome criteria are general; more specific outcomes may need to be determined for each patient.

INTERVENTIONS

1. Elevate the head of the bed.

2. *Monitor for and report signs of hypoxemia,** such as restlessness, irritability, and confusion. Observe oral mucosa, fingernail beds, palmar creases, and conjunctivae for pallor or cyanosis.

RATIONALES

1. This position allows for greater lung expansion, promoting alveolar gas exchange.

2. Baseline and serial assessments of these signs of hypoxemia help individualize care. Neurologic signs reflect cerebral ischemia. Skin color changes are observed best in unpigmented sites. Because cyanosis indicates the presence of 5 g/dl or more of desaturated hemoglobin and hemoglobin levels may be so depressed that the patient can't accumulate 5 g/dl of desaturated hemoglobin without decompensating, cyanosis may be absent or a late sign.

*Italics indicate key interventions.

3. *Monitor respirations before and after activity.* Assess breath sounds at least every 8 hours and promptly report crackles, gurgles, or decreased breath sounds to the physician.

3. Dyspnea and tachypnea may be present in mild to moderate anemia. The exact cause of dyspnea is unclear. One hypothesis suggests that decreased oxygen pressure plays an important role. Heart failure may develop with severe anemia if the heart can't handle the increased cardiac output necessary to compensate for the lower oxygen saturation of the blood.

4. *Monitor the patient's pulse, noting strength and rate.* Report a pulse that doesn't fall within normal limits for the patient.

4. To compensate for the decreased hemoglobin level, cardiac rate and output increase. Pulse weakness, threadiness, and rapidity are more pronounced as anemia becomes more severe.

5. *Note chest pain or palpitations.*

5. Angina pectoris may develop in severe anemia from ischemia of the heart muscle. Palpitations reflect increased myocardial irritability secondary to hypoxemia.

6. *Monitor ABG measurements,* as ordered, and report the results to the physician.

6. ABG measurements document the degree of hypoxemia. Inadequate hemoglobin saturation decreases the oxygen-carrying capacity of the blood.

7. *Administer oxygen,* as ordered.

7. Supplemental oxygen helps prevent tissue hypoxia by elevating the arterial oxygen content.

8. *Administer whole blood or packed RBCs,* as ordered.

8. Transfusions elevate the RBC count, hemoglobin level, and hematocrit. An increased hemoglobin level improves arterial oxygen content, lessening signs and symptoms of hypoxemia.

9. *Monitor hemoglobin level and hematocrit.*

9. These tests provide objective evidence of the degree of anemia and the efficacy of treatment.

10. *Maintain a warm room temperature.* Provide extra blankets if the patient desires.

10. The body compensates for chronic hypoxemia by lowering the metabolic rate and shunting blood to vital organs, making the patient more sensitive to cold. A cold room temperature induces vasoconstriction, which further impairs the release of oxygen to tissues.

11. Additional individualized interventions: _____
_____

11. Rationales: _____
_____

Nursing diagnosis

Imbalanced nutrition: Less than body requirements related to stomatitis, glossitis, anorexia, fatigue, lack of knowledge, or sociocultural factors

NURSING PRIORITY

Maintain adequate nutritional intake.

PATIENT OUTCOME CRITERIA

By the time of discharge, the patient will:
- show signs of improving nutritional deficiencies (manifested by improved hematocrit and hemoglobin, serum albumin, and folic acid levels)
- have less tongue, mouth, and esophagus soreness
- increase weight toward normal for age, height, and body type
- have increased energy level
- follow the recommended diet
- verbalize the ability to obtain recommended diet after discharge or have appropriate referrals made.

INTERVENTIONS

1. *Provide mouth care before and after meals, or assist the patient in performing mouth care.* (Use a soft or sponge toothbrush to minimize trauma to the gums.)

2. *Observe for soreness of the tongue, mouth, and esophagus.*

3. Recommend a bland diet (avoidance of hot, spicy, or acidic foods).

4. Serve six small meals a day, providing foods that appeal to the patient and meet specific dietary needs. Consult the dietitian for a specific diet. Specific needs vary with the type of anemia and may include the following:
– for iron deficiency — red meat, organ meats, green vegetables, and enriched breads and cereals
– for vitamin B_{12} deficiency — meat, chicken, liver, shellfish, dairy products, egg yolks, and legumes
– for folic acid deficiency — green and leafy vegetables, fruits, meats, and whole grain breads and cereals
– for vitamin C deficiency — citrus fruits and juices.

5. *Administer vitamins and minerals,* as ordered (for example, iron preparations, vitamin B_{12}, folic acid, and vitamin C). Use the Z-track method to administer I.M. iron. If parenteral iron is ordered, a test dose must be given to screen for allergies. Be alert for adverse effects of parenteral iron. If oral iron is prescribed, monitor the patient and teach these precautions:
– Take iron with meals.
– Avoid taking iron with dairy products, eggs, coffee, tea, or antacids.
– Increase vitamin C intake.
– If iron is in liquid form, dilute it, drink it through a straw, and rinse the mouth afterward.

6. *Teach the patient the importance of a well-balanced diet,* including specific dietary needs. Emphasize the importance of adequate intake. Relate dietary recommendations to the patient's signs and symptoms.

7. Document the patient's food intake.

8. *Weigh the patient daily,* or, as ordered.

9. If the patient's nutritional needs aren't met by dietary intake, consult the physician about enteral or parenteral feeding.

RATIONALES

1. A patient with pernicious anemia or severe iron-deficiency anemia may have a sore mouth, tongue, or esophagus. Mouth care soothes and refreshes irritated tissues and can stimulate the patient's appetite. Frequent mouth care also decreases bacterial growth, thereby decreasing the risk of infection.

2. Stomatitis and glossitis may be present in pernicious anemia.

3. Spicy and acidic foods can further irritate the mouth, tongue, and esophagus. Hot foods have stronger odors than cold foods and may not appeal to the patient with a poor appetite.

4. Small portions require less energy to consume and digest. Large meals shunt blood to the GI tract, further contributing to fatigue. Foods that appeal to the patient are more likely to be eaten. The dietitian is best qualified to plan a diet that meets the patient's needs.

5. Iron, vitamin B_{12}, and folic acid are needed to synthesize hemoglobin. The patient taking either folic acid or vitamin B_{12} may have allergic signs and symptoms of wheezing and itching. Possible adverse reactions to parenteral iron can include tachycardia, muscle pain, chest pain, backache, headache, chills, dizziness, fever and nausea. The Z-track method minimizes leakage of iron into surrounding tissues (thus minimizing pain) or out through the injection site (thus minimizing medication loss and tissue staining). Precautions for oral iron maximize absorption and minimize gastric distress and tooth staining. Vitamin C promotes iron absorption and influences folic acid metabolism.

6. Lack of knowledge can contribute to poor dietary intake. Stressing the importance of diet may enlist the patient's cooperation despite fatigue or discomfort. Using personal examples makes recommendations more meaningful.

7. Accurate documentation helps determine daily calorie needs.

8. The patient's weight can be used as part of the ongoing nutritional assessment and can help monitor fluid status.

9. Tube feedings or parenteral nutrition may be indicated to improve nutritional status.

10. Before discharge: – Assess the patient's understanding of the importance of proper nutrition. – Evaluate the patient's ability to obtain the prescribed diet and medications. – Make referrals to social services or community agencies as indicated.	**10.** Poor nutrition may result from ignorance, poverty, or limited ability to shop for food, as in the debilitated older person who depends on public transportation.
11. Additional individualized interventions: _____	**11.** Rationales: _____

Suggested NIC Interventions
Diet staging; Nutrition management; Weight gain assistance; Nutritional monitoring

Suggested NOC Outcomes
Nutritional status; Nutritional status: Food and fluid intake; Nutritional status: Nutrient intake; Weight control

---

Nursing diagnosis

Risk for impaired skin integrity related to tissue hypoxia, decreased mobility, and bed rest

NURSING PRIORITY

Maintain skin integrity.

PATIENT OUTCOME CRITERION

Throughout the hospital stay, the patient will maintain dry, intact skin.

INTERVENTIONS	RATIONALES
1. *Assess the patient's skin,* including bony prominences, for redness and induration at every position change.	**1.** Mechanical pressure and decreased hemoglobin availability increase the risk of tissue hypoxia and cell damage. Abnormally red skin, especially over a pressure point, may indicate reactive hyperemia after relief of pressure-induced ischemia. Induration results from cellular changes that occur with ischemia.
2. *Keep the skin clean and dry;* keep the bed linen dry and wrinkle-free.	**2.** The skin is the first line of defense against infection. Moisture provides a good medium for bacterial growth and can lead to maceration. Wrinkle-free linens distribute pressure evenly over the skin.
3. *Reposition the patient at least every 2 hours.* Apply lotion to and massage pressure points. Increase the frequency of position changes if redness or induration occurs. Avoid weight bearing on reddened areas.	**3.** Hypoxemia increases the risk of tissue breakdown. Frequent turning relieves pressure and reestablishes blood flow. Massaging pressure points with lotion keeps the skin soft and increases circulation. Redness results from reactive hyperemia when pressure is relieved. Weight bearing on reddened areas may worsen ischemia.
4. *Teach active range-of-motion (ROM) exercises,* and instruct the patient to do them hourly while awake, if tolerated. (If the patient can't tolerate active ROM exercises, substitute passive ones.)	**4.** Movement stimulates circulation and maintains muscle tone and joint mobility.
5. Assess the patient's need for a pressure-relieving device, such as a foam mattress or alternating pressure mattress, and obtain the device if indicated. (A physician's order may be required to ensure insurance reimbursement.)	**5.** Pressure-relieving devices eliminate, change, or decrease the amount of pressure on the skin, improving or maintaining circulation.

6. Additional individualized interventions: _____

6. Rationales: _____

Suggested NIC Interventions
Pressure management; Pressure ulcer care; Skin surveillance; Incision site care; Wound care

Suggested NOC Outcomes
Tissue integrity: Skin and mucus membranes; Wound healing: Primary intention; Wound healing: Secondary intention

---

Nursing diagnosis

Activity intolerance related to weakness and fatigue

NURSING PRIORITY

Increase the patient's independence in activities of daily living (ADLs) while minimizing weakness and fatigue.

PATIENT OUTCOME CRITERIA

By the time of discharge, the patient will:
- perform simple ADLs, such as eating, washing face and hands, and toileting, independently without reporting fatigue
- identify priority tasks on which to expend energy.

INTERVENTIONS

1. *Provide rest periods between activities and an environment that promotes rest.* Get a description of the patient's room at home, and try to simulate it if possible. Teach the importance of rest.

2. *Assess the patient's normal ADLs,* and offer help in prioritizing them. Help the patient establish a realistic activity level. Teach the patient to:
– avoid energy-taxing activities
– eliminate nonessential activities
– perform priority and necessary activities at times when the patient has the most energy.

3. *Help the patient ambulate.* Observe for and teach signs and symptoms of activity intolerance, such as dizziness, fainting, shortness of breath, chest pain, and worsened fatigue. Monitor orthostatic vital signs.

4. Allow as much self-care as possible, and assist as needed.

5. Place personal items (such as a water pitcher and tissues) within the patient's reach.

6. Provide safe environment. Consider obtaining a home safety evaluation by a physical therapist.

7. Additional individualized interventions: _____

RATIONALES

1. Rest decreases oxygen demand. Simulating features of the patient's room at home contributes to relaxation.

2. Initially, the patient may need to limit activities to a few. Involving the patient in selecting these activities gives a sense of self-control.

3. Orthostatic hypotension may aggravate cerebral ischemia or cardiac ischemia. The patient may need encouragement to change his position slowly and to pace activities according to tolerance.

4. Self-care encourages independence and helps promote and maintain self-esteem.

5. Placing personal items within the patient's reach encourages independence while conserving energy.

6. These measures decrease the patient's risk of injury.

7. Rationales: _____

Hematologic and immunologic disorders

Nursing diagnosis

Hopelessness related to chronic fatigue, activity intolerance, and lack of independence

NURSING PRIORITY

Provide emotional support and guidance in solving practical problems.

PATIENT OUTCOME CRITERIA

By the time of discharge, the patient will:
- identify personal support systems
- identify pertinent community resources.

INTERVENTIONS	RATIONALES
1. Actively listen while the patient expresses personal feelings and frustrations.	**1.** Active listening provides empathic support.
2. *Identify and assess the patient's personal resources.* Assist with problem solving.	**2.** The patient's participation in identifying personal resources represents a significant step in actively coping with problems.
3. Provide information about available community agencies and the services offered by each. With the patient's consent, make appropriate referrals.	**3.** The patient may require help to meet basic needs. Community assistance may be available for preparing meals, performing light household duties, assisting with ADLs, and counseling.
4. Additional individualized interventions: _____	**4.** Rationales:_____

Discharge planning

DISCHARGE CHECKLIST

Before discharge, the patient shows evidence of:
- ❒ stable vital signs
- ❒ absence of fever
- ❒ hemoglobin level and hematocrit within acceptable parameters
- ❒ ABG measurements within normal parameters
- ❒ absence of cardiovascular and pulmonary complications, such as dyspnea and angina
- ❒ ability to tolerate adequate nutritional intake
- ❒ stabilizing weight
- ❒ ability to obtain recommended diet
- ❒ ability to perform ADLs and ambulate the same as or better than before hospitalization
- ❒ adequate home support system or referral to home care (as indicated by a lack of a home support system, inability to follow diet and medication regimen, or inability to perform ADLs and tolerate moderate activities).

State professional review organizations have specific parameters for acceptable hemoglobin levels upon discharge. Parameters vary by state. A hospital can receive a citation for discharging a patient whose hemoglobin level is less than 10 g/dl, especially if the patient is readmitted within 15 days of discharge. Therefore, the patient's blood work results should be examined closely at discharge, and any abnormal findings should appear in the discharge summary.

TEACHING CHECKLIST

Document evidence that the patient and his family demonstrate an understanding of:
❑ type of anemia and its implications
❑ discharge medications, including their purpose, dosage, administration schedule, and adverse effects requiring medical attention
❑ special dietary needs
❑ community resources
❑ signs and symptoms indicating a need for medical attention
❑ dates, times, and location of follow-up appointments
❑ how to contact the physician.

DOCUMENTATION CHECKLIST

Using outcome criteria as a guide, document:
❑ clinical status on admission
❑ significant changes in clinical status
❑ pertinent laboratory and diagnostic test findings
❑ nutritional intake
❑ activity tolerance
❑ patient and family teaching
❑ discharge planning.

Associated care plans

- Acute pain
- Geriatric care
- Ineffective individual coping
- Knowledge deficit

References

Holcomb, S.S. "Anemias: Road Signs to the Real Problems," *Dimensions of Critical Care Nursing* 20(3):2-8, May-June 2001.

Ignatavicius, D.D., and Workman, M.L., eds. *Medical-Surgical Nursing: Critical Thinking for Collaborative Care,* 4th ed. Philadelphia: W.B. Saunders Co., 2002.

Thompson, J., et al. *Mosby's Clinical Nursing,* 5th ed. St. Louis: Mosby–Year Book, Inc., 2002.

Disseminated intravascular coagulation

DRG INFORMATION
DRG 397   Coagulation Disorders.
          Mean LOS = 5.2 days
   Principal diagnoses include all types of coagulation
defects or disorders, including disseminated intravascular coagulation (DIC).

Introduction
DEFINITION AND TIME FOCUS
DIC is a complex, acquired hematologic disorder characterized by a paradoxical blend of coagulation and hemorrhage. One or more procoagulants — such as bacterial toxins, exposure of collagen in damaged blood vessel walls, or tissue fragments — provoke uncontrolled microcirculatory coagulation through the intrinsic clotting pathway, extrinsic clotting pathway, or both.

   The explosive production of thrombin causes widespread microcirculatory deposition of fibrin and rapid consumption of clotting factors. It also triggers the body's fibrinolytic system, a homeostatic mechanism that limits coagulation. Fibrin split products, a by-product of fibrinolysis, exacerbate bleeding because they function as anticoagulants. Because of the anticoagulants and the scarcity of clotting factors, the patient can't form stable clots and bleeding occurs throughout the body. This care plan focuses on the patient in the critical care unit with acute DIC. (See *Clinical snapshot: Disseminated intravascular coagulation.*)

ETIOLOGY AND PRECIPITATING FACTORS
- Shock
- Cardiac arrest and cardiopulmonary resuscitation
- Acute respiratory distress syndrome (ARDS)
- Septicemia
- Neoplasms
- Transfusion reactions or other hemolytic conditions
- Trauma, lengthy cardiopulmonary bypass operations, or other tissue injury
- Tissue necrosis
- Fat or amniotic fluid emboli
- Burns

Focused assessment guidelines
NURSING HISTORY
(FUNCTIONAL HEALTH PATTERN FINDINGS)
Health-perception–health-management pattern
Patient reports are relatively unimportant in the diagnosis of DIC. Usually, the patient is too ill from the primary disorder to be aware of or report subjective manifestations. Even if the patient is alert, the widespread manifestations of DIC may cause variable, nonspecific symptoms.

Nutritional-metabolic pattern
- Nausea or vomiting

Activity-exercise pattern
- Dyspnea
- Fatigue or weakness

Cognitive-perceptual pattern
- Confusion, headache, or sudden localized pain

PHYSICAL FINDINGS
Physical findings vary greatly, depending on the underlying disorder, degree of organ involvement, and stage of DIC.

Cardiovascular
- Blood oozing from multiple sites, such as I.V. insertion sites, incisions, and nasal mucosa around endotracheal or nasogastric tubes
- Repeated episodes of minor bleeding
- Frank hemorrhage
- Hypotension
- Tachycardia

Integumentary
- Acral cyanosis (irregularly shaped, patchy cyanosis of fingers, toes, or ears), considered diagnostic of DIC
- Petechiae
- Purpura
- Ecchymoses
- Hematomas
- Necrosis over digits, nose, or genitals

Pulmonary
- Tachypnea, dyspnea, or both
- Epistaxis
- Hemoptysis

Gastrointestinal
- Hematemesis
- Melena

Neurologic
- Coma
- Seizures
- Confusion

Renal
- Hematuria
- Oliguria or anuria

DIAGNOSTIC STUDIES
DIC is a laboratory diagnosis based on a characteristic pattern of abnormal values.

- Prothrombin time/international normalized ratio — prolonged, indicating dysfunction of the extrinsic clotting pathway
- Partial thromboplastin time (PTT) — prolonged, indicating dysfunction of the intrinsic clotting pathway
- Fibrinogen level — decreased because of fibrinogen consumption
- Platelet count — diminished because of platelet consumption
- Fibrin split products — increased because of fibrinolysis
- Antithrombin III levels — decreased, indicating consumption by excessive thrombin formation

- D-dimer — increased, indicating excessive breakdown of fibrin bonds; highly predictive of DIC
- Peripheral blood smear — reveals large platelets, reflecting rapid platelet usage, and red blood cell (RBC) fragments, reflecting damage during RBC passage through fibrin webs

POTENTIAL COMPLICATIONS
- Organ necrosis
- Acute renal failure
- ARDS

CLINICAL SNAPSHOT

Disseminated intravascular coagulation

Major nursing diagnoses and collaborative problems	Key patient outcomes
CP: Risk for hemorrhage	Maintain stable vital signs, typically: heart rate, 60 to 100 beats/minute; systolic blood pressure, 90 to 140 mm Hg; and diastolic blood pressure, 50 to 90 mm Hg.
CP: Ischemia	Produce more than 60 ml/hour of urine.
CP: Risk for hypoxemia	Maintain ABG values within normal limits: pH, 7.35 to 7.45; $Paco_2$, 35 to 45 mm Hg; and HCO_3^-, 23 to 28 mEq/L.
ND: Impaired skin integrity	Maintain warm, dry, intact skin.
ND: Acute pain	State that pain (with pain medication) is less than 3 on a 0 to 10 pain rating scale.

Collaborative problem

Risk for hemorrhage related to consumption of clotting factors, increased fibrinolysis, and presence of endogenous anticoagulants

NURSING PRIORITY
Control clotting and bleeding.

PATIENT OUTCOME CRITERIA
Within 72 hours of the onset of bleeding, the patient will:
- have no further episodes of oozing or frank hemorrhage
- maintain vital signs within normal limits, typically: heart rate, 60 to 100 beats/minute; systolic blood pressure, 90 to 140 mm Hg; and diastolic blood pressure, 50 to 90 mm Hg
- exhibit coagulation laboratory values within normal limits.

INTERVENTIONS	RATIONALES
1. *Collaborate with the physician to identify and treat the cause of DIC;* * for example, administer I.V. fluids to correct hypovolemia or antibiotics to combat sepsis, as ordered.	1. Removing or controlling the underlying cause of DIC is essential to effective treatment.

*Italics indicate key interventions.

Hematologic and immunologic disorders

2. *Monitor the presence and degree of hemorrhage.* Observe for persistent oozing of blood at multiple sites, petechiae, purpura, ecchymoses, hematuria, and hemorrhagic gingivitis. Note bleeding from wounds, drains, and chest tubes. In the female patient, check for vaginal bleeding. Test all drainage for occult blood.

3. *Monitor trends in coagulation panels,* as ordered.

4. *Administer heparin,* if ordered. Monitor PTT, as ordered, and report values exceeding two times normal.

5. *Administer transfusion therapy* (typically fresh whole blood, fresh frozen plasma, platelet concentrate, cryoprecipitate, or antithrombin III), as ordered. Monitor trends in blood values, and anticipate the need for replacement blood products.

6. *Monitor vital signs.* Report systolic blood pressure below 90 mm Hg or a heart rate above 100 beats/minute.

7. Maintain a normal blood pressure by giving fluid and medications, as ordered.

8. *Monitor for fluid overload.* Observe for crackles, jugular vein distention, or increased pulmonary artery pressure (PAP) and pulmonary artery wedge pressure (PAWP). If indicated, collaborate with the physician to reduce fluid volume such as by administering diuretics.

9. Additional individualized interventions:_____

_____

2. The presence and degree of bleeding provide a rough indicator of the severity of DIC.

3. Coagulation values document the degree of DIC. They may be abnormal even if the patient doesn't show clinical signs of the disorder.

4. Heparin disrupts the vicious cycle of clotting and bleeding in DIC. Although it can't lyse existing clots, it can prevent further clot formation. Heparin therapy during intense bleeding is controversial; however, it may be indicated when signs of thrombosis are present and blood component therapy is underway. Heparin inhibits thrombin (therefore limiting platelet aggregation and conversion of fibrinogen to fibrin) and factor X (therefore blocking both intrinsic and extrinsic pathways that lead to thrombin formation). Monitoring the PTT allows the physician to adjust the heparin dose to maintain a therapeutic blood level. The use of heparin is contraindicated in patients with bleeding in the cranium.

5. Transfusion therapy replaces depleted clotting factors. Some physicians order it only after initiating heparinization, theorizing that replacing factors before interrupting the clotting cycle will only potentiate DIC. Antithrombin III inhibits the thrombin activation that triggers fibrin deposits.

6. Hypotension and tachycardia signal blood loss, requiring such interventions as fluid or blood replacement or medications to maintain blood pressure.

7. Both hypotension and hypertension are detrimental to the DIC patient. Hypotension contributes to the disease, while hypertension can dislodge precarious blood clots and initiate fresh bleeding.

8. The patient with DIC usually receives large amounts of fluid and frequent transfusions in an attempt to maintain optimal blood volume and cardiac output. Also, pulmonary capillary fragility increases the risk of interstitial edema. Untreated, fluid overload can progress to pulmonary edema.

9. Rationales:_____

_____

Collaborative problem
Ischemia related to microcirculatory thrombosis

NURSING PRIORITY
Restore tissue perfusion.

PATIENT OUTCOME CRITERIA
Within 72 hours, the patient will:
- produce more than 60 ml/hour of urine
- exhibit a balanced fluid intake and output
- maintain vital signs within normal limits, typically: heart rate, 60 to 100 beats/minute; systolic blood pressure, 90 to 140 mm Hg; and diastolic blood pressure, 50 to 90 mm Hg.

INTERVENTIONS	RATIONALES
1. *Evaluate the status of organ systems at least every 4 hours* by assessing: – neurologic function, including level of consciousness, pupils, and sensorimotor function of the arms and legs – cardiovascular function, including heart rate and volume, blood pressure, strength and symmetry of peripheral pulses, electrocardiogram pattern, and PAP and PAWP – GI function, including bowel sounds and abdominal girth – skin condition (especially fingers and toes) for petechiae, bruising, and necrosis.	1. Tissue ischemia and necrosis can occur in any body system from the widespread deposition of thrombi in the microcirculation. In addition, hypotension activates the complement system, resulting in increased vascular permeability and blood cell lysis, and the kallikrein system, resulting in increased vascular permeability and vasodilation. The net results are arteriolar vasoconstriction, capillary dilation, and arteriovenous shunting. Stagnant blood accumulates in the dilated, bypassed capillaries and becomes acidotic, further damaging tissue and contributing to clotting.
2. *Monitor renal function closely.* Document hourly urine output, noting and reporting any decreasing trend. Summarize fluid intake and output every 8 hours, noting and reporting undesirable fluid retention.	2. The renal system is most likely to suffer from thrombosis, resulting in acute tubular necrosis. Decreasing hourly urine outputs or oliguria may reflect this development. Because oliguria may also reflect other factors common in DIC, such as hypotension, cardiac failure, or hypovolemia, it must be interpreted in the context of the patient's overall condition.
3. *Implement measures* (such as fluid administration) *to treat the underlying cause of tissue ischemia,* as ordered.	3. Tissue ischemia is best treated by attacking its cause such as hypovolemia.
4. Additional individualized interventions: _____ _____	4. Rationales:_____ _____

Collaborative problem
Risk for hypoxemia related to increased pulmonary shunting, anemia, and acidosis

NURSING PRIORITY
Optimize oxygenation.

PATIENT OUTCOME CRITERIA
Within 72 hours, the patient will:
- display arterial blood gas (ABG) levels within normal limits: pH, 7.35 to 7.45; partial pressure of arterial carbon dioxide, 35 to 45 mm Hg; and HCO_3^-, 23 to 28 mEq/L
- display a eupneic respiratory pattern
- have a respiratory rate between 18 and 24 breaths/minute
- display pink nail beds and buccal mucosa.

INTERVENTIONS	RATIONALES
1. *Monitor ABG values,* as ordered, for hypoxemia and acidosis. Monitor oxygen saturation, interpreting the percentage in relation to the current hemoglobin level; don't use the oxygen saturation percentage as the sole indicator of oxygenation.	1. Ischemic damage to the pulmonary parenchyma increases pulmonary shunting, impairing oxygen uptake in the lungs. RBC destruction produces a hemolytic anemia. These factors lessen arterial oxygen content. Also, acidosis and decreased tissue perfusion impair oxygen delivery to the tissues. Oxygen saturation measures only the percentage of available hemoglobin that's saturated with oxygen. The bleeding in DIC lowers hemoglobin levels, decreasing oxygen delivery to tissue even when hemoglobin is fully saturated.
2. *Assess physical indicators of pulmonary status at least every 4 hours.* Note increasing respiratory rate, abnormal respiratory rhythm, and crackles or other abnormal breath sounds. Observe nail beds and buccal mucosa for pallor and central cyanosis.	2. The respiratory rate accelerates to compensate for hypoxemia. Rhythm changes may reflect medullary hypoxemia. Adventitious breath sounds may reflect alveolar accumulation of fluid as the heart fails from ischemia. Pallor and cyanosis reflect arterial oxygen desaturation.
3. *Administer supplemental oxygen, positive end-expiratory pressure (PEEP), or mechanical ventilation,* as ordered.	3. Supplemental oxygen alone may be insufficient to raise low arterial oxygen content from pulmonary shunting. PEEP and mechanical ventilation may be necessary to improve functional residual capacity enough to combat hypoxemia.
4. Additional individualized interventions:_____ _____	4. Rationales:_____ _____

Nursing diagnosis

Impaired skin integrity related to capillary fragility

NURSING PRIORITY

Prevent further bleeding.

PATIENT OUTCOME CRITERIA

Within 72 hours of the onset of DIC, the patient will:
- have no new hematoma formation
- maintain warm, dry, intact skin.

INTERVENTIONS	RATIONALES
1. *Avoid needle punctures,* whenever possible. If a needle puncture is essential, use the smallest gauge needle possible and apply pressure to the site for 10 minutes afterward. Whenever possible, administer medications I.V., as ordered.	1. These measures may help reduce hematoma formation. In addition, because of poor tissue perfusion, medication deposited I.M. may be absorbed erratically, if at all. Administering medications I.V. promotes absorption and avoids creating a puncture site from which the patient may bleed.
2. *Handle the patient gently.* Be particularly careful to avoid disturbing healing areas. Provide meticulous skin care.	2. Gentle handling minimizes skin trauma. Being particularly careful around healing sites minimizes the risk of dislodging unstable clots.
3. *Use an air flotation bed or cushioning and pressure-relieving devices* such as sheepskin. Pad the bed rails.	3. These devices decrease pressure and the risk of trauma and minimize the risk of hematoma development from extreme capillary fragility.

4. *Provide gentle mouth care* with swabs and diluted mouthwash.

5. Additional individualized interventions: _____

4. A toothbrush may damage fragile capillaries and result in gingival bleeding.

5. Rationales:_____

> ### *Suggested NIC Interventions*
> *Pressure management; Skin surveillance; Pressure ulcer care; Wound care*

> ### *Suggested NOC Outcomes*
> *Tissue integrity: Skin and mucous membranes; Wound healing: Secondary intention*

Nursing diagnosis
Acute pain related to tissue ischemia, hematomas, or bleeding into organ or joint capsules

NURSING PRIORITY
Relieve pain.

PATIENT OUTCOME CRITERIA
Within 1 hour of pain onset, the patient will:
- have a relaxed facial expression and body posture
- if able to communicate, rate pain (with pain medication) as less than 3 on a 0 to 10 pain rating scale.

INTERVENTIONS

1. *Assess for pain frequently.* Use various pain-relieving measures, such as ice packs for hematomas or soothing music. Promote rest and provide emotional support. Consult the "Acute pain" care plan, page 32, for details.

2. *Administer pain medications* I.V.; if the patient's pain lasts for most of a 24-hour period, give him around-the-clock medication.

3. Additional individualized interventions:_____

RATIONALES

1. The "Acute pain" care plan contains additional interventions for any patient in pain. This care plan contains interventions specific to DIC. Soothing music helps relieve tension and lessen pain perception.

2. DIC may cause erratic absorption of I.M. medications. Around-the-clock administration can provide better pain control.

3. Rationales:_____

> ### *Suggested NIC Interventions*
> *Medication management; Analgesic administration; Patient-controlled analgesia (PCA) assistance; Conscious sedation*

> ### *Suggested NOC Outcomes*
> *Comfort level; Pain control; Pain: Disruptive effects; Pain level*

Discharge planning

DISCHARGE CHECKLIST
Before discharge, the patient shows evidence of:
- ❏ stable vital signs
- ❏ laboratory coagulation panel within normal limits
- ❏ no bleeding episodes for at least 24 hours.

TEACHING CHECKLIST
Document evidence that the patient and his family demonstrate an understanding of:
- ❏ basic pathophysiology and implications of DIC
- ❏ rationale for therapy
- ❏ pain-relief measures.

Hematologic and immunologic disorders

DOCUMENTATION CHECKLIST

Using outcome criteria as a guide, document:

☐ clinical status on admission
☐ significant changes in status
☐ pertinent diagnostic test findings
☐ bleeding episodes
☐ transfusion and fluid replacement therapy
☐ pain-relief measures
☐ patient and family teaching
☐ discharge planning.

Associated care plans

- Acute pain
- Acute renal failure
- Acute respiratory distress syndrome
- Cardiac surgery
- Hypovolemic shock
- Impaired physical mobility
- Ineffective individual coping
- Liver failure
- Major burns
- Mechanical ventilation
- Multiple trauma
- Nutritional deficit
- Septic shock

References

Dice, R.D. "Intraoperative Disseminated Intravenous Coagulopathy," *Critical Care Nursing Clinics of North America* 12(2):175-79, June 2000.

Maxson, J.H. "Management of Disseminated Intravascular Coagulation," *Critical Care Nursing Clinics of North America* 12(3):341-52, September 2000.

Todres, L., et al. "On the Receiving End: A Hermeneutic-Phenomenological Analysis of a Patient's Struggle to Cope While Going Through Intensive Care," *Nursing in Critical Care* 5(6):277-87, November-December 2000.

Urden, L.D., et al. *Thelan's Critical Care Nursing: Diagnosis and Management*, 4th ed. St. Louis: Mosby–Year Book, Inc., 2002.

Wargo, C.A. "Blood Clot: Gaming to Reinforce Learning about Disseminated Intravascular Coagulation," *Journal of Continuing Education in Nursing* 31(4):149-51, July-August 2000.

Leukemia

DRG INFORMATION

DRG 403 Lymphoma or Non-Acute Leukemia with Complication or Comorbidity (CC).
Mean LOS = 8.1 days

DRG 404 Lymphoma or Non-Acute Leukemia without CC.
Mean LOS = 4.3 days

DRG 405 Acute Leukemia without Major Operating Room (OR) Procedure; Ages 0 to 17.
Mean LOS = 0 days

DRG 473 Acute Leukemia without Major OR Procedure; Age 17+.
Mean LOS = 12.8 days

DRG 409 Radiotherapy
Mean LOS = 5.9 days

These DRGs are used for the patient with leukemia admitted for either radiation or chemotherapy treatment.

Introduction

DEFINITION AND TIME FOCUS

Leukemia is the proliferation and accumulation of abnormal blood cells in the bone marrow or lymph tissue. The malignant cells prevent normal hematopoiesis in the blood marrow and migrate to other organs and tissues, causing the disease's symptoms. The leukemias may be classified according to several criteria, such as the cell and tissue type involved, the duration and course of the disease, or the number of leukocytes in the blood and bone marrow.

Leukemia is classified as *acute* if the bone marrow is infiltrated with undifferentiated, immature cells (blasts) and as *chronic* if the cells are primarily differentiated and mature. The most common types of leukemia involve abnormalities of white blood cells (WBCs), specifically granulocytes and lymphocytes.

Acute monoblastic leukemia is characterized by increased monoblasts (monocyte precursors). Adults with monoblastic leukemia have a poor prognosis, surviving about 1 year.

Acute myeloid (granulocytic) leukemia (AML) involves uncontrolled proliferation of myeloblasts, the precursors of granulocytes. The incidence of AML increases with age. The overall prognosis is poor, with a high mortality from infection and hemorrhage, usually within 1 year.

In *acute lymphoblastic leukemia (ALL)*, immature lymphocytes proliferate in the bone marrow. ALL is primarily a children's disease, with peak incidence between ages 2 and 4. Approximately 50% to 60% of patients survive 5 years.

Chronic myelogenous leukemia (CML) shows abnormal development of granulocytes in the bone marrow, blood, and tissues. An initial chronic phase is followed by an acute phase known as the blastic crisis. The disease occurs most commonly in patients ages 30 to 50. Patients survive 2 to 4 years after the initial phase but live only 3 to 6 months after the blastic crisis phase starts.

Chronic lymphocytic leukemia is the production and accumulation of functionally inactive but long-lived and mature-appearing lymphocytes. Patients (usually ages 50 to 70) typically survive 2 to 10 years.

This care plan focuses on the adult patient admitted for the diagnosis and treatment for leukemia. (See *Clinical snapshot: Leukemia*, page 773.)

ETIOLOGY AND PRECIPITATING FACTORS

The exact cause of leukemia isn't known. Possible causes include:

- exposure to carcinogenic chemicals, such as benzene, alkylating agents, or chloramphenicol
- ionizing radiation
- viruses such as the Epstein-Barr virus
- familial tendency, congenital disorders such as Down syndrome, chromosomal abnormalities, ataxia-telangiectasia, and congenital immune deficiencies
- risk factors associated with: prior chemotherapy with mechlorethamine hydrochloride (Mustargen), procarbazine (Matulane), chlorambucil (Leukeran), etoposide (VePesid, Etopophos) or cyclophosphamide (Cytoxan) hereditary syndromes: Fanconi's anemia and Bloom, Klinefelter's, or Li-Fraumeni syndromes.

Focused assessment guidelines

NURSING HISTORY (FUNCTIONAL HEALTH PATTERN FINDINGS)

Health-perception–health-management pattern

- Gradual or sudden onset of fever, fatigue, weakness and lassitude, or headache
- Evidence of bleeding tendencies related by patient, such as gingival bleeding, purpura, petechiae, ecchymoses and easy bruising, epistaxis, and prolonged menstruation
- Identification as a monozygotic (identical) twin
- Positive family history for leukemia or chromosomal abnormalities

- Exposure to carcinogenic agents or ionizing radiation

Nutritional-metabolic pattern
- Nausea, anorexia, or weight loss
- Complaints of sore throat or dysphagia

Elimination pattern
- Blood in urine
- Tarry stools

Activity-exercise pattern
- Fatigue and weakness
- Dyspnea and palpitations on exertion
- Diminished activity because of bone and joint pain
- Abnormal bruising after minor trauma

Sleep-rest pattern
- Increased desire or need for sleep and rest

Cognitive-perceptual pattern
- Discomfort from mouth ulcers; abdominal, bone, and joint pain; and chills

Role-relationship pattern
- Verbalized difficulty in maintaining role function because of fatigue

Sexuality-reproductive pattern
- Decreased libido secondary to extreme fatigue
- Menorrhagia, if female

Coping–stress tolerance pattern
- Initial denial of diagnosis

Value-belief system
- Diagnosis of cancer as punishment
- Passive, fatalistic philosophy of life and death

PHYSICAL FINDINGS

General
- Elevated temperature
- Fatigued appearance

Cardiovascular
- Tachycardia
- Systolic ejection murmur

Respiratory
- Labored breathing
- Rapid breathing
- Wheezing
- Gurgles
- Decreased breath sounds
- Nosebleeds

Gastrointestinal
- Gingival hypertrophy or bleeding
- Mouth ulcers
- Hepatosplenomegaly
- Increased abdominal girth
- Vomiting
- Oral or rectal mucosal ulceration

Neurologic
- Confusion
- Visual changes

Integumentary
- Pallor

- Purpura
- Petechiae
- Pale mucous membranes
- Ecchymoses
- Erythema
- Rash
- Poor turgor

Genitourinary
- Hematuria

Lymphoreticular
- Lymphadenopathy

Musculoskeletal
- Joint swelling
- Decreased exercise tolerance

DIAGNOSTIC STUDIES

- Complete blood count (CBC) — reflects bone marrow suppression by WBC infiltration
  –WBC count usually greater than 50,000/µl but may be low
  –differential shows increased number of lymphocytes or increased number of polymorphonuclear cells
  –red blood cell (RBC) count, hemoglobin level, and hematocrit below normal; platelet count very low, may be less than 50,000/mm³
- Prothrombin time/international normalized ratio and activated partial thromboplastin time — may be prolonged
- Histochemistry — specific chemistry tests for leukemia show Sudan black or peroxidase; stains are positive in AML
- Uric acid and lactate dehydrogenase levels — elevated in acute leukemia; may indicate extensive bone marrow infiltration
- Liver enzyme levels — may be elevated, showing hepatic infiltration
- Leukocyte alkaline phosphatase levels — may be decreased
- Blood cultures — may show general sepsis
- Urinalysis — may show bacteria and WBCs (indicating infection) or RBCs (indicating bleeding)
- Blood urea nitrogen and creatinine levels — may be elevated in renal infiltration and failure
- Bone marrow aspiration — shows domination by leukemia blast cells of the affected cell line, may show abnormalities specific to leukemia, such as Auer bodies; shows decreased RBC levels and decreased platelet formation
- Lumbar puncture — may detect central nervous system (CNS) infiltration and meningeal irritation
- Liver-spleen scan — shows hepatosplenomegaly and enlarged abdominal lymph nodes
- Chest X-ray — may show lung infiltration, infection, or mediastinal adenopathy
- Computed tomography (CT) scan — may show enlarged lymph nodes or areas of consolidation

- Chromosome analysis — may help in the classification of leukemia by showing abnormal, translocated, extra, or missing chromosomes (such as the Philadelphia chromosome in CML) in the patient's blood cells

POTENTIAL COMPLICATIONS

- Infection, including sepsis
- Hemorrhage, especially of the CNS
- Immunosuppression
- Meningeal irritation
- Cardiotoxicity secondary to chemotherapy
- Hyperuricemia
- Mouth ulcers
- Constipation or diarrhea secondary to chemotherapy
- Arrhythmias secondary to electrolyte imbalance
- Malnutrition, including protein-calorie imbalances

CLINICAL SNAPSHOT

Leukemia

Major nursing diagnoses and collaborative problems	Key patient outcomes
ND: Deficient knowledge (therapeutic modality and choice and care of vascular access device)	State an understanding of and the correct responses to vascular access device complications.
ND: Risk for infection	Maintain stable WBC count and absolute neutrophil count.
CP: Risk for hemorrhage	Maintain stable vital signs, typically: heart rate, 60 to 100 beats/minute; systolic blood pressure, 90 to 140 mm Hg; and diastolic blood pressure, 50 to 90 mm Hg.
ND: Activity intolerance	Ambulate 20% further each day.
ND: Imbalanced nutrition: Less than body requirements	Retain 75% or more of food intake.
ND: Impaired oral mucous membrane	Have no frank bleeding from gums.
ND: Ineffective protection	Remain free from infection.
ND: Ineffective coping	Express feelings, if desired.

Nursing diagnosis

Deficient knowledge (therapeutic modality and choice and care of vascular access device) related to lack of exposure to information

NURSING PRIORITY

Teach the patient and his family about the different types of vascular access devices, including how to care for the device and the site and how to identify complications.

PATIENT OUTCOME CRITERIA

Within 3 days of admission, the patient will:
- identify the type of vascular access device selected
- state an understanding of the rationale for using the device
- state an understanding of insertion procedure.
  Within 5 days of admission, the patient and his family will:
- state and demonstrate site care and the basic technique for flushing the device.
  Within 7 days of admission, the patient and his family will:
- state the correct responses to vascular access device complications, including catheter occlusion, site infection, catheter damage or dislodgment, and infiltration or extravasation of I.V. fluids.

INTERVENTIONS	RATIONALES
1. *Explain the rationale for and the different types of vascular access devices** available for the patient with leukemia.	**1.** Treatment for leukemia requires ongoing antineoplastic chemotherapy, I.V. antibiotics, fluids and nutrition, I.V. infusions, blood and blood product transfusions, and venous blood sampling. Therapy is ongoing, and chemotherapy can have potentially devastating effects on the skin and vasculature, so a vascular access device, such as a tunneled catheter (Hickman, Groshong) or an implanted port (Port-A-Cath, Groshong), is inserted. This device consists of a vascular catheter whose tip is placed in the superior vena cava, allowing delivery of medication, blood and blood products, and parenteral nutrition. It avoids the irritating effects these substances would have if peripheral veins were used and allows for rapid absorption and higher blood concentrations.
2. *Assess the functional abilities, competency level, dexterity and coordination, visual acuity, motivation, and anxiety level of the patient and his family.*	**2.** After discharge, the patient and his family will need to take responsibility for the device, including flushing the catheter and caring for the site. To prevent such complications as infection and catheter occlusion, they must be capable of performing the necessary level of care. Your assessment helps determine their capabilities.
3. *Provide care for the vascular access device,* and teach the patient and his family how to care for it and the site and recognize and manage complications. Refer to the "Lymphoma" care plan, page 789, for more information.	**3.** Teaching helps prepare the patient and his family to care for the vascular access device. The "Lymphoma" care plan provides interventions and rationales for teaching the patient and family about vascular access devices.
4. Additional individualized interventions: _____ _____	**4.** Rationales: _____ _____

> **Suggested NIC Interventions**
> *Teaching: Procedure/treatment*

> **Suggested NOC Outcomes**
> *Knowledge: Treatment regimen*

Nursing diagnosis
Risk for infection related to incompetent bone marrow and immunosuppressive effects of chemotherapy treatment

NURSING PRIORITIES
- Recognize early signs of infection.
- Minimize local and systemic infection.

PATIENT OUTCOME CRITERIA
Within 8 hours of admission, the patient will:
- have potential sites of infection identified and monitored
- present a temperature below 100° F (37.8° C)
- exhibit pulse and respirations within normal limits.
  Within 1 day of admission, the patient will:
- increase fluid intake to at least eight 8-oz (237-ml) glasses daily.
  Within 3 days of admission, the patient will:
- exhibit no septicemia
- exhibit no dysuria

---

*Italics indicate key interventions.

- have normal breath sounds.
  Within 7 days of admission, the patient will:
- have intact oral mucous membranes
- have no skin or rectal abscesses
- maintain a stable WBC count and absolute neutrophil count (ANC)
- maintain normal temperature
- display negative urine, vaginal, blood, and sputum cultures.

INTERVENTIONS

1. *Assess the CBC, noting a WBC count below 2,000/μl and any sudden rise or fall in neutrophil level.* Calculate the ANC using the formula

ANC = total WBC count × (% polys + % bands)

where polys are polymorphonuclear neutrophils and bands are immature neutrophils.

2. *Place the patient in a private room or in protective isolation, according to protocol and the patient's condition.* Maintain the immediate environment free from bacterial contamination, disinfect or sterilize equipment, keep equipment at the bedside, and don't use such items for other patients. Prohibit visitors or staff with known infections, such as a cold or influenza, from the room.

3. *Monitor, report, and document any sign or symptom of infection:* temperature above 100.4° F (38° C) lasting longer than 24 hours; chills; pulse above 100 beats/minute; crackles or gurgles; cloudy, foul-smelling urine; urgency or burning upon urination; redness; swelling; drainage from any orifice; perineal, rectal, or vaginal pain or discharge; and painful skin lesions.

4. *Monitor and record fluid intake and output.* Encourage fluid intake of up to twelve 8-oz (237-ml) glasses daily, unless contraindicated.

5. *Use strict aseptic technique when starting an I.V. or accessing the patient's vascular access device.* Consult the facility's policy manual for the frequency of and procedure for I.V. site, I.V. tubing, peripheral site, and central line dressing changes.

6. *Provide a low-bacteria diet.* Avoid raw fruits and vegetables, and use only cooked and processed or pasteurized foods.

RATIONALES

1. A decreased WBC count places the patient at increased risk for infection, a major cause of morbidity and mortality in the immunosuppressed patient. Such a decrease in the WBC count results from the disease and the chemotherapy. A sudden change in the neutrophil level indicates impending infection. The largest component of granulocytes, neutrophils are responsible for the body's early response to infection, especially bacterial infection. Because the patient can have neutropenia even when the WBC count is normal, the ANC must be calculated to show the number of WBCs that are actually mature and able to fight infection. If the ANC is less than 1,000/μl, the patient has neutropenia.

2. The patient must be protected from potential sources of infection.

3. An elevated temperature unrelated to drug or blood product administration indicates infection in about 80% of patients with leukemia. The immunosuppressed patient can't mount a normal response to infection, so an infection that would be harmless in a patient with a normal WBC count can cause septicemia in the leukopenic patient. Early treatment of any infection is essential to prevent complications and death.

4. Adequate fluid balance is essential to prevent dehydration from fever and fluid shift in septic shock.

5. Strict aseptic technique and following infection-control guidelines minimize the risk of bacterial contamination of the system and possible sepsis. The dressings on nontunneled central venous catheters are typically changed every 48 to 72 hours; dressings on tunneled catheters, every 5 to 7 days. Implanted ports don't need a dressing unless a continuous or intermittent infusion device is accessing the port.

6. These measures minimize potential sources of bacterial contamination from food.

Hematologic and
immunologic disorders

7. *Take measures to prevent respiratory tract infections.* Instruct the patient to turn, cough, deep-breathe, and use the incentive spirometer every 2 hours. Document respiratory assessment every 4 hours.

8. *Avoid invasive procedures,* such as urinary catheterization, injections, and venipunctures, when possible. Examine the sites of earlier invasive procedures (such as bone marrow aspiration or venipuncture) for signs of inflammation.

9. *Provide meticulous skin care,* paying close attention to any alteration in skin integrity. Wash the skin at least twice daily with antibacterial solutions. Monitor and document skin condition every shift.

10. *Avoid trauma to the rectal mucosa;* take the patient's temperature orally, and prevent constipation by ensuring adequate hydration and administering stool softeners, as ordered.

11. *Observe for and report clinical signs of septicemia,* such as tachycardia, hyperventilation, hypotension, or subtle mental changes. Obtain cultures and institute I.V. antibiotic therapy with cephalosporins (as ordered) within 1 hour of identifying signs and symptoms. Monitor fibrin degradation product (FDP) levels if the patient is septicemic.

12. *Reduce temperature higher than 100° F (37.8° C).* Administer acetaminophen (Tylenol) 650 mg every 4 hours, as ordered. Use tepid sponge baths, remove unnecessary clothing and linens, and apply a hypothermia blanket, as ordered. Prevent chilling and encourage oral fluid intake.

13. Prepare the patient for granulocyte transfusion if the WBC count is consistently below 500/µl and the patient has signs of infection. Infuse granulocytes slowly over 2 to 4 hours, as ordered. Observe for and document signs of a serious transfusion reaction, such as hypotension, allergic response, or wheezing. Discontinue the transfusion and notify the physician immediately if a reaction occurs.

14. Administer sargramostim (granulocyte-macrophage colony-stimulating factor [Leukine]) or filgrastim (granulocyte colony-stimulating factor [Neupogen]) subcutaneously or I.V. when ordered for neutropenia. Watch for adverse effects. Report and document any that occur.

7. Immobility promotes stasis of respiratory secretions, increasing the risk of pneumonia and atelectasis.

8. Any invasive procedure is a potential source of bacterial invasion. Take care to minimize trauma to the skin because of impaired healing abilities.

9. The skin is the body's first line of defense against infection. Any break in skin integrity is a source of potentially lethal bacterial contamination. The leukemic patient is as susceptible to infection from normal flora as from outside contamination. Frequent skin care minimizes the possibility of superficial skin breakdown and resultant infection.

10. Damage to rectal mucosa from frequent rectal temperatures or hard, dry stools may cause rectal abscesses.

11. Septicemia may occur without fever. Symptoms reflect initial stages of insufficient tissue perfusion. Prompt recognition and treatment of septic shock are crucial to prevent irreversible hypovolemia and decreased cardiac output. The septicemic patient is at increased risk for disseminated intravascular coagulation (DIC). Elevated FDP levels are seen in DIC.

12. Several measures may be necessary to reduce fever to a manageable level in the immunosuppressed patient. Untreated, high temperatures contribute to fluid imbalance, discomfort, and CNS complications.

13. Granulocyte transfusions are usually effective in the patient with granulocytopenia and progressive infections that don't respond to antibiotics or in the patient whose bone marrow doesn't recover after chemotherapy. Granulocytes are slightly contaminated with RBCs from the donor, so granulocyte transfusions must be ABO compatible to the recipient. Febrile reactions — shaking chills and temperature elevations — aren't considered serious reactions to a WBC transfusion and should not prompt discontinuation of the transfusion. WBC transfusion can cause pulmonary symptoms, transmit cytomegalovirus, and contribute to the development of graft-versus-host disease.

14. Sargramostim and filgrastim are naturally occurring glycoproteins that increase granulocyte production. The usual dosage of sargramostim is 250 mcg/m² of body surface area daily for up to 21 days. The usual dosage of filgrastim is 5 mcg/kg daily for up to 14 days. Common adverse effects include flulike symptoms, generalized rash, and bone and muscle pain.

15. Additional individualized interventions: _____

15. Rationales: _____

> **Suggested NIC Interventions**
> *Infection control; Infection protection; Incision site care; Wound care*

> **Suggested NOC Outcomes**
> *Infection status; Wound healing: Primary intention*

Collaborative problem
Risk for hemorrhage related to incompetent bone marrow and the immunosuppressive effects of chemotherapy

NURSING PRIORITY
Minimize the potential for life-threatening hemorrhage.

PATIENT OUTCOME CRITERIA
Within 1 day of admission, the patient will:
- exhibit a platelet count above 50,000/mm³
- maintain stable vital signs, typically: heart rate, 60 to 100 beats/minute; systolic blood pressure, 90 to 140 mm Hg; and diastolic blood pressure, 50 to 90 mm Hg.
  Within 3 days of admission, the patient will:
- exhibit no frank bleeding in stool, urine, vomitus, or sputum
- present minimal extension of ecchymoses
- present minimal bleeding from puncture sites, gums, and nose
- have stable or improved hemoglobin level, hematocrit, and platelet count
- exhibit minimal or no restlessness, confusion, lethargy, or other CNS symptoms.

INTERVENTIONS

1. *Monitor, report, and document signs and symptoms of bleeding problems:*
– platelet count less than 50,000/mm³
– petechiae, especially on distal portions of upper and lower extremities
– ecchymotic areas
– bleeding gums
– prolonged oozing from minor cuts or scratches
– frank or occult blood in urine, stool, vomitus, or sputum
– prolonged heavy menstruation
– decline in hematocrit and hemoglobin level
– narrowing pulse pressure with increased pulse rate
– restlessness, confusion, or lethargy.

2. *Implement measures to prevent bleeding during invasive procedures:*

– Use the smallest gauge needle possible when performing venipuncture or giving injections. Apply firm, direct pressure to the injection site for 3 to 5 minutes after the injection. If bleeding doesn't stop after 5 minutes, apply a sandbag to the site and notify the physician.
– Monitor and document the condition of old puncture sites (such as from venipuncture, lumbar puncture, or I.V. infusion).

RATIONALES

1. Normal platelet levels are required to maintain vascular integrity, platelet plug formation, and stabilized clotting. A decrease leads to local or systemic hemorrhage. With a platelet count of less than 20,000/mm³, the patient is prone to spontaneous life-threatening bleeding. The patient with leukemia is prone to platelet deficiency because of the proliferation of WBCs, which interfere with normal platelet production, and because of the immunosuppressive effects of drug treatment.

2. Even minor invasive procedures can cause excessive bleeding, especially when the platelet count falls below 50,000/mm³.
– The patient with thrombocytopenia may continue to bleed excessively even after minor invasive procedures. Firm pressure minimizes further blood loss and hematoma formation. Pressure dressings may be necessary if bleeding continues.
– Spontaneous bleeding from old puncture sites may occur at platelet levels below 20,000/mm³.

3. *Provide a soft, bland diet,* avoiding foods that are thermally, mechanically, or chemically irritating. Use only a soft-bristle or sponge toothbrush and an alcohol-free mouthwash (such as normal saline) every 4 to 8 hours.

3. The oral mucous membrane is very delicate in the leukemic patient and prone to hemorrhage with even minor irritation. Minimizing irritation decreases bleeding and promotes comfort.

4. *Administer* docusate sodium (Colace) or another *stool softener daily,* as ordered. Monitor and document the frequency of bowel movements. Avoid using enemas, suppositories, harsh laxatives, and rectal thermometers.

4. Constipation and straining during defecation must be avoided to prevent trauma to the rectal mucosa as well as increased intracranial pressure, which could cause spontaneous CNS bleeding. Rectal bleeding may develop with minimal trauma.

5. *Instruct the patient to avoid activities that may cause bleeding,* such as forcefully blowing the nose, using a straight-edged razor, cutting nails, and wearing tight, restrictive clothing.

5. The patient may be unaware that some common actions can be dangerous when platelet counts are severely decreased.

6. Prepare the patient for a platelet transfusion, as ordered, when platelet counts drop below 20,000/mm³. Obtain baseline vital signs before initiating the transfusion. Infuse each unit over approximately 10 minutes. Observe, report, and document signs and symptoms of transfusion reactions: nausea, vomiting, fever, chills, urticaria, or wheezing. Discontinue the transfusion immediately if symptoms develop, keep the vein open with normal saline, and notify the physician. Be prepared to administer diphenhydramine (Benadryl), hydrocortisone (Solu-Cortef), or acetaminophen, as ordered.

6. Platelet transfusions reduce the risk of hemorrhage. A platelet transfusion can be made up of platelets taken from random donors or from a single donor. A random-donor platelet transfusion increases the risk of antibody development and sensitization reactions; a transfusion from a single donor decreases the chance of sensitivity and transfusion reactions. Special leukocyte reduction filters should be used for patients at risk for or with a history of febrile nonhemolytic reactions. If a transfusion reaction occurs, the physician must evaluate the patient. If diphenhydramine and acetaminophen adequately control signs and symptoms, the remaining platelets can be transfused.

7. *Monitor hemoglobin level and hematocrit* and test stools, urine, and sputum for occult blood, noting and reporting positive findings.

7. Decreasing hemoglobin level and hematocrit indicate hemorrhage. Occult bleeding must be detected and monitored to prevent hypovolemia.

8. *Avoid administering aspirin, anticoagulants, indomethacin (Indocin), and medications containing alcohol.* Give phenothiazines cautiously.

8. These medications induce or prolong bleeding.

9. *Force fluid intake of eight to twelve 8-oz* (237-ml) *glasses daily,* if tolerated. Check for elevated uric acid levels and acidic urine. Administer acetazolamide (Diamox), sodium bicarbonate, and allopurinol (Lopurin), as ordered. Monitor and record fluid intake and output. Provide appropriate patient teaching for measures to be continued after discharge.

9. Hyperuricemia can result from rapid chemotherapy-induced leukemic cell lysis. Proper hydration and medication therapy are essential to prevent obstruction of the renal pelvis and ducts and subsequent renal failure. Acetazolamide is a diuretic, sodium bicarbonate maintains alkaline urine pH, and allopurinol inhibits uric acid synthesis.

10. Additional individualized interventions:_____

10. Rationales:_____

Nursing diagnosis

Activity intolerance related to fatigue secondary to rapid destruction of leukemic cells, tissue hypoxia secondary to anemia, and depressed nutritional status

NURSING PRIORITIES

- Minimize energy-depleting activities.
- Maximize energy resources.
- Decrease tissue hypoxia.

PATIENT OUTCOME CRITERIA

Within 1 day of admission, the patient will:

- exhibit no adverse effects or toxic effects of blood transfusion, such as elevated temperature or urticaria.

Within 3 days of admission, the patient will:

- show improved ability to participate in self-care, bathing, and hygiene measures
- sleep 1 hour before and after treatments
- sleep 8 hours at night
- ambulate 20% further each day
- participate in diversionary activities, such as reading, doing puzzles, and watching television
- maintain hemoglobin level at 8 g/dl or higher
- maintain hematocrit at 25% or higher.

INTERVENTIONS	RATIONALES
1. *Assess, monitor, and document the cause, pattern, and impact of fatigue on the patient's ability to engage in activities of daily living (ADLs).*	**1.** Causes of fatigue in the patient with leukemia commonly have an additive effect. To treat the problem effectively, the nurse must use a holistic approach.
2. *Monitor and document the degree of anemia present.* Assess for pallor, weakness, dizziness, headache, and dyspnea. Evaluate and report hemoglobin level, hematocrit, and RBC count, especially a significant or consistent drop in hemoglobin (below 8 g/dl) or hematocrit (below 25%). Prepare for a blood transfusion, as ordered.	**2.** The degree of anemia significantly affects the level of fatigue. Decreased RBC count and the resulting decrease in the blood's oxygen-carrying ability cause severe weakness, exhaustion, and inability to mobilize energy. The values given indicate severe anemia and require therapy with blood transfusions.
3. *Monitor and document vital signs before, during, and after blood transfusion.* Use a 19G or larger needle and tubing with a standard blood filter. Use standard Y-tubing with normal saline solution, filling the entire surface area of the filter with blood. Use a leukocyte reduction filter if the patient has a history of febrile nonhemolytic reactions.	**3.** Knowledge of baseline and ongoing vital signs is imperative to monitor for signs and symptoms of transfusion reaction. A large needle allows a suitable flow rate and prevents clumping and destruction of RBCs. The filter screens fibrin clots and particulate matter. Normal saline is the only solution suitable for use with RBCs because dextrose solutions cause hemolysis.
4. *Infuse blood slowly* (20 drops/minute) for 15 minutes. Complete the transfusion within 1½ to 2 hours if the patient's condition remains stable.	**4.** Blood is administered slowly during the first 15 minutes because transfusion reactions typically occur during this time. A slow rate minimizes the volume of cells transfused. However, blood should be transfused within 4 hours after leaving the blood bank, to prevent bacterial proliferation and RBC hemolysis.
5. *Stop the transfusion at the first sign or symptom of a transfusion reaction:* fever, chills, headache, low back pain, urticaria, wheezing, or hypotension. Keep the vein open with normal saline, and notify the physician.	**5.** Transfusion reactions must be recognized immediately to prevent death or organ damage.
6. Prepare the patient for the possible use of erythropoietin (Procrit, Epogen).	**6.** Erythropoietin helps stimulate red blood cell production and may help the red blood cell count recover more rapidly.
7. *Implement measures to improve activity tolerance,* such as the following: – Provide uninterrupted rest periods before and after meals, procedures, and diagnostic tests. – Instruct the patient to sit rather than stand when performing hygiene and daily care. – Limit the number of visitors. – Minimize environmental activity and noise.	**7.** Quiet, restful periods before and after meals, procedures such as chemotherapy, and diagnostic procedures help increase activity tolerance and promote a rested feeling. Conserving energy and improving activity tolerance usually help the patient participate more actively in care and treatment.

Hematologic and immunologic disorders

– Assist the patient with activities.
– Keep supplies and personal articles within easy reach.

8. Assess, report, and document the patient's tolerance for progressive activity. Stop the activity if the patient's pulse rate increases more than 20 beats/minute above the resting rate, if the blood pressure increases more than 40 mm Hg systolic or 20 mm Hg diastolic, or if dyspnea, chest pain, dizziness, or syncope occurs.

8. The patient's response should guide any plan of progressive activity. The cited changes in baseline vital signs indicate that the patient is being pushed beyond therapeutic levels, and activity should be stopped.

9. Reassure the patient that fatigue is an expected effect of chemotherapy.

9. The patient may fear that fatigue is related to extension of the disease. The patient should be reassured that fatigue is common after chemotherapy and doesn't necessarily reflect disease extension.

10. Additional individualized interventions:_____

10. Rationales:_____

Suggested NIC Interventions
Activity therapy; Energy management; Exercise promotion; Strength training; Nutrition management; Self-care assistance; Home maintenance assistance

Suggested NOC Outcomes
Activity intolerance; Endurance; Energy conservation; Self-care: Activities of daily living (ADL); Self-care: Instrumental activities of daily living (IADL)

Nursing diagnosis

Imbalanced nutrition: Less than body requirements related to anorexia, nausea, vomiting, taste perception changes, and alterations in cellular metabolism secondary to disease and chemotherapy

NURSING PRIORITIES
- Maximize oral intake of foods and fluids.
- Minimize catabolism and protein and vitamin deficiencies.

PATIENT OUTCOME CRITERIA
Within 3 days of admission, the patient will:
- exhibit no weight loss
- maintain serum electrolyte levels within normal limits
- tolerate nutritional supplements between meals
- maintain intake equal to output
- have no nausea or vomiting
- retain 75% or more of food intake.

INTERVENTIONS

1. *Provide standard nursing care related to nutritional deficit.* Refer to the "Nutritional deficit" care plan, page 138, for details.

2. *Provide high-calorie, high-protein snacks,* such as milk shakes, puddings, and eggnog.

3. Administer medications such as metoclopramide (Reglan) and megestrol (Megace) to counter anorexia associated with illness and treatment.

RATIONALES

1. The "Nutritional deficit" care plan presents general nursing care for this problem. This care plan presents additional information related to leukemia.

2. Protein-calorie malnutrition is common in leukemia. Increased protein intake facilitates repair and regeneration of cells, and increased calories help fight the body's tendency toward cancer-induced catabolism.

3. Metoclopramide may aid nutrition because it helps avoid early satiety by increasing gastric emptying and gastric transit time. Megestrol acetate may help stimulate appetite.

4. Provide nutritional supplements between meals, as ordered. Serve them cold in a glass or other container, not in the can. Observe for and document undesirable adverse effects, such as gastric distention, cramping, or diarrhea.

5. *Take steps to decrease or prevent nausea and vomiting.* Obtain a history of the patient's susceptibility to nausea and vomiting and determine the potential emetic effects of the chemotherapeutic agents prescribed. Administer antiemetics before the chemotherapy infusion begins. Antiemetics include benzodiazepines (such as lorazepam), butyrophenones (such as droperidol), cannabinoids (such as dronabinol), phenothiazines (such as prochlorperazine), substitute benzamides (such as metoclopramide), steroids (such as dexamethasone), antihistamines (such as diphenhydramine), and serotonin inhibitors (such as ondansetron or granisetron). Begin therapy 30 minutes to 2 hours before chemotherapy and continue for 24 to 72 hours, as ordered. Monitor the patient, and report and document the effectiveness of the therapy

6. Additional individualized interventions: _____

_____

4. Oral supplements are high in protein and are a valuable supplement to nutritious food. Many patients experience a metallic taste secondary to leukemia, and the sight of the can may aggravate this feeling. The adverse effects listed result from the high osmolality of supplemental liquids.

5. Antiemetic medications block stimulation of the true vomiting center and the chemoreceptor trigger zone in the brain, thus decreasing nausea and vomiting and promoting relaxation. Because they have different mechanisms of action, antiemetics are often given in combination to enhance their effectiveness. Benzodiazepines depress the CNS and help treat anticipatory nausea and vomiting. Butyrophenones work as dopamine antagonists in the chemoreceptor trigger zone, thereby reducing the nausea and vomiting stimulus. Cannabinoids are believed to act by suppressing pathways to the vomiting and higher CNS centers. Phenothiazines block dopamine receptors in the chemoreceptor trigger zone and inhibit the vomiting center activities. Substitute benzamides work as dopamine antagonists at the chemoreceptor trigger zone and help suppress nausea by stimulating the motility of the GI tract. Steroids enhance the effectiveness of the other antiemetics and decrease the effects of prostaglandin activity. Antihistamines block neurotransmitters in the chemoreceptor zone. The serotonin inhibitors work as selective antagonists of the 5-hydroxytryptamine$_3$ serotonin receptors in the chemoreceptor trigger zone and have been successful as part of the protocols for nausea and vomiting. To maintain a therapeutic blood level, antiemetic medications must be given around the clock rather than as needed.

6. Rationales:_____

_____

Suggested NIC Interventions
Diet staging; Nutrition management; Weight-gain assistance; Fluid monitoring; Nutritional monitoring

Suggested NOC Outcomes
Nutritional status; Nutritional status: Food and fluid intake; Nutritional status: Nutrient intake; Weight control

Hematologic and immunologic disorders

Nursing diagnosis
Impaired oral mucous membrane related to decreased nutrition and immunosuppression secondary to disease and cytotoxic effects of chemotherapy

NURSING PRIORITIES
■ Minimize pain and discomfort from stomatitis.
■ Prevent further trauma to and infection of the oral mucous membrane.

PATIENT OUTCOME CRITERIA
Within 3 days of admission, the patient will:
■ have no frank bleeding from gums

- show an improved ability to swallow
- have decreased viscosity and improved amount of saliva.
  Within 5 days of admission, the patient will:
- exhibit a decreased number of oral open ulcers
- exhibit a decreased number of oral white patches.

INTERVENTIONS	RATIONALES
1. *Assess for signs and symptoms of stomatitis,* such as dry and ulcerated oral mucosa, pain, viscous saliva, or difficulty swallowing. Document and report the condition of the oral mucous membrane—including the lips, tongue, and gums—on a scale of 1 to 4, with 1 being normal and 4 being ulcerated, bleeding, irritated, and infected. Observe the amount and viscosity of saliva. Obtain a culture of suspicious lesions; note results.	1. Stomatitis is both a sign of decreased immunocompetence and an adverse effect of chemotherapy that develops 7 to 10 days after treatment begins. Objective assessment is imperative for early identification of stomatitis so that appropriate therapy can be instituted.
2. *Teach an appropriate mouth care regimen.*	2. Preventing accumulation of food debris and bacteria is essential to preventing breakdown of the oral mucous membrane.
– If platelet levels are above 40,000/mm^3 and leukocyte levels above 1,500/µl, recommend the following: Brush the teeth with a soft, nylon-bristle toothbrush 30 minutes after meals and every 4 hours while awake. Place the brush at a 45-degree angle between the gums and the teeth, and move it in short, horizontal strokes. Floss between teeth twice daily.	– Take care to observe specified laboratory values because even this regimen will cause severe bleeding if platelet counts are low. If the WBC count is low, mouth care could cause local infection.
– If platelet or leukocyte levels are below the parameters specified, recommend rinsing only (using water or saline) until the values return to safer levels.	– For the patient with low platelet or leukocyte levels, this regimen removes debris while minimizing the risks of bleeding or infection.
3. Provide hydrogen peroxide and water solution (1:2 or 1:4), baking soda and water (1 tsp to 500 ml), or normal saline to rinse the mouth during and after brushing.	3. Many commercial mouthwashes contain alcohol, which dries and irritates the oral mucosa.
4. Administer lidocaine (Xylocaine) viscous solution as needed, 1 tsp swished in the mouth every 3 to 4 hours, or acetaminophen with codeine elixir as needed, as ordered.	4. Lidocaine is a topical anesthetic that relieves pain from mouth ulcers. Acetaminophen with codeine works systemically to control pain, and the elixir is easily swallowed.
5. *Lubricate lips with petroleum jelly or water-soluble lubricant* (K-Y Lubricating Jelly), lip balm (ChapStick), or mineral oil. Use gauze with petroleum jelly to protect the lips when the patient drinks from a cup.	5. Severe dryness, sores, and ulcers on the lips cause pain when the patient drinks from a cup or glass. This pain further discourages the patient from drinking adequate fluids and maintaining an adequate fluid balance.
6. *Encourage the use of an artificial saliva product* (Salivart).	6. Severe dryness of the oral mucous membrane increases the risk of tissue breakdown and impairs optimal nutritional intake. Artificial saliva eases dryness, buffers acidity, and lubricates and soothes mucous membranes.
7. *Monitor, report, and document the appearance of white patches on the tongue and oral mucosa.* Administer nystatin (Mycostatin) oral suspension or a gentian violet preparation, as ordered. Document the patient's response.	7. These white patches indicate yeast infection. (The immunosuppressed patient is prone to opportunistic infections such as candidiasis.) Prompt treatment of oral infection will prevent undue discomfort.

8. Apply a substrate of magnesium hydroxide (Milk of Magnesia) or a kaolin preparation (Kaopectate) with a swab or a gauze-covered tongue blade. (To prepare the substrate, allow the bottle to stand for several hours; then pour off the supernatant liquid.) Rinse with normal saline after 15 minutes.

9. Additional individualized interventions: _____

8. Topical protective agents soothe irritated areas and promote healing.

9. Rationales: _____

Suggested NIC Interventions Skin surveillance	**Suggested NOC Outcomes** Oral health; Tissue integrity: Skin and mucus membranes; Wound healing: Primary intention

---

Nursing diagnosis

Ineffective protection related to severe immunosuppression associated with bone marrow transplantation (BMT) or peripheral stem cell transplantation protocol

NURSING PRIORITY

Assess, prioritize, and intervene in problems related to transplantation procedures.

PATIENT OUTCOME CRITERIA

Within 7 days of transplantation, the patient will:
- have stable liver function tests
- maintain vital signs within normal limits, typically: heart rate, 60 to 100 beats/minute; systolic blood pressure, 90 to 140 mm Hg; and diastolic blood pressure, 50 to 90 mm Hg
- respond positively to symptom management and comfort measures.
  Within 14 days of transplantation, the patient will:
- be able to take foods and fluids by mouth
- obtain relief from nausea and vomiting
- maintain a stable body weight and a balanced intake and output
- remain free from infection
- have no signs of stomatitis, such as ulcerated or bleeding lips, tongue, and gums
- have no evidence of veno-occlusive disease, such as right upper quadrant pain or jaundice.

INTERVENTIONS

1. *Reinforce the physician's explanation for BMT or peripheral stem cell transplantation.*

RATIONALES

1. Because in the past these treatments were considered experimental and commonly resulted in poor outcomes, the patient and his family may be anxious about their effectiveness. After many decades of research and clinical trials, bone marrow or stem cell transplantation is successfully used to cure leukemia in patients who are at high risk for relapse, who respond poorly to conventional chemotherapy regimens, or who relapse after traditional treatment.

2. Explain the difference between BMT and peripheral stem cell transplantation, including the implications of each treatment.

2. BMT can be either allogenic (from another person) or autologous (from the patient's own bone marrow). In allogenic transplantation, a human leukocyte antigen (HLA) test is performed on the patient and his family members to find a compatible bone marrow donor. Because of the complexity of the HLA system, which is composed of more than 100 antigens, a compatible family member may not be found. If so, the patient may register with the National Bone Marrow Donor Registry to find a compatible donor. The process of finding such a donor can be expensive, time consuming, and stressful.

Autologous BMT involves aspirating large volumes of the patient's own bone marrow for purging and then reinfusing. Peripheral stem cell transplantation involves transplantation of blood-forming components taken from the peripheral blood, not the bone marrow. The patient himself is usually the source of the stem cells, eliminating the need for a donor. Autologous BMT may cause relapses in the disease because reinfused marrow may contain residual tumor cells. Bone marrow (hematopoietic progenitors that restore blood function) is stored and reinfused after chemotherapy.

3. Help the patient through the extensive diagnostic and psychosocial evaluation that takes place before transplantation, providing teaching and emotional support.

3. Transplantation is an aggressive treatment that has potentially life-threatening complications and requires vigorous physical and diagnostic evaluation before the procedure. The patient must undergo extensive laboratory testing; tissue typing; evaluation of renal, hepatic, cardiovascular, and respiratory function; bone marrow studies to determine the stage of the disease; CT scans, magnetic resonance imaging, and bone scans; lumbar puncture; gynecologic examination (if the patient is female); and dental examination. The patient and his family must also undergo fertility counseling (if appropriate) and comprehensive psychological evaluation to determine if the patient has sufficient support systems and coping mechanisms. All this is physically and emotionally exhausting for the patient, who already has symptoms of the disease; waiting for the results of tests adds to the patient's and family's stress. Teaching and emotional support play a crucial role in helping the patient and family cope.

4. *Explain to the patient and his family the rationale for and implications of preparations for transplantation,* adverse effects of chemotherapy, symptom management, neutropenic precautions, care of the vascular access device, and comfort measures.

4. The patient and his family need to understand that, for transplantation to be successful, all malignant cells must be killed. The patient's immune system must be suppressed, and space in the bone marrow must be created for the new cells. The patient must undergo high-dose, disease-specific chemotherapy with such drugs as cyclophosphamide (Cytoxan), busulfan, or cytosine arabinoside; the patient who needs an allogenic transplant must also undergo total body irradiation. Specific interventions for managing adverse effects, neutropenic precautions, vascular access device care, and comfort measures are given in previous nursing diagnoses.

5. As ordered, administer antipyretics (such as acetaminophen), diuretics (such as mannitol), antihistamines (such as diphenhydramine), and corticosteroids (such as dexamethasone) before gravity or I.V. push infusion of bone marrow or peripheral stem cells. Check the patient's vital signs every 5 minutes during the infusion, and watch for and report such adverse effects as elevation in temperature or pulse and hypertension or hypotension.

6. *Watch for, report, document, and treat complications of bacterial, fungal, or viral infections* that occur during the acute phase of BMT. Maintain strict neutropenic precautions in a protective environment. Monitor and report results of chest X-rays, blood counts, and blood, tissue, urine, stool, wound, and sputum cultures.

7. *Watch for, report, document, and treat complications of transplantation,* including bleeding tendencies, hepatic dysfunction, cutaneous problems, GI problems, renal insufficiency, pulmonary toxicity, and acute graft-versus-host (GVH) disease. Monitor laboratory test results, especially hematocrit; platelet count; hemoglobin, creatinine, BUN, and bilirubin levels; liver enzymes; and chest X-rays.

5. The most common adverse effects of bone marrow or stem cell transfusion include fever, chills, shortness of breath, rash, pruritus, hives, and hypertension or hypotension. Premedication can help combat these effects. Patients who receive autologous BMT or peripheral stem cell transplantation may also experience a bitter taste and an odd smell. These result from the chemical dimethylsulfoxide, used as a preservative in these transplant procedures.

6. The patient's immune system is wiped out, so he's at risk for overwhelming, life-threatening infection. From days 0 to 30, the patient needs close monitoring for signs of gram-negative and gram-positive bacterial, fungal, and herpes infections of the GI system, oropharynx, lungs, skin, and indwelling catheter sites. From days 30 to 90, the patient is at risk for cytomegalovirus and fungal, gram-positive bacterial, and *Pneumocystis carinii* infections.

7. Because of the intense nature of this aggressive therapy, failure to recognize the start of complications can be life-threatening. Active or occult bleeding episodes and signs of anemia may require blood or blood product transfusions. Veno-occlusive disease — as evidenced by hepatomegaly, elevated serum bilirubin levels, right upper quadrant pain, jaundice, and encephalopathy — can occur as a complication of treatment-induced (radiation or chemotherapy) liver damage; treatment is symptomatic. Stomatitis, mucositis, nausea, vomiting, or diarrhea may lead to malnutrition, fluid and electrolyte imbalance, and skin breakdown.

Renal complications can result from nephrotoxicity caused by certain transplantation drugs, hypovolemic states, infection, or hemorrhagic cystitis from high-dose cyclophosphamide administration. Symptoms of renal complications include anuria, elevated creatinine levels, and electrolyte and fluid imbalance.

Pulmonary complications from bacterial, viral, or fungal pneumonias; interstitial pneumonia; or fibrotic changes may occur in the acute or later phases after BMT. These complications result in a high incidence of morbidity and mortality. Signs and symptoms include cough, shortness of breath, and fever.

GVH disease occurs in allogenic BMT when the donor T lymphocytes attack the recipient's cells and organs. Acute GVH disease affects the patient's integumentary and GI systems and liver and causes effects that range from mild to life-threatening; symptoms include erythematous maculopapular rash; intense, watery diarrhea; and altered liver function (jaundice, ascites, and increased liver enzymes).

Hematologic and immunologic disorders

8. *Throughout the transplantation process, provide ongoing emotional support and education* about the complications and long-term implications for the patient and his family.

8. Although the complications from autologous stem cell transplantation are less severe than those from allogenic BMT, every patient needs intensive education and emotional support to learn how to manage self-care. Education includes the prevention and recognition of infection, comfort measures, nutrition guidelines, body-image management and self-concept alterations, concerns about sexuality, and role changes. Follow-up care includes weekly laboratory testing, throat and urine cultures, and chest X-rays and periodic pulmonary function tests, bone marrow studies, skin biopsies, and lumbar puncture.

9. Additional individualized interventions: _____

9. Rationales:_____

Suggested NIC Interventions
Infection control; Infection protection; Incision site care; Wound care

Suggested NOC Outcomes
Infection status; Wound healing: Primary intention

Nursing diagnosis

Ineffective coping related to uncertain prognosis and multiple disease- and treatment-induced losses

NURSING PRIORITY

Promote healthy coping behavior.

PATIENT OUTCOME CRITERIA

Throughout the hospital stay, the patient will:
- use healthy coping behaviors
- express feelings, if desired.

INTERVENTIONS

1. Inform the patient of the constant development of new drugs and treatment modalities as well as the availability of clinical trials. New developments include Interferon-alpha, imatinib mesylate (Gleevec), all trans-retinoic acid, arsenic trioxide, and monoclonal antibodies. Extensive information is available on the Internet for patients wishing to learn more about treatment and management options. Stress to the patient that only reputable agencies' web sites should be consulted to explore different treatment options. Recommended Web sites: American Cancer Society: *www.cancer.org,* Cancer Care: *www.cancercare.org,* the Leukemia and Lymphoma Society: *www.leukemia-lymphoma.org,* the National Cancer Institute's Cancer Information Service: *www.cancer-net.nci.nih.gov* and *www.cis.nci.nih.gov.*

RATIONALES

1. Treatments for all forms of leukemia are constantly undergoing improvement. Success rates have improved steadily with the introduction of a wider range of modalities. There's a tremendous amount of information that can be obtained from the Internet. In order to assure accuracy and appropriateness, information needs to be obtained only from credible resources.

2. *See the "Dying" care plan,* page 78, *"Grieving" care plan,* page 105, and *"Ineffective individual coping" care plan,* page 124.

2. The patient with leukemia suffers multiple losses, and his self-care ability, social contact, and energy level are reduced. Additionally, adverse effects from chemotherapy may cause body-image changes that are difficult to accept. Weakness, dependence on others, and an uncertain prognosis may create anxiety or contribute to depression. These care plans provide specific interventions helpful in dealing with the psychosocial aspects of caring for a patient with leukemia.

3. Additional individualized interventions: _____

3. Rationales: _____

Suggested NIC Interventions
Coping enhancement; Family involvement promotion

Suggested NOC Outcomes
Coping; Social support

Discharge planning
DISCHARGE CHECKLIST
Before discharge, the patient shows evidence of:
- ❒ absence of fever
- ❒ absence of cardiovascular or pulmonary complications such as crackles, gurgles, arrhythmias, or atelectasis
- ❒ stabilizing weight
- ❒ WBC count greater than 2,000/μl
- ❒ platelet count greater than 50,000/mm³
- ❒ hemoglobin level above 8 g/dl
- ❒ hematocrit above 25%
- ❒ absence of signs and symptoms of infection
- ❒ ability to tolerate adequate nutritional intake
- ❒ absence of gingival bleeding and sores
- ❒ absence of hematuria or other bladder or bowel dysfunction
- ❒ ability to control pain using oral medications
- ❒ ability to manage care of vascular access device
- ❒ ability to follow BMT or peripheral stem cell transplantation protocol
- ❒ ability to perform ADLs, transfers, and ambulation independently or with minimal assistance
- ❒ adequate home support system or referral to home care or nursing home if indicated by an inadequate home support system or the patient's inability to perform ADLs, transfer, ambulate, and follow medication regimen.

Note: All patients with leukemia must be referred to the social service department. Leukemia is a financially draining disease, commonly requiring long-term and expensive treatment, so the patient is likely to have financial concerns. For terminal leukemia, refer the patient for hospice care.

TEACHING CHECKLIST
Document evidence that the patient and his family demonstrate an understanding of:
- ❒ diagnosis and course of treatment
- ❒ discharge medications, including their purpose, dosage, administration schedule, and adverse effects requiring medical attention (Usual chemotherapy medications include alkylating agents, such as busulfan [Myleran] and chlorambucil [Leukeran]; antibiotics, such as daunorubicin [Cerubidine] and doxorubicin [Adriamycin]; antimetabolites, such as methotrexate and 6-mercaptopurine [Purinethol]; and plant alkaloids, such as vincristine [Oncovin] and vinblastine [Velban].)
- ❒ ways of preventing and identifying infections
- ❒ appropriate modifications of activity-rest patterns
- ❒ proper care of vascular access device
- ❒ ways of preventing, identifying, and reporting abnormal bleeding tendencies
- ❒ techniques to control nausea, vomiting, and anorexia
- ❒ recommended dietary modifications
- ❒ techniques to prevent urinary calculi formation
- ❒ appropriate oral hygiene techniques and procedures
- ❒ signs and symptoms indicating relapse or exacerbation of disease
- ❒ frequency of follow-up laboratory tests
- ❒ schedule for future diagnostic tests, chemotherapy administration, and appointments with health care providers
- ❒ how to contact the physician
- ❒ community resources for home management, lifestyle modifications, and support
- ❒ emotional response to chronic or terminal illness
- ❒ changes in family role patterns.

Hematologic and immunologic disorders

DOCUMENTATION CHECKLIST
Using outcome criteria as a guide, document:
❐ clinical status on admission
❐ significant changes in status, especially development of CNS symptoms and septicemia
❐ pertinent laboratory and diagnostic test findings
❐ response to chemotherapy treatments
❐ management of chemotherapy adverse reactions
❐ response to transfusions of RBCs, WBCs, or platelets
❐ nutritional intake
❐ fluid-electrolyte balance
❐ activity-rest pattern
❐ emotional coping patterns
❐ condition of skin and mucous membranes
❐ signs and symptoms of infection or bleeding tendencies
❐ I.V. line patency, condition of veins, and status of vascular access device
❐ tolerance of diagnostic procedures
❐ response to anti-infection measures
❐ patient and family teaching

Associated care plans

- Anemia
- Disseminated intravascular coagulation
- Dying
- Grieving
- Ineffective individual coping
- Lymphoma
- Nutritional deficit
- Parenteral nutrition
- Septic shock

References

Blast, R., et al. *Holland-Frie Cancer Medicine,* 5th ed. Ontario, Canada: B.C. Decker Inc., 2000.

Casciato, D., and Lowitz, B. *Manual of Clinical Oncology,* 4th ed. Philadelphia: Lippincott Williams & Wilkins, 2000.

DeVita, V., et al. *Cancer: Principles and Practice of Oncology,* 6th ed. Philadelphia: Lippincott Williams & Wilkins, 2001.

Gordon, M. *Manual of Nursing Diagnosis,* 10th ed. St. Louis: Mosby–Year Book, Inc., 2002.

Jenkins, J., et al. "Applications of Advances in Molecular Biology and Genomics to Clinical Cancer Care," *Cancer Nursing* 25(2):110-22, April 2002.

Medoff, E. "Oncology Today: Leukemia," *RN* 63(9):42-49, September 2000.

Thompson, J., et al. *Mosby's Clinical Nursing,* 5th ed. St. Louis: Mosby–Year Book, Inc., 2002.

Weinstein, S. *Plumer's Principles and Practice of Intravenous Therapy,* 7th ed. Philadelphia: Lippincott Williams & Wilkins, 2001.

Wilkes, G. "Nutrition: The Forgotten Ingredient in Cancer Care," *AJN* 100(4):46-51, April 2000.

Yarbro, C., et al. *Cancer Nursing: Principles and Practice,* 5th ed. Boston: Jones & Bartlett Pubs., Inc., 2000.

Lymphoma

DRG INFORMATION

DRG 400 Lymphoma or Leukemia with Major Operating Room (OR) Procedure.
Mean LOS = 9.1 days

Major OR procedures include biopsy, excision, or incision.

DRG 401 Lymphoma or Non-Acute Leukemia with Other OR Procedure with Complication or Comorbidity (CC).
Mean LOS = 11.3 days

DRG 402 Lymphoma or Non-Acute Leukemia with Other OR Procedure without CC.
Mean LOS = 4.1 days

DRG 403 Lymphoma or Non-Acute Leukemia with CC.
Mean LOS = 8.1 days

DRG 404 Lymphoma or Non-Acute Leukemia without CC.
Mean LOS = 4.3 days

Additional DRG information: After hospitalization for the staging workup and initial course of therapy, the patient would most likely receive ongoing chemotherapy as an outpatient.

Introduction

DEFINITION AND TIME FOCUS

Lymphoma is the abnormal, malignant proliferation and enlargement of lymph nodes, spleen, and other lymphoid tissue, resulting in impaired cellular and humoral immunity, obstruction and infiltration of adjacent structures, and systemic involvement. Lymphomas are classified as Hodgkin's (commonly called Hodgkin's disease) or malignant.

Hodgkin's disease is characterized by contiguous node involvement. Extranodal spread at the time of diagnosis is uncommon. Staging is important in Hodgkin's disease, as in other cancers, because it helps determine the treatment and estimate a prognosis. (See *Staging classification [Ann Arbor] for Hodgkin's disease,* page 791, for staging and treatment guidelines.) Commonly, the disease is localized; fever, weight loss, and night sweats (termed "B" symptoms in staging classification) are seen in about 40% of patients at presentation. Hodgkin's disease occurs most commonly between ages 15 and 35, with a second peak between ages 50 and 75.

Malignant lymphomas comprise many histologic variations. They're characterized by noncontiguous nodal spread, commonly with extranodal involvement in the GI tract, testes, central nervous system (CNS), or bone marrow. The disease is usually disseminated; "B" symptoms occur in only about 20% of patients. Malignant lymphoma is three times more common than Hodgkin's disease in the United States and can occur at any age.

Both types of lymphoma are more common in males than in females, and males tend to have a worse prognosis.

Hodgkin's disease and malignant lymphoma are considered together here because their clinical presentations, diagnostic workups, treatments, and nursing management are similar. This care plan focuses on the undiagnosed, symptomatic patient with lymphoma who is admitted for a staging workup and initial therapy. (See *Clinical snapshot: Lymphoma,* page 791.)

ETIOLOGY AND PRECIPITATING FACTORS

- Viral etiology (suggested for some lymphomas; may involve a herpeslike virus related to the Epstein-Barr virus)
- Family history (increased incidence among family members suggests genetic and environmental factors)
- Environmental exposure to certain herbicides (such as phenoxyacetic acid) linked to an increased risk of malignant lymphoma

Focused assessment guidelines

NURSING HISTORY (FUNCTIONAL HEALTH PATTERN FINDINGS)

Health-perception–health-management pattern
- Fever — highest in the afternoon; twice-daily peaks greater than 101° F (38.3° C) are common
- Drenching night sweats
- Pruritus — more intense at night, worse with bathing
- General malaise and fatigue
- Painless, swollen lymph nodes (typically in the cervical chain)

Nutritional-metabolic pattern
- Unexplained weight loss
- Anorexia
- Pain in nodes immediately after drinking alcohol (cause unknown)

Activity-exercise pattern
- General fatigue: "I'm unable to do the things I want to do"
- Shortness of breath if ascites, pleural effusion, or anemia is present

Sleep-rest pattern
- Sleep disturbances due to night sweats

Self-perception–self-concept pattern
- Fear regarding prognosis and progression of disease
- Difficulty coping with changes in lifestyle, self-esteem, and body image

Cognitive-perceptual pattern
- Interest or disinterest in knowing prognosis and expected progression of disease

Role-relationship pattern
- Concern regarding role reversals at home and inability to fulfill previous roles

Sexuality-reproductive pattern
- Concern regarding adverse effects of chemotherapy on fertility and sexual performance
- Decreased libido from chemotherapy, radiation, or general fatigue

Coping–stress tolerance pattern
- Increased anxiety

PHYSICAL FINDINGS
Lymphoreticular
- Lymphadenopathy
- Tonsillar enlargement
- Edema and cyanosis of face and neck (rare)

Pulmonary
- Shortness of breath (rare)
- Cough (rare)
- Stridor (rare)
- Signs of pleural effusion (rare)

Gastrointestinal
- Splenomegaly
- Hepatomegaly
- Ascites (uncommon)
- Jaundice (rare)

DIAGNOSTIC STUDIES
Extensive testing is necessary to diagnose and stage lymphoma.
- Complete blood count and platelet count — may reveal neutrophilic leukocytosis and mild normochromic anemia, lymphopenia, or increased eosinophil sedimentation rate
- Serum alkaline phosphatase values — increased values indicate liver or bone involvement
- Direct Coombs' (antiglobulin) test — detects autoimmune hemolytic anemia (more common in malignant lymphoma)
- Immunoglobulin studies — may show overproduction of immunoglobulin by proliferating B-cell lymphocytes
- Lymph node biopsy (performed on the most central node of the involved group) — Hodgkin's disease shows Reed-Sternberg cells and malignant lymphoma reveals destruction of lymph node architecture; normal cellular elements are replaced by increased lymphocytes and lymphoblasts

- Excretory urography — detects unsuspected renal involvement and ureteral deviation and obstruction by involved nodes
- Chest X-ray — with computed tomography (CT) scan, may reveal hilar lymphadenopathy; mediastinal masses in lymphoma usually appear as dense rounded masses (occurring as commonly in the anterior mediastinum as in the middle mediastinum)
- Lymphangiography — may show enlarged, foamy-looking nodes (number of nodes affected, unilateral or bilateral involvement, and extent of extranodal involvement help determine stage); less useful in malignant lymphoma because it doesn't visualize mesenteric nodes, which are usually involved; occasionally, nodes are so enlarged they can't be visualized
- Abdominal CT scan — may detect intra-abdominal, intrapelvic nodal involvement as well as liver involvement
- Bone scan — used to detect bone involvement
- Bone marrow aspirate and biopsy — elevated lymphocyte values indicate bone marrow involvement, more common in malignant lymphoma
- Bilateral bone marrow biopsies — commonly performed because of spotty bone marrow involvement; chances of identifying bone marrow involvement are increased by 15% to 20% with bilateral procedure
- Laparotomy and splenectomy — undertaken only if outcome will affect a therapeutic decision; may detect splenic involvement

POTENTIAL COMPLICATIONS
- Intestinal obstruction and perforation
- Ureteral obstruction
- Sepsis (treatment-related)
- Anemia
- Thrombocytopenia (treatment-related)
- Hyperuricemia (treatment-related)
- Superior vena cava syndrome (airway occlusion related to edema from impaired superior vena cava drainage)
- Spinal cord compression (rare)
- Hypercalcemia (rare)
- Sterility (treatment-related)
- Secondary cancers (treatment-related)
- Pleural, pericardial, or abdominal effusions

Staging classification (Ann Arbor) for Hodgkin's disease

Stage	Description
I	Nodal involvement within one region
IE	Single extralymphatic organ or site
II	Nodal involvement within two or more regions, limited by the diaphragm
II E	Localized extranodal site and nodal involvement within one or more regions, limited by the diaphragm
III	Nodal involvement of regions above and below the diaphragm
III E	With localized extralymphatic site
III S	With spleen involvement
III ES	Localized extralymphatic site with spleen involvement
IV	Diffuse or disseminated involvement of one or more extralymphatic organs or tissues, with or without lymph node involvement

From Carbone, P., et al. "Report of the Committee on Hodgkin's Disease Staging," *Cancer Research* 31:1860, 1971. Adapted with permission.

CLINICAL SNAPSHOT ☀

Lymphoma

Major nursing diagnoses and collaborative problems	Key patient outcomes
CP: Risk for hypoxemia	Demonstrate effective, regular use of breathing techniques.
ND: Risk for infection	Show no signs of systemic or localized infection.
CP: Pruritus	List three self-care measures to reduce pruritus.
CP: Risk for hemorrhage	Show no signs or symptoms of hemorrhage.
ND: Imbalanced nutrition: Less than body requirements	Participate in planning and implementing a dietary regimen.
ND: Deficient knowledge (self-care)	List three possible complications of a vascular access device and identify appropriate interventions for each.
ND: Disturbed body image	List measures to minimize effects of chemotherapy and radiation therapy.

Hematologic and immunologic disorders

Collaborative problem

Risk for hypoxemia related to enlarged mediastinal nodes, pulmonary compression and, for malignant lymphoma only, superior vena cava syndrome

NURSING PRIORITY

Optimize alveolar ventilation.

PATIENT OUTCOME CRITERIA

Within 48 hours of admission, the patient will:
- demonstrate effective, regular use of breathing techniques

■ rate pain as less than 3 on a 0 to 10 pain rating scale
■ tolerate increased activity level
■ show relaxed posture and facial expression
■ exhibit no head or neck cyanosis.

INTERVENTIONS	**RATIONALES**
1. *Position the patient comfortably when he's short of breath:* * Elevate the upper torso at least 45 degrees, tilt the shoulders forward, support the arms away from the sides, and support the feet.	**1.** This position promotes maximum aeration by taking weight off the shoulders and arms, allowing the accessory muscles to be used solely for breathing.
2. *Teach and supervise therapeutic breathing techniques:* – pursed-lip breathing – abdominal breathing.	**2.** Breathing techniques minimize respiratory impairment. – Pursed-lip breathing has two benefits: It creates back pressure, holding the airways open, and the prolonged expiration time slows the flow of air, preventing premature closure of the airways and allowing more complete emptying of the lungs. – The abdominal muscles can aid the diaphragm during expiration. As the patient inhales, the abdominal muscles relax. During expiration, they contract and help the diaphragm move upward to expel air.
3. *Limit activity according to respiratory capabilities.*	**3.** Decreased activity decreases the need for oxygen.
4. Plan activities to allow minimal energy expenditure and adequate rest periods: provide bed baths, assist the patient with meals as needed, and limit visitors.	**4.** Fatigue is a symptom of hypoxemia and a cause of increased dyspnea. As respiratory muscles tire, respiratory excursion and alveolar ventilation drop, worsening hypoxemia and reinforcing the vicious circle of fatigue and dyspnea.
5. *Decrease anxiety associated with dyspnea:* Explain all procedures in a calm, supportive manner; provide a quiet environment to promote adequate rest; and use relaxation techniques, music, and other diversionary activities.	**5.** Anxiety and fear increase the heart rate, increasing the need for oxygen.
6. *Control pain with analgesics,* as ordered. Use non-pharmacologic pain-control techniques as appropriate. See the "Acute pain" care plan, page 32.	**6.** Pain may be present if enlarged nodes are compressing adjacent structures or nerve roots. Pain control will help decrease anxiety, thereby reducing associated shortness of breath. The "Acute pain" care plan contains specific information and detailed interventions.

7. *Monitor for signs and symptoms of superior vena cava syndrome,* as follows:
– early — thoracic and jugular vein distention (especially on arising), change in collar size, and headache
– advanced — progressive periorbital and facial edema, dizziness, cough, stridor, dysphagia, and dyspnea.
    Report such findings to the physician immediately, and transport the patient to the radiation therapy department, as ordered, if superior vena cava syndrome is identified.
    After radiation therapy, assess for indications of improvement: reduced edema, increased ease in swallowing, and improved respiratory parameters.
	7. In superior vena cava syndrome, enlarged nodes press on the superior vena cava, impairing normal venous drainage from the head and neck. The resulting progressive edema may lead to tracheal deviation and airway occlusion. Rapid onset of superior vena cava syndrome is considered an oncologic emergency. Radiation therapy is the treatment of choice: immediate therapy of 300 to 400 rads daily for 3 to 4 days, then a full course of 3,000 to 6,000 rads. In most patients, symptoms should decrease rapidly, usually within a few days.

*Italics indicate key interventions.

8. *Administer tranquilizers, as ordered.*

8. Physiologic reactions to anxiety include stimulation of the autonomic nervous system, such as increased heart and respiratory rates. Tranquilizers relieve anxiety without inducing sleep. The benzodiazepines appear to depress the CNS at the limbic and subcortical levels of the brain, producing sedation and relaxing skeletal muscles.

9. Additional individualized interventions: _____

9. Rationales: _____

Nursing diagnosis

Risk for infection related to leukopenia, lymphopenia from bone marrow involvement, chemotherapy, and radiation therapy effects

NURSING PRIORITIES

Prevent or promptly detect and treat superinfection.

PATIENT OUTCOME CRITERIA

After a full course of antibiotic therapy (5 to 10 days) and return of adequate immunity, or 14 days after completion of the chemotherapy cycle, the patient will:
- be afebrile
- show no signs of systemic or localized infection.

INTERVENTIONS

1. Prioritize patient care assignments. Care for the neutropenic patient first.

2. *Observe good hand-washing technique.*

3. *Monitor daily white blood cell (WBC) counts and differentials.* Inform the patient and physician of results.

4. *Take protective precautions when the patient's absolute granulocyte count is dangerously depressed,* typically when less than 1,000/µl. Protective measures should include:
– serving only cooked foods
– avoiding raw, unpeeled fruits and vegetables
– removing sources of standing water (such as vases of flowers)
– not handling live flowers or plants.
Institute further protective measures according to facility protocol, as appropriate to the patient's condition.

RATIONALES

1. This minimizes the risk of cross-contamination by the caregiver.

2. The most important way to protect against infection is meticulous hand washing. Improper or infrequent hand washing is a well-known contributor to cross-contamination.

3. The degree of granulocytopenia indicates the patient's susceptibility to infection and is the most important factor in determining the risk of sepsis.

4. The risk of infection increases significantly when the absolute granulocyte count ranges from 500 to 1,000/µl and persists for more than a few days. The absolute granulocyte count indicates the number of mature WBCs (the cells most effective in fighting infection). To calculate the absolute granulocyte count, add the percentage of polys (mature neutrophils) to the percentage of bands (slightly immature neutrophils); multiply the result by the WBC count. Protective precautions may decrease the number of pathogenic organisms the immunosuppressed patient contacts. Raw fruits and vegetables are sources of gram-negative bacilli; live plants and soil are sources of fungi. Standing water may provide a medium for microorganisms, particularly *Pseudomonas*.

Hematologic and immunologic disorders

5. *Assess actual and potential infection sites at least every 8 hours,* including the lungs, mouth, rectum, I.V. sites, vagina, and surgical incisions. Monitor urine culture results. Observe carefully for subtle changes in skin and mucous membrane color, texture, or sensation. Note new complaints of pain.

5. Early detection may prevent serious complications and spread of infection. In the immunocompromised patient, however, an altered inflammatory response complicates early detection. Classic signs and symptoms of infection (such as erythema, pus, and fever) may be masked in a neutropenic patient or in a patient taking steroids (a factor in many lymphoma protocols). Localized pain may indicate a site of infection.

6. *Screen and limit visitors.* Prohibit visits by those with recent or current infections.

6. Minimizing the patient's exposure to microorganisms may help avert sepsis.

7. *Institute an appropriate oral hygiene protocol.* Monitor for oral herpes lesions and *Candida* stomatitis.

7. The patient with lymphoma is at increased risk for viral and fungal infections because of impaired cell-mediated immunity. (T lymphocytes protect against viruses, fungi, and parasites.)

8. *Avoid invasive measures,* such as injections, enemas, rectal temperatures, suppositories, and indwelling urinary catheters whenever possible.

8. Intact skin is the body's first line of defense. Sweat glands and sebaceous glands keep bacteria under control. Lysozymes, enzymes secreted by the sweat glands, attack the cell walls of bacteria. Sebum, secreted by the sebaceous glands, has antifungal and antibacterial properties. Skin and blood infections may occur when invasive measures damage the skin.

9. *Measure the patient's temperature at least every 4 hours;* if it's higher than 101.3° F (38.5° C) and the patient develops signs and symptoms of septic shock (tachycardia, tachypnea, restlessness, confusion, cough, decreased pulse pressure, and cool extremities), notify the physician.

9. Septic shock (a medical emergency) is reversible in its early stages. Massive infection, usually from gram-negative bacteria, causes septic shock. As the body fights the infection, the bacteria die, releasing endotoxins that in turn impair cell metabolism and damage surrounding tissue. Lysozomal enzymes, bradykinin, and histamine cause peripheral vasodilation and increased capillary permeability, resulting in peripheral blood pooling, inadequate venous return, and severely reduced cardiac output.

10. *Obtain blood, urine, throat, and sputum cultures, using correct technique,* as ordered. Ensure that cultures are obtained before antibiotic therapy begins.

10. Cultures must be uncontaminated to permit accurate diagnosis. Current culture results determine appropriate antibiotic therapy.

11. *Report all positive blood cultures,* even if the patient is already taking antibiotics.

11. When specific organisms are identified, therapy should be modified according to antibiotic sensitivity.

12. Administer antibiotics only after obtaining blood and urine cultures, ideally within 60 minutes of detecting sepsis. Give subsequent doses on time.

12. Prompt, timely administration of antibiotics increases the survival rate in neutropenic patients. Therapeutic blood levels of medication must be maintained to treat sepsis effectively.

13. Additional individualized interventions: _____
_____

13. Rationales:_____
_____

Suggested NIC Interventions
Infection control; Infection protection; Incision site care; Wound care

Suggested NOC Outcomes
Infection status; Wound healing; Primary intention

Collaborative problem

Pruritus related to histamine or leukopeptidase release from WBCs and to effects of radiation therapy

NURSING PRIORITIES
- Relieve discomfort.
- Prevent or minimize skin injury.

PATIENT OUTCOME CRITERIA
Throughout the hospital stay, the patient will:
- present intact skin
- verbalize reduced discomfort
- on request, list three self-care measures to minimize pruritus.

INTERVENTIONS	RATIONALES
1. *Promote adequate hydration:* twelve 8-oz (237-ml) glasses of fluid daily, unless contraindicated.	**1.** Adequate hydration is essential to minimize skin dryness.
2. Use emollient creams on the skin (if allowed during radiation therapy).	**2.** Emollient creams are oil-in-water emulsions. Water keeps the skin moist while the oil creates a film that slows normal evaporation.
3. Provide tepid, cooling baths.	**3.** Regular bathing helps protect the immunosuppressed patient from infection. Additionally, tepid water promotes vasoconstriction. Proteases are sensitive to heat, and the cutaneous nerve endings that mediate the scratch impulse are made more sensitive by vasodilation.
4. Keep the patient's fingernails short. Provide clean cotton gloves at night.	**4.** These measures may prevent damage to the skin if the patient can't control scratching.
5. Use soap designed for sensitive or dry skin.	**5.** Soaps for sensitive skin have a large proportion of emollient oils and contain no detergents or dyes to strip the skin. They liquefy instantly and leave no irritating residue.
6. *Administer antihistamines, antibiotics, tar extracts, or chemotherapeutic agents,* as ordered.	**6.** Antihistamines will help if the underlying cause of pruritus is increased histamine release. Tar extracts and topical steroids may inhibit protease release. If infection is the underlying cause, antibiotics are indicated. If a tumor is releasing enzymes, chemotherapy may shrink the tumor and proportionately reduce enzyme release.
7. Instruct the patient to avoid harsh cold and wind.	**7.** Exposure to cold and wind dries the skin.
8. Remove excessive clothing or bedding; instruct the patient not to wear restrictive clothing.	**8.** A cool environment promotes vasoconstriction. Restrictive clothing may irritate the skin.
9. Instruct the family to launder the patient's clothing with a nondetergent cleanser, and rinse thoroughly.	**9.** These precautions help prevent chemical irritation of the skin.
10. Additional individualized interventions:_____	**10.** Rationales:_____

Hematologic and immunologic disorders

Collaborative problem

Risk for hemorrhage related to decreased platelet count secondary to chemotherapy or radiation therapy effects

NURSING PRIORITY

Maximize the patient's available protective mechanisms.

PATIENT OUTCOME CRITERIA

Throughout the hospital stay, the patient will:
- have regular, soft, formed stools
- show no signs or symptoms of hemorrhage.

INTERVENTIONS	RATIONALES
1. *Don't administer aspirin or aspirin-containing products.*	**1.** The acetyl group in the aspirin compound inhibits platelet aggregation, thereby impairing fibrin strand formation. A single dose of aspirin produces an effect that remains for days, long after the aspirin has been metabolized and excreted.
2. *Administer stool softeners,* as ordered, and monitor the frequency of stools to detect constipation.	**2.** Straining at stool produces excessive pressure on the anal orifice; the rectal area is highly vascular and can hemorrhage.
3. *Avoid invasive measures* such as I.M. injections, enemas, and rectal suppositories.	**3.** Intact skin reduces the risk of bleeding. A decreased platelet count means that even minor trauma may result in significant bleeding.
4. *Use an electric razor when shaving the patient.* Avoid activities with the potential for physical injury.	**4.** These measures minimize the risk of skin trauma.
5. *Administer steroids,* as ordered, with milk products or antacids.	**5.** Coating the stomach helps prevent gastric irritation.
6. *Maintain optimal nutritional status,* encouraging protein intake.	**6.** Protein is needed to produce megakaryocytes, precursors of platelets.
7. *Test all stool, vomitus, and urine for occult blood.*	**7.** Early detection of bleeding promotes early and effective treatment.
8. *Apply direct pressure to venipuncture sites for at least 5 minutes.*	**8.** Decreased platelet levels delay clot formation.
9. *Administer platelet infusions,* as ordered.	**9.** A platelet count below 20,000/mm³ increases the risk of spontaneous hemorrhage. Active bleeding is an indication for platelet administration.
10. Use a soft-bristle toothbrush, and avoid flossing the patient's teeth.	**10.** These measures decrease the risk of physical irritation to oral mucous membranes.
11. *Instruct the patient to avoid strenuous activity,* Valsalva's maneuver, and lifting heavy objects.	**11.** These activities increase intracranial pressure and may cause cerebrovascular hemorrhage.
12. *Teach the patient self-protection measures* related to the above interventions, such as avoiding aspirin, taking stool softeners, and using an electric razor.	**12.** The knowledgeable patient's active involvement in self-care minimizes the risk of hemorrhage, especially after discharge.
13. Additional individualized interventions: _____	**13.** Rationales:_____

Nursing diagnosis

Imbalanced nutrition: Less than body requirements related to anorexia, taste alterations, fatigue, nausea and vomiting, and altered oral mucous membrane

NURSING PRIORITY

Promote adequate nutrition to enhance response to therapy and prevent complications.

PATIENT OUTCOME CRITERIA

Throughout the hospital stay, the patient will:
- participate in planning and implementing a dietary regimen
- maintain an adequate nutritional status to facilitate therapy, as evidenced by stable weight, nonemaciated appearance, and nutrition-related laboratory values within normal limits.

INTERVENTIONS	RATIONALES
1. Arrange for a dietary consultation *to* address the patient's calorie and protein needs. Explore the patient's food preferences and attempt to obtain the foods requested. Explain prescribed dietary recommendations and help the patient set goals for meeting them. Consult the "Nutritional deficit" care plan, page 138.	1. The dietitian's expertise may be helpful in planning a diet that meets the patient's needs while incorporating the patient's preferences. Including the patient in planning and goal-setting enhances compliance and promotes a sense of self-control. The "Nutritional deficit" care plan contains detailed information on assessing and managing the problem. This care plan provides additional information pertinent to lymphoma.
2. Offer sandwiches and other cold foods.	2. The odor of hot foods commonly aggravates nausea.
3. *Avoid giving liquids with meals.*	3. Fluids contribute to gastric distention and may reduce the intake of solid foods.
4. Avoid offering favorite foods during peak periods of nausea and vomiting or while the patient is receiving chemotherapy.	4. The patient can develop an aversion to foods served during periods of nausea and vomiting. During anorexic periods, favorite foods may supply the patient's only intake, so maintaining positive associations is essential.
5. Offer salty foods (such as broth or crackers) and tart foods (such as lemons or dill pickles) unless the patient has stomatitis.	5. These foods increase salivation and stimulate the taste buds. In the patient with stomatitis, however, salt and acidity will further irritate open mucous membranes.
6. Offer small, frequent meals, and encourage the patient to eat and drink slowly.	6. Small meals and eating slowly minimize gastric distention and help prevent early satiety.
7. Avoid offering greasy foods.	7. High-fat foods prolong gastric emptying time, causing feelings of overfullness and distention.
8. *Provide mouth care before meals and after vomiting* episodes.	8. Regular mouth care refreshes the mouth and enhances the flavor of foods.
9. If taste alterations are present, consult with the dietary department and advise the patient to: – use plastic utensils instead of metal silverware – eat protein in the form of eggs, cheese, beans, and peanut butter instead of meat – experiment with spices and flavorings to enhance taste sensation (such as mint, vanilla, lemon, and basil), unless contraindicated by stomatitis.	9. The presence of actively dividing cells in the oral mucous membrane that excrete amino acid–like substances enhances the bitter taste sensation. Large tumor mass also increases the degree and duration of any taste sensation. Beef and pork have high amino acid levels. A negative nitrogen balance also decreases the patient's threshold for the bitter taste sensation. Certain chemotherapy agents used in lymphoma protocols, specifically mechlorethamine (Mustargen), cyclophosphamide (Cytoxan), vincristine (Oncovin), and dacarbazine (DTIC-Dome) contribute further to taste alterations.

10. Advise the patient to increase his intake of sugar and sweet foods.

10. Taste alterations associated with the disease and chemotherapy commonly include decreased sensitivity to sweetness, although this is sometimes accompanied by an aversion to sweet foods. Increased sugar also boosts caloric intake.

11. Teach the patient how to use viscous lidocaine (Xylocaine) to reduce stomatitis pain (swish and swallow 15 ml, 15 minutes before or after meals). If ineffective, try dyclonine (Dyclone).

11. A topical anesthetic decreases sensitivity to pain, enabling the patient to eat without discomfort. Using the anesthetic after meals decreases food-induced discomfort.

12. Offer soft, moist foods, such as custards, ice cream, gelatins, cottage cheese, and ground meats with sauces and gravies.

12. Soft foods minimize mechanical irritation to the oral mucous membrane and are easier to swallow.

13. Encourage the patient to eat liquid and pudding supplements.

13. High-calorie supplements may compensate for decreased intake.

14. *Consult the physician regarding temporary enteral or parenteral feedings* if other interventions are ineffective.

14. The patient may need a temporary alternative to oral nutrition to prevent severe malnutrition, which may affect the outcome of therapy.

15. Additional individualized interventions: _____

15. Rationales:_____

Suggested NIC Interventions
Diet staging; Nutrition management; Weight gain assistance; Fluid monitoring; Nutritional monitoring

Suggested NOC Outcomes
Nutritional status; Nutritional status: Food and food intake; Nutritional status: Nutrient intake; Weight control

Nursing diagnosis

Deficient knowledge (self-care of vascular access device, including peripherally or centrally inserted venous catheters or subcutaneous ports) related to lack of exposure to information

NURSING PRIORITY

Teach self-care techniques and measures for home management of the vascular access device.

PATIENT OUTCOME CRITERIA

By the time of discharge, the patient will:
- list signs of infection
- demonstrate dressing change and irrigation techniques as taught
- list three possible complications of a vascular access device and identify appropriate interventions for each.

INTERVENTIONS

1. Teach the patient the name of the catheter or port and its purpose and anatomic placement.

RATIONALES

1. Central venous catheters or subcutaneous ports may be used to administer chemotherapy. The patient who's knowledgeable about all aspects of care is better prepared to use good judgment in decision making and to teach others about care needs. Assuming greater responsibility for the device helps the patient develop an increased sense of control, easing incorporation of the device into the patient's body image.

2. *Teach the patient how to change dressings at home* (usually a clean, occlusive dressing changed when wet or soiled or according to protocol). Have the patient demonstrate the proper technique before discharge; arrange for home care follow-up. If the patient has a subcutaneous port, explain that a dressing isn't necessary because the device is completely under the skin.

3. *Teach the patient to identify early signs and symptoms of local or generalized infection,* such as redness, swelling, purulent drainage, fever, increased fatigue, and malaise.

4. *Teach the patient the importance of proper irrigation technique,* including frequency and solution used, specified by the manufacturer and facility policy.

5. *Inform the patient of potential complications* and appropriate interventions, as follows:

– clot formation (catheter won't irrigate): Avoid forcing irrigation if resistance is felt. Contact the physician.
– catheter displacement (catheter pulled out): Apply a pressure dressing and call the physician. If bleeding is present, apply direct manual pressure until it stops.

6. Give the patient the names and telephone numbers of appropriate resource persons, such as the physician, emergency squad, and the home health nurse.

7. Additional individualized interventions: _____
_____

2. Because the catheter exit site is a break in skin integrity, the risk of opportunistic infections increases. A clean occlusive dressing can decrease the potential for microbial contamination. The frequency of dressing changes varies among institutions.

Anxiety may interfere with learning by decreasing the patient's ability to concentrate. Written materials and home care follow-up reinforce earlier learning and allow the patient to learn in a less-threatening environment.

3. Early detection of infection results in more timely and effective treatment.

4. Although catheters and subcutaneous ports are in place continuously, chemotherapy administration is intermittent. Catheter or port patency must be maintained for the device to function. Proper technique decreases the risk of contamination.

5. Recognizing complications may prevent a potentially hazardous situation, such as infection, tissue damage, catheter migration, or loss of the device.
– Forcing irrigation may push a clot out the end of the catheter and into the circulatory system.
– Pressure controls bleeding if the catheter is accidentally removed.

6. A health care provider can speed resolution of a patient problem or concern. Knowing how and where to contact resource persons may help decrease anxiety and promote a sense of control.

7. Rationales: _____
_____

Suggested NIC Interventions *Teaching: Procedure/treatment*	***Suggested NOC Outcomes*** *Knowledge: Treatment regimen*

Nursing diagnosis
Disturbed body image related to effects of chemotherapy or radiation therapy

NURSING PRIORITIES
■ Prepare the patient for therapy.
■ Promote a positive self-concept.

PATIENT OUTCOME CRITERIA
Throughout the hospital stay, the patient will:
■ verbalize feelings freely, if desired
■ participate in decision making related to care.
   By the time of discharge, the patient will:
■ identify personal concerns that may affect self-concept
■ identify personal or external resources to deal with concerns
■ list measures to minimize effects of chemotherapy or radiation therapy.

Hematologic and
immunologic disorders

INTERVENTIONS

1. *Inform the patient of anticipated adverse effects of chemotherapy or radiation* that will affect body image and role performance. Suggest measures to prevent or lessen their impact. (See *Suggestions for minimizing chemotherapeutic adverse effects*.)

2. *Inform the male patient of the availability of sperm banking before beginning chemotherapy.*

3. Provide adequate time to discuss the patient's concerns and feelings. Strive to maintain a nonjudgmental attitude. See the "Grieving" care plan, page 105, "Compromised family coping" care plan, page 67, and "Ineffective individual coping" care plan, page 124.

4. *Include the patient in decision making.* Allow the patient to plan the day's events (within facility limitations).

5. Instruct the patient and his spouse (or partner) on specific sexual adverse effects of chemotherapy and radiation therapy: for example, decreased libido, decreased vaginal lubrication, and temporary impotence. Provide written material for specific interventions related to each. Encourage the couple to share concerns and ask questions. Refer them to the social services department or other resources for ongoing counseling and support, if needed.

6. Additional individualized interventions: _____

_____

RATIONALES

1. Chemotherapy protocols for lymphoma are aggressive and cause many adverse effects. Radiation therapy may also cause severe adverse effects. Teaching the patient about specific preventive or palliative measures before therapy begins increases the patient's sense of control, decreases powerlessness, and promotes self-image.

2. Because the peak incidence of Hodgkin's disease corresponds with peak childbearing years, fertility is a major concern. Chemotherapy may cause permanent sterility. For a male patient, sperm banking can help offset this adverse effect of treatment. The well-informed patient is able to base decisions on sound judgment after considering available options.

3. The patient is more likely to discuss personal concerns if a trusting relationship is developed. Judgmental responses that reflect the caregiver's personal biases may inhibit open discussion. These care plans provide interventions helpful in addressing emotional needs.

4. Promoting maximum patient participation in care planning conveys respect and increases the patient's sense of control.

5. The couple may be comforted to know that many adverse effects of therapy are temporary. Fatigue, fear, anxiety, and lack of privacy may also contribute to problems. Many patients (and many health care professionals) aren't well educated about sex or are uncomfortable discussing sexual problems. Written information is a less threatening but effective means of providing this information. Sharing concerns may reduce the couple's anxiety.

6. Rationales: _____

_____

> **Suggested NIC Interventions**
> *Body image enhancement; Grief work facilitation; Anticipatory guidance; Coping enhancement; Self-esteem enhancement*

> **Suggested NOC Outcomes**
> *Body image; Grief resolution; Self-esteem*

Discharge planning

DISCHARGE CHECKLIST
Before discharge, the patient shows evidence of:
❑ stable vital signs
❑ absence of fever
❑ absence of cardiovascular or pulmonary complications
❑ ability to control pain using oral medications

❑ absence of bowel or bladder dysfunction
❑ WBC count within expected parameters
❑ absence of signs and symptoms of infection
❑ ability to tolerate adequate nutritional intake
❑ ability to perform activities of daily living and to ambulate independently or with minimal assistance
❑ ability to care appropriately for vascular access device, if present
❑ adequate home support system or referral to home care or a nursing home if indicated by inadequate

Suggestions for minimizing chemotherapeutic adverse effects

Alopecia
- Shampoo only one or two times weekly.
- Use a mild, protein shampoo.
- Avoid using an electric hair dryer or electric curlers.
- Avoid using hair spray or other drying products.
- Try a satin pillowcase to minimize tangling.
- Avoid excessive hair brushing or combing.
- Use a wide-tooth comb.
- Avoid using scalp hypothermia devices, which may reduce flow of medication to the head.

Weight gain
- Exercise regularly.
- Follow prescribed dietary guidelines.
- Select flattering, loose-fitting clothing.

Nausea and vomiting
- Avoid fatty, salty, or spicy foods.
- Use diversionary activities.
- Avoid eating or drinking for at least 1 hour before and after chemotherapy.
- Use a sedative that has an amnesic effect, such as lorazepam (Ativan), before chemotherapy, if prescribed.
- Suggest that family members avoid perfumes, aftershaves, and other aromatic toiletries.

Constipation
- Maintain a diet high in fiber, bulk, and fluids.
- Exercise regularly.
- Use stool softeners.

Diarrhea
- Try adding nutmeg to foods.
- Avoid milk or milk products (except yogurt, which may be helpful).
- Ensure adequate replacement of fluid and potassium.

Depression
- Understand that depression is normal and usually temporary.
- Identify and use resources for emotional support.

Sore throat or dysphagia
- Watch for difficulty swallowing or sore throat while eating.
- Eat soft foods.
- Use topical anesthetics as prescribed.

Dermatitis
- Avoid using deodorants, cosmetics, or creams, unless prescribed.
- Avoid hot baths or use of heat.

---

home support system or the patient's inability to care for himself.

TEACHING CHECKLIST
Document evidence that the patient and his family demonstrate an understanding of:
- ❏ disease and its progression
- ❏ signs and symptoms of infection and preventive measures
- ❏ discharge medications, including their purpose, dosage, administration schedule, and adverse effects requiring medical attention (usual discharge medications may include antineoplastics, analgesics, stool softeners, antiemetics, and others, depending on symptoms)
- ❏ purpose and results of radiation therapy, schedule for future treatments, and management of anticipated adverse effects
- ❏ maintenance of a vascular access device
- ❏ indications for seeking emergency medical care
- ❏ services available from local American Cancer Society chapter
- ❏ availability of home health care and ancillary support services
- ❏ date, time, and location of next scheduled appointment
- ❏ how to contact the physician.

DOCUMENTATION CHECKLIST
Using outcome criteria as a guide, document:
- ❏ clinical status on admission
- ❏ significant changes in clinical status
- ❏ teaching about and response to diagnostic and staging workups
- ❏ chemotherapy administration—I.V. line patency and site status, name of medication, dosage, and response (include teaching about protocol and the patient's response)
- ❏ skin integrity over irradiated areas
- ❏ transfusion therapy and response or reactions
- ❏ nutritional status
- ❏ status and maintenance of vascular access device
- ❏ referrals initiated
- ❏ patient and family teaching
- ❏ discharge planning.

Associated care plans
- Acute pain
- Compromised family coping
- Dying
- Grieving
- Ineffective individual coping
- Knowledge deficit
- Nutritional deficit

References

Devita, V. *Cancer: Principles and Practice of Oncology,* 6th ed. Philadelphia: Lippincott Williams & Wilkins, 2001.

Galassi, A. "Follow-up Care of Cancer Survivors," *Primary Care Practice* 4(4):359-70, July-August 2000.

Gates, R., and Finks, R. *Oncology Nursing Secrets,* 2nd ed. Philadelphia: Lippincott Williams & Wilkins, 2001.

Otto, S. *Oncology Nursing,* 4th ed. St. Louis: Mosby–Year Book, Inc., 2001.

Sainio, C. "Patient Participation in Decision Making about Care: The Cancer Patient's Point of View," *Cancer Nursing* 24(3):172-79, June 2001.

Reproductive disorders

PART

12

Hysterectomy

DRG INFORMATION

DRG 353   Pelvic Evisceration, Radical Hysterectomy, and Radical Vulvectomy.
Mean LOS = 6.5 days

DRG 354   Uterine and Adnexa Procedure for Non-Ovarian, Adnexal Malignancy with Complication or Comorbidity (CC).
Mean LOS = 5.9 days

DRG 355   Uterine and Adnexa Procedure for Non-Ovarian, Adnexal Malignancy without CC.
Mean LOS = 3.3 days

DRG 357   Uterine and Adnexa Procedures for Ovarian or Adnexal Malignancy.
Mean LOS = 8.5 days

DRG 358   Uterine and Adnexa Procedures for Non-Malignancy with CC.
Mean LOS = 4.3 days

DRG 359   Uterine and Adnexa Procedures for Non-Malignancy without CC.
Mean LOS = 2.7 days

Introduction

DEFINITION AND TIME FOCUS

Hysterectomy is the surgical removal of the uterus. Several surgical variations exist. Subtotal hysterectomy (supracervical hysterectomy), which is seldom performed, is the surgical removal of the corpus (body) of the uterus, leaving the cervical stump in place. Total hysterectomy is the surgical removal of the uterus and cervix. Total hysterectomy (simple hysterectomy) with bilateral salpingo-oophorectomy is the surgical removal of the uterus, cervix, uterine (fallopian) tubes, and ovaries. (Salpingectomy is the surgical removal of the uterine tube or tubes; oophorectomy is the removal of an ovary or ovaries.) Radical hysterectomy is the surgical removal of the uterus, cervix, upper portion of the vagina, connective tissue, and lymph nodes.

All hysterectomy procedures result in permanent sterilization. If performed in conjunction with bilateral oophorectomy in the premenopausal woman, abrupt menopause results.

The surgical approach for a hysterectomy may be vaginal or abdominal. However, the vaginal approach is increasing in popularity and, when combined with laparoscopic assistance, may be used for other disease states. The abdominal approach is commonly used for pelvic exploration of cancer, endometriosis, or infection; removal of an enlarged uterus; or removal of tubes and ovaries.

This care plan focuses on preoperative assessment and postoperative care for a patient undergoing total abdominal hysterectomy. (See *Clinical snapshot: Hysterectomy.*)

ETIOLOGY AND PRECIPITATING FACTORS

- Recent diagnosis of cervical, endometrial, or ovarian cancer
- Irreparable rupture or perforation of the uterus
- Severe (life-threatening) pelvic infection
- Myoma or nonmalignant tumor of the uterus (fibroid)
- History of endometriosis
- Hemorrhage, metrorrhagia (dysfunctional uterine bleeding), postmenopausal bleeding, perimenopausal menometrorrhagia (excessive, prolonged vaginal bleeding at irregular intervals), menorrhagia (excessive uterine bleeding occurring during regular menstruation), or postcoital bleeding with pelvic pain

Focused assessment guidelines

NURSING HISTORY
(FUNCTIONAL HEALTH PATTERN FINDINGS)

Health-perception–health-management pattern
- Postmenopausal with sudden uterine bleeding
- Abnormal Papanicolaou (Pap) test results in the past (if cervical or endometrial cancer is present)
- History of prolonged postmenopausal estrogen replacement therapy (if endometrial cancer is present)
- History of prolonged, heavy, or painful menstruation (if uterine myoma, endometriosis, or endometrial cancer is present)
- History of fibroids (myomas) in the uterus

Nutritional-metabolic pattern
- Obesity

Elimination pattern
- Pattern of frequent urination related to presence and proximity of tumor

Activity-exercise pattern
- Fatigue-related decrease in activity level if excessive vaginal bleeding has caused anemia

Sleep-rest pattern
- Sleep disturbance related to nocturia
- Sleep disturbance related to emotional stress of planned hospital stay and surgery

Cognitive-perceptual pattern
- History of abdominal, pelvic, back, or leg pain
- Fear of anticipated discomfort and pain from abdominal incision

Self-perception–self-concept pattern
- Concerns expressed about abdominal scar and removal of uterus
- Concerns expressed about femininity
- Concerns expressed about infertility

Role-relationship pattern
- Concerns expressed about spouse's or partner's acceptance of infertility

Sexuality-reproductive pattern
- Concerns expressed about resuming sexual intercourse after surgery

Value-belief pattern
- Delay in seeking medical attention if perimenopausal (because irregular menses are normal during early menopause)

PHYSICAL FINDINGS
Gastrointestinal
- Lower abdominal distention (with ovarian cancer)
- Abdominal discomfort (with uterine myoma)
- Adnexal mass (with ovarian cancer)

Genitourinary
- Leukorrhea (with infection)
- Vaginal bleeding (with uterine myoma)

Musculoskeletal
- Leg edema (less common)

DIAGNOSTIC STUDIES
- Hemoglobin level — may reveal decreased hemoglobin concentration, indicating anemia
- Hematocrit — may reveal a decrease in volume percentage of red blood cells in whole blood, indicating blood loss

- White blood cell (WBC) count — may be elevated because of severe pelvic infection
- D&C (cervical dilatation and fractional curettage) and four-quadrant endometrial biopsy — provides endometrial tissue for a histopathologic study, which may reveal endometrial cancer
- Wedge biopsy or conization biopsy of the cervix (removal of tissue for microscopic examination) — may reveal cervical cancer
- Pap test (removal of exfoliated cervical cells) — may reveal cellular dysplasia
- Colposcopy (visualization of the cervix with a colposcope) — may identify abnormal cell growth
- Schiller's test (staining of the cervix with iodine) — identifies abnormal cells
- Ultrasound or computed tomography scan — may reveal size and location of mass

POTENTIAL COMPLICATIONS
- Hemorrhagic shock
- Peritonitis
- Emboli
- Pneumonia
- Perforated bladder
- Ligation of ureter
- Wound infection
- Atelectasis
- Thrombophlebitis
- Urine retention
- Urinary tract infection (UTI)

CLINICAL SNAPSHOT ☀

Hysterectomy

Major nursing diagnoses and collaborative problems	Key patient outcomes
CP: Risk for thromboembolic and hemorrhagic complications	Show no signs or symptoms of thromboembolic or hemorrhagic complications.
ND: Risk for infection	Have clean, dry, intact wound.
ND: Urinary retention	Void at least once (greater than 100 ml) within 8 hours after catheter removal.
ND: Acute pain	Rate pain as less than 3 on a 0 to 10 pain rating scale.
ND: Disturbed body image	Verbalize beginning acceptance of possible alterations in body appearance and function.
ND: Sexual dysfunction	Verbalize strategies to manage temporary alteration in sexual functioning.

Reproductive disorders

Collaborative problem

Risk for thromboembolic and hemorrhagic complications related to immobility, venous stasis, pelvic congestion, or possible predisposing factors

NURSING PRIORITY

Prevent or promptly treat thromboembolic and hemorrhagic complications.

PATIENT OUTCOME CRITERIA

Throughout the hospital stay, the patient will:
- show no signs or symptoms of significant postoperative bleeding, such as tachycardia, hypotension, or pallor
- show no signs or symptoms of thromboembolic complications, such as calf pain or swelling or difficulty breathing.

INTERVENTIONS

1. *Monitor for signs of bleeding. Check vital signs and the surgical site according to standard postoperative protocol** (see the "Perioperative care " care plan, page 146, for details), and report tachycardia, decreasing blood pressure, increasing drainage, restlessness, pallor, diaphoresis, or any other sign of hemorrhage immediately. Institute fluid replacement therapy, as ordered. (See the "Hypovolemic shock" care plan, page 424 for details.)

2. *Institute measures to prevent and assess for thromboembolic phenomena:* Help the patient change position frequently; tell the patient to avoid placing pressure under the knee, to avoid prolonged sitting, and to apply antiembolic hose or pneumatic compression devices; and assist the patient with range-of-motion exercises. Administer anticoagulant medication, as ordered. (See the "Perioperative care" care plan, page 146 and "Thrombophlebitis" care plan, page 459, for further details.)

3. Before discharge, instruct the patient to promptly report any bleeding and to avoid heavy lifting, prolonged sitting, and wearing constrictive clothes.

4. Additional individualized interventions: _____
_____

RATIONALES

1. The proximity of the surgical site to large vessels may increase the risk of significant postoperative bleeding. Additionally, a patient with a presurgical diagnosis of cancer may have clotting factor abnormalities that increase the risk of hemorrhage. Untreated, such bleeding rapidly progresses to hypovolemic shock; death may result. The "Perioperative care" care plan provides further details about standard postoperative monitoring, while the "Hypovolemic shock" care plan covers assessment and management of that complication.

2. The postoperative patient is always at increased risk for thromboembolic complications because of circulatory disruption, immobility, and edema. The posthysterectomy patient may be at additional risk because of pelvic congestion. The "Perioperative care" and "Thrombophlebitis" care plans contain further details regarding this potential postoperative problem.

3. Postoperative hemorrhage may occur as late as 14 days after surgery. Avoiding activities that put stress on the operative site or cause venous stasis or pelvic congestion helps minimize the risk of bleeding or thromboembolic phenomena after discharge.

4. Rationales: _____
_____

Nursing diagnosis

Risk for infection related to abdominal incision, urinary tract proximity, contamination of peritoneal cavity, hypoventilation, anesthesia, or preoperative infection

NURSING PRIORITY

Prevent or promptly detect and treat infection.

PATIENT OUTCOME CRITERIA

Throughout the postoperative period, the patient will:

---

*Italics indicate key interventions.

- have clean, dry, intact wound
- perform pulmonary hygiene measures correctly and regularly
- show no symptoms of peritonitis, such as abdominal pain and rigidity
- show no signs of UTI, such as cloudy, foul-smelling urine.

INTERVENTIONS

1. *Monitor for signs and symptoms of peritonitis,* such as a significant increase in abdominal pain or a change in pain quality, abdominal rigidity or tenderness, nausea and vomiting, absent bowel sounds, or tachycardia. Report abnormal findings to the physician immediately.

2. *Implement standard postoperative nursing measures to prevent or detect other infections:*

– atelectasis and pneumonia

– UTI

– incisional infection.

See the "Perioperative care" care plan, page 146 for further details.

3. Before discharge, teach the patient about signs and symptoms indicating infection, such as cough or respiratory congestion, urinary pain or burning or cloudy urine, or redness, swelling, or purulent wound drainage. Emphasize the importance of promptly reporting such findings to the physician.

4. Additional individualized interventions: _____
_____

RATIONALES

1. The uterus is a peritoneal organ, so tissue oozing after its removal drains into the peritoneal cavity. Significant contamination from tissue, bleeding, or infection may result in potentially life-threatening peritonitis if not promptly treated.

2. The hysterectomy patient may be at increased risk for infection compared to other surgical patients because of the surgery site and the predisposing factors that may be involved.
– Ciliary depression from anesthesia, decreased mobility, and hypoventilation from abdominal incision pain contribute to stasis of pulmonary secretions, thus increasing the risk of infection.
– The urinary tract's proximity to the surgical area makes it prone to surgical trauma, edema, and resultant urine retention, which may predispose the patient to infection.
– Wound infection can be a complication of any surgery, but if the hysterectomy is performed because of cancer, the patient's immune response may be impaired, further increasing the risk.
Nursing measures related to these problems are standard postoperative interventions.

3. Prompt detection facilitates early treatment.

4. Rationales: _____
_____

Suggested NIC Interventions
Infection control; Infection protection; Incision site care; Wound care

Suggested NOC Outcomes
Infection status; Wound healing: Primary intention

Nursing diagnosis
Urinary retention related to decreased bladder and urethral muscle tone from anesthesia and mechanical trauma

NURSING PRIORITY
Promote optimal urine elimination.

PATIENT OUTCOME CRITERIA
Within 8 hours after catheter removal, the patient will:

Reproductive disorders

- void at least once
- produce adequate output (at least 100 ml per voiding)
- evidence clear, pale yellow urine.

INTERVENTIONS	RATIONALES
1. *Monitor for signs of urine retention* after catheter removal, such as small, frequent voidings; bladder distention; intake greater than output; or restless behavior.	**1.** Small, frequent voidings (less than 100 ml) may indicate urine retention, possibly related to edema, decreased muscle tone, or nerve damage to the bladder or urethra during surgery. Urine retention appears most commonly during the first 24 hours after surgery or catheter removal.
2. *Implement measures to resolve retention,* if it occurs. Encourage voiding. Obtain an order for catheterization if no voiding occurs within 8 hours after surgery. (See the "Perioperative care" care plan, page 146, for details.)	**2.** The "Perioperative care" care plan contains specific information about this common postoperative problem.
3. Additional individualized interventions: _____	**3.** Rationales: _____

> **Suggested NIC Interventions**
> *Urinary bladder training; Urinary catheterization: Intermittent; Urinary elimination management; Urinary retention care*

> **Suggested NOC Outcomes**
> *Urinary continence; Urinary elimination*

Nursing diagnosis

Acute pain related to abdominal incision and distention

NURSING PRIORITY

Minimize and relieve abdominal pain.

PATIENT OUTCOME CRITERIA

Within 1 hour of pain onset, the patient will:
- report pain level as less than 3 on a scale of 0 to 10, with pain medication.
  Within 3 days after surgery, the patient will:
- need analgesics less frequently or in lower doses
- pass flatus.

INTERVENTIONS	RATIONALES
1. *Implement measures for pain control.* See the "Acute pain" care plan, page 32 and "Perioperative care" care plan, page 146.	**1.** These care plans contain measures applicable to any patient in pain.
2. Offer application of heat to the abdomen 48 hours after surgery, as ordered.	**2.** Heat increases the elasticity of collagen tissue; lessens pain; relieves muscle spasms; helps resolve inflammatory infiltration, edema, and exudates; and increases blood flow. Heat applied less than 48 hours after surgery may cause undesirable edema.
3. Additional individualized interventions: _____	**3.** Rationales: _____

Nursing diagnosis

Disturbed body image related to changes in body appearance and function as a result of surgery

NURSING PRIORITY

Assist the patient in recognizing and accepting possible alteration in body appearance and function.

PATIENT OUTCOME CRITERIA

By the time of discharge, the patient will:
- verbalize understanding of body changes
- verbalize ability to cope with possible alterations in body appearance and function.

INTERVENTIONS

1. *Assess the patient's level of understanding regarding hysterectomy and the recovery period.*

2. Acknowledge the patient's feelings of loss and dependency and fears of complications. Provide reassurance that these concerns are normal.

3. Provide opportunities, every shift, for the patient to discuss concerns about symptoms associated with recovery. Encourage discussion of possible fatigue, wound problems, discomfort, urinary problems, and weight gain. Clarify misconceptions of such posthysterectomy myths as growing fat and flabby, developing facial hair, becoming wrinkled or masculine in appearance, or becoming depressed and nervous.

4. Encourage the patient to discuss plans for recovery at home.

5. Additional individualized interventions: _____

RATIONALES

1. Evaluating the patient's level of understanding allows the caregiver to individualize patient teaching according to the patient's preexisting knowledge base.

2. Loss of the uterus commonly triggers grief over lost fertility and concerns about femininity. Acknowledgment validates the patient's feelings and encourages communication to alleviate fears and anxieties.

3. Frequent, short teaching sessions enhance learning through repetition and by preventing information overload. Factual discussion prepares the patient to accept common symptoms. Such information does *not* act as a self-fulfilling prophecy. Clarifying misconceptions and myths reduces fears and anxiety during the recovery period.

4. Such discussion allows the patient to make plans incorporating appropriate limitations in physical activities. It also demonstrates the patient's acceptance and understanding of physical abilities.

5. Rationales: _____

Reproductive disorders

Nursing diagnosis

Sexual dysfunction (decreased libido or dyspareunia) related to fatigue, pain, grieving, altered body image, decreased estrogen levels, loss of vaginal sensations, sexual activity restrictions, or concerns about acceptance by spouse or partner

NURSING PRIORITY

Facilitate healthy coping with sexual alterations.

PATIENT OUTCOME CRITERION

By the time of discharge, the patient will verbalize strategies to manage temporary alteration in sexual functioning.

INTERVENTIONS	RATIONALES
1. Encourage the patient to explore perceptions of how surgery will affect sexual function. Listen sensitively.	**1.** Identifying current perceptions is the first step in coping with concerns. Sensitive listening allows the caregiver to identify appropriate and inappropriate perceptions.
2. *Discuss the potential impact of surgery on sexuality* by explaining: – the predictability of temporarily decreased libido	**2.** Providing factual information clarifies misconceptions and reduces fears of sexual loss. – Abdominal hysterectomy is major surgery that can have profound emotional implications. Fatigue, pain, and grieving may require so much coping energy that little remains for dealing with sexuality. The patient may need gentle "permission" to allow time to recover.
– the temporary nature of loss of vaginal sensations and of activity restrictions (sexual intercourse is discouraged for 4 to 6 weeks, then may be resumed gradually); also explain that return to full function is likely in approximately 4 months – the rationale for avoiding douching during the recovery.	– Vaginal sensory loss from surgical trauma resolves typically over a period of weeks to months. Activity restrictions allow time for tissues to heal. – Douching may increase the risk of infection or bleeding.
3. Explain that decreased libido and vaginal dryness may result from hormone loss and that hormone replacements are available.	**3.** The patient may not recognize that changes in sexual feelings and function can have a physiologic basis.
4. Suggest ways to ease sexual adjustment during the immediate postoperative period, such as holding hands, kissing, massage, and other methods of expressing love and sexuality.	**4.** Continued physical affection provides reassurance that a spouse's or partner's sexual interest continues after the hysterectomy.
5. Discuss options for conserving energy and preventing discomfort during return to sexual functioning, such as using a vaginal lubricant, scheduling sex for periods of peak energy, and avoiding positions that put pressure on the incision.	**5.** Sexual activity during the recovery period may be modified temporarily, but a return to full sexual function is expected.
6. Encourage the patient and her spouse or partner, if present, to share concerns and feelings with each other.	**6.** Mutual loving support is a positive factor in the couple's adjustment to sexual alterations.
7. Additional individualized interventions: _____	**7.** Rationales: _____

> ***Suggested NIC Interventions***
> *Sexual counseling*

> ***Suggested NOC Outcomes***
> *Sexual functioning*

Discharge planning

DISCHARGE CHECKLIST

Before discharge, the patient shows evidence of:
❏ stable vital signs
❏ hemoglobin level and WBC count within normal parameters
❏ absence of cardiovascular and pulmonary complications
❏ bowel function same as before surgery
❏ absence of dysuria, hematuria, pyuria, burning, frequency, or urgency
❏ absence of fever
❏ absence of signs and symptoms of infection
❏ ability to control pain using oral medications
❏ ability to ambulate and perform activities of daily living (ADLs) the same as before surgery
❏ healing surgical incision without redness, inflammation, or drainage
❏ ability to perform wound care independently or with minimal assistance
❏ ability to tolerate adequate nutritional intake
❏ adequate home support or referral to home care if indicated by inadequate home support system or inability to perform ADLs and wound care.

TEACHING CHECKLIST

Document evidence that the patient and her family demonstrate an understanding of:
❏ implications of total abdominal hysterectomy
❏ discharge medications, including their purpose, dosage, administration schedule, and adverse effects requiring medical attention
❏ incision care (aseptic technique, dressing changes, irrigations, cleaning procedures, hand-washing technique, and proper disposal of soiled dressings)
❏ signs and symptoms of possible infection
❏ dietary requirements and restrictions, if any
❏ activity and exercise restrictions
❏ date, time, and location of follow-up appointment
❏ how to contact the physician.

DOCUMENTATION CHECKLIST

Using outcome criteria as a guide, document:
❏ clinical status on admission
❏ postoperative clinical assessment
❏ significant changes in status
❏ appearance of incision and wound drainage
❏ I.V. line patency and condition of site
❏ assessment of pain and relief measures
❏ nutritional intake
❏ fluid intake and output
❏ patient and family teaching
❏ discharge planning.

Associated care plans

- Acute pain
- Grieving
- Ineffective individual coping
- Knowledge deficit
- Perioperative care
- Thrombophlebitis

References

Brook, N. "Nurse-led Discharge Planning Improves Quality of Care," *Nursing Times* 97(19):40, May 2001.

Brooks-Brunn, J.A. "Risk Factors Associated with Postoperative Pulmonary Complications Following Total Abdominal Hysterectomy," *Clinical Nursing Research* 9(1):27-46, February 2000.

Lindberg, C.E., and Nolan, L.B. "Women's Decision Making Regarding Hysterectomy," *Journal of Obstetrical, Gynecological, and Neonatal Nursing* 30(6):607-16, November 2001.

Moreira, V. "Hysterectomy: Nursing the Physical and Emotional Wounds," *Nursing Times* 96(20):41-42, May 2000.

Paniscotti, B.M. "Cancer of the Endometrium," in *Women and Cancer: A Gynecologic Oncology Nursing Perspective,* 2nd ed. Edited by Moore-Higgs, G.J., et al. Sudbury, Mass.: Jones & Bartlett Pubs., Inc., 2000.

Sharts-Hopko, N.C. "Hysterectomy for Nonmalignant Conditions," *AJN* 101(9):32-40, 2001.

Wade, J., et al. "Hysterectomy: What Do Women Need and Want to Know?" *Journal of Obstetrical, Gynecological, and Neonatal Nursing* 29(1):33-42, January 2000.

Williams, R.D., and Clark, A.J. "A Qualitative Study of Women's Hysterectomy Experience," *Journal of Women's Health and Gender Based Medicine* 9 (Suppl.2):S15-S25, 2000.

Reproductive disorders

Mastectomy

DRG INFORMATION

DRG 257 Total Mastectomy for Malignancy with Complication or Comorbidity (CC).
           Mean LOS = 2.7 days
   Principal diagnoses include:
- carcinoma in situ, breast
- neoplasm, breast, malignant, secondary
- neoplasm, breast, uncertain behavior
- neoplasm, female
- male breast, malignant (primary)
- neoplasm, skin, malignant, secondary.

DRG 258 Total Mastectomy for Malignancy without CC.
           Mean LOS = 1.9 days

DRG 259 Subtotal Mastectomy for Malignancy with CC.
           Mean LOS = 2.7 days

DRG 260 Subtotal Mastectomy for Malignancy without CC.
           Mean LOS = 1.4 days

Introduction

DEFINITION AND TIME FOCUS

Mastectomy is the surgical removal of mammary tissue and, in some cases, the pectoral muscles. Although usually used to treat breast cancer, subcutaneous mastectomy (with preservation of chest muscles, skin, nipple, and areola) may be appropriate in male gynecomastia and severe fibrocystic breast disease requiring multiple biopsies. Subcutaneous mastectomy may also be performed to prevent breast cancer in women at increased risk. Mastectomy commonly is followed by chemotherapy or radiation therapy. However, if the tumor is large or the cancer is advanced (with skin or chest wall involvement), such treatments may be administered before surgery.

Breast tissue is affected by several cancers, including carcinoma of the secreting glands (ductal carcinoma), carcinoma of the glandular epithelium (breast adenomas), breast sarcomas, and lymphomas. Infiltrating intraductal carcinoma accounts for 80% of all breast cancers; it has a poor prognosis. Breast cancer is responsible for 36% of all new cancer cases and 18% of all cancer deaths in women; the high mortality rate hasn't changed significantly in 60 years.

The mastectomy performed depends on tumor size, nodal involvement, and evidence of metastasis. The patient's age and desire for breast reconstruction is also considered. Procedures include:

- lumpectomy — a complete excision of the tumor (usually followed by local irradiation to destroy microscopic cancer cells)
- partial (segmental) mastectomy — removal of tumor and adjacent tissue, leaving nipple, areola, and remaining breast tissue intact
- total (simple) mastectomy — removal of all breast and mammary tissue; pectoral muscles remain intact
- subcutaneous mastectomy — a variation of simple mastectomy in which the skin, nipple, areola, and chest muscles are preserved in preparation for breast reconstruction
- modified radical mastectomy (Patey method) — removal of all breast tissue, overlying skin, nipple and areola, minor pectoral muscle, and samples of adjacent and axillary lymph nodes
- radical mastectomy (Halsted method) — removal of tissue as in the modified radical mastectomy plus removal of the major pectoral muscle (rarely performed in the United States).

This care plan focuses on the care of the female breast cancer patient before and after mastectomy. (See *Clinical snapshot: Mastectomy,* page 817, and *Clinical pathway: Managing Mastectomy,* pages 814 and 815.)

ETIOLOGY AND PRECIPITATING FACTORS

Although the exact cause of breast cancer is unknown, risk factors have been identified.

Factors associated with greatest risk
- Age — only 15% of cases occur before age 40; the greatest percentage occur between ages 45 and 60
- Personal history of previous breast cancer
- Family history of breast cancer — risk is 3 to 5 times higher if mother, sister, or daughter had the disease
- Hormones — peak incidence between ages 45 and 49 probably related to ovarian estrogen problems; between ages 65 and 69, probably related to adrenal estrogen problems
- Gene defect — a mutation or injury to the BRCA 1 gene or mutation of the p53 gene (located on chromosome 17) may increase a woman's risk of developing breast cancer with metastasis; 13% of breast cancers are thought to be from genetic defects

Factors associated with increased risk
- History of breast cancer in a maternal or paternal grandmother or aunt
- Personal history of endometrial, ovarian, or colon cancer

- History of fibrocystic breast disease
- Nulliparity
- Birth of first child after age 30
- Early onset of menstruation and late menopause
- Estrogen replacement therapy
- Culture — at increased risk if white in the upper socioeconomic levels of a Western society
- Obesity
- Diet high in animal fats
- Daily alcohol consumption
- Exposure to ionizing radiation — radon or naturally occurring nuclear fallout; excessive medical or dental X-rays; previous radiation therapy or fluoroscopy examinations (1% increase in risk per rad)

Focused assessment guidelines
NURSING HISTORY
(FUNCTIONAL HEALTH PATTERN FINDINGS)
Health-perception–health-management pattern
- Painless, firm to hard lump or nodule that has indistinct boundaries and isn't easily movable; may be found anywhere in breast tissue or axilla but most commonly in the left breast, upper outer quadrants, or just below the nipple
- Delay in seeking treatment after tumor discovery
- Focal, constant pain unrelated to menstrual cycle (advanced disease)
- Spontaneous discharge of bloody, clear, or milky secretions from nipple or nipple inversion, retraction, elevation, ulceration, or scaliness (advanced disease)

Nutrition-metabolic pattern
- Weight loss, anorexia, early satiety, and taste alterations, such as reduced sensitivity to sweetness or decreased desire for beef, pork, chocolate, coffee, and tomatoes (related to cancer or protein-calorie malnutrition)
- Nausea, vomiting, stomatitis, and mucositis (related to chemotherapy or radiation therapy)

Elimination pattern
- Constipation (related to anorexia, depression, immobility, or narcotic administration)
- Diarrhea (related to increased bacterial growth from decreased GI tract motility)

Activity-exercise pattern
- General malaise
- Weariness, weakness, or lack of physical energy
- Physical and emotional withdrawal related to depression
- Complaints of shoulder and arm immobility related to pain

Sleep-rest pattern
- Insomnia from pain, anxiety, or fear of cancer or the unknown
- Increased desire for sleep (withdrawal behavior)

Self-perception–self-concept pattern
- Grief related to perceived or actual loss
- Body-image disturbance related to impending loss of breast or lymphedema
- Guilt, anger, hostility, or denial related to diagnosis
- Breast loss with loss of femininity, desirability, and maternal instincts
- Self-concept problem related to hair loss (if alopecia is present)

Role-relationship pattern
- Hostility toward health care providers as a result of anger over role loss or sense of injustice
- Withdrawal from family and friends to avoid anticipated rejection
- Inability to assume family or work roles

Sexuality-reproductive pattern
- Concern over need for additional surgery (hysterectomy with oophorectomy or adrenalectomy) if the tumor is estrogen receptive
- Concern over adverse effects of androgenic drugs, including excessive facial hair (hirsutism), male pattern baldness, deepening voice, or increased libido

Coping–stress tolerance pattern
- Anxiety, fear, restlessness, and depression related to unknown extent of tumor and resulting prognosis
- Need for counseling
- Dependency
- Extreme independence related to fears of becoming dependent or a burden to others
- Financial, child care, and job concerns, especially if a single parent
- Demonstrated depression and despondency

Value-belief pattern
- Social conditioning leads patient to believe that personal worth and value are measured by the size and shape of breasts
- Adoption of a fatalistic attitude, equating cancer with death
- Disease perceived as punishment for past actions or indiscretions or fear of passing cancer to the next generation
- Belief that external factors control personal life
- Feelings of being forsaken by source of spiritual strength

PHYSICAL FINDINGS
Integumentary
- Painless tumor, mass, lesion, thickening, or unusual growth in breast tissue
- Palpable medial, supraclavicular, cervical or axillary nodes; isolated skin nodules; solitary, unilateral lesions; purplish color; heat and redness; ulcerations with secondary infection; or peau d'orange (skin of the orange) appearance resulting from lymphatic invasion and edema (advanced disease)
- Alopecia (from chemotherapy)

Managing mastectomy

Patient problem	Preadmission teaching	Early morning admission (EMA)
Cardiopulmonary • Altered hemodynamics related to surgery • Increased risk of atelectasis related to surgery • Increased risk for DVT & PE	• Goal: NSR on ECG – Assess C/P status. ECG if >40 yr & not done in past 30 days. CBC, survey 27, CXR • Goal: Verbalizes understanding of postop pulmonary toilet regimen. – Instruct on T, C, DB. • Goal: Verbalizes understanding of TED stockings and SCD. – Instruct on TEDS & SCD.	• Goal: NSR on ECG – Assess C/P status. ECG if >40 yr & not done. in past 30 days. Instruct re T, C, DB. • Goal: Maintains adequate venous return. – Apply TEDS. Apply SCD per physician's order.
Fluid balance • Risk for altered fluid balance or diet	• Goal: Verbalizes understanding of preop NPO instructions. – Instruct re NPO. • Goal: Verbalizes understanding postop diet progression. – Instruct re postop diet regimen.	• Goal: Compliance with NPO preop status. – NPO
Pain • Alteration in comfort related to surgery	• Goal: Verbalizes understanding of pain management. – Discuss pain management vs. absence of pain.	• Goal: Verbalizes understanding of pain management. – Discuss pain management vs. absence of pain.
Integumentary • Risk for infection at operative site or drain site	• Goal: Verbalizes understanding of incision location & purpose of drains. – Instruct re: surgical incision & postop drains.	• Goal: Verbalizes understanding of incision location & purpose of drains. – Reinforce preop instruction.
Activity • Alteration in mobility related to surgical procedure • Self-care deficit related to decreased mobility and pain with movement	• Goal: Verbalizes understanding of postop activity progression & restrictions. – Instruct re plan of postop activity/mobility restrictions with progression.	
Psychosocial/spiritual • Fear related to cancer diagnosis and future implications • Fear related to change in sexual self-concept	• Goal: Verbally acknowledges feelings of anxiety related to surgery. – Encourage expression of feelings. Assess patient and family support system. Discuss available services (social service, pastoral care).	• Goal: Verbally acknowledges feelings of anxiety related to surgery. – Encourage expression of feelings. – Pastoral care visit.
Knowledge deficit • R/T surgical procedure • R/T preop preparation • R/T acquisition of prosthesis • R/T discharge/home care	• Goal: Verbalize understanding of EMA admitting process & surgical procedure. – Instruct re admission process, preop procedures, and use of home meds. • Goal: Verbalize understanding of plan for prosthesis acquisition. – Notify Reach for Recovery, Breast Care Team. – Instruct re available resources	• Goal: Verbalizes understanding of EMA admitting process & surgical procedure. – Reinforce instructions.

Day of surgery	Postoperative day 1	Postoperative day 2
• Goal: SBP>90, DBP>50, HR>50, R>12 – VS q 15 min × 4, q 30 min × 2, q 1 hr × 4, q 4 hr • Goal: Clear bilateral breath sounds – Auscultate lungs q 8 hr – Assist with T, C, DB q 2 hr × 4 • Goal: No s/s of DVT or PE – Apply TEDS; SCD per physician's order. – Assess left extremity for temp, redness, & calf tenderness q 8 hr – Dangle legs & out of bed with help 4 to 6 hr postop	• Goal: SBP>90, DBP>50, HR>50, R>12 – VS q 4 hr • Goal: Clear bilateral breath sounds – Auscultate lungs q 8 hr • Goal: No s/s of DVT or PE – Remove TEDS for bath; then reapply – Maintain SCD when in bed • Goal: Independent ambulation q.i.d. – Assist with first walk in hall then amb q.i.d.	• Goal: SBP>90, DBP>50, HR>50, R>12 – VS q 8 hr • Goal: No s/s of DVT or PE – Remove TEDS for bath; then reapply – D/C SCD • Goal: Compliance with ambulation – Up ad lib; assess compliance
• Goal: Tolerates 500 ml P.O. 8 hr, postop without nausea and vomiting. – Sips of clear liquid; advance diet as tol – Measure & record amt q 8 hr – Heplock I.V. or maintain I.V. KVO if PCA • Goal: Voids freely, urine output of 250ml q 8 hr for 24 hr. – Measure & record urine output q 8 hr	• Goal: Tolerates regular diet – Regular diet; record % taken – Encourage 6-8 glasses fluids per 24 hr • Goal: Voids freely, urine output of 250 ml q 8 h 24 hr – Measure & record urine output q 8 hr	• Goal: Tolerates regular diet – Regular diet; record % taken – Encourages 6 to 8 glasses fluids per 24 hr • Goal: Voids freely, urine output of 250 ml q 8 hr for 24 hr – Measure & record urine output q 8 hr
• Goal: Pain controlled at level <7 – Assess pain level q 4 hr – Reinforce instructions R/T PCA pump mgt if ordered – Elevate arm on operative side on 1 to 2 pillows	• Goal: Pain controlled with P.O. meds & without adverse drug reactions – Assess pain level q 4 hr – Offer P.O. analgesics p.r.n. – D/C PCA pump if ordered – Elevate arm on operative side on 1 to 2 pillows	• Goal: Pain controlled with P.O. meds & without adverse drug reactions – Assess pain level q 4 hr – Offer p.c. analgesics p.r.n. – Elevate arm on operative side on 1 to 2 pillows
• Goal: Dressing dry & intact – Assess dressing q 4 hr; reinforce p.r.n. • Goal: Drains patent & compressed. – Assess drains for patency and compression q 2 hr × 4 – Measure & record drainage q 8 hr & p.r.n.	• Goal: Dressing dry & intact – Assess dressing q 4 hr. Reinforce p.r.n. • Goal: Drains patent & compressed – Assess drains for patency and compression q 2 hr × 4 – Measure & record drainage q 8 hr & p.r.n.	• Goal: Wound & s/s of infection – Dressing change per physician • Goal: Drains patent & compressed – Measure and record drainage q 8 hr & p.r.n. • Goal: Describe s/s of infection – Instruct re s/s of infection with patient & significant other
• Goal: Compliant with activity restrictions – Encourage arm activity within levels of comfort or as ordered per physician	• Goal: Compliant with postmastectomy exercise regimen – Instruct re limitations & restrictions • Goal: Participates in self-care activities – Assess need for assistance with bath	• Goal: Compliant with postmastectomy exercise regimen – Reinforce instructions • Goal: Perform ADLs with minimal assistance – Assess need for assistance with bath
• Goal: Verbalizes thoughts/feelings re surgery & future implications. – Encourage expression of thoughts & feelings – Assess need for inpt. support services	• Goal: Verbalizes thoughts/feelings re surgery & future implications – Encourage expression of thoughts & feelings – Assess need for inpt support services	• Goal: Verbalizes thoughts & feelings re surgery & future implications – Encourage expression of thoughts & feelings; assess need for inpt support services • Goal: Verbalizes feelings of self-worth – Actively listen; provide positive reinforcement; instruct re postop support services
• Goal: Decreased anxiety related to postop process & procedures	• Goal: Verbalizes understanding of post-op drain management – Instruct & demonstrate drain management • Goal: Verbalize understanding of BSE postop – Instruct re BSE of operative site	• Goal: Patient or significant other demonstrates ability to manage drain – Reinforce instructions of POD 1; provide measuring cup; observe technique • Goal: Verbalize understanding of plan for medical follow-up – Review discharge instructions

- Scalded skin syndrome (a debilitating condition in the immunosuppressed patient in which a *Staphylococcus aureus* infection produces epidermolytic toxins)

Hematologic
- Hypercalcemia
- Thromboembolic infarction related to hypercoagulability from cancer and tumor lysis

Cardiovascular
- Hypertension related to effect of hypercalcemia on smooth muscle
- Bradycardia or premature ventricular contractions caused by digitalis toxicity from increased calcium level
- Compensatory tachycardia with decreasing blood pressure
- Distended jugular veins
- Peripheral edema

Neurologic
- Confusion, restlessness, or disorientation (resulting from serum calcium level above 15 mg/dl)
- Muscle weakness and proximal myopathy
- Diminished deep tendon reflexes

Renal
- Polyuria or renal calculi, if hypercalcemia is present

Gastrointestinal
- Polydipsia from polyuria
- Nausea, vomiting, and anorexia as a result of hypercalcemia, chemotherapy, or radiation therapy

Musculoskeletal
- Pathologic fractures with bony metastases

DIAGNOSTIC STUDIES

- Hemoglobin level and hematocrit — if low, may be related to anemia or blood loss during surgery; before surgery, the patient should donate 2 to 3 units of blood which later can be transfused to maintain postoperative hemoglobin level and hematocrit and to aid healing
- Serum calcium level — level above 11 mg/dl indicates hypercalcemia, a common complication of cancer
- Serum phosphate level — hypophosphatemia is commonly associated with hypercalcemia
- Platelet counts, prothrombin time/international normalized ratio (PT/INR), and partial thromboplastin time (PTT) — a depressed platelet count, PT/INR, and PTT may indicate disseminated intravascular coagulation (DIC)
- Carcinoembryonic antigen titer — increases 75% with metastatic disease
- Human chorionic gonadotropin — presence in blood or urine of nonpregnant females indicates cancer; declining amounts indicate treatment effectiveness
- Serum ferritin level — may be low, indicating anemia
- Serum albumin level — may be low from fluid shifting to interstitial spaces
- Serum alkaline phosphatase level — if elevated, may indicate metastatic activity in bone and liver

- Flow cytometry studies (cellular deoxyribonucleic acid content) — identify the 40% to 50% of patients at risk for recurrence
- Estrogen receptor assay — estrogen-sensitive tumors are more susceptible to hormone therapy; non-estrogen-sensitive tumors have a low response rate to hormonal manipulation and a high recurrence rate
- Mammography — may detect nonpalpable lesions (80% to 90% accurate); 50% of breast cancers appear as a cluster of microcalcifications
- Magnetic resonance imaging — differentiates benign and malignant lesions; accurately identifies premalignant tissue changes; detects tumors in dense breast tissue; is unique in defining tumor extent; also used for staging for treatment planning
- Breast-specific positron emission tomography
- Ultrasound — differentiates fluid from solid tumor; cannot detect very small tumors
- Open biopsy — surgery differentiates benign from malignant lesions
- Closed biopsy — image-guided needle biopsy (for women with nonpalpable lesions) and fine needle aspiration biopsy (for women with palpable lesions) differentiates fluid-filled cyst from solid tumor
- Liver and bone scans (indicated if liver chemistries are elevated) — may reveal metastatic disease
- Electrocardiography (ECG) — T-wave changes, bundle-branch block, P-wave notching, or other abnormalities may result from chemotherapy

POTENTIAL COMPLICATIONS
From breast cancer
- Hypercalcemia
- Lymphedema
- Hypophosphatemia
- Thrombophlebitis
- DIC

From metastasis
- Pathological fractures
- Obstructive uropathy
- Metabolic acidosis (lactic acid increase)
- Thrombocytopenia
- DIC
- Superior vena cava syndrome
- Spinal cord compression
- Meningeal carcinomatosis
- Intracerebral metastasis
- Pleural effusion
- Pulmonary embolism
- Spontaneous pneumothorax

From metastasis or radiation therapy
- Inflammatory constrictive pericarditis
- Pericardial effusion and tamponade
- Scalded skin syndrome

From chemotherapy
- Alopecia
- Anaphylaxis
- Amyloidosis
- Hyperuricemia
- GI hemorrhage
- Paralytic ileus
- Cardiomyopathy or cardiotoxicity

- Neurotoxicity
- Pulmonary toxicity
- Sepsis
- Bone marrow suppression
- Renal tubular necrosis

Other
- Reactive depression
- Suicidal ideation

CLINICAL SNAPSHOT ✳

Mastectomy

Major nursing diagnoses and collaborative problems	Key patient outcomes
CP: Risk for lymphedema	Display circumference equal in both arms.
ND: Disturbed body image	Be able to touch and look at the wound.
CP: Risk for hypercalcemia	Maintain a serum calcium level of 8.5 to 10.8 mg/dl.

Collaborative problem

Risk for lymphedema related to interrupted lymph circulation from axillary node dissection during mastectomy.

NURSING PRIORITY
Prevent or minimize lymph stasis.

PATIENT OUTCOME CRITERIA
By the time of discharge, the patient will:
- list signs and symptoms of lymphedema and the appropriate responses to them
- demonstrate exercises to promote lymph circulation and minimize postoperative lymphedema
- display circumference equal in both arms
- remain free from infection and injury
- demonstrate increased mobility from range-of-motion (ROM) exercises.

INTERVENTIONS

1. Determine if the patient is to have a radical or modified radical mastectomy.

2. *Before surgery, measure and record the circumference of each arm 2¼" (5.7 cm) above and below the elbow. After surgery, repeat the measurements each morning until discharge.* *
– If lymphedema is noted, obtain an antiembolism sleeve for the patient to wear from morning to night (some patients wear the sleeve only at night).
– If lymphedema is severe, consult the physician about using a mechanical pressure pump every 2 to 3 hours, as needed.

RATIONALES

1. Radical mastectomy and modified radical mastectomy are the major cause of secondary lymphedema. During axillary node dissection, lymph channels are blocked or removed, shifting lymph fluid to soft tissue and decreasing lymphatic circulation.

2. Baseline measurements allow for later comparison. Lymphedema is present if the circumference of the affected arm is 1¼" (3.2 cm) larger than the unaffected arm.
– Compression of vein walls increases tissue perfusion and prevents venous stasis and edema.

– A mechanical pressure pump stimulates circulation more aggressively.

*Italics indicate key interventions.

3. *Immediately after mastectomy, position the affected arm on a pillow with the elbow higher than the shoulder, and the wrist and hand higher than the elbow.*

4. *Protect the affected arm from injury.*

– Place the patient on an air mattress or sheepskin pad; pad the side rails.
– Keep the patient's fingernails short and smooth.
– Don't allow the patient to wear a name band, watch, or similar items on the affected arm.

5. *Monitor laboratory data.* Alert the physician to deviations from these normal ranges:
– Serum albumin level — 3.5 to 5 g/dl
– Serum sodium level — 135 to 145 mEq/L
– White blood cell (WBC) count — 4,500 to 11,500/μl

6. *Check peripheral pulses daily.*

7. *Inspect the skin for color, translucency, temperature, or breakdown daily.*

8. *Assess the arm for edema* daily by pressing a thumb into the tissue for 5 to 10 seconds and observing for a depression after removing thumb.

9. Administer diuretics and salt-poor albumin, as indicated.

10. *Elevate and massage the affected arm daily* with lotion, beginning at the wrist and advancing to the shoulder.

11. Administer pain medication 30 to 45 minutes before beginning exercises.

12. *Instruct the patient to elevate the affected arm for 30 to 45 minutes every 2 hours for 2 to 3 weeks after discharge, then 2 to 3 times daily for 6 weeks.*
One day after surgery, have the patient perform the following exercises as often as the surgeon recommends:
– ball squeezing
– making a tight fist and then flexing and extending the fingers.
Two to three days after surgery, have the patient perform the following exercises as often as recommended:
– raising the affected arm to a 45- to 90-degree side angle
– walking the fingers up a wall to move the arm and shoulder
– bending over at the waist and letting the affected arm dangle, making small circular motions from the shoulder.
At discharge, provide a copy of the American Cancer Society pamphlet *Reach for Recovery, Exercises After Mastectomy: Patient Guide.*
Suggested postdischarge exercises include, but aren't limited to:

3. Positioning the arm above the apex of the heart facilitates lymph and blood movement by gravity flow.

4. Eliminating possible sources of trauma decreases the risk of infection.
– Padding cushions the affected arm.

– Short fingernails are less likely to damage the skin.
– Removing constricting bands prevents ischemia.

5. A low serum albumin level promotes lymphedema. A high serum sodium level promotes fluid retention. An abnormal WBC count may indicate infection (lymph node dissection increases the risk of infection).

6. A pulse deficit may occur in the edematous arm.

7. Lymph stasis promotes infection and decreases arterial and venous circulation.

8. Arm lymphedema usually presents as indurated (hardened) skin and, except in the early phase, is non-pitting.

9. Diuretics promote fluid excretion. Albumin maintains osmotic pressure and prevents fluid shifting to the interstitial spaces of soft tissue.

10. Elevation and compression increase lymph flow.

11. Pain relief promotes exercising.

12. Exercise is essential to prevent muscle deformities, shortening, contractures, stiffness, and "frozen shoulder." Specific postoperative exercises depend on the extent of the surgery and whether skin grafting was necessary. Exercise regimens must have the surgeon's approval.

– rope pulley — Toss a rope over the top of a door. Sit with both legs bent at the knees and feet planted firmly on the floor. Hug both sides of the door with the knees. Holding the ends of the knotted rope, slowly raise the affected arm as far as comfortable by pulling down on the rope with the unaffected arm. Keeping the raised arm close to the head, reverse the motion; rest and repeat as tolerated.
– elbow pull — Stand with arms extended sideways at shoulder level. With bent elbows, clasp the fingers at the back of the neck and pull the elbows in toward each other until they touch. Relax, rest, and repeat as tolerated.

13. Refer the patient to Reach for Recovery or a similar support group.

13. Reach for Recovery volunteers have experienced breast cancer. Their "I've been there" approach aids the mastectomy patient's rehabilitation. They encourage the patient to use the affected arm and shoulder, and can facilitate psychological and emotional adaptation to the diagnosis of cancer, loss of a breast, and changes in body image and interpersonal relationships.

14. *Teach the patient and her family the signs and symptoms of lymphedema* and when it's most likely to occur. Advise the patient to seek medical care if any of the following occur in the affected arm:
– pain
– tingling or tightness
– loss of sensation
– increased circumference
– muscle weakness.

14. The knowledgeable patient is more likely to obtain early treatment. Acute lymphedema occurs 4 to 6 weeks after surgery, can be transient, and is usually self-limiting; chronic lymphedema may occur weeks, months, or years after surgery.

15. *Teach the patient how to maintain lymphatic circulation in the affected arm and prevent infection and injury.* Reinforce teaching with written instructions.
– Use padded mitts around the oven, grill, or fireplace. Limit skin exposure to the sun and use a strong sunscreen when outdoors.
– Carry purses, packages, luggage, and other heavy objects on the unaffected side.
– Stop smoking.
– Avoid clothes with elastic or tight sleeves. Never allow blood pressure to be taken on the affected arm.
– Don't allow injections to be given in or blood to be drawn from the affected arm.

15. Maintaining effective lymphatic circulation and preventing infection and injury require the patient's active participation.
– These measures prevent burns.

– Carrying heavy items with the affected arm creates pressure that can lead to lymph stasis.
– Smoking constricts vessels.
– Tight sleeves and constricting bands impede lymph flow.
– Such measures prevent irritation and injury.

16. Additional individualized interventions: _____

16. Rationales:_____

Nursing diagnosis
Disturbed body image related to loss of a body part

NURSING PRIORITY
Assist patient to cope with the loss of a breast.

PATIENT OUTCOME CRITERIA
According to individual readiness, the patient will:

- be able to touch and look at the wound
- participate in decision making
- verbalize loss and work through the grief of an altered body image
- seek out community resources as necessary
- be able to talk about changes that impact sexuality with her partner
- experience no complications if choosing reconstruction
- agree to share information about reconstruction with at least two friends or a group of women, if the patient desires.

INTERVENTIONS	RATIONALES
1. Provide empathetic emotional support. Encourage the patient to express feelings. Listen actively, use therapeutic touch, and be available to sit with the patient as needed. Also refer to the "Grieving" care plan, page 105.	1. The patient is experiencing a time of intense personal crisis, and grieving is a normal part of emotional adjustment. Empathetic emotional support can facilitate healthy grieving and crisis resolution. The diagnosis of cancer, hospitalization, and surgery all present losses the patient may need to grieve for. The "Grieving" care plan contains interventions helpful for any patient experiencing grief.
2. Assess the patient's feelings about the mastectomy.	2. Attitudes, values, and beliefs influence physical and psychological adjustment.
3. *Monitor the patient's comments about and willingness to look at and touch the incision site.* Be alert for mood swings, continued tearfulness, expressions of overwhelming sadness, or withdrawal from family or friends.	3. Comments and behaviors can help the nurse assess the patient's level of acceptance.
4. Counsel the spouse or partner to hold and touch the patient.	4. The patient with a recent mastectomy has altered tactile perception over the operative site and over part of the upper arm. Touching creates intimacy and affirms that she is loved and lovable.
5. Encourage the patient to wear makeup (if appropriate), nightgowns, and soft, front-closing brassieres (if dressings don't interfere).	5. Some women adjust to breast surgery immediately; others need weeks or months. Attention to appearance may be a sign of recovering self-worth. The nurse's affirmation of the patient's continued femininity may bolster a shaky self-concept.
6. Offer to refer the patient to a mastectomy support group, a member of the clergy, a social worker, or a psychiatric or oncology clinical nurse specialist.	6. Other patients and professionals can help the patient accept an altered body image and return to wellness. However, such referrals should supplement nursing interventions, not substitute for the nurse's caring and empathy. The American Cancer Society offers services to patients and their families, including "I Can Cope," an 8-week group program on learning how to live with cancer, and "I Can Surmount," a support group facilitated by trained patients with cancer. Other local support groups facilitated by professionals also are available. Information about these services is available at all local offices of the American Cancer Society as well as through community hospitals.
7. Assess the patient's suitability for reconstructive surgery.	7. Contraindications to reconstructive breast surgery include inflammatory carcinomas, high-dose radiation therapy, extensive systemic metastases, and unrealistic attitudes and expectations regarding the surgery's outcome.

8. If reconstruction is an option, support the patient in the decision-making process.
– Encourage the patient to share thoughts and feelings related to breast reconstruction.

– Teach the patient about reconstruction procedures, the need for skin or muscle flap grafting, and the possibility of nipple and areolar reconstruction. Help the patient obtain information about the procedure's cost and the likelihood of insurance coverage. If possible, provide a copy of the American Cancer Society pamphlet *Breast Reconstruction Following Mastectomy from Cancer.*
– Validate the patient's decision even if you believe it wouldn't be appropriate for you.

9. If reconstruction isn't an option or will be delayed, provide information about external breast prostheses when the patient asks about them.

10. *After reconstruction, provide appropriate interventions to preserve the reconstructed breast.*

– Assess the incision site. Note its appearance and the presence of any pain or tenderness to touch. Monitor WBC counts as ordered. If the suture line doesn't appear to be healing by primary intention, request a WBC count from the surgeon. Assess surgical drains daily.
– Be alert to pallor, cyanosis, coolness, or increased capillary refill time at the surgical site. If these occur, notify the physician promptly. Protect the reconstructed breast from pressure. Assess the tightness of the dressing.
– Elevate the head of the bed to Fowler's or semi-Fowler's position.
– Monitor the patient's verbal comments and willingness to look at and touch the reconstructed breast.
– Provide psychological support. Encourage the patient to wear make-up (if appropriate), nightgowns, and soft, front-closing brassieres (if dressings don't interfere).

– Counsel the patient's spouse or partner about the importance of expressing satisfaction with the reconstructed breast.
– Instruct the patient to begin daily, vigorous massage of the implant or graft 6 weeks after surgery.
– Educate the patient about the value of sharing information about reconstruction with other women.

8. The nurse can help the patient make an informed decision.
– Some patients immediately accept reconstruction, while others may believe a desire for reconstruction is vain.
– Reconstruction is an accepted option in the management of breast cancer. The patient should have the opportunity to talk and read about breast reconstruction.

– Clarifying and validating feelings conveys respect for the patient's values and beliefs.

9. Queries indicate emotional readiness to focus on this area. A breast prosthesis may boost the patient's self-esteem by providing a natural-appearing substitute for the lost breast.

10. Loss of the reconstructed breast will provide a further blow to the patient's body image and jeopardize emotional recovery.
– Drainage, a darkening suture line, pain and tenderness to touch, and a WBC count over $11,000/\mu l$ indicate infection. Infection prolongs healing and promotes dependency on family members and health care professionals, which may result in decreased self-esteem and depression.
– These signs may indicate inadequate blood flow. If circulation isn't restored, graft or implant rejection or flap necrosis may occur. Preventing pressure at the site promotes adequate blood flow.
– Elevating the head of the bed reduces edema and stress on the reconstructed breast.
– Comments and behaviors can help the nurse evaluate the patient's acceptance of the reconstructed breast.
– Some women adjust to a reconstructed breast immediately; others need weeks or months. Attention to appearance may be a sign of recovering self-worth. The nurse's affirmation of the patient's continued femininity may bolster a shaky self-concept.
– The spouse's or partner's attitude plays a powerful role in the patient's acceptance of the reconstructed breast.

– Massage helps prevent capsular contraction, maintain breast softness, and permit a more natural contour.
– If women are aware that reconstruction is an option, they may seek help when a lump or abnormality is first discovered, rather than delaying diagnosis and treatment for fear of disfigurement.

11. Encourage the patient to talk about sexual concerns. Suggestions to initiate conversation may include, "Tell me about any sexual concerns you might have as a result of your mastectomy." Or, "Some women have anxiety and fears about their sexual relationships following a mastectomy. Is there something you would like to discuss, or questions I might help you with?" Or, "Some women have anxiety about their sexual relationships following this surgery. I'll be happy to talk with you now, or later if you prefer. Here's my card with my phone number if you need to get in touch with me at another time."

11. Body image is intimately related to sexuality. Breast cancer patients require continuing education, support, and encouragement in dealing with the emotional trauma and sexual sequelae of treatment. Many patients will desire information but won't initiate the discussion with a physician or nurse. Such information is essential to emotional healing.

12. Maintain a hopeful and positive outlook when discussing sexuality. Clarify any misconceptions. Encourage the patient to talk with members of mastectomy support groups.

12. Maintaining a positive outlook conveys hope. Clarifying misconceptions (such as a mastectomy destroying sexual attractiveness) can gently challenge beliefs that otherwise might become self-fulfilling prophecies. Women who have "been there" may provide more credible reassurance than a health professional.

13. Inform the patient that the drug tamoxifen may be prescribed for 4 to 5 years, especially in women with estrogen positive receptor tumors.

13. Tamoxifen is an antiestrogen drug that blocks the effect of estrogen on breast tissue. After an average of 4 to 5 years of tamoxifen therapy 45% of women taking the drug had fewer recurrences than those women presenting with the same risk factors who didn't take the drug.

14. A few weeks after discharge, make a home call. Inquire about visits the patient has made away from home and the resumption of social activities as well as physiological status. Reintroduce the subject of sexuality and ask about concerns the woman might have encountered since surgery.

14. Some patients remain at home to avoid their friends and hesitate to resume social activities. Reasons for withdrawal may include a fear of rejection by others. Fear of rejection from a spouse or significant other commonly manifests in withdrawal. Home calls provide an excellent opportunity for the nurse to ask questions about sex or sexuality and allow the patient to share any fears, concerns, or questions that might have arisen since discharge.

15. Additional individualized interventions: _____

15. Rationales:_____

Suggested NIC Interventions
Body image enhancement; Grief work facilitation; Anticipatory guidance; Coping enhancement; Self-esteem enhancement

Suggested NOC Outcomes
Body image; Grief resolution; Self-esteem

Collaborative problem
Risk for hypercalcemia related to abnormal calcium transport or skeletal metastases

NURSING PRIORITY
Maintain normal serum calcium levels and prevent complications of hypercalcemia.

PATIENT OUTCOME CRITERIA
Within 48 hours, calcium levels of 12 mg/dl or more will:
- decrease to 8.5 to 10.8 mg/dl.
  By the time of discharge, the patient with controllable hypercalcemia and her family will:
- verbalize signs and symptoms of blood calcium increase and appropriate interventions.

INTERVENTIONS

1. *Monitor for hypercalcemia* (serum calcium level greater than 11 mg/dl). Early signs and symptoms include nausea, vomiting, and anorexia.

2. *Monitor blood pressure and heart rate every 2 hours.*

3. *Auscultate for heart sounds and rhythms in four sites and record daily.*

4. *Assess ECG changes.* Observe for prolonged PR intervals, lengthening QT intervals, lengthening and widening T waves, atrioventricular (AV) block, and asystole.

5. *If the patient is receiving a cardiac glycoside, measure the apical pulse rate before administering;* if below 60 beats/minute, withhold the drug and check with the physician.

6. *Assess the patient's level of consciousness* every 4 to 8 hours. Assess for confusion, restlessness, disorientation, drowsiness, profound weakness, and personality changes. Orient to time, place, and person. Elevate and pad side rails, as indicated.

7. *Document fluid intake and output* every 2 hours to monitor fluid balance. Obtain baseline weight on admission. Weigh daily thereafter.

8. *Assess amount and color of urine, and note specific gravity* (normal range is 1.010 to 1.035).

9. *Assess for flank pain and strain all urine for calculi.*

10. Anticipate I.V. administration of saline, 250 to 300 ml/hour, and a loop diuretic such as furosemide (Lasix), 80 to 100 mg every 2 hours, as tolerated.

11. Anticipate administration of calcitonin (Calcimar), glucocorticoids, phosphates, plicamycin (Mithracin), or gallium nitrate (Ganite). Be alert to adverse reactions, which may include headache, anorexia, nausea and vomiting, hepatic and renal impairment, and hemorrhage from thrombocytopenia.

12. Apply an ice collar to the patient's neck if nauseated. Administer an antiemetic, if appropriate.

RATIONALES

1. Hypercalcemia, a metabolic complication, develops in 10% to 20% of all cancer patients; in breast cancer with metastasis, the incidence increases to 50%. Although the majority of patients with hypercalcemia have skeletal metastases, not all patients with metastases develop hypercalcemia.

2. Increased calcium levels can affect smooth muscle, causing hypertension.

3. Hypercalcemia may cause arrhythmias or extra heart sounds.

4. Changes in PR or QT intervals or T-wave configuration indicate a serum calcium level of 16 mg/dl or more. AV block and asystole may occur at serum calcium levels of 18 mg/dl.

5. Increased serum calcium levels enhance the action of cardiac glycosides, possibly causing toxicity; the physician may withhold the drug to prevent bradycardia, premature ventricular contractions, or paroxysmal atrial tachycardia.

6. If serum calcium levels are 15 mg/dl or more, central nervous system depression may alter mental status or thought processes, creating a risk for injury.

7. Effects of hypercalcemia include defective water conservation, leading to dehydration, sodium excretion, potassium wasting, and severe weight loss.

8. Hypercalcemia may interfere with antidiuretic hormone, limiting the kidney's ability to concentrate urine and resulting in polyuria.

9. Hypercalcemia may cause renal calculi to form.

10. Saline and furosemide diuresis usually causes calcium excretion, decreasing the serum calcium level.

11. These drugs may increase urinary calcium excretion and decrease intestinal calcium absorption by inhibiting bone resorption or inhibiting tumor production of prostaglandins.

12. Hypercalcemia and the drugs used to treat it can cause nausea and vomiting through vagal nerve stimulation in the upper GI tract or through activation of the brain's chemoreceptor trigger zone. Vagal nerve stimulation produces vasodilation; an ice collar causes vasoconstriction, providing temporary relief from nausea. Antiemetics inhibit stimulation of the chemoreceptor trigger zone.

Reproductive disorders

13. *Provide mouth care every 4 hours,* after vomiting, and before meals. Clean the teeth daily with baking soda and hydrogen peroxide or a similar solution.

14. *Auscultate for bowel sounds daily in four quadrants, and record changes in pitch and frequency.* Be alert to high-pitched, diminished, or absent sounds. Increase fluid intake to four 8-oz (237-ml) glasses every 8 hours, as tolerated.

15. In the first weeks of androgen therapy, monitor serum calcium levels.

16. *Teach the patient and her family signs and symptoms of hypercalcemia and appropriate interventions.*

17. If hypercalcemia doesn't respond to interventions, alert the family and help them prepare for the patient's death.

18. Additional individualized interventions: _____
_____

13. Oral cleaning and antiseptics refresh the mouth. Baking soda and hydrogen peroxide neutralize mouth acids.

14. Hypercalcemia depresses smooth-muscle contractility, delays gastric emptying, and decreases intestinal motility, leading to constipation, obstipation, and paralytic ileus. Dehydration exacerbates obstipation and paralytic ileus.

15. Endocrine therapy may precipitate hypercalcemia in premenopausal or early menopausal women.

16. Hypercalcemia may recur. Being aware of its signs and symptoms may cause the patient and her family to seek early medical intervention.

17. Uncontrollable hypercalcemia is a sign of impending death.

18. Rationales:_____
_____

Discharge planning

DISCHARGE CHECKLIST
Before discharge, the patient shows evidence of:
❒ hemoglobin level and hematocrit within normal limits
❒ serum calcium and serum phosphate levels within normal limits
❒ platelet count, PT/INR, and PTT within normal limits
❒ ferritin levels within normal limits
❒ serum albumin–serum globulin ratio normal (1.5:1)
❒ normal total protein values
❒ absent or low serum levels of carcinoembryonic antigen
❒ absence of HCG in serum or urine
❒ absence of metabolic complications
❒ absence of cardiac arrhythmias, and neuromuscular, renal, and GI complications
❒ absence of secondary lymphedema
❒ arms equal in circumference
❒ radial pulses equal bilaterally
❒ affected arm free from injury
❒ ability to perform ROM exercises
❒ absence of "frozen shoulder"
❒ support from family and spouse or partner
❒ referral to other health care professionals, if indicated.

TEACHING CHECKLIST
Document evidence that the patient and her family demonstrate an understanding of:
❒ nature of cancer and its implications — patients and families need to be alert to signs and symptoms of ovarian and bowel cancers; there's a moderate association between breast cancer and cancers of the ovary and bowel (fiber-optic colonoscopy aids in early detection of bowel cancer)
❒ signs and symptoms of oncologic emergencies
❒ importance of support for the patient's decision regarding reconstructive surgery
❒ signs and symptoms of graft rejection
❒ activity recommendations and limitations
❒ community or professional resources and support groups
❒ need for follow-up appointments
❒ need for long-term emotional support as a result of cancer diagnosis.

DOCUMENTATION CHECKLIST
Using outcome criteria as a guide, document:
❒ clinical status on admission
❒ changes in status
❒ presence of adequate support systems
❒ need for knowledge of endocrine therapies
❒ activity and exercise tolerance and recommendations
❒ patient and family teaching
❒ discharge planning.

Associated care plans
■ Acute pain
■ Cancer
■ Compromised family coping
■ Dying
■ Grieving
■ Ineffective individual coping
■ Perioperative care

References

Dow, K. *"Pocket Guide to Breast Cancer."* Sudbury, Mass:
   Jones & Bartlett, Pubs. Inc., 1999.

"How Is Breast Cancer Treated." American Cancer Society
   2002. Yahoo 2002.

Jordan, K. (ed). *Emergency Nursing Core Curriculum.* Emergency Nurses Association. Philadelphia: W.B. Saunders
   Co., 2000.

Lynn-McHale, D.J., and Carlson, K.K. American Association
   of Critical Care Nurses *AACN Procedure Manual for Critical
   Care,* 4th ed. Philadelphia: W.B. Saunders Co., 2001.

Shoemaker, W.C., et al. *Textbook of Critical Care,* 4th ed.
   Philadelphia: W.B. Saunders Co., 2002.

Prostatectomy

DRG INFORMATION
DRG 334 Major Male Pelvic Procedure with Complication or Comorbidity (CC).
         Mean LOS = 4.9 days
DRG 335 Major Male Pelvic Procedure without CC.
         Mean LOS = 3.3 days
DRG 336 Transurethral Prostatectomy with CC.
         Mean LOS = 3.5 days
DRG 337 Transurethral Prostatectomy without CC.
         Mean LOS = 2.1 days

Introduction
DEFINITION AND TIME FOCUS
Prostatectomy is the surgical removal of the prostate, a gland (in males) located in line with the urethra and positioned between the bladder and rectum. There are three types of prostatectomies: a partial resection removes only enlarged tissue, a simple prostatectomy removes the prostate and its capsule, and a radical prostatectomy removes the prostate, its capsule, the seminal vesicles, and a portion of the bladder neck.

Four surgical approaches are used: transurethral, suprapubic, retropubic, and perineal. (See *Surgical approaches to prostatectomy*.) The surgery's extent and approach depend on the patient's general condition and the specific problem requiring treatment. The transurethral approach is suitable for a partial resection; the suprapubic for a simple prostatectomy; and the retropubic and perineal for simple and radical prostatectomies.

Transurethral resection of the prostate (TURP), in which prostatic tissue is removed through the urethra, is performed most commonly. It's indicated for benign prostatic hyperplasia that can't be managed medically and for small cancerous lesions. Because this approach requires a lithotomy position, it isn't suitable for the patient with a hip problem or prior surgery of the hip joint.

The suprapubic approach involves a lower abdominal suprapubic incision and then a bladder incision. It's indicated for prostatic obstruction and removal of bladder calculi or diverticula.

In the retropubic approach, the gland is entered directly through an abdominal incision, without an incision into the bladder. It's used to remove a gland too large for a TURP, to remove large cancerous lesions, and for the patient who can't tolerate a lithotomy position. A nerve-sparing technique may be used to prevent or minimize impotence.

With the perineal approach, an incision is made in the perineum, the area between the scrotum and anus. This approach is used for removal of a large gland when an abdominal approach is contraindicated such as in an obese patient.

TURP usually has the shortest recovery period; the suprapubic approach, somewhat longer; and the retropubic and perineal approaches, the longest.

This care plan focuses on preoperative and postoperative care for the patient undergoing prostatectomy.

Although the collaborative problems and nursing diagnoses discussed in this care plan apply to all types of prostatectomies, their relative importance varies with the specific surgical approach, as indicated in each problem. (See *Clinical snapshot: Prostatectomy*, page 829.)

ETIOLOGY AND PRECIPITATING FACTORS
■ Age — men age 50 and over usually experience some prostate enlargement
■ Benign prostatic hyperplasia — usually associated with hormonal changes of aging
■ Prostate cancer — unknown cause; most common tumor is adenocarcinoma. Risk factors include:
– age (peak incidence averages at age 65)
– race (progresses faster in black men)
– marital status (lowest incidence in single men)
– occupation (increased incidence among workers employed in the rubber and cadmium industries)
– hormonal factors (altered androgen and estrogen metabolite levels may contribute).

Focused assessment guidelines
NURSING HISTORY
(FUNCTIONAL HEALTH PATTERN FINDINGS)
Health-perception–health-management pattern
■ Preexisting cardiac or pulmonary disorders or diabetes
■ Preoperative urinary tract infection (UTI) and bladder outlet obstruction
■ Antibiotics taken for UTIs
Nutritional-metabolic pattern
■ Weight loss, nausea and vomiting, or anorexia (from impaired renal function because of obstruction or chronic UTI)
Elimination pattern
■ Urine retention, dysuria, frequency, hesitancy, nocturia, urgency, decreased stream, postvoid dribbling, urinary incontinence, or hematuria (rare)

Surgical approaches to prostatectomy

Transurethral approach: Instrument inserted into the urethra for prostate resection; no visible scar

Suprapubic approach: Incision made into lower abdomen and bladder neck

Retropubic approach: Incision made into lower abdomen; bladder neck not resected

Perineal approach: Incision made anterior to rectum

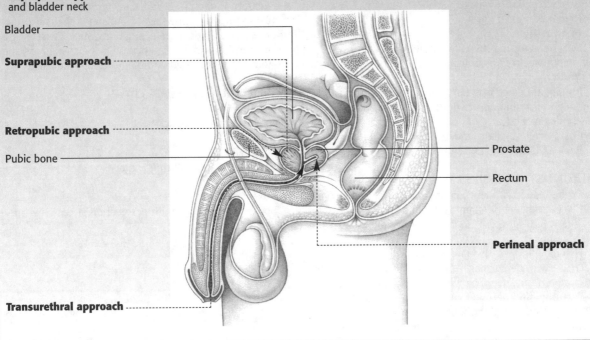

- Bladder
- **Suprapubic approach**
- **Retropubic approach**
- Pubic bone
- **Transurethral approach**
- Prostate
- Rectum
- **Perineal approach**

■ Constipation or epigastric discomfort (from pressure of the bladder on the GI tract)

Activity-exercise pattern
■ Decreased activity coinciding with pain
■ Fatigue and weakness from anorexia or nocturia, with associated sleep deprivation
■ Preexisting age-related cardiopulmonary disorders influencing exercise tolerance

Sleep-rest pattern
■ Sleep pattern disturbances from pain, nocturia, frequency, or urinary incontinence

Cognitive-perceptual pattern
■ Lack of knowledge about disease (benign prostatic hyperplasia or cancer) or surgical procedure and expected outcomes

Self-perception–self-concept pattern
■ Fears and anxieties about alterations in body image, retrograde ejaculation, or impotence from nerve transection or injury
■ Feelings of hopelessness, powerlessness, and lowered self-esteem associated with diagnosis of cancer

Role-relationship pattern
■ Disturbed role performance

■ Fear of social isolation associated with diagnosis of cancer
■ Experiences of family or friends who died from cancer or during surgery, reported by patient

Sexuality-reproductive pattern
■ Preexisting impotence as adverse effect of cardiac medications
■ Concerns about possible impotence expressed by patient
■ Spouse or sexual partner may express concerns about postoperative sexual performance

Coping–stress tolerance pattern
■ Fears and anxieties associated with diagnosis of cancer
■ Appearance of depression

Value-belief pattern
■ Disbelief (denial) about diagnosis of cancer
■ Increased reliance on spiritual support system as coping mechanism

PHYSICAL FINDINGS
Patients with localized prostatic cancer commonly have no signs or symptoms; signs and symptoms indicate advanced disease.

Genitourinary
- Enlarged prostate on rectal examination
– smooth, elastic, nonfixed gland suggests benign prostatic hyperplasia
– hard, irregular, fixed nodule suggests cancer
- Postvoid dribbling or incontinence
- Urine retention
- Hematuria (rare)

Cardiovascular
- Peripheral edema (in renal failure or in hydroureteronephrosis from obstruction)

Pulmonary
- Pulmonary edema (in renal failure or in hydroureteronephrosis from obstruction)

Musculoskeletal
- Costovertebral angle tenderness (in renal failure)
- Back pain or stiffness (with bony metastasis)

DIAGNOSTIC STUDIES
- White blood cell (WBC) count and sedimentation rate — increase with inflammation and infection (preoperative values for these laboratory tests should be within normal limits)
- Hemoglobin level, hematocrit, and platelet count — decrease with hemorrhage (preoperative values for these laboratory tests should be within normal limits)
- Prothrombin time/international normalized ratio (PT/INR) and partial thromboplastin time (PTT) — increase with hemorrhage (preoperative values for these laboratory tests should be within normal limits)
- Blood typing and crossmatching — may be done in the event transfusion is needed
- Acid phosphatase — increases in about 25% of patients with early prostatic cancer when total serum level is measured and in the majority of patients when specific enzymes are used
- Prostate-specific antigen (PSA) — increases in about 73% to 96% of patients with prostate cancer but may also be elevated in 55% to 80% of patients with benign prostatic hyperplasia; useful in monitoring patients for cancer metastasis after radical prostatectomy
- Digital rectal examination — early screening examination for prostate cancer; performed in conjunction with PSA
- Alkaline phosphatase level — increases when cancer metastasizes to bone
- Blood urea nitrogen and creatinine levels — increase may indicate renal failure
- Urinalysis — increase in WBCs suggests infection; increase in red blood cells indicates hematuria, which may delay surgery
- Culture and sensitivity testing — defines microorganisms responsible for UTIs or other infections
- Cystoscopy — evaluates degree of prostate gland fixation, especially when cancerous; evaluates bladder problems and allows direct assessment of obstruction

- Prostate biopsy — provides differential diagnosis of cancer
- Excretory urography — helps determine presence and severity of kidney obstruction
- Chest X-ray — indicates lung status before surgery, may reveal lung metastasis
- Electrocardiography — indicates preoperative cardiac status; used as baseline for comparison if changes occur
- Bone scan — aids in detecting bony metastasis
- Transrectal ultrasound — determines internal prostatic anatomy and its related pathology; guides biopsies

POTENTIAL COMPLICATIONS
- Hemorrhage
- Hypovolemic or septic shock
- Infection
- Epididymitis
- Rectal perforation during surgery
- Pulmonary embolism
- Atelectasis
- Bowel incontinence with perineal prostatectomy (rare)

Prostatectomy

Major nursing diagnoses and collaborative problems	Key patient outcomes
CP: Risk for hypovolemia	Show stable vital signs, typically: heart rate, 60 to 100 beats/minute; systolic blood pressure, 90 to 140 mm Hg; and diastolic blood pressure, 50 to 90 mm Hg.
ND: Risk for infection	Present a clean, dry incision with well-approximated edges.
ND: Acute pain	Rate pain as less than 3 on a 0 to 10 pain rating scale.
ND: Urinary retention	Have no suprapubic distention.
ND: Urge urinary incontinence	Have no postvoid residual volume.
ND: Sexual dysfunction	Identify available community resources to help with altered sexuality patterns.
ND: Risk for situational low self-esteem	Participate in ADLs.

Collaborative problem

Risk for hypovolemia related to prostatic or incisional bleeding after surgery

NURSING PRIORITY

Prevent or promptly detect internal or external bleeding.

PATIENT OUTCOME CRITERIA

Within 24 hours after surgery, the patient will:
- show stable vital signs, typically: heart rate, 60 to 100 beats/minute; systolic blood pressure, 90 to 140 mm Hg; and diastolic blood pressure, 50 to 90 mm Hg
- have normal laboratory values.
    Within 3 days after surgery, the patient will:
- have regular bowel movements
- avoid straining the abdominal and perineal muscles.

INTERVENTIONS

1. *Monitor and document the amount of blood collecting on incisional dressings and in the urinary drainage system hourly for the first 12 to 24 hours after surgery, then every 4 hours.* * Typical drains and catheters include the following:
– for TURP, a urethral catheter
– for the suprapubic approach, a urethral catheter, a suprapubic tube, and an abdominal drain
– for the retropubic approach, a urethral catheter and an abdominal drain
– for the perineal approach, a urethral catheter and a perineal drain.
    Observe the frequency of clots in the urine. Use standard precautions. Consult the surgeon concerning the amount of bleeding anticipated. Alert the surgeon if any of the following occur:

RATIONALES

1. The amount of bleeding expected after surgery varies with the reason for and extent of the surgery. Heavy bleeding is expected for the first 24 hours after a TURP or a suprapubic or retropubic prostatectomy. Minimal bleeding is expected with the perineal approach.
    Blood loss from incisional drainage usually is minimal, while blood loss through the urinary catheter may range from minimal to life-threatening. Bright red blood indicates arterial bleeding; dark blood suggests venous bleeding.
    Hemorrhage may occur with any surgical approach, but it's a particular problem with TURP. Venous bleeding during the early postoperative period is common. If necessary, traction may be placed on the catheter for 6 to 8 hours.

*Italics indicate key interventions.

Reproductive disorders

– bright red drainage
– persistent burgundy-colored drainage
– persistent clot formation.

Hemorrhage may occur with a suprapubic or perineal approach, but usually it isn't a major problem. With the retropubic approach, the risk of hemorrhage usually is minimal because this approach affords better control of bleeding.

Blood volume loss may decrease cardiac output, arterial and venous blood pressure, and hemoglobin level, decreasing the blood's oxygen-carrying capacity. A blood volume loss of 20% or more can cause hypovolemic shock.

Expected removal times for urinary catheters are discussed later in this care plan; abdominal drains are usually removed after 4 to 7 days (occasionally after 10 days with a radical perineal prostatectomy).

2. *Evaluate and document pulse rate, blood pressure, respirations, skin color, and level of consciousness* according to unit protocol — typically every 4 hours for 24 hours or until stable, then every 8 hours.

2. An increased pulse rate, a blood pressure 20 mm Hg below normal or 80 mm Hg or less, rapid and deep respirations, cold and clammy skin, pallor, and restlessness indicate shock.

3. *Monitor hemoglobin level, hematocrit, platelet count, and coagulation studies daily.* Compare current values with preoperative values. Alert the physician to abnormal values. Administer blood transfusions as ordered, using standard precautions.

3. A sudden decrease in hemoglobin level, hematocrit, and platelet count or an increase in PT/INR or PTT may indicate the need for a transfusion.

4. Consult the surgeon about applying traction to the catheter or preparing the patient for surgery if bleeding persists.

4. Applying traction pulls the catheter balloon against the bladder neck. The resulting pressure compresses bleeding vessels in the prostatic fossa. For prolonged or excessive bleeding, sutures or cauterization may be necessary.

5. *Teach the patient to avoid straining during bowel movements.* Avoid using rectal thermometers or tubes or giving enemas.

5. Straining to defecate or introducing objects into the rectum may cause bleeding, especially after the retropubic or perineal approach for radical prostatectomy.

6. *Administer and document stool softeners and laxatives,* as ordered. Use alternatives, such as increased fiber, fluids, and prune juice in the diet. Monitor the frequency and consistency of bowel movements.

6. Preventing constipation is important to decrease the risk of bleeding or rectal tearing.

7. Teach the patient to avoid lifting heavy objects for 6 to 8 weeks after surgery to allow time for internal and external wound healing.

7. Undue strain on the abdominal and perineal muscles places stress on the bladder and prostate and may cause bleeding.

8. Additional individualized interventions: _____

_____

8. Rationales: _____

_____

Nursing diagnosis

Risk for infection (postoperative) related to preoperative status or urinary catheter or abdominal drain placement

NURSING PRIORITY

Prevent or promptly detect infection.

PATIENT OUTCOME CRITERIA

Within 24 hours after surgery, the patient will:
- have no fever
- have no urinary clots
- ambulate.

Within 3 days after surgery, the patient will:
- present a clean, dry incision with well-approximated edges
- have clear urine.

INTERVENTIONS	RATIONALES
1. *Monitor and record vital signs* according to unit protocol, typically every 4 hours for 24 hours or until stable, then every 8 hours. Notify the physician of significant changes from the patient's baseline values.	**1.** The risk of infection varies with the procedure used. The risk is high with the suprapubic approach, in which a bladder incision can allow urine to leak into surrounding tissue. The presence of catheters or drains also increases the risk of infection. Sudden fever, chills, hypotension, and tachycardia are signs and symptoms of septic shock, a particular risk after prostatectomy.
2. *Monitor the incision site daily for induration, erythema, and purulent or odorous drainage.* Document all findings. Send drainage samples for culture and sensitivity testing, as ordered.	**2.** The skin is the first line of defense against infection. Testing drainage samples will identify the causative microorganism.
3. *Monitor drains and catheters for patency, and irrigate* as ordered, using standard precautions.	**3.** Catheter obstruction commonly occurs from blood clots at the tip of the indwelling urinary catheter. This may cause urine retention, stasis, and infection. Irrigation usually relieves obstruction.
4. *Provide and document meticulous urinary catheter care* at least once daily. Send urine samples for culture and sensitivity testing, as ordered, using standard precautions.	**4.** Although questioned by some, most authorities believe that cleaning with soap and water is essential to prevent microbial growth. Analysis of urine samples will identify any microorganisms.
5. *Administer I.V. fluids,* as ordered. Beginning on the first postoperative day, encourage oral fluid intake of eight to twelve 8-oz (237-ml) glasses daily (unless contraindicated) to maintain a urine output of at least 1,500 ml daily. Record fluid intake and output.	**5.** Adequate hydration promotes renal blood flow and flushes out bacteria in the urinary tract. The I.V. line is usually removed on the first postoperative day if the patient is tolerating oral fluids.
6. Encourage the patient to ambulate the day after surgery.	**6.** Immobility contributes to urinary stasis and creates a reservoir for microorganisms.
7. Administer and document prophylactic antibiotics, as ordered.	**7.** Antibiotics combat and control microbial growth. They're ordered prophylactically because of the high risk of infection with prostatectomy.
8. If the patient is discharged to home with a catheter in place, consider a home health referral.	**8.** Providing support services after discharge allows follow-up and continuation of care.
9. Additional individualized interventions: _____	**9.** Rationales: _____

> **Suggested NIC Interventions**
> *Infection control; Infection protection; Incision site care; Wound care*

> **Suggested NOC Outcomes**
> *Infection status; Wound healing: Primary intention*

Nursing diagnosis

Acute pain related to urethral stricture, catheter obstruction, bladder spasms, or surgical intervention

NURSING PRIORITY

Relieve pain.

PATIENT OUTCOME CRITERIA

Within 30 minutes after surgery, the patient will:
- have stable vital signs, typically: heart rate, 60 to 100 beats/minute; systolic blood pressure, 90 to 140 mm Hg; and diastolic blood pressure, 50 to 90 mm Hg
- have no urinary obstruction.
   Within 1 hour after surgery, the patient will:
- rate pain as less than 3 on a scale of 0 to 10, with pain medication
- find a relaxed position in bed.

INTERVENTIONS	RATIONALES
1. *See the "Acute pain" care plan,* page 32.	1. General interventions for pain management are included in the "Acute pain" care plan. Measures specific to prostatectomy are covered below.
2. *Observe for signs and symptoms of bladder spasms,* such as sharp intermittent pain, a sense of urgency, or urine around the catheter.	2. Bladder spasms occur when catheter placement or surgical manipulation irritate the bladder stretch receptors. Pain from bladder spasms can be severe in the transurethral and suprapubic approaches, in which the bladder is entered surgically. Spasm-induced pain is minimal with the retropubic and perineal approaches because they don't involve a bladder incision.
3. Irrigate, using standard precautions, and check the urinary catheter and tubing for kinks, blood clots, and mucus plugs, as needed.	3. Urine retention from catheter obstruction causes abdominal distention and pain, and may trigger bladder spasms. When the patient complains of suprapubic pain, this intervention is usually all that's needed.
4. *Assess for incisional pain.* Have patient rate pain on a scale of 0 to 10, with 0 indicating no pain, and 10 indicating severe pain.	4. Incisional pain is usually moderate with the suprapubic and retropubic approaches; with the perineal approach, it's usually mild. Using a pain scale helps monitor the patient's perception of the pain.
5. For severe or persistent pain, *administer analgesics or antispasmodics* such as oxybutynin (Ditropan). Administer medication at the pain's onset. Monitor vital signs before and after administering medication, and evaluate pain relief after 30 minutes.	5. Early medication administration prevents severe pain. Oxybutynin directly relaxes smooth muscle and inhibits acetylcholine's parasympathetic-stimulating action on the bladder.
6. Provide alternative pain-relief measures and teach them to the patient. If appropriate, help the patient take a sitz bath and apply heat to the rectal area with a heat lamp after a perineal prostatectomy. Position the patient comfortably.	6. Alternative pain-relief measures may enhance relief in conjunction with analgesics. Heat application reduces inflammation. Proper positioning may decrease discomfort from the urinary catheter.
7. Additional individualized interventions: _____	7. Rationales: _____

Nursing diagnosis

Urinary retention related to urinary catheter obstruction

NURSING PRIORITY

Prevent or minimize urine retention.

PATIENT OUTCOME CRITERIA

Within 24 hours after surgery, the patient will:
- have no urinary clots
- show approximately equal fluid intake and output
- have no suprapubic distention.
  Within 48 hours after surgery, the patient will:
- have stable weight.

INTERVENTIONS

1. *Monitor and record continuous bladder irrigation,* as ordered. Adjust the irrigating solution's flow rate, as ordered, to maintain pink-tinged urine.

2. *If the patient isn't on continuous bladder irrigation, irrigate the urinary catheter with 30 to 60 ml of normal saline solution every 3 to 4 hours or as needed* and as ordered, using gentle pressure. Use aseptic technique and standard precautions.

3. *Monitor and document fluid intake and output.* Encourage fluid intake of eight to twelve 8-oz (237-ml) glasses daily.

4. *Weigh the patient daily.* Compare with preoperative weight, and document.

5. *Observe for suprapubic distention and discomfort every 4 hours* while the patient is awake. If a suprapubic catheter is in place, monitor and record urine outflow. Use standard precautions.

6. Additional individualized interventions: _____

RATIONALES

1. Continuous irrigation dilutes blood clots and decreases obstruction. Urine normally remains pink-tinged for 3 to 4 days.

2. Blood clots or mucus plugs may adhere to the tip of the catheter and obstruct urine flow. This occurs most commonly when continuous irrigation isn't used.

3. Hydration increases urine flow. Urine output less than 60 ml/hour suggests obstruction or decreased renal perfusion.

4. Increasing weight suggests urine retention.

5. Increased distention may signal urine retention. A suprapubic catheter is commonly placed after suprapubic prostatectomy or urethral trauma or stricture.

6. Rationales: _____

Reproductive disorders

Nursing diagnosis

Urge urinary incontinence related to urinary catheter removal, trauma to the bladder neck, or decrease in detrusor muscle or sphincter tone

NURSING PRIORITY

Relieve or minimize incontinence.

PATIENT OUTCOME CRITERIA

Within 24 hours after surgery, the patient will:
- exercise perineal muscles as instructed
- void no more than once every 2 hours
- have no postvoid residual volume
- present a clean, dry perineal area.

INTERVENTIONS

1. *Before surgery, teach the patient to tighten buttock and perineal muscles for 5 to 10 seconds, then relax them, repeating 10 to 20 times/hour.* Instruct the patient to perform this exercise before and after surgery.

2. *Monitor and document the patient's urination pattern after catheter removal.* Instruct the patient to void with each urge, but no more than once every 2 hours during the first 24 hours after surgery and no more than once every 4 hours subsequently.

3. *If a suprapubic catheter is present after the urethral catheter is removed, measure residual volume after each voiding,* using standard precautions. Alert the physician if the residual volume exceeds 50 ml.

4. *Obtain one urine sample with each voiding during the first 24 hours after catheter removal, and note its color, amount, and specific gravity.* Use standard precautions.

5. Provide absorbent incontinence pads. Keep the perineal area clean and dry. Condom catheters may be used to promote dryness, especially at night.

6. Additional individualized interventions: _____

_____

RATIONALES

1. Urinary incontinence is more common with perineal incisions and takes longer to resolve. With a TURP, temporary incontinence results from trauma to the urinary sphincter. With the suprapubic approach, temporary incontinence may result from the bladder neck incision.

Strengthening the bladder sphincter promotes bladder control after urinary catheter removal. Normal urinary function usually returns in 2 to 3 weeks, although complete urinary control may take as long as 6 months to return after a perineal incision.

2. Catheter removal occurs 3 to 5 days after TURP and as long as 12 days after other procedures. Voiding with each urge prevents urine retention, and spacing voidings aids in bladder retraining.

3. When urethral and suprapubic catheters are present, the urethral catheter is usually removed on the first postoperative day to minimize the risk of stricture formation. The suprapubic catheter is usually clamped for 24 hours before its removal, 7 to 10 days after surgery. If the residual volume exceeds 50 ml, the catheter may be left in place until complete emptying is achieved through the urethra.

4. Analysis of a urine specimen helps indicate renal function. Hematuria should gradually decrease, and volume should increase. Specific gravity reflects urine concentration.

5. Keeping the perineal area clean and dry promotes comfort and reduces the risk of infection.

6. Rationales: _____

_____

Nursing diagnosis

Sexual dysfunction (decreased libido) related to fear of incontinence and decreased self-esteem; infertility related to retrograde ejaculation (from TURP and suprapubic prostatectomy); or impotence related to parasympathetic nerve damage (from radical prostatectomy)

NURSING PRIORITY
Prevent or minimize impact of altered sexuality patterns.

PATIENT OUTCOME CRITERIA
Within 24 hours before discharge, the patient will:
- identify impact of surgery or disease on sexuality
- express feelings about masculinity and changes in sexuality
- verbalize understanding of anticipated sexual capacity
- identify available community resources.

INTERVENTIONS

1. *Teach the patient before surgery, and reinforce after surgery, the expected effects of prostatectomy on sexual functioning.* Include the patient's spouse or partner in the discussion.

2. Encourage the patient and his spouse or partner to verbalize feelings of loss, grief, anxiety, and fear.

3. Encourage the patient and his spouse or partner to discuss feelings about and expectations of the sexual relationship.

RATIONALES

1. Providing correct information may decrease threats to the patient's sexual self-esteem and body image by clarifying misconceptions. TURP and suprapubic prostatectomy will produce some degree of retrograde ejaculation secondary to opening of the bladder neck during surgery: Seminal fluid flows into the bladder and is excreted in the urine. Retrograde ejaculation doesn't interfere with sexual activity but does cause infertility. Ejaculation should return to normal within a few months. Sexual function is unaffected by suprapubic prostatectomy; a patient with erectile capability can usually resume intercourse in 4 to 6 weeks. In the past, impotence always resulted from a radical prostatectomy because perineal nerves are cut. However, newer surgical techniques may be performed that spare the nerve bundles that are responsible for erections.

2. Loss of the prostate gland commonly causes feelings of loss and grief similar to those that women experience after hysterectomy. The patient with prostate cancer may also fear transmitting cancer to his sexual partner.
  Some men feel that impotence and sterility make them less manly. Verbalizing these feelings decreases anxiety and may assist in identifying ways to deal with losses.

3. Promoting open communication between sexual partners may prevent misunderstandings, enhance the relationship, and increase the patient's feelings of self-worth.

Reproductive disorders

4. Provide information about a penile prosthesis, if appropriate.

4. A penile prosthesis restores erectile capacity and may increase the patient's feelings of self-worth and sexual self-esteem after radical prostatectomy, which causes impotence, unless a nerve-sparing surgical approach is used. The patient should be totally healed (2 to 3 months after prostatectomy) before pursuing prosthetic surgery.

5. Provide information and refer the patient for sexual counseling, as needed after surgery.

5. The patient may need a sexual counselor if the prostatectomy exacerbates preexisting sexual problems. Follow-up may be needed after discharge.

6. Additional individualized interventions: _____

6. Rationales: _____

Suggested NIC Interventions	*Suggested NOC Outcomes*
Sexual counseling	Sexual functioning

Nursing diagnosis

Risk for situational low self-esteem related to incontinence, potential impotence, or sexual alterations

NURSING PRIORITY

Maximize feelings of self-esteem.

PATIENT OUTCOME CRITERIA

By the time of discharge, the patient will:
- identify effective coping behaviors
- express satisfaction with personal appearance
- express positive feelings of self-worth
- participate in daily care and activities of daily living (ADLs).

INTERVENTIONS

1. Encourage the patient to verbalize feelings about postoperative changes in body functioning and how these changes will affect lifestyle.

2. Assist the patient in identifying and using effective coping behaviors. If problems arise, see the "Ineffective individual coping" care plan, page 124. Patients experiencing prostate cancer may benefit from local community support groups (such as those sponsored by various cancer support services).

3. Encourage the patient to continue perineal and buttock exercises to decrease incontinence. Reassure the patient that incontinence is temporary. Instruct the patient to use absorbent pads to prevent embarrassment.

4. Compliment the patient on personal appearance. Instruct his spouse or partner and family to provide compliments and positive feedback to the patient.

5. Encourage the patient to participate in ADLs and in decisions affecting care.

RATIONALES

1. As with sexual alterations discussed in the previous problem, verbalizing feelings about other changes in body function is the first step in identifying healthful coping methods.

2. Promoting positive coping behavior increases adaptation to change and increases self-esteem.

3. Incontinence may cause the patient to avoid social activities and neglect self-care. See "Urge urinary incontinence," page 834.

4. Knowledge that a person is perceived by others as attractive and sexually desirable fosters self-esteem. Positive feedback reinforces a positive self-image.

5. Participating in care activities fosters independence. Decision making increases self-control and self-confidence.

6. Additional individualized interventions: _____

6. Rationales: _____

> **Suggested NIC Interventions**
> Body image enhancement; Role enhancement; Self-esteem enhancement; Sexual counseling

> **Suggested NOC Outcomes**
> Body image; Role performance; Self-esteem; Sexual identity: Acceptance

---

Discharge planning

DISCHARGE CHECKLIST

Before discharge, the patient shows evidence of:
- ❏ absence of urinary obstruction
- ❏ absence of urine retention
- ❏ urine output of at least 800 ml for 24 hours before discharge
- ❏ absence of gross hematuria or large clots
- ❏ absence of infection
- ❏ absence of pulmonary complications
- ❏ absence of cardiovascular complications (including thrombophlebitis)
- ❏ stable vital signs (oral temperature below 100° F [37.8° C] for 24 hours before discharge, without antipyretics, and blood pressure within preoperative limits)
- ❏ ability to control pain using oral medications
- ❏ ability to perform ADLs independently
- ❏ ability to perform catheter care
- ❏ ability to tolerate diet
- ❏ adequate home support or referral to home health agency or extended care facility.

TEACHING CHECKLIST

Document evidence that the patient and his family demonstrate an understanding of:
- ❏ surgical outcome and disease
- ❏ discharge medications, including their purpose, dosage, administration schedule, and adverse effects requiring medical attention (usual discharge medications include analgesics, antispasmodics if a urinary catheter is present, and antibiotics)
- ❏ urinary catheter care techniques and supplies
- ❏ signs and symptoms indicating obstruction, bleeding, or infection
- ❏ supplies to manage incontinence
- ❏ exercises to regain urinary control
- ❏ common postoperative feelings
- ❏ appropriate activity level to prevent muscle straining
- ❏ resumption of sexual activity and community resources for sexual counseling
- ❏ community or interagency referral
- ❏ need for consultation with an oncology specialist (if the diagnosis of cancer is confirmed)
- ❏ availability of cancer support groups
- ❏ date, time, and location of follow-up appointments
- ❏ how to contact the physician.

DOCUMENTATION CHECKLIST

Using outcome criteria as a guide, document:
- ❏ clinical status on admission
- ❏ significant changes in status after surgery
- ❏ pertinent laboratory and diagnostic test findings
- ❏ episodes of hemorrhage
- ❏ transfusion with blood products
- ❏ infection and treatment
- ❏ fluid intake and output
- ❏ urinary obstruction episodes
- ❏ urine retention
- ❏ urinary incontinence
- ❏ patient and family teaching
- ❏ discharge planning
- ❏ community or interagency referral.

Associated care plans

- Acute pain
- Compromised family coping
- Grieving
- Ineffective individual coping
- Perioperative care
- Septic shock
- Thrombophlebitis

References

Black, J.M., et al. *Medical Surgical Nursing: Clinical Management for Positive Outcomes,* 6th ed. Philadelphia: W.B. Saunders Co., 2001.

Butler, N. "Behind the Scenes: Partners' Perceptions of Quality of Life Post Radical Prostatectomy," *Urologic Nursing* 20(4):254-59, August 2000.

Butler, N. "Quality of Life Post-radical Prostatectomy: A Male Perspective," *Urologic Nursing* 21(4):2838-39, August 2001.

Handbook of Diseases, 2nd ed. Springhouse, Pa.: Springhouse Corp., 2000.

Hewitt, A. "Early Catheter Removal Following Radical Perineal Prostatectomy: A Randomized Clinical Trial," *Urologic Nursing* 21(1):37-39, February 2001.

Shekarriz, B., et al. "Intraoperative, Perioperative, and Long-term Complications of Radical Prostatectomy," *Urologic Clinics of North America* 28(3):639-53, August 2001.

Sokoloff, M.H., and Brendler, C.B. "Indications and Contraindications for Nerve-sparing Radical Prostatectomy," *Urologic Clinics of North America* 28(3):535-43, August 2001.

Reproductive disorders

Radioactive implant for cervical cancer

DRG INFORMATION

DRG 357   Uterine and Adnexa Procedures for Ovarian or Adnexa Malignancy.
Mean LOS = 8.5 days

DRG 363   Dilatation and Curettage (D&C), Conization, and Radio-Implant for Malignancy.
Mean LOS = 3.5 days

Many patients now receive radioactive implants as outpatients, although in the past such patients were routinely hospitalized. A patient who receives an implant during removal of the malignant neoplasm is always hospitalized.

Introduction

DEFINITION AND TIME FOCUS

The primary treatment for inoperable cervical cancer, radioactive implant therapy usually combines internal irradiation (low dose rate brachytherapy given as inpatient therapy) with external irradiation (usually given as outpatient therapy). Cancers of the vagina and endometrium may also be treated in this manner with a similar nursing care plan.

The implant may be inserted before, during, or after external radiation therapy. With the patient in the operating room and anesthetized, an applicator is inserted into the vagina. The stainless steel applicator consists of a central hollow tube, passed through the cervical os into the uterine cavity, and two hollow ovoids, placed in the vagina next to the cervix. After correct placement is confirmed by X-ray, the patient is brought back to a private room on the unit, where the physician threads the radioactive material (radium or cesium is most common) into the central cylinder and ovoids to radiate the cervix and the paracervical tissue, the usual area into which cervical cancer spreads.

During implant therapy, radiation exposure of the nursing staff is minimized by efficiently organizing care, wearing radiation monitoring devices, rotating staff assignments, and not allowing pregnant staff to care for these patients.

The implant stays in place for 2 to 4 days. Computer calculations determine the radiation dose to the tumor and the dose absorbed by normal tissues, such as the bladder and rectum. After the dose has been delivered, the physician removes the radioactive material and then the applicator. An analgesic or sedative may be required before removal. This care plan focuses on inpatient management of the patient receiving a radioactive implant for cervical cancer. (See *Clinical snapshot: Radioactive implant for cervical cancer.*)

ETIOLOGY AND PRECIPITATING FACTORS

Risk factors associated with the development of squamous cell carcinoma of the cervix include:
- early age of first intercourse
- multiple sexual partners
- multiparity
- history of human papillomavirus infection (condylomata or genital warts)
- cigarette smoking
- history of an abnormal Papanicolaou (Pap) test.

Most of these risk factors are related to early or repeated exposure of the cervix to an oncogenic virus that's probably transmitted sexually.

Focused assessment guidelines

NURSING HISTORY
(FUNCTIONAL HEALTH PATTERN FINDINGS)

Health-perception–health-management pattern
- Abnormal vaginal bleeding, commonly occurring after intercourse or douching
- History of an abnormal Pap test that was never adequately evaluated

Nutritional-metabolic pattern
- Unexplained weight loss (not usually seen with early cancers)

Elimination pattern
- Feelings of pelvic pressure with resulting constipation or frequent urination
- Decreased urine output if the tumor has caused ureteral obstruction
- Incontinence of stool or urine if rectovaginal or vesicovaginal fistulae are present

Activity-exercise pattern
- Weakness or fatigue, especially if anemic from vaginal blood loss

Cognitive-perceptual pattern
- Pelvic pain or pressure, sometimes experienced as low back pain
- Leg or hip pain as the tumor encroaches on nerve roots

Self-perception–self-concept pattern
- Anxiety or depression over the diagnosis of cancer and perceived threat of death

Role-relationship pattern
- Isolation from family, friends, or coworkers

Sexuality-reproductive pattern
- Fear of sexual intercourse because of bleeding or concern about transmitting cancer to partner
- Grief related to loss of reproductive function

Coping–stress tolerance pattern
- Feelings of powerlessness and decreased ability to cope with other stresses
- Need for education and support from community resources

Value-belief pattern
- Guilt over delaying early detection behaviors (regular Pap tests) or evaluation of early symptoms

PHYSICAL FINDINGS
Reproductive
- Vaginal bleeding
- Cervical tumor that may:
- be exophytic (growing outward on the cervix) or endophytic (growing inside the endocervical canal, making the cervix barrel shaped)
- extend down the vagina
- extend to the pelvic side wall
- invade the bladder or rectum

Gastrointestinal
- Constipation
- Passage of stool through vagina (rare)

Urinary
- Frequent urination
- Decreased urine output or anuria (rare)
- Passage of urine through vagina (rare)

DIAGNOSTIC STUDIES
Initial laboratory data may reflect no significant abnormalities.
- Blood urea nitrogen and creatinine levels — may be elevated, indicating ureteral obstruction and diminished renal function
- Hemoglobin level and hematocrit — may be lowered if vaginal bleeding has been heavy
- Excretory urography — may show ureteral obstruction by pelvic tumor
- Cystoscopy — may show bladder wall invasion by tumor
- Barium enema or proctoscopy — may show extrinsic pressure by pelvic tumor or invasion into rectal wall
- Lymphangiogram or computed tomography scan — may indicate spread of tumor outside the pelvis to para-aortic lymph nodes or other organs

POTENTIAL COMPLICATIONS
- Deep vein thrombosis or pulmonary embolus
- Peritoneal or uterine perforation by the implant apparatus
- Hemorrhage
- Atelectasis or pneumonia

CLINICAL SNAPSHOT

Radioactive implant for cervical cancer

Major nursing diagnoses	Key patient outcomes
Risk for injury	Show no signs or symptoms of perforation such as abdominal pain.
Risk for disuse syndrome	Show no signs of pulmonary or vascular complications of bed rest, such as calf or chest pain.
Social isolation	Encourage visitors' compliance with radiation safety principles.
Ineffective sexuality patterns	Verbalize on request purpose and methods of maintaining vaginal patency.

Nursing diagnosis
Risk for injury related to dislodgment of the implant

NURSING PRIORITY
Minimize risk of dislodgment and resulting perforation and peritonitis.

PATIENT OUTCOME CRITERIA
While the implant is in place, the patient will:

Reproductive disorders

- have no bowel movements
- show no signs or symptoms of perforation.
  After the implant is removed, the patient will:
- have normal bowel movements.

INTERVENTIONS	**RATIONALES**
1. *Administer preoperative laxatives or enemas,* * as ordered. Document your actions.	**1.** Evacuating the lower colon minimizes the likelihood that stool will contaminate the field during the insertion procedure. Bowel movements or bedpan placement while the implant is in place may dislodge it or cause perforation by the implant apparatus.
2. Provide a low-residue diet with adequate fluid intake.	**2.** Low-residue foods minimize bulk formation in the colon. Adequate oral fluid intake lessens the need for I.V. hydration.
3. *Administer medications* as ordered to decrease peristalsis, such as diphenoxylate (Lomotil), loperamide (Imodium), or codeine.	**3.** Medications that slow bowel function induce the constipation necessary for maintaining optimal placement and effectiveness of the implant.
4. *Document the presence and position of the implant.* When the patient returns from the operating room, place a small ink mark on the leg at the bottom of the applicator as a baseline indicator in case the applicator is dislodged. Also note the position of the handles on the applicator (vertical, horizontal, or oblique).	**4.** Accurate ongoing assessment of the implant's position detects dislodgment, which may lead to uterine perforation or other tissue injury.
5. *Assess for signs and symptoms of perforation,* including vaginal bleeding, abdominal pain or distention, fever, nausea, and vomiting. Notify the physician immediately.	**5.** The uterine cavity may be perforated at the time of insertion or with considerable pelvic movement. Prompt medical intervention is required because perforation can lead to peritonitis.
6. *Document placement of an indwelling urinary catheter* (may be done at the time of implant insertion) and connection to bedside drainage; record output.	**6.** Continuous urinary drainage allows the patient to keep her hips positioned as recommended and avoids the movement necessary for bedpan use. The catheter also helps decrease the risk of bladder injury during the procedure.
7. *Raise the head of the bed slightly* (usually no more than 30 degrees); place a trapeze bar over the bed. Limit side-to-side movement.	**7.** Because the implant apparatus may protrude slightly from the vagina, raising the patient's head more than 30 degrees may change the angle of her hips and could dislodge the implant. Changing the angle of her head will allow the patient to sleep, eat, or read more comfortably. A trapeze bar may allow the patient to move her upper body more easily. Side-to-side movement may dislodge the implant.
8. *Encourage the patient to perform grooming and personal hygiene activities.* Don't change bed linen unless necessary.	**8.** Self-care increases the patient's involvement and decreases the caregiver's radiation exposure. Changing linens may cause pelvic movement that could dislodge the implant.
9. After the implant is removed, administer (and document the use of) laxatives or enemas, begin regular diet, and discontinue constipating medications.	**9.** Normal bowel function is restored after the implant is removed so that the patient can be discharged with normal functions intact.
10. Additional individualized interventions: _____ _____	**10.** Rationales: _____ _____

***Italics indicate key interventions.**

Suggested NIC Interventions
Surveillance; Surveillance: Safety; Risk identification

Suggested NOC Outcomes
Risk control

Nursing diagnosis

Risk for disuse syndrome related to imposed bed rest

NURSING PRIORITY

Minimize risks of bed rest.

PATIENT OUTCOME CRITERIA

While the implant is in place, the patient will:
- exercise lower extremities every 2 hours while awake
- perform deep-breathing exercises every 2 hours while awake.
  Throughout the hospital stay, the patient will:
- show no signs of pulmonary or vascular complications of bed rest, such as calf pain, chest pain, or dyspnea.

INTERVENTIONS

1. *Attach a footboard to the foot of the bed; teach the patient foot and leg exercises,* and encourage her to perform them every 2 hours while awake to increase blood flow. Also, apply antiembolism stockings.

2. *Assess for signs and symptoms of thromboembolic phenomena,* including calf pain, redness, and warmth; positive Homans' sign; and sudden onset of chest pain and dyspnea. See the "Thrombophlebitis" care plan, page 459 for details. Report abnormalities promptly.

3. *Administer anticoagulants as prescribed,* and monitor for excessive bleeding around the implant.

4. *Teach deep-breathing exercises* and encourage the patient to perform them every 2 hours while awake.

5. *Assess for signs and symptoms of lung infection* every shift, such as crackles, bronchial breath sounds, fever, productive cough, and pleuritic chest pain. Report abnormalities.

6. Additional individualized interventions: _____

RATIONALES

1. Deep vein thrombophlebitis or pulmonary embolism may occur in the patient on bed rest. The patient with gynecologic cancer is at increased risk from the pressure of the pelvic tumor on large vessels. Measures to decrease venous pooling lessen this risk.

2. These signs and symptoms reflect inflammation of the vein wall and clot formation. The "Thrombophlebitis" care plan contains detailed information on thromboembolic phenomena.

3. Anticoagulants, such as heparin or warfarin (Coumadin), inhibit blood clotting, thus decreasing the risk of a thromboembolic event but increasing the risk of hemorrhage.

4. Bed rest contributes to poor lung expansion. Stasis of secretions leads to airway obstruction and atelectasis and provides a medium for bacterial growth. Deep-breathing exercises prevent pooling of secretions.

5. Systematic assessment improves the likelihood of prompt detection and treatment of developing infection.

6. Rationales: _____

Suggested NIC Interventions
Activity therapy; Energy management; Cognitive stimulation; Environmental management; Exercise therapy: Ambulation; Exercise therapy: Balance; Exercise therapy: Joint mobility; Exercise therapy: Muscle control

Suggested NOC Outcomes
Endurance; Immobility consequences: Physiological; Immobility consequences: Psycho-cognitive; Mobility level

Reproductive disorders

Nursing diagnosis

Social isolation related to implant radioactivity

NURSING PRIORITY

Minimize feelings of social isolation while the radioactive implant is in place.

PATIENT OUTCOME CRITERIA

While the implant is in place, the patient will:
- encourage visitors' compliance with radiation safety principles
- verbalize understanding of why nursing time must be limited
- pass time with diversionary activities.

INTERVENTIONS

1. *Explain to the patient and her family the reasons for isolation from other patients and the nursing staff.* Limit time spent with the patient and remind her family to remain behind the lead shields as much as possible. Limit the number of visitors, and don't allow children or pregnant women into the room.

2. *Organize patient care into multiple short interactions* instead of spending a lot of time in the room. Arrange the room so that items are within the patient's reach. Check on the patient frequently from the door.

3. Encourage diversionary activities, such as reading, handwork, talking on the phone, or watching television.

4. Additional individualized interventions: _____

RATIONALES

1. Time, distance, and lead shielding are the three components of safe care for a patient with a radioactive implant. The areas of lowest radiation levels are at the foot and the head of the bed. The lead shields are placed at the patient's sides where the radiation dose is higher.

2. Limiting time spent near the implant, maximizing distance from the implant, and staying behind the lead shields when providing bedside care will protect the nurse from excessive radiation exposure. Because of the limited number of visitors permitted, the patient will welcome frequent contact with the nurse.

3. A patient with cancer commonly experiences social isolation. Add to this mandatory physical isolation, and the patient may feel disoriented, with lowered self-esteem. Performing meaningful activities will help the patient pass the time and lend some sense of normalcy to the situation. Support and encouragement from the nurse may boost the patient's spirits.

4. Rationales: _____

Suggested NIC Interventions
Recreation therapy; Activity therapy; Socialization enhancement; Family integrity promotion; Behavior modification: Social skills; Caregiver support; Family process maintenance; Family therapy

Suggested NOC Outcomes
Leisure participation; Family environment: Internal

Nursing diagnosis

Ineffective sexuality patterns related to vaginal tissue changes or fear of radioactivity

NURSING PRIORITY

Minimize the physical and psychosexual effects of a vaginal implant.

PATIENT OUTCOME CRITERIA

By the time of discharge, the patient will:

- on request, verbalize awareness of potential problems after radioactive implant removal
- on request, verbalize purpose and methods of maintaining vaginal patency.

INTERVENTIONS	RATIONALES
1. Allow the patient to explore concerns and fears about the radioactive implant and resumption of sexual activity. Reassure the patient that after the implant has been removed, the tissues don't retain any radioactivity and, therefore, can't harm anyone.	**1.** The patient (and her partner) may be concerned with the risk of radiation exposure during intercourse.
2. Discuss with the patient and her spouse or partner (if present) the value of resuming intercourse (if the patient has a partner) or the use of vaginal dilators when postimplant discomfort has abated (usually after 2 to 4 weeks).	**2.** Radiation can cause scarring, narrowing, or fibrosis of the vaginal tissues. Regular dilation of the vagina through intercourse or the use of dilators will help minimize these effects. Vaginal flexibility facilitates vaginal examination and the taking of Pap tests to monitor the disease.
3. Discuss with the patient and her spouse or partner (if present) fears and concerns related to pain and bleeding during intercourse. Encourage the use of lubrication during intercourse.	**3.** Atrophy and the resulting dryness of the vaginal tissues can occur after radioactive implant insertion. Tissues may be thin and easily traumatized, leading to pain or bleeding. Lubrication with a water-soluble lubricant may make the patient and partner more comfortable. Don't recommend petroleum-based products; they're too thick and may cause greater irritation.
4. Additional individualized interventions: _____	**4.** Rationales: _____

> ### *Suggested NIC Interventions*
> *Body image enhancement; Role enhancement; Self-esteem enhancement; Sexual counseling*

> ### *Suggested NOC Outcomes*
> *Body image; Role performance; Self-esteem; Sexual identity: Acceptance*

Discharge planning

DISCHARGE CHECKLIST

Before discharge, the patient shows evidence of:

- ❏ ability to perform activities of daily living (ADLs) independently
- ❏ ability to ambulate the same as before surgery
- ❏ absence of dysuria
- ❏ stable vital signs
- ❏ absence of pulmonary or cardiovascular complications
- ❏ ability to have a bowel movement
- ❏ absence of infection
- ❏ ability to control pain with oral medications
- ❏ no need for I.V. support (preferably discontinued for at least 24 hours)
- ❏ hemoglobin within therapeutic levels
- ❏ minimal vaginal discharge and absence of gross bleeding
- ❏ knowledge of how to contact a cancer support group
- ❏ adequate home support, or referral to home care if indicated by an inadequate home support system or inability to perform ADLs.

TEACHING CHECKLIST

Document evidence that the patient and her family demonstrate an understanding of:

- ❏ the cancer and its implications
- ❏ treatment administered
- ❏ discharge medications, including their purpose, dosage, administration schedule, and adverse effects requiring medical attention (generally, medications aren't ordered routinely, but pain medication, antibiotics, or medications for constipation or diarrhea may be prescribed, depending on special problems)
- ❏ need to call the physician if abdominal pain or temperature above 100° F (37.8° C) develops
- ❏ likelihood of weakness or fatigue for 7 to 10 days after discharge

- ❐ likelihood of vulvovaginal discomfort for a few days
- ❐ possibility of some discharge (possibly bloody) for up to 2 weeks (Tell the patient to call the physician if bleeding becomes heavy, requiring one or more pads every hour. Tampons are usually discouraged because of the increased risk of toxic shock syndrome.)
- ❐ ability to resume intercourse after tenderness and discharge decrease
- ❐ community resources for cancer education and support
- ❐ date, time, and location of follow-up appointments
- ❐ how to contact the physician.

DOCUMENTATION CHECKLIST
Using outcome criteria as a guide, document:
- ❐ clinical status on admission
- ❐ significant changes in clinical status
- ❐ pertinent laboratory and diagnostic test findings
- ❐ preimplant patient teaching
- ❐ results of preimplant laxatives or enemas
- ❐ application of antiembolism stockings and teaching of lower extremity exercises
- ❐ function of indwelling urinary catheter
- ❐ head of bed elevated no more than 45 degrees
- ❐ correct placement of radioactive implant
- ❐ nutritional intake
- ❐ teaching of deep-breathing exercises
- ❐ results of postimplant laxatives or enemas
- ❐ patient and family teaching
- ❐ discharge planning.

Associated care plans

- Acute pain
- Compromised family coping
- Grieving
- Ineffective individual coping
- Knowledge deficit
- Thrombophlebitis

References

Brown, D., et al. "Use of Radiation in Gynecologic and Breast Malignancies," in *Women and Cancer: A Gynecologic Oncology Nursing Perspective*, 2nd ed. Edited by Moore-Higgs, G.J., et al. Sudbury, Mass.: Jones & Bartlett Pubs., Inc., 2000.

Gosselin, T.K., and Waring, J.S. "Nursing Management of Patients Receiving Brachytherapy for Gynecologic Malignancies," *Clinical Journal of Oncology Nursing* 5(2):59-63, March/April 2001.

Velji, K. "The Experience of Women Receiving Brachytherapy for Gynecologic Cancer," *Oncology Nursing Forum* 28(4): 743-51, May 2001.

Appendices
and index

Appendix A
Monitoring standards

This appendix outlines generally accepted standards for implementing selected hemodynamic monitoring techniques for critically ill patients. It should be individualized according to a specific patient's needs and unit protocol. For all monitoring techniques, remember that the trend of values is more significant than isolated readings. (*Note:* Monitoring of clinical signs and symptoms, laboratory tests, and diagnostic procedures are presented within the specific care plans in this book.)

ECG MONITORING

- Monitor electrocardiogram (ECG) continuously. Observe for arrhythmias, ST-segment changes, and T-wave abnormalities.
- Monitor in MCL_1 or MCL_6 whenever possible, because they best differentiate ectopy from aberrancy. Monitor in Lead II for atrial arrhythmias.
- Keep rate alarms on at all times.
- Mount rhythm printouts in the patient's record routinely at least once every 8 hours and as needed for significant arrhythmias.
- Evaluate and document atrial and ventricular rate, rhythm, PR interval, QRS duration, QT interval, and appearance of P waves, QRS complex, ST segment, and T waves at least once every 8 hours and as needed for significant changes.

VITAL SIGN MONITORING

- Monitor apical pulse, blood pressure, and respiratory rate every 15 minutes until stable, then every 1 to 2 hours.
- Monitor temperature at least every 4 hours.

INTAKE AND OUTPUT MONITORING

- Monitor hourly and 8-hour or 24-hour cumulative intake and output levels.
- In addition to standard nursing intake and output measures (for example, including gelatin in intake total), record the amount of all I.V. flush solutions administered.
- Measure urine specific gravity hourly or as indicated.
- Measure fingerstick blood glucose levels every 6 hours in patients with diabetes, patients on parenteral nutrition, postoperative cardiac surgery patients, and others, as indicated.

ARTERIAL PRESSURE MONITORING

- Monitor arterial pressure continuously in patients with arterial lines.
- Keep pressure alarms on at all times.
- Keep all connections in constant view; the patient can exsanguinate in a matter of minutes if a disconnection occurs.
- Balance and calibrate the transducer according to the manufacturer's directions at least every 8 hours to negate the influence of atmospheric pressure on readings and to confirm the measuring accuracy.
- Use a constant low-flow closed heparinized flush solution to maintain patency.
- Periodically observe for the characteristic arterial waveform on the oscilloscope; investigate damping or abnormal appearance promptly.
- Compare to sphygmomanometer pressure every 8 hours; investigate significant discrepancies between the two.
- Check pulse, skin temperature, and skin color distal to the insertion site at least every 2 hours.

PULMONARY ARTERY MONITORING

- Measure right atrial pressure (central venous pressure) and pulmonary artery (PA) systolic, diastolic, and mean pressures every hour or as needed.
- Use consistent baseline position for obtaining readings.
- Level the transducer's air-fluid interface with the phlebostatic axis.
- Follow unit protocol for removing patients from ventilators to record readings. If recording pressures while the patient is on the ventilator, read pressures at end-expiration to minimize respiratory influences on hemodynamic values. Document whether pressures are recorded when the patient is on or off the ventilator.
- Balance and calibrate the transducer according to the manufacturer's directions at least every 8 hours to negate the influence of atmospheric pressure on readings and to confirm accuracy of measurement.
- Use a constant low-flow closed heparinized flush solution to maintain patency.
- Before readings, confirm patency by observing the oscilloscope for characteristic PA waveforms.

■ Usually, when the previously described standards are followed, regard a change in values of more than 5 mm Hg as clinically significant.

PAWP MONITORING

■ Measure pulmonary artery wedge pressure (PAWP) as ordered.

■ To read PAWP, inflate the balloon until the characteristic PAWP waveform appears, using no more than the specified amount of air for that size balloon. After reading the pressure, make sure the balloon is deflated by removing the syringe used for inflation, releasing the lever if used to lock air in the balloon for the reading, and confirming on the oscilloscope the return to the usual PA waveform.

■ To avoid frequent wedging, which damages the balloon and can cause pulmonary infarction, and to monitor left ventricular filling pressure constantly, consider continuous monitoring of PA diastolic pressure. Verify correlation with PAWP every 4 to 8 hours by confirming that the pressures are within 5 mm Hg of each other.

CARDIAC OUTPUT MONITORING

■ Measure cardiac output, as ordered.

■ Obtain at least three readings at a time. Discard any readings that deviate significantly from each other and average the remaining readings.

■ Use injectate at room temperature. Use iced injectate if room temperature injectate readings consistently deviate more than 15% from each other.

■ Monitor cardiac index electronically or by dividing cardiac output by the patient's body surface area, obtainable from a DuBois nomogram.

■ Monitor systemic vascular resistance electronically or by dividing cardiac output into mean arterial pressure (MAP) minus mean right atrial pressure.

ICP MONITORING

■ Monitor intracranial pressure (ICP) continuously in patients with ICP monitoring catheters.

■ Use a consistent baseline position for obtaining readings, usually a 20- to 30-degree elevation of the head of the bed.

■ Level the air-fluid interface of the transducer with the reference point for the foramen of Monro, usually considered to be the outer corner of the eye, top of the ear, or the external auditory meatus.

■ Verify patency of the line by observing the characteristic waveform on the oscilloscope.

■ Don't read pressures while the patient is moving, coughing, or has the head turned to one side or the other; all will falsely elevate pressures.

■ Never aspirate an ICP line; doing so may draw brain tissue into the catheter or screw.

■ Don't flush an ICP line unless specifically ordered to do so by the patient's doctor.

■ Monitor cerebral perfusion pressure by subtracting ICP from MAP.

■ Balance and calibrate the transducer at least every 8 hours.

REFERENCES

Lynn-McHale, D.J., and Carlson, K.K. American Association of Critical Care Nurses *AACN Procedure Manual for Critical Care*, 4th ed. Philadelphia: W.B. Saunders Co., 2001.

Phipps, W.J., et al. *Medical-Surgical Nursing. Health and Illness Perspectives*, 7th ed. St. Louis: Mosby–Year Book, Inc., 2003.

Shoemaker, W.C., et al. *Textbook of Critical Care*, 4th ed. Philadelphia: W.B. Saunders Co., 2002.

Thompson, J.M., et al. *Mosby's Clinical Nursing*, 5th ed. St. Louis: Mosby–Year Book, Inc., 2002.

Appendix B
Acid-base imbalances

Imbalance	ABG findings	Patho-physiology	Possible causes	Signs and symptoms	Compensatory mechanisms
Respiratory acidosis	• Decreased pH • Increased $Paco_2$ • Compensatory decrease in HCO_3^-	• Decreased alveolar ventilation, which leads to retention of carbon dioxide	• Depression of medullary respiratory center from drugs, injury, or disease • Pulmonary diseases • Inadequate tidal volume or respiratory rate on ventilator	• Decreased mentation • Restlessness • Combativeness • Headache • Diaphoresis • Anxiety • Tachycardia	Renal compensation via HCO_3^- retention, acid elimination, and increased ammonia production
Respiratory alkalosis	• Increased pH • Decreased $Paco_2$ • Compensatory decrease in HCO_3^-	• Increased alveolar ventilation, which results in a loss of carbon dioxide	• Hyperventilation from anxiety, pain, or excessive tidal volume or respiratory rate on ventilator • Respiratory-center stimulation by drugs, injury, or disease • Fever or high ambient temperature • Sepsis	• Increased rate and depth of respirations • Numbness and tingling • Light-headedness, syncope • Anxiety	Renal compensation via HCO_3^- elimination, acid retention, and decreased ammonia production
Metabolic acidosis	• Decreased pH • Decreased HCO_3^- • Compensatory decrease in $Paco_2$	• Loss of HCO_3^- • Increased acid formation	• Diarrhea • Diabetes • Shock • Renal failure • Azotemia • Small-bowel fistulas	• Increased rate and depth of respirations • Fatigue • Lethargy • Acetone odor to breath • Unconsciousness	Rapid pulmonary compensation via hyperventilation, renal metabolic compensation (except in renal failure) by HCO_3^- retention, acid elimination, increased ammonia production
Metabolic alkalosis	• Increased pH • Increased HCO_3^- • Compensatory increase in $Paco_2$	• Increased HCO_3^- retention • Loss of acids or potassium	• Vomiting • Gastric suctioning • Prolonged use of diuretics • Excessive HCO_3^- ingestion	• Decreased rate and depth of respirations • Hypertonicity • Twitching, tetany • Seizures • Irritability • Restlessness • Combativeness • Unconsciousness	Rapid pulmonary compensation via hypoventilation, renal metabolic compensation by HCO_3^- elimination, acid retention, decreased ammonia production

Appendix C
Fluid and electrolyte imbalances

Imbalance	Possible causes	Signs and symptoms	Laboratory results	Treatment
Hypovolemia	• Hemorrhage • Diabetes insipidus (DI) • Renal disease • Vagal stimulation • Drug reactions • Hyperosmolar hyperglycemic nonketotic syndrome	• Tachycardia • Weak pulse • Hypotension • Oliguria • Pallor • Decreased level of consciousness (LOC)	• Decreased central venous pressure (CVP) • Decreased hematocrit and hemoglobin	• Correct the underlying cause. • Administer appropriate I.V. fluids.
Hypervolemia	• Excessive I.V. fluid administration	• Hypertension • Edema • Bounding pulse • Pulmonary edema • Venous distention	• Increased CVP • Decreased hemoglobin and hematocrit • Decreased blood urea nitrogen (BUN)	• Treat with diuretics and dialysis as ordered. • Keep in mind that no treatment may be needed and that prevention is the best treatment.
Intravascular to interstitial shift	• Hemorrhage • Decreased water intake • Concentrated tube feedings • Vomiting • Diarrhea • Burns • Prolonged gastric suctioning • Soft-tissue injury • Intestinal obstruction • Fever	• Shock state • Tachycardia • Weak pulse • Oliguria • Dry mucous membranes • Hypotension	• Decreased LOC • Increased hemoglobin and hematocrit • Increased BUN	• Correct the underlying cause. • Administer appropriate I.V. fluids.
Interstitial to intravascular shift	• Burns • Soft-tissue injury • Excessive colloid or hypertonic I.V. administration	• Hypertension • Bounding pulse • Venous distention • Weakness • Hyponatremia	• Increased CVP • Decreased hemoglobin and hematocrit • Decreased BUN	• No treatment is usually needed for otherwise healthy patients. • Administer diuretics to patients with abnormal heart, liver, or kidney function.
Hyponatremia	• Excessive sweating or water intake • Decreased salt intake • Heart failure • Renal failure • Diuretic therapy • Fresh water near drowning • Vomiting • Diarrhea • Burns • Nasogastric (NG) tube suctioning	• Confusion • Headache • Abdominal cramps • Apathy • Hypotension • Weakness • Hyperactive reflexes • Seizures • Oliguria	• Decreased serum sodium • Decreased chloride • Decreased urine specific gravity	• Decrease water intake or increase sodium intake.

Imbalance	Possible causes	Signs and symptoms	Laboratory results	Treatment
Hypernatremia	• Decreased water intake • Increased sodium intake • Prolonged watery diarrhea • Prolonged hyperventilation • Salt water near drowning • DI	• Dehydration • Thirst • Dry mucous membranes • Weakness • Fever • Warm, flushed skin • Muscle pain	• Increased serum sodium level • Increased serum chloride level • Increased urine specific gravity	• Correct the underlying cause, if possible. • Restrict sodium intake. • Increase fluid intake.
Hypokalemia	• Decreased potassium intake • Diuretics • Vomiting or diarrhea • Burns • Heart failure • Fistulas • Colitis • Steroids • NG tube suctioning	• Diminished reflexes • Irregular pulse • Thirst • Hypotension • Electrocardiography (ECG) changes • Muscular weakness or irritability	• Decreased serum potassium level • Decreased serum chloride level	• Increase dietary potassium intake. • Administer P.O. or I.V. potassium supplements.
Hyperkalemia	• Increased potassium intake • Burns • Soft tissue injury • Advanced kidney disease • Adrenal insufficiency • Hemorrhagic shock • Excessive I.V. administration • Irritability	• Diarrhea • Nausea • Confusion • Flaccid muscles • ECG changes • Hypotension • Abdominal cramping	• Increased serum potassium level	• Decrease dietary potassium intake. • Treat with dialysis. • Administer a sodium polystyrene sulfonate enema. • Administer sodium bicarbonate, glucose, and insulin together I.V.
Hypocalcemia	• Diarrhea • Burns • Renal failure • Draining wounds • Citrated blood administration • Overcorrection of acidosis • Vitamin D deficiency	• Carpopedal spasms • Tetany • Seizures • Tingling in fingers, toes, lips • Muscle cramps • ECG changes	• Decreased serum calcium level	• Administer calcium P.O., I.V., or I.M.
Hypercalcemia	• Vitamin D overdose • Renal disease • Excessive antacid use • Excessive calcium intake	• Pathologic fractures • Deep-bone or flank pain • Lethargy • Nausea • Vomiting • ECG changes • Osteoporosis • Renal calculi • Kidney infections	• Increased serum calcium level	• Correct the underlying cause. • Administer disodium phosphate, sodium sulfate, and diuretics.
Hypomagnesemia	• Alcohol abuse • Vomiting • Decreased intake • Malnutrition • Diuretics • Prolonged GI suctioning • Diarrhea • Pancreatitis • Kidney disease	• Tetany • Lethargy • Nausea • Vomiting • Tachyarrhythmias • Hypotension • Confusion • Hyperactive reflexes	• Decreased serum magnesium level	• Increase dietary magnesium intake. • Administer I.V. magnesium.

Imbalance	Possible causes	Signs and symptoms	Laboratory results	Treatment
Hypermagnesemia	• Excessive magnesium intake • Kidney disease • Severe dehydration • Repeated magnesium-containing enemas • Magnesium antacids in renal failure	• Lethargy • Flushing • Depressed respirations • Hypotension • Flaccid muscles or paralysis • Arrhythmias	• Increased serum magnesium level	• Decrease dietary magnesium intake. • Administer I.V. 10% calcium gluconate. • Treat renal failure patients with dialysis.

Appendix D
Nursing diagnostic categories

This list represents nursing diagnostic categories approved by the North American Nursing Diagnosis Association (NANDA) for clinical use and testing as of 2002.

HEALTH-PERCEPTION–HEALTH-MANAGEMENT PATTERN

Effective therapeutic regimen management
Disturbed energy field
Health-seeking behaviors
Ineffective community therapeutic regimen management
Ineffective family therapeutic regimen management
Ineffective health maintenance
Ineffective protection
Ineffective therapeutic regimen management
Noncompliance
Risk for falls
Risk for infection
Risk for injury
Risk for perioperative-positioning injury
Risk for poisoning
Risk for suffocation

NUTRITIONAL-METABOLIC PATTERN

Adult failure to thrive
Deficient fluid volume
Effective breast-feeding
Excess fluid volume
Hyperthermia
Hypothermia
Imbalanced nutrition: Less than body requirements
Imbalanced nutrition: More than body requirements
Impaired dentition
Impaired oral mucous membrane
Impaired skin integrity*
Impaired swallowing
Impaired tissue integrity
Ineffective breast-feeding
Ineffective infant feeding pattern
Ineffective thermoregulation
Interrupted breast-feeding
Latex allergy response
Nausea
Risk for aspiration

Risk for deficient fluid volume
Risk for imbalanced body temperature
Risk for imbalanced fluid volume
Risk for imbalanced nutrition: More than body requirements
Risk for impaired skin integrity
Risk for latex allergy response

ELIMINATION PATTERN

Bowel incontinence
Constipation
Diarrhea
Functional urinary incontinence
Impaired urinary elimination
Perceived constipation
Reflex urinary incontinence
Risk for constipation
Risk for urinary urge incontinence
Stress urinary incontinence
Total urinary incontinence
Urge urinary incontinence
Urinary retention

ACTIVITY-EXERCISE PATTERN

Activity intolerance
Autonomic dysreflexia
Bathing or hygiene self-care deficit
Decreased cardiac output*
Decreased intracranial adaptive capacity
Delayed growth and development
Delayed surgical recovery
Disorganized infant behavior
Dressing or grooming self-care deficit
Dysfunctional ventilatory weaning response
Fatigue
Feeding self-care deficit
Impaired bed mobility
Impaired gas exchange
Impaired home maintenance

---

* The author believes these diagnoses represent renaming of commonly accepted medical terms and recommends that they not be used for nursing diagnoses guiding independent nursing care. Interdependent nursing care related to these problems is included in the collaborative problems in this book and labeled with familiar terms (such as shock and ischemia).

Impaired physical mobility
Impaired spontaneous ventilation
Impaired transfer ability
Impaired walking
Impaired wheelchair mobility
Ineffective airway clearance
Ineffective breathing pattern
Ineffective tissue perfusion (specify type)
Readiness for enhanced organized infant behavior
Risk for activity intolerance
Risk for autonomic dysreflexia
Risk for delayed development
Risk for disorganized infant behavior
Risk for disproportionate growth
Risk for disuse syndrome
Risk for peripheral neurovascular dysfunction
Toileting self-care deficit
Wandering

SLEEP-REST PATTERN
Disturbed sleep pattern
Sleep deprivation

COGNITIVE-PERCEPTUAL PATTERN
Acute confusion
Acute pain
Chronic confusion
Chronic pain
Decisional conflict (specify)
Deficient knowledge
Disturbed thought processes
Impaired environmental interpretation syndrome
Impaired memory
Unilateral neglect

SELF-PERCEPTION–SELF-CONCEPT PATTERN
Anxiety
Chronic low self-esteem
Death anxiety
Disturbed body image
Disturbed personal identity
Fear
Hopelessness
Powerlessness
Risk for loneliness
Risk for powerlessness
Risk for self-directed violence
Risk for situational low self-esteem
Situational low self-esteem

ROLE-RELATIONSHIP PATTERN
Anticipatory grieving
Caregiver role strain
Chronic sorrow

Dysfunctional family process: Alcoholism
Dysfunctional grieving
Impaired parenting
Impaired social interaction
Impaired verbal communication
Ineffective role performance
Interrupted family processes
Parental role conflict
Relocation stress syndrome
Risk for caregiver role strain
Risk for impaired parent/infant/child attachment
Risk for impaired parenting
Risk for other-directed violence
Risk for relocation stress syndrome
Social isolation

SEXUALITY-REPRODUCTIVE PATTERN
Ineffective sexuality patterns
Rape-trauma syndrome
Rape-trauma syndrome: Compound reaction
Rape-trauma syndrome: Silent reaction
Sexual dysfunction

COPING–STRESS-TOLERANCE PATTERN
Compromised family coping
Defensive coping
Disabled family coping
Impaired adjustment
Ineffective community coping
Ineffective coping
Ineffective denial
Posttrauma syndrome
Readiness for enhanced community coping
Readiness for enhanced family coping
Risk for posttrauma syndrome
Risk for self-mutilation
Risk for suicide
Self-mutilation

VALUE-BELIEF PATTERN
Readiness for enhanced spiritual well-being
Risk for spiritual distress
Spiritual distress

Appendix E
Critical care transfer criteria guidelines

Although the decision to transfer a patient is a medical one, the critical care nurse commonly has input in the decision. This appendix presents general criteria for transferring a patient from a critical care unit to a telemetry unit or a medical-surgical unit. These transfer criteria guidelines should be individualized according to the patient's needs and unit protocol. (Additional disease-specific criteria are presented within the care plans in this book.)

GENERAL CONSIDERATIONS
- Patient no longer requires constant surveillance.
- Resuscitation status is specified in medical order.
- Discharge planning has been initiated (with assessments made of patient's living arrangements before admission, discharge prognosis, anticipated length of stay, ability to perform activities of daily living, educational goals, and family or friend's ability and willingness to assist the patient after discharge).
- Referrals to appropriate ancillary services have been initiated.

NEUROLOGIC SYSTEM
- Level of consciousness and other neurologic vital signs have improved or remained stable for 12 hours.
- Patient doesn't require intracranial pressure monitoring line.

PULMONARY SYSTEM
- Pulmonary status has been stable for 12 hours.
- If patient still requires mechanical ventilation, he's stable and being transferred to caregivers experienced with this therapy.
- PaO_2 is greater than 80 mm Hg (except in chronic obstructive pulmonary disease).
- $PaCO_2$ is less than 10 mm Hg above patient's normal value.

CARDIOVASCULAR SYSTEM
- Patient no longer needs I.V. therapy requiring continuous cardiac monitoring.
- Blood pressure is within 20 mm Hg of patient's normal value (or has an otherwise acceptable value) for 12 hours, without I.V. drugs, such as inotropes, vasodilators, or vasoconstrictors; or mechanical assist devices, such as intra-aortic balloon pump.

- Patient doesn't require an arterial line or pulmonary artery catheter.

RENAL SYSTEM
- Urine output is at least 0.5 ml/kg/hour, except in chronic renal failure.
- If patient is receiving concentrated potassium infusion greater than 20 mEq/hour, transfer him to a monitored bed.

Appendix F
Quick-reference guide to laboratory test results

A

Acetylcholine receptor antibodies, serum
  Negative or ≤0.03 nmol/L
Acid mucopolysaccharides, urine
  < 13.3 µg glucuronic acid/mg creatinine
Acid phosphatase, serum
  0.5 to 1.9 U/L
Activated partial thromboplastin time
  25 to 36 seconds
Adrenocorticotropic hormone, plasma
  < 60 pg/ml
Adrenocorticotropic hormone, rapid, plasma
  Cortisol rises 7 to 18 µg/dl above baseline 60 minutes after injection
Alanine aminotransferase
  Males: 10 to 35 U/L
  Females: 9 to 24 U/L
Albumin, peritoneal fluid
  50% to 70% of total protein
Albumin, serum
  3.3 to 4.5 g/dl
Aldosterone, urine
  2 to 16 µg/24 hours
Alkaline phosphatase, peritoneal fluid
  Males > 18 years: 90 to 239 U/L
  Females < 45 years: 76 to 196 U/L; ≥45 years: 87 to 250 U/L
Alkaline phosphatase, serum
  Males
  18 years: 113 to 482 U/L
  ≥19 years: 98 to 251 U/L
  Females
  17 to 23 years: 114 to 312 U/L
  24 to 45 years: 81 to 213 U/L
  46 to 50 years: 84 to 218 U/L
  51 to 55 years: 90 to 234 U/L
  56 to 60 years: 99 to 257 U/L
  61 to 65 years: 108 to 282 U/L
  ≥65 years: 119 to 309 U/L
Alpha-fetoprotein, amniotic fluid
  ≤18.5 µg/ml at 13 to 14 weeks
Alpha-fetoprotein, serum
  Males and nonpregnant females: 0 to 6.4 IU/ml
Ammonia, peritoneal fluid
  < 50 µg/dl

Ammonia, plasma
  < 50 µg/dl
Amniotic fluid analysis
  Lecithin-sphingomyelin ratio: > 2
  Meconium: absent
  Phosphatidylglycerol: present
Amylase, peritoneal fluid
  138 to 404 U/L
Amylase, serum
  ≥18 years: 35 to 115 U/L
Amylase, urine
  10 to 80 amylase units/hour
Androstenedione (radioimmunoassay)
  Males
  ≥18 years: 0.3 to 3.1 ng/ml
  Females
  ≥18 years: 0.2 to 3.1 ng/ml
Angiotensin-converting enzyme
  17 to 19 years: 7.2 to 26.6 U/L
  ≥20 years: 6.1 to 21.1 U/L
Anion gap
  8 to 14 mEq/L
Antibodies to extractable nuclear antigens
  Negative
Antibody screening, serum
  Negative
Antideoxyribonucleic acid antibodies, serum
  < 7 IU/ml
Antidiuretic hormone, serum
  1 to 5 pg/ml
Antiglobulin test, direct
  Negative
Antimitochondrial antibodies, serum
  Negative at titer < 20
Antinuclear antibodies, serum (Hep-2 substrate)
  Negative at ≤1:40
Anti-Smith antibodies
  Negative
Anti–smooth-muscle antibodies, serum
  Normal titer < 1:20
Antistreptolysin-O, serum
  < 120 Todd units/ml
Antithrombin III
  > 50% of normal control values
Antithyroid antibodies, serum
  Normal titer < 1:100

Arginine test
  Human growth hormone levels increase to > 10 ng/ml in men, to > 15 ng/ml in women
blood gases
  pH: 7.35 to 7.45
  PaO_2: 75 to 100 mm Hg
  $PaCO_2$: 35 to 45 mm Hg
Arterial blood gases (continued)
  O_2CT: 15% to 23%
  SaO_2: 94% to 100%
  HCO_3^-: 22 to 26 mEq/L
Arylsulfatase A, urine
  Males: 1.4 to 19.3 U/L
  Females: 1.4 to 11 U/L
Aspartate aminotransferase
  Males: 8 to 20 U/L
  Females: 5 to 40 U/L
Aspergillosis antibody, serum
  Normal titer < 1:8
Atrial natriuretic factor, plasma
  20 to 77 pg/ml

B

Bacterial meningitis antigen
  Negative
Bence Jones protein, urine
  Negative
Beta-hydroxybutyrate
  < 0.4 mmol/L
Bilirubin, amniotic fluid
  Absent at term
Bilirubin, serum
  Adults: direct, < 0.5 mg/dl; indirect, ≤1.1 mg/dl
  Neonates: total, 1 to 12 mg/dl
Bilirubin, urine
  Negative
Blastomycosis antibody, serum
  Normal titer < 1:8
Bleeding time
  Template: 2 to 8 minutes
  Modified template: 2 to 10 minutes
  Ivy: 1 to 7 minutes
  Duke: 1 to 3 minutes
Blood urea nitrogen
  8 to 20 mg/dl
B-lymphocyte count
  270 to 640/µl

C

Calcitonin, plasma
Baseline: males, ≤40 pg/ml; females, ≤20 pg/ml
Calcium infusion: males, ≤190 pg/ml; females, ≤130 pg/ml

Pentagastrin infusion: males, ≤110 pg/ml; females, ≤30 pg/ml
Calcium, serum (atomic absorption)
Males
19 to 21 years: 9.3 to 10.3 mg/dl
≥22 years: 8.9 to 10.1 mg/dl
Females
≥19 years: 8.9 to 10.1 mg/dl
Calcium, urine
Males: <275 mg/24 hours
Females: <250 mg/24 hours
Calculi, urine
None
Candida antibodies, serum
Negative
Capillary fragility

Petechiae per 5 cm:	Score:
0 to 10	1 +
10 to 20	2 +
0 to 50	3 +
50	4 +

Carbon dioxide, total, blood
22 to 34 mEq/L
Carcinoembryonic antigen, serum
<5 ng/ml
Cardiac pressures (mm Hg)
Right atrial mean: 2 to 8
Right ventricle peak systolic/end-diastolic: 15 to 30/2 to 8
Pulmonary artery
Peak systolic/end-diastolic: 15 to 30/4 to 12
Mean: 9 to 18
Left atrial (or pulmonary capillary wedge)
Mean: 2 to 10
Left ventricle
Peak systolic/end-diastolic: 100 to 140/3 to 12
Cardiolipin antibodies
1:2 titer: negative
1:4 titer: borderline
1:8 titer: positive
Carotene, serum
48 to 200 µg/dl
Catecholamines, plasma
Supine: epinephrine, 0 to 110 pg/ml; norepinephrine, 70 to 750 pg/ml; dopamine, 0 to 30 pg/ml
Standing: epinephrine, 0 to 140 pg/ml; norepinephrine, 200 to 1,700 pg/ml; dopamine, 0 to 30 pg/ml

Cerebrospinal fluid
Pressure: 50 to 180 mm H_2O
Appearance: clear, colorless
Gram stain: no organisms
Ceruloplasmin, serum
Males
≥19 years: 22.9 to 43.1 mg/dl
Females
≥19 years: 22.9 to 43.1 mg/dl
Chloride, cerebrospinal fluid
118 to 130 mEq/L
Chloride, serum
100 to 108 mEq/L
Chloride, sweat
10 to 35 mEq/L
Chloride, urine
110 to 250 mEq/24 hours
Cholesterol, total, serum
170 to 240 mg/dl
Cholinesterase (pseudocholinesterase)
8 to 18 U/ml
Clot retraction
50%
Coccidioidomycosis antibody, serum
Normal titer <1:2
Cold agglutinins, serum
Normal titer <1:32
Complement, serum
Total: 25 to 110 U
C1: esterase inhibitor: 8 to 24 mg/dl
C3: 70 to 150 mg/dl
C4: 14 to 40 mg/dl
Complement, synovial fluid
10 mg protein/dl: 3.7 to 33.7 U/ml
20 mg protein/dl: 7.7 to 37.7 U/ml
Copper, urine
15 to 60 µg/24 hours
Copper reduction test, urine
Negative
Coproporphyrin, urine
Males: 0 to 96 µg/24 hours
Females: 1 to 57 µg/24 hours
Cortisol, free, urine
24 to 108 µg/24 hours
Cortisol, plasma
Morning: 7 to 28 µg/dl
Afternoon: 2 to 18 µg/dl
C-reactive protein, serum
Negative
Creatine, serum
Males: 0.2 to 0.6 mg/dl
Females: 0.6 to 1 mg/dl
Creatine kinase
Total
Males
≥18 years: 52 to 336 U/L
Females
≥18 years: 38 to 176 U/L

Creatine kinase *(continued)*
Isoenzymes
CK-BB: undetectable
CK-MB: 0 to 7 U/L
CK-MM: 5 to 70 U/L
$CK-MB_2$: <1 U/L
$CK-MB_2/CK-MB_1$ ratio: <1.5
Creatinine, serum
Males: 0.8 to 1.2 mg/dl
Females: 0.6 to 0.9 mg/dl
Creatinine, urine
Males: 0 to 40 mg/24 hours
Females: 0 to 80 mg/24 hours
Creatinine clearance
Males (age 20): 85 to 146 ml/min/1.73 m²
Females (age 20): 81 to 134 ml/min/1.73 m²
Cryoglobulins, serum
Negative
Cryptococcosis antigen, serum
Negative
Cyclic adenosine monophosphate, urine
Parathyroid hormone infusion: 3.6- to 4-µmol increase
Cytomegalovirus antibodies, serum
Negative

D

Delta-aminolevulinic acid, urine
1.5 to 7.5 mg/dl/24 hours
D-xylose absorption
Blood: adults, 25 to 40 mg/dl in 2 hours; children, >30 mg/dl in 1 hour
Urine: adults, >3.5 g excreted in 5 hours; children, 16% to 33% excreted in 5 hours

E

Epstein-Barr virus antibodies
Negative
Erythrocyte distribution, fetal-maternal
No fetal red blood cells
Erythrocyte sedimentation rate
Males: 0 to 10 mm/hour
Females: 0 to 20 mm/hour
Esophageal acidity
pH >5.0
Estriol, amniotic fluid
16 to 20 weeks: 25.7 ng/ml
Term: <1,000 ng/ml
Estrogens, serum
Menstruating women: days 1 to 10 of menstrual cycle, 24 to 68 pg/ml; days 11 to 20, 50 to 186 pg/ml; days 21 to 30, 73 to 149 pg/ml
Males: 12 to 34 pg/ml

Estrogens, total urine
  Menstruating women: follicular
      phase, 5 to 25 µg/24 hours; ovu-
      latory phase, 24 to 100 µg/24
      hours; luteal phase, 12 to
      80 µg/24 hours
  Postmenopausal women: < 10 µg/
      24 hours
  Males: 4 to 25 µg/24 hours
Euglobulin lysis time
  2 to 4 hours

F

Factor assay, one-stage
  50% to 150% of normal activity
Febrile agglutination, serum
  Salmonella antibody: < 1:80
  Brucellosis antibody: < 1:80
  Tularemia antibody: < 1:40
  Rickettsial antibody: < 1:40
Ferritin, serum
  Males: 20 to 300 ng/ml
  Females: 20 to 120 ng/ml
Fibrinogen, peritoneal fluid
  0.3% to 4.5% of total protein
Fibrinogen, plasma
  195 to 365 mg/dl
Fibrinogen, pleural fluid
  Transudate: absent
  Exudate: present
Fibrin split products
  Screening assay: < 10 µg/ml
  Quantitative assay: < 3 µg/ml
Fluorescent treponemal antibody
      absorption, serum
  Negative
Folic acid, serum
  3 to 16 ng/ml
Follicle-stimulating hormone, serum
  Menstruating women: follicular
      phase, 5 to 20 mIU/ml; ovulatory
      phase, 15 to 30 mIU/ml; luteal
      phase, 5 to 15 mIU/ml
  Menopausal women: 5 to
      100 mIU/ml
  Males: 5 to 20 mlU/ml
Free thyroxine, serum
  0.8 to 3.3 ng/dl
Free triiodothyronine
  0.2 to 0.6 ng/dl

G

Galactose-1-phosphate uridyltrans-
      ferase
  Qualitative: negative
  Quantitative: 18.5 to 28.5 mU/g of
      hemoglobin

Gamma-glutamyltransferase
  Males: 8 to 37 U/L
  Females < 45 years: 5 to 27 U/L;
      ≥45 years: 6 to 37 U/L
Gastric acid stimulation
  Males: 18 to 28 mEq/hour
  Females: 11 to 21 mEq/hour
Gastric secretion, basal
  Males: 1 to 5 mEq/hour
  Females: 0.2 to 3.8 mEq/hour
Gastrin, serum
  < 300 pg/ml
Globulin, peritoneal fluid
  30% to 45% of total protein
Globulin, serum
  Alpha$_1$: 0.1 to 0.4 g/dl
  Alpha$_2$: 0.5 to 1.0 g/dl
  Beta: 0.7 to 1.2 g/dl
  Gamma: 0.5 to 1.6 g/dl
Glucagon, fasting, plasma
  < 250 pg/ml
Glucose, amniotic fluid
  < 45 mg/dl
Glucose, cerebrospinal fluid
  50 to 80 mg/dl
Glucose, peritoneal fluid
  70 to 100 mg/dl
Glucose, plasma, fasting
  70 to 100 mg/dl
Glucose, plasma, 2-hour postprandial
  < 145 mg/dl
Glucose, synovial fluid
  70 to 100 mg/dl
Glucose, urine
  Negative
Glucose-6-phosphate dehydrogenase
  8.6 to 18.6 U/g of hemoglobin
Glucose tolerance, oral
  Peak at 160 to 180 mg/dl 30 to 60
      minutes after challenge dose
Glutathione reductase activity index
  0.9 to 1.3
Growth hormone suppression
  0 to 3 ng/ml after 30 minutes to
      2 hours

H

Ham test
  Negative red blood cell hemolysis
Haptoglobin, serum
  38 to 270 mg/dl
Heinz bodies
  Negative
Hematocrit
  Males: 42% to 54%
  Females: 38% to 46%
Hemoglobin (Hb), glycosylated
  Total: 5.5% to 9%
  Hb A$_{1a}$: 1.6% of total Hb

Hemoglobin (Hb), glycosylated
  (continued)
  Hb A$_{1b}$: 0.8% of total Hb
  Hb A$_{1c}$: 5% of total Hb
Hemoglobin, total
  Males: 14 to 18 g/dl
  Males after middle age: 12.4 to
      14.9 g/dl
  Females: 12 to 16 g/dl
  Females after middle age: 11.7 to
      13.8 g/dl
Hemoglobin, unstable
  Heat stability: negative
  Isopropanol: stable
Hemoglobin, urine
  Negative
Hemoglobin (Hb) electrophoresis
  Hb A: > 95%
  Hb A$_2$: 2% to 3%
  Hb F: < 1%
Hemosiderin, urine
  Negative
Hepatitis B surface antigen, serum
  Negative
Herpes simplex antibodies, serum
  Negative
Heterophil agglutination, serum
  Normal titer < 1:56
Hexosaminidase A and B, serum
  Total: 5 to 12.9 U/L; hexosaminidase
      A, 55% to 76% of total
Histoplasmosis antibody, serum
  Normal titer < 1:8
Homovanillic acid, urine
  < 8 mg/24 hours
Human chorionic gonadotropin, serum
  < 4 IU/L
Human chorionic gonadotropin, urine
  Pregnant women: first trimester,
      ≤500,000 IU/24 hours; second
      trimester, 10,000 to 25,000 IU/24
      hours; third trimester, 5,000 to
      15,000 IU/24 hours
Human growth hormone, serum
  Males: 0 to 5 ng/ml
  Females: 0 to 10 ng/ml
Human immunodeficiency virus anti-
      body, serum
  Negative
Human placental lactogen, serum
  Pregnant women 5 to 27 weeks:
      < 4.6 µg/ml
  28 to 31 weeks: 2.4 to 6.1 µg/ml
  32 to 35 weeks: 3.7 to 7.7 µg/ml
  36 weeks to term: 5 to 8.6 µg/ml
Hydroxybutyric dehydrogenase (HBD)
  Serum HBD: 114 to 290 U/ml
  Lactate dehydrogenase–HBD ratio:
      1.2 to 1.6:1

17-hydroxycorticosteroids, urine
  Males: 4.5 to 12 mg/24 hours
  Females: 2.5 to 10 mg/24 hours
5-hydroxyindoleacetic acid, urine
  < 6 mg/24 hours
Hydroxyproline, total, urine
  14 to 45 mg/24 hours

IJ

Immune complex, serum
  Negative
Immunoglobulins (Ig), serum
  IgG
    Males and females: 700 to
      1,500 mg/dl
  IgA
    Males and females: 60 to
      400 mg/dl
  IgM
    Males
    ≥ 18 years: 60 to 300 mg/dl
    Females
    ≥ 18 years: 60 to 300 mg/dl
Insulin, serum
  0 to 25 μU/ml
Insulin tolerance test
  10- to 20-ng/dl increase over base-
    line levels of human growth hor-
    mone and adrenocorticotropic
    hormone
Iron, serum
  Males: 70 to 150 μg/dl
  Females: 80 to 150 μg/dl
Iron, total binding capacity, serum
  Males: 300 to 400 μg/dl
  Females: 300 to 450 μg/dl
Isocitrate dehydrogenase
  1.2 to 7 U/L

K

17-ketogenic steroids, urine
  Males: 4 to 14 mg/24 hours
  Females: 2 to 12 mg/24 hours
Ketones, urine
  Negative
17-ketosteroids, urine
  Males: 6 to 21 mg/24 hours
  Females: 4 to 17 mg/24 hours

L

Lactate dehydrogenase (LD)
  Total: 48 to 115 IU/L
  LD$_1$: 14% to 26%
  LD$_2$: 29% to 39%
  LD$_3$: 20% to 26%
  LD$_4$: 8% to 16%
  LD$_5$: 6% to 16%
Lactic acid, blood
  0.93 to 1.65 mEq/L

Leucine aminopeptidase
  < 50 U/L
Leukoagglutinins
  Negative
Lipase, serum
  < 300 U/L
Lipids, amniotic fluid
  > 20% of lipid-coated cells stain
    orange
Lipids, fecal
  Constitute < 20% of excreted solids;
    < 7 g excreted in 24 hours
Lipoproteins, serum
  High-density lipoprotein cholesterol:
    29 to 77 mg/dl
  Low-density lipoprotein cholesterol:
    62 to 185 mg/dl
Long-acting thyroid stimulator, serum
  Negative
Lupus erythematosus cell preparation
  Negative
Luteinizing hormone, serum
  Menstruating women: follicular
    phase, 5 to 15 mIU/ml; ovulatory
    phase, 30 to 60 mIU/ml; luteal
    phase, 5 to 15 mIU/ml
  Postmenopausal women: 50 to
    100 mIU/ml
  Males: 5 to 20 mIU/ml
  Children: 4 to 20 mIU/ml
Lyme disease serology
  Nonreactive
Lysozyme, urine
  < 3 mg/24 hours

M

Magnesium, serum
  1.5 to 2.5 mEq/L
  Atomic absorption: 1.7 to 2.1 mg/dl
Magnesium, urine
  < 150 mg/24 hours
Manganese, serum
  0.04 to 1.4 μg/dl
Melanin, urine
  Negative
Myoglobin, urine
  Negative

N

5′-Nucleotidase
  2 to 17 U/L

O

Occult blood, fecal
  < 2.5 ml/24 hours
Ornithine carbamoyltransferase, serum
  0 to 500 sigma U/ml
Oxalate, urine
  ≤ 40 mg/24 hours

PQ

Parathyroid hormone, serum
  Intact: 210 to 310 pg/ml
  N-terminal fraction: 230 to
    630 pg/ml
  C-terminal fraction: 410 to
    1,760 pg/ml
Pericardial fluid
  Amount: 10 to 50 ml
  Appearance: clear, straw-colored
  White blood cell count: < 1,000/μl
  Glucose: approximately whole blood
    level
Peritoneal fluid
  Amount: ≤ 50 ml
  Appearance: clear, straw-colored
Phenylalanine, serum
  < 2 mg/dl
Phosphate, tubular reabsorption, urine
  and plasma
  80% reabsorption
Phosphates, serum
  1.8 to 2.6 mEq/L; in children, up to
    4.1 mEq/L
  Atomic absorption: 2.5 to 4.5 mg/dl;
    in children, up to 7 mg/dl
Phosphates, urine
  < 1,000 mg/24 hours
Phospholipids, plasma
  180 to 320 mg/dl
Plasma renin activity
  Sodium-depleted, peripheral vein
    (upright position)
    18 to 39 years: 2.9 to 24 ng/ml/
      hour (range); 10.8 ng/ml/hour
      (mean)
    ≥ 40 years: 2.9 to 10.8 ng/ml/hour
      (range); 5.9 ng/ml/hour (mean)
  Sodium-replete, peripheral vein
    (upright position)
    18 to 39 years: ≤ 0.6 to 4.3 ng/ml/
      hour (range); 1.9 ng/ml/hour
      (mean)
    ≥ 40 years: ≤ 0.6 to 3 ng/ml/hour
      (range); 1 ng/ml/hour (mean)
Plasminogen, plasma
  Immunologic method: 10 to
    20 ng/ml
  Functional method: 80 to 120 U/ml
Platelet aggregation
  3 to 5 minutes
Platelet count
  Adults: 140,000 to 400,000/μl
Platelet survival
  50% tagged platelets disappear with-
    in 84 to 116 hours; 100% disap-
    pear within 8 to 10 days
Porphobilinogen, urine
  ≤ 1.5 mg/24 hours

Porphyrins, total
16 to 60 mg/dl of packed red blood cells
Potassium, serum
3.8 to 5.5 mEq/L
Potassium, urine
25 to 125 mEq/24 hours
Pregnanediol, urine
Males: 1.5 mg/24 hours
Nonpregnant females: 0.5 to 1.5 mg/24 hours
Postmenopausal women: 0.2 to 1 mg/24 hours
Pregnanetriol, urine
Males
≥16 years: 0.2 to 2 mg/24 hours
Females
≥16 years: 0 to 1.4 mg/hours
Progesterone, plasma
Menstruating women: follicular phase, <150 ng/dl; luteal phase, 300 ng/dl; midluteal phase, 2,000 ng/dl
Pregnant women: first trimester, 1,500 to 5,000 ng/dl; second and third trimesters, 8,000 to 20,000 ng/dl
Prolactin, serum
0 to 23 ng/ml
Prostate-specific antigen
40 to 50 years: 2 to 2.8 ng/ml
51 to 60 years: 2.9 to 3.8 ng/ml
61 to 70 years: 4 to 5.3 ng/ml
≥71 years: 5.6 to 7.2 ng/ml
Protein, cerebrospinal fluid
15 to 45 mg/dl
Protein, pleural fluid
Transudate: <3 g/dl
Exudate: >3 g/dl
Protein, serum
Total: 6.6 to 7.9 g/dl
Albumin: 3.3 to 4.5 g/dl
Alpha$_1$-globulin: 0.1 to 0.4 g/dl
Alpha$_2$-globulin: 0.5 to 1 g/dl
Beta globulin: 0.7 to 1.2 g/dl
Gamma globulin: 0.5 to 1.6 g/dl
Protein, total, peritoneal fluid
0.3 to 4.1 g/dl
Protein, total, synovial fluid
<10.7 to 21.3 mg/dl
Protein, urine
≤150 mg/24 hours
Protein C, plasma
70% to 140%
Prothrombin consumption
20 seconds

Prothrombin time
10 to 14 seconds; International Normalized Ratio for patients on warfarin therapy, 2.0 to 3.0 (those with prosthetic heart valves, 2.5 to 3.5)
Protoporphyrins
16 to 60 mg/dl
Pyruvate kinase
Ultraviolet: 9 to 22 U/g of hemoglobin
Low substrate assay: 1.7 to 6.8 U/g of hemoglobin
Pyruvic acid, blood
0.08 to 0.16 mEq/L

R
Red blood cell count
Males: 4.5 to 6.2 million/µl venous blood
Females: 4.2 to 5.4 million/µl venous blood
Red blood cell survival time
25 to 35 days
Red blood cells, pleural fluid
Transudate: few
Exudate: variable
Red blood cells, urine
0 to 3 per high-power field
Red cell indices
Mean corpuscular volume: 84 to 99 fl
Mean corpuscular hemoglobin: 26 to 32 fl
Mean corpuscular hemoglobin concentration: 30 to 36 g/dl
Respiratory syncytial virus antibodies, serum
Negative
Reticulocyte count
Adults: 0.5% to 2% of total red blood cell count
Rheumatoid factor, serum
Negative or titer <1:20
Ribonucleoprotein antibodies
Negative
Rubella antibodies, serum
Titer of 1:8 or less indicates little or no immunity

S
Semen analysis
Volume: 0.7 to 6.5 ml
pH: 7.3 to 7.9
Liquefaction: within 20 minutes
Sperm: 20 million to 150 million/ml
Sickle cell test
Negative

Sjögren's antibodies
Negative
Sodium, serum
135 to 145 mEq/L
Sodium, sweat
10 to 30 mEq/L
Sodium, urine
30 to 280 mEq/24 hours
Sodium chloride, urine
5 to 20 g/24 hours
Sporotrichosis antibody, serum
Normal titers <1:40
Synovial fluid
Color: colorless to pale yellow
Clarity: clear
Quantity (in knee): 0.3 to 3.5 ml
Viscosity: 5.7 to 1,160
pH: 7.2 to 7.4
Mucin clot: good
Pao$_2$: 40 to 80 mm Hg
Paco$_2$: 40 to 60 mm Hg

T
Terminal deoxynucleotidyl transferase, serum
<2% in bone marrow; undetectable in blood
Testosterone, plasma or serum
Males: 300 to 1,200 ng/dl
Females: 30 to 95 ng/dl
Thrombin time, plasma
10 to 15 seconds
Thyroid-stimulating hormone, neonatal
≤2 days: 25 to 30 µIU/ml
>2 days: <25 µIU/ml
Thyroid-stimulating hormone, serum
0 to 15 µIU/ml
Thyroid-stimulating immunoglobulin, serum
Negative
Thyroxine, total, serum
5 to 13.5 µg/dl
Thyroxine-binding globulin, serum
Electrophoresis: 10 to 26 µg thyroxine (binding capacity)/dl
Immunoassay: 12 to 25 mg/L (males); 14 to 30 mg/L (females)
T-lymphocyte count
1,400 to 2,700/µl
Tolbutamide tolerance
Plasma glucose drops to one-half fasting level for 30 minutes and recovers in 1 to 3 hours
Transferrin, serum
200 to 400 mg/dl
Triglycerides, serum
Males: 40 to 160 mg/dl
Females: 35 to 135 mg/dl

Triiodothyronine, serum
90 to 230 ng/dl

U

Urea clearance
Maximal clearance: 64 to 99 ml/minute
Uric acid, serum
Males: 4.3 to 8 mg/dl
Females: 2.3 to 6 mg/dl
Uric acid, synovial fluid
Males: 2 to 8 mg/dl
Females: 2 to 6 mg/dl
Uric acid, urine
250 to 750 mg/24 hours
Urinalysis, routine
Color: straw to dark yellow
Appearance: clear
Specific gravity: 1.005 to 1.035
pH: 4.5 to 8.0
Epithelial cells: 0 to 5 per high-power field
Casts: occasional hyaline casts
Crystals: present
Urine osmolality
24-hour urine: 300 to 900 mOsm/kg
Random urine: 50 to 1,400 mOsm/kg
Urobilinogen, fecal
50 to 300 mg/24 hours
Urobilinogen, urine
Males: 0.3 to 2.1 Ehrlich units/2 hours
Females: 0.1 to 1.1 Ehrlich units/2 hours
Uroporphyrin, urine
Males: 0 to 42 µg/24 hours
Females: 1 to 22 µg/24 hours
Uroporphyrinogen I synthase
≥7 nmol/second/L

V

Vanillylmandelic acid, urine
0.7 to 6.8 mg/24 hours
Venereal Disease Research Laboratory test, cerebrospinal fluid
Negative
Venereal Disease Research Laboratory test, serum
Negative
Vitamin A, serum
Adults: 30 to 95 µg/dl
Vitamin B_1, urine
100 to 200 µg/24 hours
Vitamin B_2, urine
0.9 to 1.3 activity index
Vitamin B_6 (tryptophan), urine
<50 µg/24 hours
Vitamin B_{12}, serum

Adults: 200 to 900 pg/ml
Vitamin C, plasma
≥0.3 mg/dl
Vitamin C, urine
30 mg/24 hours
Vitamin D_3, serum
10 to 55 ng/ml

WXY

White blood cell count, blood
4,000 to 10,000/µl
White blood cell count, cerebrospinal fluid
0 to 5/µl
White blood cell count, peritoneal fluid
<300/µl
White blood cell count, pleural fluid
Transudate: few
Exudate: many (may be purulent)
White blood cell count, synovial fluid
0 to 200/µl
White blood cell count, urine
0 to 4 per high-power field
White blood cell differential, blood
Adults
Neutrophils: 47.6% to 76.8%
Lymphocytes: 16.2% to 43%
Monocytes: 0.6% to 9.6%
Eosinophils: 0.3% to 7%
Basophils: 0.3% to 2%
White blood cell differential, synovial fluid
Lymphocytes: 0 to 78/µl
Monocytes: 0 to 71/µl
Clasmatocytes: 0 to 26/µl
Polymorphonuclears: 0 to 25/µl
Other phagocytes: 0 to 21/µl
Synovial lining cells: 0 to 12/µl
Whole blood clotting time
5 to 15 minutes

Z

Zinc, serum
60 to 150 µg/dl

Index

A

Abdominal aortic aneurysm repair, 328-336
  bleeding related to, 333
  breathing pattern and, 332-333
  complications of, 329, 333-334
  decreased cardiac output and, 331-332
  description of, 328
  diagnostic studies for, 329
  discharge checklist for, 335
  documentation checklist for, 335
  DRG information for, 328
  knowledge deficit and, 330-331
  nursing history for, 328
  pain and, 335
  physical findings in, 328-329
  precipitating factors for, 328
  teaching checklist for, 335
  techniques used for, 328
Abdominal breathing, benefits of, 792
Abdominal pain, surgery and, 155
Abdominal trauma, interventions for, 587. *See also* Trauma, multiple.
Absolute granulocyte count, calculating, 793
Access to health care, 4
ACE inhibitors. *See* Angiotensin-converting enzyme inhibitors.
Acetaminophen overdose, 182t
Acid-base imbalances, 848t
Acidosis, diabetic ketoacidosis and, 641-642
Acquired immunodeficiency syndrome, 732-754
  categories of, 732
  complications of, 735
  confusion and, 743-744
  coping and, 740-742
  definition of, 732
  diagnostic criteria for, 735
  diagnostic studies for, 734-736
  discharge checklist for, 754
  disorders associated with, 732-733
  documentation checklist for, 754
  DRG information for, 732
  fluid volume deficit and, 748
  home care of patient with, 753
  hypoxemia and, 742-743
  infection and, 736-740

Acquired immunodeficiency syndrome (*continued*)
  knowledge deficit and, 752-754
  lymphocyte categories in, 733t
  nursing history for, 733-734
  nutritional deficit and, 747-748
  oral mucous membrane and, 749-750
  physical findings in, 734
  physical mobility and, 746-747
  precipitating factors for, 733
  resources for, 746
  sexual dysfunction and, 751
  skin integrity and, 750
  social isolation and, 745-746
  teaching checklist for, 754
  transmission of, 733, 745
  treatment of, 733
Acquired immunodeficiency syndrome-related complications, signs and symptoms of, 752
Activated charcoal, 186
Activity intolerance
  anemia and, 761-762
  angina and, 360-361
  cancer and, 58-59
  cardiogenic shock and, 389-390
  chronic obstructive pulmonary disease and, 276-277
  heart failure and, 416-418
  leukemia and, 778-780
  obesity and, 663
Acute alcohol withdrawal, 24-31
  complications of, 26
  diagnostic studies for, 25-26
  discharge checklist for, 30
  documentation checklist for, 31
  etiology of, 24
  injury and, 26-28
  nursing history for, 24-25
  nutritional deficit and, 28-29
  physical findings in, 25
  precipitating factors for, 24
  sensory perception and, 29-30
  signs of, 24
  teaching checklist for, 30-31
  thought processes and, 30
  time focus for, 24
Acute coronary syndrome, 355

Acute pain, 32-39. *See also* Chronic pain.
  abdominal aortic aneurysm repair and, 335
  amputation and, 552-553
  analgesic regimen for, 35
  angina and, 357-358
  behavior control strategies for, 36
  cholecystectomy and, 527-528
  complications of, 33
  diagnostic studies for, 32
  discharge checklist for, 39
  disseminated intravascular coagulation and, 769
  documentation checklist for, 39
  dying and, 86-87
  etiology of, 32
  femoral popliteal bypass and, 409
  hysterectomy and, 808-809
  indicators of, 33
  laminectomy and, 211-212
  major burns and, 576
  management of, 32, 35
  myocardial infarction and, 344, 346
  nephrectomy and, 709
  nonpharmacologic control strategies for, 35-36
  nursing history for, 32
  osteomyelitis and, 595-596
  pancreatitis and, 544-545
  percutaneous transluminal coronary angioplasty and, 437-438
  physical findings in, 32
  pneumonia and, 303-304
  precipitating factors for, 32
  preparing patient for, 34
  prostatectomy and, 832-833
  rating systems for, 33, 34i
  renal dialysis and, 717, 721-722
  surgery and, 149
  teaching checklist for, 39
  thrombophlebitis and, 462
  urolithiasis and, 725-726
Acute renal failure, 668-679. *See also* Chronic renal failure.
  as abdominal aortic aneurysm repair complication, 334
  complications of, 670
  definition of, 668

i refers to an illustration; t refers to a table.

Index

Acute renal failure *(continued)*
  diagnostic studies for, 669-670
  discharge checklist for, 678
  documentation checklist for, 679
  DRG information for, 668
  electrolyte imbalance and, 671-672
  etiology of, 668
  fluid volume excess and, 672-673
  hypovolemic shock as cause of, 430
  infection and, 676-677
  injury related to, 674-676
  knowledge deficit and, 678
  nursing history for, 668-669
  nutritional deficit and, 677-678
  physical findings in, 669
  as septic shock complication, 457
  signs and symptoms of, 430
  stages of, 668
  teaching checklist for, 679
Acute respiratory distress syndrome, 252-258
  chemical mediators involved in, 252
  clinical features of, 252
  complications of, 253
  definition of, 252
  diagnostic studies for, 252-253
  discharge checklist for, 258
  documentation checklist for, 258
  DRG information for, 252
  etiology of, 252
  hypovolemic shock as complication of, 430
  hypoxemia and, 253-256
  ineffective coping and, 257-258
  nursing history for, 252
  organ failure related to, 256-257
  physical findings in, 252
  septic shock as risk factor for, 455
  signs and symptoms of, 254
  teaching checklist for, 258
Adenocarcinomas, 48. *See also* Cancer.
Advance directive, 79-80
Advanced practice nursing, 8
Aging. *See also* Geriatric patient.
  changes associated with, 92
  cognitive decline and, 162
Aging population, health care delivery and, 3
AIDS. *See* Acquired immunodeficiency syndrome.
Air embolism
  as dialysis complication, 715
  signs and symptoms of, 513
Airway clearance, ineffective
  impaired physical mobility and, 113-115
  drug overdose and, 184-185
  mechanical ventilation and, 288-289

Airway clearance, ineffective *(continued)*
  seizures and, 230-231
  stroke and, 241-242
Albumin level, nutritional assessment and, 139
Alcohol overdose, 182t
Alcohol withdrawal delirium, 24. *See also* Acute alcohol withdrawal.
Alcohol withdrawal syndrome, indications of, 547
Alkylating agents, 51t
Alternative care, 6
Alzheimer's disease, 160-169
  caregiver role strain and, 168-169
  complications of, 161
  confusion and, 162-165
  constipation and, 167-168
  definition of, 160
  diagnostic studies for, 161
  discharge checklist for, 169
  documentation checklist for, 169
  DRG information for, 160
  etiology of, 160
  injury and, 166-167
  nursing history for, 160-161
  nutrition and, 165-166
  physical findings in, 161
  stages of, 164t
  teaching checklist for, 169
Aminoglycosides, minimizing adverse effects of, 599t
Amputation, 550-558
  body image disturbance and, 556-557
  complications of, 551
  definition of, 550
  diagnostic studies for, 550-551
  discharge checklist for, 557
  disuse syndrome and, 554-556
  documentation checklist for, 558
  DRG information for, 550
  hemorrhage and, 551-552
  infection and, 553-554
  muscle-strengthening exercises for, 555
  nursing history for, 550
  pain and, 552-553
  physical findings in, 550
  precipitating factors for, 550
  teaching checklist for, 557-558
Amrinone, 389
Anemia, 755-763
  activity intolerance and, 761-762
  as chronic renal failure complication, 686-687
  classifying, 755
  complications of, 756
  diagnostic studies for, 756
  discharge checklist for, 762-763

Anemia *(continued)*
  documentation checklist for, 763
  DRG information for, 755
  etiology of, 755
  hopelessness and, 762
  hypoxemia and, 757-758
  nursing history for, 755-756
  nutritional deficit and, 758-760
  physical findings in, 756
  precipitating factors for, 755
  skin integrity and, 760-761
  teaching checklist for, 763
Angina pectoris, 355-365
  activity intolerance and, 360-361
  arrhythmias related to, 358-360
  chest pain in, 355, 357-358
  classifying, 355
  complications of, 356
  definition of, 355
  diagnostic studies for, 356
  discharge checklist for, 364
  documentation checklist for, 364
  DRG information for, 355
  drug therapy for, 359t
  etiology of, 355
  knowledge deficit and, 363-364
  myocardial infarction related to, 358-360
  nursing history for, 355-356
  physical findings in, 356
  precipitating factors for, 361
  teaching checklist for, 364
  therapeutic regimen management and, 361-363
Angioplasty as revascularization technique, 404
Angiotensin-converting enzyme inhibitors, 414
Anorexia, nutritional deficit and, 141-142
Antacids, 484
Antiarrhythmic agents, 348, 359-360
Antibiotic therapy, minimizing adverse effects of, 599-600t
Anticholinergics, 481
Anticoagulant therapy
  patient teaching for, 247-248
  as prophylactic measure, 116
  risk for complications related to, 311-312
  thrombophlebitis and, 461
Antidiarrheals, 481
Antiembolism stockings, 116, 151
Antiemetics, 480, 781
Antihyperlipidemic agents, 358, 359t
Antihypertensives, 686
Anti-inflammatory agents, thrombophlebitis and, 461
Antimetabolites, 51t

Antitumor antibiotics, 51t
Anxiety, 40-47
    cancer and, 52-53
    complications of, 41
    definition of, 40
    diagnostic information and, 42-43
    discharge checklist for, 46
    documentation checklist for, 46
    etiology of, 40
    fear of dying and, 43-44
    fear of unknown and, 43-44
    knowledge deficit and, 44-45
    levels of, 40
    nursing history for, 40-41
    percutaneous transluminal coronary
        angioplasty and, 433-434
    physical findings in, 41
    precipitating factors for, 40
    substance abuse or drug reactions
        and, 45-46
    teaching checklist for, 46
Aortic valve replacement, arrhythmias
        associated with, 370t. *See also*
        Cardiac surgery.
Appetite stimulants, 747
Aprotinin, 377
ARDS. *See* Acute respiratory distress
        syndrome.
ARF. *See* Acute renal failure.
Arrhythmias
    as inflammatory bowel disease com-
        plication, 500-501
    as myocardial infarction complication,
        348-349
    as permanent pacemaker insertion
        complication, 441-443
    risk for, angina and, 358-360
Arterial insufficiency, femoral popliteal
        bypass and, 406-407
Arterial pressure monitoring, standards
        for, 846
Ascites, liver failure and, 537-538
Aspirin, 345t
Asterixis, 535
Asthma, 259-266
    characteristics of, 259
    complications of, 261
    diagnostic studies for, 260-261
    discharge checklist for, 265
    documentation checklist for, 266
    DRG information for, 259
    etiology of, 259
    knowledge deficit and, 263-265
    nursing history for, 259-260
    physical findings in, 260
    pulmonary arrest and, 261-263
    status asthmaticus and, 261-263
    symptoms of attack of, 264
    teaching checklist for, 265-266

Asthma (*continued*)
    triggers for attacks of, 265t
    types of, 259
Atelectasis
    as nephrectomy complication, 710
    as thoracotomy complication, 324
Atherectomy, 363
Atherosclerosis
    as cause of carotid disease, 392
    risk factors for, 328
Autografts, 577, 602. *See also* Skin
        grafts.
Autotransfusion, 585

B
Bacteremia, 452
Barbiturate coma therapy, 196
Barbiturate overdose, 182t
Bathing self-care deficit, permanent
        pacemaker insertion and, 444-445
Bed rest
    effects of, on cardiovascular function,
        113
    liver failure and, 537
    pulmonary complications associated
        with, 114-115
    skin breakdown and, 117
    thrombophlebitis and, 460, 463
    venous stasis and, 417
Benzodiazepine overdose, 182t
Beta-adrenergic blockers, 345t, 358,
        359t
Biological response modifiers, 51t
Bladder perforation as dialysis compli-
        cation, 718-719
Bladder retraining, 244
Bleeding
    as abdominal aortic aneurysm repair
        complication, 333
    as anticoagulant and thrombolytic
        therapy complication, 312
Blood loss
    assessing, 489-490
    guidelines for, in multiple trauma, 586
Blood pressure lability, carotid
        endarterectomy and, 394-396
Blood products as fluid replacement
        therapy, 428, 490
Blood transfusion, 779
Body image disturbance
    amputation and, 556-557
    colostomy and, 474-475
    craniotomy and, 177-178
    hysterectomy and, 809
    ileal conduit urinary diversion
        and, 703
    lymphoma and, 799-800
    major burns and, 579-580
    mastectomy and, 819-822

Body image disturbance (*continued*)
    obesity and, 664-665
    permanent pacemaker and, 447
    skin grafts and, 608
Body mass index, calculating, 139, 656
Body temperature, imbalanced, surgery
        and, 156
Bone marrow transplantation, 783-786
Bowel function, maintaining, impaired
        physical mobility and, 100
Bowel ischemia as abdominal aortic
        aneurysm repair complication,
        334
Bowel perforation as dialysis complica-
        tion, 718-719
Bowel retraining, 244
Brain attack. *See* Stroke.
Brain tumors, seizures and, 232
Breast cancer, 812. *See also* Mastectomy.
    risk factors for, 812-813
Breast reconstruction, 820-821
Breathing, effective, measures to
        promote, 114
Breathing pattern, ineffective
    abdominal aortic aneurysm repair
        and, 332-333
    cholecystectomy and, 529-530
    chronic obstructive pulmonary
        disease and, 274-275
    renal dialysis and, 719-720
Breathing strategies for coughing
        episode, 264
Bricker procedure. *See* Ileal conduit
        urinary diversion.
Bronchopleural fistula as pneumonecto-
        my complication, 325
Bullet wounds, 588
Bundle-branch block as myocardial
        infarction complication, 350-351
Burns, major, 567-581
    body image disturbance and, 579-580
    classifying, 567
    complications of, 569
    definition of, 567
    diagnostic studies for, 568-569
    discharge checklist for, 580
    documentation checklist for, 581
    DRG information for, 567
    estimating area affected by, 567
    fluid volume deficit and, 572-573
    impaired gas exchange and, 570-571
    infection and, 574-575
    injury related to, 569-570
    nursing history for, 567-568
    nutritional deficit and, 578
    pain and, 576
    physical findings in, 568
    physical mobility and, 579
    precipitating factors for, 567

Burns, major *(continued)*
skin integrity and, 576-578
teaching checklist for, 580
tissue perfusion and, 573-574
treatment setting for, 567

C

Calcium channel blockers, 345t, 358, 359t
Cancer, 48-62
activity intolerance and, 58-59
anxiety and, 52-53
categories of, 48
complications of, 49
constipation and, 57
definition of, 48
diagnostic studies for, 49
discharge checklist for, 61-62
documentation checklist for, 62
hemorrhage and, 49-50, 52
incidence and prevalence of, 48
infection and, 53-54
nursing history for, 48
nutritional deficit and, 55-56
pain and, 53
peripheral neurovascular dysfunction and, 54-55
physical findings in, 48-49
risk factors for, 48
sexuality patterns and, 60-61
situational low self-esteem and, 59-60
sleep deprivation and, 59
staging, 48
teaching checklist for, 62
urinary elimination and, 57-58
Carcinomas, 48. *See also* Cancer.
Cardiac catheterization, 363
Cardiac glycosides, 387
Cardiac glycoside toxicity, 414
Cardiac index, 385
calculating, 369
Cardiac injury, blunt, signs of, in multiple trauma, 587
Cardiac output, decreased
abdominal aortic aneurysm repair and, 331-332
cardiogenic shock and, 387-389
heart failure and, 413-415
mechanical ventilation and, 291
Cardiac output monitoring, standards for, 847
Cardiac surgery, 366-381
arrhythmias associated with, 370t
cardiopulmonary bypass and, 366
clinical pathway for, 372-374t
complications of, 367
confusion and, 379
description of, 366
diagnostic studies for, 367

Cardiac surgery *(continued)*
discharge checklist for, 381
documentation checklist for, 381
DRG information for, 366
endocarditis risk and, 371, 374-375
fluid volume deficit and, 376-378
impaired gas exchange and, 378-379
interstitial edema and, 375-376
knowledge deficit and, 380
low cardiac output syndrome and, 368-371
nursing history for, 366-367
precipitating factors for, 366
teaching checklist for, 381
Cardiac tamponade
as chronic renal failure complication, 684-685
indicators of, 371, 587
Cardiogenic shock, 382-390
activity intolerance and, 389-390
complications of, 383
decreased cardiac output and, 387-389
definition of, 382
diagnostic studies for, 382-383
discharge checklist for, 390
documentation checklist for, 390
DRG information for, 382
etiology of, 382
impaired gas exchange and, 383-386
as myocardial infarction complication, 349
nursing history for, 382
physical findings in, 382
risk for, myocardial infarction and, 339, 342-343
risk for, pulmonary embolism and, 310-311
teaching checklist for, 390
Cardiopulmonary bypass, cardiac surgery and, 366, 375, 378
Caregiver role strain, Alzheimer's disease and, 168-169
Care plans, how to use, 16-18
Carotid angioplasty with stenting, 392. *See also* Carotid endarterectomy.
Carotid endarterectomy, 392-403
blood pressure lability and, 394-396
complications of, 394
cranial nerve injury and, 398-399
description of, 392
diagnostic studies for, 393-394
discharge checklist for, 402
documentation checklist for, 403
DRG information for, 392
impaired gas exchange and, 400-402
indicators for, 392
myocardial infarction risk and, 399-400
nursing history for, 392-393

Carotid endarterectomy *(continued)*
physical findings in, 393
teaching checklist for, 402
tissue perfusion and, 396-397
Cast care, 589
Cathartics, 186
Central venous pressure monitoring, 427
Cephalosporins, minimizing adverse effects of, 599t
Cerebral blood flow, promoting, after carotid surgery, 397
Cerebral hemorrhage, seizures and, 233
Cerebral ischemia
as abdominal aortic aneurysm repair complication, 334
increased intracranial pressure and, 192-196
risk for, craniotomy and, 173
Cerebral metabolism, increased, increased intracranial pressure and, 198
Cerebrospinal fistula, laminectomy and, 210-211
Cerebrovascular accident. *See* Stroke.
Cervical cancer, radioactive implant for, 838-844
complications of, 839
description of, 838
diagnostic studies for, 839
discharge checklist for, 843
disuse syndrome and, 841
documentation checklist for, 844
DRG information for, 838
injury related to, 839-841
nursing history for, 838-839
physical findings in, 839
sexuality patterns and, 842-843
social isolation and, 842
teaching checklist for, 843-844
Cervical cancer, risk factors for, 838. *See also* Cervical cancer, radioactive implant for.
Chemical burn, interventions for, 570. *See also* Burns, major.
Chemotherapeutic adverse effects, 49-50, 52, 53-55, 56-58, 60-61
minimizing, 801
Chemotherapeutic agents, 51t
Chest pain, angina and, 355, 357-358
Chest physiotherapy
as airway clearance measure, 114
asthma and, 263
Chest trauma, interventions for, 587. *See also* Trauma, multiple.
Chest tube, caring for, 322-323
Cholecystectomy, 524-532
breathing pattern and, 529-530
complications of, 525

Cholecystectomy *(continued)*
  description of, 524
  diagnostic studies for, 525
  discharge checklist for, 532
  documentation checklist for, 532
  DRG information for, 524
  hemorrhage and, 527
  infection and, 528-529
  nursing history for, 525
  nutritional deficit and, 530-531
  oral mucous membrane and, 531-532
  pain and, 527-528
  peritonitis and, 526
  physical findings in, 525
  precipitating factors for, 524
  teaching checklist for, 532
Cholecystitis, 524
Cholelithiasis, 524
Cholesterol levels, nutritional assess-
    ment and, 140
Chronic bronchitis, 267. *See also* Chron-
    ic obstructive pulmonary disease.
Chronic care, health care delivery and,
    3-4
Chronic obstructive pulmonary disease,
    267-280
  activity intolerance and, 276-277
  breathing pattern in, 274-275
  clinical features of, 267
  clinical pathway for, 270-272t
  complications of, 268
  definition of, 267
  diagnostic studies for, 268
  discharge checklist for, 279
  documentation checklist for, 280
  DRG information for, 267
  etiology of, 267
  impaired gas exchange and, 268,
    273-274
  knowledge deficit and, 278
  nursing history for, 267-268
  nutritional deficit and, 275-276
  physical findings in, 268
  sexuality patterns and, 279
  sleep pattern disturbance and,
    277-278
  teaching checklist for, 279-280
Chronic pain, 63-66. *See also* Acute
    pain.
  analgesic regimen for, 64-65
  cancer and, 53, 64-66
  characteristics of, 63
  complications of, 64
  controlling, 63, 64-66
  diagnostic studies for, 63
  duodenal ulcer and, 482-483
  esophagitis and, 482, 483-484
  etiology of, 63
  gastroenteritis and, 482, 483-484

Chronic pain *(continued)*
  inflammation and, 64-66
  inflammatory bowel disease and,
    504-505
  nursing history for, 63
  physical findings in, 63
  tissue or nerve injury and, 64-66
Chronic renal failure, 680-696. *See also*
    Acute renal failure.
  anemia related to, 686-687
  complications of, 682, 684-685
  creatinine ranges in, 682t
  definition of, 680
  diagnostic studies for, 681-682
  discharge checklist for, 695
  documentation checklist for, 696
  DRG information for, 680
  etiology of, 680
  hyperkalemia related to, 683-684
  hypertension related to, 685-686
  knowledge deficit and, 694-695
  noncompliance and, 692-693
  nursing history for, 680-681
  nutritional deficit and, 688-689
  oral mucous membrane and, 690
  osteodystrophy and, 687-688
  peripheral neuropathy and, 690-691
  physical findings in, 681
  sexual dysfunction and, 693-694
  skin integrity and, 691
  teaching checklist for, 695-696
  thought processes and, 692
Clinical Institute Withdrawal Assess-
    ment-Alcohol, revised, 27
Clinical pathways, 19-21
  benefits of, 19
  for cardiac surgery, 372-374t
  for chronic obstructive pulmonary
    disease, 270-272t
  as complement to care plans, 19
  contents of, 19-20
  for coronary artery bypass grafting,
    372-374t
  developing, 20
  elements of, 20
  evaluating effectiveness of, 20
  for gastrointestinal hemorrhage,
    494-495t
  goal of, 19
  implementing, 21
  for mastectomy, 814-815t
  for myocardial infarction, 340-342t
  for nonhemorrhagic stroke, 238-240t
  patient teaching and, 20
  for pneumonia, 300-301t
  for total joint replacement in lower
    extremity, 616-617t
  variances of, 20-21
Cocaine overdose, 183t

Cognitive impairment as dementia type,
    162
Collaboration, emphasis on, 6
Colloid solutions as fluid replacement
    therapy, 428, 572
Colostomy, 468-476
  body image disturbance and, 474-475
  construction of, 468
  description of, 468
  diagnostic studies for, 469-470
  discharge checklist for, 476
  documentation checklist for, 476
  DRG information for, 468
  duration of, 468
  flatulence and, 474
  irrigating, 473
  knowledge deficit and, 473
  location of, 468
  nursing history for, 468-469
  odor control and, 474
  precipitating factors for, 468
  sexual dysfunction and, 475
  skin integrity and, 472
  stomal necrosis and, 470-471
  stomal retraction and, 471
  teaching checklist for, 476
  types of, 468
Community-based programs, health
    care delivery and, 5
Compartment syndrome, 562, 592
Complementary care, 6
Complete heart block as myocardial
    infarction complication, 351
Compression balloon tubes, 491
Confusion, 71-77
  acquired immunodeficiency syndrome
    and, 743-744
  Alzheimer's disease and, 162-165
  cardiac surgery and, 379
  classifying, 71
  complications of, 73
  definition of, 71
  diagnostic studies for, 72-73
  as dialysis complication, 716
  discharge checklist for, 77
  documentation checklist for, 77
  geriatric patient and, 95-96
  long-term care and, 71
  nursing history for, 72
  physical findings in, 72
  physiological or psychological cause
    and, 73-77
  precipitating factors for, 71
  teaching checklist for, 77
Constipation
  Alzheimer's disease and, 167-168
  as chemotherapy adverse effect, 57
  factors that increase risk of, 120

Index

Constipation *(continued)*
impaired physical mobility and, 120-121
indications of, 121
multiple sclerosis and, 222-223
myocardial infarction and, 347
as narcotic analgesic adverse effect, 37t
surgery and, 155
Continuous positive airway pressure, 284
COPD. *See* Chronic obstructive pulmonary disease.
Coping with stress, anxiety related to, 44-45
Coronary artery bypass graft surgery, 363. *See also* Cardiac surgery.
arrhythmias associated with, 370t
clinical pathway for, 372-374t
Coughing as airway clearance measure, 114
Cranial nerve function, assessing, 398
Cranial nerve injury, risk for, carotid endarterectomy and, 398-399
Craniotomy, 170-180
body image disturbance and, 177-178
cerebral ischemia and, 173
complications of, 171
definition of, 170
diagnostic studies for, 171
discharge checklist for, 179
documentation checklist for, 180
DRG information for, 170
fluid volume deficit and, 177
imbalanced fluid volume related to, 176
infection and, 174-175
injury related to, 176
knowledge deficit and, 172-173, 178-179
nursing history for, 170
physical findings in, 170-171
precipitating factors for, 170
respiratory failure and, 175
surgical approaches for, 170
teaching checklist for, 179-180
Creatinine, ranges of, in renal failure, 682t
Creatinine height index, 139
CRF. *See* Chronic renal failure.
Critical care transfer criteria guidelines, 854
Crohn's disease, 498. *See also* Inflammatory bowel disease.
Crystalloid solutions as fluid replacement therapy, 428, 490, 572
Cultural diversity, health care delivery and, 2-3

Culture and sensitivity testing, obtaining specimens for, 452

D

Death, definition of, 78. *See also* Dying.
Decisional conflict, dying and, 79-80
Decortication. *See* Thoracotomy.
Deep breathing as airway clearance measure, 114
Deep vein thrombosis, common sites of, 459. *See also* Thrombophlebitis.
Dehydration
diabetic ketoacidosis and, 637
dying patient and, 87
hyperosmolar hypoglycemic nonketotic syndrome and, 647
Delirium tremens, 24. *See also* Acute alcohol withdrawal.
Dementia, 160
types of, 162
Diabetes mellitus, 624-634
clinical hallmark of, 624
complications of, 626
definition of, 624
diabetic neuropathy and, 632
diagnostic studies for, 625-626
dietary guidelines for, 628-629
discharge checklist for, 633
documentation checklist for, 634
DRG information for, 624
etiology of, 624
eye complications of, 632
home management of, 631
hyperglycemia and, 624, 626-629
infection susceptibility and, 631
knowledge deficit and, 629-632
nursing history for, 624-625
physical findings in, 625
renal and urinary complications of, 632
"sick day" management techniques and, 631, 642
teaching checklist for, 633-634
therapeutic regimen management and, 632-633
types of, 624
vascular complications of, 631
Diabetes neuropathy, 632
Diabetic ketoacidosis, 629, 635-643. *See also* Diabetes mellitus.
acidosis related to, 641-642
clinical features of, 635
complications of, 636
definition of, 635
diagnostic studies for, 636
discharge checklist for, 643
documentation checklist for, 643
DRG information for, 635
etiology of, 635

Diabetic ketoacidosis *(continued)*
hyperglycemia and, 638-640
hypovolemia and, 636-638
injury related to, 640
knowledge deficit and, 642-643
nursing history for, 635
pathophysiology of, 635
physical findings in, 635-636
teaching checklist for, 643
Diagnosis-related groups. *See also* Prospective payment system.
assignment of, 9-10
factors that affect success under, 10-11
role of, in delivery quality, 9-12
use of, 10
Dialysis, indicators for, 674, 675. *See also specific type of dialysis.*
Diarrhea as acquired immunodeficiency syndrome complication, 748
Diazepam, 231
DIC. *See* Disseminated intravascular coagulation.
Difficulty chewing and swallowing, nutritional deficit and, 140-141
Digestion of nutrients, nutritional deficit and, 142-144
Disseminated intravascular coagulation, 764-770
complications of, 765
definition of, 764
diagnostic studies for, 764-765
discharge checklist for, 769
documentation checklist for, 770
DRG information for, 764
etiology of, 764
hemorrhage and, 765-766
hypovolemic shock as risk factor for, 430
hypoxemia and, 767-768
ischemia and, 766-767
nursing history for, 764
pain and, 769
as pancreatitis complication, 546
pathophysiology of, 764
physical findings in, 764
septic shock as risk factor for, 457
signs and symptoms of, 430
skin integrity and, 768-769
teaching checklist for, 769
Distal symmetrical sensorimotor neuropathy as acquired immunodeficiency syndrome complication, 744
Distraction as pain-control strategy, 36
Distributive shock, septic shock as form of, 449. *See also* Septic shock.

Disuse syndrome
  amputation and, 554-556
  as cervical cancer treatment complication, 841
  impaired physical mobility and, 121-122
  interventions for, 121-122
  osteomyelitis and, 598, 600
Dobutamine, 371, 388
Dopamine, 371, 388, 389, 544
DRGs. *See* Diagnosis-related groups.
Drug overdose, 181-189. *See also specific drug.*
  airway clearance and, 184-185
  definition of, 181
  diagnostic studies for, 181, 184
  discharge checklist for, 189
  documentation checklist for, 189
  DRG information for, 181
  hopelessness and, 187-188
  multiple organ dysfunction syndrome and, 185-187
  nursing history for, 181
  precipitating factors for, 181
  teaching checklist for, 189
Drug resistance, 453
Duodenal ulcer, 477-486
  complications of, 479
  diagnostic studies for, 479
  discharge checklist for, 486
  documentation checklist for, 486
  DRG information for, 477
  etiology of, 477
  fluid volume deficit and, 480-482
  nursing history for, 477-478
  nutritional deficit and, 485
  pain and, 482-483
  physical findings in, 478
  teaching checklist for, 486
Durable power of attorney for health care, 79-80
Dying, 78-91
  anxiety related to fear of, 43-44
  decisional conflict and, 79-80
  discharge checklist for, 90
  documentation checklist for, 91
  family processes and, 87-89
  fear and, 80-81
  fluid volume deficit and, 87
  grieving and, 89-90
  nursing history for, 78
  pain and, 86-87
  physical findings in, 78
  powerlessness and, 82-83
  precipitating factors for, 78
  situational low self-esteem and, 83-84
  spiritual distress and, 84-85
  teaching checklist for, 90
Dyspnea, 309

E
Eating difficulties, nutritional deficit and, 140-141
Electrocardiogram monitoring, standards for, 846
Electrolyte levels, nutritional assessment and, 140
Electrolytes as component in parenteral nutrition, 512
Electromagnetic power sources, pacemakers and, 446
Emphysema, 267. *See also* Chronic obstructive pulmonary disease.
  subcutaneous, 320
Encephalopathy syndrome, liver failure and, 535
Endocarditis
  as cardiac surgery complication, 371, 374-375
  signs and symptoms of, 375
Endometrial cancer treatment. *See* Cervical cancer, radioactive implant for.
Endotracheal tube, monitoring position of, 288
Endovascular stenting, 328. *See also* Abdominal aortic aneurysm repair.
End-stage renal disease, 680. *See also* Chronic renal failure.
Enhanced external counterpulsation, 364
Escharotomy, 573
Esophageal varices, liver failure and, 538
Esophagitis, 477-486
  complications of, 479
  definition of, 478
  diagnostic studies for, 479
  discharge checklist for, 486
  documentation checklist for, 486
  DRG information for, 477
  etiology of, 477
  fluid volume deficit and, 480-482
  nursing history for, 478
  nutritional deficit and, 485
  pain and, 482, 483-484
  physical findings in, 478-479
  teaching checklist for, 486
Ethanol overdose, 182t
Evidence-based practice, 7

F
Falls, geriatric patient and, 96-97
Family coping, compromised, 67-70
  complications of, 67
  definition of, 67
  discharge checklist for, 70
  documentation checklist for, 70
  etiology of, 67

Family coping, compromised (*continued*)
  illness of family member and, 68-70
  multiple sclerosis and, 225-226
  nursing history for, 67
  pulmonary embolism and, 313-314
  teaching checklist for, 70
Family coping, ineffective, acute respiratory distress syndrome and, 257-258
Family processes, interrupted, dying and, 87-89
Fat embolism, 150
  as fractured femur complication, 563
  as total joint replacement complication, 615
  as trauma complication, 592
Fat emulsions, 516, 517
Fear
  dying and, 80-81
  gastrointestinal hemorrhage and, 493
  mechanical ventilation and, 293-294
  of unknown, anxiety related to, 43-44
Femoral artery occlusion, risk for, percutaneous transluminal coronary angioplasty and, 434
Femoral popliteal bypass, 404-410
  arterial insufficiency and, 406-407
  complications of, 405
  description of, 404
  diagnostic studies for, 405
  discharge checklist for, 409
  documentation checklist for, 410
  DRG information for, 404
  indicators for, 404
  nursing history for, 404-405
  pain and, 409
  physical findings in, 405
  physical mobility and, 408-409
  skin integrity and, 407-408
  teaching checklist for, 409
Fever, risk for, liver failure and, 536-537
Filgrastim, 776
First-degree atrioventricular block as myocardial infarction complication, 351
Fluid and electrolyte imbalance, 849-851t
  acute renal failure and, 671-672
  diabetic ketoacidosis and, 637-638
  hyperosmolar hypoglycemic nonketotic syndrome and, 647
  liver failure and, 537-538
  major burns and, 572
  as nephrectomy complication, 709-710
  pancreatitis and, 543
  parenteral nutrition and, 516
  renal dialysis and, 720
  seizures and, 232

t refers to a table.

Fluid loss, signs and symptoms of, 427
Fluid overload, signs and symptoms of, 97, 673
Fluid replacement therapy
  diabetic ketoacidosis and, 638
  hyperosmolar hypoglycemic nonketotic syndrome and, 647
  hypovolemic shock and, 426-428
  inflammatory bowel disease and, 501
  major burns and, 572-573
Fluid retention, mechanical ventilation and, 292
Fluid shifting
  liver failure and, 537
  pancreatitis and, 543
Fluid status, assessing, 414-415
Fluid volume deficit
  acquired immunodeficiency syndrome and, 748
  cardiac surgery and, 376-378
  craniotomy and, 177
  duodenal ulcer and, 480-482
  dying and, 87
  esophagitis and, 480-482
  gastroenteritis and, 480-482
  hypovolemic shock and, 425-426
  increased intracranial pressure and, 200-201
  laminectomy and, 213-214
  major burns and, 572-573
Fluid volume excess
  acute renal failure and, 672-673
  craniotomy and, 176
  heart failure and, 415-416
  increased intracranial pressure and, 201-203
  inflammatory bowel disease and, 501-502
  parenteral nutrition and, 518-519
Fluoroquinolones, minimizing adverse effects of, 600t
Fractured femur, 559-566
  classifying, 559
  complications of, 560
  diagnostic studies for, 559-560
  discharge checklist for, 565
  documentation checklist for, 565-566
  DRG information for, 559
  etiology of, 559
  injury related to, 562-564
  knowledge deficit and, 564-565
  nursing history for, 559
  physical findings in, 559
  preoperative complications related to, 560-561
  teaching checklist for, 565
Frank-Starling curve, 387
Frontotemporal dementia, 162

G

Gas exchange, impaired
  cardiac surgery and, 378-379
  cardiogenic shock and, 383-386
  carotid endarterectomy and, 400-402
  chronic obstructive pulmonary disease and, 269, 273-274
  hypovolemic shock and, 428-429
  major burns and, 570-571
  mechanical ventilation and, 282-288
  multiple trauma and, 584-585
  myocardial infarction and, 343-344
  obesity and, 659-660
  pulmonary embolism and, 309-310
  septic shock and, 455-456
  surgery and, 149-150
  thoracotomy and, 319-321
Gastric lavage, 186, 490
Gastroenteritis, 477-486
  complications of, 479
  definition of, 477
  diagnostic studies for, 479
  discharge checklist for, 486
  documentation checklist for, 486
  DRG information for, 477
  etiology of, 477
  fluid volume deficit and, 480-482
  nursing history for, 478
  nutritional deficit and, 485
  pain and, 482, 483-484
  physical findings in, 478-479
  teaching checklist for, 486
Gastrointestinal bleeding, mechanical ventilation and, 292. *See also* gastrointestinal hemorrhage.
Gastrointestinal hemorrhage, 487-497
  clinical pathway for, 494-495t
  complications of, 488
  diagnostic studies for, 488
  discharge checklist for, 496
  documentation checklist for, 496-497
  DRG information for, 487
  fear related to, 493
  hypovolemic shock and, 488-492
  injury related to, 492-493
  knowledge deficit and, 496
  liver failure and, 538
  nursing history for, 487
  physical findings in, 487-488
  precipitating factors for, 487
  teaching checklist for, 496
Geriatric patient
  caring for, 92-104
  changes associated with aging and, 92
  confusion and, 95-96
  definition of, 92
  discharge checklist and, 104
  documentation checklist and, 104
  injury and, 96-97

Geriatric patient *(continued)*
  nursing history for, 92
  nutrition and, 97-99
  physical findings in, 92-93
  physical mobility and, 99-100
  renal impairment and, 97
  situational low self-esteem and, 101-102
  sleep pattern and, 100-101
  social isolation and, 102-103
  spiritual distress and, 103-104
  teaching checklist and, 104
  thought processes and, 94-95
Glucose as parenteral nutrition component, 512, 515
Glucose levels, monitoring, 627, 639
Glycoprotein inhibitors, 345t, 358, 359t
Government regulation, health care and, 4
Graft-versus-host disease, 785
Granulocyte transfusion, 776
Grief. *See* Grieving.
Grieving, 105-109
  anticipatory, 105, 106-108
  complications of 106
  diagnostic studies for, 106
  discharge checklist for, 109
  documentation checklist for, 109
  dying and, 89-90
  etiology of, 105
  nursing history for, 105
  physical findings in, 105-106
  teaching checklist for, 109
  time focus for, 105
Guided imagery as pain-control strategy, 36
Gut lavage, 186

H

Hair loss as chemotherapy adverse effect, 60
Harris-Benedict equation, height-weight ratio and, 139
Head trauma. *See also* Trauma, multiple.
  interventions for, 586
  seizures and, 232
Health care
  changes in delivery of, 2-8
  evolution of, 4-5
Health patterns, categories of, 17
Health status, anxiety related to major change in, 42-43
Heart failure, 411-423
  activity intolerance and, 416-418
  classification of, by hemodynamic subsets, 387t
  complications of, 412
  decreased cardiac output and, 413-415
  definition of, 411

Heart failure *(continued)*
discharge checklist for, 422
documentation checklist for, 422-423
DRG information for, 411
etiology of, 411
fluid volume excess and, 415-416
knowledge deficit and, 418-420
as myocardial infarction complication, 349
nursing history for, 411-412
nutritional deficit and, 418
physical findings in, 412
teaching checklist for, 422
therapeutic regimen management and, 420-422
Height-weight ratio as malnutrition indicator, 139
Helicobacter pylori infection, treatment of, 483
Hemodialysis, 713
assessing site of, 674
Hemorrhage. *See also* Gastrointestinal hemorrhage.
amputation and, 551-552
cancer and, 49-50, 52
cholecystectomy and, 527
disseminated intravascular coagulation and, 765-766
as hysterectomy complication, 806
leukemia and, 777-778
lymphoma and, 796
as surgical complication, 324
Heparin therapy, 312
disseminated intravascular coagulation and, 766
Herniated disk, laminectomy and, 205-217
Heterografts, 577, 602. *See also* Skin grafts.
HHNS. *See* Hyperosmolar hyperglycemic nonketotic syndrome.
Histamine-2 receptor antagonists, 484
Hodgkin's disease, 789. *See also* Lymphoma.
staging classification for, 791t
Homans' sign, 460
Homografts, 577, 602. *See also* Skin grafts.
Hopelessness
anemia and, 762
drug overdose and, 187-188
Hormonal agonists/antagonists, 51t
Human immunodeficiency virus infection, 732. *See also* Acquired immunodeficiency syndrome.
preventing exposure to, 738
Humidification as airway clearance measure, 114

Hygiene self-care deficit, permanent pacemaker insertion and, 444-445
Hypercalcemia, 850t
breast cancer and, 822-824
Hyperglycemia
diabetic ketoacidosis and, 638-640
diabetes mellitus and, 624, 626-629
hyperosmolar hypoglycemic nonketotic syndrome and, 648
pancreatitis and, 543
parenteral nutrition and, 515
seizures and, 232
Hyperkalemia, 850t
as chronic renal failure complication, 683-684
Hypermagnesemia, 851t
Hypermetabolic state, nutritional deficit and, 142-144
Hypermetabolism, 143
Hypernatremia, 850t
Hyperosmolar hyperglycemic nonketotic syndrome, 645-650
clinical features of, 645
complications of, 646
definition of, 645
diabetes mellitus and, 629
diagnostic studies for, 646
discharge checklist for, 650
documentation checklist for, 650
DRG information for, 645
hyperglycemia and, 648
hypovolemia and, 646-648
injury related to, 649
knowledge deficit and, 649-650
nursing history for, 645
parenteral nutrition and, 516
physical findings in, 645-646
precipitating factors for, 645
teaching checklist for, 650
Hypertension as chronic renal failure complication, 685-686
Hypervolemia, 849t
Hypocalcemia, 850t
Hypoglycemia, 651-655
complications of, 652
as diabetes mellitus complication, 651
diagnostic studies for, 651
discharge checklist for, 655
documentation checklist for, 655
DRG information for, 651
injury related to, 652-653
knowledge deficit and, 653-654
nursing history for, 651
physical findings in, 651
precipitating factors for, 651
seizures and, 232
signs and symptoms of, 652
teaching checklist for, 655
treatment of, 653

Hypoglycemia unawareness, 651
Hypokalemia, 850t
as cardiac surgery complication, 376
Hypomagnesemia, 850t
Hyponatremia, 849t
Hypothermia blanket, precautions for, 198
Hypovolemia, 849t
diabetic ketoacidosis and, 636-638
hyperosmolar hypoglycemic nonketotic syndrome and, 646-648
percutaneous transluminal coronary angioplasty and, 435-436
as prostatectomy complication, 829-830
Hypovolemic shock, 424-431
complications of, 425
coping related to, 431
definition of, 424
diagnostic studies for, 425
discharge checklist for, 431
documentation checklist for, 431
DRG information for, 424
etiology of, 424
fluid replacement and, 426-428
fluid volume deficit and, 425-426
as gastrointestinal hemorrhage complication, 488-492
impaired gas exchange and, 428-429
injury related to, 429-430
as multiple trauma complication, 585
nursing history for, 424
as pancreatitis complication, 543-544
pathophysiology of, 424
physical findings in, 424
as risk factor for septic shock, 454-455
teaching checklist for, 431
as total joint replacement complication, 613-614
Hypoxemia
acquired immunodeficiency syndrome and, 742-743
acute respiratory distress syndrome and, 253-256
anemia and, 757-758
asthma and, 261
disseminated intravascular coagulation and, 767-768
lymphoma and, 791-793
myocardial infarction and, 343
pneumonia and, 299, 302-303
preventive measures for, 402
Hypoxia, seizures and, 232
Hysterectomy, 804-811
body image disturbance and, 809
complications of, 805, 806
description of, 804
diagnostic studies for, 805
discharge checklist for, 811

Hysterectomy *(continued)*
documentation checklist for, 811
DRG information for, 804
hemorrhage and, 806
infection and, 806-807
nursing history for, 804-805
pain and, 808-809
physical findings in, 805
precipitating factors for, 804
sexual dysfunction and, 810
surgical approaches for, 804
teaching checklist for, 811
thromboembolic phenomena and, 806
urinary retention and, 807-808
variations of, 804

I

Ileal conduit urinary diversion, 697-706
body image disturbance and, 703
care of, 699
complications of, 698
description of, 697
diagnostic studies for, 698
discharge checklist for, 706
documentation checklist for, 706
DRG information for, 697
indications for, 697
knowledge deficit and, 699-700,
703-705
nursing history for, 697-698
physical findings in, 698
postoperative peritonitis and, 700
sexual dysfunction and, 705
stoma ischemia and necrosis and, 701
stoma retraction and, 701-702
teaching checklist for, 706
urinary elimination and, 702
Illness and hospitalization as stressors,
ineffective individual coping and,
126-128
Illness of family member, compromised
family coping related to, 68-70
Immunomodulators, 51t
Immunosuppression, risk for infection
and, 53-54, 775-776
Incentive spirometry as airway clearance measure, 114
Individual coping, ineffective, 124-128
acquired immunodeficiency syndrome
and, 740-742
acute respiratory distress syndrome
and, 257-258
complications of, 125
definition of, 124
diagnostic studies for, 125
discharge checklist for, 128
documentation checklist for, 128
etiology of, 124
hypovolemic shock and, 431

Individual coping, ineffective
(continued)
leukemia and, 786-787
myocardial infarction and, 346-347
nursing history for, 124
physical findings in, 125
precipitating factors for, 124
septic shock and, 457-458
stress of illness and hospitalization
and, 126-128
teaching checklist for, 128
Infarct extension as myocardial infarction complication, 349
Infection, risk for
acquired immunodeficiency syndrome
and, 736-740
acute renal failure and, 676-677
amputation and, 553-554
cancer and, 53-54
cardiac surgery and, 371, 374-375
cholecystectomy and, 528-529
craniotomy and, 174-175
hysterectomy and, 806-807
increased intracranial pressure and,
196-198
inflammatory bowel disease and,
503-504
leukemia and, 774-777
lymphoma and, 793-794
major burns and, 574-575
osteomyelitis and, 596-597
parenteral nutrition and, 520-522
permanent pacemaker insertion and,
443-444
pneumonia and, 299
prostatectomy and, 830-831
renal dialysis and, 720-721
seizures and, 233
septic shock and, 451-453
skin grafts and, 606
surgery and, 152-153
thoracotomy and, 325-326
Infection control measures, 452
acquired immunodeficiency syndrome
and, 752
Inflammatory bowel disease, 498-509
arrhythmias and, 500-501
complications of, 500
definition of, 498
diagnostic studies for, 499-500
discharge checklist for, 509
documentation checklist for, 509
DRG information for, 498
etiology of, 498
fluid volume excess and, 501-502
infection and, 503-504
nursing history for, 498-499
nutritional deficit and, 502-503
pain and, 504-505

Inflammatory bowel disease *(continued)*
physical findings in, 499
sexuality patterns and, 508
skin integrity and, 506
sleep pattern disturbance and,
505-506
social isolation and, 507
teaching checklist for, 509
Injection sclerotherapy, 491
Injury, risk for
acute alcohol withdrawal and, 26-28
acute renal failure and, 674-676
Alzheimer's disease and, 166-167
craniotomy and, 176
diabetic ketoacidosis and, 640
fractured femur and, 562-564
gastrointestinal hemorrhage and,
492-493
geriatric patient and, 96-97
hyperosmolar hypoglycemic nonketotic syndrome and, 649
hypoglycemia and, 652-653
hypovolemic shock and, 429-430
increased intracranial pressure and,
203-204
major burns and, 569-570
mechanical ventilation and, 289-293
multiple trauma and, 586-588,
591-592
myocardial infarction and, 347-352
as narcotic analgesic adverse effect,
37t
osteomyelitis and, 597-598
pancreatitis and, 545-547
parenteral nutrition and, 511-513
percutaneous transluminal coronary
angioplasty and, 435
pulmonary embolism and, 308-309
radioactive implant for cervical cancer
and, 839-841
renal dialysis and, 716-717, 718-719
seizures and, 233-234
septic shock and, 456-457
surgery and, 151-152
Insulin reactions, 628, 640. *See also* Hypoglycemia.
Insulin shock. *See* Hypoglycemia.
Insulin therapy, 627-628, 639
Intake and output monitoring, standards
for, 846
Interstitial edema, cardiac surgery and,
375-376
Interstitial to intravascular shift, 849t
Intra-aortic balloon pump counterpulsation, 389
Intracoronary stenting, 363
Intracranial pressure, increased, 190-204
cerebral ischemia and, 192-196
complications of, 192

Intracranial pressure, increased
  (continued)
  craniotomy and, 173
  definition of, 190
  diagnostic studies for, 191-192
  discharge checklist for, 204
  documentation checklist for, 204
  DRG information for, 190
  etiology of, 190
  fluid volume deficit and, 200-201
  fluid volume excess and, 201-203
  head of bed position and, 195
  increased cerebral metabolism
    and, 198
  infection and, 196-198
  injury related to, 203-204
  monitoring, 193, 194
  nursing history for, 190
  physical findings in, 190-191
  respiratory failure and, 199-200
  teaching checklist for, 204
Intracranial pressure monitoring, standards for, 847
Intravascular stent placement, 404
Intravascular to interstitial shift, 849t
Intravenous antibiotics, minimizing
  adverse effects of, 600t
Ipecac syrup, 186
Ischemia as disseminated intravascular
  coagulation complication, 767

J
Job expectations, changes in, 6

K
Kaposi's sarcoma, 732
Ketone levels, monitoring, 639
Kidney stones. *See* Urolithiasis.
Knowledge deficit, 129-137
  abdominal aortic aneurysm repair
    and, 330-331
  acquired immunodeficiency syndrome
    and, 752-754
  acute renal failure and, 678
  angina and, 363-364
  asthma and, 263-265
  cardiac surgery and, 380
  chronic obstructive pulmonary
    disease and, 278
  chronic renal failure and, 694-695
  colostomy and, 473
  craniotomy and, 172-173, 178-179
  definition of, 129
  diabetes mellitus and, 629-632
  diabetic ketoacidosis and, 642-643
  discharge checklist for, 137
  documentation checklist for, 137
  fractured femur and, 564-565
  gastrointestinal hemorrhage and, 496

Knowledge deficit *(continued)*
  heart failure and, 418-420
  hyperosmolar hypoglycemic nonketot-
    ic syndrome and, 649-650
  hypoglycemia and, 653-654
  ileal conduit urinary diversion and,
    699-700, 703-705
  implementation of teaching plan and,
    134-136
  inappropriate teaching program and,
    132-134
  lack of modification in teaching and,
    136-137
  lack of readiness to learn and,
    130-132
  laminectomy and, 207-208, 215-217
  leukemia and, 773-774
  lymphoma and, 798-799
  myocardial infarction and, 353
  nephrectomy and, 708-709
  nursing history for, 129
  parenteral nutrition and, 519-520
  percutaneous transluminal coronary
    angioplasty and, 438
  perioperative routines and, 146-147
  permanent pacemaker insertion and,
    445-447
  pneumonia and, 304-305
  precipitating factors for, 129
  pulmonary embolism and, 312-313
  seizure management and, 234-235
  skin grafts and, 609-610
  stroke management and, 246-248
  teaching checklist for, 137
  teaching strategies for, 133t
  thoracotomy and, 317-319
  thrombophlebitis and, 463-464
  urolithiasis and, 728

L
Laboratory test results, quick-reference
  guide to, 855-858
Lactulose, 535
Laminectomy, 205-217
  cerebrospinal fistula and, 210-211
  complications of, 206
  definition of, 205
  diagnostic studies for, 206
  discharge checklist for, 217
  documentation checklist for, 217
  DRG information for, 205
  fluid volume deficit and, 213-214
  indications for, 205
  knowledge deficit and 207-208,
    215-217
  nursing history for, 205
  pain and, 211-212
  paralytic ileus and, 212-213
  physical findings in, 205-206

Laminectomy *(continued)*
  precipitating factors for, 205
  sensory and motor deficits and,
    208-209
  teaching checklist for, 217
  tissue perfusion and, 214-215
Left ventricular end-diastolic pressure,
  cardiogenic shock and, 384
Leukemia, 48, 771-788. *See also* Cancer.
  activity intolerance and, 778-780
  classifying, 771
  complications of, 773
  coping and, 786-787
  definition of, 771
  diagnostic studies for, 772-773
  discharge checklist for, 787
  documentation checklist for, 788
  DRG information for, 771
  etiology of, 771
  hemorrhage and, 777-778
  immunosuppression and, 783-786
  infection and, 774-777
  knowledge deficit and, 773-774
  nursing history for, 771-772
  nutritional deficit and, 780-781
  oral mucous membrane and, 781-783
  physical findings in, 772
  teaching checklist for, 787
  types of, 771
Level of consciousness as neurologic
  indicator, 193
Lewy body dementia, 162
Liver failure, 533-540
  complications of, 534
  definition of, 533
  diagnostic studies for, 534
  discharge checklist for, 540
  documentation checklist for, 540
  DRG information for, 533
  etiology of, 533
  fever related to, 536-537
  fluid and electrolyte imbalance and,
    537-538
  gastrointestinal hemorrhage and, 538
  hypovolemic shock as cause of, 430
  neurologic deterioration and, 535-536
  nursing history for, 533
  nutritional deficit and, 538-539
  physical findings in, 533-534
  as septic shock complication, 457
  signs and symptoms of, 430
  skin integrity and, 539-540
  symptoms of, 533
  teaching checklist for, 540
Liver, functions of, 533
Living will, 79-80
Lobectomy. *See* Thoracotomy.
Long-term care, growth in, 4-5
Loss, grieving as response to, 105-109

t refers to a table.

Low blood sugar. *See* Hypoglycemia.
Low cardiac output syndrome, risk for, cardiac surgery and, 368-371
Lumpectomy, 812. *See also* Mastectomy.
Lymphedema as mastectomy complication, 817-819
Lymphoma, 48, 789-801. *See also* Cancer.
  body image disturbance and, 799-800
  classifying, 789
  complications of, 790
  definition of, 789
  diagnostic studies for, 790
  discharge checklist for, 800-801
  documentation checklist for, 801
  DRG information for, 789
  etiology of, 789
  hemorrhage and, 796
  hypoxemia and, 791-793
  infection and, 793-794
  knowledge deficit and, 798-799
  nursing history for, 789-790
  nutritional deficit and, 797-798
  physical findings in, 790
  precipitating factors for, 789
  pruritus and, 795
  staging for, 791t
  teaching checklist for, 801

M

Magnesium as parenteral nutrition component, 512
Malignant hyperthermia, surgery and, 156
Malignant lymphoma, 789. *See also* Lymphoma.
Mastectomy, 812-824. *See also* Breast cancer.
  body image disturbance and, 819-822
  clinical pathway for, 814-815t
  complications of, 816-817
  definition of, 812
  diagnostic studies for, 816
  discharge checklist for, 824
  documentation checklist for, 824
  DRG information for, 812
  hypercalcemia and, 822-824
  indications for, 812
  lymphedema and, 817-819
  nursing history for, 813
  physical findings in, 813, 816
  teaching checklist for, 824
  types of, 812
Mean arterial pressure monitoring, 428
Mechanical ventilation, 281-296
  airway clearance and, 288-289
  complications of, 282
  definition of, 281
  diagnostic studies for, 281

Mechanical ventilation *(continued)*
  discharge checklist for, 296
  documentation checklist for, 296
  DRG information for, 281
  fear related to, 293-294
  impaired gas exchange and, 282-288
  injury related to, 289-293
  nursing history for, 281
  physical findings in, 281
  precipitating factors for, 281
  teaching checklist for, 296
  ventilatory weaning response and, 294-295
Mediastinal shift, excessive, as pneumonectomy complication, 325
Medicare, DRGs and, 9
Medication reactions, anxiety related to, 45-46
Memory, assessing, 75
Meningitis
  craniotomy as risk factor for, 175
  laminectomy as risk factor for, 210
Mental status examination
  acute alcohol withdrawal and, 27, 30
  confusion and, 74
  geriatric patient and, 94
Metabolic acidosis, 848t
Metabolic alkalosis, 848t
Metastatic calcifications as chronic renal failure complication, 687-688
Metered-dose inhaler, medication adverse effects with use of, 264
Midarm muscle circumference, muscle protein stores and, 139
myocardial infarction. *See* Myocardial infarction, acute.
Mitoxantrone, 222
Mitral valve repair or replacement, arrhythmias associated with, 370t. *See also* Cardiac surgery.
Morphine, 386
Motor deficits, risk for, laminectomy and, 208-209
Multi-infarct dementia, 162
Multiple organ dysfunction syndrome, drug overdose and, 185-187
Multiple sclerosis, 218-227
  complications of, 219
  constipation and, 222-223
  definition of, 218
  diagnostic studies for, 219
  discharge checklist for, 226
  documentation checklist for, 227
  DRG information for, 218
  etiology of, 218
  family coping and, 225-226
  incidence and prevalence of, 218
  nursing history for, 218-219
  physical findings in, 219

Multiple sclerosis *(continued)*
  physical mobility and, 220-222
  sexual dysfunction and, 223-224
  situational low self-esteem and, 224-225
  teaching checklist for, 226-227
Muscle protein stores, assessing, 139
Myocardial infarction, acute, 337-354
  as angina risk factor, 358-360
  cardiogenic shock and, 339, 342-343
  as carotid endarterectomy complication, 399-400
  clinical pathway for, 340-342t
  complications of, 338
  constipation and, 347
  definition of, 337
  diagnostic studies for, 338
  discharge checklist for, 354
  documentation checklist for, 354
  DRG information for, 337
  drug therapy for, 345t
  etiology of, 337
  hypovolemic shock as complication of, 430
  impaired gas exchange and, 343-344
  individual coping and, 346-347
  injury related to, 347-352
  knowledge deficit and, 353
  nursing history for, 337
  pain and, 344, 346
  physical findings in, 337-338
  as septic shock complication, 457
  signs and symptoms of, 360
  teaching checklist for, 354
Myocardial ischemia, indicators of, 370
Myocardial rupture as myocardial infarction complication, 350
Myoglobinuria as trauma complication, 592

N

Narcotic analgesics
  pain control and, 35, 38, 65
  preventing adverse effects of, 37t, 65
Nasotracheal suctioning, 303
Nausea and vomiting
  as chemotherapeutic adverse effects, 56
  as narcotic analgesic adverse effect, 37t
  surgery and, 157
Nephrectomy, 707-712
  atelectasis and, 710
  complications of, 708
  diagnostic studies for, 707-708
  discharge checklist for, 711
  documentation checklist for, 711-712
  DRG information for, 707

Nephrectomy *(continued)*
  fluid and electrolyte imbalance and, 709-710
  knowledge deficit and, 708-709
  nursing history for, 707
  pain and, 709
  paralytic ileus and, 711
  physical findings in, 707
  precipitating factors for, 707
  surgical approaches for, 707
  teaching checklist for, 711
Neurologic status
  assessing, 242, 396
  liver failure and, 535-536
Neurovascular damage
  interventions for, 209
  as total joint replacement complication, 614-615
Nitrogen balance, nutritional assessment and, 139
Nitroglycerin, 346, 358, 386
Nitroprusside sodium, 386, 389
Nitrosureas, 51t
Noncardiogenic pulmonary edema. *See* Acute respiratory distress syndrome.
Noncompliance, chronic renal failure and, 692-693
Nonnarcotic analgesics, pain control and, 35, 65
Non-nucleoside reverse transcriptase inhibitors, 739
Nonsteroidal anti-inflammatory drugs, pain control and, 65
North American Nursing Diagnosis Association terminology, 13-14, 852-853
Nosocomial infection, risk factors for, 450t. *See also* Septic shock.
Nucleoside reverse transcriptase inhibitors, 739
Nucleotide reverse transcriptase inhibitor, 740
Nurse-patient relationship
  changes in, 6
  pros and cons of, 7
Nursing education, increased need for, 7-8
Nursing Interventions Classification, 14
Nursing languages, 13-15
Nursing Outcomes Classification, 14-15
Nursing shortage, 6
Nutrition, imbalanced: less than body requirements. *See also* Nutritional deficit.
  acquired immunodeficiency syndrome and, 747-748
  acute alcohol withdrawal and, 28-29
  acute renal failure and, 677-678

Nutrition, imbalanced: less than body requirements *(continued)*
  Alzheimer's disease and, 165-166
  anemia and, 758-760
  cancer and, 55-56
  cholecystectomy and, 530-531
  chronic obstructive pulmonary disease and, 275-276
  chronic renal failure and, 688-689
  duodenal ulcer and, 485
  esophagitis and, 485
  gastroenteritis and, 485
  geriatric patient and, 97-99
  heart failure and, 418
  inflammatory bowel disease and, 502-503
  leukemia and, 780-781
  liver failure and, 538-539
  lymphoma and, 797-798
  major burns and, 578
  pancreatitis and, 547-548
  parenteral nutrition and, 514-518
  renal dialysis and, 722-723
  skin grafts and, 607-608
Nutrition, imbalanced: more than body requirements, obesity and, 660-661
Nutritional deficit, 138-144. *See also* Nutrition, imbalanced: less than body requirements.
  anorexia and, 141-142
  complications of, 138
  definition of, 138
  diagnostic studies for, 139-140
  discharge checklist for, 144
  documentation checklist for, 144
  eating difficulties and, 140-141
  hypermetabolic state and, 142-144
  inability to digest nutrients and, 142-144
  nursing history for, 138
  physical findings in, 138
  precipitating factors for, 138
  teaching checklist for, 144
Nutritional replacement methods, 143-144

O

Obesity, 656-666
  activity intolerance and, 663
  body image disturbance and, 664-665
  classifying, 656
  complications of, 656, 658
  definition of, 656
  diagnostic studies for, 658
  discharge checklist for, 665-666
  documentation checklist for, 666
  DRG information for, 656
  impaired gas exchange and, 659-660

Obesity *(continued)*
  nursing history and, 656-657
  nutritional excess and, 660-661
  physical findings in, 657-658
  physical mobility and, 662
  precipitating factors for, 656
  skin integrity and, 661-662
  social isolation and, 664
  teaching checklist for, 666
Opiate overdose, 183t
Oral antibiotic, minimizing adverse effects of, 600t
Oral hypoglycemics, 627
Oral mucous membrane, impaired
  acquired immunodeficiency syndrome and, 749-750
  cholecystectomy and, 531-532
  chronic renal failure and, 690
  leukemia and, 781-783
Organ donation, dying patient and, 85
Organ dysfunction syndrome, acute respiratory distress syndrome and, 256-257
Orthostatic hypotension, 152
Osteodystrophy as chronic renal failure complication, 687-688
Osteomyelitis, 594-601
  classifying, 594
  complications of, 595
  definition of, 594
  diagnostic studies for, 594-595
  discharge checklist for, 600-601
  disuse syndrome and, 598, 600
  documentation checklist for, 601
  DRG information for, 594
  etiology of, 594
  injury related to, 597-598
  nursing history for, 594
  pain and, 595-596
  physical findings in, 594
  repeat infection and, 596-597
  teaching checklist for, 601
Outpatient services, 4
Overflow incontinence, 154
Oxygen toxicity, 287

PQ

Pacemaker codes, 443. *See also* Permanent pacemaker insertion.
Pain medication for terminally ill patient, 53
Pain. *See* Acute pain *and* Chronic pain.
Pancreatic fistulas, 546
Pancreatitis, 541-548
  complications of, 542
  definition of, 541
  diagnostic studies for, 542
  discharge checklist for, 548
  documentation checklist for, 548

Index

Pancreatitis *(continued)*
  DRG information for, 541
  etiology of, 541
  forms of, 541
  hypovolemic shock and, 543-544
  injury related to, 545-547
  nursing history for, 541
  nutritional deficit and, 547-548
  pain and, 544-545
  physical findings in, 541-542
  teaching checklist for, 548
Paradoxical pulse, assessing, 685
Paralytic ileus, risk for
  hypovolemic shock and, 430
  laminectomy and, 212-213
  as major burn complication, 578
  as nephrectomy complication, 711
  septic shock and, 456
  surgery and, 155
Parenteral nutrition, 510-522
  complications of, 511
  definition of, 510
  discharge checklist for, 522
  documentation checklist for, 522
  DRG information for, 510
  fluid volume excess and, 518-519
  indications for, 510
  infection and, 520-522
  injury related to, 511-513
  knowledge deficit and, 519-520
  major elements monitored in, 512
  nursing history for, 510
  nutritional deficit and, 514-518
  physical findings in, 510-511
  teaching checklist for, 522
Parkland formula for fluid replacement, 572
Patient-controlled analgesia, 38
Patient education, changes in, 5
Patient satisfaction, evaluating, 5
Patient teaching
  implementing plan for, 134-136
  knowledge deficit and, 129-137
  modifying plan for, 136-137
  strategies for, 133t
Peak flow meter, asthma patient and, 264
PEEP. *See* Positive end-expiratory pressure.
Peer review organizations, 11-12
Penetrating wounds, interventions for, 588. *See also* Trauma, multiple.
Penicillins, minimizing adverse effects of, 599t
Percutaneous nephrolithotomy with ultrasonic lithotripsy, 724

Percutaneous transluminal coronary angioplasty, 363, 432-439
  anxiety related to, 433-434
  assessment guidelines for, 432
  complications of, 432
  description of, 432
  discharge checklist for, 439
  documentation checklist for, 439
  DRG information for, 432
  femoral artery occlusion and, 434
  hypovolemia related to, 435-436
  injury related to, 435
  knowledge deficit and, 438
  pain and, 437-438
  precipitating factors for, 432
  sheath removal after, 437t
  teaching checklist for, 439
Pericardial effusion as chronic renal failure complication, 684-685
Pericarditis
  as acute renal failure complication, 675
  as chronic renal failure complication, 684-685
  as myocardial infarction complication, 349
Perioperative care, 146-158
  body temperature imbalance and, 156
  discharge checklist for, 157
  documentation checklist for, 158
  impaired gas exchange and, 149-150
  infection and, 152-153
  injury risk and, 151-152
  lack of familiarity with hospital procedures and, 146-147
  nausea and vomiting and, 157
  pain and, 149
  postoperative paralytic ileus and, 155
  shock and, 147-148
  teaching checklist for, 157
  thromboembolic phenomena and, 150-151
  urinary retention and, 154-155
Peripheral neuropathy, chronic renal failure and, 690-691
Peripheral neurovascular dysfunction, risk for, cancer and, 54-55
Peripheral perfusion, indicators of adequacy of, 370
Peripheral stem cell transplantation, 783-786
Peripheral tissue perfusion, decreased, as abdominal aortic aneurysm repair complication, 334
Peritoneal dialysis, 713
  assessing catheter site for, 675

Peritonitis
  cholecystectomy and, 526
  as hysterectomy complication, 807
  as ileal conduit complication, 700
Permanent pacemaker insertion, 440-448
  arrhythmias as complication of, 441-443
  bathing self-care deficit and, 444-445
  body image disturbance and, 447
  complications of, 441
  description of, 440
  diagnostic studies for, 441
  discharge checklist for, 448
  documentation checklist for, 448
  DRG information for, 440
  hygiene self-care deficit and, 444-445
  indications for, 440
  infection and, 443-444
  knowledge deficit and, 445-447
  nursing history for, 440
  physical findings in, 440-441
  teaching checklist for, 448
Phantom limb pain, 553
Phantom limb sensation, 553
Phenobarbital, 232
Phenytoin, 232
Phosphorus as parenteral nutrition component, 512
Physical mobility, impaired, 111-123
  airway clearance and, 113-115
  complications of, 112
  constipation and, 120-121
  definition of, 111
  diagnostic studies for, 112
  discharge checklist for, 123
  disuse syndrome and, 121-122
  documentation checklist for, 123
  femoral popliteal bypass and, 408-409
  geriatric patient and, 99-100
  major burns and, 579
  multiple sclerosis and, 220-222
  multiple trauma and, 588-590
  nursing history for, 111
  obesity and, 662
  physical findings in, 112
  precipitating factors for, 111
  pulmonary embolism and, 115-116
  renal dialysis and, 717-718
  situational low self-esteem and, 122-123
  skin care and, 99
  skin grafts and, 607
  skin integrity and, 117-118
  stroke and, 243-245
  teaching checklist for, 123
  tissue perfusion and, 118-120
  total joint replacement and, 615, 618-619

---

t refers to a table.

Plant alkaloids, 51t
Platelet activation inhibitors, 358, 359t
Platelet transfusion, 778
Pleural effusion as thoracotomy complication, 324
Pneumocystis carinii pneumonia, 732, 742-743
Pneumonectomy, complications of, 325. *See also* Thoracotomy.
Pneumonia, 297-305
  clinical pathway for, 300-301t
  complications of, 298
  diagnostic studies for, 298
  discharge checklist for, 305
  documentation checklist for, 305
  DRG information for, 297
  etiology of, 297
  hypoxemia and, 299, 302-303
  infection and, 299
  knowledge deficit and, 304-305
  as liver failure complication, 536
  nursing history for, 297-298
  pain and, 303-304
  physical findings in, 298
  teaching checklist for, 305
  as thoracotomy complication, 325
Pneumothorax as thoracotomy complication, 324
Positioning as pain-control strategy, 36
Positive end-expiratory pressure
  acute respiratory distress syndrome and, 255
  as mechanical ventilation mode, 284, 287, 288, 289
Positive inotropic agents, 371, 388
Postpump lung. *See* Acute respiratory distress syndrome.
Posttrauma syndrome, risk for, multiple trauma and, 590-591
Postural hypotension, 152
Powerlessness, dying and, 82-83
PPS. *See* Prospective payment system.
Preoperative complications, risk for, fractured femur and, 560-561
Prospective payment system. *See also* Diagnosis-related groups.
  evolution of, 9
  nurse's role in, 11
Prostatectomy, 826-837
  complications of, 828
  definition of, 826
  diagnostic studies for, 828
  discharge checklist for, 837
  documentation checklist for, 837
  DRG information for, 826-837
  hypovolemia and, 829-830
  infection and, 830-831
  nursing history for, 826-827
  pain and, 832-833

Prostatectomy *(continued)*
  physical findings in, 827-828
  precipitating factors for, 826
  sexual dysfunction and, 835-836
  situational low self-esteem and, 836-837
  surgical approaches for, 826, 827i
  teaching checklist for, 837
  types of, 826
  urge urinary incontinence and, 834-835
  urinary retention and, 833
Prosthesis
  for amputated body part, 557
  dislocation of, 618
Protease inhibitors, 739
Protection, ineffective, severe immunosuppression and, 783-786
Protein malnutrition as infection risk factor, 453
Pruritus
  liver failure and, 540
  lymphoma and, 795
Pseudocysts, pancreatitis and, 546
PTCA. *See* Percutaneous transluminal coronary angioplasty.
Pulmonary arrest, risk for, asthma and, 261-263
Pulmonary artery monitoring, standards for, 846-847
Pulmonary artery wedge pressure monitoring, 385, 427
  standards for, 847
Pulmonary capillary hydrostatic pressure, 384
Pulmonary contusion, signs of, in multiple trauma, 587
Pulmonary edema as thoracotomy complication, 324
Pulmonary embolism, 306-314
  cardiogenic shock and, 310-311
  clinical features of, 306
  complications of, 307
  deep vein thrombosis as risk factor for, 463
  definition of, 306
  diagnostic studies for, 307
  discharge checklist for, 314
  documentation checklist for, 314
  DRG information for, 306
  etiology of, 306
  family coping and, 313-314
  as fractured femur complication, 563
  impaired gas exchange and, 309-310
  injury related to, 308-309
  knowledge deficit and, 312-313
  nursing history for, 306
  physical findings in, 306-307
  physical mobility and, 115-116

Pulmonary embolism *(continued)*
  risk factors for, 115
  risks associated with therapy for, 311-312
  signs and symptoms of, 116
  teaching checklist for, 314
Pulmonary infection, mechanical ventilation and, 292
Pulmonary status, factors that affect, 113
Pursed-lip breathing, benefits of, 792

R

Readiness to learn, knowledge deficit and, 130-132
Regional enteritis, 498
Reimbursement, reduced, 4
Reimplantation, maintaining severed body part for, 589
Relaxation techniques as pain-control strategy, 36
Remicade, 504
Renal calculi. *See* Urolithiasis.
Renal dialysis, 713-723
  air embolism and, 715
  breathing pattern and, 719-720
  complications of, 714
  confusion related to, 716
  description of, 713
  diagnostic studies for, 714
  discharge checklist for, 723
  documentation checklist for, 723
  DRG information for, 713
  fluid and electrolyte imbalance and, 720
  indications for, 713
  infection and, 720-721
  injury related to, 716-717, 718-719
  nursing history for, 713
  nutritional deficit and, 722-723
  pain and, 717, 721-722
  physical findings in, 713-714
  physical mobility and, 717-718
  teaching checklist for, 723
  transfusion reaction and, 716
  types of, 713
Renal impairment
  geriatric patient and, 97
  as pancreatitis complication, 546
Renin-angiotensin-aldosterone system, 414
Reperfusion injury, 407
Respiratory acidosis, 848t
Respiratory alkalosis, 848t
Respiratory distress
  mechanical ventilation and, 290-291
  thoracotomy and, 321-323

Index

i refers to an illustration; t refers to a table.

Respiratory failure, risk for
  craniotomy and, 175
  increased intracranial pressure and,
    199-200
Revascularization techniques, 404
Reversible ischemic neurologic deficits
    as indicator for carotid surgery,
    392
Right ventricular infarction as myocar-
    dial infarction complication,
    351-352

S

Safe sex practices, 751
Salicylate overdose, 183t
Sarcomas, 48. *See also* Cancer.
Sargramostim, 776
Second-degree atrioventricular block as
    myocardial infarction complica-
    tion, 351
Segmental resection. *See* Thoracotomy.
Seizures, 228-235
  airway clearance and, 230-231
  assessment guidelines for, 228-229
  classifying, 228
  complications of, 230
  definition of, 228
  diagnostic studies for, 229
  discharge checklist for, 235
  documentation checklist for, 235
  DRG information for, 228
  etiology of, 228
  increased intracranial pressure
    and, 203
  injury related to, 233-234
  knowledge deficit and, 234-235
  phases of, 228, 229t
  physical findings in, 229t
  precautions for, 203
  status epilepticus and, 231-233
  teaching checklist for, 235
Sengstaken-Blakemore tube, 491
Sensory deficits
  laminectomy and, 208-209
  multiple sclerosis and, 221
Sensory perception, disturbed
  acute alcohol withdrawal and, 29-30
  stroke and, 245
Septicemia, signs and symptoms of, 776
Septic shock, 449-458
  clinical features of, 449
  complications of, 451
  coping and, 457-458
  definition of, 449
  diagnostic studies for, 450-451
  discharge checklist for, 458
  documentation checklist for, 458
  DRG information for, 449
  etiology of, 449

Septic shock *(continued)*
  hypovolemic shock and, 454-455
  impaired gas exchange and, 455-456
  infection and, 451-453
  injury related to, 456-457
  nursing history for, 449
  pathophysiology of, 449
  physical findings in, 449-450
  signs and symptoms of, 454, 455
  teaching checklist for, 458
Sexual dysfunction
  acquired immunodeficiency syndrome
    and, 751
  chronic renal failure and, 693-694
  colostomy and, 475
  hysterectomy and, 810
  ileal conduit urinary diversion and,
    705
  multiple sclerosis and, 223-224
  prostatectomy and, 835-836
Sexuality patterns, ineffective
  cancer and, 60-61
  cervical cancer treatment and,
    842-843
  chronic obstructive pulmonary
    disease and, 279
  inflammatory bowel disease and, 508
Shock lung. *See* Acute respiratory
    distress syndrome.
Shock. *See also specific type.*
  multiple trauma and, 585-586
  surgery and, 147-148
Sinus bradycardia as myocardial infarc-
    tion complication, 351
Sites of care, 4-5
Situational low self-esteem, risk for
  cancer and, 59-60
  dying and, 83-84
  geriatric patient and, 101-102
  impaired physical mobility and,
    122-123
  multiple sclerosis and, 224-225
  prostatectomy and, 836-837
Skin breakdown
  risk factors for, 117
  signs and symptoms of, 117
Skin care, impaired physical mobility
    and, 99, 244
Skin-fold measurements, nutritional as-
    sessment and, 140
Skin grafts, 602-611
  body image disturbance and, 608
  caring for, 609
  complications of, 603
  definition of, 602
  diagnostic studies for, 603
  discharge checklist for, 610
  documentation checklist for, 610
  DRG information for, 602

Skin grafts *(continued)*
  infection and, 606
  knowledge deficit and, 609-610
  nonadherence of, 604-606
  nursing history for, 602-603
  nutritional deficit and, 607-608
  physical findings in, 603
  physical mobility and, 607
  precipitating factors for, 602
  teaching checklist for, 610
  types of, 602
Skin integrity, impaired
  acquired immunodeficiency syndrome
    and, 750
  acute renal failure and, 676
  anemia and, 760-761
  chronic renal failure and, 691
  colostomy and, 472
  disseminated intravascular coagula-
    tion and, 768-769
  femoral popliteal bypass and, 407-408
  impaired physical mobility and,
    117-118
  inflammatory bowel disease and, 506
  liver failure and, 539-540
  major burns and, 576-578
  obesity and, 661-662
  total joint replacement and, 619-620
Skin-test antigens as malnutrition
    indicator, 140
Sleep deprivation
  cancer, and, 59
  effects of, 100
Sleep pattern, disturbed
  chronic obstructive pulmonary
    disease and, 277-278
  geriatric patient and, 100-101
  inflammatory bowel disease and,
    505-506
Social isolation
  acquired immunodeficiency syndrome
    and, 745-746
  geriatric patient and, 102-103
  inflammatory bowel disease and, 507
  obesity and, 664
  radioactive implant and, 842
Speech deficits, stroke and, 246
Spinal cord injury, mechanisms of, 588.
    See also Trauma, multiple.
Spinal cord ischemia as abdominal aor-
    tic aneurysm repair complication,
    334
Spiritual distress, risk for
  dying and, 84-85
  geriatric patient and, 103-104
Squamous cell carcinomas, 48. *See also*
    Cancer.
Stab wounds, 588
Starvation, characteristics of, 143

Status asthmaticus, 259, 261-263
  signs of, 262
Status epilepticus, 231-233
Sterility as chemotherapy adverse
    effect, 61
Stimulation as pain-control strategy, 36
Stoma care
  for colostomy, 472
  for ileal conduit, 699, 701-702
Stoma ischemia as ileal conduit compli-
    cation, 701
Stomal necrosis
  as colostomy complication, 470-471
  as ileal conduit complication, 701
Stomal retraction
  as colostomy complication, 471
  as ileal conduit complication, 701-702
Stomatitis
  as narcotic analgesic adverse
      effect, 37t
  signs and symptoms of, 782
Streptokinase, 312
Stroke, 236-249
  airway clearance and, 241-242
  as cardiac surgery complication, 379
  cerebral injury related to, 242-243
  complications of, 237, 240
  definition of, 236
  diagnostic studies for, 237
  discharge checklist for, 248-249
  documentation checklist for, 249
  DRG information for, 236
  etiology of, 236
  as indicator for carotid surgery, 392
  inhibiting progression of, 243
  knowledge deficit and, 246-248
  nonhemorrhagic, clinical pathway for,
      238-240t
  nursing history for, 236-237
  physical findings in, 237
  physical mobility and, 243-245
  precipitating factors for, 236
  rehabilitation and, 248
  risk factors for, 236
  sensory perception and, 245
  signs and symptoms of, 248
  teaching checklist for, 249
  verbal communication and, 245-246
Stump care, 553-554
Subcutaneous emphysema, 320
Substance abuse, anxiety related to,
    45-46
Sucralfate, 484
Suctioning as airway clearance measure,
    114
Suicide potential, assessing, 110t, 125
Sulfonamides, minimizing adverse ef-
    fects of, 599t
Sundowning, 96

Superior vena cava syndrome, 792
Supraventricular arrhythmias as myo-
    cardial infarction complication,
    348
Surfactant, alveolar surface tension and,
    310
Surgery. *See also specific procedure.*
  complications of, 146
  diagnostic studies for, 146
  perioperative care and, 146-158
Synchronized intermittent mandatory
    ventilation, 283
Syndrome of inappropriate antidiuretic
    hormone, 202
Systemic vascular resistance, calculat-
    ing, 369

T

Tachypnea, 309
Tamoxifen, 822
Therapeutic regimen management,
    ineffective
  angina and, 361-363
  diabetes mellitus and, 632-633
  heart failure and, 420-422
Thoracoplasty. *See* Thoracotomy.
Thoracotomy, 315-326
  complications of, 316, 324-325
  definition of, 315
  diagnostic studies for, 316
  discharge checklist for, 326
  documentation checklist for, 326
  DRG information for, 315
  impaired gas exchange and, 319-321
  infection and, 325-326
  knowledge deficit and, 317-319
  nursing history for, 315
  physical findings in, 315-316
  precipitating factors for, 315
  respiratory distress and, 321-323
  surgical approaches for, 315
  teaching checklist for, 326
  types of, 315
Thought processes, disturbed
  acute alcohol withdrawal and, 30
  chronic renal failure and, 692
  geriatric patient and, 94-95
Thromboembolic complications, signs
    and symptoms of, 116
Thromboembolic phenomena, 116
  as cervical cancer treatment complica-
      tion, 841
  as hysterectomy complication, 806
  surgery and, 150-151
  as total joint replacement complica-
      tion, 614, 615

Thromboembolism
  thrombophlebitis and, 462-463
  as total joint replacement complica-
      tion, 615
Thrombolytic therapy, risk for complica-
    tions related to, 311-312
Thrombophlebitis, 459-465
  acute venous insufficiency and,
      460-461
  common sites for, 459
  complications of, 459
  definition of, 459
  diagnostic studies for, 459
  discharge checklist for, 464-465
  documentation checklist for, 465
  DRG information for, 459
  etiology of, 459
  factors that increase risk of recurrence
      of, 464
  as fractured femur complication, 564
  knowledge deficit and, 463-464
  nursing history for, 459
  pain and, 462
  physical findings in, 459
  signs and symptoms of, 116, 460
  teaching checklist for, 465
  thromboembolism and, 462-463
Tidalling, 322
Tissue perfusion, ineffective
  carotid endarterectomy and, 396-397
  impaired physical mobility and,
      118-120
  laminectomy and, 214-215
  major burns and, 573-574
Topoisomerase inhibitors, 51t
Total hip replacement. *See* Total joint
    replacement in lower extremity.
Total iron-binding capacity, nutritional
    assessment and, 140
Total joint replacement in lower extrem-
    ity, 612-621
  clinical pathway for, 616-617t
  complications of, 613-615
  description of, 612
  diagnostic studies for, 613
  discharge checklist for, 620
  documentation checklist for, 621
  DRG information for, 612
  nursing history for, 612-613
  physical findings in, 613
  physical mobility and, 615, 618-619
  precipitating factors for, 612
  rehabilitation plan for, 619
  skin integrity and, 619-620
  teaching checklist for, 620-621
Total knee replacement. *See* Total joint
    replacement in lower extremity.
Total lymphocyte count, nutritional as-
    sessment and, 139

t refers to a table.

Index

Toxins, seizures and, 233

Trace mineral deficiencies, signs and symptoms of, 518t

Tracheal trauma, mechanical ventilation and, 293

Tracheoesophageal injury, signs and symptoms of, 587

Transcutaneous electrical nerve stimulation, 38

Transferrin level, nutritional assessment and, 139

Transfusion reaction as dialysis complication, 716

Transfusion therapy for disseminated intravascular coagulation, 766

Transient ischemic attacks as indicator for carotid surgery, 392

Transurethral resection of the prostate, 826, 827i

Trauma, multiple, 582-593
  complications of, 583, 591-592
  diagnostic studies for, 583
  discharge checklist for, 592
  documentation checklist for, 593
  DRG information for, 582
  impaired gas exchange and, 584-585
  injury related to, 586-588
  nursing history for, 582
  physical findings in, 582-583
  physical mobility and, 588-590
  posttrauma syndrome and, 590-591
  precipitating factors for, 582
  shock related to, 585-586
  teaching checklist for, 592-593

Trauma bed, types of, 589

Tricuspid valve repair or replacement, arrhythmias associated with, 370t. *See also* Cardiac surgery.

Tricyclic antidepressant overdose, 183t

T-tube care, 528-529

Tube feedings, nursing measures for, 144

24-hour urine urea nitrogen excretion, protein catabolism and, 139

U

Ulcerative colitis, 498

Uremic syndrome as acute renal failure complication, 674, 676

Urge urinary incontinence, prostatectomy and, 834-835

Urinary diversion. *See* Ileal conduit urinary diversion.

Urinary elimination, impaired
  cancer and, 57-58
  ileal conduit urinary diversion and, 702
  impaired physical mobility and, 118-120

Urinary elimination, impaired *(continued)*
  stroke and, 244
  urolithiasis and, 726-727

Urine retention
  laminectomy and, 214-215
  hysterectomy and, 807-808
  prostatectomy and, 833
  signs of, 154
  surgery and, 154-155

Urokinase, 312

Urolithiasis, 724-729
  complications of, 725
  definition of, 724
  diagnostic studies for, 725
  discharge checklist for, 728-729
  documentation checklist for, 729
  DRG information for, 724
  knowledge deficit and, 728
  nursing history for, 724
  pain and, 725-726
  physical findings in, 724-725
  precipitating factors for, 724
  teaching checklist for, 729
  urinary elimination and, 726-727

Urostomy. *See* Ileal conduit urinary diversion.

V

Vaginal cancer treatment. *See* Cervical cancer, radioactive implant for.

Valsalva's maneuver, 417

Vancomycin, minimizing adverse effects of, 600t

Vascular access device
  caring for, 694-695
  types of, 774

Vascular dementia, 162

Vasodilators, 345t, 358, 359t, 371

Vasopressin, 490

Venous insufficiency
  acute, thrombophlebitis and, 460-461
  chronic, signs of, 461

Venous return, measures to promote, 115-116, 461, 464

Ventilators, types of, 282-284

Ventilatory weaning response, dysfunctional, mechanical ventilation and, 294-295

Ventricular aneurysm as myocardial infarction complication, 349

Ventricular arrhythmias as myocardial infarction complication, 348

Verbal communication, impaired, stroke and, 245-246

Vinca alkaloids, 51t

Visual field deficits, stroke and, 245

Vital sign monitoring, standards for, 846

Vitamin deficiencies, signs and symptoms of, 518t

Vomiting. *See* Nausea and vomiting.

WXYZ

Weaning from ventilator, 294-295

Wedge resection. *See* Thoracotomy.

Weight loss, assessing, 139

Wheezing, 309

Wong-Baker Faces Pain Rating Scale, 34i

Worrying, setting limits on, 44

Wound classification, 153

i refers to an illustration; t refers to a table.

PHP AND MYSQL® 24-HOUR TRAINER

INTRODUCTION xvii

▶ **SECTION I**   **GETTING STARTED WITH PHP**

LESSON 1   Setting Up Your Workspace 3

LESSON 2   Adding PHP to a Web Page 23

LESSON 3   Learning PHP Syntax 33

LESSON 4   Working with Variables 45

LESSON 5   Debugging Code 57

LESSON 6   Working with Complex Data 71

▶ **SECTION II**   **WORKING WITH PHP CONTROLS, FUNCTIONS, AND FORMS**

LESSON 7   Making Decisions 91

LESSON 8   Repeating Program Steps 107

LESSON 9   Learning about Scope 119

LESSON 10   Reusing Code with Functions 125

LESSON 11   Creating Forms 141

▶ **SECTION III**   **OBJECTS AND CLASSES**

LESSON 12   Introducing Object-Oriented Programming 161

LESSON 13   Defining Classes 167

LESSON 14   Using Classes 177

LESSON 15   Using Advanced Techniques 187

▶ **SECTION IV**   **PREVENTING PROBLEMS**

LESSON 16   Handling Errors 205

LESSON 17   Writing Secure Code 217

▶ **SECTION V**   **USING A DATABASE**

LESSON 18   Introducing Databases 227

LESSON 19   Introducing MySQL 239

Continues

LESSON 20   Creating and Connecting to the Database .263

LESSON 21   Creating Tables. 275

LESSON 22   Entering Data 295

LESSON 23   Selecting Data 313

LESSON 24   Using Multiple Tables 331

LESSON 25   Changing Data 343

LESSON 26   Deleting Data 361

LESSON 27   Preventing Database Security Issues. 387

▶ **SECTION VI** **PUTTING IT ALL TOGETHER**

LESSON 28   Creating User Logins. 399

LESSON 29   Turn the Case Study into a Content Management System. 419

LESSON 30   Creating a Dynamic Menu 443

LESSON 31   Next Steps. 461

APPENDIX   What's on the DVD?. 463

INDEX. 467

PHP and MySQL®

24-HOUR TRAINER

Andrea Tarr

John Wiley & Sons, Inc.

PHP and MySQL® 24-Hour Trainer

Published by
John Wiley & Sons, Inc.
10475 Crosspoint Boulevard
Indianapolis, IN 46256
www.wiley.com

Published by John Wiley & Sons, Inc., Indianapolis, Indiana

Published simultaneously in Canada

ISBN: 978-1-118-06688-1
ISBN: 978-1-118-17291-9 (ebk)
ISBN: 978-1-118-17293-3 (ebk)
ISBN: 978-1-118-17291-9 (ebk)

Manufactured in the United States of America

10 9 8 7 6 5 4 3 2 1

For general information on our other products and services please contact our Customer Care Department within the United States at (877) 762-2974, outside the United States at (317) 572-3993 or fax (317) 572-4002.

Wiley also publishes its books in a variety of electronic formats and by print-on-demand. Not all content that is available in standard print versions of this book may appear or be packaged in all book formats. If you have purchased a version of this book that did not include media that is referenced by or accompanies a standard print version, you may request this media by visiting http://booksupport.wiley.com. For more information about Wiley products, visit us at www.wiley.com.

Library of Congress Control Number: 2011932086

For my parents, who gave me the feeling that it was perfectly natural for a girl to have a passion for math.

CREDITS

ABOUT THE AUTHOR

 ANDREA TARR has been a programmer and IT manager for 30 years and now works for Tarr Consulting and 4Web Inc. writing custom extensions, templates, and websites with the open source content management system Joomla! She is currently a member of the Joomla Production Leadership Team and is active in the Joomla Bug Squad. Andrea was involved in the development of Joomla 1.6 and created the accessible administrator template Hathor. She wrote the first computerized library circulation system in the state of New Hampshire and holds a Master of Science in Information Technology from Marlboro College Graduate School.

ABOUT THE TECHNICAL EDITOR

 WIM MOSTREY has 10 years' experience in PHP development and is a long-time Drupal developer. He's passionate about enabling corporate, non-profit, and governmental organizations to switch to free and open-source software.

ACKNOWLEDGMENTS

Thanks to my executive editor, Carol Long, and my project editor, Charlotte Kughen, for their suggestions and helpfulness during this process.

Thanks to Jen Kramer for her inspiration, support, and encouragement in the writing of this book.

Thanks to Bob Ross and Karen Augusta for giving me a glimpse of their fascinating business and allowing me to use wonderful photographs from their website: www.augusta-auction.com.

Finally, thanks to Bill Tomczak, my fellow geek. Everyone needs someone they can turn to with the truly stupid questions.

CONTENTS

INTRODUCTION   *xvii*

SECTION I: GETTING STARTED WITH PHP

LESSON 1: SETTING UP YOUR WORKSPACE   **3**

Installing XAMPP   3
   Installing XAMPP on a Windows PC   4
   Installing XAMPP on Mac OS X   6
   Troubleshooting Your XAMPP Installation   8
   Configuring XAMPP   9
Installing Your Editor   11
Configuring Your Workspace   12
   Preparing a Place to Put Your Files   12
   Using Eclipse for the First Time   14
Try It   18
   Lesson Requirements   19
   Hints   19
   Step-by-Step   19

LESSON 2: ADDING PHP TO A WEB PAGE   **23**

Writing Your First PHP Page   23
Introducing the Case Study   25
Using echo and include   27
Try It   29
   Lesson Requirements   29
   Hints   30
   Step-by-Step   30

LESSON 3: LEARNING PHP SYNTAX   **33**

Picking a Formatting Style   33
Learning PHP Syntax   35
Entering Comments   39
Using Best Practices   40
Try It   40
   Lesson Requirements   41
   Hints   41
   Step-by-Step   41

LESSON 4: WORKING WITH VARIABLES   45

Introduction to Variables   45
Working with Text   46
    Working with the Concatenation Operator   48
    Working with String Functions   48
Understanding Different Types of Numbers   50
Working with Numbers   50
Changing between Text and Numbers   52
Try It   52
    Lesson Requirements   53
    Hints   53
    Step-by-Step   53

LESSON 5: DEBUGGING CODE   57

Troubleshooting Techniques   57
    Display Errors while Developing   57
    Common Issues   59
    Seeing What's What   60
Using Xdebug   61
    Configuring Xdebug   62
    Using Xdebug   66
Try It   67
    Lesson Requirements   68
    Hints   68
    Step-by-Step   68

LESSON 6: WORKING WITH COMPLEX DATA   71

Working with Arrays   71
Working with Logical Variables   73
Working with Constants   74
Working with Dates   74
    Time Zone Functions   74
    Date/Time Functions   75
Working with Built-in Functions   80
    $_GET   80
    $_POST   81
    Cookies   82
    filter_var()   84
Working with Objects   86
Try It   86
    Lesson Requirements   86
    Hints   86
    Step-by-Step   86

SECTION II: WORKING WITH PHP CONTROLS, FUNCTIONS, AND FORMS

LESSON 7: MAKING DECISIONS
91

If/Else — **91**
Basic If Statements — **91**
Comparison Operators for If/Else Statements — **94**
If/Else with Ternary Operator — **96**
Logical Operators — **97**
Switch Statements — **100**
Alternative Syntax — **102**
Try It — **103**
Lesson Requirements — **103**
Hints — **103**
Step-by-Step — **103**

LESSON 8: REPEATING PROGRAM STEPS
107

While Loops — **107**
Do/While Loops — **109**
For Loops — **110**
Foreach Loops — **112**
Continue/Break — **114**
Try It — **115**
Lesson Requirements — **115**
Hints — **115**
Step-by-Step — **116**

LESSON 9: LEARNING ABOUT SCOPE
119

Learning about Local Variables — **119**
Learning about Global Variables — **120**
Try It — **122**
Lesson Requirements — **122**
Hints — **122**
Step-by-Step — **122**

LESSON 10: REUSING CODE WITH FUNCTIONS
125

Defining Functions — **126**
Passing Parameters — **127**
Getting Values from Functions — **131**
Using Functions — **132**
Including Other Files — **137**
Try It — **137**
Lesson Requirements — **137**
Step-by-Step — **138**

LESSON 11: CREATING FORMS — 141

Setting Up Forms — 141
Processing Forms — 146
Redirecting with Headers — 153
Try It — 154
  Lesson Requirements — 154
  Hints — 154
  Step-by-Step — 154

SECTION III: OBJECTS AND CLASSES

LESSON 12: INTRODUCING OBJECT-ORIENTED PROGRAMMING — 161

Understanding the Reasons for Using OOP — 161
Introducing OOP Concepts — 162
  Objects and Classes — 162
  Extending Classes — 163
Learning Variations in Different PHP Releases — 163
Try It — 164
  Lesson Requirements — 164
  Hints — 164
  Step-by-Step — 164

LESSON 13: DEFINING CLASSES — 167

Defining Class Variables (Properties) — 168
Defining Class Functions (Methods) — 169
Try It — 173
  Lesson Requirements — 173
  Hints — 174
  Step-by-Step — 174

LESSON 14: USING CLASSES — 177

Instantiating the Class — 177
Using Objects — 178
Try It — 181
  Lesson Requirements — 182
  Hints — 182
  Step-by-Step — 182

LESSON 15: USING ADVANCED TECHNIQUES — 187

Initializing the Class — 187
Understanding Scope — 188
  Properties — 188
  Methods — 191
  Classes — 192

Understanding Inheritance 192
Understanding Static Methods and Properties 197
Try It 199
    Lesson Requirements 199
    Hints 199
    Step-by-Step 199

SECTION IV: PREVENTING PROBLEMS

LESSON 16: HANDLING ERRORS 205

Testing for Errors 205
Using Try/Catch 210
Try It 211
    Lesson Requirements 211
    Hints 212
    Step-by-Step 212

LESSON 17: WRITING SECURE CODE 217

Understanding Common Threats 217
Using Proper Coding Techniques 218
Try It 221
    Lesson Requirements 221
    Hints 221
    Step-by-Step 221

SECTION V: USING A DATABASE

LESSON 18: INTRODUCING DATABASES 227

What Is a Database? 227
Gathering Information to Define Your Database 228
Designing Your Tables 229
Setting up Relationships between Tables 229
Instituting the Business Rules 230
Normalizing the Tables 231
Try It 232
    Lesson Requirements 232
    Hints 233
    Step-by-Step 233

LESSON 19: INTRODUCING MYSQL 239

Using phpMyAdmin 239
    Creating Databases 241
    Defining Tables and Columns 244
    Entering Data 248
    Backing Up and Restoring 250

Learning the Syntax 253
  Literal Values 253
  Identifiers 254
  Comments 255
Try It 255
  Lesson Requirements 255
  Hints 255
  Step-by-Step 256

LESSON 20: CREATING AND CONNECTING TO THE DATABASE 263

Connecting with mysql/mysqli 263
Connecting with PDO 269
Creating the Database 270
Try It 271
  Lesson Requirements 271
  Hints 272
  Step-by-Step 272

LESSON 21: CREATING TABLES 275

Understanding Data Types 275
  Strings 275
  Numeric 277
  Date and Time 278
  Other Data Types 279
Using AUTO_INCREMENT 279
Understanding Defaults 280
Creating Tables in phpMyAdmin 281
Using .sql Script Files 283
Adding MySQL Tables to PHP 287
Try It 288
  Lesson Requirements 288
  Hints 289
  Step-by-Step 289

LESSON 22: ENTERING DATA 295

Understanding the INSERT Command 295
Executing MySQL Commands in PHP 297
Processing Data Entry Forms in PHP 302
Try It 305
  Lesson Requirements 305
  Hints 305
  Step-by-Step 306

LESSON 23: SELECTING DATA

313

Using the SELECT Command	314
Using WHERE	317
Selecting Data in PHP	319
Try It	321
Lesson Requirements	322
Hints	322
Step-by-Step	322

LESSON 24: USING MULTIPLE TABLES

331

Using the JOIN Clause	332
Using Subqueries	335
Try It	336
Lesson Requirements	336
Hints	337
Step-by-Step	337

LESSON 25: CHANGING DATA

343

Using the UPDATE Command	344
Updating Data in PHP	345
Using Prepared Statements	347
MYSQLI	348
PHP Data Objects (PDO)	350
Try It	352
Lesson Requirements	352
Hints	352
Step-by-Step	353

LESSON 26: DELETING DATA

361

Using the DELETE Command	361
Deleting Data in PHP	364
Try It	365
Lesson Requirements	365
Hints	366
Step-by-Step	366

LESSON 27: PREVENTING DATABASE SECURITY ISSUES

387

Understanding Security Issues	387
Using Best Practices	389
Filtering Data	391

Try It 393
    Lesson Requirements 393
    Hints 393
    Step-by-Step 393

SECTION VI: PUTTING IT ALL TOGETHER

LESSON 28: CREATING USER LOGINS 399

Understanding Access Control 399
Protecting Passwords 400
Using Cookies and Sessions 402
Putting Logins to Work 403
Try It 404
    Lesson Requirements 405
    Hints 405
    Step-by-Step 405

LESSON 29: TURN THE CASE STUDY INTO A CONTENT MANAGEMENT SYSTEM 419

Designing and Creating the Table 419
Creating the Class 420
    Properties 420
    Methods 420
Creating the Maintenance Pages 422
Creating the Display Page 422
Try It 425
    Lesson Requirements 425
    Hints 425
    Step-by-Step 425

LESSON 30: CREATING A DYNAMIC MENU 443

Setting up the Menu Table 443
Adding the Menu to the Website 444
Try It 445
    Lesson Requirements 446
    Hints 446
    Step-by-Step 446

LESSON 31: NEXT STEPS 461

APPENDIX : WHAT'S ON THE DVD? 463

INDEX 467

INTRODUCTION

PHP IS A POPULAR PROGRAMMING LANGUAGE that powers many websites. It originally started out as a way to make dynamic websites by generating HTML. Today it stands on its own as a general-purpose programming language and is available on most web hosting sites. Because of its roots, it is very easy to insert bits and pieces of PHP inside of standard HTML/XHTML code.

MySQL is a popular relational database management system. It is the standard database system available on web hosting sites. Although it works with many different programming languages, it is frequently paired with PHP.

WHO THIS BOOK IS FOR

This book is for beginners who have never programmed before or who have never worked with databases. It's also for those who have copied a few lines of PHP into their HTML pages and want to know more. General programming concepts are explained while you learn to program PHP and manipulate data with MySQL. If you already program other languages, this book may be too basic for you.

To get the most out of this book, you need to understand HTML and the basic concept of CSS. Much of the PHP that you do is aimed at creating HTML, so you need to know what you are trying to create.

WHAT THIS BOOK COVERS

This book teaches you to take a static website and turn it into a dynamic website run from a database using PHP and MySQL. You start by preparing your computer to run PHP and MySQL by downloading and installing free software. Next, you write your first PHP by including some PHP code on an HTML page. Then you dive into PHP, learning what variables are, how to work with them, and how to debug your programs. You learn how to have your programs make decisions and loop through code.

The modern PHP is object oriented. You learn what that means and how to use it to make your programs less buggy and error prone, and easier to maintain. Along with that you learn best practices and how to write secure code.

You learn how databases work and how to design one, as well as how to use phpMyAdmin to work with MySQL. You learn different ways of connecting to MySQL through PHP, and how to create tables, enter data, select data, change data, and delete data. Finally, you learn how to combine all of these things into creating a mini content management system with a dynamic menu.

PHP is a general-purpose language that isn't limited to running websites. However, this beginning book is concentrated on programming websites because that is a natural extension for those who have been coding in HTML and CSS. By the same token, database programming can be quite complex. This book teaches the fundamentals needed to work with databases and how to do it safely.

HOW THIS BOOK IS STRUCTURED

This book consists of short lessons, each focusing on a particular aspect of PHP and/or MySQL. The lessons are arranged in a logical order of study. Although you can study the lessons in any order, you often need to know what is taught in the early lessons before the later ones make sense. It is not meant as an exhaustive resource or as an in-depth look at technical aspects of the language. The goal is to teach you what you need to know in order to start using PHP and MySQL in your web pages and applications.

This book consists of 31 lessons, broken into six sections:

➤ **Section I, "Getting Started with PHP":** In this section you set up your computer to run PHP and MySQL. You learn the fundamentals of programming as you learn the fundamentals of programming in PHP.

➤ **Section II, "Working with PHP Controls, Functions, and Forms":** In this section you learn how to control what lines your programs will process and how to loop through repeating program steps. You learn about creating your own functions and how to process HTML forms.

➤ **Section III, "Objects and Classes":** In this section you learn what object-oriented programming is and why you want to use it. Then you learn how to use it.

➤ **Section IV, "Preventing Problems":** In this section you learn how to handle errors and how to write secure code.

➤ **Section V, "Using a Database":** In this section you are introduced to databases and how to design a database. You learn the basics of how MySQL works and then how to integrate it with PHP. You learn how to take static information on your HTML page and put it in a database and retrieve it.

➤ **Section VI, "Putting It All Together":** In this last section you take what you have learned and create user logins, a mini content management system, and a menu based on database information.

The lessons end with a tutorial called "Try It." Each tutorial applies concepts from the lesson.

A Case Study is used in most of the Try It sections. This Case Study starts as a static website created from HTML and CSS. As the lessons progress, you replace parts of it with PHP and MySQL until at the end you have a website that takes its information from a database that you maintain through pages on the website.

As you work through the Case Study, you start most Try It sections with the Case Study that you finished in the previous Try It section. However, at any time you can download the Case Study code as it should be at the beginning of each Try It section and also download the code as it should be at the end of the Try It section.

You can watch the DVD to see the Try It sections from the lesson done by the author. After you've finished reading the book and watching the DVD, you can visit Wrox's P2P forums, where your author offers support.

WHAT YOU NEED TO USE THIS BOOK

To get the best results from this book, you should perform the examples and do the Try It sections. In order to do that, you need the following resources:

➤ PHP and MySQL need to run on a web server. You have two options: You can turn your computer into a local web server or you can use an online web host that runs PHP 5.3 and MySQL 5. This book assumes that you will be running a local web server and the first lesson steps you through the process of downloading free software and configuring your computer.

➤ You need a text editor that can produce plain-text files. The first lesson shows you how to download and install the Eclipse PDT, which is a very helpful editor for writing PHP. However, other text editors such as Adobe's Dreamweaver in code mode, Notepad, TextWrangler, or NetBeans also work. A word processing program such as Microsoft Word does not work.

INSTRUCTIONAL VIDEOS ON DVD

Some people learn better with a visual and audio aid. That is why a DVD that includes a video tutorial for each lesson accompanies this book. So if seeing something done and hearing it explained help you understand a subject better than just reading about it, this book-and-DVD combination is just the thing for you.

CONVENTIONS

To help you get the most from the text and keep track of what's happening, this book uses a number of conventions.

Boxes like this one hold important, not-to-be forgotten information that is directly relevant to the surrounding text.

Notes, tips, hints, tricks, and asides to the current discussion are offset and placed in italic like this.

References like this one point you to watch the instructional video on the DVD with the print book or watch online at www.wrox.com/go/24phpmysql.

As for styles in the text:

➤ New terms and important words are *italicized* when introduced.

➤ Code appearing in text looks like this: `document.body`.

➤ URLs look like the following when inside text: `www.wrox.com`.

➤ Code blocks are presented in the following way:

```
A monofont type on its own line(s)
denotes code examples.
```

➤ Important or changed parts of code blocks are highlighted in the following way:

```
Some code examples have
sections that are highlighted which
illustrate different or key parts.
```

SUPPORTING PACKAGES AND CODE

As you work through the lessons in this book, you can choose to type the code and create all the files manually or you can use the supporting code files that accompany the book. All the code and other support files used in this book are available for download at `www.wrox.com`. On the site, simply locate the book's title (either by using the Search box or by using one of the title lists), and then click the Download Code link on the book's detail page to obtain all the source code for the book.

> *Because many books have similar titles, you may find it easiest to search by ISBN; this book's ISBN is 978-1-118-06688-1.*

After you download the code, just decompress it with your favorite compression tool. Alternatively, you can go to the main Wrox code download page at `www.wrox.com/dynamic/books/download.aspx` to see the code available for this book and all other Wrox books.

ERRATA

Every effort is made to ensure that there are no errors in the text or in the code. However, no one is perfect, and mistakes do occur. If you find an error in this book or any Wrox book for that matter, such as a spelling mistake or faulty piece of code, your feedback is appreciated. By sending in errata, you can save a reader hours of frustration, and at the same time, you can help your author and Wrox provide even higher-quality information.

To find the errata page for this book, go to `www.wrox.com` and locate the title using the Search box or one of the title lists. Then, on the Book Search Results page, click the Errata link. On this page, you can view all errata that have been submitted for this book and posted by Wrox editors.

> *A complete book list, including links to errata, is also available at* www.wrox.com/misc-pages/booklist.shtml.

If you don't spot "your" error on the Errata page, click the Errata Form link and complete the form to send us the error you have found. We'll check the information and, if appropriate, post a message to the book's Errata page and fix the problem in subsequent editions of the book.

P2P.WROX.COM

For author and peer discussion, join the P2P forums at p2p.wrox.com. The forums are a Web-based system you can use to post messages relating to Wrox books and related technologies and interact with other readers and technology users. The forums offer a subscription feature to email you topics of interest of your choosing when new posts are made to the forums. Wrox authors and editors, other industry experts, and your fellow readers are present on these forums.

At http://p2p.wrox.com you can find a number of different forums that help you not only as you read this book, but also as you develop your own applications. To join the forums, just follow these steps:

1. Go to p2p.wrox.com and click the Register link.

2. Read the terms of use and click Agree.

3. Complete the required information for joining as well as any optional information you want to provide and click Submit.

4. You receive an e-mail with information describing how to verify your account and complete the joining process.

> *You can read messages in the forums without joining P2P, but in order to post your own messages, you must join.*

After you join, you can post new messages and respond to messages other users post. You can read messages at any time on the Web. If you would like to have new messages from a particular forum emailed to you, click the Subscribe to This Forum icon by the forum name in the forum listing.

For more information about how to use the Wrox P2P, be sure to read the P2P FAQs for answers to questions about how the forum software works as well as many common questions specific to P2P and Wrox books. To read the FAQs, click the FAQ link on any P2P page.

SECTION I
Getting Started with PHP

- ▶ **LESSON 1:** Setting Up Your Workspace

- ▶ **LESSON 2:** Adding PHP to a Web Page

- ▶ **LESSON 3:** Learning PHP Syntax

- ▶ **LESSON 4:** Working with Variables

- ▶ **LESSON 5:** Debugging Code

- ▶ **LESSON 6:** Working with Complex Data

In this section, you learn the basics of working with PHP. In the first lesson, you learn what PHP requires on your computer before PHP will run. If your computer does not have the necessary software, you can use the instructions provided to download the free software, install it, and configure it to work. In the next lesson, you learn how HTML and PHP work together as you add your first PHP code to a web page. You are also introduced to the Case Study website you use throughout the book.

You learn in the third lesson about the syntax of PHP and how to write PHP statements. In the fourth lesson, you learn what variables are and how to use them. At this point, you will have learned enough to start making mistakes, so in the next lesson you learn about how to find your errors and debug your code. You need to know about debugging as you work with more complex data in the final lesson of this section.

1

Setting Up Your Workspace

Your computer needs to be able to run as a web server with PHP and MySQL. XAMPP is a package of software that installs the web server, PHP, and MySQL for you. You learn how to download and install XAMPP in this lesson.

If you already have a web server with PHP and MySQL running on your computer, you do not need XAMPP. Other packages that fulfill the same need are WAMPServer and MAMP.

You also need a text editor that can produce plain-text files. You learn how to download and install Eclipse PDT in this lesson. Some other text editors that you can use are Adobe's Dreamweaver in code mode, Notepad, TextWrangler, or NetBeans.

INSTALLING XAMPP

XAMPP stands for whatever operating system you have: (X), Apache (A), MySQL (M), PHP (P), and Perl (P). Separate packages are available for each of the different operating systems such as Windows, Mac OS X, or Linux. This lesson covers installing the Windows and Mac versions.

> *Perl is another programming language. It's popular for housekeeping tasks and for communications between different programs and programming languages. You won't need to use it for the lessons in this book.*

XAMPP is intended for local development work. It is not set up for running production websites.

Do not use XAMPP to host websites on the Internet. Although it uses the same building blocks as production hosts, it is not set up to be secure. You will get hacked if you try it.

Installing XAMPP on a Windows PC

This section walks you through downloading the proper XAMPP package and installing it on your Windows PC. If you have a Mac, skip forward to the section "Configuring XAMPP on Mac OS X."

1. Go to the Apache Friends website at `www.apachefriends.org/en/xampp.html`.

2. Locate the section labeled XAMPP for Windows and click the title. Scroll down to the Download section that lists the versions available for download. See Figure 1-1.

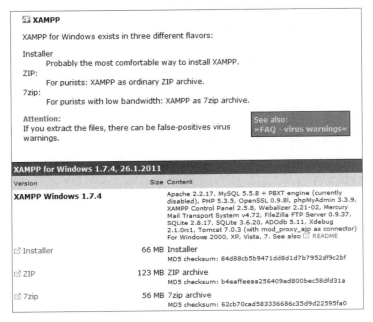

FIGURE 1-1

3. You have a choice of three ways to install this package: via the installer, via a ZIP file, or via a 7zip file. The easiest way to change options is to use the installer, but you are more likely to encounter problems. Because you are using the defaults, use the ZIP version. Click the ZIP link and save the ZIP file.

4. Unzip all the files to `c:\`. The ZIP file contains a folder called xampp that holds all the folders and files so unzipping to the `c:` drive creates the `c:\xampp` folder.

5. The program you use is `c:\xampp\xampp-control.exe`. In Windows Explorer, right-click the file and select Create Shortcut. Drag that shortcut to your desktop.

6. Double-click the XAMPP Control desktop icon you just created. The Control Panel is displayed. See Figure 1-2.

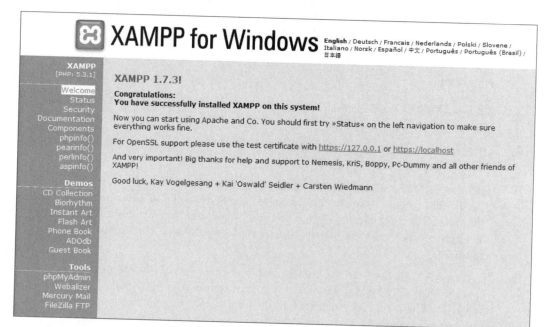

FIGURE 1-2

7. To start XAMPP, first start the Apache web service by clicking the Start button next to Apache. Then start MySQL by clicking the Start button next to MySQL. You do not need to start FileZilla or Mercury. When you click the Start buttons, they change to Stop buttons to indicate that the processes are running.

8. To stop XAMPP, click the Stop button next to MySQL and then click the Stop icon next to Apache.

9. To test that XAMPP is properly working, go to your browser and enter **http://localhost/xampp**. You should see a screen similar to Figure 1-3.

FIGURE 1-3

If the installation is successful, skip to the "Configuring XAMPP" section later in this lesson. Otherwise, check out the "Troubleshooting Your XAMPP Installation" section that follows the "Installing XAMPP on Mac OS X" section.

Installing XAMPP on Mac OS X

This section walks you through downloading the proper XAMPP package and installing it on your Mac OS X system. If you are using a Windows PC, you used the prior section to install XAMPP so you can jump forward to the "Configuring XAMPP" section.

1. Go to the Apache Friends website at `www.apachefriends.org/en/xampp.html`.

2. Locate the section labeled XAMPP for Mac OS X and click the title. Scroll down to find the section labeled Installation in 4 Steps. See Figure 1-4.

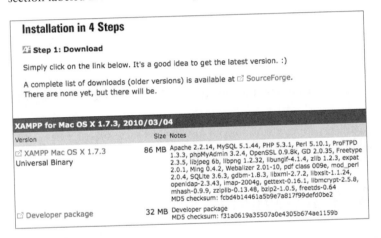

FIGURE 1-4

3. Click XAMPP Mac OS X. You want the Universal Binary, not the Developer Package. Click OK to save the file when asked.

4. Open the `.dmg` file you just saved. Drag the XAMPP icon over to the Applications icon as shown in Figure 1-5.

5. Find the XAMPP `Control.app` in `/Applications/XAMPP/Xamppfiles`. This is the application file that you use to start and stop XAMPP and you will find it convenient to add it to your dock. The first time you open it you receive the standard warning about using files from the Internet. Click the Open button to start the Control Panel. The Control Panel looks like Figure 1-6.

6. To start XAMPP, first start the Apache web service by clicking the Start button next to Apache. Then start MySQL by clicking the Start button next to MySQL. You do not need to start FTP. When you click the Start buttons, they change to Stop buttons to indicate that the processes are running.

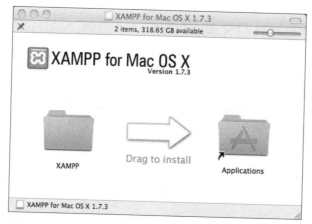

FIGURE 1-5

FIGURE 1-6

7. To stop XAMPP, click the Stop button next to MySQL and then click the Stop button next to Apache.

> Apache needs to be running for http://localhost and PHP to work. If you get an error that the server cannot be found, check that you've started Apache.

8. To test that XAMPP is properly working, go to your browser and enter **http://localhost/ xampp**. You should see a screen similar to Figure 1-7.

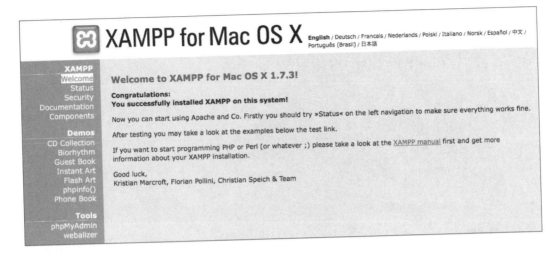

FIGURE 1-7

Troubleshooting Your XAMPP Installation

Usually, XAMPP installs easily. Sometimes, however, you can run into issues. The Apache Friends have a forum where you can find answers to many problems at `www.apachefriends.org/f/ viewforum.php?f=34`.

The Mac OS X ships with Apache. Apache works by listening on a specific port. If you run two copies of Apache, both listening to the same port, you will have problems. The default port is 80 and the common alternate port to use is 8080. If you need both, change the port on one of them and restart Apache.

If you want to change the port in XAMPP, go to `/Applications/XAMPP/xamppfiles/etc/httpd .conf` and change `Listen 80` to **`Listen 8080`**. Stop and restart Apache for the change to take effect. If you cannot get into the XAMPP control to stop and start Apache, shut down your Mac and restart it.

If you want to change the port in the pre-installed Apache, go to `etc/Apache2/http.conf` and change `Listen 80` to **`Listen 8080`**. To get to this hidden file, go to Finder and press Shift+Command+G and then enter **`\etc`**. You need to restart the pre-installed Apache. The easiest way to do that is to shut down your Mac and restart it.

> *If you changed the port that Apache listens to, you need to enter it as part of the address. If you changed the port to 8080, the address is* `http://localhost:8080/xampp.`

Skype is another program that might conflict with port 80. If you have problems, look in the Skype Advanced section of Tools/Options (on the PC) or Preferences (on the Mac) and be sure it isn't using port 80 for incoming or alternative ports.

Configuring XAMPP

Now that you have successfully installed XAMPP on your Windows PC or Mac, make sure XAMPP is running and then call up XAMPP in your browser. The address to call up XAMPP is `http://localhost/xampp`. A screen similar to Figure 1-8 displays.

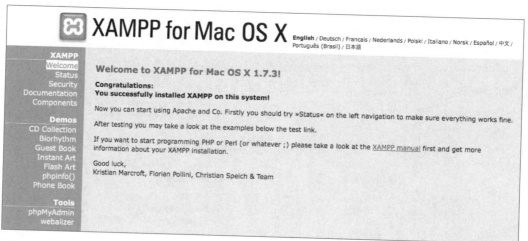

FIGURE 1-8

You need to create a password on MySQL. Some programs do not allow you to use MySQL unless MySQL has a password, for security reasons. Click the phpMyAdmin link on the left-side navigation under Tools to open the page shown in Figure 1-9.

Click Privileges on the top menu. You see a table of the users. Click the Edit icons next to the users. Scroll down to find the Change Password box as shown in Figure 1-10.

Enter a password and click Go. Do this for each of the users with All Privileges.

Now that you've added a password to MySQL, you need to change the configuration in XAMPP for phpMyAdmin so that it can access the database. The configuration file is in `c:\xampp\phpMyAdmin\config.inc.php` on the Windows PC or in `/Applications/XAMPP/xamppfiles/phpmyadmin/config.inc.php` on the Mac. Find the following code:

```
/* Authentication type */
$cfg['Servers'][$i]['auth_type'] = 'config';
/* Server parameters */
$cfg['Servers'][$i]['host'] = 'localhost';
$cfg['Servers'][$i]['user'] = 'root';
$cfg['Servers'][$i]['password'] = '';
```

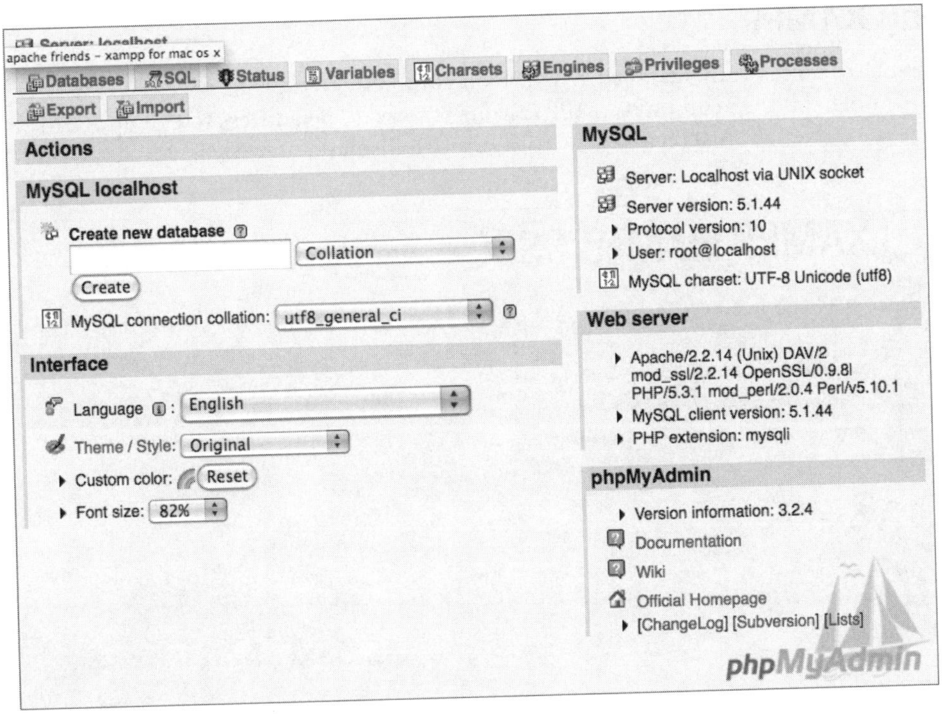

FIGURE 1-9

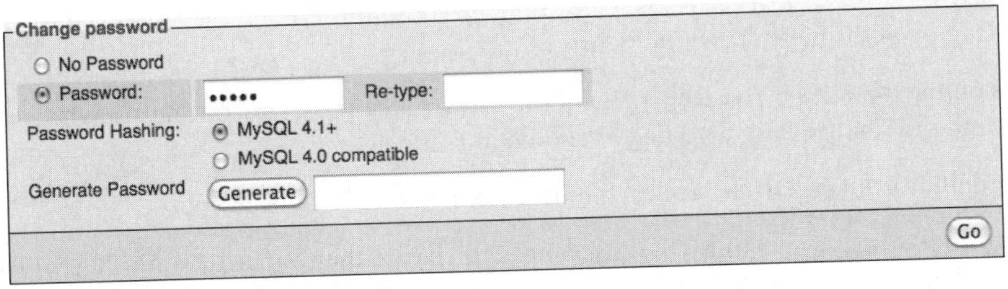

FIGURE 1-10

Change the password to your new password. For instance, if your new password is `!xYz72g`, the change looks like the following:

```
$cfg['Servers'][$i]['password'] = '!xYz72g';
```

Restart the XAMPP server by going into the Control Panel and stopping first MySQL and then Apache. Restart by starting Apache and then restarting MySQL.

Call up XAMPP in your browser and see that you can open phpMyAdmin.

INSTALLING YOUR EDITOR

You need a text editor for programming. Word processing editors such as Word change your code and add extraneous codes and characters that invalidate your program, so you should not use them. Possible text editors are Notepad, TextWrangler, Dreamweaver in the code mode, NetBeans, or Eclipse.

A good text editor for PHP is Eclipse PDT. It has syntax checking, auto-completion for commands, color syntax coding, debugging, and other features that become important as you do more complex PHP programming.

To install Eclipse PDT, go to `http://www.eclipse.org/pdt/downloads/` to download the program. You see a screen similar to Figure 1-11.

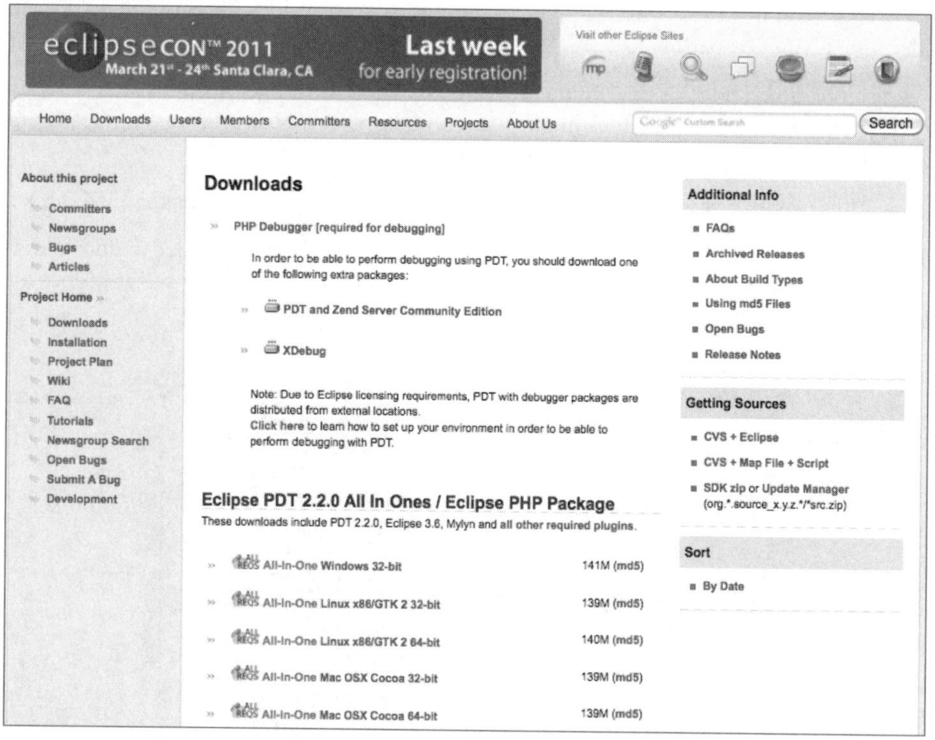

FIGURE 1-11

Find the All-in-One package for your operating system and click it. You are given a choice of mirrors from which you can download the package, as shown in Figure 1-11. Click the mirror displayed (which in this figure is Georgia Tech) and save the file when requested.

Unzip the file in an appropriate folder. In Windows a good folder is `c:\eclipse`. It does not need to be installed. On the Mac, put it in the Applications directory.

The program file is `eclipse.exe` in the `eclipse` folder. Make a shortcut on your desktop or add it to your dock (on the Mac) so you can find it easily.

CONFIGURING YOUR WORKSPACE

Now that you've installed the programs, you need to do some configuring.

Preparing a Place to Put Your Files

The first thing you need to do is decide where you are going to put your files. By default the Apache web server looks for web files in the htdocs folder. On a Windows PC, this is directly off where you installed XAMPP. If you installed XAMPP in `c:/xampp`, then your htdocs file is in the `c:/xampp/htdocs` folder. On a Mac the path is `/Applications/XAMPP/xamppfiles/htdocs`.

If you are going to be doing a lot of development work, you should change this default and set up virtual hosts so that you can put your files in more convenient places. However, setting up virtual hosts is beyond the scope of this book, so use the default htdocs folder.

If you are on a Windows PC, skip forward to the next section, "Using Eclipse for the First Time."

On the Mac OS X you need to change the permissions to the htdocs folder in order to add folders and files to it. Open Finder, browse to `/Applications/XAMPP/xamppfiles`, and select htdocs as shown in Figure 1-12.

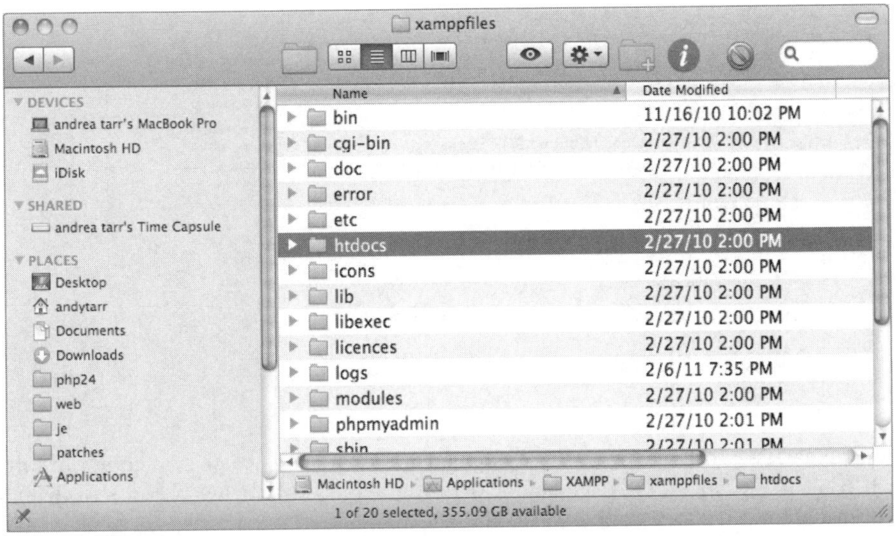

FIGURE 1-12

Press Command+I to display the htdocs Info as shown in Figure 1-13.

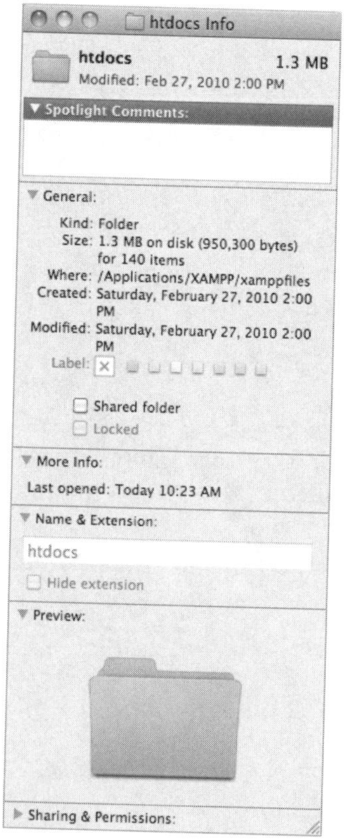

FIGURE 1-13

Click the arrow next to Sharing & Permissions to expand the section as shown in Figure 1-14.

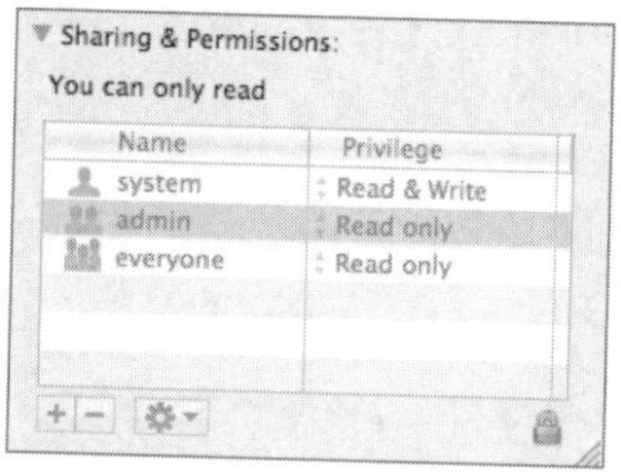

FIGURE 1-14

You need to unlock the padlock before you are allowed to make changes to the permissions. Click the padlock in the lower-right corner. Enter your administrator password for the Mac when asked.

Now you can click the Privilege drop-down for the admin. Change from Read Only to Read & Write. Your permissions should look similar to Figure 1-15.

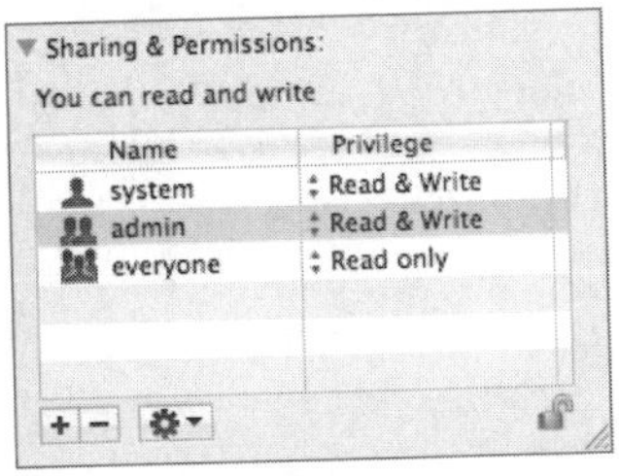

FIGURE 1-15

Click the padlock again to relock the permissions.

Using Eclipse for the First Time

The first time you go into Eclipse, you have to identify an Eclipse workspace. See Figure 1-16. This workspace is the place that you put your files. You use the htdocs folder.

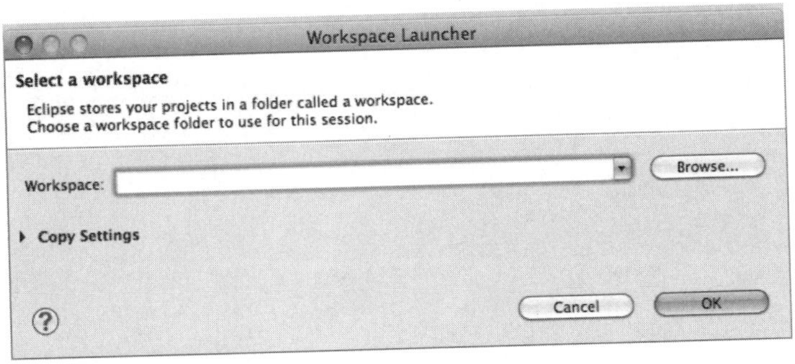

FIGURE 1-16

Use the Browse button to locate and accept the htdocs folder. On the PC, if you installed XAMPP in `c:/xampp`, your htdocs file is in the `c:/xampp/htdocs` folder. On a Mac, the path is `/Applications/XAMPP/xamppfiles/htdocs`. See Figure 1-17. Click OK.

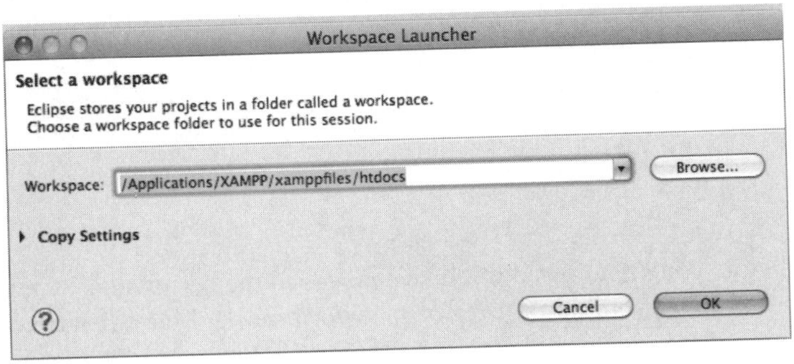

FIGURE 1-17

Eclipse displays a splash screen along with a request for permission for Eclipse to collect and send usage information, as shown in Figure 1-18.

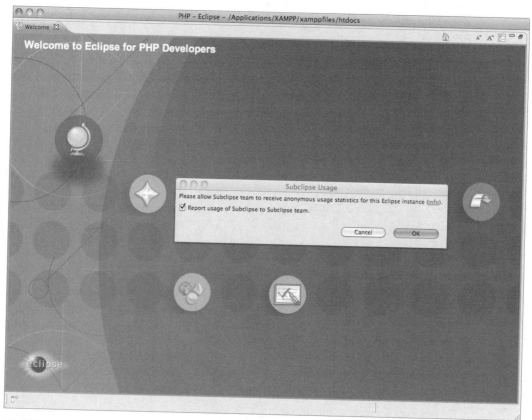

FIGURE 1-18

Uncheck the box if you do not want to have this information collected and sent. Click OK and then close the tab for the splash screen. You see the main workspace for Eclipse, as shown in Figure 1-19.

Across the top of the window, Eclipse lists the path to the workspace you are in. If you use virtual hosts you can create multiple workspaces, although you can have only one open at a time. To switch between workspaces, or to add a new workspace, use File ➪ Switch Workspaces. You use only one workspace in this book.

Within the workspace, you have projects. All your folders and files are created inside these projects. To create a project for this book, click File ➪ New ➪ PHP Project. You see a screen similar to Figure 1-20.

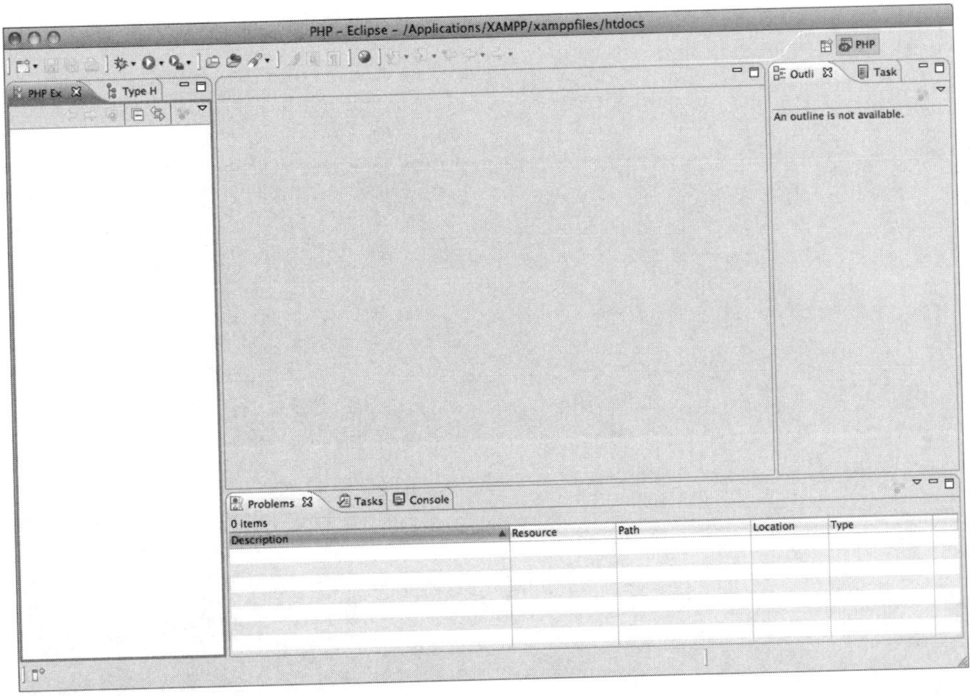

FIGURE 1-19

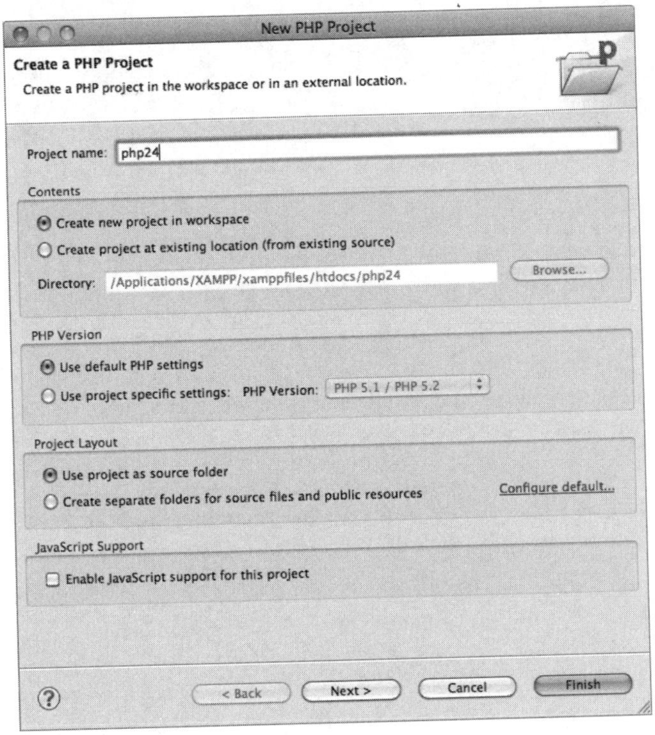

FIGURE 1-20

Type in a project name of **php24**. You can use what you want here, but this is part of the address you use to call your programs, so short and uncomplicated is best. Leave all the rest as the defaults and click Finish. You should see a screen similar to Figure 1-21.

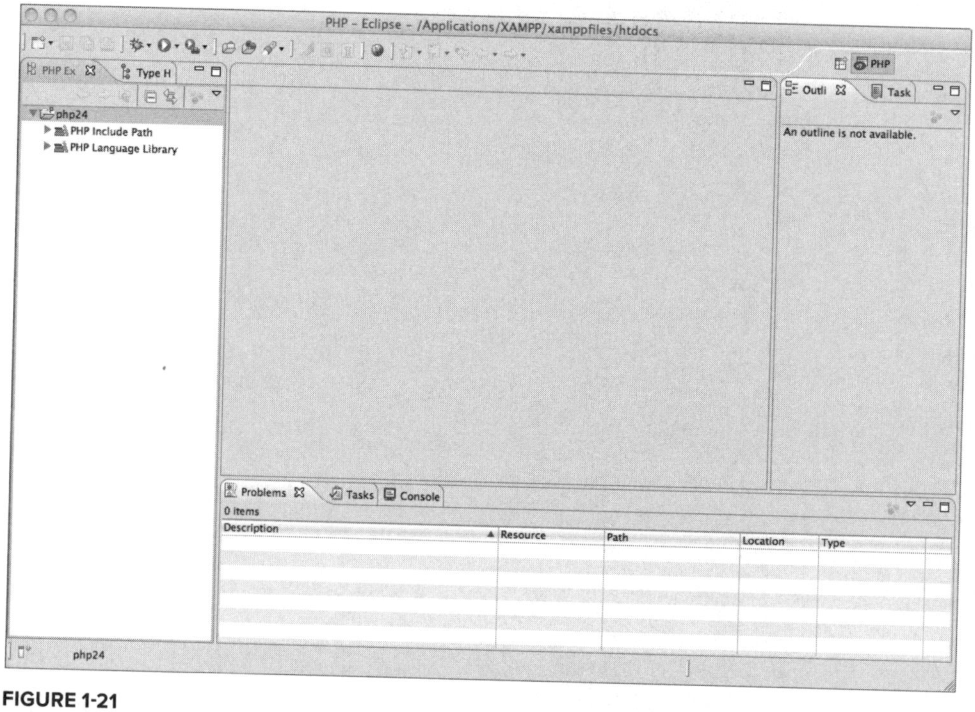

FIGURE 1-21

Notice that you now have the project php24 listed in the left window. This is the PHP Explorer. It works like the Windows Explorer, showing a hierarchical view of the folders and files within the different projects. Just as in Windows Explorer, you use this to open and select files and perform other actions on them. Right-clicking php24 displays a menu as shown in Figure 1-22.

Here's what some of these options do:

➤ **New:** Use this to create new folders and files.

➤ **Copy/Paste/Delete:** These work as you would expect.

➤ **Refactor:** This is where Rename and Move are hidden.

➤ **Refresh:** Use this if you've added, renamed, or moved files outside of Eclipse.

➤ **Debug As:** You learn more about this in Lesson 5.

➤ **Validate:** This is for validating files without needing to open them.

➤ **Compare With:** This compares files either with another file or with an earlier version of the same file. Files are automatically posted to Local History so you can roll back to a prior version. See Options (in Windows) or Preferences (Mac) if you want to change how many copies and how long they are kept.

➤ **Properties:** This is for quite a bit of Meta information.

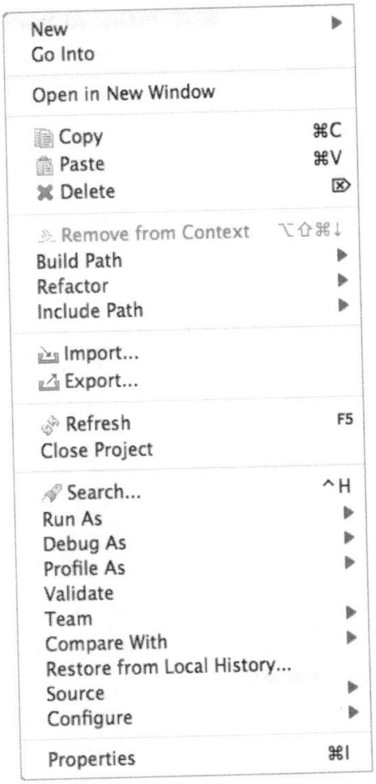

New	▶
Go Into	
Open in New Window	
📄 Copy	⌘C
📄 Paste	⌘V
✖ Delete	⌦
🔌 Remove from Context	⌥⇧⌘↓
Build Path	▶
Refactor	▶
Include Path	▶
📥 Import...	
📤 Export...	
🔄 Refresh	F5
Close Project	
🔍 Search...	^H
Run As	▶
Debug As	▶
Profile As	▶
Validate	
Team	▶
Compare With	▶
Restore from Local History...	
Source	▶
Configure	▶
Properties	⌘I

FIGURE 1-22

In the center of the screen is a blank window. This is where you edit your files. Over to the right is another window with tabs in it. The Outline tab shows you the outline of whatever file you have open and selected and can be used to navigate to various sections in the file. The bottom of the screen has another window with tabs. The Problems tab shows validation errors and the Tasks tab lists to-do's you have put inside your files and enables you to navigate directly to them.

This full screen that you see is called by Eclipse a "perspective." This particular perspective is the PHP perspective. Later you use a Debug perspective. Perspectives, which can be customized in Windows ⇨ Customize Perspectives, enable you tailor your work area to best suit the project you are working on.

TRY IT

In this Try It, you create a .php file and run it to test your PHP setup. This program runs a very handy function to see how you have your PHP configured. This is even handier for hackers so it is good practice not to have a file running it on your system. For a local system it is not a problem however, because you delete it when you are done.

Lesson Requirements

To run PHP files locally, you need to set up your computer so it can process PHP and run MySQL. This lesson shows you how to do that using XAMPP.

You also need to be able to create the PHP files themselves. You can do this with any editor that can produce plain-text files, including Notepad, TextWrangler, Dreamweaver in the code mode, NetBeans, or Eclipse. You learned in this lesson how to install the Eclipse PDT.

You should have a folder called php24 in the htdocs folder where you put your code files. If you created the Eclipse workspace, the folder was created for you automatically.

> *You can download the code and resources for this Try It from the book's web page at* www.wrox.com. *You can find them in the Lesson01 folder in the download. You will find code for both before and after completing the exercises.*

Hints

This is the code you need in the .php file:

```
<?php phpinfo();
```

Be sure that the Apache server is running when you run the program.

Step-by-Step

> *In this lesson I am giving detailed instructions using Eclipse PDT for those new to Eclipse. You can use a different text editor if you chose not to install Eclipse PDT.*

1. Create a blank .php file called test.php. In Eclipse, create it with the following steps:

    a. Right-click your project in the PHP Explorer.

    b. Select New ⇨ PHP File. Note that this is a PHP file, not a PHP project.

    c. Leave Source Folder as /php24 (your project name).

    d. Type **test.php** as the name of the file in the File Name field.

    e. Click Finish. You see a screen similar to Figure 1-23.

    f. The center window contains a file called test.php. This file is also showing on the left in the PHP Explorer window. If you don't see it below your project, click the triangle next to your project to expand the list.

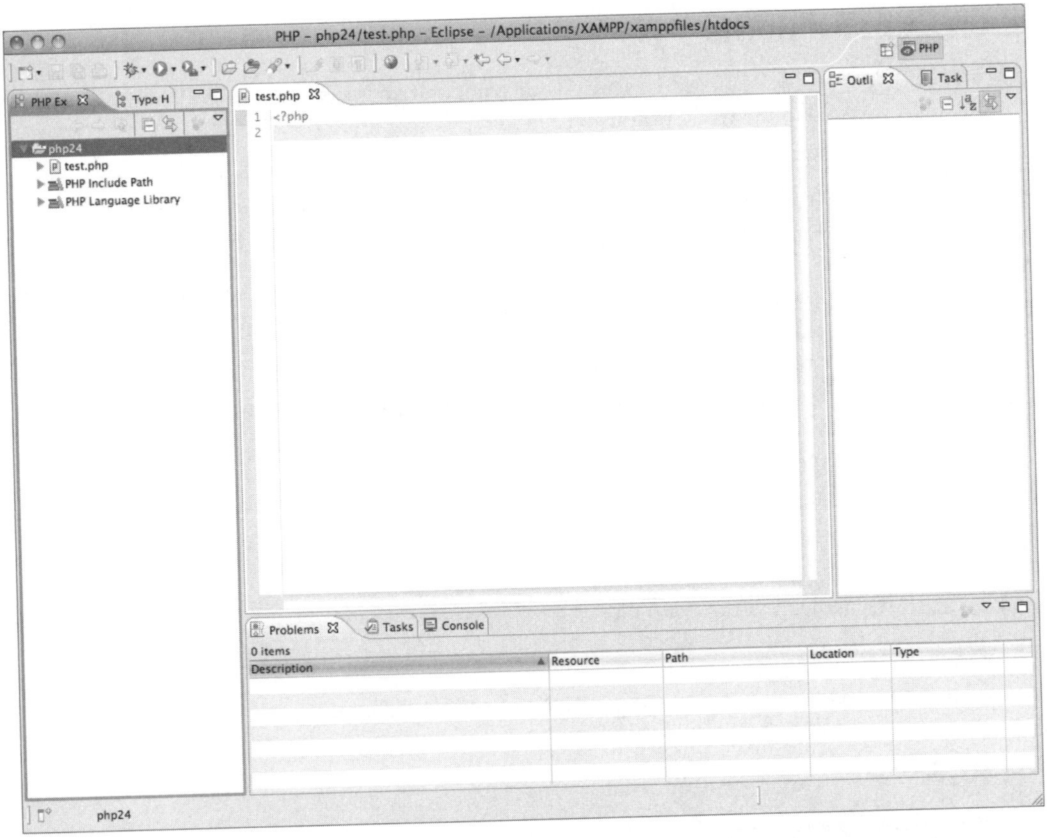

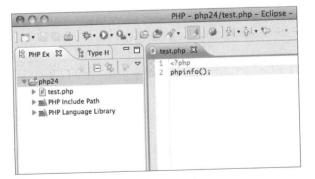

FIGURE 1-23

2. Your text editor may have already typed in `<?php` for you. If it did, do not retype it in step 3.

3. Type in **`<?php phpinfo();`**.

4. Your screen should look like Figure 1-24.

FIGURE 1-24

5. Save the file. In Eclipse you save by pressing Ctrl+S on the PC or Command+S on the Mac. You can also save the file by selecting File ⇨ Save.

6. To run the program, go to your browser and enter `localhost/php24/test.php`.

a. **localhost:** This identifies the web server, which in our case points to the htdocs folder.

b. **php24:** This is the folder that was automatically created to hold your project if you use Eclipse, or, if you are not using Eclipse, it is a folder you created to contain your code files.

c. **test.php:** This is the PHP file to run.

7. Your screen should look similar to Figure 1-25.

PHP Version 5.3.1	
System	Darwin mbpro.local 10.6.0 Darwin Kernel Version 10.6.0: Wed Nov 10 18:13:17 PST 2010; root:xnu-1504.9.26~3/RELEASE_I386 i386
Build Date	Feb 27 2010 12:28:52
Configure Command	'./configure' '--prefix=/Applications/XAMPP/xamppfiles' '--program-suffix=-5.3.1' '--libdir=/Applications/XAMPP/xamppfiles/lib/php/php-5.3.1' '--includedir=/Applications/XAMPP /xamppfiles/include/php/php-5.3.1' '--with-apxs2=/Applications/XAMPP/xamppfiles/bin/apxs' '--with-config-file-path=/Applications/XAMPP/xamppfiles/etc' '--with-mysql=/Applications /XAMPP/xamppfiles' '--disable-debug' '--enable-cli' '--enable-cgi' '--enable-bcmath' '--enable-calendar' '--enable-ctype' '--enable-discard-path' '--enable-filepro' '--enable-filter' '--enable-force-cgi-redirect' '--enable-fastcgi' '--enable-ftp' '--enable-hash' '--enable-ipv6' '--enable-json' '--enable-odbc' '--enable-path-info-check' '--enable-gd-imgstrttf' '--enable-gd-native-ttf' '--with-ttf' '--enable-magic-quotes' '--enable-memory-limit' '--enable-safe-mode' '--enable-shmop' '--enable-sysvsem' '--enable-sysvshm' '--enable-track-vars' '--enable-trans-sid' '--enable-reflection' '--enable-session' '--enable-spl' '--enable-tokenizer' '--enable-wddx' '--enable-yp' '--enable-xmlreader' '--enable-xmlwriter' '--enable-zlib' '--enable-zts' '--with-simplexml' '--with-iconv' '--with-libxml' '--with-wddx' '--with-xml' '--with-ftp' '--with-ncurses=/Applications/XAMPP /xamppfiles' '--with-gdbm=/Applications/XAMPP/xamppfiles' '--with-jpeg-dir=/Applications /XAMPP/xamppfiles' '--with-png-dir=/Applications/XAMPP/xamppfiles' '--with-freetype-dir=/Applications/XAMPP/xamppfiles' '--without-xpm' '--with-zlib=shared' '--with-zlib-dir=/Applications/XAMPP/xamppfiles' '--with-openssl=/Applications/XAMPP/xamppfiles' '--with-expat-dir=/Applications/XAMPP/xamppfiles' '--enable-xslt=shared,/Applications/XAMPP /xamppfiles' '--with-xsl=shared,/Applications/XAMPP/xamppfiles' '--with-dom=shared,/Applications/XAMPP/xamppfiles' '--with-ldap=shared,/Applications/XAMPP /xamppfiles' '--with-gd=shared' '--with-mysql-sock=/Applications/XAMPP/xamppfiles/var/mysql /mysql.sock' '--with-mcrypt=/Applications/XAMPP/xamppfiles' '--with-mhash=/Applications /XAMPP/xamppfiles' '--enable-sockets' '--enable-zend-multibyte' '--with-libxml-dir=/Applications /XAMPP/xamppfiles' '--enable-pcntl' '--enable-dbx=shared' '--with-mysqli=shared,/Applications /XAMPP/xamppfiles/bin/mysql_config' '--with-pear=/Applications/XAMPP/xamppfiles/lib/php /pear' '--with-mssql=/Applications/XAMPP/xamppfiles' '--with-imap-dir=/Applications/XAMPP /xamppfiles' '--with-imap=shared,/Applications/XAMPP/xamppfiles' '--enable-mbstring=shared,all' '--with-pgsql=shared,/Applications/XAMPP/xamppfiles' '--with-gettext=/Applications/XAMPP/xamppfiles' '--enable-apache2-2filter=shared' '--enable-apache2-2handler=shared' '--with-bz2=shared' '--with-curl=shared' '--with-dba=shared' '--enable-dbase=shared' '--with-fdf=shared' '--enable-mbregex' '--enable-mbregex-backtrack' '--with-mime-magic=shared' '--with-mysql=shared,/Applications/XAMPP/xamppfiles' '--enable-shmop=shared' '--with-snmp=shared' '--enable-sockets=shared' '--enable-pdo' '--with-sqlite=shared' '--enable-zip=shared,/Applications/XAMPP/xamppfiles' '--enable-exif=shared' '--with-pdo-mssql=shared,/Applications/XAMPP/xamppfiles' '--with-pdo-mysql=shared,/Applications/XAMPP/xamppfiles/bin/mysql_config' '--with-pdo-pgsql=shared,/Applications/XAMPP/xamppfiles' '--with-pdo-sqlite=shared' '--with-pdo-sqlite-external=shared' '--enable-soap=shared' '--with-xmlrpc=shared' '--with-oracle=shared' '--with-pdf=shared' '--with-sqlite3=shared,/Applications/XAMPP/xamppfiles'
Server API	Apache 2.0 Handler
Virtual Directory Support	disabled
Configuration File (php.ini) Path	/Applications/XAMPP/xamppfiles/etc
Loaded Configuration	/Applications/XAMPP/xamppfiles/etc/php.ini

FIGURE 1-25

TROUBLESHOOTING

If you're having trouble, verify the following things:

➤ There should be a space between `<?php` and `phpinfo()`.

➤ There should be no space between `phpinfo` and the `()`.

➤ Don't forget the final semicolon.

➤ Don't forget to use `localhost:8080` if you changed your XAMPP port to 8080.

8. Go back to your text editor.

9. Close the file. In Eclipse, click the X on the tab with the `test.php` filename to close the file.

10. Delete the file. In Eclipse, delete your file by doing the following:

    a. Expand your project by clicking the triangle next to the project name if it is not already expanded.

    b. Right-click `test.php`.

    c. Click Delete.

    d. Confirm that you want to delete the file.

 Watch the video for Lesson 1 on the DVD or watch online at `www.wrox.com/ go/24phpmysql`.

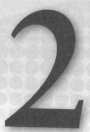

Adding PHP to a Web Page

PHP is a programming scripting language that was first developed to generate HTML statements. Even programs written totally in PHP are ultimately displayed as ordinary HTML.

You can also write programs that are mostly HTML with just the occasional PHP statement. In this lesson you start with an HTML page and learn how to add PHP statements to it.

You are also introduced to the Case Study website. By the end of this book, you will have changed it from a static HTML/CSS site to a dynamic website. In this lesson you add the first bit of dynamic code.

WRITING YOUR FIRST PHP PAGE

You start with a simple HTML page that looks like Figure 2-1. The file is called `lesson2a.html`.

Here's the HTML for that page:

```
<html>
<head>
    <title>Lesson 2a</title>
</head>

<body>

<h1>Welcome</h1>
<p>Today is Sep 27, 2011</p>

</body>
</html>
```

Welcome
Today is Sep 27, 2011

FIGURE 2-1

Now you turn this into a PHP page. All you do is change the file extension from `.html` to `.php` and it becomes a PHP file. When you call that in your browser it still looks just like Figure 2-1.

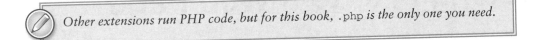

You can display standard HTML in your browser by entering the file path. An example of a file path is `c:/xamppfiles/htdocs/lesson2a.html`. *With* `.php` *files, you enter the address that starts with the web root. An example of an address is* `http://localhost/lesson2a.php`.

The difference is that, because of the `.php` extension, the PHP processor reads through the file to see if there is any PHP to process. Any HTML that it finds it prints to the screen. Because all it found was HTML, the results were just the same as the `.html` file.

So the first rule of writing PHP code is to use the file extension `.php`.

Other extensions run PHP code, but for this book, `.php` *is the only one you need.*

Today isn't really Sep 27, 2011, so you can add PHP code to dynamically display today's date. Make a copy of the previous file, call it `lesson2b.php`, change the title to **Lesson 2b** and replace `Sep 27, 2011` with the following code:

```
<?php echo date('M j, Y'); ?>
```

The file now looks like the following:

```
<html>
<head>
    <title>Lesson 2b</title>
</head>

<body>

<h1>Welcome</h1>
<p>Today is <?php echo date('M j, Y'); ?></p>

</body>
</html>
```

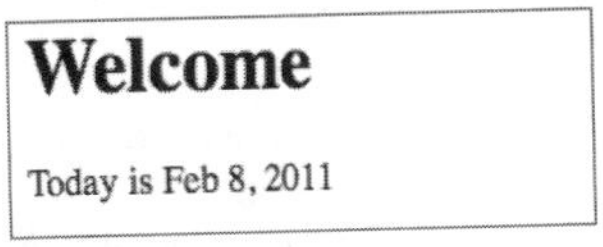

When you run this code in your browser it looks similar to Figure 2-2. Of course your screen displays the current date.

Welcome

Today is Feb 8, 2011

FIGURE 2-2

The PHP processor looks for blocks of code that start with `<?php`. It interprets everything after that as PHP code until it gets to a `?>`. The `echo date('M j, Y')` tells the processor to find today's date;

format it with a three-character month, the day without leading zeros followed by a comma, and a four-digit year; and then output it. The program continues to output the HTML that it finds, but also processes the new PHP code.

You learn more about echo later in this lesson and about processing dates in Lesson 6.

INTRODUCING THE CASE STUDY

To give you a feel for how PHP code can make a website dynamic, you take a static HTML/CSS website and replace sections of it with PHP code as you work through the lessons. The site is for a fictitious company called Smithside Auctions. This company holds auctions of historic clothing throughout the year. Figure 2-3 shows the Home page.

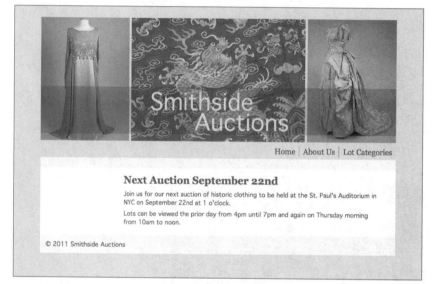

FIGURE 2-3

The About Us page lists the employees, as shown in Figure 2-4.

Smithside Auctions assigns the clothing into lots for the auctions and then puts those lots into appropriate categories. The categories are shown in Figure 2-5 and a sample of the detail of one of the categories is shown in Figure 2-6.

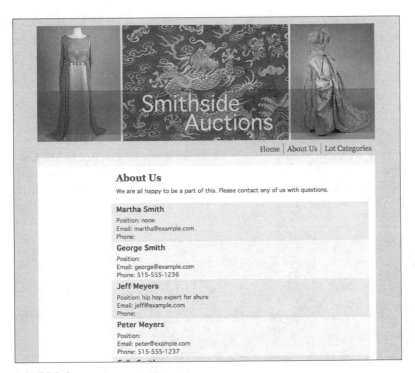

FIGURE 2-4

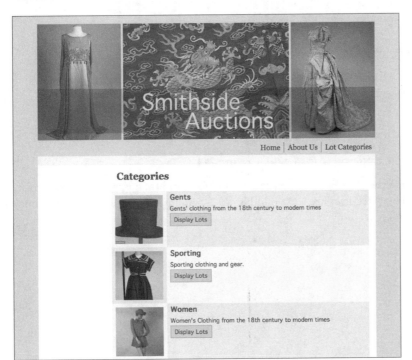

FIGURE 2-5

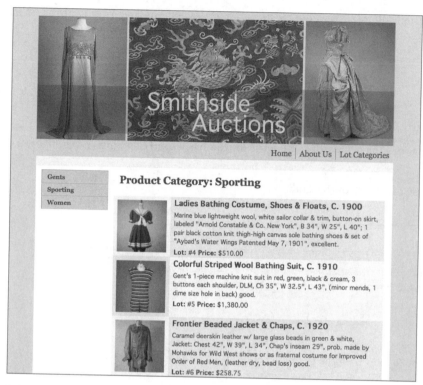

FIGURE 2-6

You can download the code for this site from the book's website at www.wrox.com. There is a version available for the start of each lesson in which you use the case study. Thus you can follow along, making the changes as you do the lessons, or you can simply download appropriate code at any point in the process if you want.

> *The photographs are from Augusta Auctions, an actual company that auctions consigned historic clothing and textiles. You can use the photographs for the exercises in this book. If you want to use them for any other purpose, contact Augusta Auctions through its website at* www.augusta-auction.com. *While there, you can browse through the rest of the 30,000 photos on the site.*

USING ECHO AND INCLUDE

The echo function tells the processor to output data. The PHP version

```
<?php echo '<p>Where is the dog?</p>'; ?>
```

is the same as the HTML version

```
<p>Where is the dog?</p>
```

You can use either a single quote (') or a double quote ("). If the text you are printing already has single or double quotes in it, use the other type of quote to surround it. For example:

```php
<?php echo "<p>Where's my dog?</p>"; ?>
```

is the same as

```
<p>Where's my dog?</p>
```

You learn about some differences between the two quote types in Lesson 4.

The `include` function tells the processor to take the file that you specify and insert it in place of the include statement.

Create the file `lesson02d.php` with this code:

```
<h1>Welcome</h1>
<p>Today is <?php echo date('M j, Y'); ?>.</p>
```

> Some text editors automatically put a `<?php` at the beginning of any PHP file you create. Just type over it if you are not starting the file with PHP code, as in this example.

Create the file `lesson02e.php` with the following code. Your output should look similar to Figure 2-7.

```
<html>
<head>
  <title>Lesson 2e</title>
</head>

<body>

<?php include('lesson02d.php'); ?>

</body>
</html>
```

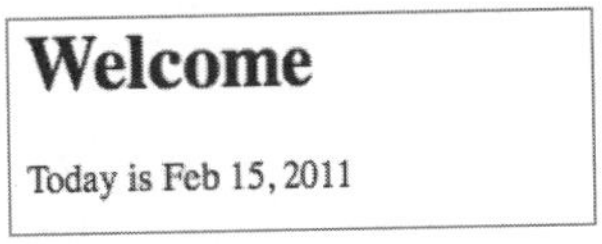

Welcome

Today is Feb 15, 2011

FIGURE 2-7

This is what the processor sees:

```
<html>
<head>
  <title>Lesson 2e</title>
</head>

<body>

<h1>Welcome</h1>
<p>Today is <?php echo date('M j, Y'); ?></p>

</body>
</html>
```

If you view the source in your browser, you see:

```
<html>
<head>
  <title>Lesson 2e</title>
</head>

<body>

<h1>Welcome</h1>
<p>Today is Feb 15, 2011.</p>

</body>
</html>
```

The `include` makes it possible to create a single file that can be called multiple times or to create a single file where you can swap different parts in and out.

TRY IT

In this Try It, you take the content out of the Home page (`index.html`), put it in a separate file, and include it into the renamed `index.php` file. This content file goes in a new folder called content. Then you change `about.html` so that the content section is called as an include in `index.php`.

Like most websites, the header information and the footer information in the Case Study site stay the same while the content on the page changes. Using the `include` enables you to create several web pages that share a single file for the header and footer information, making changes easier.

> *You can download the code and resources for this Try It from the book's web page at* www.wrox.com. *You can find them in the Lesson02 folder in the download. You will find code for both before and after completing the exercises.*

Lesson Requirements

Your computer needs to be able to run as a web server with PHP and MySQL. XAMPP is a package of software that installs the web server, PHP, and MySQL for you. You can find instructions for downloading and installing XAMPP in Lesson 1.

You need a text editor that can produce plain-text files. You can find instructions for downloading and installing Eclipse PDT in Lesson 1. Other text editors that you can use are Adobe's Dreamweaver in code mode, Notepad, TextWrangler, or NetBeans.

If you are following along with the Case Study, you need your files from the end of the previous lesson. Alternatively, you can download the files from the book's website at www.wrox.com.

Hints

Remember to rename the files to `.php`.

Remember to use the localhost address to call the website locally.

Step-by-Step

1. Start with the HTML Case Study code. You can download it from the Lesson02/lesson02cs folder on the book's web page at www.wrox.com. This exercise could also be done on any simple HTML site.

2. Rename the `index.html` file to **`index.php`**.

3. Create a folder called content.

4. Create a blank file **`content/home.php`**.

5. Cut the following code from `index.php` and put it in `contents/home.php`:

    ```
    <h1>Next Auction September 22nd</h1>
    <p>Join us for our next auction of historic clothing
    to be held at the St. Paul's Auditorium in NYC on September 22nd at
    1 o'clock.</p>

    <p>Lots can be viewed the prior day from 4pm until 7pm and again on Thursday
    morning from 10am to noon.</p>
    ```

6. Replace that code in `index.php` with the following:

    ```
    <?php include 'content/home.php';?>
    ```

7. Change the menu to look for the `.php` file instead of the `.html` file. The code should look like this:

    ```
    <li><a href="index.php">Home</a></li>
    ```

8. Call up the Home page in your browser. It should still look like Figure 2-3.

9. Rename `about.html` to **`about.php`**.

10. Move `about.php` to the content folder.

11. Remove all the code except the code in the `<div class="content">` div.

12. Check that the remaining code in `content/about.php` is

    ```
    <h1>About Us</h1>
    <p>We are all happy to be a part of this. Please contact any of us
    with questions.</p>

    <ul class="ulfancy">
    <li class="row0">
    ```

```
        <h2>Martha Smith</h2>
        <p>Position: none<br />
        Email: martha@example.com<br />
        Phone: <br /></p>
    </li>

    <li class="row1">
        <h2>George Smith</h2>
        <p>Position: <br />
        Email: george@example.com<br />
        Phone: 515-555-1236<br /></p>
    </li>

    <li class="row0">
        <h2>Jeff Meyers</h2>
        <p>Position: hip hop expert for shure<br />
        Email: jeff@example.com<br />
        Phone: <br /></p>
    </li>

    <li class="row1">
        <h2>Peter Meyers</h2>
        <p>Position: <br />
        Email: peter@example.com<br />
        Phone: 515-555-1237<br /></p>
    </li>

    <li class="row0">
        <h2>Sally Smith</h2>
        <p>Position: <br />
        Email: sally@example.com<br />
        Phone: 515-555-1235<br /></p>
    </li>

    <li class="row1">
        <h2>Sarah Finder</h2>
        <p>Position: Lost Soul<br />
        Email: finder@a.com<br />
        Phone: 555-123-5555<br /></p>
    </li>

</ul>
```

13. Go to the index.php file and change the include statement from `<?php include 'content/home.php';?>` to **`<?php include 'content/about.php';?>`**.

14. Change the menu to look for the index.php file instead of the about.html file. The code should look like this:

```
<li><a href="index.php">About Us</a></li>
```

15. Call up the About Us page in your browser. It should still look like Figure 2-4.

> *Both the Home page and the About Us page are called by the* index.php *file. At the moment, you need to change the* include *statement in the* index.php *file to switch between the pages. In Lesson 7 you learn how to make them change automatically.*

16. Go back to the index.php file and change the include statement from `<?php include 'content/about.php';?>` to **`<?php include 'content/home.php';?>`**.

> *Watch the video for Lesson 2 on the DVD or watch online at* www.wrox.com/ go/24phpmysql.

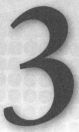

Learning PHP Syntax

You've seen how PHP can work on a web page. Now it's time to learn some basics of coding in PHP before you get into the detail of the language.

In this lesson you find out about formatting styles for PHP. You learn the general rules of PHP syntax and how to create comments. You learn the specific syntax of different PHP elements as you go over them in subsequent chapters.

Finally, you learn some best practices to make life easier and your code better.

PICKING A FORMATTING STYLE

When you read a book or type a letter you are used to certain conventions. For instance, each paragraph might have the first line indented and a space before the next paragraph. Each chapter might start with the first letter enlarged.

Styling makes the text easier to understand because it organizes the information and tells you what to expect. If there are no paragraphs, if all the sentences continue one after the other without a break, you can read it but it is more difficult.

Programming uses formatting styles in the same way. The program runs fine without using any formatting but it is more difficult for a human being to read. It is harder to see what is happening and harder to find errors.

A computer has no trouble reading this code:

```
<?php $messages='';$task=filter_input(INPUT_POST,'task',FILTER_SANITIZE_
STRING);if ($task=='product.maint'):$results=maintProduct();$a==true;$mess
ages .=$results;endif;if ('contact.maint'):$results=maintContact();$messa
ges .=$results;endif;if ('category.maint'):$results=maintCategory();$messages
.=$results;endif;?>
```

However, even if you don't know PHP, the following is much easier to understand:

```php
<?php
$messages = '';
$task = filter_input(INPUT_POST,'task', FILTER_SANITIZE_STRING);

if ($task == 'product.maint') :
    $results = maintProduct();
    $a == true;
    $messages .= $results;
endif;
if ('contact.maint')   :
$results = maintContact();
    $messages .= $results;
endif;

if ('category.maint') :
    $results = maintCategory();
    $messages .= $results;
endif;

?>
```

Formatting styles address the following issues:

➤ **Indention:** What should be indented? How big is the indentation? Do you use spaces or a tab?

➤ **Line length:** Do you restrict how long a single line can be before you use more than one line? How many characters is it?

➤ **Whitespace:** What additional whitespace (that is, spaces, new or blank rows) do you add for readability?

➤ **Use of {} (curly braces):** If these are optional in the syntax, do you use them anyway or leave them off?

Just as one book might have a different style than another, there are different PHP formatting styles. It's more important that you are consistent in your coding style than the particular style that you use.

Two popular styles are the Zend Framework (http://framework.zend.com/manual/en/coding-standard.html) and the Pear Coding Standards (http://pear.php.net/manual/en/standards.php).

LEARNING PHP SYNTAX

As you saw in the preceding lesson, the first step to using PHP is to put your PHP code in a file with the extension of `.php`. This warns the server to be on the lookout for a PHP block.

A block of PHP code starts with `<?php` and ends with `?>`. So an example code block looks like this:

```
<?php
some php code here
?>
```

You can have one PHP block that encompasses an entire file or a number of PHP blocks interspersed with HTML. If your file contains only PHP, or if it ends with a PHP block, leave off the final `?>`.

> The final `?>` is omitted because if there is any information, including blanks or an extra line, after that final `?>`, it is interpreted as HTML and the system sends that data to the browser. This results in extraneous whitespace and possible header errors.

> Some servers permit you to use the short tag version of `<?` to start a PHP block. Don't do this. Your code will not be accepted on all servers and is open to misinterpretation.

Each statement ends with a semicolon:

```
<?php
$first_name = 'Andrea';
?>
The end of a statement is often at the end of a line, but not always. This is
  particularly noticeable when mixing PHP with HTML.<p>Hello, <?php echo
$first_name; ?></p>
```

The official manual for PHP located on the php.net website is a great resource, although it can be confusing. As an example, look up information on the function `echo` that you used in the previous lesson.

Go to `www.php.net/manual/en/index.php`. You see a table of contents as shown in Figure 3-1.

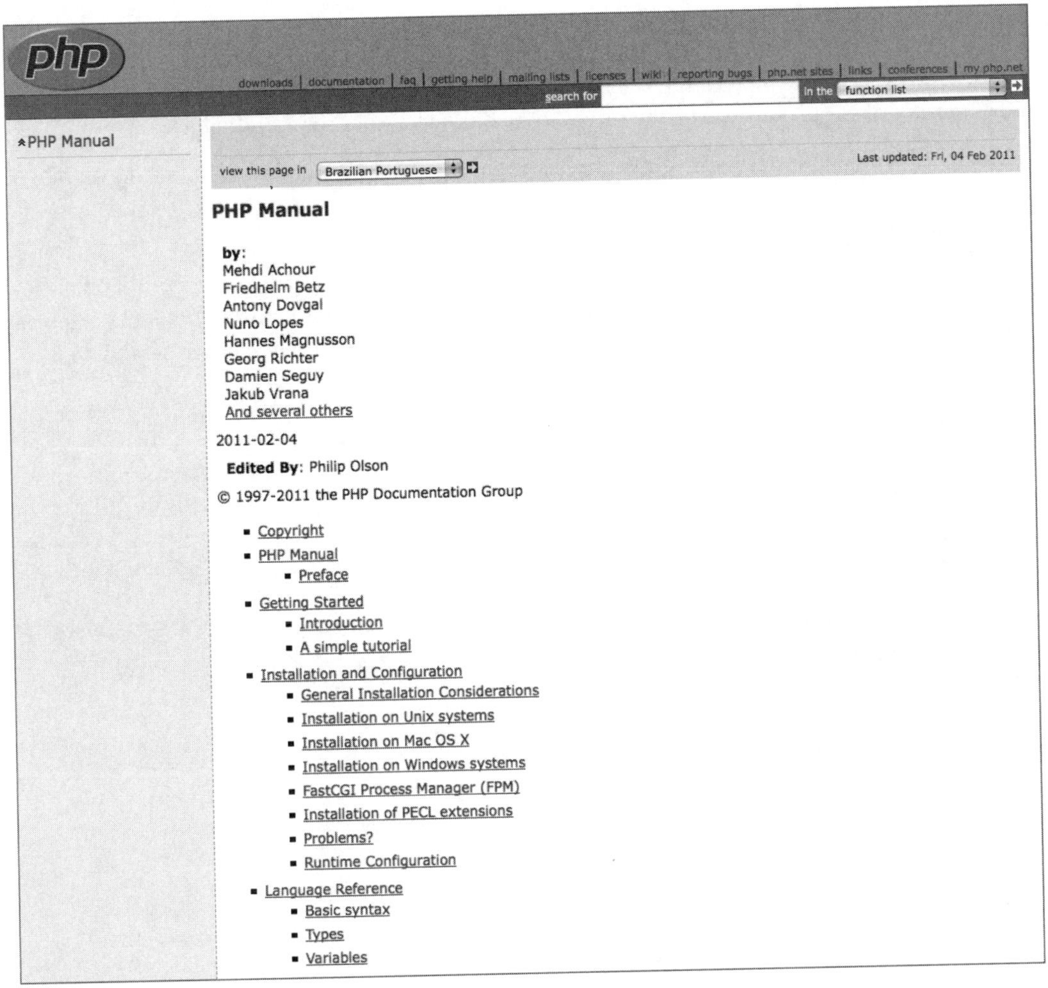

FIGURE 3-1

You could use the table of contents to locate what you are looking for, but there's a quicker way. In the upper-right corner, type **echo** in the Search For box and press Enter. Your window should look like Figure 3-2.

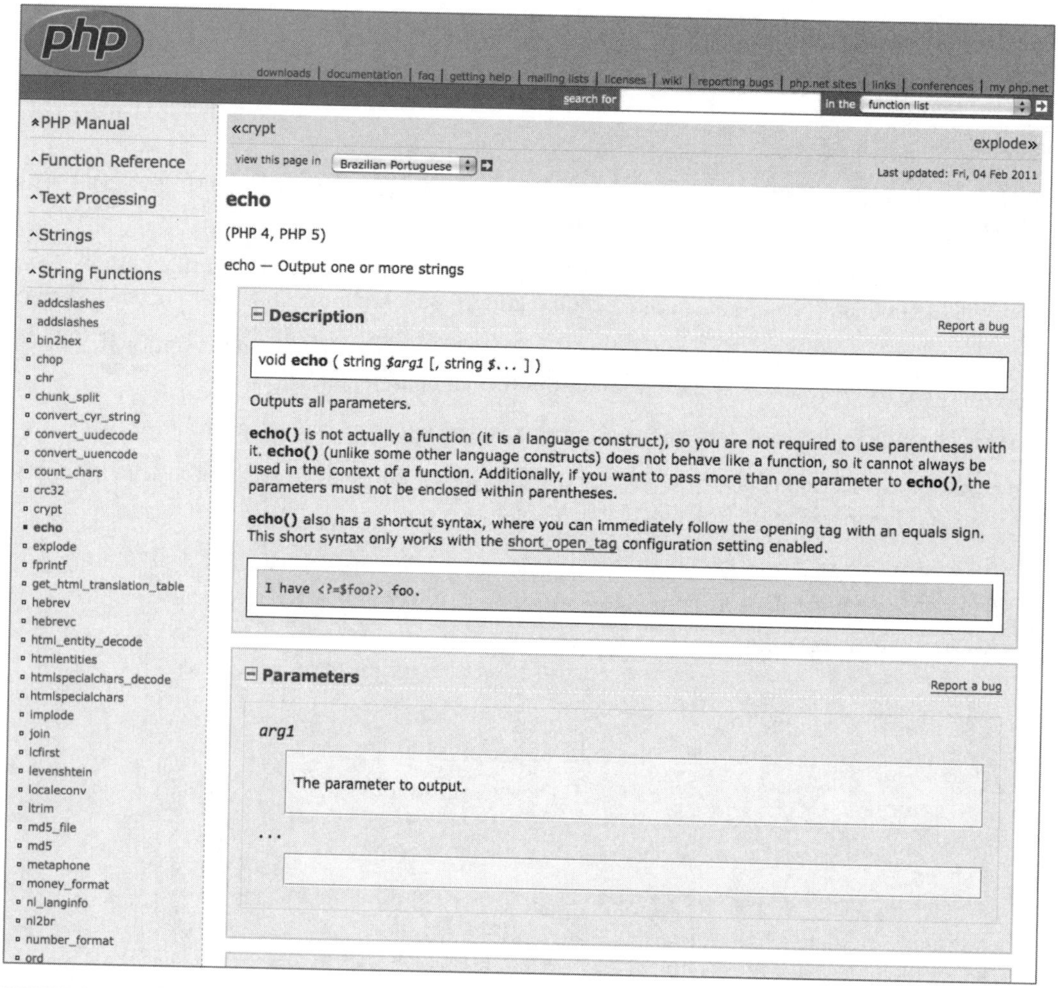

FIGURE 3-2

You may be thinking it's a good thing that you know what echo does because the explanation here doesn't help much. The following explanation should help you make more sense of it.

The first section contains a description that starts with the syntax of the element. See Figure 3-3.

```
void echo ( string $arg1 [, string $... ] )
```

FIGURE 3-3

The element is in bold text.

The keywords `void` and `string` tell you what the type is. You learn about types in Lesson 4. This is just informational and you don't type those words.

The parameters are shown in italic. Parameters are the changeable data that the function uses. Detail about the parameters is contained in the second section. You learn more about parameters in Lesson 6.

The square brackets around the second parameter indicate that the parameter is optional. The ellipsis (...) means that you can have more than one additional parameter.

The third section gives the return values. You learn more about return values in Lesson 10.

The most helpful section is often the next one: Examples. Here you can see how the function is actually used, as shown in Figure 3-4.

Report a bug

⊟ Examples

Example #1 echo() examples

```php
<?php
echo "Hello World";

echo "This spans
multiple lines. The newlines will be
output as well";

echo "This spans\nmultiple lines. The newlines will be\noutput as well.";

echo "Escaping characters is done \"Like this\".";

// You can use variables inside of an echo statement
$foo = "foobar";
$bar = "barbaz";

echo "foo is $foo"; // foo is foobar

// You can also use arrays
$baz = array("value" => "foo");

echo "this is {$baz['value']} !"; // this is foo !

// Using single quotes will print the variable name, not the value
echo 'foo is $foo'; // foo is $foo

// If you are not using any other characters, you can just echo variables
echo $foo;          // foobar
echo $foo,$bar;     // foobarbarbaz

// Some people prefer passing multiple parameters to echo over concatenation.
echo 'This ', 'string ', 'was ', 'made ', 'with multiple parameters.', chr(10);
echo 'This ' . 'string ' . 'was ' . 'made ' . 'with concatenation.' . "\n";
```

FIGURE 3-4

Programmers are allowed to add notes directly to the bottom of the page. These often consist of tips and techniques in using the function.

ENTERING COMMENTS

Comments are an important part of PHP coding. Although you might remember tomorrow what you were trying to do with a certain bit of code, you probably won't remember in six months. Document what you are trying to do as you do it.

Comments are not sent on to the browser so they don't slow down your system. If you look at the source code of a web page, the only comments you see are HTML comments, not PHP comments.

There are two main types of PHP comments. The first type is for commenting a single line or partial line. The comment starts with a // and ends at the end of the line:

```php
<?php

// This is a single line comment
$temperature = 65;
$celsius = ($temperature - 32)* (5/9); // this is also a valid comment
echo '<p>The answer is ' . $celsius . '</p>';

// You can, of course, have multiple lines
// of single line comments.

?>
```

The second type of comment is a block comment. The block comment starts with a /* and ends with a */:

```php
<?php

/* This is an example of using a multiple line comment. With
this type of comment you don't need to keep repeating
the comment code. */
$temperature = 65;
$celsius = ($temperature - 32)* (5/9); /* this is also a valid comment */
echo '<p>The answer is ' . $celsius . '</p>';

/* You can also use different techniques
 * to make your comments stand out
 * because everything is ignored until the */

?>
```

Note that, unlike the single-line comments, you need to indicate when the block comment ends.

There is a special type of multiple-line comment called a PHPDoc block comment. Automated tools, including Eclipse PDT, pick up comments that use this specific style.

The PHPDoc comment starts with /**, has a * at the beginning of each line, and ends with */. This is an example that documents the file itself:

```
/**
 * Short description for file
 *
 * Long description for file (if any)...
 *
 * @version    1.2 2011-02-03
 * @package    Your Project Name
 * @copyright  Copyright (c) 2011 Your company name
 * @license    GNU General Public License
 * @since      Since Release 1.0
 */
```

There are specific setups for PHPDoc comments depending on what you are documenting. You learn the common blocks as you learn about the different elements in later lessons. You can find details about the PHPDoc comment at the phpDocumentor site at `http://manual .phpdoc.org/HTMLSmartyConverter/HandS/phpDocumentor/tutorial_phpDocumentor .howto.pkg.html`.

USING BEST PRACTICES

Following best practices makes your code less error prone, easier to maintain, and more secure.

You've already learned some of the best practices earlier in this lesson:

➤ Don't use the `<? ?>` short tag.

➤ Comment your code.

➤ Be consistent within your own code but recognize that other developers may have their own styles.

➤ If you are working on a project with other developers, use the style adopted by the project rather than your personal preference.

Additionally, you should

➤ Create the ending tag, bracket, or parenthesis when you create the beginning tag, bracket, or parenthesis. You save a lot of headaches this way.

➤ Use extra lines to separate related blocks of code for improved readability.

➤ Indent nested elements.

➤ Be consistent with naming conventions and use meaningful names.

➤ Leave error reporting on while developing and turn it off when your code goes into production. This enables you to locate errors, but protects the user from strange error messages. If you are using XAMPP, error reporting is turned on by default.

⬇ TRY IT

In this Try It you add comments to `.php` files. You use all three types of comments.

> You can download the code and resources for this Try It from the book's web page at www.wrox.com. You can find them in the Lesson03 folder in the download. You will find code for both before and after completing the exercises.

Lesson Requirements

Your computer needs to be able to run as a web server with PHP and MySQL. XAMPP is a package of software that installs the web server, PHP, and MySQL for you. You can find instructions for downloading and installing XAMPP in Lesson 1.

You need a text editor that can produce plain-text files. You can find instructions for downloading and installing Eclipse PDT in Lesson 1. Other text editors that you can use are Adobe's Dreamweaver in code mode, Notepad, TextWrangler, or NetBeans.

If you are following along with the Case Study, you need your files from the end of the previous lesson. Alternatively, you can download the files from the book's website at www.wrox.com.

Hints

Remember that the comments need to be within `<?php ?>` tags.

Step-by-Step

Add comments to the given code.

1. Open Eclipse or your text editor.

2. Create a blank .php file called **exercise03a.php**.

3. Type in the following code:

```
<!DOCTYPE html PUBLIC "-//W3C//DTD XHTML 1.0 Transitional//EN"
"http://www.w3.org/TR/xhtml1/DTD/xhtml1-transitional.dtd">
<html xmlns="http://www.w3.org/1999/xhtml">
<head>
 <meta http-equiv="Content-Type" content="text/html; charset=UTF-8" />
 <title>Lesson 3</title>
</head>

<body>
 <?php
 echo '<h1>Lesson 3</h1>';
 echo '<p>This is the first paragraph</p>' ;
 echo '<p>This is the second paragraph</p>';
 ?>
</body>
</html>
```

4. To enter the PHPDoc block at the beginning, you need to go into PHP, so go to the start of the file and press Enter to get a new line.

5. Type the beginning and ending PHP tags of `<?php ?>`. Your editor may auto-complete the commands once you start typing.

6. Put your cursor between the tags and press Enter twice to make space to enter the PHPDoc block.

7. Type in the following code:

```
/**
 * Try it Lesson 3
 *
 * This program creates a php file demonstrating PHPDoc blocks
 * and basic PHP syntax
 *
 * @version    1.0 2011-02-03
 * @package    PHP & MySQL 24-hr Trainer
 * @subpackage Lesson 3
 * @copyright  Copyright (c) 2011 Your company name
 * @license    GNU General Public License
 * @since      Since Release 1.0
 */
```

8. On a new line above `echo '<h1>Lesson 3</h1>';` add the following code:

```
/* This is a long comment about
 * the h1 command
 */
```

9. On a new line above `echo '<p>This is the first paragraph</p>'` ; add the following code:

```
// This is a comment about the first paragraph
```

10. Add the following comment on the same line after `echo '<p>This is the second paragraph</p>';`:

```
// Comment about paragraph 2
```

11. Save the file.

12. In your browser enter `http://localhost/exercise03a.php`.

You should see the results shown in Figure 3-5. None of your comments show.

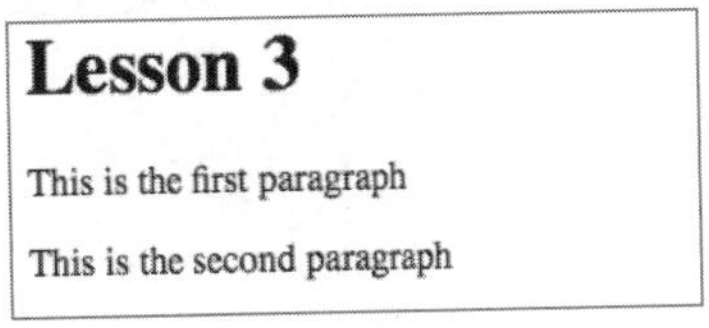

Add the PHPDoc blocks to the beginning of the .php files in the Case Study.

1. Copy the program you created in Lesson 2.

2. Open `index.php`.

3. At the beginning of the file, add `<?php ?>` tags.

4. Enter the following code between those tags. Leave the beginning and ending tags on their own lines.

```
/**
 * index.php
 *
 * Main file
```

Lesson 3

This is the first paragraph

This is the second paragraph

FIGURE 3-5

```
 *
 * @version    1.2 2011-02-03
 * @package    Smithside Auctions
 * @copyright  Copyright (c) 2011 Smithside Auctions
 * @license    GNU General Public License
 * @since      Since Release 1.0
 */
```

5. Open content/home.php.

6. At the beginning of the file, add `<?php ?>` tags.

7. Enter the following code between those tags. Leave the beginning and ending tags on their own lines.

```
/**
 * home.php
 *
 * Content for the home page
 *
 * @version    1.2 2011-02-03
 * @package    Smithside Auctions
 * @copyright  Copyright (c) 2011 Smithside Auctions
 * @license    GNU General Public License
 * @since      Since Release 1.0
 */
```

8. Open the Case Study in your browser. You should not be able to see the comments on the Home page. See Figure 3-6.

9. Open content/about.php.

10. At the beginning of the file, add `<?php ?>` tags.

11. Enter the following code between those tags. Leave the beginning and ending tags on their own lines.

```
/**
 * about.php
 *
 * Content for About Us page
 *
 * @version    1.2 2011-02-03
 * @package    Smithside Auctions
 * @copyright  Copyright (c) 2011 Smithside Auctions
 * @license    GNU General Public License
 * @since      Since Release 1.0
 */
```

12. In order to see the About Us page, you need to change the content page from home.php to about.php.

a. Open index.php.

b. Find this code: `<?php include 'content/home.php';?>`.

c. Change home to **about**.

d. Save the file.

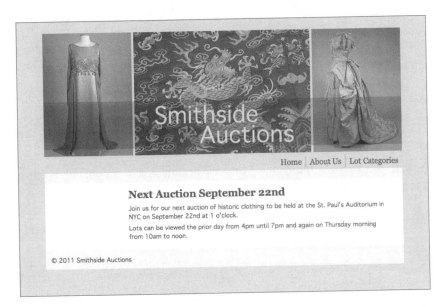

FIGURE 3-6

13. Open the Case Study in your browser. The About Us page displays. You should not be able to see the comments. See Figure 3-7.

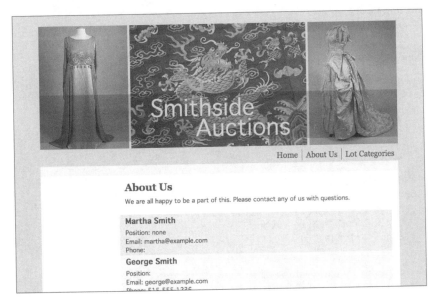

FIGURE 3-7

 Watch the video for Lesson 3 on the DVD or watch online at www.wrox.com/go/24phpmysql.

4

Working with Variables

In this lesson you learn what variables are, how to define them, and how to use them in several ways. You learn how PHP treats text and numbers differently.

INTRODUCTION TO VARIABLES

Variables are used to store information that can change. By creating variables, you have a way to write a program that can be used again and again with different data.

Say you want to calculate the tip at a restaurant. You normally give 20 percent. You know that to calculate a 20 percent tip you multiply the cost of the dinner by .20. You then add the tip to the cost of the dinner to get the total you pay. Your formula stays the same every time you go out to eat (well, unless the service is exceptionally bad or good, of course), but the cost of the dinner is different each time. You can think of the cost of the dinner as a variable.

In PHP, variables start with a dollar sign and you assign the variable a value using the = sign:

```
$costOfDinner = 15.95;
```

The following list includes rules for naming variables (after the $):

➤ You must start variables with a letter or an underscore. By convention, underscores are used only at certain times. You learn about when to use underscores in Lesson 15. For now, always start with a letter.

➤ You can use only alphanumeric characters and underscores (a–z, A–Z, 0–9 and _).

➤ You cannot use dashes or spaces.

➤ If the variable is more than one word, you should separate the words with capitalization or underscores.

> *PHP is case sensitive, which means that it sees lowercase and uppercase letters as totally different characters. So $myVar and $myvar are not the same. They are two separate variables. Remember this when you are trying to troubleshoot problems.*

In some programming languages you have to declare the variable ahead of time and say what type of information you are putting in the variable, such as whether it is text or numeric. In PHP you don't need to do this for simple variables. The variable takes on the type of the information you assign to it. You do need to assign a value to the variable before you can use it or you get an undefined variable error, however.

Complex variables, such as arrays and objects, should be declared. You learn about the arrays in Lesson 6 and objects in Lesson 13.

WORKING WITH TEXT

In programming, another term for text is *string*. Variables that contain text are called string variables. "Hello, world!" is a string. To assign that string to a variable, use the equal sign (=). This is actually called the *assignment operator*. Try not to think of it as an equal sign because that might cause you trouble later on. The = takes what is on the right side and uses that to set the value on the left side. This piece of code assigns a value to $myVar and then displays it.

```php
<?php
$myVar = 'Hi, my name is Andy';
echo $myVar;
?>
```

You can use either the single quote or the double quote when assigning a string value.

You can create a file and run that piece of code in your browser. You don't actually need any HTML at all. However, if you write a real program, you should wrap code that you are displaying to the browser in HTML such as this:

```php
<?php
$myVar = 'Hi, my name is Andy';
?>
<html>
<head>
    <title>Lesson 4b</title>
</head>

<body>

<h1>Welcome</h1>
<p><?php echo $myVar; ?></p>

</body>
</html>
```

Technically, if you want your HTML to validate, you also need a Doctype declaration. To add a Doctype, replace <html> with

```
<!DOCTYPE html PUBLIC "-//W3C//DTD XHTML 1.0 Transitional//EN"
"http://www.w3.org/TR/xhtml1/DTD/xhtml1-transitional.dtd">
<html xmlns="http://www.w3.org/1999/xhtml">
```

To keep the examples simple, I am not using a Doctype declaration in most of them.

Up to now, single and double quotes have been used interchangeably. There is a difference in how the two act. If you use double quotes, the PHP parser converts variables into their value within the string. The following code will interpret $myVar as "Hi, my name is Andy":

```php
<?php
$myName = 'Andy';
$myVar = "Hi, my name is $myName";
echo $myVar;
?>
```

If, however, you use single quotes, $myVar is interpreted as "Hi, my name is $myName." The PHP parser does not *expand* the variable; that is, it does not replace the variable with the value inside the variable.

```php
<?php
$myName = 'Andy';
$myVar = 'Hi, my name is $myName';
echo $myVar;
?>
```

Sometimes with double quotes there is some ambiguity about what exactly the parser should interpret as a variable to be translated. This can happen if text starts immediately after the variable. You can put curly braces ({}) around the variable to delineate it. The following code interprets $myVar as "There are 5 cats":

```php
<?php
$myAnimal = 'cat';
$myVar = "There are 5 {$myAnimal}s";
echo $myVar;
?>
```

It can happen that you have both single quotes and double quotes in the data that you need to quote. At that point you need to *escape* the quote. To escape something is to tell the PHP parser that the character is a data character and is not to be used as a *control character*, such as the ending quote. To escape, type a backslash (\) before the character that needs to be escaped:

```php
<?php
$saying1 = 'She said, "I didn\'t hear what you said."';
$saying2 = "She said, \"I didn't hear what you said.\"";
echo $saying1;
echo '<br />';
echo $saying2;
?>
```

Working with the Concatenation Operator

You can attach two string values together. They can either be actual strings or variables that have strings in them. This is called *concatenation.* You use a period (.) to concatenate the different strings:

```php
<?php
$myName = 'Andy';
$myVar = 'Hi, my name is ' . $myName;
echo $myVar;
?>
```

Notice that there is a space after the word `is`. All the spaces are ignored after the single quote until you get to the variable. So if you do not have the space after `is` and before the single quote, `$myVar` would be "Hi, my name isAndy." The spaces are optional around the concatenation operator and are there to make the code easier to read.

If you are concatenating two variables and need a space between them, you concatenate a string that consists of just a space:

```php
<?php
$firstName = 'Andy';
$lastName = 'Tarr';
$myVar = 'Hi, my name is ' . $firstName. ' ' . $lastName . '.';
echo $myVar;
?>
```

The last`.`is not a concatenation period, but the period at the end of the sentence. So `$myVar` is equal to "Hi, my name is Andy Tarr."

In PHP you often have different ways of doing the same thing. You could accomplish the same thing using double quotes and no concatenation:

```php
<?php
$firstName = 'Andy';
$lastName = 'Tarr';
$myVar = "Hi, my name is $firstName $lastName.";
echo $myVar;
?>
```

Notice that you don't need curly braces around `$lastName`. Even though it is immediately followed by text, a period cannot be part of a variable name so the parser knows to stop with `$lastName`. It would not hurt anything to use curly braces, however. Notice also that the space between the two variables shows in the final result.

Working with String Functions

You can think of *functions* as little programs that perform tasks for you. PHP has a number of functions for manipulating strings. Often you pass the function a variable by putting the variable in the parentheses that are suffixed to the function. In addition to performing tasks, a function can *return* a value; that is, the value of the function is the value that is returned by the function.

Functions do not start with a dollar sign and they are immediately followed by parentheses.

> *For a complete list of string functions, see the PHP manual at* `http://php.net/manual/en/ref.strings.php`. *This also contains more detail and examples of the functions you are about to learn.*

strlen()

String Length returns the length of the string. The following function returns a result of 4:

```php
<?php
$myName = 'Andy';
echo strlen($myName);
?>
```

htmlspecialchars()

HTML Special Characters takes a string and converts &, <, >, and double quotes to proper HTML entities.

```php
<?php
$myName = 'Andy & Amos';
echo htmlspecialchars($myName);
?>
```

This code displays "Andy & Amos," but if you look at the source for the browser page, you see "Andy & Amos."

ucfirst()

Upper Case First changes the first character to uppercase. The following function returns a result of "The book of days":

```php
<?php
$myVar = 'the book of days';
echo ucfirst($myVar);
?>
```

ucwords()

Upper Case Words changes the first character of each word to uppercase. The following function returns "The Book Of Days":

```php
<?php
$myVar = 'the book of days';
echo ucwords($myVar);
?>
```

trim()

Trim removes any blank characters from the beginning and end of the string. The following function returns "the book of days":

```php
<?php
$myVar = '   the book of days   ';
echo trim($myVar);
?>
```

strtolower()

String to Lower converts any uppercase letters to lowercase. The following function returns "the book of days":

```php
<?php
$myVar = 'THE BOOK OF DAYS';
echo strtolower($myVar);
?>
```

strtoupper()

String to Upper converts any lowercase letters to uppercase. The following function returns "THE BOOK OF DAYS":

```php
<?php
$myVar = 'the book of days';
echo strtoupper($myVar);
?>
```

You can nest the functions as well. The following code converts the text to lowercase and then capitalizes the first letter of each word, resulting in "The Book of Days":

```php
<?php
$myVar = 'THE BOOK OF daYs';
echo ucwords(strtolower($myVar));
?>
```

UNDERSTANDING DIFFERENT TYPES OF NUMBERS

PHP works with two different types of numbers: *integer* and *floating-point* numbers.

Integers are whole numbers. They have no decimal points and can be positive, negative, or zero.

Floating-point numbers are numbers that have decimals. Arguably one of the strangest concepts of working with numbers in computers is that after you introduce decimals you introduce rounding errors. You may not always notice it because the error may be small enough that it does not affect what you are doing. The most likely place you will get tripped up is if you try to determine if two numbers are equal and at least one of them is a floating point. The two numbers might print out looking identical, but one could be 6.599999991234 while the other is 6.599999992236.

Integers do not have the rounding issue.

When you perform arithmetic with integers, they could turn into floating-point numbers if the results require decimals.

WORKING WITH NUMBERS

You can assign values to numeric variables with the = sign. This is called the *assignment operator*. Try not to think of it as an equal sign because that might cause you trouble later on. The = takes what is on the right side and uses that to set the value on the left side. The following code sets $result to 2. Notice that, unlike strings, there are no quotes around the number.

```php
<?php
$result = 2;
echo $result;
?>
```

The following code sets `$result` to 1.45:

```php
<?php
$result = 1.45;
echo $result;
?>
```

Besides assigning a specific value in the same way that you assign a value to a text variable, numeric variables have additional ways to assign values, as shown in Table 4-1.

TABLE 4-1: Assignment Operators

OPERATOR	EXAMPLE	EQUALS
=	$a = 3;	$a = 3;
+=	$a += 3;	$a = $a + 3;
-=	$a -= 3;	$a = $a - 3;
*=	$a *= 3;	$a = $a * 3;
/=	$a /= 3;	$a = $a / 3;
%=	$a %= 3;	$a = $a % 3;

The *numeric operators* should look very familiar to you. `$a` is equal to 3 in Table 4-2.

TABLE 4-2: Numeric Operators

OPERATOR	DESCRIPTION	EXAMPLE	RESULT
+	Addition	$a + 2;	5
-	Subtraction	$a - 2;	3
*	Multiply	$a * 2;	6
/	Divide	$a / 2;	1.5
%	Remainder	$a%2;	1
++	Increment	$a++;	$a equals 4
--	Decrement	$a--;	$a equals 2

CHANGING BETWEEN TEXT AND NUMBERS

Various functions and operations require that the variables be of a particular type. For instance, you can multiply only numeric variables. PHP quietly converts variables to the right data type if it can. In the following code, `$stringNumber` is automatically converted to a number and 15 is displayed:

```
<?php
$stringNumber = '3';
$number = 5;
echo $stringNumber * $number;
?>
```

Here, the `$stringNumber` is converted to 15, giving 75 as the result:

```
<?php
$stringNumber = '15a4';
$number = 5;
echo $stringNumber * $number;
?>
```

And here, the `$stringNumber` is converted to 0, giving the result as 0 as well:

```
<?php
$stringNumber = 'aaa';
$number = 5;
echo $stringNumber * $number;
?>
```

The following code uses concatenation, which expects string variables. The variables are converted to strings and the result displayed is 35.

```
<?php
$stringNumber = 3;
$number = 5;
echo $stringNumber . $number;
?>
```

Here's another string function that takes a float number and displays it as a formatted string. Because it expects `$number` to be a floating-point number, it converts it from a string to a float:

```
<?php
$number = '15';
echo number_format($number, 2);
?>
```

TRY IT

In this Try It, you start changing static information in the Case Study website to variables. You work with the page that displays the gents category of lots.

You start by moving the information in the content `<div>` from the `gents.html` file into a PHP file in the content folder and then deleting the HTML page. You also change the link references to `gent.html` in `index.php`.

You create and assign values to variables for the data used on the page. You use those variables to display the data. Use the string functions to automatically change the & to & for you in the text.

Finally, you replace the odd/even row class with a calculated formula.

> *You can download the code and resources for this Try It from the book's web page at* www.wrox.com. *You can find them in the Lesson04 folder in the download. You will find code for both before and after completing the exercises.*

Lesson Requirements

Your computer needs to be able to run as a web server with PHP and MySQL. XAMPP is a package of software that installs the web server, PHP, and MySQL for you. You can find instructions for downloading and installing XAMPP in Lesson 1.

You need a text editor that can produce plain-text files. You can find instructions for downloading and installing Eclipse PDT in Lesson 1. Other text editors that you can use are Adobe's Dreamweaver in code mode, Notepad, TextWrangler, or NetBeans.

If you are following along with the Case Study, you need your files from the end of Lesson 3. Alternatively, you can download the files from the book's website at www.wrox.com.

Hints

Remember that you moved the home.php and about.php into the content folder in Lesson 2.

The string function htmlspecialchars() encodes & characters into the proper HTML entities.

Use number_format() to display the price with two decimals.

Step-by-Step

Move the content in gents.html to the new file content/gents.php.

1. Move gents.html to the content folder. If you are using Eclipse, right-click the gents.html file in the list on the left, select Refactor ⇨ Move, and select the content folder.

2. Rename gents.html to **gents.php**. If you are using Eclipse, right-click and then select Refactor ⇨ Rename and change the .html to .php.

3. Open content/gents.php.

4. Delete all the code up to and including <div class="content">. Your first line is now the h1 tags.

5. Delete </div><!--end content --> and all code below it. Your last line is an ending </ul> tag.

6. Open `index.php` and change the line `<?php include 'content/about.php';?>` to **`<?php include 'content/gents.php';?>`**.

7. Open the Case Study. The first page that shows should be the Gents lots page similar to Figure 4-1.

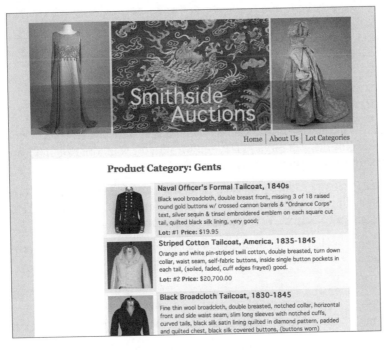

FIGURE 4-1

Change the image, name, description, price, and lot (`lot_number`) to variables and assign values to the variables.

1. Add the following variable assignments to the top of the `gents.php` file:

```php
<?php
// Get the lot information
$lot_number   = '1';
$image        = "naval-19-173.jpg";
$name         = "Naval Officer's Formal Tailcoat, 1840s";
$description  = 'Black wool broadcloth, double breast front, missing
 3 of 18 raised round gold buttons w/crossed cannon barrels &
"Ordnance Corps" text, silver sequin & tinsel embroidered emblem
on each square cut tail, quilted black silk lining, very good; ';
$price        = 5700.00;
$lot_number2  = '2';
$image2       = "gents-striped-8-26.jpg";
```

```
$name2        = "Striped Cotton Tailcoat, America, 1835-1845";
$description2 = 'Orange and white pin-striped twill cotton, double
breasted, turn down collar, waist seam, self-fabric buttons, inside
single button pockets in each tail, (soiled, faded, cuff edges
frayed) good. ';
$price2       = 20700.00;
$lot_number3  = '3';
$image3       = "gents-black-8-27.jpg";
$name3        = "Black Broadcloth Tailcoat, 1830-1845";
$description3 = 'Fine thin wool broadcloth, double breasted, notched collar,
horizontal front and side waist seam,
slim long sleeves with notched cuffs, curved tails, black silk satin lining
quilted in diamond pattern, padded and quilted chest, black silk covered
buttons, (buttons worn) excellent. ';
$price3       = 3450.00;
?>
```

a. Notice that the descriptions with single quotes have double quotes around them and descriptions with double quotes have single quotes around them. Also notice that the HTML entities & are changed to a simple &. You automatically convert these before they are output, so you don't need to manually translate them ahead of time.

b. The commas in the prices have been removed.

2. Replace the hardcoded data with the variables.

a. **Images:** Use the same variable for the thumbnail and the full size image with this code:

```
<div class="list-photo"><a href="images/<?php echo $image; ?>">
  <img src="images/thumbnails/<?php echo $image; ?>" alt="" /></a>
</div>
```

b. **Name:** Add the ucwords() string function to be sure that the first letter of each word is capitalized:

```
<h2><?php echo ucwords($name); ?></h2>
```

c. **Description:** Because the data now might have &'s in it, use the string function htmlspecialchars() to automatically turn them into &:

```
<p><?php echo htmlspecialchars($description); ?></p>
```

d. **Lot:** Use the variable $lot_number for the lot:

```
<p><strong>Lot:</strong> #<?php echo $lot_number; ?>
```

e. **Price:** Use number_format() to format the price:

```
<strong>Price:</strong> $<?php echo number_format($price,2); ?></p>
```

3. Repeat step 2 for the second and third lots.

4. Save the file.

5. Open the Case Study. You should see the Gents list of lots still looking like Figure 4-1.

> *When you learn about databases you will be able to load the variables from the database. You will also be able to loop around and fill all three lots from one set of variables.*

Replace the hardcoded `row0`, `row1` classes with a calculated class in `gents.php`.

1. Initialize a variable for counting the number of rows. Put this at the end of the list of variables at the top of the file:

    ```
    $i = 0; // for counting line number
    ```

2. Take the row number and divide it by 2. The remainder, either 0 or 1, is then appended to the class row. To do this, replace `<li class="row0">` with

    ```
    <li class="row<?php echo $i % 2; ?>">
    ```

3. You need to add 1 to the number of rows after printing each row. Use the increment operator. The following code is added just after displaying the price:

    ```
    <?php $i++; ?>
    ```

4. Repeat steps 2 and 3 for the next two rows.

5. Save the file.

6. Open the Case Study. You should see the Gents list of lots still looking like Figure 4-1.

> *Watch the video for Lesson 4 on the DVD or watch online at* www.wrox.com/ go/24phpmysql.

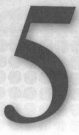

Debugging Code

From Grace Hopper and her moth in the 1940s to the present day, programmers have been debugging to locate errors. No one writes perfect code the first time, and the better you are at finding your errors, the less frustrated you will be and the better your code will be.

Your first line of defense is using a good editor that validates syntax for you. That catches many possible errors.

In this lesson you learn techniques for locating problems and identifying common issues. You are also introduced to a debugging program you can use to facilitate your debugging.

TROUBLESHOOTING TECHNIQUES

In this section you learn when and how to display PHP errors in order to get automatic feedback on PHP problems. You also learn what many of the common problems are and how to avoid them. Finally, you are introduced to various ways to see what is happening inside your program as it processes.

Display Errors while Developing

You want errors to be displayed for you while you are developing your code. To do this, make sure that display_errors is on in your php.ini file. You can check this by running phpinfo(). If you are using XAMPP, display_errors is on by default because it is set up for development, not production. This is the code for running phpinfo():

```php
<?php
phpinfo();
```

> *In the earlier lessons, I included the ending PHP tag of ?> to make it easier and clearer. However, it is good practice not to use the ending tag at the end of a file, so from now on I leave off the ending tag where it is not needed.*

Find the section called Core. It should look similar to Figure 5-1.

Core

Directive	Local Value	Master Value
PHP Version		5.3.1
allow_call_time_pass_reference	On	On
allow_url_fopen	On	On
allow_url_include	Off	Off
always_populate_raw_post_data	Off	Off
arg_separator.input	&	&
arg_separator.output	&	&
asp_tags	Off	Off
auto_append_file	no value	no value
auto_globals_jit	On	On
auto_prepend_file	no value	no value
browscap	no value	no value
default_charset	no value	no value
default_mimetype	text/html	text/html
define_syslog_variables	Off	Off
detect_unicode	On	On
disable_classes	no value	no value
disable_functions	no value	no value
display_errors	On	On
display_startup_errors	Off	Off
doc_root	no value	no value
docref_ext	no value	no value
docref_root	no value	no value
enable_dl	On	On
error_append_string	no value	no value
error_log	no value	no value
error_prepend_string	no value	no value
error_reporting	30711	30711
exit_on_timeout	Off	Off

FIGURE 5-1

If your `display_errors` is not on, edit the `php.ini` file so `display_errors` is on. If you are using XAMPP, the `php.ini` file is located at `c:\xampp\php` on a Windows PC and at `/Applications/XAMPP/Xamppfiles/etc` on a Mac OS X.

```
display_errors = on
```

`display_errors` determines if reported errors are displayed. `error_reporting` determines which errors should be reported. Errors have different levels, from minor notices to warning to severe. Your error reporting level is also listed on the `phpinfo()` report, but it is in machine-readable code, so it is easier to look in your `php.ini` file. A good level for developing is to show all errors except for notices. The tilde (~) prefixed to `E_NOTICE` provides direction to not show those errors.

```
error_reporting = E_ALL & ~E_NOTICE
```

If you want to make sure you get all notices, including if you have a defined variable, do not exclude the notices. This is helpful if you have typos or problems remembering the right cases.

```
error_reporting = E_ALL
```

If you want to go one step further, you can also display errors that don't meet very strict PHP standards. The pipe symbol (|) means to display if the error violates `E_ALL` or `E_STRICT`.

```
error_reporting  =  E_ALL | E_STRICT
```

If you make changes to php.ini, be sure to stop your Apache web server and start it again.

Take a look at what the errors look like when they are reported. Can you find the error in the following code?

```php
<?php
$firstName = 'Andy';
$nameLength = str_len($firstName);
$myVar = 'Hi, my name is ' . $nameLength. ' letters long.';
echo $myVar;
```

If you run the code, you see an error message similar to Figure 5-2. The error message starts out with the error level, which in this case is "Fatal error." It then says what the error is, which is a "Call to undefined function." Then it gives the name of the function, which is str_len(). Then it says what file contains the error, which is lesson05b.php, and finally what line the system was on when it realized there was an error, which is line 3.

You know the problem is that str_len() in line 3 doesn't exist. Oops. That should be strlen(). So you remove the underscore and successfully rerun.

⚠ Fatal error: Call to undefined function str_len() in /Users/andytarr/Documents/php24/wphp24/php24/lesson05code/lesson05b.php on line 3			
Call Stack			
# **Time**	**Memory**	**Function**	**Location**
1 0.0003	324236	{main}( )	../lesson05b.php:0

FIGURE 5-2

> Note that the line number is when the system realizes the problem. Your actual error could be on another line. For instance, a common error is a missing semicolon, which often results in a parse error on the following line. A parse error means that the PHP parser just threw up its hands and said, "I have no idea what you are trying to tell me."

Common Issues

Here are things to check when your code isn't working:

➤ **Typos:** Did you type what you meant to?

➤ **Missing echo:** One of the most common errors, even for experienced programmers, is forgetting to echo a variable when you need to display it. `<p>$myVar</p>` displays nothing.

➤ **Case:** PHP is case sensitive, so $firstname is not the same as $firstName.

➤ **Semicolons:** Check that you have not missed ending a statement with a semicolon.

➤ **Misplaced or missing closing braces:** You'll use parentheses, curly braces, and even square brackets. Make sure they all begin and end when you want them to and make sure you are using the right type of brace.

➤ **= versus ==:** This is assignment versus comparison. You learn about comparisons in Lesson 7. For now, realize that the question "Is x equal to y?" uses a double equal sign (==) or, sometimes, a triple equal sign (===). If you use a single equal sign for comparison, you won't get any errors but the code does not work the way you think it does. Instead of comparing, it assigns. So, in this example, x is made equal to y instead of checking to see if it is equal to y.

➤ **$ on variables:** Don't forget that variables have to start with a $ sign.

➤ **Quotes:** Check your single quotes, double quotes, nested quotes, and escaped quotes, and also your use of MySQL backticks (`) with regard to the following.

> ➤ Double quotes expand enclosed variables and single quotes do not.

> ➤ Use curly braces ({}) around variables if there is any ambiguity.

> ➤ If you have one type of quotes in your text, enclose with the other type.

> ➤ If you have both types or need to enclose with the same type of quote, escape the quote by prefixing with a backslash (\).

> ➤ When concatenating a mix of PHP and HTML, it can be helpful to replace the PHP with the values and then replace each block of PHP code one at a time.

> ➤ MySQL uses backticks (`) around database, table, and column names. You learn about this in Lesson 19.

➤ **Array number:** Arrays in PHP start counting with 0, not 1. So the third element is number 2. You learn about arrays in Lesson 6.

Seeing What's What

So how do you see what's going on inside a program before it displays to your browser?

If your web page does not look right, first check the source for the browser page. Is the HTML showing you what you expect? If it is, you have an HTML issue to fix. If it is not, you can see what PHP is actually outputting.

The echo command that you have been using throughout these lessons can be used to display the value of a variable. You can use it to trace where you are in a program by echoing a variable or even just echoing here:

```php
<?php
$number = 42;
if ($number > 2) {
   // some code here
} else {
   // some other code here
}
```

This code does something if $number is greater than 2 and something else if $number is not greater than 2. In this instance you are setting $number to 42 just before this statement, but pretend that that was several lines up and not so obvious. You learn about the if statement in Lesson 7.

You want to know what the number is just before the if statement and which of the two paths it follows. So you add an echo statement before the if statement to display $number and add an echo statement in each of the branches. Now when you run the program you know what is in the variable

and which path it took. Obviously you remove these after you don't need them anymore. Running the following code looks similar to Figure 5-3:

```php
<?php
$number = 42;
echo $number.'<br />';
if ($number > 2) {
  echo 'here 1';
} else {
  echo 'here 2';
}
```

```
42
here 1
```

FIGURE 5-3

Arrays are lists of variables that you learn about in Lesson 6. The print_r() function works like echo but is used for arrays because arrays are too complex for the echo statement. The syntax for print_r() is different but you can use it in the same way as the echo statement. The following code displays output similar to Figure 5-4:

```
Array ( [0] => Mon [1] => Tue [2] => Wed [3] => Thu [4] => Fri )
```

FIGURE 5-4

```php
<?php
$myArray = array("Mon", "Tue", "Wed", "Thu", "Fri");
print_r($myArray);
```

var_dump() is another function that displays a variable. It also displays the complex data types such as the arrays you learn about in Lesson 6 and objects that you learn about in Section III. The following code displays output similar to Figure 5-5:

```php
<?php
$myArray = array("Mon", "Tue", "Wed", "Thu", "Fri");
var_dump($myArray);
```

If you want processing to stop when you reach a certain point, you can use the die() function. Notice that the following code never gets to the echo statement, as shown in Figure 5-6:

```php
<?php
$myArray = array("Mon", "Tue", "Wed", "Thu", "Fri");
var_dump($myArray);
die('Stop here');
echo 'We never get here.';
```

```
array
  0 => string 'Mon' (length=3)
  1 => string 'Tue' (length=3)
  2 => string 'Wed' (length=3)
  3 => string 'Thu' (length=3)
  4 => string 'Fri' (length=3)
```

FIGURE 5-5

```
array
  0 => string 'Mon' (length=3)
  1 => string 'Tue' (length=3)
  2 => string 'Wed' (length=3)
  3 => string 'Thu' (length=3)
  4 => string 'Fri' (length=3)
Stop here
```

FIGURE 5-6

USING XDEBUG

If you are working with complex PHP programs, you will find that echos and var_dumps can be cumbersome. At that point, you should use a debugger program. A debugger program does not tell you what is wrong with your program, but it does let you step through your code line by line so you can see where it goes. It enables you to see the value of all the variables whenever you want.

Eclipse PDT comes with two debugger programs. They can be tricky to configure but it is well worth the time to set one up. If you don't use Eclipse, your text editor may have its own debugger or you can use the methods you learned earlier in this lesson.

Configuring Xdebug

In Eclipse, go to Tools ➪ Option (Windows) or Eclipse ➪ Preferences (Mac). You see a window similar to Figure 5-7. You take several steps in this window.

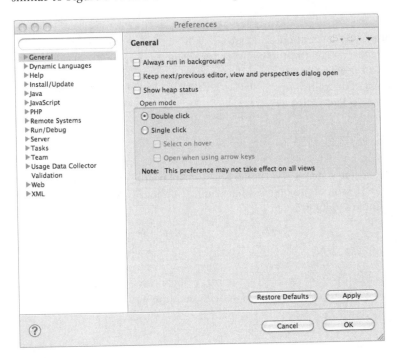

FIGURE 5-7

Go to PHP ➪ Debug and change PHP Debugger to Xdebug as shown in Figure 5-8. Click Apply to save the change.

Click PHP ➪ Debug ➪ Installed Debuggers. Select each of the debuggers in turn and click the Configure link to change the ports so they match Figure 5-9. Zend Debugger is Port 10001 and Xdebug is Port 10000. Click Apply to save the change.

Go to General ➪ Web Browser. Select the Use External Web Browser function. The window looks similar to Figure 5-10.

If you don't use http://localhost as your root, you need to change your PHP server. So if you didn't change your port, and you aren't using virtual hosts (if you don't know what they are, you are not using them), you can skip this next step.

To change your PHP server, go to PHP ➪ PHP Servers. The window looks similar to Figure 5-11.

Select the Default PHP Web Server, click Edit, and change the URL to your root. If your root is http://localhost:8080, your resulting window looks similar to Figure 5-12. Click Apply to save the change.

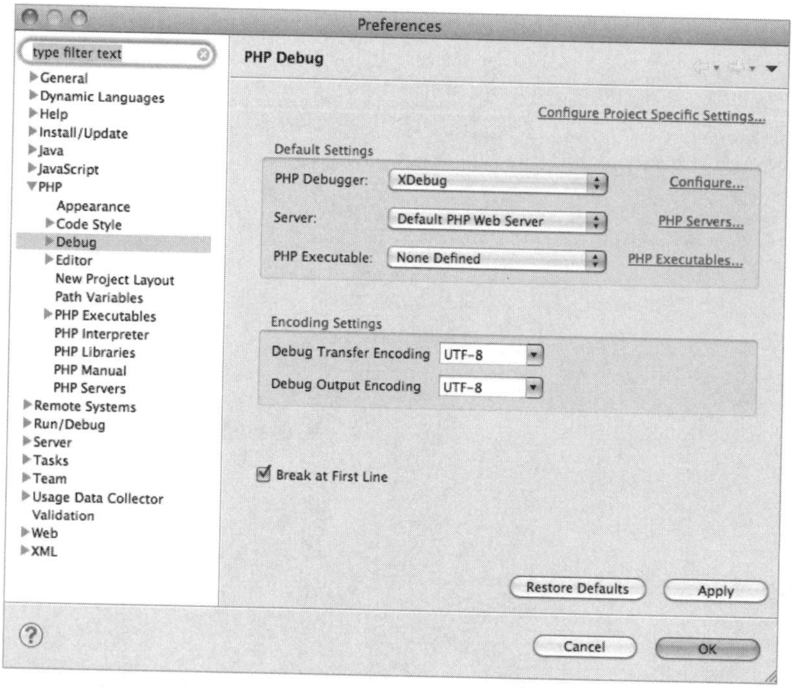

FIGURE 5-8

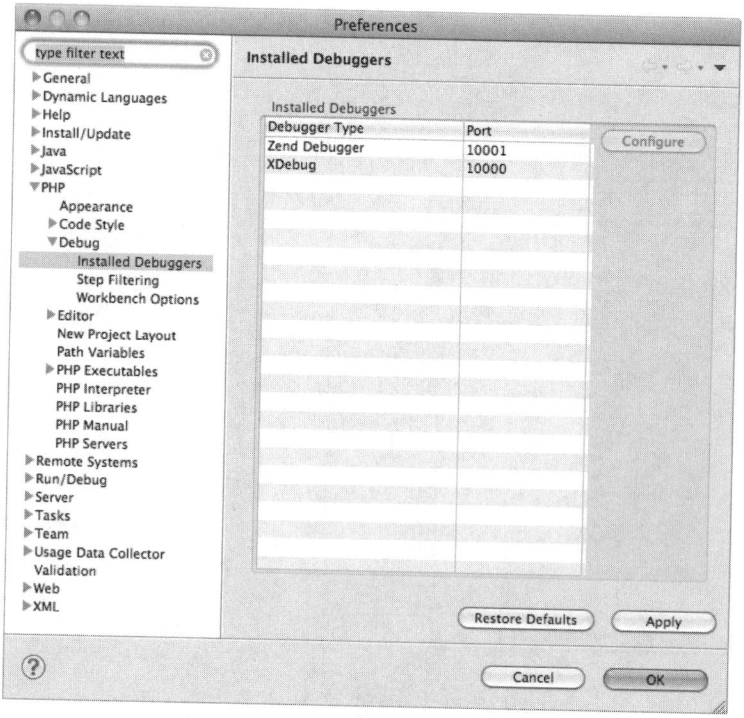

In Figure 5-9, the Installed Debuggers table shows:

Debugger Type	Port
Zend Debugger	10001
XDebug	10000

FIGURE 5-9

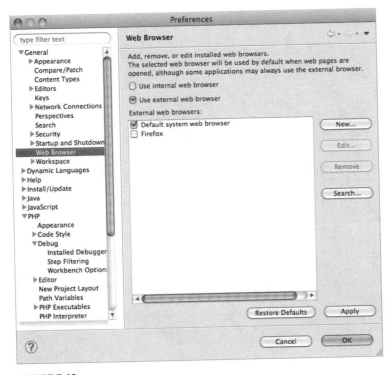

FIGURE 5-10

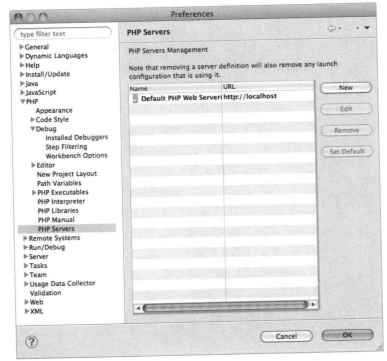

FIGURE 5-11

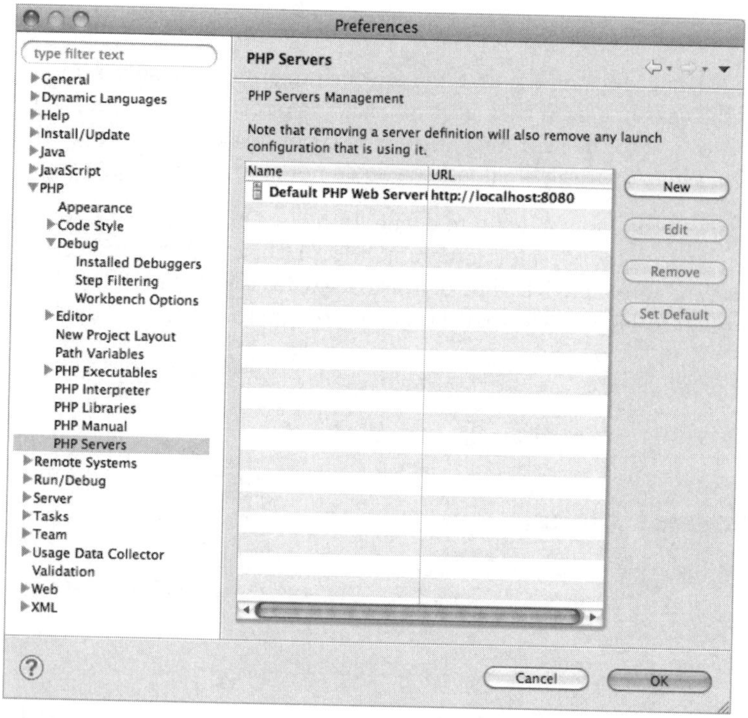

FIGURE 5-12

Click OK to exit.

The last task to configuring is to change the `php.ini` file. XAMPP sets up the debug configuration needed, though depending on the exact install you may need to change the `xdebug.remote_port`. The following code is an example of the Xdebug configuration code on the Mac:

```
;xdebug Configuration starts

zend_extension="/Applications/XAMPP/xamppfiles/lib/php/php-5.3.1/extensions/
no-debug-non-zts-20090626/xdebug.so"

xdebug.profiler_output_dir = "/tmp/xdebug/"
xdebug.profiler_enable = On
xdebug.remote_enable=On
xdebug.remote_host="localhost"
xdebug.remote_port=10000
xdebug.remote_handler="dbgp"

;xdebug Configuration ends
```

You need to exit Eclipse, stop and restart Apache, then restart Eclipse.

Using Xdebug

When you start the debugger, Xdebug stops on the first line of your program by default. From there you can choose to go to the next line or, if the line is an `include` or calls another file, you can choose to step into that file or just to the next line. You can also put breakpoints on PHP lines, which pause the program on that line. By using breakpoints you do not need to pause on every line.

To use Xdebug, you right-click the program you want to debug. If this is a program that is dependent on other programs, you start with the top-most program. Select Debug ⇨ Debug as Web Page. If you get a dialog box, confirm the starting URL. The perspective switches to the PHP Debug perspective. You see a window similar to Figure 5-13 that shows your program.

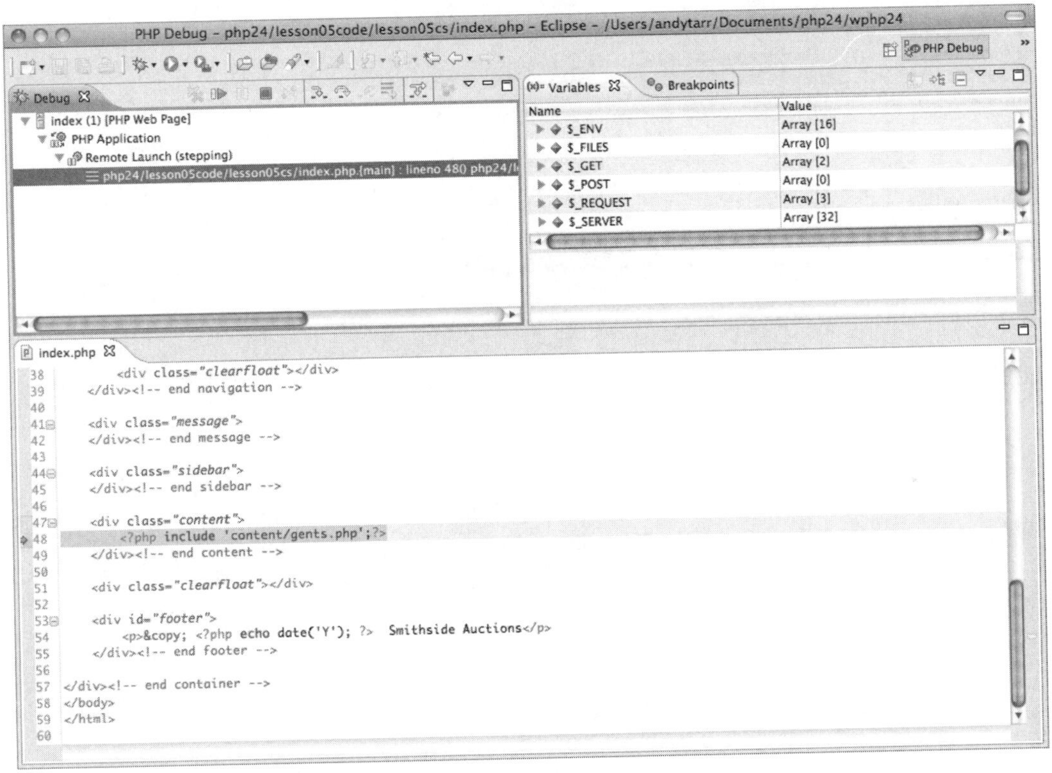

FIGURE 5-13

Perspectives are the different prearranged groupings of screens that show for the editor. If the PHP Debug perspective does not automatically appear, look at the upper-right corner where the name of the current perspective shows. Click the >> symbol and choose PHP Debug from the list to switch to that perspective. If the perspective does not appear in the list, go to Window ⇨ Open Perspective ⇨ Other. Click PHP Debug and click Open. It now appears in your list of perspectives.

The main screen shows the source code for the file you are debugging with the current line highlighted.

In the upper right are the tabs that show you the variables and a list of the breakpoints. The Variable tab shows all the current variables and their values.

In the upper left you see the Debug tab. See Figure 5-14. This shows you which file you are in along with the files you went through to get there. Along the top of this window are icons that you use to control the debugger.

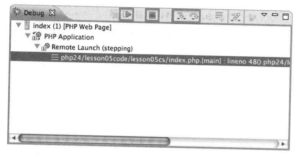

FIGURE 5-14

➤ **Resume:** This arrow tells the program to continue processing. It pauses at the next break-point or the end of the program.

➤ **Stop:** This square ends the debugging.

➤ **Step into:** This arrow pointing between two dashes steps into the current line. For instance, if the line you are on is an `include` statement, clicking this icon jumps you into the included file.

➤ **Step over:** The arrow pointing past the dash takes you to the next statement in the same file.

It is easy to create breakpoints. All you need to do is double-click in the column to the left of the line numbers in the file. Breakpoints are remembered even after you close a file.

TRY IT

In this Try It, you use the techniques learned in this lesson to debug a code sample. You have numerous other opportunities to debug as you complete the rest of the lessons.

You also use Xdebug to explore the Case Study files.

> You can download the code and resources for this Try It from the book's web page at www.wrox.com. You can find them in the Lesson05 folder in the download. You will find code for both before and after completing the exercises.

Lesson Requirements

Your computer needs to be able to run as a web server with PHP and MySQL. XAMPP is a package of software that installs the web server, PHP, and MySQL for you. You can find instructions for downloading and installing XAMPP in Lesson 1.

You need a text editor that can produce plain-text files. You can find instructions for downloading and installing Eclipse PDT in Lesson 1. Other text editors that you can use are Adobe's Dreamweaver in code mode, Notepad, TextWrangler, or NetBeans.

If you are following along with the Case Study you need your files from the end of Lesson 4. Alternatively, you can download the files from the book's website at www.wrox.com.

Hints

Remember to go through the list of common errors.

Step-by-Step

Find the error in the following code:

```php
<?php
$firstName = 'Andy';
$nameLength = str_len($firstName);
$myVar = 'Hi, my name is ' . $namelength. ' letters long.';
echo $myVar;
```

1. If you have Notices printing, you see a message saying that $namelength is uninitialized. If you are not displaying Notices, you still see that you are missing the number of letters. See Figure 5-15.

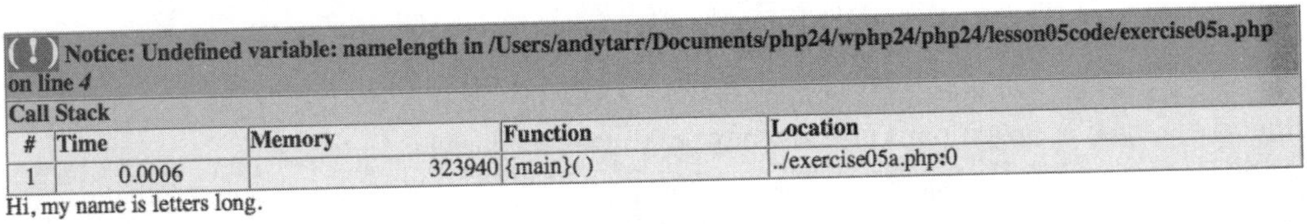

(!) Notice: Undefined variable: namelength in /Users/andytarr/Documents/php24/wphp24/php24/lesson05code/exercise05a.php on line *4*

#	Time	Memory	Function	Location
1	0.0006	323940	{main}( )	../exercise05a.php:0

Call Stack

Hi, my name is letters long.

FIGURE 5-15

2. The variable that you initialized was $nameLength not $namelength. Change $namelength to **$nameLength** to fix.

The following code should print out the name and number of characters. They are missing, as shown in Figure 5-16. The correct result is shown in Figure 5-17. Find the error.

```php
<?php
$firstName = 'Andy';
$nameLength = strlen($firstName);
?>
<html>
<head>
```

Welcome

My name is and it is characters long.

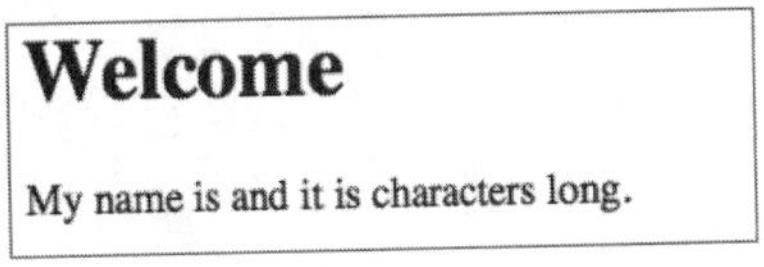

FIGURE 5-16

```
    <title>Exercise 5b</title>
</head>
<body>

<h1>Welcome</h1>
<p>My name is <?php $firstName; ?>
and it is <?php $nameLength; ?> characters long.</p>

</body>
</html>
```

3. Go through the list of the common errors. This is the corrected code:

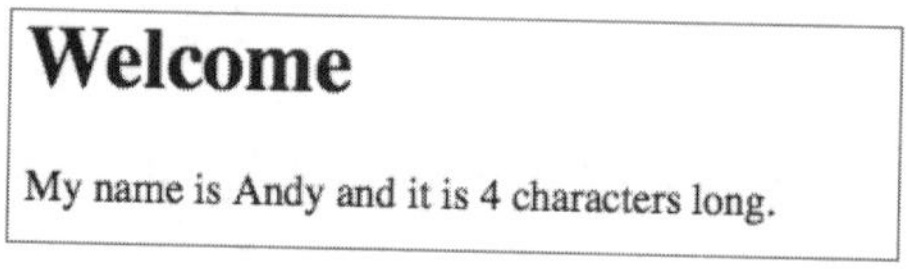

Welcome

My name is Andy and it is 4 characters long.

FIGURE 5-17

```
<?php
$firstName = 'Andy';
$nameLength = strlen($firstName);
?>
<html>
<head>
    <title>Exercise 5bfinal</title>
</head>
<body>

<h1>Welcome</h1>
<p>My name is <?php echo $firstName; ?>
and it is <?php echo $nameLength; ?> characters long.</p>

</body>
</html>
```

Use Xdebug to explore the Case Study files.

1. Right-click the `index.php` file from the Case Study.

2. Select Debug ⇨ Debug as Web Page. The program stops on the first PHP line, which happens to be the include line to the `gents.php` file.

3. Click the Step Into icon twice to go into that file.

4. Step Into or Step Over several times and then scroll through the Variable tab. You see the variables for those that have been given a value. Variables not assigned a value are uninitialized. See Figure 5-18.

5. Try creating a breakpoint by double-clicking the column to the left of the numbers. Remember that only lines with PHP code can be debugged.

6. Click the Resume icon to jump to the breakpoint.

7. When you are done exploring, click the red square Stop icon to terminate the debugger.

8. If the perspective does not change automatically, you can return to the PHP perspective by clicking the >> in the upper-right corner and choosing PHP.

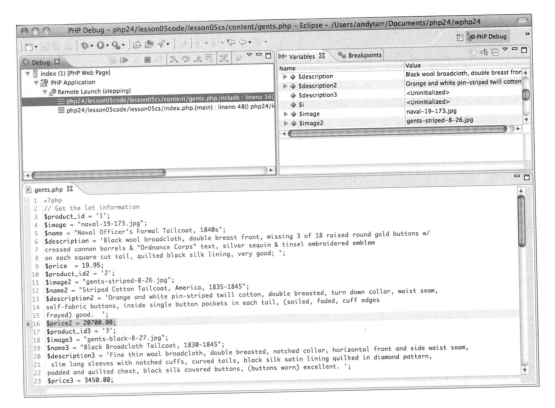

FIGURE 5-18

Watch the video for Lesson 5 on the DVD or watch online at www.wrox.com/go/24phpmysql.

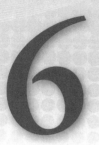

Working with Complex Data

You have learned how to work with variables that store text and numbers. This works well for simple data, but what if you have a list you need to manipulate or you want to know how many days there are between January 15, 2011, and March 2, 2011?

In this lesson you learn how to use special variables that are designed for specific types of data.

WORKING WITH ARRAYS

An *array* holds multiple values in a single variable. Within one variable you have an entire list of values. You refer to and access the entire array just by the array name as you would a regular variable, or you can use indexes to access the individual values. You can even nest arrays within arrays. These nested arrays are called *multi-dimensional* arrays.

Let's display a list of employees on a web page. You could assign each employee to a regular variable and then display each of those variables. Your results look similar to Figure 6-1.

```
<?php
// Assign Value
$employee1 = 'Sally Meyers';
$employee2 = 'George Smith';
$employee3 = 'Peter Hengel';
?>
<html>
<head>
  <title>Lesson 6a</title>
</head>

<body>

<h1>Employee List</h1>
  <p><?php echo $employee1; ?></p>
  <p><?php echo $employee2; ?></p>
  <p><?php echo $employee3; ?></p>

</body>
</html>
```

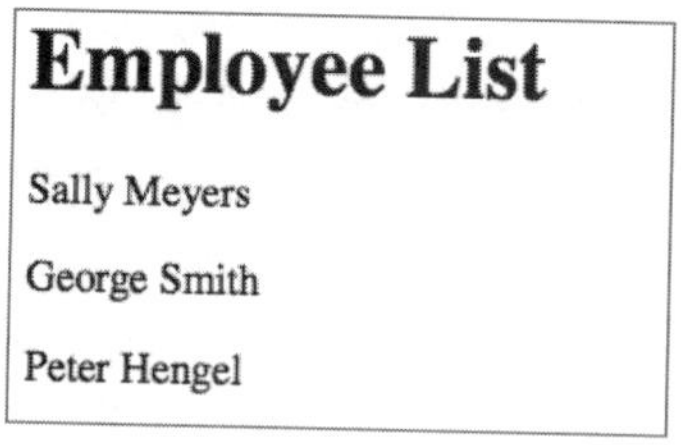

Employee List

Sally Meyers

George Smith

Peter Hengel

FIGURE 6-1

Now try it using an array. There are two types of arrays in PHP. The first type is a numeric array where the index is the position of the value in an array. You can assign the values in the array just by telling PHP this variable is an array and then listing the values:

```php
$employee = array('Sally Meyers', 'George Smith', 'Peter Hengel');
```

Just like regular variables, you need quotes around text and not around numbers. To reference a single value, add the index in square brackets to the array variable name. Your results look like Figure 6-2.

```php
<?php
$employee = array('Sally Meyers', 'George Smith', 'Peter Hengel' );
echo $employee[1];
```

Not quite what you were expecting? Unlike normal counting where you start with 1, PHP uses standard computer geek counting and starts with 0. Therefore index 1 displays the second value, which happens to be George Smith.

George Smith

FIGURE 6-2

You can also assign values using the same syntax you used to display the array element:

```php
$employee[0] = 'Sally Meyers';
$employee[1] = 'George Smith';
$employee[2] = 'Peter Hengel';
```

To see what is in an array use the `print_r()` function instead of the echo statement you are familiar with. If you echo an array it displays the word "array" instead of the values in the array. Add the following line of code to display the values in the array $employee. See Figure 6-3.

```php
print_r($employee);
```

Array ([0] => Sally Meyers [1] => George Smith [2] => Peter Hengel)

FIGURE 6-3

The second type of array is the associative array. In addition to being able to access the element values by their position, you can assign a name (key) to each value, which you can use to reference the element. Instead of a list of employees, make a list of information about a particular employee:

```php
$employee = array('name'=>'Sally Meyers', 'position'=>'President',
                  'yearEmployed'=>2001 );
```

Alternatively, you can assign the values with the same syntax you use to display the elements:

```php
$employee['name'] = 'Sally Meyers';
$employee['position'] = 'President';
$employee['yearEmployed'] = 2001;
```

Either way, if you `print_r()` the employee array you see a result similar to Figure 6-4.

```php
print_r($employee);
```

Array ([name] => Sally Meyers [position] => President [yearEmployed] => 2001)

FIGURE 6-4

You can combine these two arrays into a multi-dimensional array that holds information on all the employees. Use the HTML `<pre>` tag around the `print_r()` so that the display is easier to read. You should see a window similar to Figure 6-5.

```php
<?php
$employees = array(
array('name'=>'Sally Meyers', 'position'=>'President', 'yearEmployed'=>2001 ),
array('name'=>'George Smith', 'position'=>'Treasurer', 'yearEmployed'=>2006 ),
array('name'=>'Peter Hengel', 'position'=>'Clerk', 'yearEmployed'=>1992 ),
);
?>
<pre>
<?php print_r($employees);  ?>
</pre>
```

If you want to reference a specific element, use both of the indexes. To reference Sally's position, for example, use the following code:

```php
echo $employees[0]['position'];
```

WORKING WITH LOGICAL VARIABLES

PHP has special types of variables to show simple true/false conditions and to indicate a variable with no value.

A Boolean variable value is either true or false. You expressly set a variable to true or false using TRUE or FALSE. The results of the following code are shown in Figure 6-6:

```php
<?php
$myVar1 = TRUE; // No quotes and case-insensitive
$myVar2 = FALSE;
?>
<p>True: <?php echo $myVar1; ?></p>
<p>False: <?php echo $myVar2; ?></p>
```

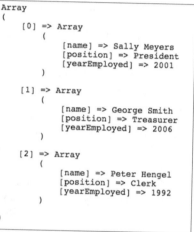

```
Array
(
    [0] => Array
        (
            [name] => Sally Meyers
            [position] => President
            [yearEmployed] => 2001
        )

    [1] => Array
        (
            [name] => George Smith
            [position] => Treasurer
            [yearEmployed] => 2006
        )

    [2] => Array
        (
            [name] => Peter Hengel
            [position] => Clerk
            [yearEmployed] => 1992
        )

)
```

FIGURE 6-5

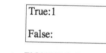

```
True:1

False:
```

FIGURE 6-6

As you see from the results, a TRUE resolves to 1 and FALSE is nothing. When PHP converts a different type of variable to Boolean, the following are false:

➤ Numeric 0 or string '0'

➤ An empty string or an array with no elements

➤ A variable with no value

Everything else evaluates to true.

 If you put quotes around the TRUE *or* FALSE, *the variable becomes a string variable and evaluates to true. So* $myVar = 'FALSE'; *is the same as* $myVar = TRUE.

PHP has a special value to represent a variable with no value. This is the null type. A variable is null if you have not assigned it to a value yet or if you assigned it to NULL. The following code displays nothing:

```php
<?php
$myVar = NULL; // No quotes and case-insensitive
echo $myVar;
```

WORKING WITH CONSTANTS

Variables are variable because they can change throughout the program. Sometimes you have a value that does not alter during the running of the program. Rather than directly using that value, you can assign it to a *constant* and use the constant instead. Constants are frequently used for configurations where different values may be assigned for different times you run the program.

In Lesson 20, you use constants to define your database name, username, and password. You can then use the constant throughout your program without having to change it if you change any of those values.

Constants use the same rules as variables for naming. They are not prefixed with a $. They are case-sensitive, but by convention constants are all uppercase. Rather than using the assignment operator (=), you use the define() function:

```php
<?php
define('DATABASE', 'mydatabase');
define('USERNAME', 'andyt');
define('PASSWORD', 's0mePassw0rd')
?>
<p>This program uses the <?php echo DATABASE;?> database with the user name
<?php echo USERNAME;?> and password <?php echo PASSWORD?>.</p>
```

As its name implies, you cannot change a constant after you have defined it. If you try to do so, you get an error message. You use the function defined() to see if the constant is already defined. defined('DATABASE') is true if the constant is already defined, and false if it is not.

WORKING WITH DATES

PHP uses *Unix timestamps* to represent dates. Unix timestamps represent a given date/time by the number of seconds since January 1, 1970. By translating dates into a number rather than actual dates, you can use ordinary math to manipulate the dates. Negative numbers show dates before January 1, 1970, but they do not work in pre-5.1.0 versions of PHP on Windows.

Time Zone Functions

It is important to be aware of time zones when dealing with dates. Your server has a time zone, which may be different from the local time zone. The following code displays your current default time zone:

```php
<?php
echo 'Current timezone: ' . date_default_timezone_get() . '<br />';
```

You can set your default time zone if it should be different. The following code changes the default time zone to that of New York City:

```php
<?php
date_default_timezone_set('America/New_York');
echo 'Current timezone: ' . date_default_timezone_get() . '<br />';
```

> *To find your time zone, check out the list of supported time zones at* http://us2.php.net/manual/en/timezones.php.

Your time zone may also be set in the php.ini file. This is a best practice. By default, XAMPP adds the UTC time zone as shown in the following code:

```
date.timezone = 'UTC'
```

You change it by supplying a different supported time zone. The following code changes the time zone to that in New York City:

```
date.timezone = 'America/New_York'
```

If you start receiving unexpected results from your dates, check what your time zone is. That could be the problem. Depending on your error reporting and your PHP version, you could receive error messages if the time zone is not set before you use the date/time functions.

Date/Time Functions

Dealing with dates and times is complex because you are dealing with arbitrary measurements. PHP has a series of functions for getting the current time, dealing with time zones, and doing calculations with dates. The following is a list of some of the common functions that you will come across.

time()

You use the time() function to get the current time as a timestamp. Your results for the following code are an integer such as that in Figure 6-7:

```php
<?php
echo time();
```

```
1299442037
```

FIGURE 6-7

date()

You use the date() function to take a timestamp and format it so it is easier to read. By default, it uses the current time. The following code displays the current date in various formats as shown in Figure 6-8. Table 6-1 has a partial listing of the format codes.

```php
<?php
echo date('c') . '<br />';
echo date('m/d/Y') . '<br />';
echo date('l, F n, Y') . '<br />';
echo date('l ga') . '<br />';
echo date('h:i a') . '<br />';
```

```
2011-03-06T15:08:58-05:00
03/06/2011
Sunday, March 3, 2011
Sunday 3pm
03:08 pm
```

FIGURE 6-8

TABLE 6-1: Date Formats for date()

FORMAT CHARACTER	DESCRIPTION
Day	
d	01 to 31
D	Mon through Sun
j	1 to 31
l (lowercase L)	Sunday through Saturday
Week	
W	Week number in the year
Month	
F	January through December
m	01 through 12
M	Jan through Dec
n	1 through 12
t	Number of days in the month
Year	
L	1 if leap year, otherwise 0
Y	Four-digit year
y	Two-digit year
Time	
a	am or pm
A	AM or PM
g	1 through 12 (hours)
G	0 through 23 (hours)
h	01 through 12 (hours)
H	00 through 23 (hours)
i	00 to 59 (minutes)
s	00 to 59 (seconds)

FORMAT CHARACTER	DESCRIPTION
Timezone	
e	Timezone Identifier (e.g., UTC, GMT)
I (Capital i)	1 for Daylight Savings Time, else 0
O	Offset from GMT in hours (e.g., +0200)
P	Offset from GMT in hours (e.g., +02:00)
T	Timezone abbreviation (e.g., EST, MDT)
Z	Timezone offset in seconds
Full Date/Time	
c	2004-02-12T15:19:21+00:00

php.net/manual/en/function.date.php

You can also specify the date you want to format. It needs to be in the timestamp format. This example takes the current time, adds seven days in seconds to it and then displays it formatted. See Figure 6-9 for sample output.

```php
<?php
echo '<p>Original date/time: ' . date('l, F j, Y g:ia T') . '</p>';
$myTime = time() + (60 * 60 * 24 * 7);
echo '<p>New date/time in different formats: </p>';
echo date('c', $myTime) . '<br />';
echo date('m/d/Y', $myTime) . '<br />';
echo date('l, F j, Y', $myTime) . '<br />';
echo date('l g:ia T', $myTime) . '<br />';
echo date('h:i a', $myTime) . '<br />';
```

Notice the automatic change from standard to daylight savings time. Programmers frequently leave the calculations for the seconds as shown for clarity.

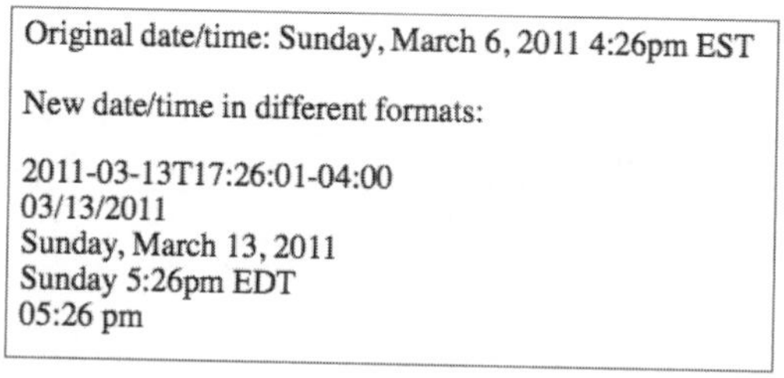

Original date/time: Sunday, March 6, 2011 4:26pm EST

New date/time in different formats:

2011-03-13T17:26:01-04:00
03/13/2011
Sunday, March 13, 2011
Sunday 5:26pm EDT
05:26 pm

FIGURE 6-9

strftime()

The strftime() function also formats dates. It has the advantage of begin able to convert based on the locale settings. However, it does not have some of the formatting options of date(). The syntax is the same, but, just to make things confusing, the formatting options are different. The following code performs the same function as the previous example for date(). See Figure 6-10 for example results. Table 6-2 has a partial listing of format codes.

```php
<?php
echo '<p>Original date/time: ' . strftime('%A, %B %e, %Y %I:%M%p %Z') . '</p>';
$myTime = time() + (60 * 60 * 24 * 7);
```

```
echo '<p>New date/time in different formats: </p>';
echo strftime('%c', $myTime) . '<br />';
echo strftime('%m/%e/%Y', $myTime) . '<br />';
echo strftime('%A, %B %e, %Y', $myTime) . '<br />';
echo strftime('%A %I:%M%p %Z', $myTime) . '<br />';
echo strftime('%I:%M %p', $myTime) . '<br />';
```

> Original date/time: Sunday, March 6, 2011 04:31PM EST
>
> New date/time in different formats:
>
> Sun Mar 13 17:31:56 2011
> 03/13/2011
> Sunday, March 13, 2011
> Sunday 05:31PM EDT
> 05:31 PM

FIGURE 6-10

TABLE 6-2: Date Formats for strftime()

FORMAT CHARACTER	DESCRIPTION
Day	
%d	01 to 31
%a	Sun through Sat
%e	1 to 31
%A	Sunday through Saturday
Week	
%U	Week number in the year
Month	
%B	January through December
%m	01 through 12
%b	Jan through Dec
Year	
%Y	Four-digit year
%y	Two-digit year
Time	
%P	am or pm

FORMAT CHARACTER	DESCRIPTION
%p	AM or PM
%I (upper case i)	01 through 12 (hours)
%H	00 through 23 (hours)
%M	00 to 59 (minutes)
%S	00 to 59 (seconds)
Timezone	
%z or %Z (depending on operating system)	Offset from GMT in hours (e.g., +0200)
%z or %Z (depending on operating system)	Timezone abbreviation (e.g., EST, MDT)
Full Date/Time	
%c	2004-02-12T15:19:21+00:00

`php.net/manual/en/function.strftime.php`

Depending on your technical specifications, your system may not support all of the formatting codes.

mktime()

You use `mktime()` to put a date into a timestamp so that you can use it in other date/time functions. The syntax is as follows:

```
mktime(hour, minute, second, month, day, is_dst)
```

The last parameter, `is_dst`, is depreciated and not to be used. It was for specifying daylight savings time. The following code displays the date 12/5/2011:

```php
<?php
$myDate = mktime(0,0,0,12,5,2011);
echo date('n/j/Y', $myDate);
```

A helpful feature of `mktime()` is that it converts out-of-bounds dates to valid dates. In other words, if you specify arithmetic that, for instance, gives you 14 months, it adds one to the year and changes the months to 2. The following code displays the date 2/5/2012:

```php
<?php
$offset = 2;
echo date('n/j/Y', mktime(0,0,0,12+$offset,5,2011));
```

strtotime()

The `strtotime()` function is another way to get a Unix timestamp. With this function you translate a string into a timestamp. This is the syntax:

```
strtotime(time, now)
```

The first parameter is the text string of the date and/or time. It can be a simple date such as 12/5/2011 or a relative term such as yesterday. See Figure 6-11 for an example of results from the following code:

```php
<?php
echo date('l, F j, Y', strtotime('12/5/2011')) . '<br />';
echo date('l, F j, Y', strtotime('yesterday', strtotime('12/5/2011')))
   . '<br />';
echo date('l, F j, Y', strtotime('yesterday')) . '<br />';
echo date('l, F j, Y', strtotime('now')) . '<br />';
echo date('l, F j, Y', strtotime('Dec 5 2011')) . '<br />';
echo date('l, F j, Y', strtotime('+4 hours')) . '<br />';
echo date('l, F j, Y', strtotime('+1 week')) . '<br />';
echo date('l, F j, Y', strtotime('+2 weeks 1 day 4 hours 10 seconds'))
   . '<br />';
echo date('l, F j, Y', strtotime('next Tuesday')) . '<br />';
echo date('l, F j, Y', strtotime('last Monday'));
```

For a complete list of the terms that can be used, see www.php.net/manual/en/datetime.formats.php.

```
Monday, December 5, 2011
Sunday, December 4, 2011
Saturday, March 5, 2011
Sunday, March 6, 2011
Monday, December 5, 2011
Sunday, March 6, 2011
Sunday, March 13, 2011
Monday, March 21, 2011
Tuesday, March 8, 2011
Monday, February 28, 2011
```

FIGURE 6-11

getdate()

The getdate() function takes a Unix timestamp and puts the date and time information in an array. If there is no timestamp it uses the current time. See Figure 6-12 as an example of the following code:

```php
<pre><?php print_r(getdate()); ?></pre>
```

To see full documentation on all the date/time functions, see http://www.php.net/manual/en/ref.datetime.php.

```
Array
(
    [seconds] => 5
    [minutes] => 45
    [hours] => 17
    [mday] => 6
    [wday] => 0
    [mon] => 3
    [year] => 2011
    [yday] => 64
    [weekday] => Sunday
    [month] => March
    [0] => 1299451505
)
```

FIGURE 6-12

WORKING WITH BUILT-IN FUNCTIONS

PHP has built-in functions for passing data and communicating.

$_GET

The $_GET function stores values from a form sent with the method="get" or added to the URL. You learn more about using forms in PHP in Lesson 11. This simple form displays like Figure 6-13:

```html
<form action="lesson06w.php" method="get">
  <label for="username">User Name:</label><br />
  <input type="text" id="username" name="username" /><br />
  <label for="password">Password</label><br />
  <input type="text" name="password" /><br />
  <button type="submit">Submit</button>
</form>
```

```
User Name:
_____

Password
_____

(Submit)
```

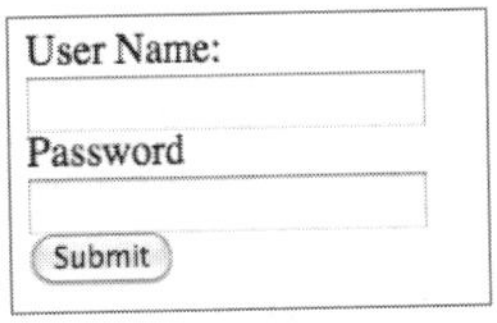

FIGURE 6-13

When you type a username and password and click Submit, the screen looks the same, but the username and password are added to the URL address. If you type in "Andy" as the username and "12345" as the password you see `?username=andy&password=12345` added to the end of your address.

The parameter section starts with a ? and each subsequent parameter starts with an &. The parameter names are taken from the `name` attribute of the input tag.

PHP reads those parameters with the `$_GET` function. `$_GET` is an associative array of the GET variables. To select the appropriate parameter, put that name surrounded by quotes in square brackets, just as you would an associative array. The following code lets you enter a username and password and then displays them. Results look similar to Figure 6-14.

```
<form action="lesson06x.php" method="get">
  <label for="username">User Name:</label><br />
  <input type="text" id="username" name="username" /><br />
  <label for="password">Password</label><br />
  <input type="text" name="password" /><br />
  <button type="submit">Submit</button>
</form>
<p>You entered <?php echo $_GET["username"] ?> as the User Name
  and <?php echo $_GET["password"] ?> as the Password.</p>
```

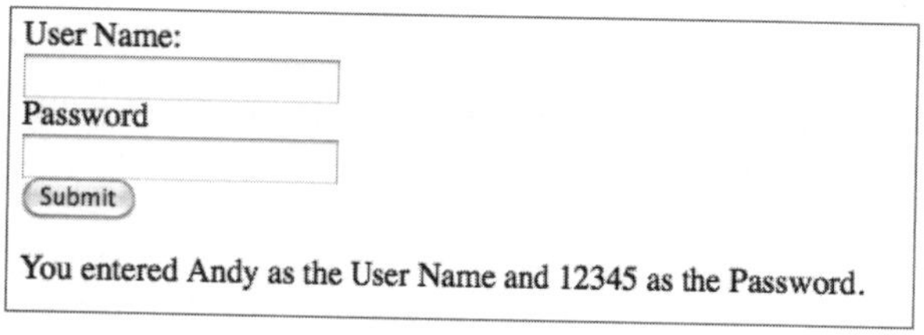

User Name:

Password

Submit

You entered Andy as the User Name and 12345 as the Password.

FIGURE 6-14

Now, obviously, you never actually use a GET for a password because everyone would be able to see it. By the same token, you should always filter the input that you receive. You learn how to filter later in this lesson.

Use the GET method when you are doing inquiries that can be repeated, if the variables are less than 2,000 characters, and the variables do not need to be private.

$_POST

The `$_POST` function stores values from a form sent with the `method="post"`. This simple form displays just like the `$_GET` did in Figure 6-13:

```
<form action="lesson06y.php" method="post">
  <label for="username">User Name:</label><br />
  <input type="text" id="username" name="username" /><br />
  <label for="password">Password</label><br />
```

```
<input type="text" name="password" /><br />
<button type="submit">Submit</button>
</form>
```

When you type a username and password and click Submit, the screen looks the same though PHP has saved them. The following code uses $_POST to retrieve the values and display them. Again, the display is the same as using the GET method shown in Figure 6-14.

```
<form action="lesson06z.php" method="post">
  <label for="username">User Name:</label><br />
  <input type="text" id="username" name="username" /><br />
  <label for="password">Password</label><br />
  <input type="text" name="password" /><br />
  <button type="submit">Submit</button>
</form>
<p>You entered <?php echo $_POST["username"] ?> as the User Name and <?php echo $_POST["password"] ?> as the Password.</p>
```

Use the $_POST method if you are adding or updating data, doing something that should not be repeated, if the variables are more than 2,000 characters, or if the variables need to be private. As with GET, you should always filter the input that you receive. You learn how to filter later in this lesson.

Cookies

Cookies are little files of data that the server puts on the user's computer. They are often used to identify a user and retain data needed in multiple screens.

setcookie()

You create a cookie with the setcookie() command and retrieve it with the $_COOKIE function that works just like $_GET and $_POST. The syntax of the setcookie() looks like:

```
setcookie(name, value, expire, path, domain);
```

The following code creates two cookies called "username" and "password" and assigns the values "andyt" and "12345" to them. It expires in one day. The setcookie() function must be before any HTML including the <html> tag.

```
<?php
setcookie("username", "andy", time()+(60*60*24));
setcookie("password", "12345", time()+(60*60*24));
```

You can view cookies in your browser. Each browser has a different way of viewing cookies. In Firefox on the PC, go to Tools ➪ Options, select Privacy, and then select Show Cookies. On the Mac, go to Preferences, select the Privacy tab, and then click Remove Individual Cookies. The cookies are displayed by the domain name. If you have used the setup in this book, your domain is "localhost." Figures 6-15 and 6-16 show what the display looks like on a Mac with the domain of wphp24.

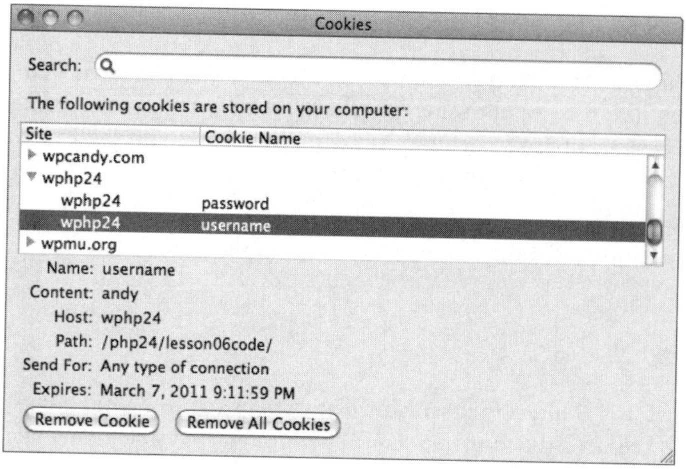

FIGURE 6-15

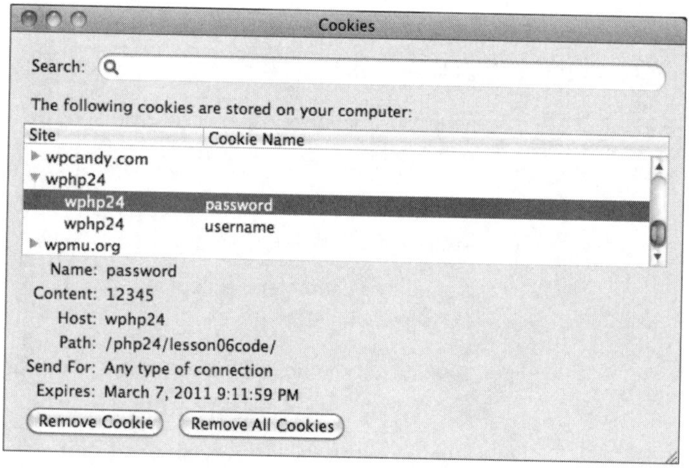

FIGURE 6-16

$_COOKIE

The following code displays the information in the two cookies with the $_COOKIE function:

```
<p>You entered <?php echo $_COOKIE["username"] ?> as the User Name
    and <?php echo $_COOKIE["password"] ?> as the Password.</p>
```

You should remember how easy it was to display the cookies in the browser when you decide what you want to save in plain text in a cookie.

filter_var()

Any time you accept input from a user or an unknown source, you need to be sure that the data is in an appropriate format both to be sure you are not using garbage and to prevent against hacking attacks. PHP has a number of filters you can use to cleanse your data. You work with the `filter_var()` function to filter the built-in functions you have just learned.

The filters can be used to either verify that you have good data (returns true or false) or to sanitize the data of particular issues (returns safe or usable data). The syntax of the `filter_var()` function is

```
filter_var(variable, filter, options)
```

Table 6-3 contains some of the most useful filters that sanitize your data by removing or changing specific characters. The function returns the sanitized data. Your original variable remains unchanged.

TABLE 6-3: Common Sanitation Filters

ID	DESCRIPTION
FILTER_SANITIZE_STRING	Strip tags, optionally strip or encode special characters
FILTER_SANITIZE_ENCODED	URL-encode string, optionally strip or encode special characters
FILTER_SANITIZE_EMAIL	Remove all characters, except letters, digits and !#$%&'*+-/=?^_`{|}~@.[]
FILTER_SANITIZE_URL	Remove all characters, except letters, digits and $-_.+!*'(),{}|\\^~[]<>#%";/?:@&=
FILTER_SANITIZE_NUMBER_INT	Remove all characters, except digits and +-
FILTER_SANITIZE_NUMBER_FLOAT	Remove all characters, except digits, +- and optionally .,eE
FILTER_SANITIZE_SPECIAL_CHARS	HTML-escape '"<>& and characters with ASCII value less than 32

Table 6-4 contains some of the most useful filters that tell you if your data is valid. The function does not make changes to your data. The function returns true or false, unless otherwise indicated.

The following code takes the `$_POST` data and sanitizes it before displaying the data:

```
<form action="lesson06zc.php" method="post">
  <label for="username">User Name:</label><br />
  <input type="text" id="username" name="username" /><br />
  <label for="password">Password</label><br />
```

```
    <input type="text" name="password" /><br />
    <button type="submit">Submit</button>
</form>
<p>You entered
<?php echo filter_var($_POST["username"],
FILTER_SANITIZE_STRING) ?>
 as the User Name and
<?php echo filter_var($_POST["password"],
FILTER_SANITIZE_STRING) ?>
 as the Password.</p>
```

TABLE 6-4: Common Validation Filters

ID	DESCRIPTION
FILTER_VALIDATE_INT	Validate value as integer, optionally from the specified range
FILTER_VALIDATE_BOOLEAN	Return TRUE for "1", "true", "on" and "yes", FALSE for "0", "false", "off", "no", and "", NULL otherwise
FILTER_VALIDATE_FLOAT	Validate value as float
FILTER_VALIDATE_URL	Validate value as URL, optionally with required components
FILTER_VALIDATE_EMAIL	Validate value as e-mail

Enter some invalid data, such as that shown in Figure 6-17.

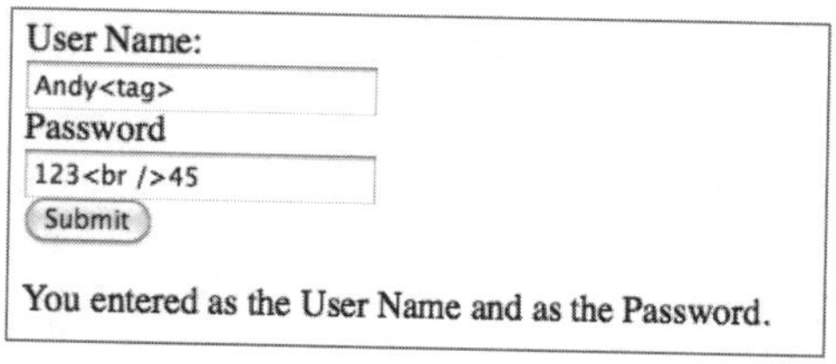

User Name:
Andy<tag>
Password
123
45
Submit

You entered as the User Name and as the Password.

FIGURE 6-17

After you click Submit, you should see that the invalid data has been stripped out, as shown in Figure 6-18.

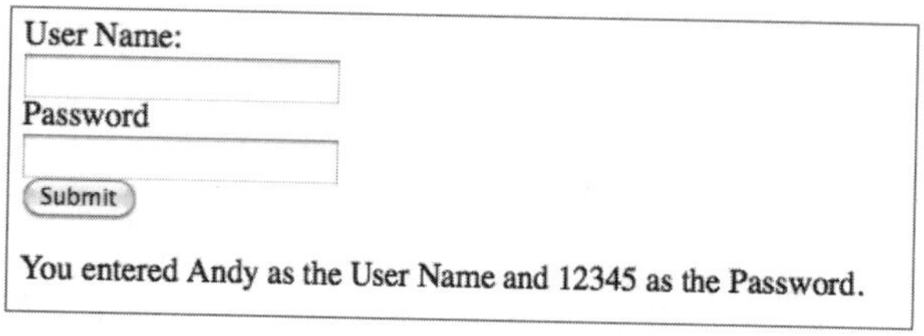

User Name:

Password

Submit

You entered Andy as the User Name and 12345 as the Password.

FIGURE 6-18

WORKING WITH OBJECTS

An object is a complex type that combines variables and functions in a single unit. You learn about objects starting with Lesson 12.

 TRY IT

In this Try It, you change the Case Study to use arrays instead of numerous individual variables in the gents.php file.

> *You can download the code and resources for this Try It from the book's web page at www.wrox.com. You can find them in the Lesson06 folder in the download. You will find code for both before and after completing the exercises.*

Lesson Requirements

Your computer needs to be able to run as a web server with PHP and MySQL. XAMPP is a package of software that installs the web server, PHP, and MySQL for you. You can find instructions for downloading and installing XAMPP in Lesson 1.

You need a text editor that can produce plain-text files. You can find instructions for downloading and installing Eclipse PDT in Lesson 1. Other text editors that you can use are Adobe's Dreamweaver in code mode, Notepad, TextWrangler, or NetBeans.

If you are following along with the Case Study you need your files from the end of Lesson 4. Alternatively, you can download the files from the book's website at www.wrox.com.

Hints

Use a numbered array for each row. Make the variables on each row the indexes for a nested associative array.

If you have trouble with the array, you can use print_r() or var_dump to see what you have.

Step-by-Step

1. Define the array at the beginning of the assignments. This clears the array if anything is in it.

```php
<?php
// Get the lot information
$lots = array();
```

2. Change the first row of variables to an associative array within the array row [0]:

```php
$lots[0]['lot_number'] = '1';
$lots[0]['image'] = "naval-19-173.jpg";
```

```
$lots[0]['name'] = "Naval Officer's Formal Tailcoat, 1840s";
$lots[0]['description'] = 'Black wool broadcloth, double breast front,
missing 3 of 18 raised round gold buttons w/crossed cannon barrels &
"Ordnance Corps" text, silver sequin & tinsel embroidered emblem
on each square cut tail, quilted black silk lining, very good; ';
$lots[0]['price'] = 5700.00;
```

3. Change the second row of variables to an associative array within the array row [1]. Notice that the associative array indexes are exactly the same in this row as the first row.

```
$lots[1]['lot_number'] = '2';
$lots[1]['image'] = "gents-striped-8-26.jpg";
$lots[1]['name'] = "Striped Cotton Tailcoat, America, 1835-1845";
$lots[1]['description'] = 'Orange and white pin-striped twill cotton,
double breasted, turn down collar, waist seam, self-fabric buttons,
inside single button pockets in each tail, (soiled, faded, cuff edges
frayed) good. ';
$lots[1]['price'] = 20700.00;
```

4. Change the third row of variables to an associative array within the array row [2]:

```
$lots[2]['lot_number'] = '3';
$lots[2]['image'] = "gents-black-8-27.jpg";
$lots[2]['name'] = "Black Broadcloth Tailcoat, 1830-1845";
$lots[2]['description'] = 'Fine thin wool broadcloth, double breasted,
  notched collar, horizontal front and side waist seam, slim long sleeves
  with notched cuffs, curved tails, black silk satin lining quilted
  in diamond pattern, padded and quilted chest, black silk covered buttons,
  (buttons worn) excellent. ';
$lots[2]['price'] = 3450.00;
```

5. Change the first display row to use the array. Use $i for the array row index.

```
<div class="list-photo"><a href="images/<?php echo $lots[$i]['image']; ?>">
  <img src="images/thumbnails/<?php echo $lots[$i]['image']; ?>"  alt="" /></a>
</div>
<div class="list-description">
  <h2><?php echo ucwords($lots[$i]['name']); ?></h2>
  <p><?php echo htmlspecialchars($lots[$i]['description']); ?></p>
  <p><strong>Lot:</strong> #<?php echo $lots[$i]['lot_number']; ?>
  <strong>Price:</strong> $<?php echo number_format($lots[$i]['price'],2); ?></p>
  <?php $i++; ?>
</div>
```

6. Copy and paste the first row over rows two and three. Because you are using a numbered array, you can let $i do all the work for you.

 Watch the video for Lesson 6 on the DVD or watch online at www.wrox.com/
go/24phpmysql.

SECTION II
Working with PHP Controls, Functions, and Forms

▶ **LESSON 7:** Making Decisions

▶ **LESSON 8:** Repeating Program Steps

▶ **LESSON 9:** Learning about Scope

▶ **LESSON 10:** Reusing Code with Functions

▶ **LESSON 11:** Creating Forms

In this section you learn how to make a program perform different actions based on different criteria. If variables are nouns, control structures are verbs.

In Lesson 7, you learn how to set up conditional statements so that code is performed only if the conditions are met. In Lesson 8, you learn how to make the program loop, performing the same action multiple times.

You discover how local and global scope work in Lesson 9. Scope refers to where a specific variable, function, or object can be seen. You create user-defined functions in Lesson 10, and in Lesson 11 you use what you have learned so far as you process forms.

Making Decisions

One of the most useful aspects of a programming language is the ability to do different actions in different situations. If it rains today I use an umbrella, but if it is sunny I wear my sunglasses. When the light is red I stop; when it is green I go; and when it is yellow I go fast.

In this lesson you learn how to use various conditional statements to make the program perform differently depending on the situation.

IF/ELSE

The most recognizable conditional statement is the `if` statement. You use the `if` statement to tell the program to execute some code if a given condition is true. Optionally, you can add an `else` statement to tell the program what to do if the condition is not true.

Basic If Statements

The most basic `if` statement consists of the condition that is being evaluated along with the code to be executed enclosed in curly braces This is how you write a basic `if` statement:

```
if (some condition) {
    some lines of PHP code here;
    that are performed;
    if the condition evaluated to true;
}
```

> ✖ *If you have only a single line of code, you can leave off the curly braces. However, this can cause errors if you later add another line and do not add the curly braces.*

Following is an example of how you could report on a rainy day. The results look similar to Figure 7-1.

```
<html>
<head>
  <title>Lesson 7a</title>
</head>
<body>
  <h1>Weather Report</h1>
  <?php
  $weather = 'rainy';
  if ($weather == 'rainy') {
    echo "<p>It will be rainy today. Use your umbrella.</p>";
  }
  ?>
</body>
</html>
```

Weather Report

It will be rainy today. Use your umbrella.

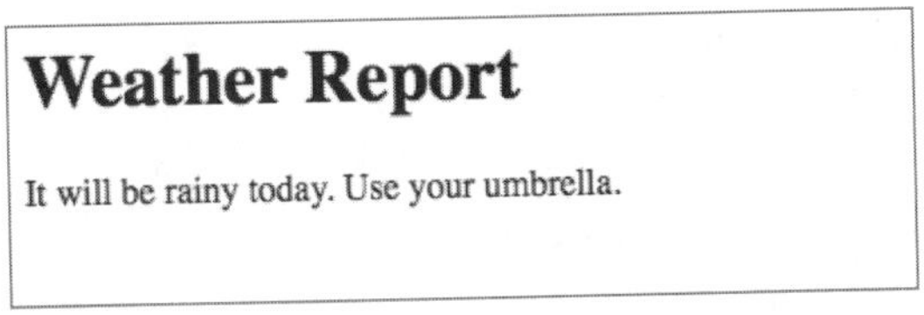

FIGURE 7-1

Notice that when you check to see if the weather is rainy, you use a double equal sign (==) and that all the PHP statements still end with a semicolon, although the `if` statement itself does not have a semicolon.

> It is a common error to use a single equal sign in a conditional statement. The single equal sign (=) is the assignment operator. It takes whatever is on the right side and makes the left side equal to it. That is usually not what you want to do. The double equal sign (==) is the equal comparison operator, which determines if the left and right sides are equal. There is also the triple equal sign (===), which checks that the two sides are even more equal. You learn about that later in this lesson.
>
> In a few instances you could use the single equal sign in a conditional statement, but the best practice is to avoid it completely because of the ambiguity of whether or not it is there in error.

Now, of course, it is always rainy with that code. If you make the day sunny, nothing displays because that code is never executed. If you want to have code execute if the condition is not met, you add an `else` statement. `else` statements never live on their own. They must always follow an `if` statement. The following code shows the syntax of an `if` statement with an `else` statement.

```
if (some condition) {
  some lines of PHP code here;
  that are performed;
```

```
      if the condition evaluated to true;
    } else {
    some lines of PHP code here;
    that are performed;
      if the condition did not evaluate to true;
    }
```

So now the code performs some action whatever the weather. If the weather is rainy then the output tells you to use your umbrella. Otherwise it tells you to wear your sunglasses. Because the variable weather is set to sunny, you are told to wear your sunglasses. See Figure 7-2.

```html
<html>
<head>
  <title>Lesson 7b</title>
</head>
<body>
<h1>Weather Report</h1>
  <?php
  $weather = 'sunny';
  if ($weather == 'rainy') {
    echo "<p>It will be rainy today. Use your umbrella.</p>";
  } else {
    echo "<p>It will be sunny today. Wear your sunglasses.</p>";
  }
  ?>
</body>
</html>
```

Weather Report

It will be sunny today. Wear your sunglasses.

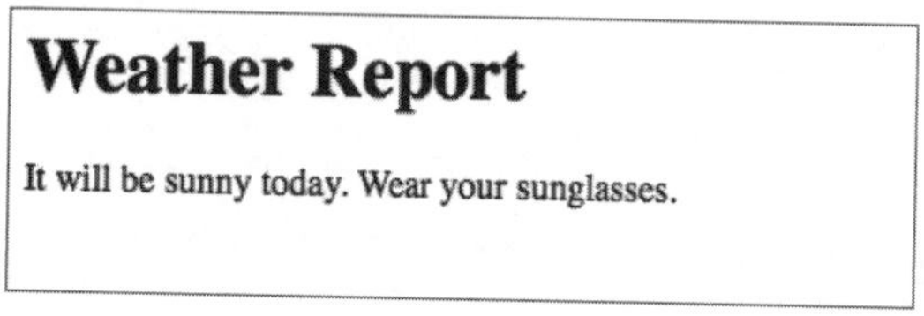

FIGURE 7-2

You can add a condition on the else statement by turning it into an elseif statement. In the following code, if it is not rainy, you check to see if it is actually sunny before you decide to wear your sunglasses. After you know it is sunny, you perform your actions and jump to the bottom of the if statement. See Figure 7-3.

```html
<html>
<head>
  <title>Lesson 7c</title>
</head>
<body>
<h1>Weather Report</h1>
  <?php
  $weather = 'sunny';
  if ($weather == 'rainy') {
    echo "<p>It will be rainy today. Use your umbrella.</p>";
  } elseif ($weather == 'sunny') {
    echo "<p>It will be sunny today. Wear your sunglasses.</p>";
  } elseif ($weather == 'snowy') {
```

```
        echo "<p>It will be snowy today. Bring your shovel.</p>";
    } else {
        echo "<p>I don't know what the weather is doing today.</p>";
    }
    ?>
</body>
</html>
```

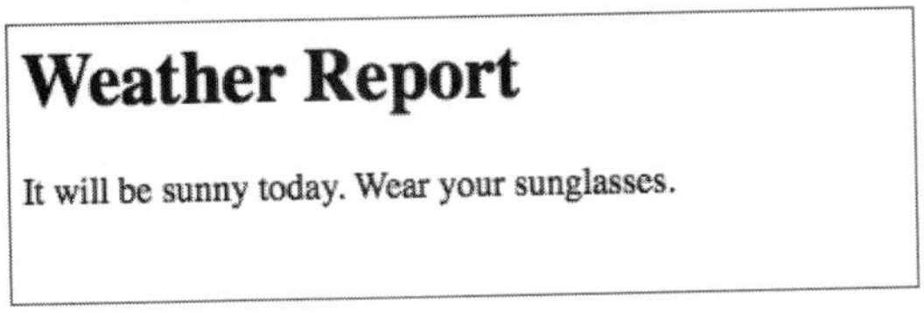

Weather Report

It will be sunny today. Wear your sunglasses.

FIGURE 7-3

Comparison Operators for If/Else Statements

So far you have just been using the equal *comparison operator*, but conditional statements are really checking to see if a statement evaluates to true, not if something is equal. You can also check to see if something is not equal to something, less than something else, more than something, and so on. Strings that consist of numbers are converted to numeric before the test except for the identical ===. Table 7-1 has a list of comparison operators.

TABLE 7-1: Comparison Operators

OPERATOR	DESCRIPTION	EXAMPLE
==	Is equal to	6=='6' returns true
===	Is identical to (including the type cast)	6==='6' returns false
!=	Is not equal to	6!=5 returns true
<>	Is not equal to	6<>5 returns true
<	Is less than	6<5 returns false
>	Is greater than	6>5 returns true
<=	Is less than or equal to	6<=5 returns false
>=	Is greater than or equal to	6>=5 returns true

Some if statements can become complex as you perform actions within the conditional statement itself. Because the conditional statement is testing for "true" and anything that is not false is true, you have a wide range of conditions that you can test for. Refer to Lesson 6 for a discussion on what is true and false.

TRUE AND FALSE

As a reminder, the following are false:

➤ Numeric 0 or string '0'.

➤ An empty string or an array with no elements.

➤ A variable with no value. Undeclared variables or variables set to NULL have no value.

Everything else is true.

The following code gives some examples of the different ways that you use if statements. See Figure 7-4 for the results.

```php
<html>
<head>
  <title>Lesson 7d</title>
</head>
<body>
  <h1>If Statements</h1>
  <?php
  $a = 5;
  $b = 8;
  $c = 58;
  $d = 40;
  $date = date('D, M d, Y');
  if ($d < 50) {

    if ($a >= strlen($data)) {
      echo "<p>Position 1: $a</p>";
    }

    echo "<p>Position 2: $d</p>";

    if (($d + $b) < ($c - $a)) {
      echo '<p>Position 3: ' . ($d + $b) .'</p>';
    } else {
      echo '<p>Position 4: ' . ($c - $a) . '</p>';
    }

  }

  ?>
  <div>
    <?php if ($date) { ?>
      <p>Today is <?php echo $date; ?>.</p>
      <p>You can check to see if there's something
```

```
          in a variable before you print it.<p>
          <p>You can also jump in and out of PHP in the
          middle of an if statement.</p>
       <?php } ?>
    </div>
  </body>
</html>
```

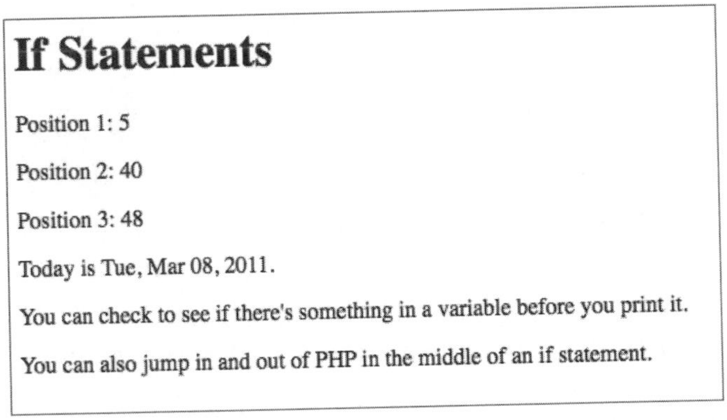

If Statements

Position 1: 5

Position 2: 40

Position 3: 48

Today is Tue, Mar 08, 2011.

You can check to see if there's something in a variable before you print it.

You can also jump in and out of PHP in the middle of an if statement.

FIGURE 7-4

If/Else with Ternary Operator

You can use a shortcut syntax with simple if-then-else statements that can make your code easier to read, especially if you are interspersing it in HTML code. The following code does a simple test for gender:

```
<?php
$gender = 'F';
if ($gender == 'M') {
  echo 'Man';
} else {
  echo 'Woman';
}
```

This same code can be written using the *ternary operator* (?) as:

```
<?php
$gender = 'F';
echo ($gender == 'M') ? 'Man' : 'Woman';
```

Ternary stands for three parts. This statement consists of the condition in parentheses followed by the ternary operator (the question mark), then the result-if-the-condition-is-true separated with a colon from the result-if-the-condition-is-false. Notice that there is no `if` in the ternary `if` statement at all as can be seen in the previous statement and in the following syntax statement:

```
(condition) ? whentrue : whenfalse;
```

This shorthand version of if/else is useful as well when assigning defaults. In the following code, if a variable is empty, you give it a value; otherwise you use whatever is in the variable:

```php
<?php
echo (empty($_GET['task'])) ? 'home' : $_GET['task'];
```

LOGICAL OPERATORS

Sometimes you need to look at multiple conditions before you decide to execute a block of code. The following example displays similar to Figure 7-5:

```php
$weather = 'sleeting';

if ($weather == 'snowing') {
  echo '<p>Something is falling from the sky.</p>';
} elseif ($weather == 'sleeting') {
    echo '<p>Something is falling from the sky.</p>';
} elseif ($weather == 'raining') {
    echo '<p>Something is falling from the sky.</p>';
} elseif ($weather == 'sunny') {
    echo '<p>I need my sunglasses.</p>';
} elseif ($weather == 'partly sunny') {
    echo '<p>I need my sunglasses.</p>';
} else {
    echo '<p>The weather is ' . $weather .'.</p>';
}
```

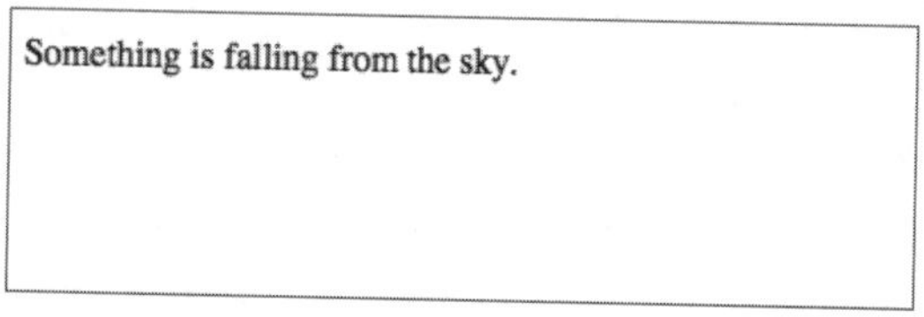

Something is falling from the sky.

FIGURE 7-5

The same actions are performed whether it is snowing, sleeting, or raining. Imagine that that code block was 20 lines long. That is a lot of extra code, not to mention there is a greater chance for errors and more work to maintain it.

Instead of the multiple `if` statements, you can link together multiple conditions. In this case, you want to say that something is falling from the sky if it is snowing, sleeting, or raining. Here is how that works. The results are shown in Figure 7-6.

```php
<?php
$weather = 'sleeting';

if ($weather == 'snowing' OR $weather == 'sleeting' OR $weather == 'raining') {
  echo '<p>Something is falling from the sky.</p>';
} elseif ($weather == 'sunny' OR $weather == 'partly sunny') {
    echo '<p>I need my sunglasses.</p>';
```

```
    } else {
        echo '<p>The weather is ' . $weather .'.</p>';
    }
```

Something is falling from the sky.

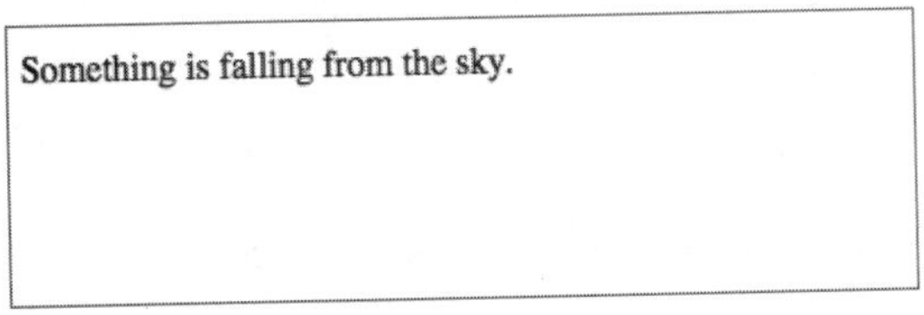

FIGURE 7-6

When using the OR operator, the condition is true if any of the conditions are true. The OR operator is case insensitive and can also be written as a | |. This vertical bar symbol is called a *double pipe* symbol. This code is identical to the preceding code as you can see in Figure 7-7:

```
<?php
$weather = 'sleeting';

if ($weather == 'snowing' || $weather == 'sleeting' || $weather == 'raining') {
    echo '<p>Something is falling from the sky.</p>';
} elseif ($weather == 'sunny' || $weather == 'partly sunny') {
    echo '<p>I need my sunglasses.</p>';
} else {
    echo '<p>The weather is ' . $weather .'.</p>';
}
```

Something is falling from the sky.

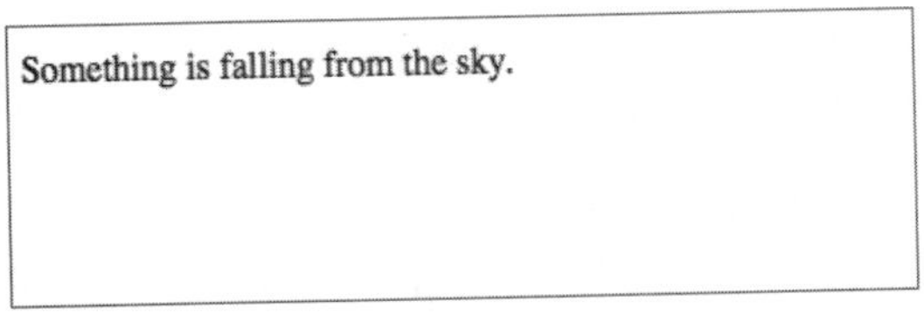

FIGURE 7-7

In the same way, you use the AND operator when you need all conditions to be true before executing a block of code. This code produces output as shown in Figure 7-8:

```
<?php
$author = 'Dodie Smith';
$title = 'I Capture the Castle';

if ($author == 'Dodie Smith' AND $title == 'I Capture the Castle') {
    echo "<p>Found the book.</p>";
} else {
    echo "<p>$title by $author is the wrong book.</p>";
}
```

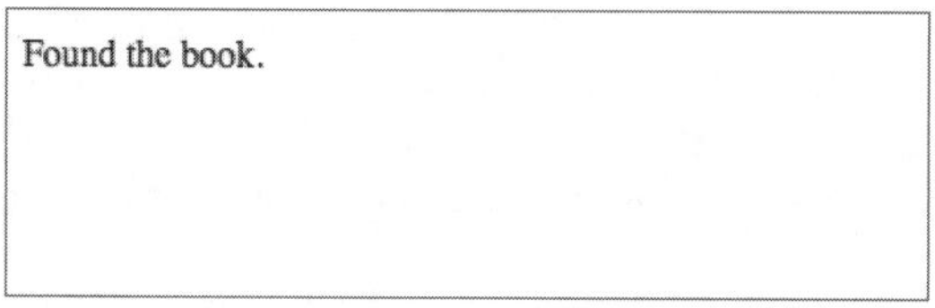

```
Found the book.
```

FIGURE 7-8

Instead of using AND you can use the symbol &&, which gives you the same result as the previous example, as shown in Figure 7-9.

```php
<?php
$author = 'Dodie Smith';
$title = 'I Capture the Castle';

if ($author == 'Dodie Smith' && $title == 'I Capture the Castle') {
  echo "<p>Found the book.</p>";
} else {
  echo "<p>$title by $author is the wrong book.</p>";
}
```

```
Found the book.
```

FIGURE 7-9

You can mix AND and OR as needed as shown here. See Figure 7-10.

```php
<?php
$city = 'Springfield';
$state = 'MA';

if ($city == 'Springfield' AND ($state == 'MA' OR $state =='VT')) {
  echo "<p>This Springfield is in Massachusetts or Vermont.</p>";
} else {
  echo "<p>$city, $state is not Springfield in MA or VT.</p>";
}
```

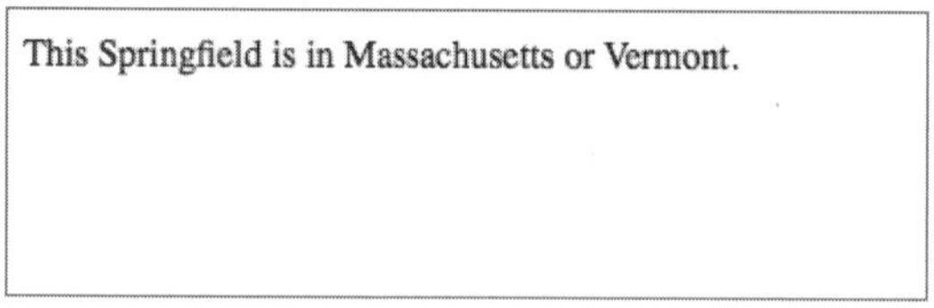

```
This Springfield is in Massachusetts or Vermont.
```

FIGURE 7-10

There is a slight difference between AND/OR and &&/||. The words AND/OR have a lower *operator precedence* than the symbols &&/||, which for practical purposes means that you do not want to mix the word version and the symbol version in the same statement or you could get unexpected results. Just as in regular mathematics, you can use parentheses to change the precedence order, to improve readability, or when there is any ambiguity.

The final logical operator is the not (!) operator. Use this to negate. The following code tells you to put away your umbrella if it's not rainy, otherwise it tells you it is raining. See Figure 7-11.

```php
<?php
$weather = 'sunny';
if (!($weather == 'rainy')) {
  echo "<p>Put away your umbrella.</p>";
} else {
  echo "<p>It's raining!</p>";
}
```

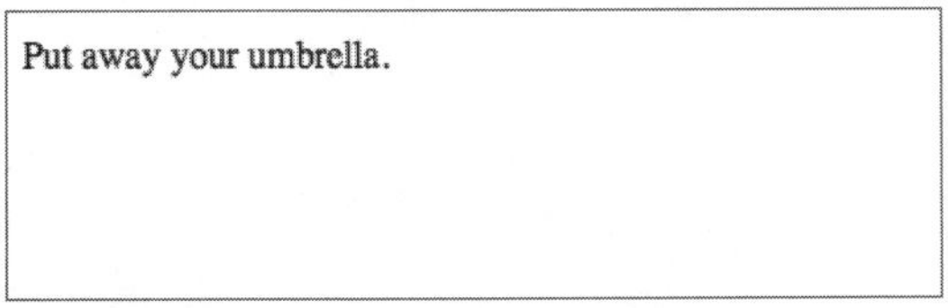

> Put away your umbrella.

FIGURE 7-11

SWITCH STATEMENTS

switch statements are also used to perform specific blocks of code depending on conditions. They are used when you want to compare the same variable or expression to several different values. Take, for example, the following series of if statements:

```php
<html>
<head>
  <title>Lesson 7m</title>
</head>
<body>
  <h1>Weather Report</h1>
  <?php
  $weather = 'sunny';
  if ($weather == 'rainy') {
    echo "<p>It will be rainy today. Use your umbrella.</p>";
  } elseif ($weather == 'sunny') {
    echo "<p>It will be sunny today. Wear your sunglasses.</p>";
  } elseif ($weather == 'snowy') {
    echo "<p>It will be snowy today. Bring your shovel.</p>";
  } else {
    echo "<p>I don't know what the weather is doing today.</p>";
  }
  ?>
</body>
</html>
```

Each `if` statement is comparing to the variable `$weather`. With a `switch` statement you write the same code in a clearer fashion. The following code performs the same functions:

```
<html>
<head>
  <title>Lesson 7n</title>
</head>
<body>
  <h1>Weather Report</h1>
  <?php
  $weather = 'sunny';

  switch ($weather) {
  case 'rainy':
    echo "<p>It will be rainy today. Use your umbrella.</p>";
    break;
  case 'sunny':
    echo "<p>It will be sunny today. Wear your sunglasses.</p>";
    break;
  case 'snowy':
    echo "<p>It will be snowy today. Bring your shovel.</p>";
    break;
  default:
    echo "<p>I don't know what the weather is doing today.</p>";
  }
  ?>
</body>
</html>
```

The syntax of the `switch` statement is as follows:

```
switch ($variable) {
case value1:
  code to be executed if $variable is equal to value1;
  break;
case value2:
  code to be executed if $variable is equal to value2;
  break;
default:
  code to be executed if $variable is different from both value1 and value2;
}
```

The `switch ($variable)` establishes what is compared. Each of the `case` statements lists a value. Notice that the `case` statements end with a colon. This is the normal practice, though a semicolon works as well. If the variable in the `switch` statement matches the value in the `case` statement, the associated block of code is performed. The `break;` tells the program to jump to the end of the `switch` block, ignoring all the rest of the `case` statements. If you want to perform some action when the value matches and then get out, use the `break;`. The `default` statement at the end is always performed unless an earlier matching `case` contained a `break`.

If you want to have two or more values perform the same actions, skip the `break` on the first value. It then drops through and executes the lines (regardless of matching any subsequent `case`

statements) until it finds a break. In the following code the state is MA, so after it gets a match, it displays "Southern New England" because it continues until it finds a break;.

```php
<?php
$state = 'MA';

switch ($state) {
case 'ME':
case 'VT':
case 'NH':
  echo "<p>Northern New England</p>";
  break;
case 'CT':
case 'MA':
case 'RI':
  echo "<p>Southern New England</p>";
  break;
default:
  echo "<p>$state is not in New England.</p>";
}
```

ALTERNATIVE SYNTAX

There is an alternative syntax for the control structures: the if and switch statements that you already know as well as the control statements you learn in the next lesson.

Curly braces have a tendency to get lost in long stretches of code, especially if you are hopping in and out of PHP and HTML. You often end up with lines that look like this:

```php
<?php } ?>
```

This alternative syntax replaces the curly braces with a colon and an end word. The syntax for an if statement is as follows:

```php
if (condition) :
  some lines of PHP code here;
  that are performed;
  if the condition evaluated to true;
elseif (condition) :
  some lines of PHP code here;
else :
  some lines of PHP code here;
endif;
```

The switch statement uses this syntax:

```php
switch ($variable) :
case value1:
  code to be executed if $variable is equal to value1;
  break;
case value2:
  code to be executed if $variable is equal to value2;
```

```
        break;
    default:
        code to be executed if $variable is different from both value1 and value2;
    endswitch;
```

The recommendation is to use this syntax if you are mixing HTML and PHP on a page and to use the curly brace syntax if you are doing straight PHP.

TRY IT

In this Try It, you finally put the case study back together so that the menus display the right content. You use the GET parameters in the URL that you learned to manipulate in Lesson 6 along with the conditional statements that you learned in this lesson to create a dynamic menuing system that tells the program what content to display.

> You can download the code and resources for this Try It from the book's web page at www.wrox.com. You can find them in the Lesson07 folder in the download. You will find code for both before and after completing the exercises.

Lesson Requirements

Your computer needs to be able to run as a web server with PHP and MySQL. XAMPP is a package of software that installs the web server, PHP, and MySQL for you. You can find instructions for downloading and installing XAMPP in Lesson 1.

You need a text editor that can produce plain-text files. You can find instructions for downloading and installing Eclipse PDT in Lesson 1. Other text editors that you can use are Adobe's Dreamweaver in code mode, Notepad, TextWrangler, or NetBeans.

If you are following along with the case study, you need your files from the end of Lesson 6. Alternatively, you can download the files from the book's website at www.wrox.com.

Hints

Lesson 6 teaches how to work with GET values.

Remember the shortcut if/else statement for setting up a default:

```
$variable = (empty($variable)) ? "default" : $variable;
```

Step-by-Step

The first task is to create a .php file in the content folder that contains the sidebar menu in the sporting.html file.

1. Create a blank file called **catnav.php** in the content folder. If `<?php` is automatically entered in the file, remove it.

2. Copy the code inside the sidebar div from the `sporting.html` file, paste it into the new `catnav.php` file, and save the file:

```
<h3 class="element-invisible">Lot Categories</h3>
  <ul class="catnav">
    <li><a href="gents.html">Gents</a></li>
    <li><a href="sporting.html">Sporting</a></li>
    <li><a href="women.html">Women</a></li>
  </ul>
```

The next task you need to do is to take the remaining HTML pages (`categories.html`, `sporting.html`, and `women.html`) and turn them into PHP content files. This process is described in more detail in the Try It sections of Lessons 2 and 4. If you want to skip this step, you can download the lesson07cs01 folder for the completed files.

1. Move `categories.html`, `sporting.html`, and `women.html` to the `content` folder.

2. Change the extensions to **.php**.

3. Delete everything in the files except the code inside the div `class="content"`.

4. Save the files.

Add a parameter called `content` to each of the menu options in the `index.php` mainnav menu.

1. Open `index.php`.

2. Find the `ul` with the `class="mainnav"`.

3. Change the `href` for each of the items to **index.php?content=contentname** where **contentname** is the name of the file in the `content` folder without the extension. This passes a GET parameter that you use in the next step. This is standard HTML, not PHP. The code should look like this:

```
<ul class="mainnav">
  <li><a href="index.php?content=categories">Lot Categories</a></li>
  <li><a href="index.php?content=about">About Us</a></li>
  <li><a href="index.php?content=home">Home</a></li>
</ul>
```

Change the include statement in the content div to `include` based on the GET parameter.

1. Find the div with `class="content"` in the `index.php` file.

2. Between the `<?php` and the `include` statement, get the content from the URL if there is one. The `isset()` function checks to see if the variable exists.

```
<?php
$content = '';
// Get the content from the url
if (isset($_GET['content'])) :
$content = $_GET['content'];
```

3. Someone could enter malicious data into a GET parameter, so sanitize the data before using it:

```
// Sanitize it for security reasons
$content = filter_var($content, FILTER_SANITIZE_STRING);
endif;
```

4. Set up the home page as a default if there is no GET parameter:

```
// Set up the home page as the default
$content = (empty($content)) ? "home" : $content;
```

5. Change the include to use the $content variable:

```
// Include the chosen page
include 'content/' . $content . '.php';
?>
```

6. Your links in the main menu should now work to take you to the Home page, the About Us page, and the Lot Categories page.

Now you change the categories.php file to also use the GET parameters on its links to the lots pages.

1. Open contents/categories.php.

2. Find the h2 tag containing the link to the Gents page and change it as you did the mainnav menu:

```
<h2><a href="index.php?content=gents">Gents</a></h2>
```

3. Find the a tag with class="button display" containing the link to the Gents page and change it the same way:

```
<a class="button display" href="index.php?content=gents">Display Lots</a>
```

4. Find the h2 tag containing the link to the Sporting page and change it the same way:

```
<h2><a href="index.php?content=sporting">Sporting</a></h2>
```

5. Find the a tag with class="button display" containing the link to the Sporting page and change it the same way:

```
<a class="button display" href="index.php?content=sporting">Display Lots</a>
```

6. Find the h2 tag containing the link to the Women page and change it the same way:

```
<h2><a href="index.php?content=women">Women</a></h2>
```

7. Find the a tag with class="button display" containing the link to the Women page and change it the same way:

```
<a class="button display" href="index.php?content=women">Display Lots</a>
```

8. Save the file and you should now be able to link to the Gents, Sporting, and Women's pages from the Lot Categories page either by clicking the titles or by clicking the Display Lots buttons.

Now you add these changes to the catnav menu and add the menu to show on the lots pages.

1. Open the `content/catnav.php` file.

2. Change the `href` link to match the links from the previous steps and then save the file:

```
<li><a href="index.php?content=gents">Gents</a></li>
<li><a href="index.php?content=sporting">Sporting</a></li>
<li><a href="index.php?content=women">Women</a></li>
```

3. Open the `index.php` file.

4. Find the div where `class="sidebar"`.

5. Include the content for the catnav if the page is Gents, Sporting, or Women and save the file. This example uses a `switch` statement, but you could use multiple `if` statements here instead.

```
<div class="sidebar">
  <?php
  switch (isset($_GET['content'])) :
  case 'gents' :
  case 'sporting' :
  case 'women' :
    include 'content/catnav.php';
  endswitch;
  ?>
</div><!-- end sidebar -->
```

6. You can now use a menu on the left to move between the different categories of lots without returning to the Lot Categories page.

Watch the video for Lesson 7 on the DVD or watch online at www.wrox.com/ go/24phpmysql.

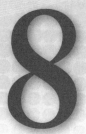

Repeating Program Steps

Loops let you repeat blocks of code multiple times. Depending on the type of loop, you can repeat the code a given amount of times or while a certain condition is true.

In this lesson you learn how to use the different types of loops:

➤ While loops repeat the code while a given condition is true.

➤ Do/While loops do the code and then repeat the code while a given condition is true.

➤ For loops repeat the code a given number of times.

➤ Foreach loops repeat the code separately for each element in an array or object.

You also learn how to break out of a loop or jump to the next iteration using break and continue.

Finally, you learn what array pointers are and how to manipulate them. This enables you to use loops more effectively with arrays.

WHILE LOOPS

While loops execute a block of while a given condition is true. This is the syntax of a while loop:

```
while (condition) {
   lines of code here;
   as many as you need;
}
```

As with the other control structures, the while loop also has the alternative syntax that is preferred if you are mixing PHP and HTML:

```
while (condition) :
   lines of code here;
   as many as you need;
endwhile;
```

A standard use of this type of loop is to set a counter and loop through until it meets the condition. Each of the loops is called an *iteration* and you often find that programmers use the variable $i as the counter. The following program sets $i to 1, then loops through printing $i and adding 1 to it until $i reaches 5 and makes the while condition false. See Figure 8-1.

```
<h1>Print 1 through 4</h1>
<?php
$i = 1;
while ($i < 5) {
  echo "<p>The counter is $i.";
  $i++;
}
```

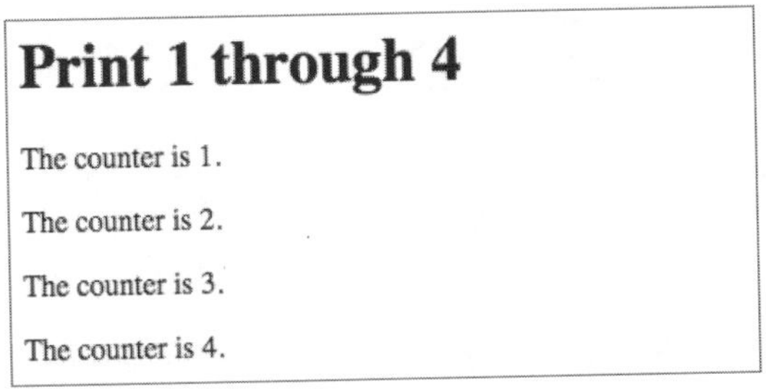

Print 1 through 4

The counter is 1.

The counter is 2.

The counter is 3.

The counter is 4.

FIGURE 8-1

The ++ attached to $i is the *increment operator*. It is used to increase $i by 1. The while loop does not automatically change the variable in the condition as it loops, so you need to remember to do that.

> You need to make sure that all this looping eventually ceases or you get an infamous infinite loop. Make sure your condition eventually goes false. A common problem is to forget to increment a counter variable.

Increment and decrement operators are convenient ways to count up and down. You can attach the operator before or after the variable depending on whether you want to increment/decrement before or after you use the original variable. Assume that $i is equal to 3 in Table 8-1.

TABLE 8-1: Increment/Decrement Operators

EXAMPLE	NAME	RESULT
echo ++$i;	Pre-increment	Adds 1 and then prints 4
echo $i++;	Post-increment	Prints 3 and then adds 1
echo --$i;	Pre-decrement	Subtracts 1 and then prints 2
echo $i--;	Post-decrement	Prints 3 and then subtracts 1

You do not need to use the increment operator. You can use any calculation that is appropriate to change the counter.

You do not even need to use a counter to run a while loop. Any statement that can evaluate to true or false can be used as the condition. Just be sure that it does not end up in an infinite loop!

DO/WHILE LOOPS

The do/while loops are the same as while loops except that the condition is checked after running the block of code instead of before. While loops that start with a false condition never run; do/while loops always run at least once.

Following is the syntax for a do/while loop. The do/while loop does not have an alternate syntax.

```
do {
  lines of code here;
  as many as you need;
} while (condition);
```

Here is the same example as the while loop, *refactored* as a do/while loop. See Figure 8-2.

```
<h1>Print 1 through 4</h1>
<?php
$i = 1;
do {
  echo "<p>The counter is $i.";
  $i++;
} while ($i < 5);
```

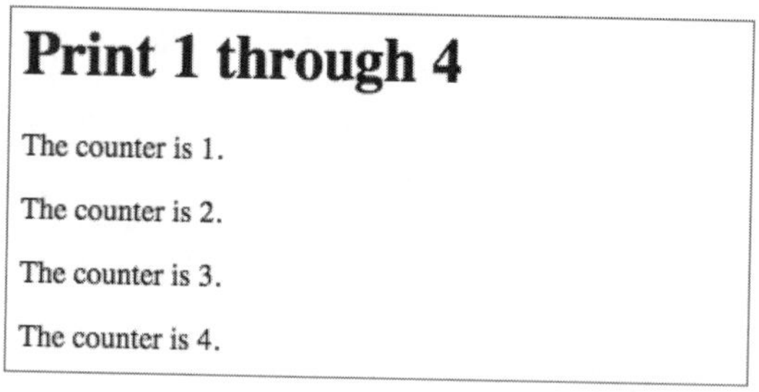

Print 1 through 4

The counter is 1.

The counter is 2.

The counter is 3.

The counter is 4.

FIGURE 8-2

 Refactoring is rewriting the same code in a different, presumably better, way. It can include restructuring to take advantage of new techniques or reworking an old program to more elegantly integrate added features. You are refactoring the Case Study as you add more advanced PHP.

FOR LOOPS

The `for` loops execute a block of code a given number of times. Unlike `while` loops, `for` loops handle the incrementing/decrementing of the counter for you. This is the syntax of the `for` loop:

```
for (init; condition; increment) {
  lines of code here;
  as many as you need;
}
```

➤ `init` is executed at the beginning of the first loop. It is usually used to initialize the counter. It can contain more than one expression (separated by commas) or be empty. It always ends with a semicolon.

➤ `condition` is evaluated at the beginning of each loop. If it is false, the looping stops. It can contain more than one expression (separated by commas) or be empty. If there is more than one expression, they are all processed, but the last one determines if the loop should continue. If this element is empty, you need to exit the loop using the `break` statement, which you learn about later in this lesson. It always ends with a semicolon.

➤ `increment` is executed at the end of each pass of the loop. It is usually used to increment the counter. It can contain more than one expression (separated by commas) or be empty. Notice that it does not end with a semicolon.

The `for` loop has alternative syntax as well:

```
for (init; condition; increment) :
  lines of code here;
  as many as you need;
endfor;
```

Following is the same function used for the `while` loop, but refactored as a `for` loop. See Figure 8-3.

```
<h1>Print 1 through 4</h1>
<?php
for ($i=1; $i < 5; $i++) {
  echo "<p>The counter is $i.";
}
```

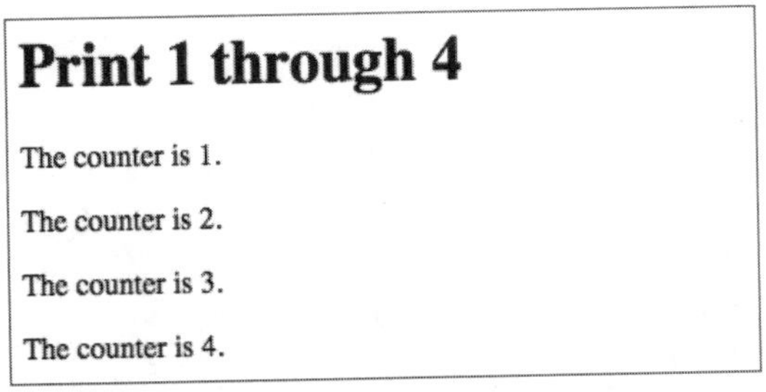

Print 1 through 4

The counter is 1.

The counter is 2.

The counter is 3.

The counter is 4.

FIGURE 8-3

As you can see, the `for` loop takes elements that you commonly used for iteration in the `while` loop and puts them tidily in one spot. `For` loops are handy for looping through arrays. The following code lists out the contacts in the array. See the display in Figure 8-4.

```
<h1>Contacts</h1>
<?php
$contacts = array(
        array('name' => 'George Smith', 'email' => 'george@example.com'),
        array('name' => 'Sally Carpenter', 'email' => 'sally@example.com'),
        array('name' => 'Peter Jason', 'email' => 'peter@example.com'),
        array('name' => 'Lila Carhausen', 'email' => 'lila@example.com')
        );
?>
<ul>
<?php for ($i=0, $size=count($contacts); $i < $size; $i++) : ?>

  <li><?php echo $contacts[$i]['name']; ?><br />
  <?php echo $contacts[$i]['email']; ?></li>

<?php endfor; ?>
</ul>
```

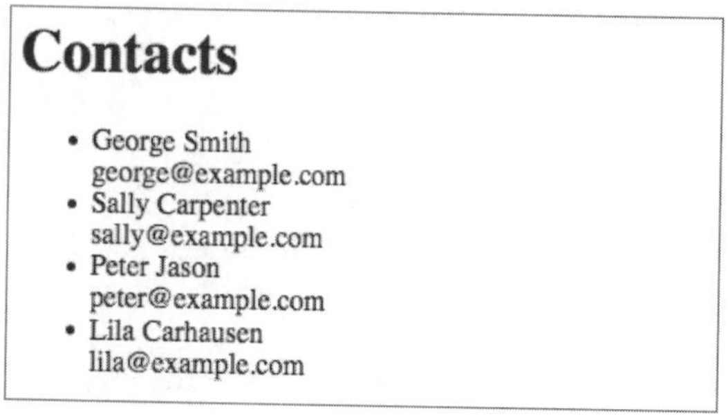

Contacts

- George Smith
  george@example.com
- Sally Carpenter
  sally@example.com
- Peter Jason
  peter@example.com
- Lila Carhausen
  lila@example.com

FIGURE 8-4

This is a typical example of how a program jumps in and out of PHP. You could have stayed in PHP and echo'd all the HTML. For clarity of the PHP, most of the examples have done that. However, generally speaking, if you are outputting to the screen, it is better to think of it as mostly HTML with PHP helping out where needed.

It's important that you understand the sequence of events for the `for` loop so here's a closer analysis of this example:

➤ You start out in HTML with the `<h1>` tag and then jump into PHP to assign values to the `$contact` array.

➤ You go briefly back into HTML to start the unordered list.

➤ Now you jump back into PHP for the start of the `for` loop.

➤ Next you define the loop. The initialization, condition, and increment of this example are more complex than the earlier examples:

  ➤ The first expression of the initialization sets the starting point of $i. By setting $i to 0 you are able to use it as the index for the array because array indexes start at 0. The second expression counts the number of elements in the array.

  ➤ The condition compares the variable containing the index of the array to the number of items in the array. Notice when the condition turns false. That is when the looping stops. It turns false when the index of the array matches the number of items in the array. Hmm. Does that mean that you miss the last person? No, because the array index is 0,1,2,3 and number of elements is 4.

  ➤ The increment is the standard increment that you have been using. It adds 1 to $i as it finishes each loop. Because this is the first time through, this statement is ignored.

➤ Now that you've finished defining the `for` loop, you get out of PHP.

➤ While in HTML, you define a list tag. You need to define only one `<li>` tag because you are using this single one as you loop through.

➤ To display the name and e-mail of this row of the array you use a PHP `echo` command.

➤ The end of the code in the loop is signaled by the `endfor` statement. At that point the following happens:

  ➤ You are sent back to the `for` statement.

  ➤ The increment statement is processed.

  ➤ The conditional statement is evaluated to see if it is now true or false:

    ➤ If it is true, you continue to do the loop again.

    ➤ If it is false, you jump to the `endfor`, which takes you out of the loop and out of PHP. You then end with the unordered list tag.

FOREACH LOOPS

The `foreach` loop is a simple way of looping through all the elements in an array or object. Although you could do the same thing with a `for` loop, using a `foreach` loop is less complex and gives you advantages. This is the standard syntax:

```
foreach ($array as $element) {
  code to be executed using $element;
}
```

As with most of the other control structures, the `foreach` has an alternative syntax that is helpful when moving in and out of PHP:

```
foreach ($array as $element) :
  code to be executed using $element;
endforeach;
```

It is a convention, when it makes sense, for the array name to be plural and the element to be the singular. The following example loops through the outer array with a `foreach` loop and gives the same results as in Figure 8-4. Here each element happens to be another array.

```php
<h1>Contacts</h1>
<?php
$contacts = array(
        array('name' => 'George Smith', 'email' => 'george@example.com'),
        array('name' => 'Sally Carpenter', 'email' => 'sally@example.com'),
        array('name' => 'Peter Jason', 'email' => 'peter@example.com'),
        array('name' => 'Lila Carhausen', 'email' => 'lila@example.com')
        );
?>
<ul>
<?php foreach ($contacts as $contact) : ?>

  <li><?php echo $contact['name']; ?><br />
  <?php echo $contact['email']; ?></li>

<?php endforeach; ?>
</ul>
```

If the array you are looping through is an associative array you can keep track of the index with the following syntax:

```php
foreach ($array as $key=>$value) {
  code to be executed using $element and/or $key;
}

foreach ($array as $key=>$element) :
  code to be executed using $element and/or ;
endforeach;
```

In the following code you loop through the array and use each key as a label for displaying the value. See Figure 8-5.

```php
<h1>Contact</h1>
<?php
$myArr = array('name' => 'George Smith',
'email' => 'george@example.com',
'phone' => '555-555-1212',
'state' => 'MA');

?>
<ul>
<?php foreach ($myArr as $key=>$value) : ?>

  <li><?php echo ucfirst($key); ?>:
  <?php echo $value; ?></li>

<?php endforeach; ?>
</ul>
```

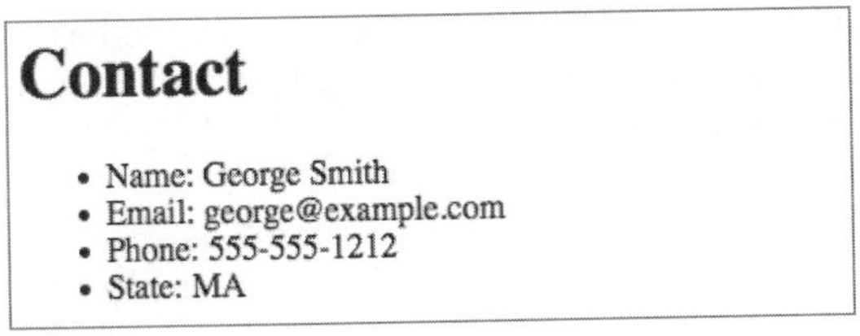

Contact

- Name: George Smith
- Email: george@example.com
- Phone: 555-555-1212
- State: MA

FIGURE 8-5

You should be aware of these behaviors:

➤ The `foreach` loop always starts on the first element of the array.

➤ The element variable is a copy of the array element so nothing you do to it affects the actual array. If you want to make changes to the actual array, prefix an `&` to the element variable as in `foreach ($array as &$value)`. The `&` makes this a reference of the array rather than a copy. The new variable is just another name for the same variable.

➤ If you reference the array, the last referenced element remains after the `foreach` finishes so it is recommended that you remove the variable by unsetting with `unset($value)`.

CONTINUE/BREAK

You use `continue` if you are done with a particular loop iteration and want to jump to the start of the next iteration. In the following example, the `email` value is skipped:

```php
<h1>Contact</h1>
<?php
$myArr = array('name' => 'George Smith',
'email' => 'george@example.com',
'phone' => '555-555-1212',
'state' => 'MA');

?>
<ul>
<?php foreach ($myArr as $key=>$value) :

  if ($key == 'email') :
    continue;
  endif; ?>

  <li><?php echo ucfirst($key); ?>:
  <?php echo $value; ?></li>

<?php endforeach; ?>
</ul>
```

If you have multiple nested loops, you can use a numeric argument to skip to the next iteration of enclosing loops.

You use `continue` to jump to the next iteration of a loop. To jump completely out of the loop, use `break`. You used `break` in Lesson 7 when learning about switches, but you can also use `break` to jump out of loops.

> *Overuse of `continue` and `break` can lead to what is called spaghetti code. This is code that is convoluted and jumps around. It is hard to read, hard to debug, and error prone. Breaks are standard on `switch` statements and a simple `continue` can be very helpful, but be cautious of more than that.*

TRY IT

In the first part of this Try It, you create a program to display the even numbers from an array using the `for` loop.

You continue improving the Case Study in the second part of the Try It. In the previous lesson you moved information from individual variables to arrays and duplicated the code for each element in the array. Now you replace the duplicated code with a loop.

> *You can download the code and resources for this Try It from the book's web page at www.wrox.com. You can find them in the Lesson08 folder in the download. You will find code for both before and after completing the exercises.*

Lesson Requirements

Your computer needs to be able to run as a web server with PHP and MySQL. XAMPP is a package of software that installs the web server, PHP, and MySQL for you. You can find instructions for downloading and installing XAMPP in Lesson 1.

You need a text editor that can produce plain-text files. You can find instructions for downloading and installing Eclipse PDT in Lesson 1. Other text editors that you can use are Adobe's Dreamweaver in code mode, Notepad, TextWrangler, or NetBeans.

If you are following along with the case study, you need your files from the end of Lesson 7. Alternatively, you can download the files from the book's website at www.wrox.com.

Hints

Remember that the first index of an array is 0, not 1.

Remember that the index of an element is not the same thing as the value of that element.

Don't forget the echo when needed.

Step-by-Step

Create a program to display the even numbers from an array using the `for` loop. See Figure 8-6 for the desired results.

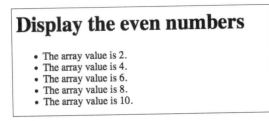

Display the even numbers

- The array value is 2.
- The array value is 4.
- The array value is 6.
- The array value is 8.
- The array value is 10.

FIGURE 8-6

1. Start by creating a file called **exercise08a.php**.

2. Enter the basic code for an HTML page:

```
<html>
<head>
    <title>Exercise 8a</title>
</head>

<body>

</body>
</html>
```

3. Initialize an array called **$myArray** with the numbers 1–10. Insert it on a line just after the `<body>` tag. Remember to go into PHP.

```
<?php
$myArray = array(1,2,3,4,5,6,7,8,9,10);
```

4. Count the total number of items in the array:

```
$total = count($myArray);
```

5. Insert a heading that says **Display the even numbers**. Use HTML, rather than PHP.

```
?>
<h1>Display the even numbers</h1>
```

6. Start an unordered list:

```
<ul>
```

7. Set up the `for` loop. You are using the index to print the value and to control the loop. Because you want the second value (2) to be the first to print, set a variable called `$i` with the

beginning value of 1. This is the index for the second value. You want the loop to continue while the index is less than the count of the items. Because you are printing only even numbers, you want to increase $i by 2 at the end of each loop. You use HTML after this statement, so get out of PHP at the end.

```
<?php for ($i=1; $i < $total; $i += 2) : ?>
```

8. Display the value of the element in a list:

```
<li>The array element value is <?php echo $myArray[$i]; ?>.</li>
```

9. End the `for` loop and the unordered list:

```
<?php endfor; ?>
</ul>
```

10. The resulting code should look like this:

```
<html>
<head>
  <title>Exercise 8a</title>
</head>

<body>

<?php
$myArray = array(1,2,3,4,5,6,7,8,9,10);
$total = count($myArray);
?>

<h1>Display the even numbers</h1>
<ul>
  <?php for ($i=1; $i < $total; $i += 2) : ?>
    <li>The array element value is <?php echo $myArray[$i]; ?>.</li>
  <?php endfor; ?>
</ul>

</body>
</html>
```

In the Case Study, add a `foreach` loop to display the list in `content/gents.php`.

1. Open `contents/gents.php`.

2. Find the `<ul class="ulfancy">` line and add the beginning of the `foreach` loop following that line. Use `$i` as a key. That will give you a counter to use for calculating alternating rows:

```
<?php foreach ($lots as $i=>$lot) : ?>
```

3. Add the `endforeach` after the `</li>`:

```
<?php endforeach; ?>
```

4. Within that loop, change `$lots[$i]` to **$lot**.

5. Remove the increment counter `<?php $i++; ?>` because you are letting the `foreach` loop key do that work.

6. Delete the next two `<li></li>` groupings.

7. The `<ul>` group should now match this:

```
<ul class="ulfancy">

<?php foreach ($lots as $lot) : ?>
  <li class="row<?php echo $i % 2; ?>">
    <div class="list-photo"><a href="images/<?php echo $lot['image']; ?>">
      <img src="images/thumbnails/<?php echo $lot['image']; ?>"  alt=""
/></a>
    </div>
    <div class="list-description">
      <h2><?php echo ucwords($lot['name']); ?></h2>
      <p><?php echo htmlspecialchars($lot['description']); ?></p>
      <p><strong>Lot:</strong> #<?php echo $lot['product_id']; ?>
      <strong>Price:</strong> $<?php echo number_format($lot['price'],2);
?></p>
    </div>
    <div class="clearfloat"></div>
  </li>
<?php endforeach; ?>

</ul>
```

8. Back at the end of the first block of PHP code is the line `$i = 0;`. You used that when you were counting the lines manually. Because the `foreach` loop is handling that, you can delete this line.

 Watch the video for Lesson 8 on the DVD or watch online at www.wrox.com/ go/24phpmysql.

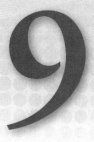

Learning about Scope

In this lesson you learn about the concept of *scope*. As you learn about user-defined functions in Lesson 10 and objects in Lesson 12, you learn the details of how scope works when you use functions and objects.

Scope refers to where a specific variable, function, or object can be seen. Scope can be local or global.

LEARNING ABOUT LOCAL VARIABLES

Think of a program as a village where the houses have blinds on all their windows. Imagine that a variable is a person taking a walk down the street. He can talk and interact with all the other people outside, but he cannot be seen by anyone inside the houses nor can he see them. If he needs to talk with someone inside a house, he has to knock on the door and be let in first.

This is the way that local scope works. Variables can be seen only where they are created. The houses are the user-defined functions you learn about in Lesson 10. If you create a variable outside a function, it cannot be seen inside the function. Conversely, if you create a variable inside a function, it can be seen only within that function.

Global scope, on the other hand, is as if that village was on a South Seas island and the houses were open-air tents. Everyone can see everyone else at all times.

Scope is local by default in PHP. Having local scope allows for *encapsulation*. Encapsulation means that you can create a function and know that nothing that goes on outside of that function will change anything inside the function unexpectedly. It also means that you are free to make changes inside the function and do not have to worry that you are messing up something outside the function. This makes your code easier to debug and more robust.

Older programming styles made extensive use of global variables so you may see programs using it, but it's not a style you should copy.

At times you may need to create and use global variables, however. In the next section you learn how to define and work with global variables.

LEARNING ABOUT GLOBAL VARIABLES

Setting a variable to global scope is very easy. Just put the word `global` before the variable before you use it:

```php
<?php
global $myVar;
$myVar = '15';
```

In addition to regular globals, PHP has predefined variables called superglobals. These variables are automatically global. You used the superglobals `$_GET`, `$_POST`, and `$_COOKIE` in Lesson 6. The rest of the superglobals work the same way. The superglobals and an explanation of each are listed in Table 9-1.

TABLE 9-1: Superglobal Variables

SUPERGLOBAL VARIABLE	CONTENTS
$GLOBALS	All global variables
$_SERVER	Server and execution environment information
$_GET	Variables passed via URL parameters
$_POST	Variables passed via the HTTP POST method
$_FILES	Items uploaded via the HTTP POST method (file uploads)
$_COOKIE	Variables passed via HTTP cookies
$_SESSION	Session variables
$_REQUEST	Contains contents of $_GET, $_POST, and $_COOKIE
$_ENV	Variables passed via environment method
$_SERVER	Server and execution environment information

Notice that `$GLOBALS` does not have an underscore. It is the superglobal that has been around for the longest time.

Globals have undergone many changes in the different versions of PHP. It is handy to be familiar with the old style so that you know not to copy it. Some of the old ways of doing things still work, but will be removed in later versions. That is another reason for moving right to the modern style.

In the old style the superglobals were prefixed with HTTP and suffixed with VARS. Table 9-2 contains a cross-reference from the current values to the terms that are being retired.

$_SERVER ELEMENTS

The $_SERVER superglobal has several predefined keys (elements) for the data it contains. Not all elements work on all servers and they might give you unexpected data depending on the server setup. Here are some that may be useful to you:

➤ PHP_SELF: Filename of the currently executing script, relative to the document root

➤ SERVER_NAME: Name of the server host

➤ DOCUMENT_ROOT: Document root directory under which the current script is executing

➤ HTTP_REFERER: Address of the page that referred the user agent to the current page (not available with all user agents)

➤ HTTP_USER_AGENT: Contents of the User-Agent such as Mozilla/4.5 [en] (X11; U; Linux 2.2.9 i586)

➤ SCRIPT_FILENAME: Absolute pathname of the currently executing script

➤ SCRIPT_NAME: Current script's path

➤ REQUEST_URI: URI used to access this page; for instance /index.html

These are some of the elements listed in the PHP manual. See the full list at www.php.net/manual/en/reserved.variables.server.php.

TABLE 9.2 Deprecated Variables

NEW STYLE	DEPRECATED OLD STYLE
$GLOBALS	This has always been $GLOBALS
$_SERVER	$HTTP_SERVER_VARS
$_GET	$HTTP_GET_VARS
$_POST	$HTTP_POST_VARS
$_FILES	$HTTP_POST_FILES
$_COOKIE	$HTTP_COOKIE_VARS
$_SESSION	$HTTP_SESSION_VARS
$_ENV	$HTTP_ENV_VARS

Variables are local by default in PHP. There is a setting in your php.ini file where you can change that. If you turn register_globals on, all your variables will be global by default. Some older

programs depended on that setting being on to work. Properly run servers do not allow `register_globals` to be on because it is a security risk, so most of those programs have been weeded out. In PHP6, `register_globals` will not exist.

TRY IT

In this Try It, you set a variable to global and use a superglobal to display information about the server.

> *You can download the code and resources for this Try It from the book's web page at* www.wrox.com. *You can find them in the Lesson09 folder in the download. You will find code for both before and after completing the exercises.*

Lesson Requirements

Your computer needs to be able to run as a web server with PHP and MySQL. XAMPP is a package of software that installs the web server, PHP, and MySQL for you. You can find instructions for downloading and installing XAMPP in Lesson 1.

You need a text editor that can produce plain-text files. You can find instructions for downloading and installing Eclipse PDT in Lesson 1. Other text editors that you can use are Adobe's Dreamweaver in code mode, Notepad, TextWrangler, or NetBeans.

This Try It does not use the Case Study.

Hints

The superglobal for the server information is `$_SERVER`.

`$_SERVER` works the same way as `$_GET`, which you learned to use in Lesson 6.

Step-by-Step

Create a program that creates a global variable, assigns a value to it, locates the document root, and concatenates the two results.

1. Create the file **exercise09a.php**.

2. Create a global variable called **$file**, set it to **exercise09a.php**, and display it:

```php
<?php
global $file;
$file = 'exercise09a.php';
echo '$file: ' . $file .'<br />';
```

3. Look up DOCUMENT_ROOT, SCRIPT_NAME, and REQUEST_URI and display them:

```
$path = $_SERVER['DOCUMENT_ROOT'];
echo 'DOCUMENT_ROOT: ' . $path .'<br />';
$script = $_SERVER['SCRIPT_NAME'];
echo 'SCRIPT_NAME: ' . $script .'<br />';
$uri = $_SERVER['REQUEST_URI'];
echo 'REQUEST_URI: ' . $uri .'<br />';
```

4. Your results should look similar to Figure 9-1. They reflect your server and documents.

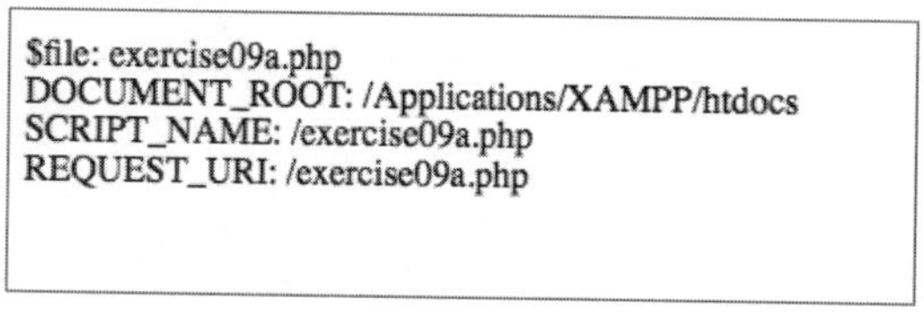

```
$file: exercise09a.php
DOCUMENT_ROOT: /Applications/XAMPP/htdocs
SCRIPT_NAME: /exercise09a.php
REQUEST_URI: /exercise09a.php
```

FIGURE 9-1

 Watch the video for Lesson 9 on the DVD or watch online at www.wrox.com/ go/24phpmysql.

10

Reusing Code with Functions

Writing code can be time-consuming and error prone. After you have written a piece of code that works well, you want to reuse that code instead of constantly rewriting it when you need to do the same thing again.

You could copy and paste that piece of code everywhere you need it, but then if you found a new bug or thought of an enhancement, you'd need to change it everywhere that you copied it — assuming you could find all the places.

PHP lets you take those pieces of code and create mini-programs called *functions* out of them. Functions make it easier to read your code because functions move extraneous detail out of the main flow of the program. You learned several PHP functions in Lesson 4, such as the function strlen() that counts the number of characters:

```php
<?php
$myName = 'Andy';
echo strlen($myName);
```

You give strlen() some information (optionally), it does something, and it (optionally) gives you something back. When it gives something back, it is said to *return* something.

In this lesson you learn how to take the valuable pieces of code that you've written and turn them into user functions of your own. You learn how to define the function, how to pass data to the functions, and how to get data back from the functions. Then you take that knowledge to learn how to use the functions in your code.

Another way of reusing code is include statements. You are using a simple include in the Case Study. In this lesson you also learn about the different types of includes, how they work, and how you can use them to organize your collection of functions.

DEFINING FUNCTIONS

You name functions with the same rules as naming variables. Functions do not have a $ before their name and they are immediately followed by parentheses. The simplest function definition looks like this:

```
function functionname() {
  // PHP code goes here;
}
```

> ✕ *PHP, in general, is very forgiving of whitespace — those blank spaces, tabs, new lines, and blank lines you put in code to make it more readable. However, one place where whitespace is not allowed is between the end of the function name and the parentheses. The () must immediately follow the name.*

It's easy to turn code into a function. This code displays "George Smith":

```
<?php
$name = "George Smith";
echo $name;
```

This is how you define a function to display "George Smith":

```
<?php
function getName() {
  $name = "George Smith";
  echo $name;
}
```

This defines the function but does not run the function. To actually run the function and display "George Smith" you need to also call the function, as shown in the following code. See Figure 10-1.

```
<?php
function getName() {
  $name = "George Smith";
  echo $name;
}
?>

<h1>Contacts</h1>
<p><?php getName(); ?></p>
```

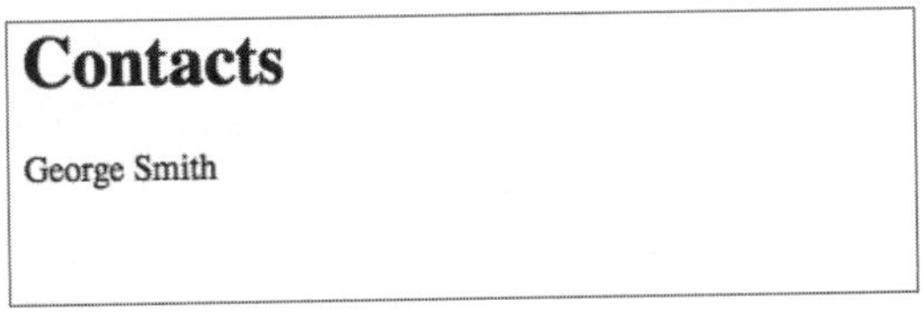

Contacts

George Smith

FIGURE 10-1

You see that the code in the function is not processed when you define it in the function. It is only when you call the function that "George Smith" is displayed. After you have defined the function you can call it as often as you need it. So if you had a need to echo out George's name three times, you could do it this way (see Figure 10-2):

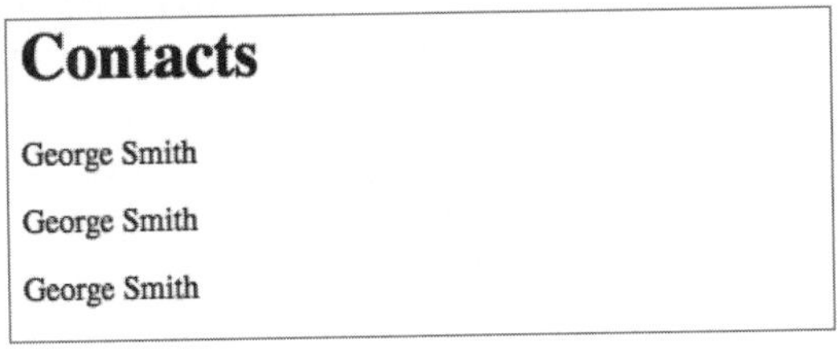

```
<?php
function getName() {
  $name = "George Smith";
  echo $name;
}
?>
```

Contacts

George Smith

George Smith

George Smith

FIGURE 10-2

```
<h1>Contacts</h1>
<p><?php getName(); ?></p>
<p><?php getName(); ?></p>
<p><?php getName(); ?></p>
```

Each time you run a function, the variables in your function are new variables. If you change the value of a variable in a function, that change does not exist the next time the function is called. Look at this code and compare it to the results in Figure 10-3:

```
<?php
function getCount() {
    $count++;
    echo "Count: " . $count. "<br />";
}
?>

<h1>Count</h1>
<?php for ($i=0; $i < 5; $i++) :
    getCount();
endfor; ?>
```

Count

Count: 1
Count: 1
Count: 1
Count: 1
Count: 1

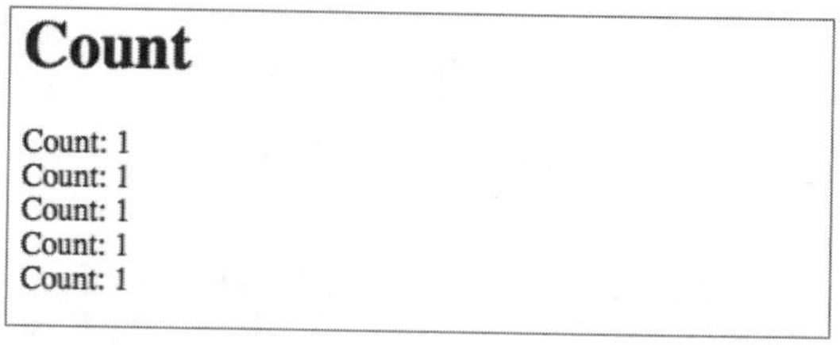

FIGURE 10-3

When the getCount() in the preceding code is called, it adds 1 to $count using the $count++ command and then prints it out. So when you loop through the for loop five times, $count prints out as 1 each time because every time getCount() is called $count is initialized to 0. This is a good thing because it keeps your functions clean and contained. You know that your variables start fresh every time you run the function.

Every so often, however, you may want to have a variable stick around through all the times you run the function in a script. Two examples of this would be if you want to do something different the first time you run a function or if you are trying to keep a counter going. To do that you declare your variable as a *static variable*. Static variables maintain their values instead of reinitializing. See how the results change when $count is declared as static in the following code. Figure 10-4 shows the results.

```
<?php
function getCount() {
    static $count;
    $count++;
    echo "Count: " . $count. "<br />";
}
?>

<h1>Count</h1>
<?php for ($i=0; $i < 5; $i++) :
    getCount();
endfor; ?>
```

Count

Count: 1
Count: 2
Count: 3
Count: 4
Count: 5

FIGURE 10-4

PASSING PARAMETERS

All this function can do is print out "George Smith," which is not very useful. If, however, you could tell it to print any name you wanted, it would more useful. The parentheses following the function name are used to hold *parameters*, which are variables that can be passed from the calling

program into the function. You pass different values to the function and the function uses those values when it processes its code. This code displays two different names as shown in Figure 10-5:

```php
<?php
function getName($name) {
  echo $name;
}
?>

<h1>Contacts</h1>
<p><?php getName("George Smith"); ?></
p>
<p><?php getName("Sally Meyers"); ?></p>
```

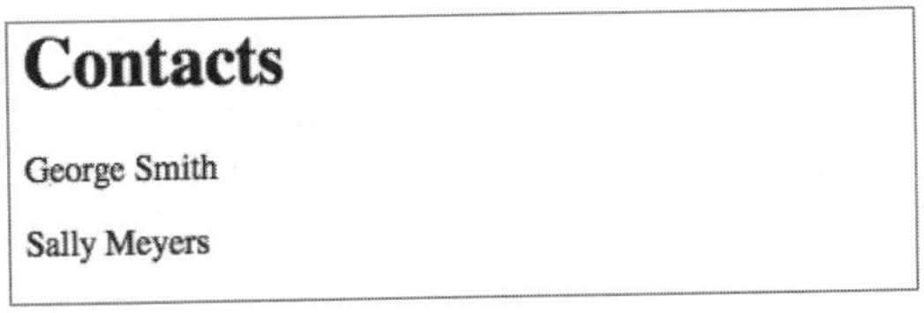

Contacts

George Smith

Sally Meyers

FIGURE 10-5

PARAMETERS AND ARGUMENTS

You often hear the terms "parameters" and "arguments" used interchangeably. Technically, parameters are the list of variables in the function definition. Arguments are the actual values that are passed to the parameters when the function is used.

You can also pass the information as a variable. This code produces the same results as the prior code:

```php
<?php
function getName($name) {
  echo $name;
}
?>

<h1>Contacts</h1>
<?php
  $name1 = "George Smith";
  $name2 = "Sally Meyers";
?>
<p><?php getName($name1); ?></p>
<p><?php getName($name2); ?></p>
```

You can use all the different arrays and loops that you have learned as well. This code is another way to get the same results:

```php
<?php
function getName($name) {
  echo $name;
}
?>

<h1>Contacts</h1>
<?php
$contacts = array("George Smith", "Sally Meyers");

foreach ($contacts as $contact) :
```

```
?>
   <p><?php getName($contact); ?></p>
<?php endforeach; ?>
```

The name of the variable that you are passing does not need to be the same as the name in the function definition. It ignores the actual name of the variable. Note that in the prior code the variable $contact was passed to the function getName(), but the function defined the parameter as $name.

You can pass more than one parameter to a function. The function loads the information you send it in the same order that the information is received. The following code passes both the name of the contact and the department he or she is in. See the results in Figure 10-6.

```
<?php
function getName($name, $department) {
  echo $name . ' - ' . $department;
}
?>

<h1>Contacts</h1>
<?php
$contacts = array("George Smith", "Sally Meyers");
$department = "Office";

foreach ($contacts as $contact) :
?>
   <p><?php getName($contact, $department); ?></p>
<?php endforeach; ?>
```

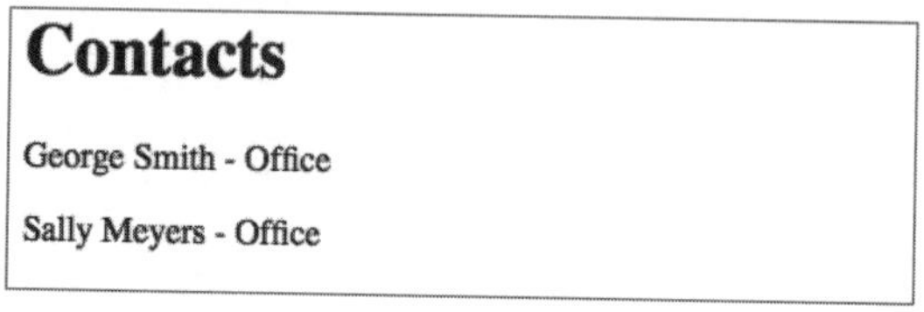

Contacts

George Smith - Office

Sally Meyers - Office

FIGURE 10-6

When variables are created within a function, they are automatically created as local variables and can be seen only within the function. Even if a variable has been declared a global variable outside of the function, within the function a variable created with the same name would be a separate local variable and would not know the value in the global variable. If you want a variable in a function to be global, you must specifically declare it as global:

```
global $myVariable;
```

The following example tries to display $department, but it shows as blank. The reason you see the value of the $name within the function is because you passed it through the parentheses. Because you did not do that with $department, you are not passed those values. See the results in Figure 10-7.

```
<?php
function getName($name) {
  echo $name . ' - ' . $department;
}
?>

<h1>Contacts</h1>
<?php
$name = "George Smith";
$department = "Office";
?>

<p><?php getName($name); ?></p>
```

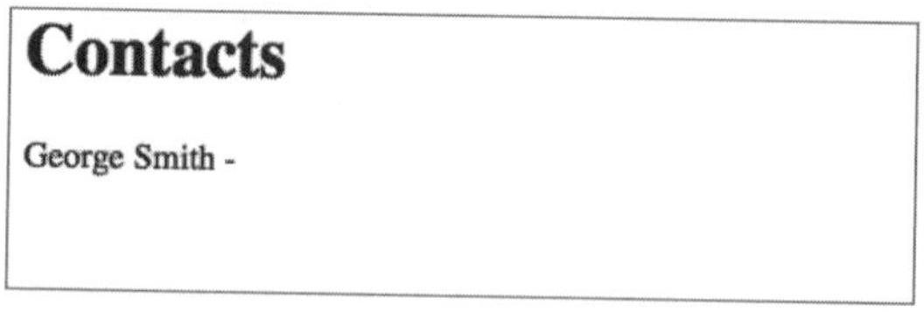

Contacts

George Smith -

FIGURE 10-7

The function is passed a copy of the argument so any changes made to the variable are not made to the original variable. The following example changes the value of $name in the function after it is displayed from within the function. However, when the $name variable is displayed outside the function, it has not changed. See Figure 10-8 for the results of the following code.

```php
<?php
function getName($name) {
  echo $name;
  $name = "Sally Meyers";
}
?>

<h1>Contacts</h1>
<?php
$name = "George Smith";
?>

<p><?php getName($name); ?></p>
<p><?php echo $name; ?>
```

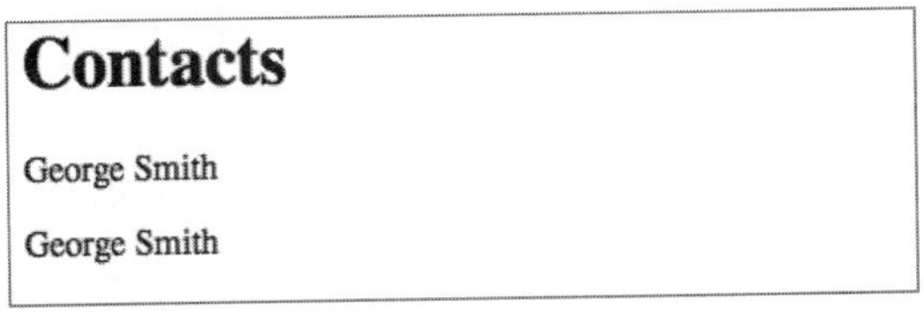

Contacts

George Smith

George Smith

FIGURE 10-8

If you want to make changes to the original variable, you need to pass it by *reference*. When you pass a variable by reference you create a link, a shortcut, or an alias to the original variable rather than making a copy of it. You are creating multiple names for the same thing. Prefix the parameter in the function definition with an ampersand (&) to indicate it should pass by reference, rather than making a copy. In the following example, $name is passed by reference. When the function is called, it prints out the passed name and department and then changes those variables. When you echo $contact after calling the function, you see that the value variable passed by reference, $contact, has changed. On the other hand, $department was not passed by reference, so it is unchanged. See Figure 10-9.

```php
?php
function getName(&$name, $department) {
  echo $name . ' - ' . $department;
  $name = "Sally Meyers";
  $department = "Techs";
}
?>

<h1>Contacts</h1>
<?php
$contact = "George Smith";
$department = "Office";
?>

<p><?php getName($contact, $department); ?></p>
<p><?php echo $contact; ?></p>
<p><?php echo $department; ?></p>
```

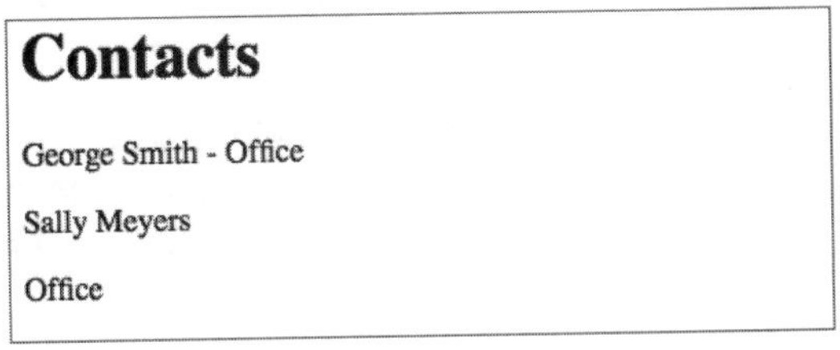

Contacts

George Smith - Office

Sally Meyers

Office

FIGURE 10-9

You can also assign a *default* to a parameter. If a parameter has a default value, that value is assigned if no argument is passed. You must pass an argument for every parameter without a default, so always put the arguments with defaults at the end. In the following code, notice that George has no department passed, so he gets the default, while Sally uses the department that is passed. See Figure 10-10.

```php
<?php
function getName($name, $department="Office") {
  echo $name . ' - ' . $department;
}
?>

<h1>Contacts</h1>
<?php
$contact = "George Smith";
$department = "Tech";
?>
<p><?php getName($contact); ?></p>

<?php
$contact = "Sally Meyers";
?>


<p><?php getName($contact, $department); ?></p>
```

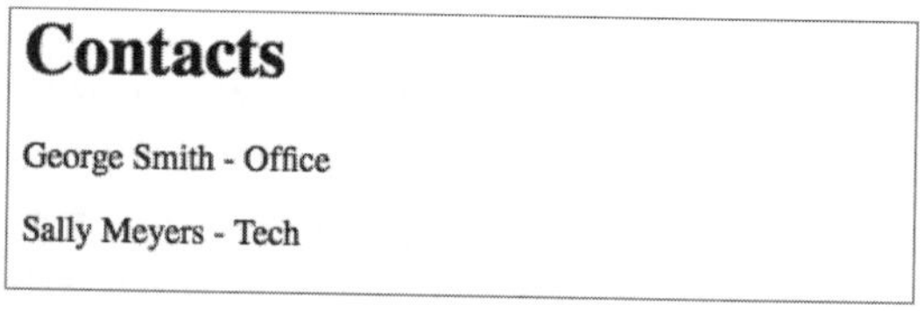

Contacts

George Smith - Office

Sally Meyers - Tech

FIGURE 10-10

GETTING VALUES FROM FUNCTIONS

Up until now, the examples of the functions in this lesson have been functions that just perform an action. They print something to the browser. Often, however, you want a function to perform an action and then give you the results back. This "giving the result back" is called *returning*. For instance, you could have a function that takes two arguments and adds them together and returns the result. Give it two and three and it returns five. This example creates a function that adds two numbers together. The result of that function is assigned to the variable $answer, which is then printed out. Here is what that code would look like:

```php
<?php
function addNumbers($number1, $number2) {
  $result = $number1 + $number2;
  return $result;
}

$answer = addNumbers('2', '3');
echo answer;
```

If you want to know if a function performed correctly and it does not have data to return, you would return true or false. You could also return false if there were errors in calculating the data. The following code creates a function that checks to be sure that it received valid numbers and returns false if it received non-numeric data. The program uses the result of the function as the condition in an if statement to determine what to do. See the results in Figure 10-11.

```php
<?php
function addNumbers($number1, $number2) {
  if (is_numeric($number1) AND is_numeric($number2)) {
    $result = $number1 + $number2;
    return $result;
  } else {
    return false;
  }
}
```

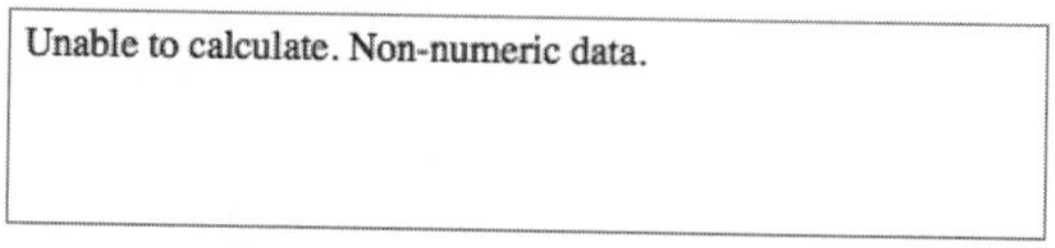

Unable to calculate. Non-numeric data.

FIGURE 10-11

```php
$answer = addNumbers('2', 'all');

if ($answer) {
  echo $answer;
} else {
  echo 'Unable to calculate. Non-numeric data.';
}
```

If you want to pass multiple bits of data, you use an array. The following code uses an associative array to return the value of the calculation and a separate value for the success or failure. Refer to Figure 10-12.

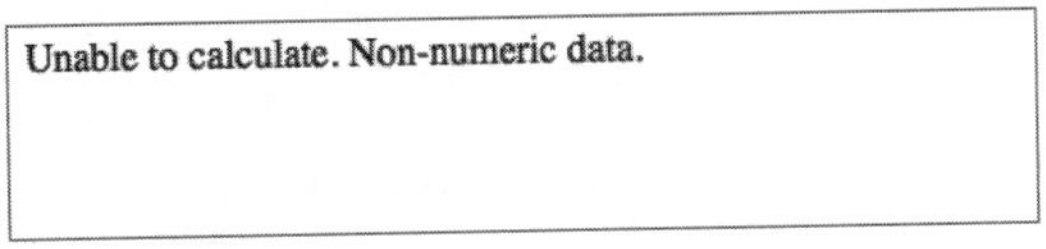

Unable to calculate. Non-numeric data.

FIGURE 10-12

```php
<?php
function addNumbers($number1, $number2) {
  if (is_numeric($number1) AND is_numeric($number2)) {
    $result['answer'] = $number1 + $number2;
    $result['status'] = true;
    $result['message'] = "The answer is ";
    return $result;
  } else {
    $result['answer'] = null;
    $result['status'] = false;
    $result['message'] = "Unable to calculate. Non-numeric data.";
    return $result;
  }
}

$answer = addNumbers('2', 'all');

if ($answer['status']) {
  echo $answer['message'] . $answer['answer'];
} else {
  echo $answer['message'];
}
```

Change `$answer = addNumbers('2', 'all');` to `$answer = addNumbers('2', '3');`, which gives you a valid result. You see a result similar to Figure 10-13.

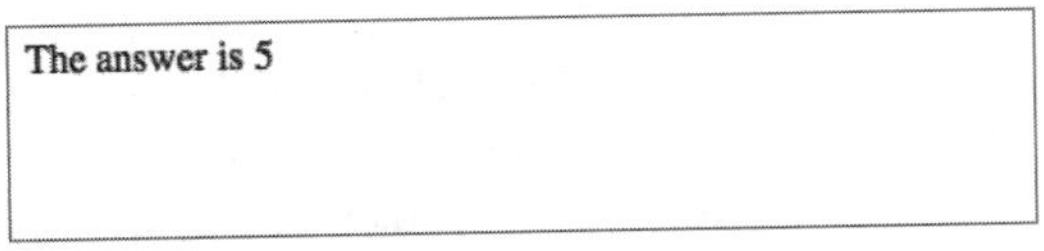

The answer is 5

FIGURE 10-13

You can use a return (with or without a value) to end a function wherever you want. If you use return without a value, it returns a NULL value.

USING FUNCTIONS

Now that you know how to define functions, how to pass data to them, and how to get data back, it is time to try using them.

You are creating a program that takes a temperature, converts it from Fahrenheit to Celsius (or vice versa), and displays it. See Figure 10-14.

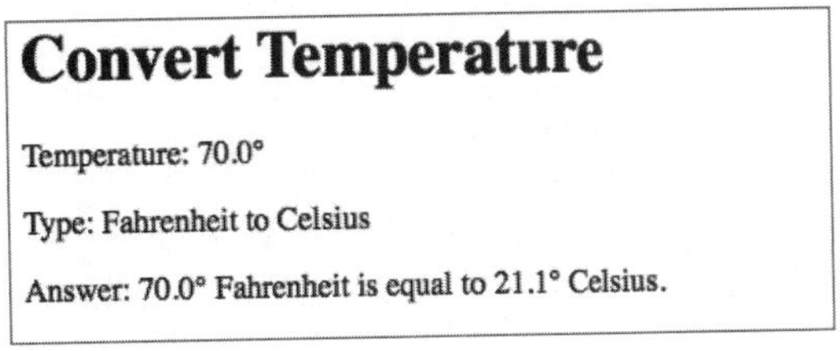

Convert Temperature

Temperature: 70.0°

Type: Fahrenheit to Celsius

Answer: 70.0° Fahrenheit is equal to 21.1° Celsius.

FIGURE 10-14

First, look at the main script for the program:

```php
<?php
// Set up the inputs
$temperature = 70; // Enter the temperature to be converted
$type = 'FtoC'; // Enter FtoC or CtoF for the type of conversion

// Display the Results
?>
<html>
<head>
  <title>Lesson 10t</title>
</head>

<body>
<h1>Convert Temperature</h1>
<p>Temperature: <?php echo formatDeg($temperature); ?></p>
<p>Type: <?php echo expandType($type); ?>
<p>Answer: <?php echo convertTemperature($temperature, $type); ?>
</body>
</html>
```

This code is just the script. If you run it, you receive errors because it is calling several functions that you have not given it yet. Let's go through the script and the functions that need to be added to the start of the program.

This script starts by setting the variables for temperature and for the type of conversion. In Lesson 11 you learn how to get this information from a form, but for now you can just hard-code it.

HARDCODING

You might come across the term hardcoding often in programming. Hardcode just means that you have directly specified the data instead of using a dynamic method of getting it. It is used for testing or when it's deemed too difficult, too time-consuming, too insecure, or just unnecessary to use a more flexible method.

Next, you display the temperature with this code: `echo formatDeg($temperature);`. You are displaying a temperature several times, so you create a function called `formatDeg()` that takes a number and returns it formatted to display with the proper number of decimals and the special HTML entity for a degree symbol. If the value received is not numeric, the function returns 0.

```php
function formatDeg($number) {
  if (is_numeric($number)) {
    return number_format($number, 1) . '&deg;';
  } else {
    return 0 . '&deg;';
  }
}
```

The next line displays the type of conversion: echo expandType($type);. You could just display FtoC or CtoF, but it is easier for the user if you spell out what that means. The expandType() does that for you:

```
function expandType($type) {
  if ($type=='CtoF') {
    return 'Celsius to Fahrenheit';
  } else {
    return 'Fahrenheit to Celsius';
  }
}
```

And now we come to the real meat of the matter where you display the following answer:

```
echo convertTemperature($temperature, $type);
```

The convertTemperature() function takes the temperature and the type of conversion and returns an answer with the converted temperature:

```
function convertTemperature($temperature, $type = "FtoC") {
  switch ($type) {
  case 'CtoF':
    $result = convertCtoF($temperature);
    break;
  case 'FtoC':
  default :
    $result = convertFtoC($temperature);
  }
  return $result;
}
```

Notice that the convertTemperature() function is really just a controlling function that calls the function that does the real work, depending on what type of conversion needs to happen. There are a few defaults happening here as well. The two valid types are CtoF and FtoC. If no type is specified when the function is called, then the type is set to FtoC. If the type that comes in is not one of the two valid types then it is processed as an FtoC.

Finally we come to the two functions that do the conversion calculations and create the answer text, convertFtoC() and convertCtoF(). Notice that these functions also call the formatDeg() function described earlier:

```
function convertFtoC($temperature) {
  $celsius = ($temperature - 32)* (5/9);
  $result = formatDeg($temperature) . ' Fahrenheit is equal to ' .
          formatDeg($celsius) . ' Celsius.';
  return $result;
}

function convertCtoF($temperature) {
  $fahren = $temperature * (9/5) + 32;
  $result = formatDeg($temperature) . ' Celsius is equal to ' .
          formatDeg($fahren) . ' Fahrenheit.';
  return $result;
}
```

Taking all the preceding code and adding comments, the final code is as follows:

```php
<?php
// FUNCTIONS
/**
 * convertTemperature
 * Convert Temperature
 * @param $temperature
 * @param $type
 */
function convertTemperature($temperature, $type = "FtoC") {
  switch ($type) {
  case 'CtoF':
    $result = convertCtoF($temperature);
    break;
  case 'FtoC':
  default :
    $result = convertFtoC($temperature);
  }
  return $result;
}

/**
 * convertFtoC
 * Convert from Fahrenheit to Celsius
 * @param $temperature
 */
function convertFtoC($temperature) {
  $celsius = ($temperature - 32)* (5/9);
  $result = formatDeg($temperature) . ' Fahrenheit is equal to ' .
            formatDeg($celsius) . ' Celsius.';
  return $result;
}

/**
 * convertCtoF
 * Convert from Celsius to Fahrenheit
 * @param unknown_type $temperature
 */
function convertCtoF($temperature) {
  $fahren = $temperature * (9/5) + 32;
  $result = formatDeg($temperature) . ' Celsius is equal to ' .
            formatDeg($fahren) . ' Fahrenheit.';
  return $result;
}

/**
 * formatDeg
 * Format the numbers to display as Degrees
 * @param unknown_type $number
 */
function formatDeg($number) {
  if (is_numeric($number)) {
```

```php
      return number_format($number, 1) . '&deg;';
    } else {
      return 0 . '&deg;';
    }
}

/**
 * expandType
 * Convert the type to a description
 * @param $type
 */
function expandType($type) {
  if ($type=='CtoF') {
    return 'Celsius to Fahrenheit';
  } else {
    return 'Fahrenheit to Celsius';
  }
}

?>

<?php
// SCRIPT

// Set up the inputs
$temperature = 70; // Enter the temperature to be converted
$type = 'FtoC'; // Enter FtoC or CtoF for the type of conversion

// Display the Results
?>
<html>
<head>
  <title>Lesson 10t</title>
</head>
<body>
<h1>Convert Temperature</h1>
<p>Temperature: <?php echo formatDeg($temperature); ?></p>
<p>Type: <?php echo expandType($type); ?>
<p>Answer: <?php echo convertTemperature($temperature, $type); ?>
</body>
</html>
```

> ✖ *If you forget and put a $ in front of a function such as* $myVar(), *PHP calls a function with the name of the value of* $myVar. *So the following code calls the function* foo():
>
> ```php
>     <?php
>     $myVar = 'foo';
>     echo $myVar();
> ```
>
> *This is called a variable function and is perfectly good PHP, but likely not what you intended to do.*

INCLUDING OTHER FILES

With user functions you have moved from just writing scripts to the more upscale *procedural* programming where your code is in reusable modules. Procedural programming cuts down on redundant code and makes debugging and maintenance easier.

You use the PHP commands `include`, `include_once`, `require`, and `require_once` to organize your files by grouping your functions in their own files and then "including" them in the code you are writing. You did this in Lesson 2 when you moved the content div into files in the content folder and then included them back in.

Includes are different from functions. You can think of an include as an automatic copy/paste. PHP goes out, grabs the file, and plops it right down where the `include` command is. Include files can contain just straight PHP and HTML, which is executed immediately, or they can contain function definitions, which are now available to be called.

These four commands, `include`, `include_once`, `require`, and `require_once`, all have the same syntax: the command and then the filename to be included:

```php
<?php
include 'content/home.php';
```

The difference between include and require is that the two require commands give you a fatal error and stop if the file is missing, whereas the two include commands just issue a warning and keep going. The "once" on the end means that PHP loads the file only once. If the file is already loaded it won't try to load it again.

> Functions and classes (which you learn about in Lesson 12) can be loaded only once because otherwise they attempt to load duplicate functions or classes, which causes a fatal error. So always use `include_once` or `require_once` with those files.

TRY IT

In this Try It, you create a new folder for the Case Study where you put your functions. You create a new function that loads content for different areas of the web page based on parameters passed and from the URL string.

> You can download the code and resources for this Try It from the book's web page at www.wrox.com. You can find them in the Lesson10 folder in the download. You will find code for both before and after completing the exercises.

Lesson Requirements

Your computer needs to be able to run as a web server with PHP and MySQL. XAMPP is a package of software that installs the web server, PHP, and MySQL for you. You can find instructions for downloading and installing XAMPP in Lesson 1.

You need a text editor that can produce plain-text files. You can find instructions for downloading and installing Eclipse PDT in Lesson 1. Other text editors that you can use are Adobe's Dreamweaver in code mode, Notepad, TextWrangler, or NetBeans.

If you are following along with the case study, you need your files from the end of Lesson 8. Alternatively, you can download the files from the book's website at www.wrox.com.

Step-by-Step

Create a function that loads content from the URL string and puts it in a file called functions.php in a new folder that contains the includes files.

1. Create a folder called **includes**.

2. Create a file called **functions.php** in that folder. You put your new functions in this file.

3. Create a new function called **loadContent()**:

```php
<?php
/**
 * loadContent
 * Load the Content
 * @param $default
 */
function loadContent() {


}
```

4. Open index.php and move the code that is in the content div inside the PHP tags to this new function. Your function should now look like this:

```php
<?php
/**
 * loadContent
 * Load the Content
 * @param $default
 */
function loadContent() {
  $content = '';
  // Get the content from the url
  if (isset($_GET['content'])) :
    $content = $_GET['content'];
    // Sanitize it for security reasons
    $content = filter_var($content, FILTER_SANITIZE_STRING);
  endif;
    // Set up the home page as the default
  $content = (empty($content)) ? "home" : $content;
  // Include the chosen page
  include 'content/' . $content . '.php'; }
```

5. In the index.php file, add a require_once command to the functions file, just below the starting comments:

```php
require_once 'includes/functions.php';
?>
```

6. In the `index.php` file, call the new `loadContent()` function. Your content div should now look like this:

```
<div class="content">
  <?php loadContent(); ?>
</div><!-- end content -->
```

7. Save the `function.php` and `index.php` files and test that the pages are showing up as they did before without errors.

Use the `loadContent` to load the catnav div menu. To do this you add the $where and $default parameters to the `loadContent` function.

1. Add a $where parameter to the function in `function.php` so you know where the request is coming from. Make it the first parameter because there is no default value for it. Add a $default parameter with the default of ''. You use the file in $default if you don't get passed a good file name in the $where parameter:

```
function loadContent($where, $default='') {
```

2. Change the call directly to the content URI parameter with one that locates the URI parameter specified in the $where passed to the function. Remove the following code:

```
if (isset($_GET['content'])) :
  $content = $_GET['content'];
  // Sanitize it for security reasons
  $content = filter_var($content, FILTER_SANITIZE_STRING);
endif;
```

3. Replace it with this code, which retrieves the GET parameter whose name is in the $where variable:

```
$content = filter_input(INPUT_GET, $where, FILTER_SANITIZE_STRING);
```

4. Filter the $default parameter:

```
$default = filter_var($default, FILTER_SANITIZE_STRING);
```

5. Change the hardcoded "home" default to the $default variable:

```
$content = (empty($content)) ? $default : $content;
```

6. Change the `include` statement so that you include a file only if there is something in $content and return the `include` statement:

```
if ($content) {
  // sanitize the data to prevent hacking.
  $html = include 'content/'.$content.'.php';
  return $html;
}
```

7. Add those same parameters where you call the function in `index.php`. Pass 'content' and 'home' as the values:

```
<?php loadContent('content', 'home'); ?>
```

8. Add the parameter **&sidebar=catnav** to the URL of the Gents, Sporting, and Women links in `contents/catnav.php`:

```
<li><a href="index.php?content=gents&sidebar=catnav">Gents</a></li>
<li><a href="index.php?content=sporting&sidebar=catnav">Sporting</a></li>
<li><a href="index.php?content=women&sidebar=catnav">Women</a></li>
```

9. Add the parameter **&sidebar=catnav** to the URL of the Gents, Sporting, and Women links in contents/categories.php:

```
<h2><a href="index.php?content=gents&sidebar=catnav">Gents</a></h2>
<p>Gents' clothing from the 18th century to modern times</p>
<a class="button display"
href="index.php?content=gents&sidebar=catnav">Display Lots</a>
...
<h2><a href="index.php?content=sporting&sidebar=catnav">Sporting</a></h2>
<p>Sporting clothing and gear.</p>
<a class="button display"
href="index.php?content=sporting&sidebar=catnav">Display Lots</a>
...
<h2><a href="index.php?content=women&sidebar=catnav">Women</a></h2>
<p>Women's Clothing from the 18th century to modern times</p>
<a class="button display"
href="index.php?content=women&sidebar=catnav">Display Lots</a>
```

10. In index.php, replace everything in the sidebar div to a loadContent(). with the first argument of 'sidebar' and the second argument of '':

```
<div class="sidebar">
        <?php loadContent('sidebar', ''); ?>
</div><!-- end sidebar -->
```

 Watch the video for Lesson 10 on the DVD or watch online at www.wrox.com/ go/24phpmysql.

Creating Forms

Forms are ubiquitous on websites. They include not only obvious "fill in the blank" forms but also are the method used to interact with the user. Search boxes and drop-down filters, for instance, are contained within forms.

In this lesson you review the HTML needed to code a form. Then you learn how to use PHP to process that form and gather the responses. Finally, you learn how to send users to the right page after they have submitted the form.

SETTING UP FORMS

Forms are set up primarily using HMTL code. This is a basic form that asks for your name (see Figure 11-1):

```
<html>
<head>
  <title>Contact</title>
</head>
<body>
<form action="index.php" method="get">
  <fieldset>
  <legend>Contact</legend>
    <label for="fullname">Name</label>
    <input id="fullname" name="fullname" type="text" />
    <input name="contactForm" type="submit" value="Submit" />
  </fieldset>
</form>
</body>
</html>
```

The `<form>` tag sets the action that occurs when the Submit button is clicked. This is the URI of the program that processes the form. It can either be a file specifically for processing forms or it can be an existing file that checks for whether form data was sent and automatically processes it. You learn how to do that later in this lesson.

FIGURE 11-1

The <form> tag also assigns the method that is used to send the form data. You learned about the two methods, GET and POST, in Lesson 6. In general, use get, which is the default, for inquiries and use post for database changes or actions that should not be repeated. GET data is appended to the end of the URL and POST data is not.

The for attribute in the <label> tag links to the <input> tag's id. The name attribute on the <input> tag is the name that is used to identify the data. The for, name, and id attributes are often the same, but only the for and the id need to match.

The <input> tag of type="submit" is the Submit button. When the user clicks that button, the form is submitted for processing. This is often used to identify the form. The data is named by the name attribute and the value is from the value attribute, which is also what is displayed on the button.

> Use the <input> tag to create the submit buttons in forms. <input type="submit"> automatically submits the form. <input type="button"> does not automatically submit the form. You need to use JavaScript to submit it.
>
> If you use the <button> tag instead of the <input> tag, be aware that Internet Explorer passes the information between the button tags and all the other browsers use the value.

To create radio buttons, you use an <input> tag of type="radio":

```
<fieldset>
<legend>What is your gender?</legend>
  <input type="radio" id="genderf" name="gender" value="f" checked="checked"/>
  <label for="genderf"> Female</label>
  <input type="radio" id="genderm" name="gender" value="m"/>
  <label for="genderm"> Male</label>
</fieldset>
```

The name attribute matches for each of the radio buttons. This groups the radio buttons together so only one value is sent for the group. The value attribute is the value that is submitted, not what is in the label. Because you cannot have duplicate id attributes, this is one place where your for and id attributes do not match your name attribute.

Checkboxes are similar to radio buttons, except that more than one box can be marked:

```
<fieldset>
<legend>Where do you live?</legend>
  <input type="checkbox" id="arearural" name="areatypes[]" value="rural" />
  <label for="arearural"> Rural</label>
  <input type="checkbox" id="areasuburb" name="areatypes[]" value="suburb"/>
  <label for="areasuburb"> Suburb</label>
  <input type="checkbox" id="areacity" name="areatypes[]" value="city"/>
  <label for="areacity"> City</label>
</fieldset>
```

Here the name attribute for all the checkmarks is the same and has square brackets prefixed to it. The square brackets tell the system to send the checked values as an array. If you leave off the square

brackets, only the last checked value is sent. You could also have each name be different and without the square brackets. In that case each name that was selected is sent as a separate value. With checkboxes, only checked values are sent.

You can also have individual checkboxes that are not part of a group. In the following instance, if the box is checked, the form field imagesonly is sent with the value of yes. If it is not checked, nothing is sent:

```
<input type="checkbox" id="imagesonly" name="imagesonly" value="yes" />
<label for="imagesonly"> Check here if you only want images.</label>
```

If you want to enter multiple lines of text, you use the <textarea> tag instead of a type of <input> tag. The following code shows what that looks like:

```
<label for="address">Address</label><br />
<textarea id="address" name="address" rows="3" cols="30"></textarea>
```

To enable a user to select from a drop-down list, you use the <select> tag with <option> tags as in the following example. This passes the value selected with the name given in the name attribute.

```
<label for="level">Level</label>
<select id="level" name="level">
  <option value="">- Select a level -</option>
  <option value="gold">Gold</option>
  <option value="silver">Silver</option>
  <option value="bronze">Bronze</option>
</select>
```

To enable multiple selections, you add the multiple attribute and add square brackets to the end of the name attribute as shown in the following code. The multiple attribute enables the user to select multiple options with his operating system's shortcut using the Shift, Control, or Command keys. The square brackets on the name attribute create an array to hold the multiple selections. The size attribute determines how many options should be displayed at a time.

```
<label for="interests">What do you like?</label>
<select id="interests" name="interests[]" multiple="multiple" size="3">
  <option value="0">Reading</option>
  <option value="1">Whitewater boating</option>
  <option value="2">Music</option>
</select>
```

If you want to let the user clear his form, you use the <input> tag of type="reset". This automatically resets the values for you, as shown in the following code.

```
<input type="reset" value="Clear" />
```

You can also send hidden values. "Hidden" just means the form field is not displayed in the form. It is still displayed in the URL. Use the <input> tag with type="hidden" to specify hidden values:

```
<input type="hidden" name="id" value="12345" />
```

When you put all these examples together you have a form that looks similar to Figure 11-2. This is the code for that program:

```
<!DOCTYPE html PUBLIC "-//W3C//DTD XHTML 1.0 Transitional//EN" "http://www.w3.org/
TR/xhtml1/DTD/xhtml1-transitional.dtd">
```

```
<html xmlns="http://www.w3.org/1999/xhtml">
<head>
  <meta http-equiv="Content-Type" content="text/html; charset=UTF-8" />
  <title>Contact</title>
  <style type="text/css">
    li {list-style:none; margin-bottom: 10px}
  </style>
</head>

<body>
<form action="lesson11b.php" method="get">
<fieldset>
<legend>Contact</legend>

<ul>

<li><label for="fullname">Name</label><br />
<input id="fullname" name="fullname" type="text" /></li>

<li><label for="address">Address</label><br />
<textarea id="address" name="address" rows="3" cols="30"></textarea></li>

<li>
<fieldset>
<legend>What is your gender?</legend>
<input type="radio" id="genderf" name="gender" value="f" checked="checked"/>
<label for="genderf"> Female</label>
<input type="radio" id="genderm" name="gender" value="m"/>
<label for="genderm"> Male</label>
</fieldset>
</li>

<li>
<input type="checkbox" id="imagesonly" name="imagesonly" value="yes" />
<label for="imagesonly"> Check here if you only want images.</label>
</li>

<li>
<fieldset>
<legend>Where do you like to live?</legend>
<input type="checkbox" id="arearural" name="areatypes[]" value="rural" />
<label for="arearural"> Rural</label>
<input type="checkbox" id="areasuburb" name="areatypes[]" value="suburb"/>
<label for="areasuburb"> Suburb</label>
<input type="checkbox" id="areacity" name="areatypes[]" value="city"/>
<label for="areacity"> City</label>
</fieldset>
</li>

<li>
<label for="level">Level</label>
<select id="level" name="level">
<option value="">- Select a level -</option>
```

```
<option value="gold">Gold</option>
<option value="silver">Silver</option>
<option value="bronze">Bronze</option>
</select>
</li>

<li>
<label for="interests">What do you like?</label>
<select id="interests" name="interests[]" multiple="multiple" size="3">
<option value="0">Reading</option>
<option value="1">Whitewater boating</option>
<option value="2">Music</option>
</select>
</li>

</ul>

<input type="submit" value="Submit" name="contactForm" />
<input type="reset" value="Clear" />

<div>
<input type="hidden" name="id" value="12345" />
</div>

</fieldset>
</form>

</body>
</html>
```

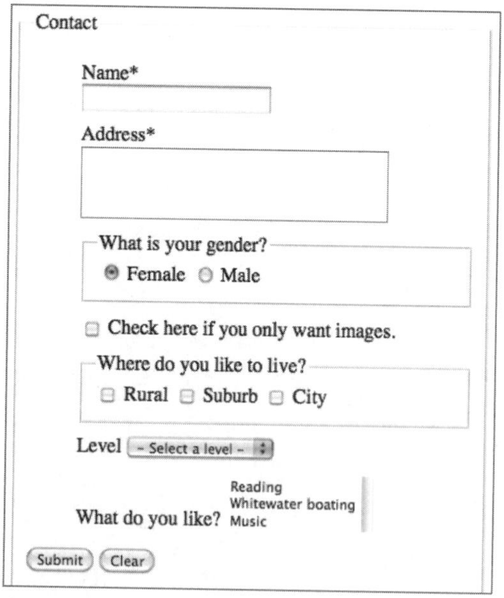

FIGURE 11-2

> You can download the preceding code in this book from the book's web page at www.wrox.com. The program is `lesson11b.php` in the Lesson11 folder in the download. "Processing Forms" starts with `lesson11c.php` for the step-by-step files, though the instructions refer to the completed file `lesson11i.php`. It is important to be aware of the name of the file because that must match the action on the `<form>` tag.

PROCESSING FORMS

You have refreshed your knowledge of coding forms in HTML and you have learned how to set up the information that is passed when the user submits the form. So now it is time to learn how to process the form using the example at the end of the previous section. Figure 11-3 shows the form just before the user submits it.

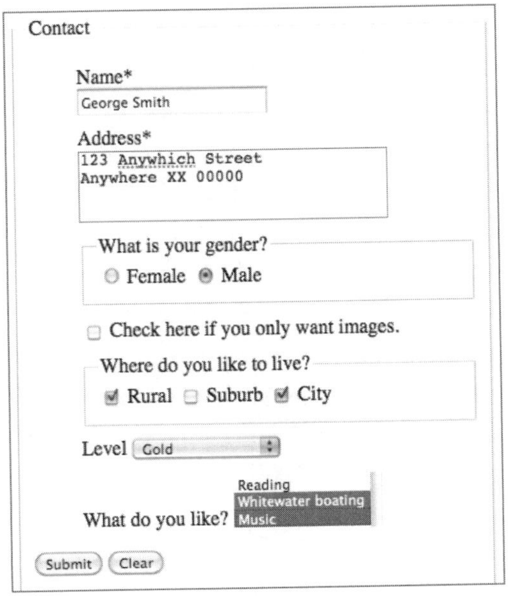

Contact

Name*

George Smith

Address*

123 Anywhich Street
Anywhere XX 00000

What is your gender?
○ Female ◉ Male

☐ Check here if you only want images.

Where do you like to live?
☑ Rural ☐ Suburb ☑ City

Level [Gold ⬦]

Reading
Whitewater boating
What do you like? Music

(Submit) (Clear)

FIGURE 11-3

When the form is submitted, the data is passed to either the GET or the POST variable, depending on the method attribute. Here is the code used for the `<form>` tag:

```
<form action="lesson11i.php" method="get">
```

Normally you use a POST because this is data that you are probably using to update a database. I used the GET method here so that you can see the data being passed. Look at the data in the address bar. You see something similar to this:

```
http://localhost/lesson11i.php?fullname=George+Smith&address=123+Anywhich+Street%0D
%0AAnywhere+XX+00000&gender=m&areatypes[]=rural&areatypes[]=city&level=gold&
interests[]=1&interests[]=2&contactForm=Submit&id=12345
```

This is dictated by the HTTP protocol, not PHP itself. Just after the filename `lesson11i.php` is a question mark. That signals the start of a *query string*. The GET variables show as key=value pairs separated by ampersands within the query string. The `name` attribute from the form fields is the key and the `value` attribute (or equivalent) is the value.

Only certain characters are allowed in a URL so characters that are not allowed are encoded to an allowable sequence. Notice that blanks are changed to + and the carriage return between the two lines of address is encoded as `%0D%0A`.

You submit the form with `<input type="submit" value="Submit" name="contactForm" />` so you should be able to find `&contractForm=Submit` in that query string. It's near the end of the string if you are having trouble locating it. You can have your program look for that value shortly.

As well as passing the data, the action on the `<form>` tag is performed. If a URL, either absolute or relative, is listed, that program is called. Your action is to call the same program that contains the form.

You add code to the top of the file to see if a form has been submitted. First, you check to see if there is a GET variable with the same name as the Submit button that contains the value of that Submit button. If you had used the POST method, you would look for it in POST. Because you are just doing a compare with this data, you do not need to worry about filtering it. If a form is submitted, you display a message to the user. It's a good idea to let the user know that she is successful in submitting the form and it also is a quick way to test your `if` statement.

```php
<?php
if($_GET['contactForm'] == "Submit") {
  echo 'Thank you for submitting the form';
}
?>
```

You should not see the message the first time you go to the page. Fill in the form and submit it. Figure 11-4 shows the form after submitting. A message is displayed across the top thanking the user for submitting the form and the form has been reset to the default values.

Next, it is time to collect the rest of the data within the form. You do this using `$_GET`, `$_POST`, and the sanitizing methods you learned at the end of Lesson 6. Normally you would do something constructive with this data, such as update a database. For this example, you just display it on the screen.

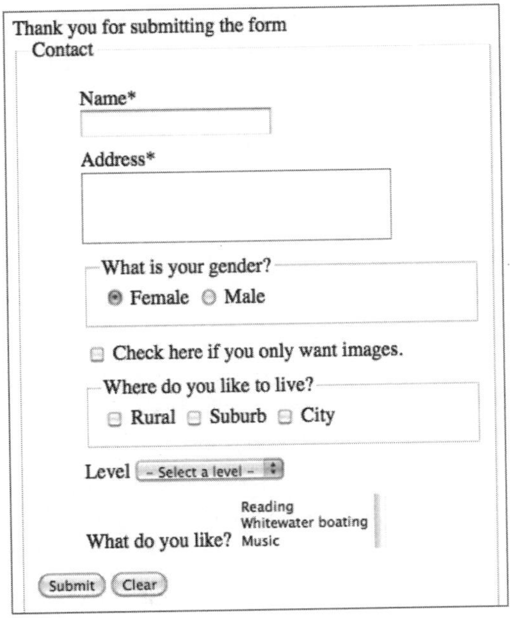

```
Thank you for submitting the form
  Contact
      Name*
      [                    ]

      Address*
      [                              ]
      [                              ]


      What is your gender?
        ● Female  ○ Male

      ☐ Check here if you only want images.
      Where do you like to live?
        ☐ Rural ☐ Suburb ☐ City

      Level [ – Select a level – ▼]
                        Reading
                        Whitewater boating
      What do you like? Music

  ( Submit ) ( Clear )
```

FIGURE 11-4

You can assign single values to a variable. The following code gets the value from the `fullname` form field, sanitizes it, and assigns it to `$name`. It does the same thing for the `address`, `gender`, and `level` form fields. You then display the data as a test. See Figure 11-5.

```php
<?php
if($_GET['contactForm'] == "Submit") {
    $name = filter_var($_GET['fullname'], FILTER_SANITIZE_STRING);
    $address = filter_var($_GET['address'], FILTER_SANITIZE_STRING);
    $gender = filter_var($_GET['gender'], FILTER_SANITIZE_STRING);
    $level = filter_var($_GET['level'], FILTER_SANITIZE_STRING);
    echo $name . '<br />';
    echo $address . '<br />';
    echo $gender . '<br />';
    echo $level . '<br />';

    echo 'Thank you for submitting the form';
}
```

Radio buttons, such as gender in the preceding example, are passed only if one is selected. In that example you preselected a choice. If you don't require your user to answer the question, when you process the form you should check first to see if a value was passed. You can do this with the `isset()` function, which is demonstrated in the discussion on checkmark boxes next.

> *Remember that the data from this form is in the address bar. If you get tired of filling in the form while you are testing, just copy and use the full URL. It simulates submitting the form.*

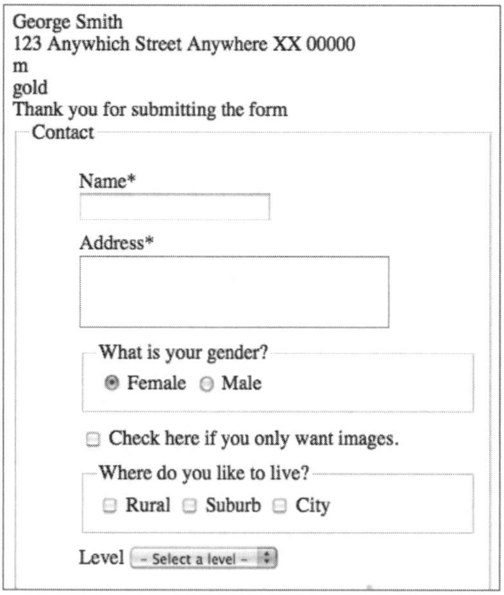

George Smith
123 Anywhich Street Anywhere XX 00000
m
gold
Thank you for submitting the form

Contact

Name*

Address*

What is your gender?
● Female ○ Male

☐ Check here if you only want images.

Where do you like to live?
☐ Rural ☐ Suburb ☐ City

Level [- Select a level - ▾]

FIGURE 11-5

Next you process the checkboxes. With checkboxes, the field itself is passed only if the box was checked, so you want to see if the field exists. Take your single checkbox named imagesonly, which has a value of Yes. You check that the parameter was set and that it is equal to the value. If not, you know the checkbox was not checked. See Figure 11-6 to see the results when the box is not checked.

```php
<?php
if (isset($_GET['imagesonly']) && $_GET['imagesonly'] == 'Yes') {
    $imagesonly = 'Yes';
} else {
    $imagesonly = 'No';
}
echo 'Images Only? ' . $imagesonly . '<br />';
```

In the example you also had a group of checkboxes that you want to process as an array. You signi-fied this by using the same name and suffixing the name with square brackets. Because the check-boxes are sent only if they are checked, you use isset() to see if any of the areatype checkboxes were selected at all. Then you loop through and filter each element of the array and build the filtered $areatypes array that you will display. See Figure 11-7 for the results.

```php
if (isset($_GET['areatypes'])) {
    $inputs = array();
    $inputs = $_GET['areatypes'];
    foreach ($inputs as $input) {
        $areatypes[] = filter_var($input, FILTER_SANITIZE_STRING);
    }
    foreach ($areatypes as $areatype) {
        echo $areatype . '<br />';
    }
} else {
    echo "You don't want to live anywhere.<br />";
}
```

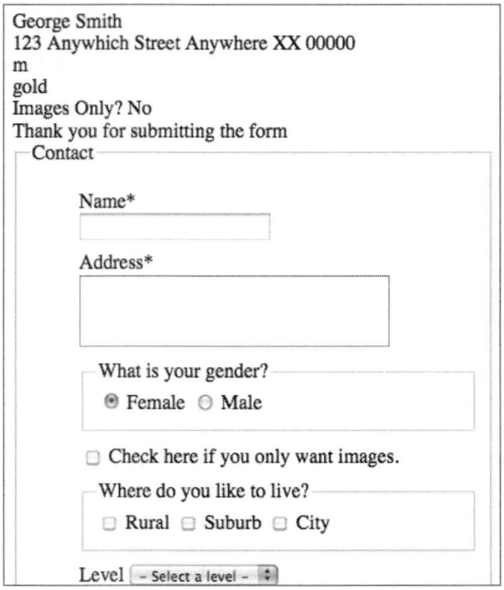

George Smith
123 Anywhich Street Anywhere XX 00000
m
gold
Images Only? No
Thank you for submitting the form

Contact

Name*

Address*

What is your gender?
◉ Female ○ Male

☐ Check here if you only want images.

Where do you like to live?
☐ Rural ☐ Suburb ☐ City

Level – Select a level – ⬍

FIGURE 11-6

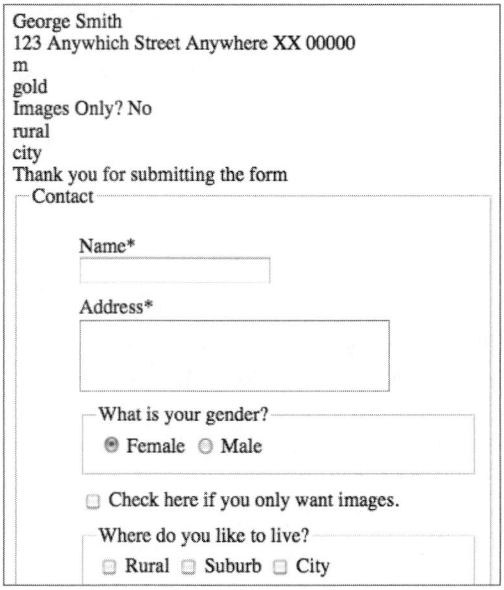

George Smith
123 Anywhich Street Anywhere XX 00000
m
gold
Images Only? No
rural
city
Thank you for submitting the form

Contact

Name*

Address*

What is your gender?
◉ Female ○ Male

☐ Check here if you only want images.

Where do you like to live?
☐ Rural ☐ Suburb ☐ City

FIGURE 11-7

You can use the same procedure for the multi-select box as well. The values here should be integers so you force them to integers as your filter. See Figure 11-8.

```
if (isset($_GET['interests'])) {
    $inputs = array();
    $inputs = $_GET['interests'];
    foreach ($inputs as $input) {
```

```
        $interests[] = (int) $input;
    }
    foreach ($interests as $interest) {
        echo $interest . '<br />';
    }
} else {
    echo "You have no interests.<br />";
}
```

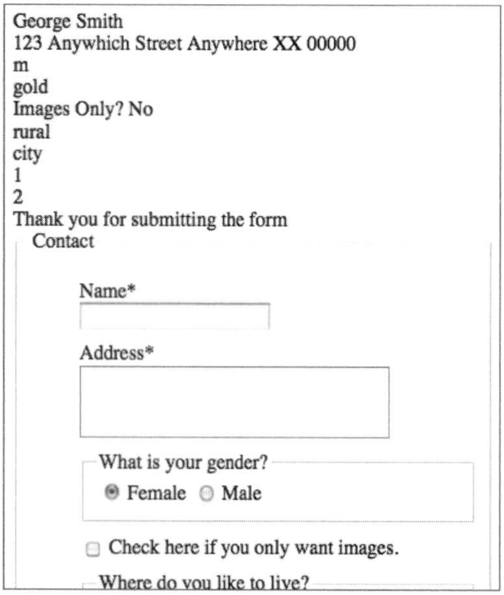

```
George Smith
123 Anywhich Street Anywhere XX 00000
m
gold
Images Only? No
rural
city
1
2
Thank you for submitting the form
  Contact

    Name*


    Address*




    ┌ What is your gender? ──────────────
    │ ◉ Female ○ Male

    ☐ Check here if you only want images.
    ┌ Where do you like to live? ─────────
```

FIGURE 11-8

Hidden parameters are processed just like regular parameters. In this case your hidden parameter field id should be an integer, so you filter it by forcing it to an integer. See Figure 11-9.

```
$id = (int) $_GET['id'];
echo $id . '<br />';
```

Now that you know how to read the data, you can run error checking to see if the form was filled out correctly. In this example, the only checking you need is to be sure that the user entered a name and address. You change the processing for the fullname and address parameters. You build an array with any errors and then loop through and display those errors. You fill in the same form, but submit it without an address. Your result should be similar to Figure 11-10.

```
// initialize error array
$errors = array();
// see if the form was submitted
if($_GET['contactForm'] == "Submit") {
  // Process required fields
  $name = filter_var($_GET['fullname'], FILTER_SANITIZE_STRING);
  if (!(trim($name))) {
    $errors[] = "You must enter a name";
  }
  $address = filter_var($_GET['address'], FILTER_SANITIZE_STRING);
```

```
if (!(trim($address))) {
  $errors[] = "You must enter an address";
}
if ($errors) {
  foreach ($errors as $error) {
    echo $error . '<br />';
  }
}
```

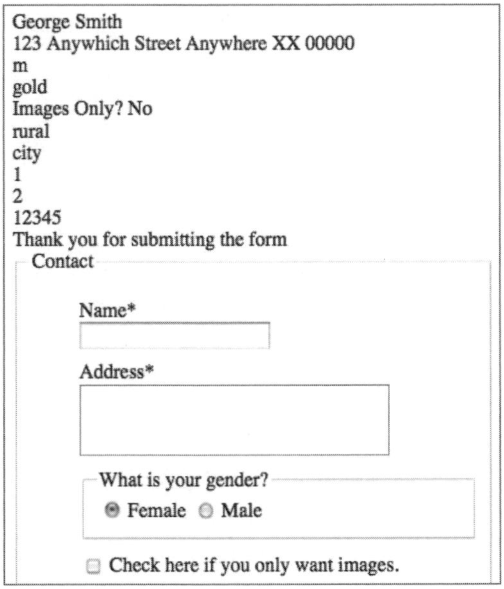

George Smith
123 Anywhich Street Anywhere XX 00000
m
gold
Images Only? No
rural
city
1
2
12345
Thank you for submitting the form

Contact

Name*

Address*

What is your gender?
◉ Female ○ Male

☐ Check here if you only want images.

FIGURE 11-9

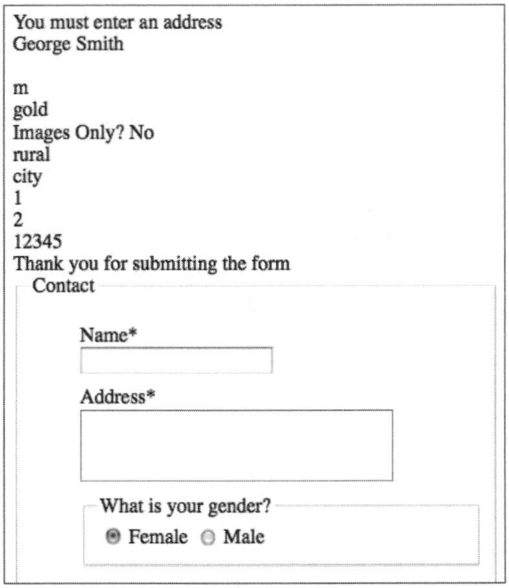

You must enter an address
George Smith

m
gold
Images Only? No
rural
city
1
2
12345
Thank you for submitting the form

Contact

Name*

Address*

What is your gender?
◉ Female ○ Male

FIGURE 11-10

REDIRECTING WITH HEADERS

Often when processing forms you need to send the user to another page, depending on the user's response. You can redirect the pages this way, using the `header()` function.

Headers are part of the HTTP protocol that the Web uses to direct traffic and carry data. You see the HTTP every time you call a web page: `http://www.example.com`. HTTP consists of two parts: the headers and the body. The headers contain the address to go to as well as the GET information. The body is where the data goes, including HTML and POST data.

HTTP sends the headers before the body of the message. If it comes across a body before it is given any headers, it automatically creates the headers. Any HTML that you create, even a blank line or an invisible newline character, is seen as part of the body. After headers have been created and the body started, any attempt to add another header results in an error. This is the reason for leaving off the final `?>` tag at the end of PHP files (so no final control characters are seen as output) and why cookies have to be set before any HTML (because setting cookies involves creating headers).

When you use the `header()` function, you are creating headers, so you need to use this before you have created any HTML or `echos` or stray blank lines. The syntax of the `header()` function is

```
header("Location: filename.php");
```

In this example you are echoing out information so you do not use the redirect. If instead you were saving the data to a database, you could choose to redirect to a different page upon successful completion or stay on the same page to allow the user to correct errors. You can also use redirects if you have a series of forms for the user to go through as in an order entry process.

In most of the examples you have been using GET rather than POST to send your data because then you then can see what is being passed. When you use POST, the parameters do not appear as part of the URL. Some of these example forms would normally have used POST. One of the decisions you need to make for every form you create is whether to use the method GET or POST. Here are some pointers on which one to select when.

Use GET when the same submission of the form can be processed multiple times, such as when making inquiries that don't change a database. GET parameters are part of the address and are displayed in the address bar so they are easily visible to users. Because they are part of the address they can be included in a bookmark.

Use POST when the same submission of the form cannot be processed multiple times without making changes. For instance, a form that is part of registering a new user should be created using POST parameters rather than GET. You may have noticed this difference when you use the back button on your browser and you get a message that warns you that you are about to reprocess POST data. POST data is not part of the address so it is not seen as easily. This also means that you cannot use POST to create different pages that can be bookmarked.

WHERE ARE THE GET PARAMETERS?

You may come across programs that are using GET but you don't see them in the address bar. All the GET parameters in the URL can look messy, which was historically a disadvantage when it came to search engine optimization (SEO). There are ways to rewrite the address so that the GET parameters don't show, but that is beyond the scope of this book.

TRY IT

In this Try It, you create a form that allows people to enter a temperature and have it converted from Fahrenheit to Celsius or vice versa. You use the temperature conversion functions you created in Lesson 10. You do not use the Case Study for this Try It.

> You can download the code and resources for this Try It from the book's web page at www.wrox.com. You can find them in the Lesson11 folder in the download. You will find code for both before and after completing the exercises.

Lesson Requirements

Your computer needs to be able to run as a web server with PHP and MySQL. XAMPP is a package of software that installs the web server, PHP, and MySQL for you. You can find instructions for downloading and installing XAMPP in Lesson 1.

You need a text editor that can produce plain-text files. You can find instructions for downloading and installing Eclipse PDT in Lesson 1. Other text editors that you can use are Adobe's Dreamweaver in code mode, Notepad, TextWrangler, or NetBeans.

Hints

The conversion from Fahrenheit to Celsius is $C = (F - 32) * (5/9)$.

The conversion from Celsius to Fahrenheit is $F = C * (9/5) + 32$.

Step-by-Step

Create a form to get the temperature. The form should have two buttons: one for Fahrenheit to Celsius and the other for Celsius to Fahrenheit.

1. Create a new file called `exercise11a.php`.

2. Enter the following code to create the form:

```
<!DOCTYPE html PUBLIC "-//W3C//DTD XHTML 1.0 Transitional//EN" "http://www.
w3.org/TR/xhtml1/DTD/xhtml1-transitional.dtd">
<html xmlns="http://www.w3.org/1999/xhtml">
<head>
  <title>Convert Temperature</title>
</head>
<body>

<form action="exercise11a.php" method="post">

<fieldset>
<legend>Fahrenheit/Celsius Converter</legend>
  <p><label for="temperature">Temperature</label>
    <input type="text" name="temperature" id="temperature" size="6" />
  </p>
  <p><input type="submit" name="FtoC" value="Fahrenheit to Celsius" /></p>
  <p><input type="submit" name="CtoF" value="Celsius to Fahrenheit" /></p>
</fieldset>
</form>
</body>
</html>
```

Create a file containing functions to convert the temperature.

1. Create a new file called **exercise11b.php**.

2. Add the `convertFtoC()` and `convertCtoF()` functions as shown in Lesson 10.

```
/**
 * convertFtoC
 * Convert from Fahrenheit to Celsius
 * @param $temperature
 */
function convertFtoC($temperature) {
  $celsius = ($temperature - 32)* (5/9);
  $result = formatDeg($temperature) . ' Fahrenheit is equal to ' .
  formatDeg($celsius) . ' Celsius.';
  return $result;
}

/**
 * convertCtoF
 * Convert from Celsius to Fahrenheit
 * @param unknown_type $temperature
 */
function convertCtoF($temperature) {
  $fahren = $temperature * (9/5) + 32;
  $result = formatDeg($temperature) . ' Celsius is equal to ' .
  formatDeg($fahren) . ' Fahrenheit.';
  return $result;
}
```

3. These functions call the `formatDeg()` function that formats the temperature for display, so add that function to the same file:

```
/**
 * formatDeg
```

```
 * Format the numbers to display as Degrees
 * @param unknown_type $number
 */
function formatDeg($number) {
  if (is_numeric($number)) {
    return number_format($number, 1) . '&deg;';
  } else {
    return 0 . '&deg;';
  }
}
```

Back in the exercise11a.php file, include the exercise11b.php file. Check to see which button was clicked. Based on that, do the conversion.

1. In the exercise11a.php file, include the file with the functions using the require_once() function:

    ```
    require_once "exercise11b.php";
    ```

2. Use an if statement to check the $_POST to see if the FtoC button was clicked:

    ```
    if ($_POST['FtoC'] =="Fahrenheit to Celsius") {
    }
    ```

3. Inside that if statement call convertFtoC() passing the $_POST['temperature'] parameter. Force a conversion to float type to prevent a malicious code from getting in.

    ```
    $answer = convertFtoC((float) $_POST['temperature']);
    ```

4. Continue the if statement with an elseif statement to check for the other button and process it:

    ```
    elseif ($_POST['CtoF']) {
        $answer = convertCtoF((float) $_POST['temperature']);
    }
    ```

Display the answer. Initialize it in the beginning so it is set to nothing.

1. In the exercise11a.php file, initialize $answer before the if statement performing the conversions:

    ```
    $answer = '';
    ```

2. In the HTML below the form, echo out $answer:

    ```
    <p><?php echo $answer; ?></p>
    ```

3. The full exercise11a.php file should look like this:

    ```
    <?php
    require_once("exercise11b.php");
    $answer = '';
    if ($_POST['FtoC']) {
        $answer = convertFtoC((float) $_POST['temperature']);
    } elseif ($_POST['CtoF']) {
        $answer = convertCtoF((float) $_POST['temperature']);
    }
    ?>
    ```

```
<!DOCTYPE html PUBLIC "-//W3C//DTD XHTML 1.0 Transitional//EN" "http://www.
w3.org/TR/xhtml1/DTD/xhtml1-transitional.dtd">
 <html xmlns="http://www.w3.org/1999/xhtml">
 <head>
   <title>Convert Temperature</title>
 </head>
 <body>

 <form action="exercise11a.php" method="post">

 <fieldset>
 <legend>Fahrenheit/Celsius Converter</legend>
   <p><label for="temperature">Temperature</label>
     <input type="text" name="temperature" id="temperature" size="6" />
   </p>
   <p><input type="submit" name="FtoC" value="Fahrenheit to Celsius" /></p>
   <p><input type="submit" name="CtoF" value="Celsius to Fahrenheit" /></p>
 </fieldset>

 </form>
 <p><?php echo $answer; ?></p>
 </body>
 </html>
```

4. Test the program. You should see results like Figure 11-11 if you enter 70 and click the Fahrenheit to Celsius button.

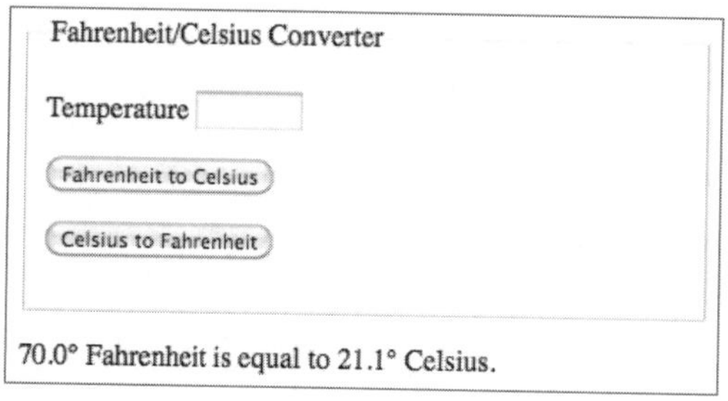

Fahrenheit/Celsius Converter

Temperature

(Fahrenheit to Celsius)

(Celsius to Fahrenheit)

70.0° Fahrenheit is equal to 21.1° Celsius.

FIGURE 11-11

 Watch the video for Lesson 11 on the DVD or watch online at www.wrox.com/go/24phpmysql.

SECTION III
Objects and Classes

- ▶ **LESSON 12:** Introducing Object-Oriented Programming

- ▶ **LESSON 13:** Defining Classes

- ▶ **LESSON 14:** Using Classes

- ▶ **LESSON 15:** Using Advanced Techniques

The first level in PHP programming is writing scripts, which is just sequential lines of PHP code or bits of PHP interspersed with HTML. The second level is procedural programming, which you learned in Lesson 10 when you started moving code into functions. The next level is object-oriented programming (OOP).

In Lesson 12, you learn the basic concepts of object-oriented programming and why you would want to use it. In the next two lessons you learn how to create classes and use them. The final lesson of this section teaches the more advanced object-oriented techniques.

Introducing Object-Oriented Programming

Programmers strive to write code that has fewer errors, is easier to read, and is easier to maintain, and they strive to write that code faster. *Object-oriented programming (OOP)* gives you more tools to do that. In this lesson you learn the reasons for using OOP and the basic concepts behind it.

UNDERSTANDING THE REASONS FOR USING OOP

Object-oriented programming is a way of coding that organizes your programs, encourages consistency, reduces redundancy and complexity, increases flexibility, and promotes better security.

It enables you to create building blocks of basic functionality. You can then reuse these blocks, add on to the blocks, or even override parts of the blocks to create more complex structures. Being able to reuse code in this flexible manner means you have fewer bugs when creating your programs, which makes them more reliable over time.

OOP also uses what is called *encapsulation*. You use encapsulation every time you use local variables in functions because the variables have local scope and can't be seen outside of the function. Encapsulation is the concept that what you do in one section of your program is not affected by and does not affect another section. OOP has similar structures that encapsulate data and actions. You are inside your house with the shades drawn and you control the door through which you receive and disseminate information.

Additionally, OOP is well suited for implementing both design patterns, which are an advanced technique for modeling program designs, and MVC (Model-View-Controller), which is a software design technique for separating database interactions, presentation, and control systems much as you separate content from presentation with HTML and CSS.

INTRODUCING OOP CONCEPTS

One reason people shy away from OOP is that it involves some advanced concepts that can be hard to grasp at first. However, good programming often incorporates OOP so you need to know how to handle it when you come across it. Besides, it is a lot of fun when you understand it.

Objects and Classes

OOP is a way of thinking about what you need to accomplish in terms of objects (nouns) that you need to define and actions (verbs) that you need to perform.

An *object* is an *instantiation* of a *class* that contains *properties* and *methods*. This sounds like so much geek-speak, but you will understand it by the time you are done with this section.

Let's use the example of a cell phone. The cell phone itself is an object. This particular phone is 4.5 inches tall by 2.3 inches wide by .37 inches thick. It has 32GB of storage and weighs 4.8 ounces. It contains specific songs, phone numbers, and ebooks. These are properties that the phone has. Properties are information.

This cell phone can do actions. You can tell it to make phone calls, take pictures, browse the Internet, or play tunes. Each of those types of actions is a method. These are the verbs, the acts that can be performed.

A class corresponds to the blueprint for creating this cell phone. A class is what defines the object.

An object, such as this particular cell phone, is an instance of the class. You can imagine a manufacturing line just churning out instances (objects) of the class. The act of making an instance from a class is called instantiation.

So you could say, "My cell phone was manufactured based on plans and it contains songs and a way for me to play them." An object is an instantiation of a class that contains properties and methods.

To illustrate the concept more clearly, here are some other examples:

Customer Class

➤ **Properties:** First name, last name, company, address, e-mail, phone number

➤ **Methods:** Place an order, inquire about an order, change an e-mail address

Product Class

➤ **Properties:** Product number, description, cost, price, quantity on hand, image of product

➤ **Methods:** Increase quantity when product received, decrease quantity when product shipped, format the price, find an extended price for a given quantity

Article Class

➤ **Properties:** Title, author, abstract, content, ratings, permanent link

➤ **Methods:** Check for proper authority to see the article, save the article to the database, delete the article from the database, format the article for display

To bring it into PHP terms, properties are variables for the class and the methods are functions that are in a class. You learn in the next lesson how to create the classes in PHP.

Extending Classes

You can create a parent class that contains common functions and properties and then build more detailed classes on top of it. For example, a Phone class is able to receive calls and make calls. A Cellphone class extends the phone class so it can automatically receive and make calls, but is also able to retrieve phone numbers from an address book. A Smartphone class extends the Cellphone class and is able to keep track of your calendar, browse the Internet, and play songs.

The classification of animals is another example. The parent class is Animal. Dog, Cat, and Bird all extend Animal, but with different properties and methods. Dog has a Tail Wagging method, whereas Cat has a Purring method and a Length of Fur property, and Bird has a Flying method.

You can also override methods in the parent class with your new class. So the Whale class can override those parts of the Mammal class that it needs to because it swims in the ocean instead of walking on land as most mammals do.

The ability to extend classes (inheritance) and override them makes OOP very powerful. It enables you to create classes that are generic enough to reuse in many programs and yet it enables you to tailor classes for very specific needs.

LEARNING VARIATIONS IN DIFFERENT PHP RELEASES

OOP features are relatively new to PHP. They existed in PHP4 but were more fully developed in PHP5, especially 5.2. Also, PHP 5.3 introduced additional features.

If you are writing your own code in 5.3, these differences are not important. If you are dipping into someone else's code you should be aware of these changes so you can recognize a remnant of an older coding style:

➤ **Pass by Reference:** When you assign an object to a variable it used to create a copy of the object. Now it creates a reference so that changes in either the original or the new object affect both.

➤ **Visibility & Final:** The ability to alter the scope of properties and functions. You learn about visibility in Lesson 15.

➤ **Constructors:** An optional method that is called when you create an object. In PHP4 this was the same name as the class. Now there is a special function, __construct(). You learn about this in Lesson 13.

➤ **Class Constants and Static Methods:** This is a way to use classes without creating an object. You learn about this in Lesson 15.

➤ **Abstract Classes:** This is a special type of parent class that you can use to define other classes. You learn about this in Lesson 15.

➤ The __autoload **Function:** This is a way to automatically load your class definitions without needing long lists of require_once statements. This is not fully implemented until PHP 5.3. You learn more about this in Lesson 15.

TRY IT

In this Try It, you analyze the contacts in the About Us page of the Case Study to decide what properties and methods you need for a Contact object.

> *You can download the code and resources for this Try It from the book's web page at* www.wrox.com. *You can find them in the Lesson12 folder in the download. This lesson does not contain any changes to the code.*

Lesson Requirements

If you want to look at the Case Study on your local computer, your computer needs to be able to run as a web server with PHP and MySQL. XAMPP is a package of software that installs the web server, PHP, and MySQL for you. You can find instructions for downloading and installing XAMPP in Lesson 1.

Hints

This is a conceptual exercise, not a PHP coding exercise.

Step-by-Step

Based on the contacts in Figure 12-1, write down the properties and methods that a Contact object might need.

1. The properties are the pieces of information about the Contact.

Properties include the following:

➤ First name

➤ Last name

➤ Position

➤ Email

➤ Phone

2. The methods are functions that the object would need.

➤ A method that assembles a full name from first name and last name

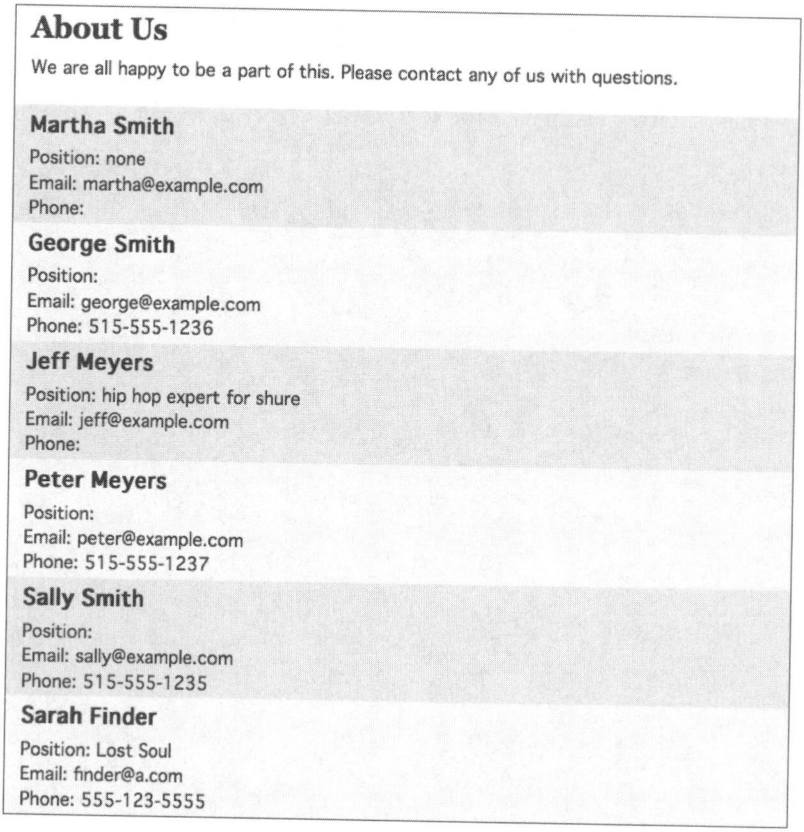

About Us

We are all happy to be a part of this. Please contact any of us with questions.

Martha Smith

Position: none
Email: martha@example.com
Phone:

George Smith

Position:
Email: george@example.com
Phone: 515-555-1236

Jeff Meyers

Position: hip hop expert for shure
Email: jeff@example.com
Phone:

Peter Meyers

Position:
Email: peter@example.com
Phone: 515-555-1237

Sally Smith

Position:
Email: sally@example.com
Phone: 515-555-1235

Sarah Finder

Position: Lost Soul
Email: finder@a.com
Phone: 555-123-5555

FIGURE 12-1

 Watch the video for Lesson 12 on the DVD or watch online at www.wrox.com/go/24phpmysql.

Defining Classes

Classes are the heart of object-oriented programming. They define what an object looks like, what information it can store, and what actions and calculations it can perform. In this lesson you learn how to create classes.

The basic syntax of a class looks like this:

```php
<?php
class MyClassname
{
  // Properties
  public $someProperty;
  public $someOtherProperty;

  // Methods
  public function someFunction($input = false) {
    // php code
  }

  public function anotherFunction() {
    // php code
  }
}
```

Begin a class declaration with the word class followed by the name of the class. The body of the class goes in curly brackets. Put property definitions next, followed by the methods.

The class name can be any combination of letters, numbers, or underscores. It can start with either a letter or an underscore, but, according to convention, a class name should begin with a capital letter. The name is case sensitive. Note that like functions, classes do not start with a $.

It is standard practice to put each class in a file with the same name as the class. So the class Myclassname would go in a file called myclassname.php. This makes it easier to find the right file while you are programming and easier to reuse selected ones in different programs.

If you document your classes with PHPDoc blocks, many editors are able to use them as help text as you program. The block for a class looks like this:

```
/**
 * Class short description
 *
 * Class longer description if needed
 *
 * @package     PackageName
 */
```

If the class is in its own file, you have both the page PHPDoc block and the class PHPDoc block.

Up until now you have been able to run the code in the lessons. Classes do not actually do anything because they are just blueprints. So you are not able to see this code in action until the next lesson.

DEFINING CLASS VARIABLES (PROPERTIES)

Class variables, called properties, are where you put information that is specific to the object. Valid property names are the same as valid variable names. This is the syntax for a property:

```
public $someProperty = 'Mine';
public $someOtherProperty = true;
```

The declaration starts with the scope keyword (public, protected, or private) followed by the property. You learn more about the scope keywords in Lesson 15. For now use public.

You can initialize the property as you do with regular variables except that you can only initialize with a constant, including the Boolean literals. The following code is not valid because you cannot use variables:

```
public $someOtherProperty = $myVar;
```

Notice that these class variables are outside the functions. The functions themselves can have ordinary variables within them, but the properties are separate. When you create an object from a class, a brand new set of properties is initialized and set aside specifically for that object.

To use a property in a method, you prefix the property name with $this->:

```
$this->someProperty
```

> *Notice that when using* $this->, *the property name does not have a* $. *If you put a* $ *in front of the property name, you are telling the program that you want to use the property name that is the value of the property, not that property.*
>
> ```
> $someProperty = 'anotherProperty';
> $anotherProperty = 'Hello';
> echo $this->someProperty; // displays 'anotherProperty'
> echo $this->$someProperty; // displays 'Hello'
> ```

It's important when you start working with methods that you recognize the difference between properties, which are defined in the class, and variables, which are defined in a method. The properties require $this and keep their value for the life of the object. Variables in methods (like variables in functions) do not use $this and start new each time the method is called.

You should document each of your properties with a PHPDoc block. The comment includes a short description, any pertinent or confusing information, the @var tag to signal that this is a variable, and the type of variable expected, such as string, integer, float, array, Boolean, or object.

```
/**
 * The phone number of this cell phone
 * @var string
 */
```

DEFINING CLASS FUNCTIONS (METHODS)

Although properties have a vital difference from ordinary variables, methods act just like functions and are often called functions. The main difference between methods and functions (other than that one is inside a class and the other is not) is that methods are defined with a scope keyword. This scope affects access to the method, not to anything within the method. You learn more about scope for methods in Lesson 15. For now use public scope. This is the syntax for a method:

```
public function myMethod($input) {
  // php code
}
```

You can put anything in this function as you would in a regular function. In addition, you can use the properties by using the $this->someProperty form. If you want to call another method in the class you use $this as well. So to call yourMethod() use $this->yourMethod().

Let's go through a complete class, including the methods. The following is a class describing a cell phone.

Start with the class name and the properties:

```
class Cellphone
{
  // Properties
  public $phoneNumber;
  public $model;
  public $color;
  public $contacts;
  public $songs;
```

Next come the methods. The first is a method to add contacts. The Contact name and Contact phone number are passed in when the method is called. They are then added to the property contacts, which is an associative array. Notice the use of $this-> to reference the property.

```
public function addContact($number, $name) {
  $this->contacts[$name] = $number;
}
```

The following method adds songs to the cell phone. A song is passed into the method when it is called. If the argument is an array, the program loops through the array and adds the songs. If it is not an array, it adds the single song. Remember that empty square brackets on an array automatically add an element with the next available numeric index.

```
public function addSongs($songs) {
  if (is_array($songs)) {
    foreach ($songs as $song) {
      $this->songs[] = $song;
    }
  } else {
    $this->songs[] = $songs;
  }
}
```

The following method displays the contacts, which are stored in the property $contacts. It uses a foreach loop that loops through the property $contacts, which is an array. Remember that this is just a class — a blueprint — so nothing runs until you create an object from it in the next lesson.

```
public function displayContacts() {
  // Notice that the property has -> and no $
  // while the array has => and a $
  foreach ($this->contacts as $name=>$number) {
    echo $name . ' - ' . $number . '<br />';
  }
}
```

It's easy to get confused between -> and => as well as when you need a $ and when you don't.

The class construction uses a dash with the greater-than sign, and constructions working with associative arrays use the equal sign with the greater-than sign.

The associative array uses the normal form for the second variable, so it has a $ in front of the second variable.

There is normally no $ following $this->. You can think of the $ as meaning "use the value of what is inside." If you want to use the property $contacts, it is $this->contacts. You use the $ only if you want to use the value of what is in a property as the name of another property. The following two echo statements both display "George Smith":

```
$this->field = 'contact';
$this->contact = 'George Smith';
echo $this->$field;
echo $this->contact;
```

The following method calls two other methods in the same class. It uses the same $this-> construction as used for properties.

```
public function addThenDisplayContacts($newname, $newnumber) {
  $this->addContacts($newnumber, $newname);
```

```
    $this->displayContacts();
  }
```

The next method counts the number of songs. It passes the result back via the `return` statement. The earlier methods did what they needed within the method so they did not need to return anything. With this method, the whole point is to return an answer.

```
  public function countSongs() {
    $result = count($this->songs);
    return $result;
  }
```

And, finally, you need the closing curly bracket for the class:

```
  }
```

Document each of the methods with a PHPDoc block. You will find this invaluable when programming if you are using one of the many editors that are able to use it as dynamic help text. This is an example:

```
  /**
   * Add contacts
   * @param string $number
   * @param string $name
   * @return integer | boolean
   */
```

The comment starts with a description. Include in the description anything about the method that might trip someone up. List all the parameters coming in, along with their type and parameter name. If you have a return in the method, document it here, along with the type. If it could be more than one type (such as a good value or false if there was an error), separate the types with a pipe symbol (|). Some of the editors even give you a skeleton of the comment. If you are using Eclipse, type a /** on the line before a method and Eclipse gives you a comment template with the parameters filled in.

This is what the full Cellphone class looks like, complete with documentation:

```
<?php
/**
 * cellphone.php
 *
 * Cellphone class file
 *
 * @version    1.2 2011-02-03
 * @package    Example
 * @copyright  Copyright (c) 2011 Myself
 * @license    GNU General Public License
 * @since      Since Release 1.0
 */
/**
 * Cellphone class
 *
 * @package    Example
 */
```

```php
class Cellphone
{
  /**
   * The phone number of this cell phone
   * @var string
   */
  public $phoneNumber;
  /**
   * The model number
   * @var string
   */
  public $model;
  /**
   * The color of the phone, using an id from the color file
   * @var int
   */
  public $color;
  /**
   * Assoc. Array with contact name as the key, the phone number as the value
   * @var array
   */
  public $contacts;
  /**
   * Array with filenames of song mp3 files
   * @var array
   */
  public $songs;

  /**
   * Create a new Contact
   * @param string $number
   * @param string $name
   */
  public function addContact($number, $name) {
    $this->contacts[$name] = $number;
  }

  /**
   * Add an array mp3 filename to the Songs array,
   * if it isn't an array, then just add the single song
   * @param array|string $songs
   */
  public function addSongs($songs) {
    if (is_array($songs)) {
      foreach ($songs as $song) {
        $this->songs[] = $song;
      }
    } else {
      $this->songs[] = $songs;
    }
  }

  /**
```

```
   * Display a list of the Contacts
   */
  public function displayContacts() {
    foreach ($this->contacts as $name=>$number) {
      echo  $name . ' - ' . $number . '<br />';
    }
  }

  /**
   * Create a new contact and then display all the contacts
   * @param string $newname
   * @param string $newnumber
   */
  public function addThenDisplayContacts($newname, $newnumber) {
    $this->addContacts($newnumber, $newname);
    $this->displayContacts();
  }

  /**
   * Count the songs
   * @return int
   */
  public function countSongs() {
    $result = count($this->songs);
    return $result;
  }


}
```

You have learned how to define a class. In the next lesson you learn how to use this class.

TRY IT

In this Try It, you create a class for the contacts in the Case Study. A contact should include first name, last name, position, email, and phone along with a method that creates a full name out of the first name and last name.

> You can download the code and resources for this Try It from the book's web page at www.wrox.com. You can find them in the Lesson13 folder in the download. You will find code for both before and after completing the exercises.

Lesson Requirements

Your computer needs to be able to run as a web server with PHP and MySQL. XAMPP is a package of software that installs the web server, PHP, and MySQL for you. You can find instructions for downloading and installing XAMPP in Lesson 1.

You need a text editor that can produce plain-text files. You can find instructions for downloading and installing Eclipse PDT in Lesson 1. Other text editors that you can use are Adobe's Dreamweaver in code mode, Notepad, TextWrangler, or NetBeans.

If you are following along with the case study, you need your files from the end of Lesson 10. Alternatively, you can download the files from the book's website at www.wrox.com.

Hints

You do not need the PHPDoc block comments for the code to work but it is good to get into a habit of entering it as you go.

Step-by-Step

Create the includes/classes/contact.php file.

1. Create a folder called **classes** in the includes folder.

2. Create a file called **contact.php** in the includes/classes folder. Enter the page-level documentation:

    ```php
    <?php
    /**
     * contact.php
     *
     * Contact class file
     *
     * @version     1.2 2011-02-03
     * @package     Smithside Auctions
     * @copyright   Copyright (c) 2011 Smithside Auctions
     * @license     GNU General Public License
     * @since       Since Release 1.0
     */
    ```

3. Define the class called **Contact**:

    ```php
    /**
     * Contact class
     *
     * @package     Smithside Auctions
     */
    class Contact
    {
    }
    ```

4. Enter the properties in between the curly braces:

    ```php
    /**
     * First name
     * @var string
     */
    public $first_name;
    /**
     * Last Name
     * @var String
    ```

```
   */
  public $last_name;
  /**
   * Position in the company.
   * @var string
   */
  public $position;
  /**
   * Email
   * @var string
   */
  public $email;
  /**
   * Phone number, formatted in string
   * @var string
   */
  public $phone;
```

5. Create a function called name that concatenates the first and last names with a space in between. Put this method after the properties.

```
  /**
   * Creates a full name by concatenating first and last names
   * @return string
   */
  public function name() {
    $name = $this->first_name . ' ' . $this->last_name;
    return $name;
  }
```

You test this class in the Try It in Lesson 14.

 Watch the video for Lesson 13 on the DVD or watch online at www.wrox.com/go/24phpmysql.

14

Using Classes

In the previous lesson you learned how to define classes. In this lesson you learn how to use them.

INSTANTIATING THE CLASS

A class is a blueprint for creating objects. When you create an object you are instantiating the class—making an instance of the class. You can create multiple objects from the same class. They all start out the same, with properties empty or equal to a default and with the capability of performing all the actions detailed by the methods. They are all independent so when you change a property in one, it does not affect the property in any of the other objects made from that class. It is just like when you enter a contact in your cell phone; no one else's cell phone is affected.

Instantiating the class is very easy. Make sure that the class code has been included. Use a `require_once` to include it. You need the file, so it should be a `require` rather than an `include`. You also want the class to be included only once because you get an error if you try to define the class a second time, even if it is identical. It is standard practice to include your common classes when you start the program. If you rarely use a class, you can include it before you create an object.

If a class called `Cellphone` is in the `cellphone.php` file, the following code creates an object called `$myPhone`:

```php
<?php
require_once 'cellphone.php';
$myPhone = new Cellphone();
```

The object called `$myPhone` is a regular variable that happens to be an object. You use all the same naming conventions for the variable as you do for other variables.

If you want to create multiple objects, create multiple variables:

```php
<?php
require_once 'cellphone.php';
$myPhone = new Cellphone();
```

```php
$sallyPhone = new Cellphone();
$georgePhone = new Cellphone();
```

You can also use a variable to contain the name of the class:

```php
<?php
$type = 'cell';
$classname = $type . 'phone';
$myPhone = new $classname();
$sallyPhone = new $classname();
$georgePhone = new $classname();
```

> Be careful that you only use the $ when using a variable to specify the class name. If you use the actual name of the class, which is usual, do not use a $.

USING OBJECTS

To access an object's properties or classes use the "dash-greater-than" construction. If `$myPhone` is an object with a property of `$phoneNumber`, the following code assigns 555-555-7777 to that property:

```php
<?php
$myPhone->phoneNumber = '555-555-7777';
```

Assuming that the object has a method called `$displayContacts()`, the following code runs that method:

```php
<?php
$myPhone->displayContacts();
```

Often the purpose of a method is to give you a value, that is, to return a value. You capture this by assigning it to a variable or by using it. Here are two ways of getting the same information from `countSongs()`:

```php
<?php
$numberSongs = $myPhone->countSongs();
echo $numberSongs;
echo $myPhone->countSongs();
```

In the previous lesson you created the class `Cellphone`, which you put in the file `cellphone.php`. You can see that code at the end of Lesson 13, just before the Try It section, or you can download it from this book's website at www.wrox.com in the Lesson14 folder. You are now ready to create code using the class so that you can run it and see results.

The first step is to include the class and create an object:

```php
<?php
require_once 'cellphone.php';
$myPhone = new Cellphone();
```

Now put some data into the object. You can put data into the properties directly. This is how you load the cell phone's own number, model, and color:

```
$myPhone->phoneNumber = '555-555-1111';
$myPhone->model = '3GS';
$myPhone->color = 'Black';
```

Echo them back to verify that it worked. The results should look like Figure 14-1. This is what the full code looks like:

```
<?php
require_once 'cellphone.php';
$myPhone = new Cellphone();
$myPhone->phoneNumber = '555-555-1111';
$myPhone->model = '3GS';
$myPhone->color = 'Black';
echo 'Phone number: ' . $myPhone->phoneNumber . '<br />';
echo 'Model: ' . $myPhone->model . '<br />';
echo 'Color: ' . $myPhone->color . '<br />';
```

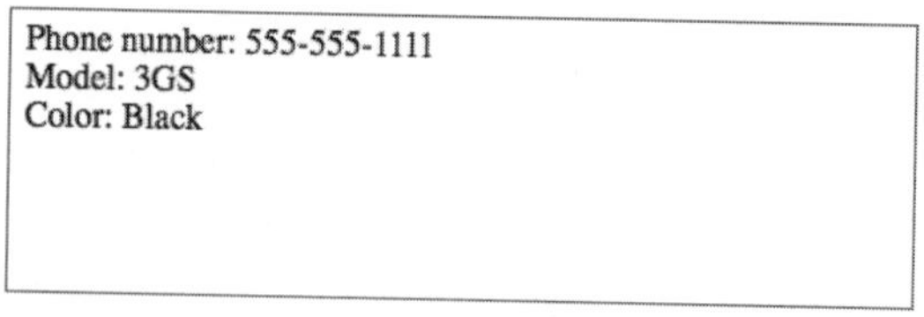

```
Phone number: 555-555-1111
Model: 3GS
Color: Black
```

FIGURE 14-1

There are also a couple of methods that enable you to enter data into the properties: addContact() and addSongs(). Use addContact() to add to the $contacts property array by giving the name and phone number of the contact. Display the array to see that the contacts were added properly. Use print_r() to display an array rather than echo. The results look like Figure 14-2.

```
$myPhone->addContact('555-555-1212', 'Sally Strange');
$myPhone->addContact('555-555-1515', 'George Mason');
print_r($myPhone->contacts);
```

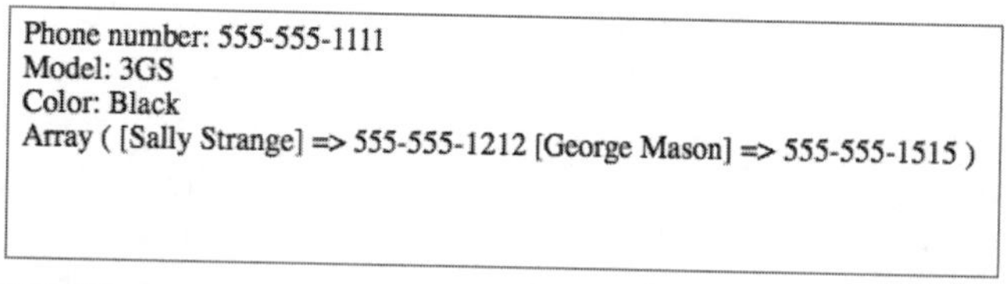

```
Phone number: 555-555-1111
Model: 3GS
Color: Black
Array ( [Sally Strange] => 555-555-1212 [George Mason] => 555-555-1515 )
```

FIGURE 14-2

Use a method that prints the contacts. Replace the print_r() statement with a call to displayContacts(). See Figure 14-3.

```
$myPhone->displayContacts();
```

```
Phone number: 555-555-1111
Model: 3GS
Color: Black
Sally Strange - 555-555-1212
George Mason - 555-555-1515
```

FIGURE 14-3

The addSongs() property is looking for either an array of filenames of songs or a single filename. Add an array of songs and then display the property to verify it. Putting the <pre> tags around print_r() makes the results easier to read when testing. See Figure 14-4.

```
$myPhone->addSongs(array('ibelieve.mp3','heaven.mp3','song3.mp3'));
echo '<pre>';print_r($myPhone->songs);echo '</pre>';
```

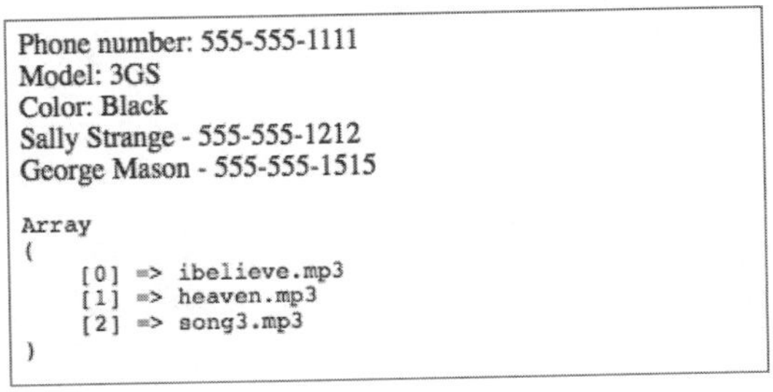

```
Phone number: 555-555-1111
Model: 3GS
Color: Black
Sally Strange - 555-555-1212
George Mason - 555-555-1515

Array
(
    [0] => ibelieve.mp3
    [1] => heaven.mp3
    [2] => song3.mp3
)
```

FIGURE 14-4

The countSongs() method counts the number of songs and returns the number. It does not display the number, though, so you need to display it so you can see that you received it. Instead of printing out the song names, display how many songs are on the phone. See Figure 14-5.

```
echo 'My phone has ' . $myPhone->countSongs(). ' songs.<br />';
```

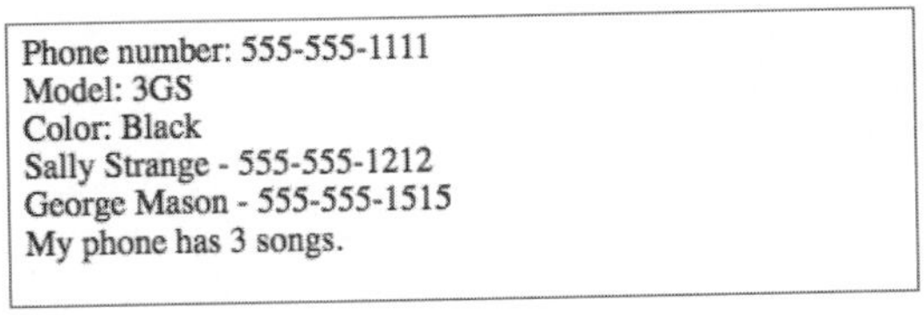

```
Phone number: 555-555-1111
Model: 3GS
Color: Black
Sally Strange - 555-555-1212
George Mason - 555-555-1515
My phone has 3 songs.
```

FIGURE 14-5

Updating a property directly is convenient but best practices recommend using a method. Using a method enables you to handle any other actions that need to be done when you change the property. This could be error checking, filtering, or adding subsidiary information. Even if you only need to change the value now, at some point in the future you might need to add filtering. If you are updating through a method, the only place you need to change is in the class. If you are updating directly, you need to locate all those places and make changes to all of them.

Two special methods help you fill in the properties when you create the object. The __construct() method is automatically called when you create an object. You pass arguments to the method, which

can be used to update the methods or perform any other initializing tasks you need. As an example, add the following method to the cellphone class definition:

```php
public function __construct($phoneNumber, $model, $color) {
  $this->phoneNumber = $phoneNumber;
  $this->model = $model;
  $this->color = $color;
}
```

Note that the method begins with a double underscore. You are taking the phone number, model, and color and using them to update those properties.

Now create a new file and create some objects from the class and then display them. See Figure 14-6.

```php
<?php
require_once 'cellphone.php';
$myPhone = new Cellphone('555-555-1111', 'iPhone', 'Black');
$yourPhone = new Cellphone('555-555-2222', 'Droid', 'Purple');
$hisPhone = new Cellphone('555-555-3333', 'Blackberry', 'Pink');
echo 'Phone number: ' . $myPhone->phoneNumber . '<br />';
echo 'Model: ' . $myPhone->model . '<br />';
echo 'Color: ' . $myPhone->color . '<br />';
echo 'Phone number: ' . $yourPhone->phoneNumber . '<br />';
echo 'Model: ' . $yourPhone->model . '<br />';
echo 'Color: ' . $yourPhone->color . '<br />';
echo 'Phone number: ' . $hisPhone->phoneNumber . '<br />';
echo 'Model: ' . $hisPhone->model . '<br />';
echo 'Color: ' . $hisPhone->color . '<br />';
```

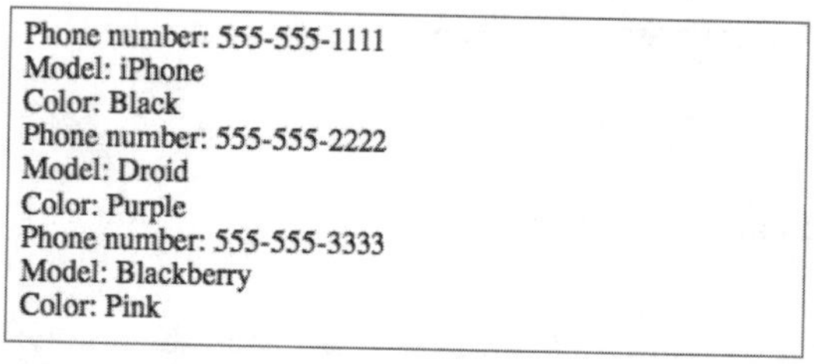

```
Phone number: 555-555-1111
Model: iPhone
Color: Black
Phone number: 555-555-2222
Model: Droid
Color: Purple
Phone number: 555-555-3333
Model: Blackberry
Color: Pink
```

FIGURE 14-6

If PHP does not find a __construct() method, it looks for a method with the same name as the class. This is the old style and you should avoid it in new coding.

TRY IT

In this Try It, you replace the static HTML code on the About Us page of the Case Study with objects for each of the contacts.

First you add the __construct() method to the Contact class that you created in Lesson 13. Then you update the properties in the objects with the names and contact information. Finally you use those objects to display them on the About Us page.

When you start using databases in Section V, you will be able to fill these objects from the database.

> You can download the code and resources for this Try It from the book's web page at www.wrox.com. You can find them in the Lesson14 folder in the download. You will find code for both before and after completing the exercises.

Lesson Requirements

Your computer needs to be able to run as a web server with PHP and MySQL. XAMPP is a package of software that installs the web server, PHP, and MySQL for you. You can find instructions for downloading and installing XAMPP in Lesson 1.

You need a text editor that can produce plain-text files. You can find instructions for downloading and installing Eclipse PDT in Lesson 1. Other text editors that you can use are Adobe's Dreamweaver in code mode, Notepad, TextWrangler, or NetBeans.

If you are following along with the Case Study, you need your files from the end of Lesson 13. Alternatively, you can download the files from the book's website at www.wrox.com.

Hints

The __construct method is called automatically when you create an object.

Because objects are just another type of variable, they can be array elements. By putting objects into an array you can use the power of the array to loop through the objects.

Step-by-Step

So that you can instantiate the Contact class, add an include to the index.php file and add a __construct() method to the class.

1. Include the contact.php file so that the class is available. In index.php, add the following code immediately following the PHPDoc block comments:

   ```
   require_once 'includes/classes/contact.php';
   ```

2. In the contact.php file, add a __construct() method as the first method. The following code shows what it should look like.

   ```
   /**
    * Initialize the Contact with first name, last name, position
    * email, and phone
    * @param array
    */
   public function __construct($input = false) {
     if (is_array($input)) {
       foreach ($input as $key => $val) {
         // Note the $key instead of key.
         // This will give the value in $key instead of 'key' itself
         $this->$key = $val;
       }
   ```

```
      }
   }
```

Create an object for each of the contacts and fill with the information on each of the contacts.

1. In about.php, just below the PHPDoc comment block, create an object called **$item** from the Contact class. Pass an associative array with the property names as the keys and the values from the first contact in the list.

```
$item = new Contact(array('first_name'=>'Martha',
'last_name'=>'Smith',
'position'=>'none',
'email'=>'martha@example.com',
'phone'=>''));
```

2. Change the first item in the unordered list to use the object instead of the hardcoded information about Martha Smith:

```
<li class="row0">
  <h2><?php echo $item->name(); ?></h2>
  <p>Position: <?php echo $item->position; ?><br />
  <?php echo $item->email; ?><br />
  Phone: <?php echo $item->phone; ?><br /></p>
</li>
```

3. Run your program and verify that your About Us page looks similar to Figure 14-7.

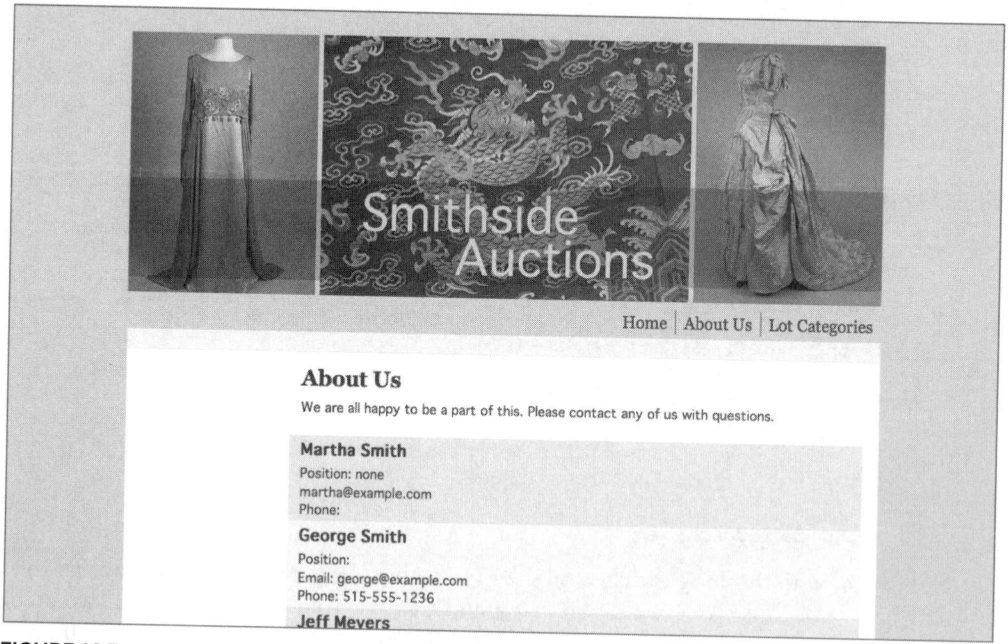

FIGURE 14-7

4. Now that you have successfully created and used your first object, you create an array of objects and loop through the array to display all the contacts. In the about.php file, just before you create the $item object, initialize the array $items:

```
$items = array();
```

5. Change the variable $item to **$items[]** where you create your object. This adds an element to the $items array instead of using a single variable. This is what the altered code looks like:

```
$items[] = new Contact(array('first_name'=>'Martha',
'last_name'=>'Smith',
'position'=>'none',
'email'=>'martha@example.com',
'phone'=>''));
```

6. Create objects for the rest of the contacts, adding them to the $items array:

```
$items[] = new Contact(array('first_name'=>'George',
'last_name'=>'Smith',
'position'=>'none',
'email'=>'george@example.com',
'phone'=>'515-555-1236'));
$items[] = new Contact(array('first_name'=>'Jeff',
'last_name'=>'Meyers',
'position'=>'hip hop expert for shure',
'email'=>'jeff@example.com',
'phone'=>''));
$items[] = new Contact(array('first_name'=>'Peter',
'last_name'=>'Meyers',
'position'=>'none',
'email'=>'peter@example.com',
'phone'=>'515-555-1237'));
$items[] = new Contact(array('first_name'=>'Sally',
'last_name'=>'Smith',
'position'=>'none',
'email'=>'sally@example.com',
'phone'=>'515-555-1235'));
$items[] = new Contact(array('first_name'=>'Sarah',
'last_name'=>'Finder',
'position'=>'Lost Soul',
'email'=>'finder@a.com',
'phone'=>'555-123-5555'));
```

7. Put a `foreach` loop around the first item in the unordered list to loop through the $items array:

```
<?php foreach ($items as $item) : ?>
  <li class="row0">
    <h2><?php echo $item->name(); ?></h2>
    <p>Position: <?php echo $item->position; ?><br />
    <?php echo $item->email; ?><br />
    Phone: <?php echo $item->phone; ?><br /></p>
  </li>
<?php endforeach; ?>
```

8. Notice that with this loop the class on the `<li>` tag is always `"row0"`. You want that to alternate between `"row0"` and `"row1"` so that your CSS background colors alternate. To do this, add the index of the array in the `foreach` loop. Because you created the array by automatically adding each element, the index counts starting from 0. You then use the formula $i % 2, which divides the index by 2 and returns the remainder, thus alternating between 0 and 1. Change your `foreach` statement and the `<li>` tag to the following code:

```
<?php foreach ($items as $i=>$item) : ?>
  <li class="row<?php echo $i % 2; ?>">
```

9. Now remove the remaining hardcoded contacts in the unordered list. Your complete `<ul>` group should look like the following:

```
<ul class="ulfancy">
  <?php foreach ($items as $i=>$item) : ?>
    <li class="row<?php echo $i % 2; ?>">
      <h2><?php echo $item->name(); ?></h2>
      <p>Position: <?php echo $item->position; ?><br />
      <?php echo $item->email; ?><br />
      Phone: <?php echo $item->phone; ?><br /></p>
    </li>
  <?php endforeach; ?>
</ul>
```

10. Your About Us page should still look the same. See Figure 14-8. You have changed the internal workings of the page but not what it looks like.

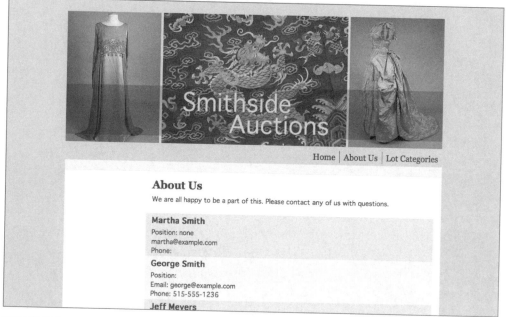

FIGURE 14-8

Watch the video for Lesson 14 on the DVD or watch online at www.wrox.com/go/24phpmysql.

Using Advanced Techniques

Now that you have a grasp of the basic concepts of using classes and objects in PHP, you are ready to learn more advanced techniques. In this lesson you learn easier ways of including the code for the class files and best practice techniques for updating and accessing properties. You learn how to use scope with classes to make your code more secure.

You also learn how to extend classes so that you can build on stable classes, and how to organize the functionality in your program by using static functions and classes.

INITIALIZING THE CLASS

Best practice dictates that you create a new file for each of your classes. You also have to include any of those files once, and only once, to define the class before you can use it. You can use different techniques to do this.

As you learned in the previous chapter, you can use `require_once` statements at the beginning of your program or just before you use your classes. This, however, can result in a lot of tedious code or a lot of extra code that might never be needed.

PHP has what are called "magic methods." These are functions that are called automatically at certain times. One magic method you are familiar with is `__contruct()`, which is called when you create a new object. Magic methods start with a double underscore.

PHP has a magic function called `__autoload()` that is automatically called if you try to use a class that has not been defined. You define this function at the beginning of your program and you can use it to include your class files when they are needed.

The `Cellphone` class was included in the previous lesson with this code:

```php
<?php
require_once 'cellphone.php';
```

The following code takes the class that is being instantiated, adds the `.php` extension, and includes that file if this is the first time it has been looked for:

```php
<?php
function __autoload($class_name) {
  require_once $class_name . '.php';
}
```

PHP calls this magic function if you have created it, but you have control over what happens when `__autoload` is called because you write the function. You need to include this function at the beginning of your code because it needs to exist or PHP will not call it.

That code works if your server is case insensitive, but `Cellphone.php` and `cellphone.php` are considered two different files on most servers. So you need to take that class name and convert it to lowercase before you use it in as a filename. This assumes that you are following the convention of using all lowercase for your filenames. The following code shows the addition of this functionality:

```php
<?php
function __autoload($class_name) {
  require_once strtolower($class_name) . '.php';
}
```

Obviously if you have one class, this is overkill. But if you have several classes using the `__autoload()` function is easier than remembering to go into your first program and adding a `require_once` for each new class. It is also more efficient in terms of performance than including all the files at the beginning of the program if you might not use them all.

UNDERSTANDING SCOPE

Scope dictates who can see what; what has *visibility*. You learned in Lesson 9 that variables have local scope (they can only been seen where they are created) unless they are declared as global. You have more options when using scope with classes.

Properties

When you create a property in a class, you can use it in any of the methods in an object using the `$this->` construction. This gives you the value for the property in the particular object you are in, as opposed to the values of the same property in other instances of the same class. You can think of it as "`$this` gives you the value in this object". Remember that variables that are not properties (those ordinary variables in the methods) do not use `$this`. You can have a property and a variable with the same name, so in a method `$this->myVar` and `$myVar` refer to different variables. The first is a property and its value is accessible anywhere in the object; it is still there the next time you go into the same object. The second is an ordinary variable and is available only in that method; it is initialized every time you use the method.

When you declare a property at the beginning of the class you preface the declaration with the scope. The scope keywords are `public`, `protected`, and `private`. So far in this book, you have been using `public` as the scope:

```php
public $phoneNumber;
```

When a property is public, it can be accessed directly from outside the class. You indicate the object that the property is in to locate it. The following code gives you the public $phoneNumber from objects created from the `Cellphone` class. See Figure 15-1.

```php
<?php
require_once 'cellphone.php';
$myPhone = new Cellphone('555-555-1111', 'iPhone', 'Black');
$yourPhone = new Cellphone('555-555-2222', 'Droid', 'Purple');
echo 'Phone number: ' . $myPhone->phoneNumber . '<br />';
echo 'Phone number: ' . $yourPhone->phoneNumber . '<br />';
```

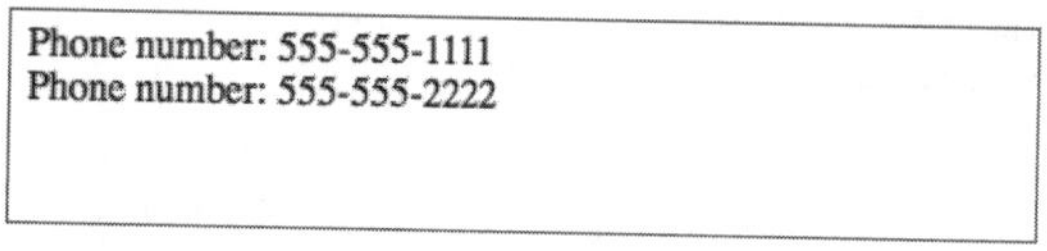

```
Phone number: 555-555-1111
Phone number: 555-555-2222
```

FIGURE 15-1

> You may see properties using the var scope. This is a holdover from PHP 4 and is the same as `public` if there is no scope keyword.

Protected properties cannot be seen outside the class except in inherited classes or parent classes. You learn about inheritance later in this lesson. The following code is how you define a protected property in the class.

```
protected $_phoneNumber;
```

Private properties are available only within the class itself. This code is an example of defining a private property:

```
private $_phoneNumber;
```

> Private and protected properties often start with a single underscore. This was the convention used in earlier versions of PHP, which did not have scope keywords. It was a signal to programmers not to use the property outside of the class. Many programmers continue the convention because it is a good reminder of which properties are private.
>
> However, just starting a variable name with an underscore does not make it private. You need to add the `protected` or `private` keyword.

The `protected` and `private` keywords are not necessarily used in the same sense that you keep your Social Security number private. They are used for control and encapsulation. As an example, say that whenever you change a customer's e-mail address, you want to send an e-mail to the old address as confirmation. If you can change the customer's address directly, you have to know and remember that you also need to send the e-mail. Instead, you can make the e-mail property private and force programmers to use a method to update the e-mail address. You send the e-mail confirmation from within that method. So then any time someone changes the e-mail, the message is automatically sent.

If you need to access these properties outside of the class, you use what are commonly called *getter* and *setter* methods. These are methods you write that return the property value (getters) or change the property value (setters). By convention, the method name begins with get or set followed by the property name with the first letter capitalized. The following is the earlier example in which you directly retrieved the public property $phoneNumber:

```php
<?php
require_once 'cellphone.php';
$myPhone = new Cellphone('555-555-1111', 'iPhone', 'Black');
$yourPhone = new Cellphone('555-555-2222', 'Droid', 'Purple');
echo 'Phone number: ' . $myPhone->phoneNumber . '<br />';
  echo 'Phone number: ' . $yourPhone->phoneNumber . '<br />';
```

This next example uses a protected phone number and retrieves the property with a getter method instead. This is the class definition that defines the protected property $phoneNumber and the new getter function getPhoneNumber():

```php
<?php
class Cellphone
{
    protected $_phoneNumber;
    public $model;
    public $color;

    public function __construct($phoneNumber, $model, $color) {
        $this->_phoneNumber = $phoneNumber;
        $this->model = $model;
        $this->color = $color;
    }

    public function getPhoneNumber() {
        return $this->_phoneNumber;
    }
}
```

The following is the script that retrieves the protected property. Remember that the method requires parentheses.

```php
<?php
require_once 'cellphone_v2.php';
$myPhone = new Cellphone('555-555-1111', 'iPhone', 'Black');
$yourPhone = new Cellphone('555-555-2222', 'Droid', 'Purple');
echo 'Phone number: ' . $myPhone->getPhoneNumber() . '<br />';
echo 'Phone number: ' . $yourPhone->getPhoneNumber() . '<br />';
```

The getter method is simply returning the value of the $_phoneNumber property. However, at a later date, you could add more functionality to that method without needing to change any of the places that are calling it and they would all get the new version.

> You may have noticed that in the previous example the require_once file was cellphone_v2.php but the class name was Cellphone. The filename and the class name do not have to be the same, although if you want to use __autoload() to load the classes for you, it's easier if they are.

Methods

Methods have the same scope keywords as properties: `public`, `protected`, and `private`. If they have no scope keyword, `public` is assumed. Older code doesn't include the scope because it has been available only since PHP 5. Get into the habit of always using a scope keyword.

If you use a method as a getter or setter for a property, the method should be public because only public methods work outside the class.

Private and protected methods are used when they are needed only within the class or they are using variables that are available only within the class. In the following example, the `_formatDeg()` method is only needed to format the information in the other class methods. See Figure 15-2 for the results. Though you usually put the classes in a separate file, for the sake of demonstration, the class and script to use the class are in one file.

```php
<?php
class Converter
{

    public function convertFtoC($temperature) {
      $celsius = ($temperature - 32)* (5/9);
      $result = $this->_formatDeg($temperature) . ' Fahrenheit is equal to '
        . $this->_formatDeg($celsius) . ' Celsius.';
      return $result;
    }

    public function convertCtoF($temperature) {
      $fahren = $temperature * (9/5) + 32;
      $result = $this->_formatDeg($temperature) . ' Celsius is equal to '
        . $this->_formatDeg($fahren) . ' Fahrenheit.';
      return $result;
    }

    private function _formatDeg($number) {
      if (is_numeric($number)) {
        return number_format($number, 1) . '&deg;';
      } else {
        return 0 . '&deg;';
      }
    }
  }

} // end of class

// script to use the class
$newTemp = new Converter;
echo $newTemp->convertFtoC(70);
```

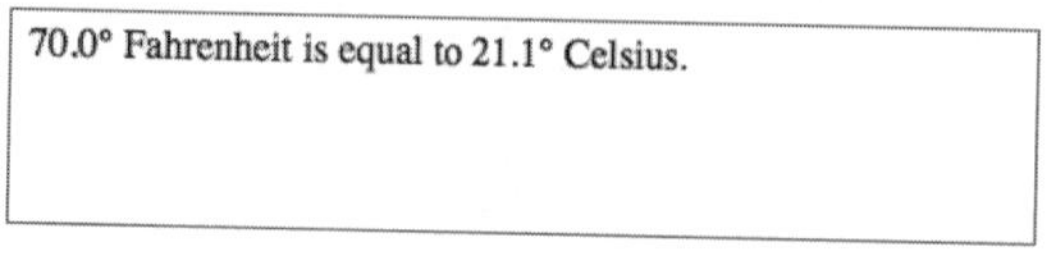

70.0° Fahrenheit is equal to 21.1° Celsius.

FIGURE 15-2

Classes

Classes do not use scope keywords, but you can prevent people from instantiating the class by making the __construct() method and the __clone() methods private or protected. The __construct() method is used to create the object so if it is not accessible, the object cannot be created. You don't need a __construct() method in your class to create an object, but if there is a __construct() method then it needs to be available. So if you don't need a __construct() method but don't want people to instantiate the class from outside the class, just create an empty protected or private __construct() method. You are still able to create an object from within itself or an inherited or parent class, depending on the scope. If you are wondering how you could create an object inside the class if you cannot create an object, you find out when you learn about static methods later in this lesson. The __clone() method is used to create a copy of an object, so if you need to prevent anyone from creating a copy you need to make that method protected or private.

UNDERSTANDING INHERITANCE

One of the powerful features of using classes is that you can extend them. You can make a base class and then create subclasses that inherit all the public and protected properties and methods in addition to their own properties and methods. You can also override existing parent methods with special ones for the child class by using the same name. Here is an example:

```
class Child extends Parent
```

> *It is the classes that are being extended, not the objects. Another way of saying it is that the blueprints are extended, and you build houses based on those extended blueprints. So inheriting properties does not inherit any property values because you have your own values.*

The terms base class and parent class are interchangeable as are subclass and child class. They are just descriptive terms that indicate that one class is the class being extended (base, parent) and the other is the extended class (subclass, child class). You may also come across talk of grandparents and siblings.

The following class, Smartphone, extends the Cellphone class. In addition to the properties and methods it inherits from the Cellphone class, it has apps and a method to list the apps. There are three files: one each for the classes and the script file. In the interest of space I have left off the documentation blocks.

The first file is the base file for the Cellphone class. This is the same file used earlier at the end of the discussion on property scope.

```php
<?php
class Cellphone
{
```

```php
        protected $_phoneNumber;
        public $model;
        public $color;

        public function __construct($phoneNumber, $model, $color) {
          $this->_phoneNumber = $phoneNumber;
          $this->model = $model;
          $this->color = $color;
        }


        public function getPhoneNumber() {
          return $this->_phoneNumber;
        }
      }
```

The following code defines the Smartphone class. You add a public property for $apps that contains the names of apps stored on the phone in an array. In the __construct() method, you bring in all four properties; the one you add in this class, plus the three inherited from the Cellphone class. You can use all the inherited properties just as if you had created them in the child class. $app should be an array, so you use the shortcut if statement to cast it to an array if it isn't already.

You also add a public function called displayApps() that creates an unordered list of the apps. The period before the = is a concatenation sign. It appends what is on the right side to the value on the left. This is a common way of building a long, complex string in an easy-to-read, easy-to-create way.

```php
      <?php
      class Smartphone extends Cellphone
      {
        public $apps;

        public function __construct($phoneNumber, $model, $color, $apps) {
          $this->_phoneNumber = $phoneNumber;
          $this->model = $model;
          $this->color = $color;
          $this->apps = is_array($apps) ? $apps : array($apps);
        }

        public function displayApps() {
          $result = '<ul>';
          foreach ($this->apps as $key=>$app) {
            $result .=  '<li>' . ($key + 1)  . ' - ' . $app . '</li>';
          }
          $result .= '</ul>';
          return $result;
        }
      }
```

TRYING TO USE UNAVAILABLE PRIVATE PROPERTIES

If the phone number were private, rather than protected, in the Cellphone class, the Smartphone class would not see the Cellphone class phone number. Because PHP does not require declarations of properties, it would create _phoneNumber as a public property in Smartphone.

This next part is a little tricky, but see if you can follow it. If you use $this->_phoneNumber in Smartphone, it works as you expect because PHP created a property. However, when you use the methods that you inherit from Cellphone you have a problem. $this-> refers to the class it is in, which in this case is Cellphone. Because you put the value into Smartphone's _phoneNumber, not Cellphone's _phoneNumber, the Cellphone method to display the phone number displays blanks.

The moral of this story is that you need to be aware of the scope of the variables and PHP's overly helpful tendencies.

The following is the script that uses the Smartphone class. First, include the code for the two classes. The parent class code must exist before the child class. Then populate two instances of Smartphone, my phone and your phone, with data. You can display the phone number using a method inherited from Cellphone and display the apps list from a method that you added in Smartphone. See the results in Figure 15-3.

```php
<?php
require_once 'cellphone_v2.php';
require_once 'smartphone_v1.php';

$applist = array("Angry Birds", "Tetris", "Pandora");
$myPhone = new Smartphone('555-555-1111', 'iPhone', 'Black', $applist);

$applist = array("CNN", "Angry Birds");
$yourPhone = new Smartphone('555-555-2222', 'Droid', 'Purple', $applist);

echo 'Phone number: ' . $myPhone->getPhoneNumber() . '<br />';
echo 'List Apps: '. $myPhone->displayApps() . '<br />';
echo 'Phone number: ' . $yourPhone->getPhoneNumber() . '<br />';
echo 'List Apps: '. $yourPhone->displayApps() . '<br />';
```

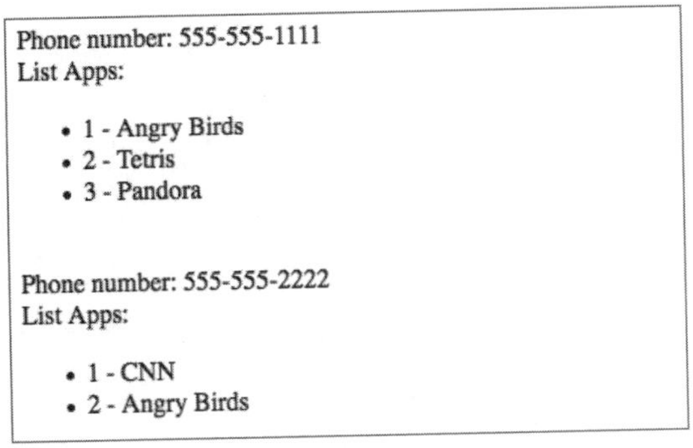

Phone number: 555-555-1111
List Apps:

- 1 - Angry Birds
- 2 - Tetris
- 3 - Pandora

Phone number: 555-555-2222
List Apps:

- 1 - CNN
- 2 - Angry Birds

FIGURE 15-3

Take another look at the __construct() methods in Cellphone and Smartphone.

From Cellphone:

```
public function __construct($phoneNumber, $model, $color) {
    $this->_phoneNumber = $phoneNumber;
    $this->model = $model;
    $this->color = $color;
}
```

From Smartphone:

```
public function __construct($phoneNumber, $model, $color, $apps) {
    $this->_phoneNumber = $phoneNumber;
    $this->model = $model;
    $this->color = $color;
    $this->apps = is_array($apps) ? $apps : array($apps);
}
```

The only thing different is that the Smartphone pulls in the $apps and updates it. What you want to do is extend the __construct() method itself. You cannot extend methods but you can call the parent's version of a method.

To call a parent's version of a method, use the scope resolution operator, which is a double colon (::), known affectionately as a *Paamayim Nekudotayim*. You may see this name in error messages. This calls a parent's __construct() method:

```
parent::__construct($phoneNumber, $model, $color);
```

You could also use the class name instead of the keyword parent, but using a generic keyword is better in case your inheritance tree changes. The only change you need to make is to change the Smartphone's __construct() to the following:

```
public function __construct($phoneNumber, $model, $color, $apps) {
    parent::__construct($phoneNumber, $model, $color);
    $this->apps = is_array($apps) ? $apps : array($apps);
}
```

You call the parent's __construct(), passing it the three parameters it is expecting. Then you use the fourth parameter to update the new property. Normally when you override a parent's method you should keep the same parameters. The __construct() method is the exception to that rule.

You can override any of the parent's methods and call the parent's version of the method as well, if you need it.

FINAL KEYWORD

If you have a method in the parent that you do not want children to override, add the final keyword to the definition in the parent class:

```
final protected MyClassMethod()
```

Because it is a protected method, the children can use it and because it is final they can't override it. As a reminder, private methods can't be seen by the children.

Often the classes that you extend are ordinary classes. When you are creating an application, however, you may find it makes sense to use *abstract* classes to extend. Abstract classes are classes that are only blueprints; you cannot create objects from them. They are there to act as a base for other classes, not to be used themselves. They are a template for creating classes. You declare a class abstract with the `abstract` keyword:

```
abstract class MyBaseClass
```

An abstract class can contain both regular and abstract methods. Child classes inherit the regular methods. Abstract classes are empty in the parent and must be defined in the child class. In the following example, `MyBaseClass` is an abstract class. It requires that child classes create a method called `getItem()` and a method called `quantity()`, which has a parameter of `$qty`. This abstract class also has a regular method that the child classes inherit called `listItem()`.

```php
<?php
abstract class MyBaseClass
{
    abstract protected function getItem();
    abstract protected function quantity($qty);

    public function listItem() {
      $result = '<p>' . $this->getItem() . '</p>';
        return $result;
    }
}
```

The child class in the example, `MyChildClass`, defines the two abstract classes, one of which it changes to public scope so that it can be called from outside the class:

```php
class MyChildClass extends MyBaseClass
{
    protected function getItem() {
        return "This is an Item";
    }

    public function quantity($qty) {
        return '<p>Your quantity is ' . $qty . '.</p>';
    }
}
```

The script that uses these classes starts by instantiating (creating an object) from the `MyChildClass`:

```php
$myObject = new MyChildClass
```

Next, the script echoes out (displays on the screen) the result from `$myObject->quantity(5)`. The object `$myObject` uses the public method in `MyChildClass` to create an HTML paragraph to display.

```php
echo $myObject->quantity(5);
```

Finally, the script displays the result from the inherited public method `listItem()`, which calls a method in the child class and creates another HTML paragraph. The results are shown in Figure 15-4.

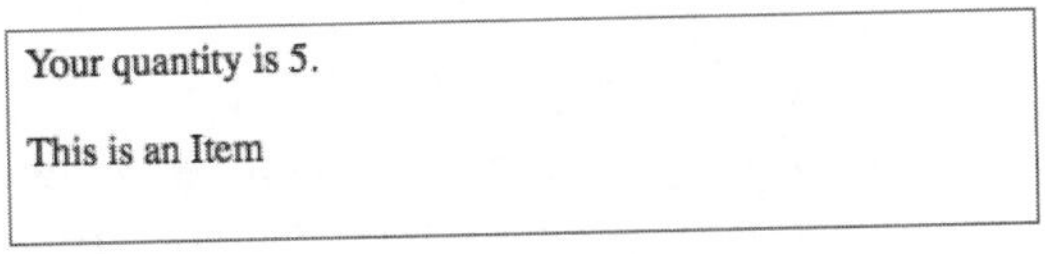

```php
echo $myObject->listItem();
```

Your quantity is 5.

This is an Item

FIGURE 15-4

UNDERSTANDING STATIC METHODS AND PROPERTIES

So far I have emphasized that the class is just a blueprint and the objects created from the class are the actual items that you use. *Static* methods and properties are accessible without creating an object. As such, they do not have access to regular properties because it is the object that holds the property values.

You might want to use static methods if you have a function that is related to a class but does not require the data from an object. For instance, take the Customer class example from Lesson 12:

➤ **Properties:** First name, last name, company, address, e-mail, phone number

➤ **Methods:** Place an order, inquire about an order, change an e-mail address

Say you have a function that pulls a list of all the customers from the database. You could just leave it as a function but if you put it in the class, you know where to find it and don't need to include more files. You do not want to make a customer object to get the list, however, because a customer object is one customer and what you want is an array with a list of customers.

To move back to the Converter class from earlier in the lesson, notice that it has no properties; all that is happening is calculations based on data that passed to it. If you turn those into static methods, you do not have to take the expense of creating objects when you want to use the methods:

```php
<?php
class Converter
{

    static public function convertFtoC($temperature) {
      $celsius = ($temperature - 32) * (5/9);
      $result = self::_formatDeg($temperature) . ' Fahrenheit is equal to '
        . self::_formatDeg($celsius) . ' Celsius.';
      return $result;
    }

    static public function convertCtoF($temperature) {
      $fahren = $temperature * (9/5) + 32;
      $result = self::_formatDeg($temperature) . ' Celsius is equal to '
        . self::_formatDeg($fahren) . ' Fahrenheit.';
      return $result;
    }

    static private function _formatDeg($number) {
      if (is_numeric($number)) {
        return number_format($number, 1) . '&deg;';
      } else {
        return 0 . '&deg;';
      }
    }

} // end of class
```

To convert this to static, you add the static keyword to the method definitions. Because you do not have an object to work with, you cannot use $this-> because that refers to the object data. You use the self construction with the scope resolution parameter self:: instead of $this->. So calling the formatting class changes from $this->_formatDeg($celsius) to self::_formatDeg($celsius).

Now that there are static methods to call, you do not need to create an object. You can reference the class itself, using the same scope resolution parameter. See the results in Figure 15-5.

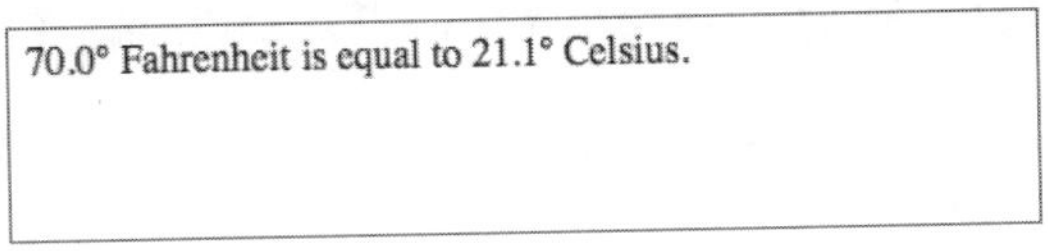

> 70.0° Fahrenheit is equal to 21.1° Celsius.

FIGURE 15-5

```
// script to use the class
echo Converter::convertFtoC(70);
```

Static properties can be used as a substitution for global variables. Because they can be accessible from anywhere and retain their values, they can hold or transfer data that needs to be available to many classes and programs. They can also be used as counters. The following is a class that is used to hold site-wide information:

```php
<?php
class Sitewide
{
  public static $copyright ='&copy; 2011';
  private static $site = 'Counting Site';
  private static $count;

  public static function getSite() {
    return self::$site;
  }
  public static function getCopyright() {
    return self::$copyright;
  }
  public static function getCount() {
    self::$count++; // add one to count
    return self::$count; // return count
  }
}
```

The following program could then reference it. You need to include the data either with a `require_once` or the autoloader. See Figure 15-6 for the results.

```html
<html>
  <title><?php echo Sitewide::getSite(); ?></title>
<body>
<h1><?php echo Sitewide::getSite(); ?></h1>
<ul>
  <li><?php echo Sitewide::getCount(); ?></li>
  <li><?php echo Sitewide::getCount(); ?></li>
  <li><?php echo Sitewide::getCount(); ?></li>
</ul>
<p><?php echo Sitewide::$copyright; ?></p>
</body>
</html>
```

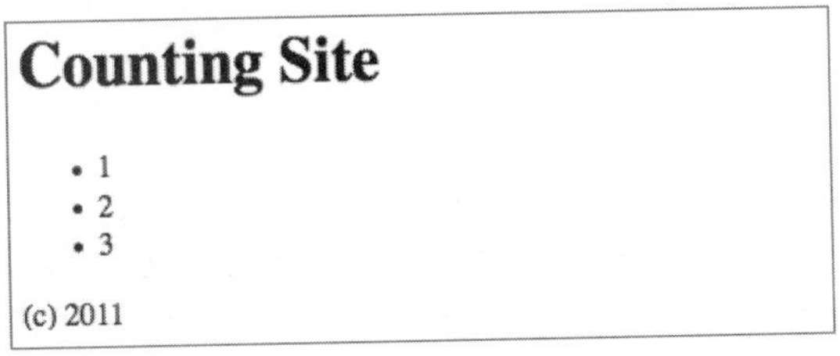

Counting Site

- 1
- 2
- 3

(c) 2011

FIGURE 15-6

You can also use the `static` keyword on variables within functions or methods as well as on properties. Static variables remember their value across multiple opens of the functions or methods. Ordinary variables are initialized each time a function or method is used, but static variables remember their value. So when you use a function again, it still remembers the value of any static variables.

TRY IT

In this Try It, you improve the Case Study by adding autoloading of the classes. With only one class this is not needed yet but you add more classes in the later lessons. Without autoloading you would need to change the initialization for each class to include a `require_once` for the class file.

You also change the scope of appropriate properties and methods, adding needed getter methods in the `Contact` class.

> *You can download the code and resources for this Try It from the book's web page at* www.wrox.com. *You can find them in the Lesson15 folder in the download. You will find code for both before and after completing the exercises.*

Lesson Requirements

Your computer needs to be able to run as a web server with PHP and MySQL. XAMPP is a package of software that installs the web server, PHP, and MySQL for you. You can find instructions for downloading and installing XAMPP in Lesson 1.

You need a text editor that can produce plain-text files. You can find instructions for downloading and installing Eclipse PDT in Lesson 1. Other text editors that you can use are Adobe's Dreamweaver in code mode, Notepad, TextWrangler, or NetBeans.

If you are following along with the Case Study, you need your files from the end of Lesson 14. Alternatively, you can download the files from the book's website at www.wrox.com.

Hints

Move the initial processing out of the `index.php` to a separate file to keep `index.php` less complex.

To autoload classes, use the magic method `__autoload()` that you used in the "Initializing the Class" section. You need to add the path to where you put the classes in the Case Study.

Step-by-Step

Create a file called `includes/init.php` to put in all the initial processing including autoloading the classes. Move the initialization code out of `index.php`.

1. Create a file `includes/init.php` with an initial PHPDoc block comment:

```php
<?php
/**
 * init.php
```

```
 *
 * Initialization file
 *
 * @version    1.2 2011-02-03
 * @package    Smithside Auctions
 * @copyright  Copyright (c) 2011 Smithside Auctions
 * @license    GNU General Public License
 * @since      Since Release 1.0
 */
```

2. Add the magic function for autoloading class files:

```
/**
 * Auto load the class files
 * @param string $class_name
 */
function __autoload($class_name) {
  require_once 'includes/classes/' . strtolower($class_name) . '.php';}
```

3. Move the `require_once` for the functions file from the `index.php` file and paste it into the `includes/init.php` file:

```
// include required files
require_once 'includes/functions.php';
```

4. In the `index.php` file, change the `require_once` for the `contact.php` file to the `init.php`. The PHP section before the `<DOCTYPE>` now looks like this:

```
<?php
/**
 * index.php
 *
 * Main file
 *
 * @version    1.2 2011-02-03
 * @package    Smithside Auctions
 * @copyright  Copyright (c) 2011 Smithside Auctions
 * @license    GNU General Public License
 * @since      Since Release 1.0
 */
require_once 'includes/init.php';
?>
```

Change the `Contact` class to use protected properties. Add the getter methods to return the values.

1. In the `includes/classes/contact.php` file change all the properties to protected. They should look like the following when you are done:

```
/**
 * First name
 * @var string
 */
protected $first_name;

/**
 * Last Name
 * @var String
```

```
    */
    protected $last_name;

    /**
     * Position in the company.
     * @var string
     */
    protected $position;

    /**
     * Email
     * @var string
     */
    protected $email;

    /**
     * Phone number, formatted in string
     * @var string
     */
    protected $phone;
```

2. In the `includes/classes/contact.php` file, add public methods to return each of the properties. Use the `getProperty` naming convention for the methods. Put the following code after the `__construct` method:

```
    /**
     * Return First Name
     * @return string
     */
    public function getFirst_name() {
      return $this->first_name;
    }

    /**
     * Return Last Name
     * @return string
     */
    public function getLast_name() {
      return $this->last_name;
    }

    /**
     * Return Position
     * @return string
     */
    public function getPosition() {
      return $this->position;
    }

    /**
     * Return Email
     * @return string
     */
    public function getEmail() {
      return $this->email;
```

```
    }

    /**
     * Return Phone
     * @return string
     */
    public function getPhone() {
      return $this->phone;
    }
```

3. In the `content/about.php` file, change `$item->position`, `$item->email`, and `$item->phone` to use the getter methods. The name is already a function so it does not change. The `<li>` group should look like this:

```
<li class="row<?php echo $i % 2; ?>">
  <h2><?php echo $item->name(); ?></h2>
  <p>Position: <?php echo $item->getPosition(); ?><br />
  <?php echo $item->getEmail(); ?><br />
  Phone: <?php echo $item->getPhone(); ?><br /></p>
</li>
```

4. Test your changes. Your About Us page should look just the same as it did in the previous lesson. See Figure 15-7.

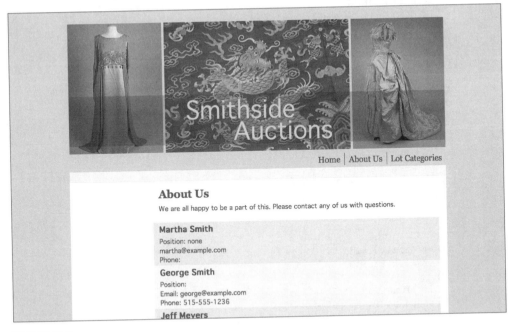

FIGURE 15-7

Watch the video for Lesson 15 on the DVD or watch online at www.wrox.com/ go/24phpmysql.

SECTION IV
Preventing Problems

▶ **LESSON 16:** Handling Errors

▶ **LESSON 17:** Writing Secure Code

You want a program that runs smoothly. To do that you need to minimize the errors that can occur and handle gracefully errors that do happen.

In the first lesson in this section, you learn how to test for possible errors so that you can fix the problem, bypass it, or gently inform the user. You learn how to set up PHP to monitor for specific error conditions and react to them. In the second lesson, you learn how to secure your code against malicious people.

16

Handling Errors

Errors come in different types and levels. The first type, which you likely have become very familiar with, is programming errors. This is when you use a wrong syntax or do something incorrectly in PHP. If you have `display_errors` set to `on` in your `php.ini` file, PHP is not shy about letting you know there is a problem. You receive big orange warnings with a lot of barely comprehensible stack information. These PHP errors have levels from minor notices where the code still works, to warnings where there is an error but the code continues to run after the error, to fatal errors where processing stops.

> You should display all of these errors while you are developing, but not when your program goes into production. You can have them posted to a log file instead where you can see them if needed but they do not inconvenience your user.

The next type is those errors that happen not because of intrinsic problems with your code, but because of data and resources outside your code. For example, the variable you want to divide by happens to be zero; the e-mail given by the user is not an e-mail address; the image file you want to display is missing; or the database is not accessible.

You learn how to handle this second type of error in the first part of this lesson. You also learn how to incorporate this in the standard error reporting of PHP. In the second part of this lesson, you learn the new error processing techniques that PHP has added to use with objects.

TESTING FOR ERRORS

Testing for errors can be divided into two groups. One is to test for conditions that will produce the errors, so you can prevent them before they happen. The other is to test whether an error has happened.

Here are conditions that could produce errors that you should check for:

➤ **Variable types and values:** Is the variable the type you expected and is the value within the range you expected? Are you trying to use a `foreach` loop on a variable that isn't an array or an object? Are you trying to divide by 0? Does the variable contain the name of a valid file?

➤ **Existence of a resource:** Are you trying to include a file that doesn't exist? Are you trying to display an image that doesn't exist? Does the parameter exist? Is the variable NULL or not set?

➤ **Validity of user supplied data:** Did the user fill in all the required inputs on the form? Did the user inject malicious code? Did the user give you data that needs to be encoded before it can be displayed in HTML?

PHP is a *loosely typed* programming language. A variable can switch between containing text or numbers. PHP automatically converts text to numbers, if it can, if the calculation requires numbers. It uses numbers as text if the operation calls for text. You were introduced to this in Lesson 6.

In the following example, $a has a value of 2 and a type of string. $b has a value of 3 and a type of integer. When you multiply them together, PHP converts $a to a type of integer because 2 is a valid integer. The result of the calculation is 6. PHP does not change the type of the variable; it just converts it while it uses it in the calculation. See Figure 16-1.

```
6

string '2' (length=1)

int 3
```

FIGURE 16-1

```php
<?php
$a = '2';
$b = 3;
echo $a * $b;
var_dump($a);
var_dump($b);
```

This works even if both of the variables are string. Change the assignment to $b = '3'; and you get the same result. In fact, change that same assignment to $b = '3xyz'; and you still get the answer 6. PHP sees the 3, converts that, and ignores the rest. However, if you change the assignment to $b = 'xyz3';, PHP uses 0 for the variable and the result is 0. It is hard to predict how a string with mixed numbers and letters will convert.

Although it is convenient that PHP automatically converts the type for you, it can make it more difficult to know if you have the right type of data for a particular situation. PHP has built-in functions that enable you to check for variable types or for certain values in the variable. The PHP function `is_numeric()` checks whether a variable is a number (2) or a valid numeric string ('2'). If it is either, then it returns true. You saw this function in use in the temperature converter. If the variable is a number, it is formatted. If it is not a number, a 0 is returned.

```php
function formatDeg($number) {
  if (is_numeric($number)) {
    return number_format($number, 1) . '&deg;';
  } else {
    return 0 . '&deg;';
  }
}
```

Table 16-1 lists other common functions for verifying types and values in variables.

TABLE 16-1: Checking Variable Values and Types

FUNCTION	DESCRIPTION
is_numeric()	True if number or numeric string
ctype_digit()	True if all digits are numeric characters
is_bool()	True if variable is a Boolean
is_null()	True if variable is NULL
is_float()	True if variable type is a float
is_double()	True if variable type is a double
is_int()	True if variable type is integer
is_string()	True if variable type is string
is_object()	True if variable is an object
is_array()	True if variable is an array

You should check that a variable is not 0 before attempting to divide by it. The following example shows different ways of checking for the condition as well as different variable values that PHP would convert to 0. See Figure 16-2.

```php
<?php
$b = 3;
$c = 0;
$d = '0';
$e = 'xyz3';
if ($c != 0) {
  echo $b/$c . '<br />';
} else {
  echo 'Cannot divide by 0. <br />';
}
echo ($c != 0) ? $b/$c : 'Cannot divide by 0.<br />';
echo ($d != 0) ? $b/$d : 'Cannot divide by 0.<br />';
echo ($e != 0) ? $b/$e : 'Cannot divide by 0.<br />';
```

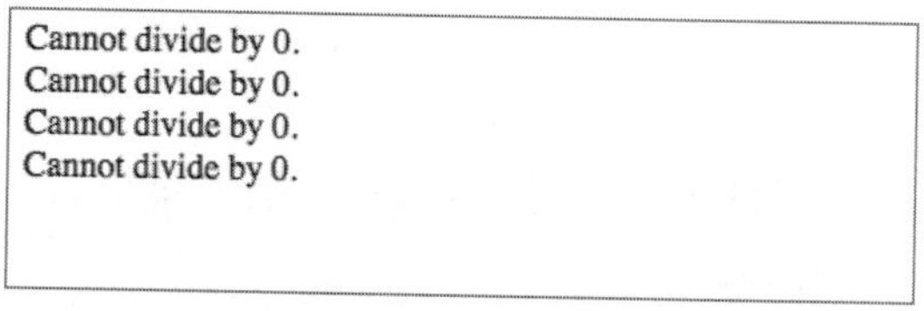

```
Cannot divide by 0.
Cannot divide by 0.
Cannot divide by 0.
Cannot divide by 0.
```

FIGURE 16-2

You can handle errors in different ways. Here you just displayed a message to the user. In the converter example, you took steps in the program to handle the error so that the user never saw it. Another option is to use the PHP error reporting system. Rather than just displaying a message, you use the trigger_error() function. This is the syntax:

```
trigger_error($error_msg, $error_level);
```

This posts your error as using the same system that PHP uses. If you have display_errors on, the user sees the error message. If you are logging errors, it is logged. You can use the E_USER_NOTICE level to post informational notices that do not affect the processing, E_USER_WARNING level for errors that allow processing to continue, or E_USER_ERROR to stop the processing. If you do not

specify a level when you create the message, the level defaults to E_USER_NOTICE. Remember that it is good practice to display errors only while testing so this would be more useful for logging. See Figure 16-3.

```php
<?php
$b = 3;
$c = 0;
$d = '0';
$e = 'xyz3';

if ($c != 0) {
  echo $b/$c . '<br />';
} else {
  trigger_error('The value of $c is ' . $c .'. You cannot divide by it ',
    E_USER_NOTICE);
}

if ($d != 0) {
  echo $b/$d . '<br />';
} else {
  trigger_error('The value of $d is ' . $d .'. You cannot divide by it ',
    E_USER_WARNING);
}

if ($e != 0) {
  echo $b/$e . '<br />';
} else {
  trigger_error('The value of $e is ' . $e .'. You cannot divide by it ',
    E_USER_ERROR);
}

echo 'You will never see this because E_USER_ERROR stops the program';
```

Notice: The value of $c is 0. You cannot divide by it in /Users/andytarr/Documents/php24/wphp24/php24/lesson16code/lesson16h.php on line 9

Call Stack

#	Time	Memory	Function	Location
1	0.0005	327588	{main}( )	../lesson16h.php:0
2	0.0005	328064	trigger_error ( )	../lesson16h.php:9

Warning: The value of $d is 0. You cannot divide by it in /Users/andytarr/Documents/php24/wphp24/php24/lesson16code/lesson16h.php on line 15

Call Stack

#	Time	Memory	Function	Location
1	0.0005	327588	{main}( )	../lesson16h.php:0
2	0.0007	328144	trigger_error ( )	../lesson16h.php:15

Fatal error: The value of $e is xyz3. You cannot divide by it in /Users/andytarr/Documents/php24/wphp24/php24/lesson16code/lesson16h.php on line 21

Call Stack

#	Time	Memory	Function	Location
1	0.0005	327588	{main}( )	../lesson16h.php:0
2	0.0008	328148	trigger_error ( )	../lesson16h.php:21

FIGURE 16-3

You can create a custom class for handling errors so all errors, including PHP errors, are processed by your custom class. You could make that class user-friendly enough that you would use it for displaying errors to the user during production. However, that is beyond the scope of this book.

Sometimes it is not the value that you are concerned about but whether the item exists. To see if a variable exists, use the isset() function. This example prints the variables if they exist. See Figure 16-4.

```
<?php
$b = 3;
$c = 0;

if (isset($a)) {
  echo '$a equals ' . $a . '<br />';
}
if (isset($b)) {
 echo '$b equals ' . $b . '<br />';
}
if (isset($c)) {
 echo '$c equals ' . $c . '<br />';
}
```

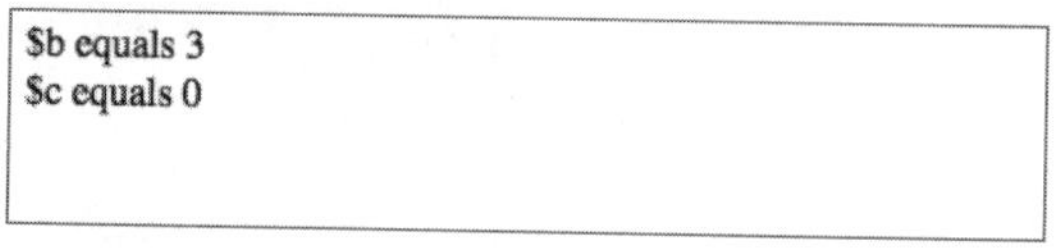

```
$b equals 3
$c equals 0
```

FIGURE 16-4

To find out if a file exists, you use either file_exists() or is_file(). file_exists() looks for either a directory or a file. is_file() is faster and works better if you are working with relative paths but fails on very large files. It only locates files. Use is_dir() as the alternative for directories. The following example checks for the existence of the image before trying to display it. See Figure 16-5.

```
<?php
$name = "Sally Meyers";
$phone = "515-555-1222";
$image = "sally-meyers-t.jpg"
?>
<html>
<head>
<title>Contact</title>
</head>
<body>

<p>
  <?php  if (file_exists($image)) : ?>
    <img src="<?php echo $image; ?>" />
  <?php endif; ?>
  <?php echo $name; ?> :
  <?php echo $phone; ?>
</p>

</body>
</html>
```

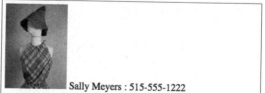

Sally Meyers : 515-555-1222

FIGURE 16-5

FILE SYSTEM PATH VERSUS URL

When dealing with files and folders, you need to remember when you are giving the location based on where it is in the folder and file structure on the computer or servers (file system path), or when based on the URL. Some functions are looking for the URL and others for the file system path. If your website does not start at your web root the relative paths are different.

You should check all data that is coming from users or gets or posts for validity or sanitize it. As a reminder, checking for validity means to see if a value meets certain parameters and sanitizing means to automatically make changes to values to render them harmless or in a proper state. See Lesson 6 for more information.

Check the data from users as early as possible in the processing so that you can try to get the proper data before you have done anything that cannot be undone. For instance, if you have required fields, check that you have data for those fields while you can still go back to the user for more information. Be specific about what the customer has to do differently when you display an error message for the user so that he has an easier time fixing it. Some people suggest that you be very non-specific to users about errors over which the user has no control. However, this can make it difficult to track down bugs. You may want the message language to be non-specific but have an error number that identifies the actual problem.

USING TRY/CATCH

With the proliferation of object-oriented abilities in PHP 5, a new type of error handling has been introduced. Most of PHP's internal errors still use the old system, but its object-oriented expressions have started using try/catch and the Exception class to handle errors.

This new system has four parts: try, throw, catch, and the Exception class. The try/catch has a syntax similar to the if/else. Your main code goes in the try block, where you throw an error if you find one. It is then caught in the catch block where you handle the error.

```php
<?php
try {
  // your code goes here that might have an error
  // when you find an error you throw an exception
  // by creating an object in Exception class,
  // passing it the error message
  throw new Exception('Divide by Zero');
} catch (Exception $e) {
  // Here's where you handle the error
  echo 'Found an error:', $e->getMessage();
}
```

Here is an example where you check to see if the number you are going to divide by is 0. If it is 0, you throw an Exception with the message "Divide by Zero". See Figure 16-6.

```php
<?php
$b = 3;
$c = 0;

try {
  if ($c != 0) {
    echo $b/$c . '<br />';
  } else {
    throw new Exception('Divide by
Zero');
  }
} catch (Exception $e) {
  echo 'Found an error: ', $e->getMessage();
}

echo '<p>And then the code continues.</p>';
```

> Found an error: Divide by Zero
>
> And then the code continues.

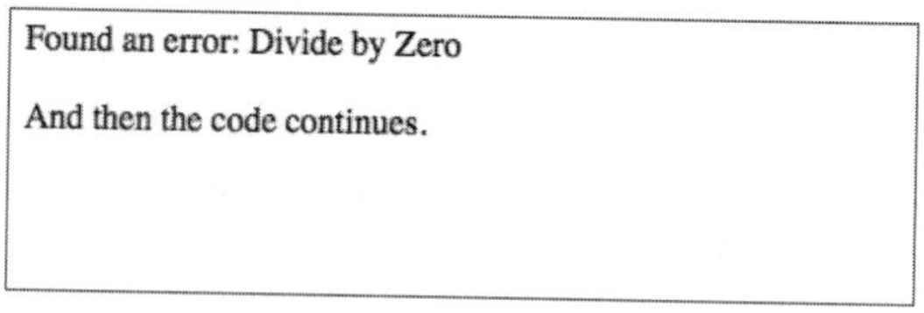

FIGURE 16-6

You throw only objects and the object must be the Exception class or a subclass that you have extended from the Exception class. If you throw an object, be sure that it will be caught or you will get an error.

TRY IT

In this Try It, you add error checking to the Case Study. You check for the existence of images files in the display of the gents lots before displaying them.

You add a try/catch block around the autoloading of classes.

> You can download the code and resources for this Try It from the book's web page at www.wrox.com. You can find them in the Lesson16 folder in the download. You find code for both before and after completing the exercises.

Lesson Requirements

Your computer needs to be able to run as a web server with PHP and MySQL. XAMPP is a package of software that installs the web server, PHP, and MySQL for you. You can find instructions for downloading and installing XAMPP in Lesson 1.

You need a text editor that can produce plain-text files. You can find instructions for downloading and installing Eclipse PDT in Lesson 1. Other text editors that you can use are Adobe's Dreamweaver in code mode, Notepad, TextWrangler, or NetBeans.

If you are following along with the Case Study, you need your files from the end of Lesson 15. Alternatively, you can download the files from the book's website at www.wrox.com.

Hints

You can use either is_file() or file_exists() to check for the existence of a file.

Try/catch only works with autoloading if you are using at least PHP 5.3. If you are still on PHP 5.2, substitute with a check for the existence of the file and a trigger_error().

Step-by-Step

Check for the existence of the image files before trying to display them in the content/gents.php file.

1. Decide what to do if you have no image files. You want something to display as a thumbnail because it is part of the design. So if you do not have a good thumbnail, you use a placeholder photo that exists in the thumbnail folder. You could check to see if that exists each time, but because that is unlikely on a production system and the result of a missing image is not catastrophic, assume your placeholder image exists.

    The larger image is a link from the thumbnail. If there is no larger image, show the thumbnail with no link.

2. Open content/gents.php.

3. Create variables to hold the calculated paths. If there is no thumbnail, replace it with the nophoto.jpg. Add the following code immediately following <div class="list-photo">:

    ```php
    <?php // Set up the images
    $image = 'images/'. $lot['image'];

    $image_t = 'images/thumbnails/'. $lot['image'];
    if (!is_file($image_t)) :
      $image_t = 'images/thumbnails/nophoto.jpg';
    endif;
    ```

4. Add an if statement to see if the larger image file exists. You can use either the is_file() or file_exists(). Get out of PHP at the end because you are going back to HTML.

    ```php
    if (is_file($image)) :
    ?>
    ```

5. Change the <a> tag and <img> tag to reference the $image and $image_t variables:

    ```php
    <a href="<?php echo $image; ?>">
    <img src="<?php echo $image_t; ?>"  alt="" />
    </a>
    ```

6. Display just the thumbnail if the larger image did not exist:

    ```php
    <?php else : ?>
      <img src="<?php echo $image_t; ?>"  alt="" />
    <?php endif; ?>
    ```

Your results should look the same as they did in the previous lesson. See Figure 16-7.

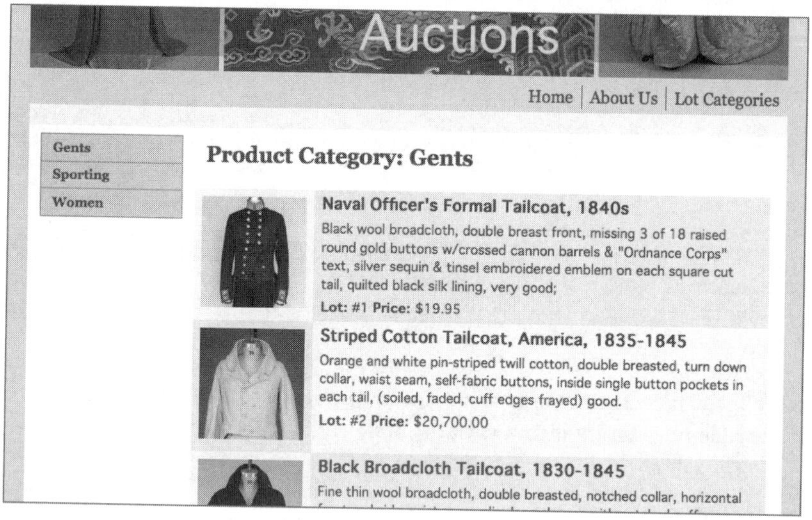

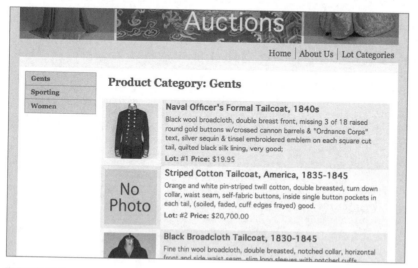

FIGURE 16-7

7. To see what it looks like if there is no photo, temporarily change one of the filenames, such as the following. Your results should look similar to Figure 16-8.

```
$lots[1]['image'] = "gents-striped-8-26XXX.jpg";
```

FIGURE 16-8

8. Change the filename back to the correct name.

Add a `try`/`catch` block to the autoloading of the classes. Note: If you are not running at least PHP 5.3, leave off the `try`/`catch` structure and use a `trigger_error()` function instead of throwing an error.

1. Open the `includes/init.php` file.

2. Add the `try`/`catch` structure around the `require_once` statement in the `__autoload()` function:

```
try {
  require_once 'includes/classes/' . strtolower($class_name) . '.php';
} catch (Exception $e) {
  echo 'Exception caught: ', $e->getMessage(), "\n";
}
```

3. Add a check to see if the file exists around the `require_once`. Because there are a lot of calculations to get the filename, assign it to a variable first:

```
$class_file = 'includes/classes/' . strtolower($class_name) . '.php';
if (is_file($class_file)) {
  require_once $class_file;
}
```

4. Add an `else` to the `if` statement to throw an error if the file was not found:

```
} else {
    throw new Exception("Unable to load class $class_name in file $class_
file.");
    }
```

5. The completed `__autoload()` function should look like this:

```
function __autoload($class_name) {
  try {
    $class_file = 'includes/classes/' . strtolower($class_name) . '.php';
    if (is_file($class_file)) {
      require_once $class_file;
    } else {
      throw new Exception("Unable to load class $class_name in file $class_
file.");
    }
  } catch (Exception $e) {
    echo 'Exception caught: ', $e->getMessage(), "\n";
  }
}
```

6. To test it, go to the About Us page. It should look similar to Figure 16-9 and contain no errors.

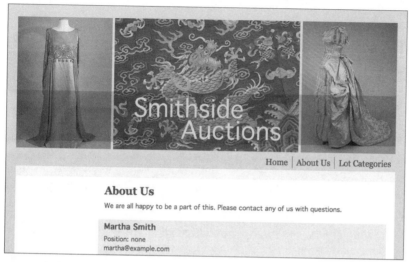

FIGURE 16-9

7. To see what an error looks like, temporarily change the path to an invalid path. Your results should look similar to Figure 16-10.

```
$class_file = 'includes/classesXXX/' . strtolower($class_name) . '.php';
```

Exception caught: Unable to load class Contact in file includes/classesx/contact.php.

Fatal error: Class 'Contact' not found in /Users/andytarr/Documents /php24/wphp24/php24/lesson16code/lesson16csfinal/content/about.php on line *15*

Call Stack

#	Time	Memory	Function	Location
1	0.0004	327880	{main}( )	../index.php:0
2	0.0011	336448	loadContent( )	../index.php:50
3	0.0014	350772	include('/Users/andytarr/Documents/php24 /wphp24/php24/lesson16code /lesson16csfinal/content/about.php')	../functions.php:17

FIGURE 16-10

8. Change your path back to the correct path.

 Watch the video for Lesson 16 on the DVD or watch online at www.wrox.com/ go/24phpmysql.

Writing Secure Code

One of the most important things you can learn about PHP and MySQL is how to prevent your code from being an easy target to those who are malicious. There is no way to make your code completely hack-proof, but you can go a long way to securing it by following certain practices. This is not an exhaustive lesson in all the ways that a hacker can get into your site, but it is the equivalent of keeping your car safe by removing your keys and locking your doors.

You might think that the chance of your site being hacked is slight, but remember that hackers can find your site and its vulnerabilities the same way that Google scans your site for search indexes.

In the first section of this lesson you learn what is meant by three common threats: cross-site scripting, cross-site request forgery, and SQL injection. You learn proper coding habits in the second part, which mitigate those and other threats.

UNDERSTANDING COMMON THREATS

Cross-site scripting (XSS), a type of code injection, embeds malicious code inside innocent code that is later output; for instance, when a user enters a search term it is usually displayed on the screen with the results. If, instead of an innocent word, the data entered were JavaScript, that code would be run when the search term was output to the screen. Hackers can install programs that track your keystrokes and track where you go.

Cross-site request forgeries (CSRF, XSRF) work by allowing an attacker to hijack a user's session so that the hacker can use an authenticated user's authority or identity. Requests from the attacker look like they are legitimate responses from forms on your website. The attacker is able to do such things as post comments as a different person, transfer funds to another person's account, or do a distributed password-guessing attack. Attackers can alter your website to trick your users into linking to their site where the hacker can then have control.

SQL Injections are where a hacker injects his own code to alter your database queries, enabling him to access, alter, or even destroy your database. The dynamic power of the PHP/MySQL combination is using PHP variables and expressions when creating queries and updates to the

database. If you use input directly from a user in creating those queries, a malicious user can effectively change your innocent queries into different queries that give him direct access to your database. You learn more specifics about preventing this type of attack starting in the next lesson.

USING PROPER CODING TECHNIQUES

The first rule of writing secure code is to never trust your users. They will give you data you do not expect, either intentionally or unintentionally. You need to check all data that a user submits or could intercept. This includes information from forms or data from POSTs, GETs, or cookies. You should check variables for the proper type of data, for malicious data, and for any character substitutions required, such as changing & to & before displaying in HTML.

You already know several ways of sanitizing your data, such as these:

```php
<?php
$myVar = htmlspecialchars($myInput); // Lesson 4
$myVar = filter_var($myInput, FILTER_SANITIZE_STRING); // Lesson 6
$myVar = filter_input(INPUT_GET, $where, FILTER_SANITIZE_STRING); // Lesson 10
$myVar = (int) $myInput; // Lesson 11
```

When displaying any user output to the browser, use `htmlspecialchars()` if you have not verified that it is an integer. Before saving any data to a database you need to escape it properly for that database. With MySQL you use `mysql_real_escape_string`, which you learn in Lesson 22.

When given an option of using quotes or not, use quotes because it makes it more difficult for a hacker to break out. You still need to sanitize the variable. Here is a case where using valid XHTML makes your code more secure. Take, for instance, the following insecure code:

```php
<?php $myClass = $_GET['class']; ?>
<div class=<?php echo $myClass; ?>>Text goes here</div>
```

Call that code with `?class=red` at the end of the URL and your source code evaluates to `<div class=red>Text goes here</div>`. However, if you call the code with `?class=g><b>BAD STUFF HERE </b>`, you see results similar to Figure 17-1.

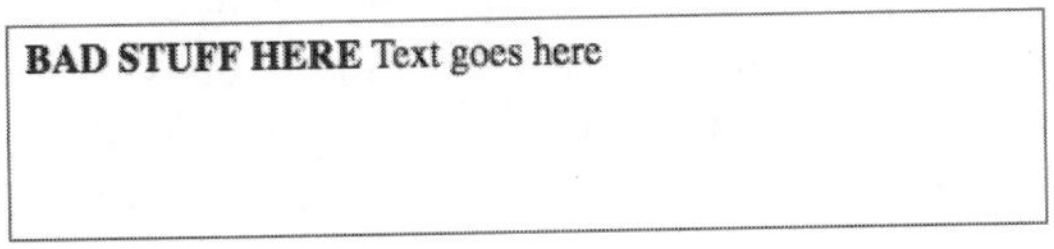

FIGURE 17-1

If you enclose the class with quotes, which is the valid method in XHTML, your results look like Figure 17-2.

```php
<?php $myClass = $_GET['class']; ?>
<div class="<?php echo $myClass; ?>">Text goes here</div>
```

FIGURE 17-2

You should also sanitize any input coming from your GET so your final code will look like this:

```php
<?php $myClass = filter_input(INPUT_GET, 'class', FILTER_SANITIZE_STRING); ?>
<div class="<?php echo $myClass; ?>">Text goes here</div>
```

If you validate forms using a client-side validation such as JavaScript, always back it up with server-side validation such as PHP. Using JavaScript enables you to create a better user experience, but it is easier to bypass than server-side validations or could be turned off, so using a combination is the better solution.

How your PHP is set up is important for security. Global variables should be off in php.ini. On a production site, turn off display_errors. You can do this via php.ini for the whole site or use .htaccess if you are using a site for both production and development.

Initialize your variables if you are not setting the variable in all cases. Do not assume they start empty because users can add variable assignments to URLs.

```php
<?php
$myVar = '';
if ($someCondition) {
  $myVar = '1';
}
```

Do not include a file directly from a get request. Use a two-step process. First verify that there is no invalid data in the name itself using filter_input or filter_var. Then you need to verify that the file is one of your files and not from some remote site. You can do this by checking against a list of valid files or only displaying files from valid folders. An example is the loadContent function in the Case Study:

```php
function loadContent($where, $default='') {
  $content = filter_input(INPUT_GET, $where, FILTER_SANITIZE_STRING);
  $default = filter_var($default, FILTER_SANITIZE_STRING);
  $content = (empty($content)) ? $default : $content;
  if ($content) {
    $html = include 'content/'.$content.'.php';
    return $html;
  }
}
```

Do not let users list your file directories. There are ways to prevent this with the .htaccess file, but if your program is run where you do not have control of the .htaccess file you should take measures yourself. The easiest way to do that is to create a skeleton index.html file and add it to each of your folders that does not have an index.php file. A typical index.html file contains this code:

```html
<!DOCTYPE html PUBLIC "-//W3C//DTD XHTML 1.0 Transitional//EN"
"http://www.w3.org/TR/xhtml1/DTD/xhtml1-transitional.dtd">
<html xmlns="http://www.w3.org/1999/xhtml">
<head>
<meta http-equiv="Content-Type" content="text/html; charset=UTF-8" />
<title></title>
</head>
<body>
</body>
</html>
```

To prevent cross-site request forgeries when using forms, use randomly generated tokens on the form and verify those tokens when you use the data.

In the following example, a token is generated on the form. That token is then passed to both the *session* and to the form as a hidden value. Remember that hidden just means that it does not display on the form page. If the form uses the GET method, the hidden field is displayed in the URL.

A session is used for storing data such as gets, posts, and cookies. The session file is stored on the server, not in the user's browser, so is not generally viewable by the user. A cookie holds a session ID that is used to link to the session file. A session lasts until you destroy it or your user closes her browser.

To start a session or access an existing session, put this code at the very beginning of your program:

```php
<?php session_start(); ?>
```

On your form, create a random value. For security, you want to *salt* that value. To salt a value is to add an additional piece to it that makes it more difficult to decode. There are many ways of creating salts. You can use a randomly created salt or put a salt constant in a configuration file. Randomly generated salts are the safest if you are using a salt with a password. This token is created by choosing a random number between 1 and 1,000,000 that is concatenated to the $salt value. That is then encrypted as a sha1() hash:

```php
<?php $token = sha1(mt_rand(1,1000000) . $salt); ?>
```

$token is assigned to both a session variable 'token' and a hidden input in the form:

```php
<?php $_SESSION['token'] = $token; ?>
<input type='hidden' name='token' value='<?php echo $token; ?>'/>
```

In the program that reads your form values, start the session and compare the session value with the POST/GET value. If the token parameter is not set in either the POST or the SESSION or if it is empty or if they do not match then do not trust the input.

```php
<?php
session_start();
if (!isset($_POST['token'])
    || !isset($_SESSION['token'])
    || empty($_POST['token'])
    || $_POST['token'] !== $_SESSION['token']) {
    die('Bad token');
} else {
    $name = filter_input(INPUT_POST, 'name', FILTER_SANITIZE_STRING);
    unset($_SESSION['token']);
}
```

For the best user experience, you want to control how you end a program. However, when dealing with security, it is sometimes better just to get out of the program entirely if you detect an insecurity. In these cases, the die() function ends the program immediately and optionally displays a message to a user. You may also want to be wary of how much information you give a user at this point because the user could use that information maliciously.

An additional security precaution against CSRF is to add a confirmation page and to check that both the original request and the confirmation page are processed.

TRY IT

In this Try It, you add an additional security feature to the Case Study. You have been using some security features already, such as sanitizing data from forms. Here you add `index.html` files to the folders in the Case Study. This prevents attackers from seeing your folders and files if they enter a folder name in the URL.

For the second part of the Try It, you create a form with a generated token and check for the valid token before processing the form.

> *You can download the code and resources for this Try It from the book's web page at* www.wrox.com. *You can find them in the Lesson17 folder in the download. You will find code for both before and after completing the exercises.*

Lesson Requirements

Your computer needs to be able to run as a web server with PHP and MySQL. XAMPP is a package of software that installs the web server, PHP, and MySQL for you. You can find instructions for downloading and installing XAMPP in Lesson 1.

You need a text editor that can produce plain-text files. You can find instructions for downloading and installing Eclipse PDT in Lesson 1. Other text editors that you can use are Adobe's Dreamweaver in code mode, Notepad, TextWrangler, or NetBeans.

If you are following along with the Case Study, you need your files from the end of Lesson 16. Alternatively, you can download the files from the book's website at www.wrox.com.

Hints

Don't forget to add the `index.html` file to subfolders.

You don't need an `index.html` file in your root directory because you already have the `index.php` file there instead. Depending on your server setup, an `index.html` file might be displayed instead of your `index.php` file.

When you use sessions, you need to do a `session_start()` at the very beginning of any file where you want to use the session variables.

Step-by-Step

Prevent users from seeing your folders and files.

1. Create a file called **index.html** that displays a blank screen using the following code:

```
<!DOCTYPE html PUBLIC "-//W3C//DTD XHTML 1.0 Transitional//EN"
"http://www.w3.org/TR/xhtml1/DTD/xhtml1-transitional.dtd">
<html xmlns="http://www.w3.org/1999/xhtml">
<head>
```

```
<meta http-equiv="Content-Type" content="text/html; charset=UTF-8" />
<title></title>
</head>
<body>
</body>
</html>
```

2. Add a copy of that file to the following folders. The only folder that doesn't need an `index.html` file is the root folder, which already has the `index.php` file.

   ➤ content

   ➤ css

   ➤ images

   ➤ images/thumbnails

   ➤ includes

   ➤ includes/classes

Create a form and then add a generated token to verify the form before processing in order to prevent CSFR.

1. Create a standard HTML input form called **exercise17a.php** that asks for a name input. The form action is **exercise17b.php** and the method is **post**. The results look like Figure 17-3.

   ```
   <!DOCTYPE html PUBLIC "-//W3C//DTD XHTML 1.0 Transitional//EN"
     "http://www.w3.org/TR/xhtml1/DTD/xhtml1-transitional.dtd">
   <html xmlns="http://www.w3.org/1999/xhtml">
   <head>
     <title>Test Form</title>
   </head>
   <body>

   <form action="exercise17b.php" method="post">

   <fieldset>
     <legend>Test Form</legend>
     <p><label for="name">Name</label>
     <input type="text" name="name" id="name"   />
     </p>
     <p><input type="submit" name="testform" value="Submit" /></p>
   </fieldset>

   </form>
   </body>
   </html>
   ```

2. Create the file **exercise17b.php** that processes the form and then displays the name. Run `exercise17a.php`, enter a name, and submit. Your results should look similar to Figure 17-4.

   ```
   <?php
   $name = filter_input(INPUT_POST, 'name', FILTER_SANITIZE_STRING);
   ?>
   ```

```
<!DOCTYPE html PUBLIC "-//W3C//DTD XHTML 1.0 Transitional//EN"
    "http://www.w3.org/TR/xhtml1/DTD/xhtml1-transitional.dtd">
<html xmlns="http://www.w3.org/1999/xhtml">
<head>
  <title>Test Form</title>
</head>
<body>

<p>My name is <?php echo $name; ?></p>

</body>
</html>
```

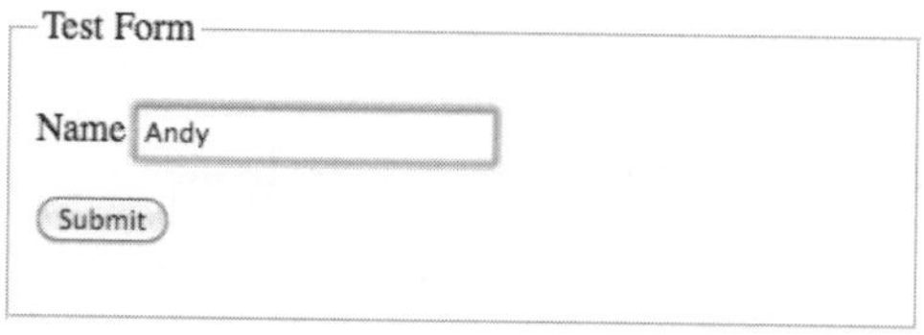

Test Form

Name Andy

Submit

FIGURE 17-3

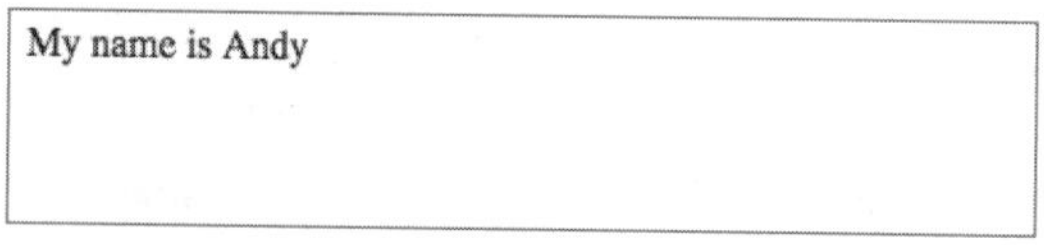

My name is Andy

FIGURE 17-4

3. Now that you have a form that works, you can add the CSFR prevention features to it. At the very beginning of exercise17a.php, start a session:

   ```
   <?php session_start(); ?>
   ```

4. Create a token just before the </fieldset>:

   ```
   <?php
   $salt = 'SomeSalt';
   $token = sha1(mt_rand(1,1000000) . $salt);
   ```

5. Add that token to the session and to a hidden input:

   ```
   $_SESSION['token'] = $token;
   ?>
   <input type='hidden' name='token' value='<?php echo $token; ?>'/>
   ```

6. In exercise17b.php, start a session at the very beginning of the file:

   ```
   <?php
   session_start();
   ```

7. Initialize $message to nothing and $badToken to true:

   ```
   $message = '';
   $badToken = true;
   ```

8. Check to see if the token parameter is missing in either the POST or the SESSION, if the token value is empty, and if the tokens from the POST and the SESSION are not equal. If any

of those conditions exist, set the "bad token" message; otherwise set $badToken to false and set up the $name variable. Unset the session token so that it cannot be used again.

```php
if (!isset($_POST['token'])
    || !isset($_SESSION['token'])
    || empty($_POST['token'])
    || $_POST['token'] !== $_SESSION['token']) {
    $message = 'Sorry, go back and try again. There was a security issue.';
    $badToken = true;
} else {
    $badToken = false;
    $name = filter_input(INPUT_POST, 'name', FILTER_SANITIZE_STRING);
    unset($_SESSION['token']);
}
?>
```

9. Change the output so that it displays the name only if there is a good token:

```php
<?php if (!$badToken) : ?>
    <p>My name is <?php echo $name; ?></p>
<?php else : ?>
    <p><?php echo $message; ?></p>
<?php endif ?>
```

10. Run `exercise17a.php` and your results should look the same as before.

11. To test what happens if a bad token is found, temporarily change the session in `exercise17a.php`. To do that, change `$_SESSION['token'] = $token;` to **`$_SESSION['token'] = '12345';`** and rerun `exercise17a.php`. Your results should look similar to Figure 17-5.

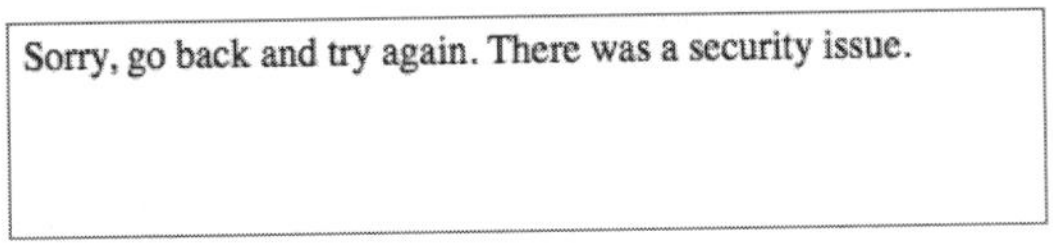

Sorry, go back and try again. There was a security issue.

FIGURE 17-5

 Watch the video for Lesson 17 on the DVD or watch online at www.wrox.com/go/24phpmysql.

SECTION V
Using a Database

▶ **LESSON 18:** Introducing Databases

▶ **LESSON 19:** Introducing MySQL

▶ **LESSON 20:** Creating and Connecting to the Database

▶ **LESSON 21:** Creating Tables

▶ **LESSON 22:** Entering Data

▶ **LESSON 23:** Selecting Data

▶ **LESSON 24:** Using Multiple Tables

▶ **LESSON 25:** Changing Data

▶ **LESSON 26:** Deleting Data

▶ **LESSON 27:** Preventing Database Security Issues

Variables in PHP hold information, but only for the length of the program. You can fill in a form to get information, but you need to store it somewhere. You need a place to hold your data that is still there after the program ends. This section introduces you to what databases are and how to design a database. You learn how to create a MySQL database, how to set up the appropriate tables, and how to use the MySQL scripting language within PHP to create, update, query, and delete information.

18

Introducing Databases

In this lesson you learn about databases, what they are, how to figure out what to put in them, and how to organize them so that you can retrieve the information you need when you need it. Most of the information is true for most databases, but the information covered is in the context of the relational database system MySQL.

WHAT IS A DATABASE?

Databases have terminology all their own. Several terms are also used interchangeably:

➤ **Database:** A database is an organized collection of data. In MySQL you often create separate databases for each of your projects.

➤ **Table:** A table is a collection of similar information. In MySQL you might have a Customers table that contains data about your customers, a Products table that has data about your products, an Order Headers table that contains header and totals about your orders, and an Order Details table that contains the line items on the orders.

➤ **Row:** Inside a table, you have rows. Each row is a related set of data. In the Customers table, each customer is in a row.

➤ **Record:** A record is another word for a row.

➤ **Column:** Inside your table you also have columns. Columns are the types of information you are storing in your table. For instance in the Customers table, name, street, and city would all be columns.

➤ **Field:** A field is another word for a column. Sometimes used to refer to a specific row's column.

➤ **Value:** A value is what is in a given cell. In the Customers table, for instance, you would have a row for George Smith where the value of the cell in the name column is "George Smith."

➤ **Relationship:** A relationship is a link between two tables. For instance, an Order Details table would link to the Order Headers so that you can associate the line items with the correct order.

➤ **Key:** A key is a field, or fields, that link the tables. In the Order Details table you have an order number field that matches an order number field in the Order Headers table. The order number field is a key or key field.

➤ **Index:** An index is an internal system that a database system uses to locate information more quickly. In MySQL you can specify that certain columns, usually keys, are indexes.

There are different types of databases. The simplest are flat files. A `.csv` file is a flat file as are `.ini` files such as the `php.ini` file you may have had to configure in the first lesson. These are in a single file, each row is a complete record, and there are no relationships. Hierarchical databases have hierarchical relationships such as you see in the Windows Explorer folders and files lists. Relational database management systems, such as MySQL, have multiple tables with dynamic relationships that you define and a query language for extracting data in different formats and groupings without having to reorganize the tables.

For your database to be successful, it needs to contain all the data that the business needs. It needs to contain the business rules for processing the data and to protect the data security and integrity. Your database also needs to be able to access the data effectively, yet be flexible enough to handle exceptions and questions you didn't think of when you first created the database. It should have the ability to allow for growth and change.

Research, and a lot of trial and error, has gone into determining the most likely way to meet these goals. The rest of this lesson shows you the best practices in designing your database.

GATHERING INFORMATION TO DEFINE YOUR DATABASE

Before you can design your tables, you need to gather certain information. This part is not technical. It is finding out about the business. You need to know the problem you are trying to solve and the scope. You need to know the purpose and objectives of the database. You need to know the data that has to be retained and what the database needs to do. Ideally, the client provides this information for you, but if he doesn't, you need to find it out.

Find out what you already have. What are people already using? Are there existing databases? What do they contain? What are they missing? Are there spreadsheets that people are using? Forms? Reports? These all give you a handle on the data that that needs to be in the database as well as the type of data it is. MySQL has data types, just as PHP does, but they are more rigid so you need to know what type of data you can expect.

If you have a chance, observing people gathering and working with the data is invaluable. It helps answer the "What did you know and when did you know it?" question. You need to know if there is a specific order when the users find out what certain data is or when they use the data, so you should be familiar with the standard workflow of the data. For instance, if you find out there is a vital required piece of data that is not known until late in the workflow, you know you won't always have access to it. You also need to understand the exceptions that can occur.

After you have all this information, you are ready to start designing your tables.

DESIGNING YOUR TABLES

At this point you have analyzed your data needs. Now it is time to organize a list of the different data pieces you have collected into tables and fields. The nouns (things) are likely to become tables. Adjectives and aspects of a thing are likely to become fields. Data that can be calculated generally does not belong in a database because you can create functions in PHP to do the calculations when they are needed.

Based on the information showing on the Case Study website, Table 18-1 shows you what a database would look like to provide the information needed:

TABLE 18-1: Tables and Fields for the Case Study

TABLE	FIELDS
Contacts	First name, last name, position, e-mail, phone
Lots	Category, lot name, description, image, lot number, price
Categories	Category, description, image

The next task is to determine the characteristics of each of the fields. For instance, which fields are text fields and which are numeric fields? How long do your text fields need to be? Is there any validation that you need? Which fields do you have to have information in from the start? MySQL assigns data types to each field. In Lesson 21, you use the information about what type of data is stored in each of the fields to assign specific data types to the fields when you create your tables. You also use this information to set up business rules such as whether an email is required for all contacts or whether a phone number is a formatted numeric field in the form xxx-xxx-xxxx or a freeform text field. This is what the Contacts table could look like:

Table: Contacts

First name: Text, up to 50 characters long, required

Last name: Text, up to 50 characters long, required

Position: Text, up to 50 characters long

Email: Text, up to 255 characters long

Phone: Text, up to 20 characters long

SETTING UP RELATIONSHIPS BETWEEN TABLES

You link between tables by including in one table a field that identifies a record in another table. For instance, in the Case Study, lots are assigned to a category. So in the Lots table you need a field that matches a uniquely identifying field in the Categories table.

Those fields are called *keys*. The key in the Lots table is called a *foreign key* because it links to something outside the table. This key in the Categories table is the *primary key*, which uniquely identifies the category record. The primary key is often referred to as the id.

Requirements exist for determining what fields can be used as primary keys. These requirements are not forced on you by the database, but if you do not follow them you will have trouble keeping your database working correctly.

➤ **Unique:** The primary key must be unique. If it is not unique then you are not able to match to a single record.

➤ **Not null and not optional:** There must always be something in the field.

➤ **Not changeable:** There should be no reason you should need to change the field. If you use a person's name for the primary key and the person changes his name, then all the tables trying to link with the old name won't work.

➤ **Should not violate security policies:** In other words, do not use something as a key that needs to be private, such as a Social Security number or a password.

Many database developers create a new field whose only purpose is to be the primary key. These are called *artificial keys*. Integers are usually used because they are fast to process and do not take up much room in the database. In MySQL, you learn how to create such keys with `auto_increment`. Because these keys are arbitrary and divorced from the business logic, there is no need for them to change. They can be assigned when the record is created, and they can be unique.

Not all foreign keys have to match to a primary key. They could match to a different field that also identifies the record.

Relationships can be one-to-one (driver to driver's license) or one-to-many (teacher to students) or many-to-many (students to courses). The most common relationship between tables is a one-to-many relationship. In a one-to-many relationship, one record in a table links to many records in a second table. In the Case Study the link between the Categories table and the Lots table is a one-to-many.

When tables have a many-to-many relationship, the relationship can be defined with a separate file that contains only the foreign keys. So if you allowed lots to be in multiple categories, your files might look like this:

Table: Lots

Fields: Lot id, lot name, description, image, lot number, price

Table: Categories

Fields: Category id, category name, description, image

Table: Categories-Lots

Fields: Category id, Lot id

There would be multiple records in the Categories-Lots table; one for each category/lot combination that exists.

INSTITUTING THE BUSINESS RULES

Business rules are policies that a business uses to make its business run smoothly and profitably. There are different ways of enforcing business rules. Some are enforced just in the way that you design your database. The Case Study has a business rule that each lot needs to be in one and only one category. By putting a foreign key in the Lots table to the Categories table, you are enforcing that rule.

Data typing is another way to enforce business rules. If a business rule is that prices have to be numeric, you set the data type for the price field to be numeric. Data types in MySQL can also include lengths or sizes. If you have a business rule that no comment can be longer than 100 characters, you can specify that the field is no more than 100 in size.

Some database systems allow you to enforce other aspects of the data. MySQL enables you to force certain fields to be unique or to not be empty. It also enables you to set a default value for fields.

You use validation files if you need to restrict a field to containing only specific values. An example is if you want to restrict a State field to the two-character abbreviation of the state. Validation files in MySQL are just like any other table. They can be a small table with one or two columns or they can be a regular table, such as the Categories table.

Then, finally, you can use program validation in place of or in addition to database validation. MySQL enforces the integrity of the database, but if you try to give it something invalid it gives you an error message. Because you do not want error messages going to your user, you want to verify that the data about to go into the database meets the criteria the database is looking for, and fix it first.

NORMALIZING THE TABLES

If you hang around with people dealing with databases, you might hear them talking about *normalization* or about *normalizing a database*. Normalization is the reorganization of the database so it meets certain design standards. Like the list of requirements for a primary key, these are rules established so that the database ends up more usable. Normalization aims to design databases that are more robust and that will be useful longer. It does this by designing for flexibility, so that you can use the database for a variety of general queries and tasks rather than designing it so that it is optimized for a single task but is unfit for handling future tasks.

Normalization reduces redundancy. Redundancy requires more storage space and introduces maintenance errors. If, instead of just having a key to the categories table in the Lots table, you had the description in all the lots records, you would use more storage. Any time the description changed, you would have to change it in each of the lots.

Normalization ensures that data that is independent in reality is independent in the database. If you have the category description in the Lots table instead of in a separate Categories table, you have to create a lot before you can have a category. If you delete all the lots in a particular category, you lose that category altogether.

To normalize a database, you apply a series of rules to the tables and change them as necessary to pass the rules. There is a balance to be maintained among flexibility, performance, and understandability. There are six levels of normalization, but most databases use only the first three levels, achieving what is called *third normal form*.

First normal form (1NF) states that a field must provide a fact about a key, that there can be no repeating elements, and no multivalued elements. Take the following table:

Table: Lots

Fields: Lots id, lot name, description, image, lot number, price, category id1, category id2, category id3

Category id1, category id2, and category id3 are repeating elements. They allow up to three categories to be assigned to the Lots table. However, if the business rule changes and you now need to assign a fourth category, you have to change the database and all the programs that use that table. Instead use the many-to-many relationship file as shown earlier in this lesson.

> Table: Lots
>
> Fields: Lot id, lot name, description, image, lot number, price
>
> Table: Categories
>
> Fields: Category id, category title, description
>
> Table: Categories-Lots
>
> Fields: Category id, Lot id

Now if a fourth category is needed, there is no problem.

Second normal form (2NF) states that you need the whole key in order to retrieve the data. You need to worry about second normal form only if you have a composite key, which is a key made up of more than one field.

Third normal form (3NF) states that you cannot have any hidden dependencies and no duplicate or calculated fields. Category description in the following table is a hidden dependency because it depends on category id rather than lot id.

> Table: Lots
>
> Fields: Lot id, Lot name, description, image, lot number, price, category id, category description

TRY IT

In this Try It, you design the three database tables for the Case Study website, contacts, categories, and lots. You use this design when you create the tables in Lesson 21. There is no coding for this exercise, but you may want to display the Case Study to see the information that you need to store.

> *You can download the code and resources for this Try It from the book's web page at* www.wrox.com. *You can find them in the Lesson18 folder in the download.*

Lesson Requirements

There is no coding in this Try It. If you use the figures in the "Step-by-Step" section, you don't need your computer. If you want to look at the Case Study on your computer, you have the following two requirements:

Your computer needs to be able to run as a web server with PHP and MySQL. XAMPP is a package of software that installs the web server, PHP, and MySQL for you. You can find instructions for downloading and installing XAMPP in Lesson 1.

If you are following along with the Case Study, you need your files from the end of Lesson 17. Alternatively, you can download the files from the book's website at www.wrox.com.

Hints

I used the Case Study tables as examples in this lesson.

Look at the About Us page, Lot Categories page, and the Display Lots pages to see the tables to be created or look at the figures in the Try It.

The lots in the Gents, Sporting, and Women pages can all be in one table.

Step-by-Step

Look at the About Us page. Based on that, design the Contacts table, showing the fields and characteristics. See Figure 18-1.

1. List the fields needed in the Contacts table, including an artificial key for the primary key: Contact id, first name, last name, position, e-mail, phone.

2. Write down characteristics to each of the fields.

> Table: Contacts
>
> Contact id: Integer, positive number, required, primary key
>
> First name: Text, up to 50 characters long, required
>
> Last name: Text, up to 50 characters long, required
>
> Position: Text, up to 50 characters long
>
> E-mail: Text, up to 255 characters long
>
> Phone: Text, up to 20 characters long

Look at the Lot Categories page. Based on that, design the Categories table, showing the fields and characteristics. See Figure 18-2.

1. List the fields needed in the Categories table, including an artificial key for the primary key: Category id, category name, category description, category image.

2. Write down the characteristics for each of the fields.

> Table: Categories
>
> Category id: Integer, positive number, required, primary key

Category name: Text, up to 50 characters long, required

Category Description: Text, up to 5 or 6 lines of text

Category Image: Text, up to 255 for the name of the file

Look at the Gents, Sporting, and Women pages. Based on that, design the lots table, showing the fields and characteristics. See Figure 18-3, Figure 18-4, and Figure 18-5.

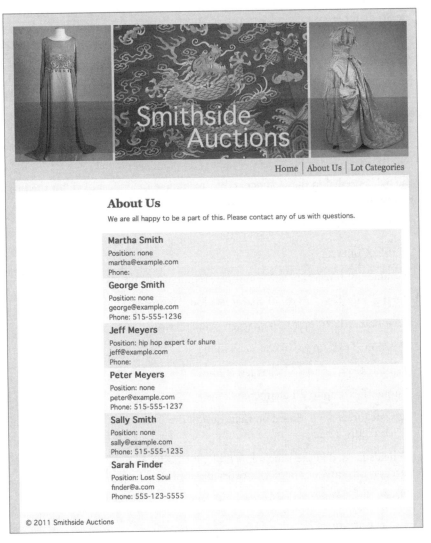

FIGURE 18-1

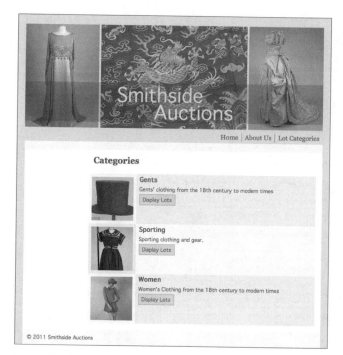

FIGURE 18-2

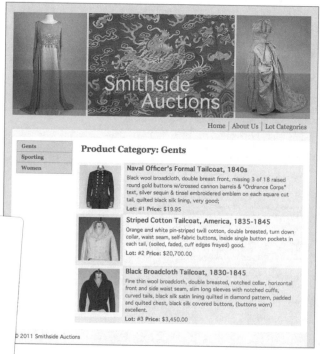

FIGURE 18-3

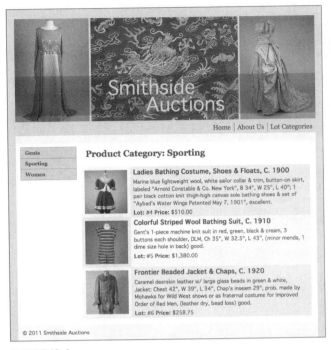

FIGURE 18-4

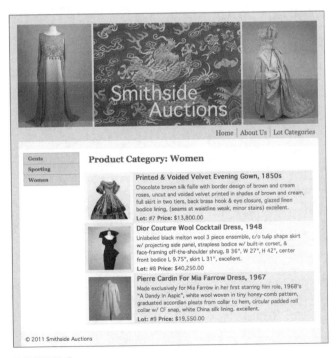

FIGURE 18-5

1. List the fields needed in the Lots table, including an artificial key for the primary key: Lot id, lot name, description, image, lot number, price. Add a key to link to the Categories table.

2. Write down the characteristics to each of the fields.

Table: Lots

Lots id: Integer, positive number, required, primary key

Lot name: Text, up to 50 characters long, required

Description: Text, up to 5 or 6 lines of text

Image: Text, up to 255 for the name of the file

Lot number: Integer, positive number

Price: Numeric, up to $100,000.00

Category id: Integer, positive number, link to categories table

 Watch the video for Lesson 18 on the DVD or watch online at `www.wrox.com/go/24phpmysql`.

19

Introducing MySQL

MySQL is a free open-source relational database management system. It's pronounced either as My S-Q-L or as My Sequel. It is a standard for many shared hosting services and is part of the standard (L)AMP stack of Apache web server, MySQL database, and PHP scripting that runs many of the Internet's sites. Access to MySQL data is based on SQL, a query language developed in the 1970s. Other SQL databases include Oracle (the current owner of MySQL), PostgreSQL, MS SQL Server, and SQLite. Although all are based on SQL, differences exist in the implementation, so the different databases and SQL commands are not interchangeable.

MySQL runs on many platforms including various Unix/Linux versions, Windows, and Mac OS X. It can be used in many different programming languages, including PHP, Java, C#, Visual Basic, ASP, and ColdFusion. Using MySQL in PHP is a combination of running the MySQL statements and using special PHP functions written to interact with MySQL.

MySQL as shipped allows for manipulation at a command line and does not have a graphical interface. The most widespread graphical interface is phpMyAdmin. Because it is generally the interface that is available and because it displays the MySQL statements for the actions you do, it is a good choice to use when learning MySQL.

In the first part of this lesson you learn your way around phpMyAdmin. As you create a database and a table with phpMyAdmin, you get exposure to MySQL statements. In the second part of this lesson you learn the basics of the SQL syntax as used by MySQL.

USING PHPMYADMIN

You installed phpMyAdmin in Lesson 1 as part of XAMPP. You run phpMyAdmin either by going to `http://localhost/xampp` and clicking the phpMyAdmin link on the left as shown in Figure 19-1, or by going directly to `http://localhost/phpMyAdmin` where you see a page similar to Figure 19-2.

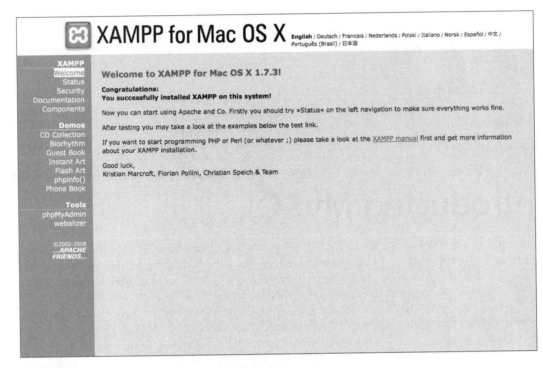

FIGURE 19-1

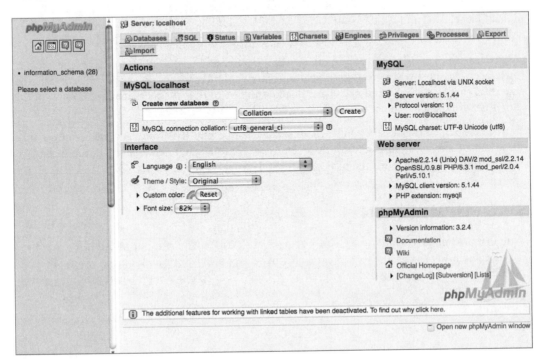

FIGURE 19-2

If you did not install XAMPP and do not have phpMyAdmin, you can freely download it from www.phpmyadmin.net.

Creating Databases

On the left in Figure 19-2 is a list of your databases. If at any point you want to return to this screen, click the icon that looks like a house just above the list. You likely have only one database showing, information_schema. This is the database that contains all the information about the MySQL databases on your server. You do not want to touch this.

There are several tabs across the top of the window. This list of tabs and what they refer to changes depending on whether you are at the base level, as you are now, in a selected database, or in a selected table.

At this level the only tab you are likely to use is called Privileges. This is where you add or remove users or change passwords as you learned in Lesson 1. When you are working with MySQL in PHP, you specify a single user for the program to use. You do not create a user for everyone who runs the PHP program. In a production program it is more secure to use a user that has only the privileges needed to run the program.

To create a new user, click on the Privileges tab. On the page that appears, find the Add a New User link as shown in Figure 19-3 and click it.

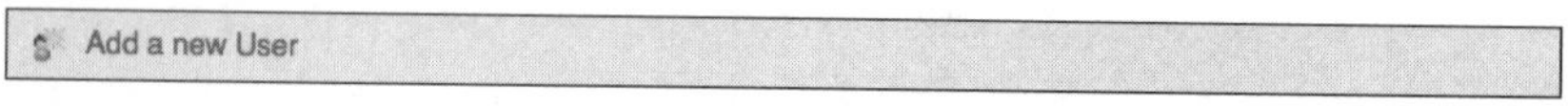

§ Add a new User

FIGURE 19-3

Fill in the screen as shown in Figure 19-4. To match the sample code, use php24sql for the User Name. Your Host is most likely localhost. To match the sample code, use hJQV8RTe5t for the Password and Re-type fields.

In the Global privileges section, check the following boxes in the Data section: SELECT, INSERT, UPDATE, DELETE. This gives your user (that is, the program you run) the ability to update the data in the database. Because you have not given the user any privileges in the Structure section, he isn't able to change the structure of your database. Because you haven't given him any privileges in the Administration section, he won't be able to do any administrative tasks. This is important because if a hacker is able to run code through your program, he is more limited in what he can do.

Click the Go button to create this user.

This is the user you use when you need to connect to the database within your program. This does not affect the user you use to run MySQL itself or when you are in phpMyAdmin, so don't change anything in your XAMPP configuration.

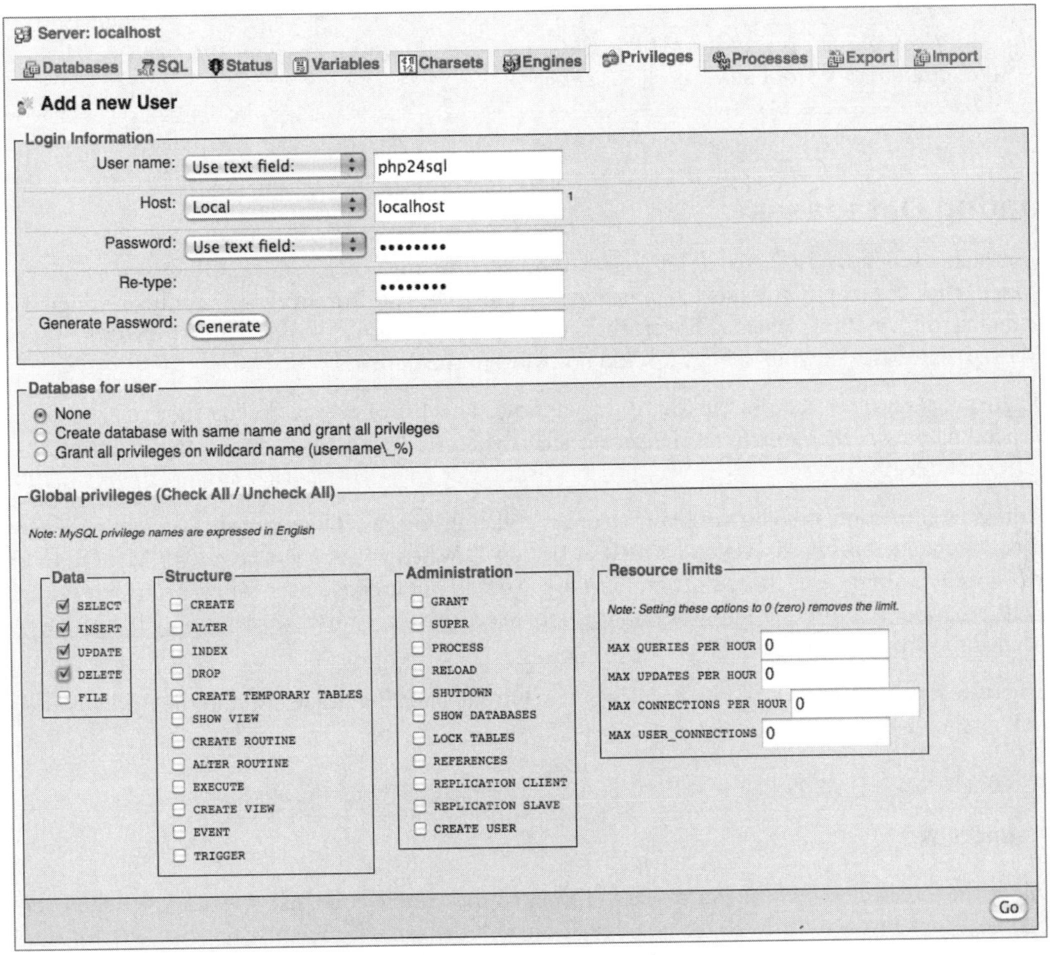

FIGURE 19-4

Next, you need to create a database. To create a database you need to know two things: the name of the database and the default *character set* and *collation* the database will use.

A character set is a list of the symbols and their internal representation. At its simplest, you can think of a character set as the alphabet, numbers, and punctuation along with the encoding of those characters. A collation is the set of rules for comparing and ordering those characters. The collation decides not only that A comes before B and 1 comes before 2, but whether or not A and a are equivalent and whether letters come first or numbers.

Character sets can contain not just the characters used in English, but also characters for accented characters used in other languages or the thousands of characters used in other systems of writing. The early common character sets were limited in scope and although they work with English, they

cannot handle many of the world's languages. Use a UTF-8 such as `utf8_general_ci` collation to allow for more languages.

The character set/collation is used only on text data. Fields that are numeric types have no character sets or collations. You can also have text data that has no character set or collation. These are called *binary* strings. An example of a binary string is a field that contains the bytes for an image.

MySQL is flexible with its use of character sets and collations. You can mix and match different character sets and collations on the same server, the same database, and even within the same table. Unless you know what you are doing, however, you can really get into trouble. If possible, use the same character set and collation at all the levels.

Follow these steps as illustrated in Figure 19-5 to create a database called `test`.

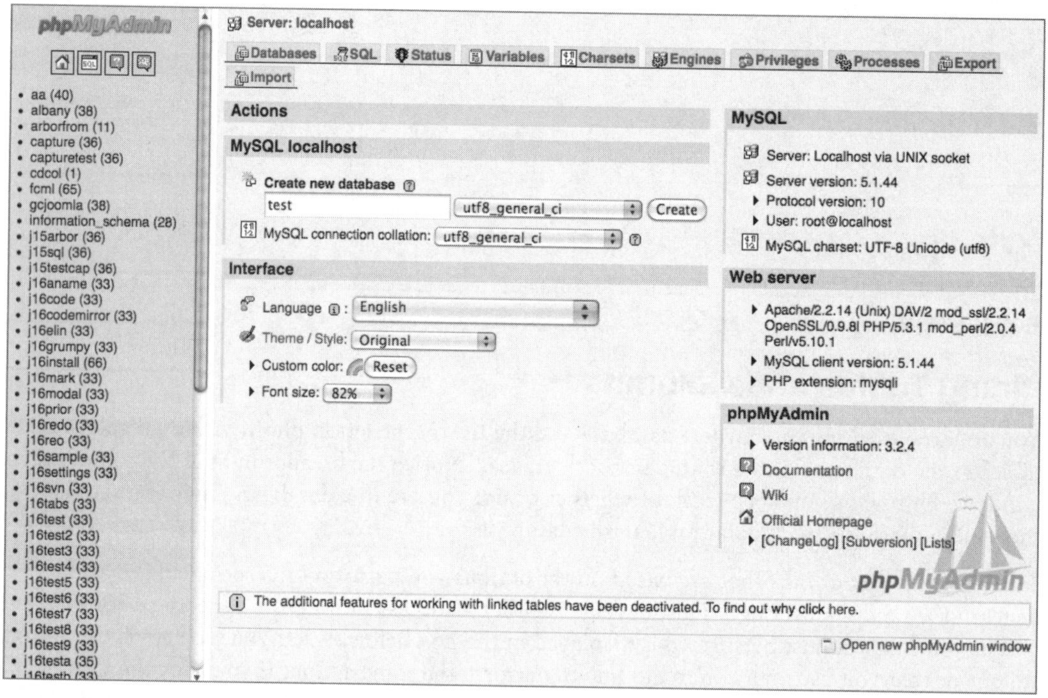

FIGURE 19-5

1. Type **test** in the input box labeled Create New Database. (If you do not see that input box, click the house icon to return to the Home page first.)

2. Click the down arrow in Collation and select `utf8_general_ci`.

3. Click the Create button.

Your results should look similar to Figure 19-6.

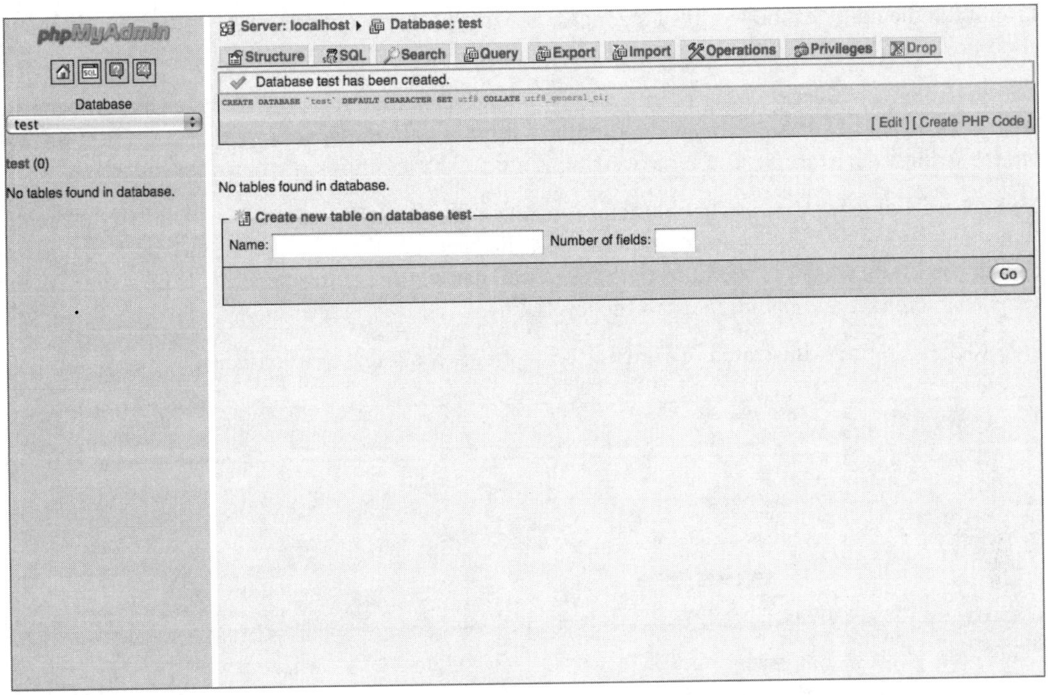

FIGURE 19-6

Defining Tables and Columns

You are now working in your test database and the list on the left in phpMyAdmin displays any tables in the database, rather than a list of databases. Notice the breadcrumbs at the top of the window. This helps you keep track of whether or not you are in a database. Later you see that it also shows if you are in a particular table in the database.

There is a new set of tabs that are based on the actions you perform on a specific database. Just beneath the tabs is a message. This message is either a success message or a specific error message. The action that you just performed is displayed in the box below. What you see here is the actual statement that you use on a command line to perform the same action. If you click the Create PHP Code link, you see the same statement transformed into an assignment to a PHP variable by adding the variable, double quotes around the statement, and a semicolon. Either version can be easily copied with the standard keyboard shortcuts of Ctrl+A, Ctrl+C (on a PC) or Command+A, Command+C (on a Mac).

> *If you click Create PHP Code and then try to return by clicking Without PHP Code, the program tries to rerun your code. Use the back arrow for the browser instead.*

Next comes a list of the tables in this database. There are no tables yet, so you need to create one now:

1. Enter **table1** as the name.

2. Enter **2** for the number of fields (columns) to create.

3. Click the Go button and a window similar to Figure 19-7 is presented.

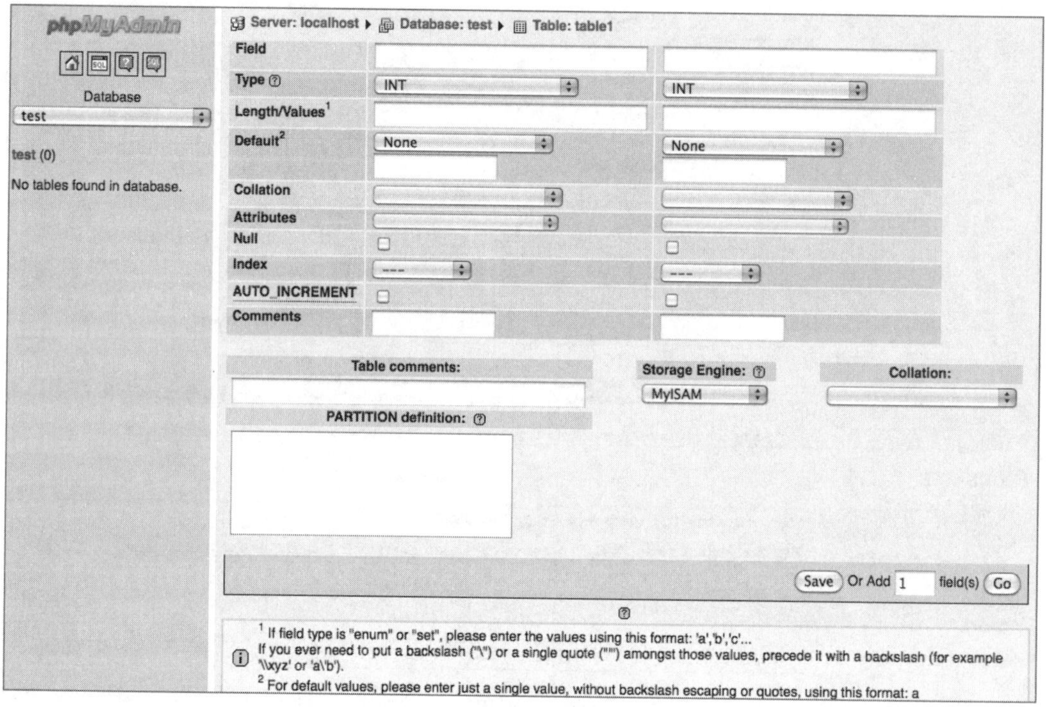

FIGURE 19-7

4. Fill in the field ID by giving it the name **id**, selecting PRIMARY from the Index drop-down, and clicking the AUTO_INCREMENT checkbox. Selecting Primary for the index tells MySQL that this is a main field that is used to identify records in the table. MySQL creates an index for the field in order to retrieve the data more quickly. Flagging the field as auto_increment means that MySQL automatically creates a unique sequential number in this field when a record is added.

5. Fill in the field description by giving it the name **description**, changing the Type drop-down to TEXT, and clicking the Null checkbox to allow nulls to exist. Allowing nulls to exist means that the field is not required. Your window looks like Figure 19-8.

6. Click the Save button to add these two columns to table1 as shown in Figure 19-9.

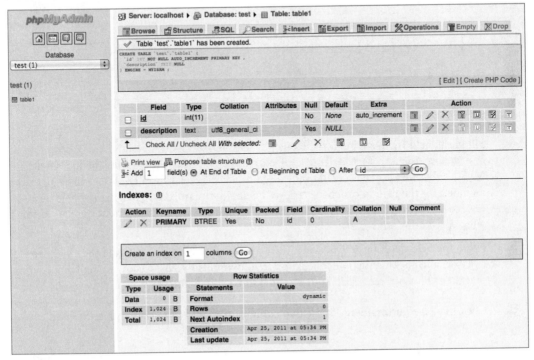

FIGURE 19-8

FIGURE 19-9

The table table1 is now listed in the left column. To work with a specific table, click that table on the left. If there are records in the table, the Browse tab is activated; otherwise, as in this case, the Structure tab is active as it was in Figure 19-7. You add or change columns (not the data in the columns) in the Structure tab. You can add a column either at the end of the table, at the beginning of the table, or after a given column as shown in Figure 19-10.

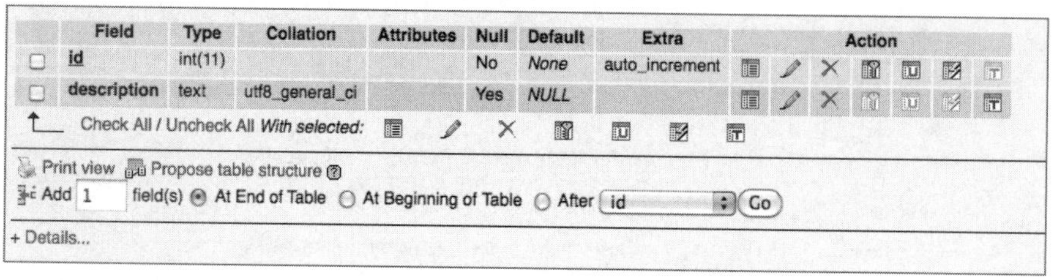

	Field	Type	Collation	Attributes	Null	Default	Extra	Action
☐	id	int(11)			No	None	auto_increment	📋 ✏ ✕ 🔲 🔟 📝 🔣
☐	description	text	utf8_general_ci		Yes	NULL		📋 ✏ ✕ 🔲 🔟 📝 🔣

↑ Check All / Uncheck All *With selected:* 📋 ✏ ✕ 🔲 🔟 📝 🔣

Print view ⬛ Propose table structure ⓐ

⧉ Add 1 field(s) ● At End of Table ○ At Beginning of Table ○ After [id] ⬥ (Go)

+ Details...

FIGURE 19-10

After you click the Go button, the window where you create your new column displays as shown in Figure 19-11. This example creates an integer column called code, where any new rows default to 42 if not set to a different number.

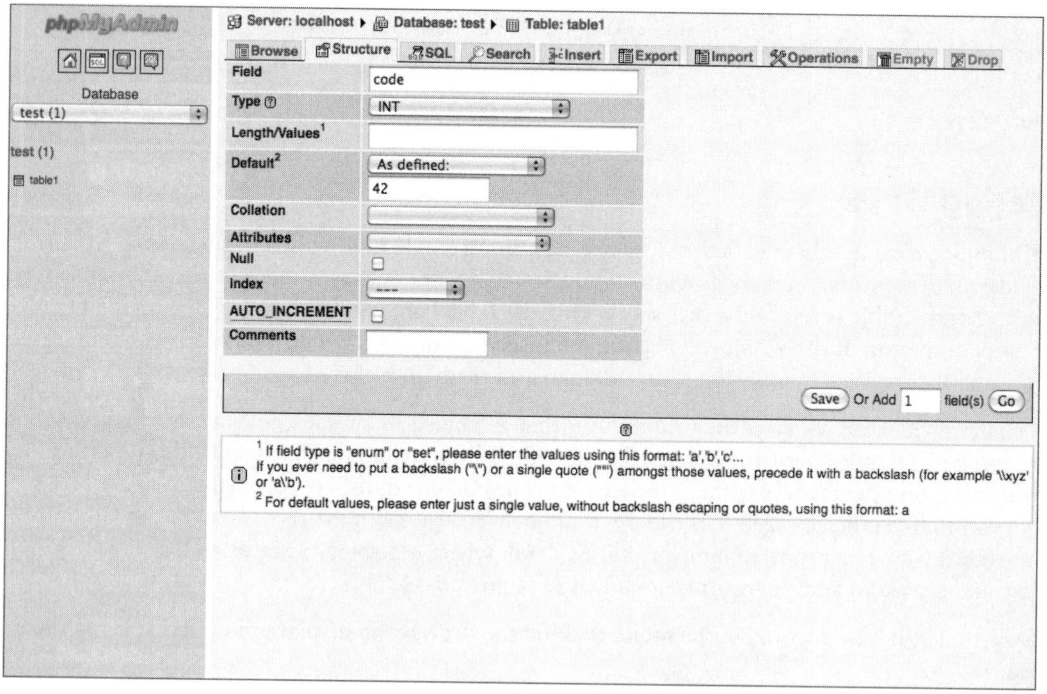

FIGURE 19-11

Clicking the Save button adds the column to table1 as shown in Figure 19-12.

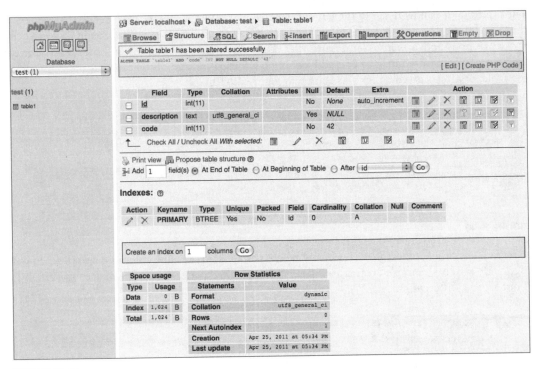

FIGURE 19-12

Entering Data

You now have a database called test, which contains a single table called table1, which has three fields: id, description, and code. At this point you can enter data into your database. To do so, be sure that the table is selected either by clicking the table name on the left or checking the bread-crumb at the top of the window. Clicking the Insert tab opens a window with forms to enter two records. Figure 19-13 shows the forms filled in and ready to be saved.

The first field is id, which is the primary key that is flagged as an `auto_increment` field. When left blank, MySQL automatically assigns the next number in sequence. The next field is description, which is a text field where text can be entered. The code field displays the default of 42 to start, but can that can be changed to a different number. To save both the records, click the Go button in either form. The program jumps to the SQL tab where it displays a status message and the SQL command used to add the records as shown in Figure 19-14.

Now that you have records in the table, clicking the Browse tab displays those records as shown in Figure 19-15.

To delete the records in a table, but leave the structure intact, click the Empty tab. You are asked if you want to TRUNCATE TABLE. Click the OK button to continue with the deletion of the records.

To delete the entire table, including the structure, click the Drop tab. You are asked if you want to DROP TABLE. Click the OK button to continue to delete the table completely.

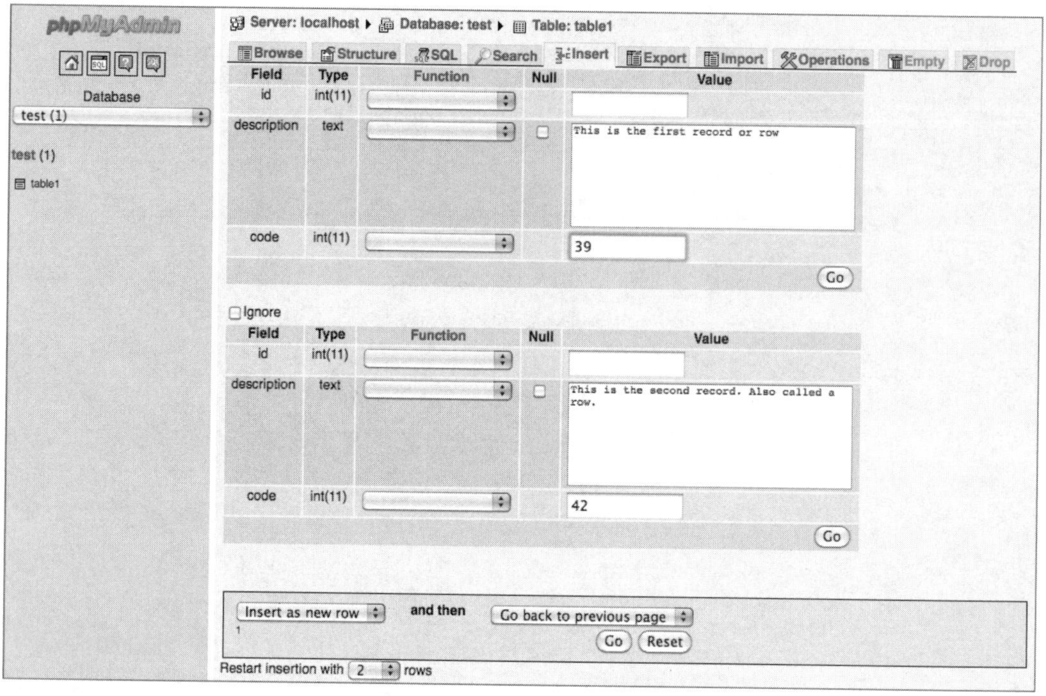

FIGURE 19-13

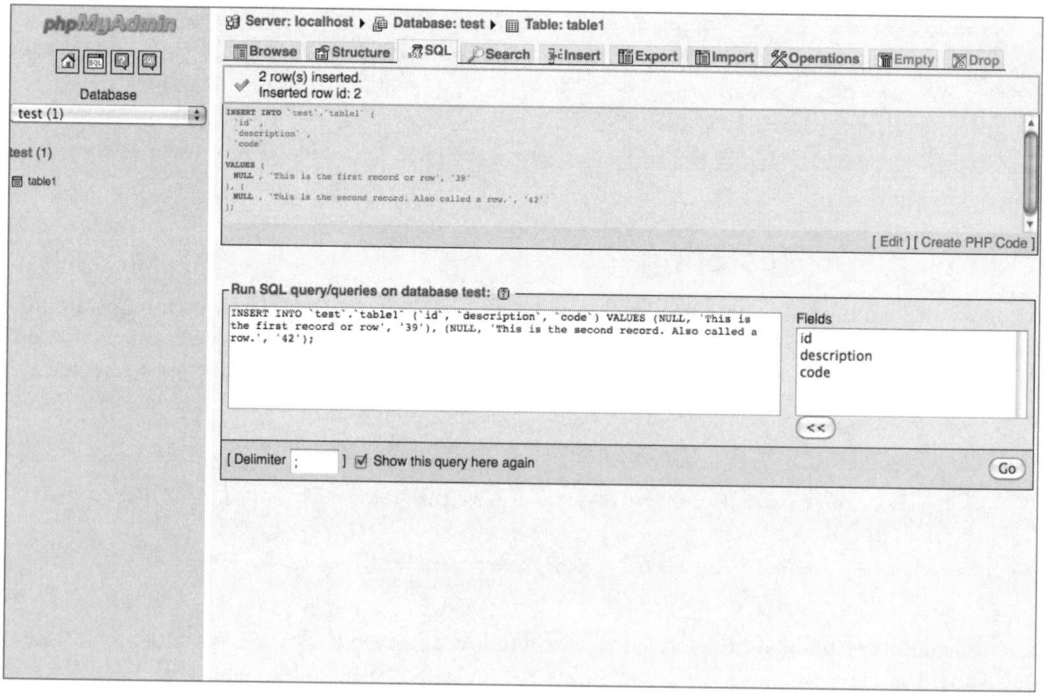

FIGURE 19-14

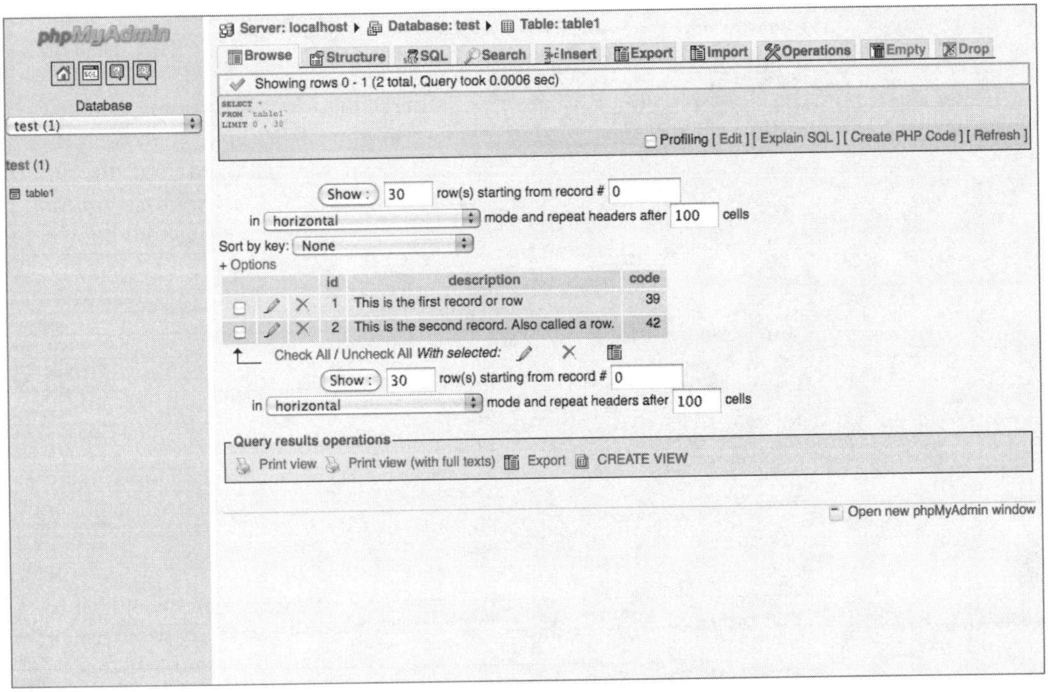

FIGURE 19-15

> Make sure that it says DROP TABLE, not DROP DATABASE. If you are at the database level instead of in a table, the Drop tab deletes the database including all the tables and all the data.

Backing Up and Restoring

After you have a database, you need to know how to back up that database. Databases are not backed up by creating a copy of a file, but by creating commands that enable you to re-create that database. In phpMyAdmin you can back up the entire database, a single table, or a selected group of tables.

> If you need to back up the entire database, be sure that you are at the database level, not in a table.

Click the database name on the left side of the window and then click the Export tab to see the window shown in Figure 19-16.

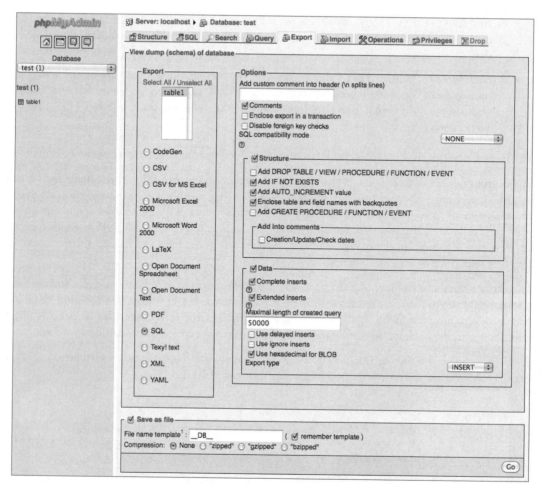

FIGURE 19-16

The form is divided into three sections. On the left is the Export fieldset that enables you select the tables to include and the format to use. On the right is the Option fieldset that lists a series of options that change depending on the format. At the bottom is where you specify how you want to save.

At the top of the Export fieldset is a list of the tables in the database. All the tables are automatically selected, but you can change that to only specific tables. Below that is a list of formats that can be used to export the database. For a normal backup you use SQL.

The Options for the SQL format are displayed on the right. The defaults work well for a standard backup. The Structure fieldset refers to setting up the table: what columns it has, how those columns are defined, and so on. It coordinates with the Structure tab. Here are explanations on common items you might change:

➤ Add DROP TABLE deletes an existing table with the same name if one exists. Check this if you want to replace an existing table.

➤ Add IF NOT EXISTS creates a table only if there is not one. If it finds a table with the same name it leaves it intact. If you use the default Export type of INSERT in the Data fieldset, the data also stays.

➤ Add AUTO_INCREMENT value copies over the current value. If you are bringing over the data as well, you usually need to bring over the `auto_increment` value so that new records start on the right value. If you are just exporting the structure, uncheck this so that new records start at the beginning value.

The Data fieldset deals with the actual data in tables—the records. Leave these at the defaults.

The bottom fieldset is where you tell the program whether you want to save the statements it creates in a file or to display them in the SQL tab box. When saving as a file you have the option of giving a specific name or of setting up a template that automatically creates a name for you. The default template is to use the database name, which is what _DB_ stands for. In this case, where you are exporting as in the SQL format, the database test is saved as `test.sql`. Files in the `.sql` format are simple text files that contain SQL statements.

To restore a database from an SQL Export, you use the Import tab at a database level. You can restore the tables to the same database or a different database. If you restore into the same database, you need to remove the tables first, either manually with the Drop tab on the table or by including the DROP table in the backup. To restore into a new database, you create a new database and select it.

To restore your test database into a new database, create a new database called testbackup. Click the Import tab. You see a window that looks similar to Figure 19-17.

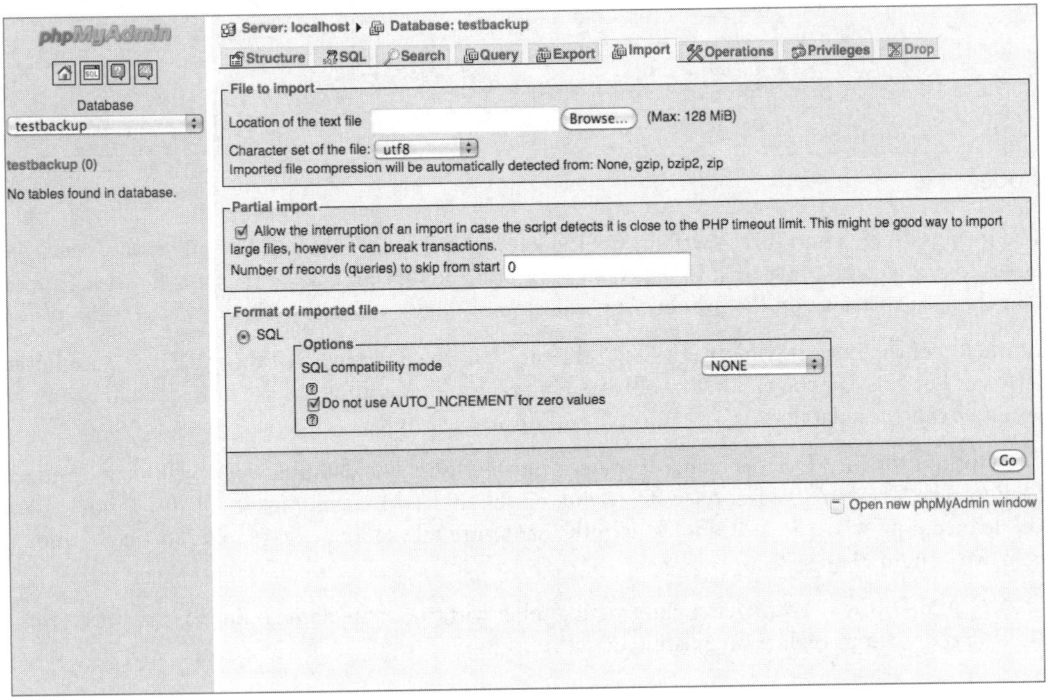

FIGURE 19-17

Click the Browse button for the Location of the Text File input, select the `.sql` file from your hard drive, and click the Go button. The results look similar to Figure 19-18. You have successfully re-created your database.

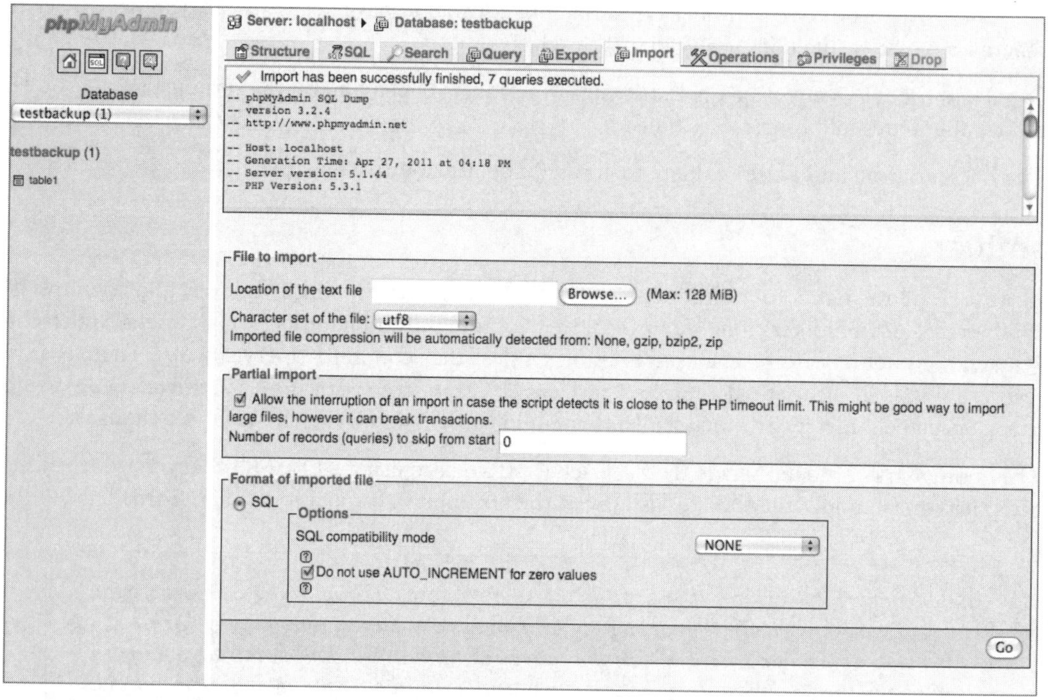

FIGURE 19-18

LEARNING THE SYNTAX

MySQL has an online reference manual for each of the versions of MySQL. You can find the manual for version 5.6 at `http://dev.mysql.com/doc/refman/5.6/en/`. The manual contains a list of all the statements, along with the syntax for each. The manual is for MySQL as used on a command line or in the SQL box of phpMyAdmin. Before trying to use a statement in PHP it can be helpful to be sure that it is a valid MySQL command that works as you expect it to. In this section you learn the common language structure for the statements and the conventions of the manual.

A command is a MySQL statement followed by a semicolon. You can have multiple commands on a single line and a single command can be on multiple lines.

There is a difference between `.sql` files and statements within PHP programs. In the .sql files the only things in the file are MySQL statements. When you use MySQL in PHP programs, the actual MySQL statement is contained within other PHP code and may have variables inside it.

Literal Values

Text strings in MySQL are quoted. You can use either single quotes or double quotes. As in PHP, single quotes and double quotes are usually, though not always, interchangeable. Standard SQL uses

only single quotes, so that is preferred. If you have a quote as part of the text, you either need to enclose the text with the other type of quote mark, escape the quote with a backslash (\), or double it.

Numbers are not enclosed in quotes. They can be preceded by a - or a + to show whether the number is negative or positive. Number types that are allowed to have decimals can also have a decimal separator (.). Scientific notation is also allowed.

Dates and times can either be quoted strings or numbers depending on the circumstances. You learn more about dates and times in Lesson 21.

The Boolean True and False evaluate to 1 and 0 and are not case sensitive.

Identifiers

Identifiers are the names of objects in MySQL such as databases, tables, indexes, and columns. They can be up to 64 characters long. Identifiers that contain only alphanumeric characters, underscores (_), and $ do not have to be enclosed in quotes unless they contain a reserved word. There is a list of reserved words in the manual at `http://dev.mysql.com/doc/refman/5.6/en/reserved-words.html`. Special characters are encoded so that could cause issues if the character set changes.

The quote mark for identifiers is the backtick (`` ` ``). If you are using a QWERTY keyboard, this is the little ticky-mark under the tilde (~) usually in the far upper-left side of your keyboard.

> *The backtick (`` ` ``) is not the same as the single quote (‘). You will get errors if you use the wrong one in the wrong place. The easiest way to remember which to use is that the backtick goes on the names of things (databases, tables, columns) whereas the single quote goes on values and around statements and commands.*

Identifiers can be qualified or unqualified as long as the unqualified identifier is unambiguous. For example, if you have a database named test and a table named table1 and a column named id it could be written as

```
id
table1.id
test.table1.id
`id`
`table1`.`id`
`test`.`table1`.`id`
```

Notice that if you quote the names in a qualified identifier, you quote each name separately. If an identifier is unqualified, the defaults are used.

Technically databases and tables are not case sensitive but they map to files in the filesystem on the host. Depending on your operating system, files in the filesystem are case sensitive. Windows is not case sensitive but if you develop on Windows and then move your work to an online host that is Linux, your code could fail. For that reason, it is recommended that you code as if your identifiers are case sensitive.

Comments

If you are using MySQL through your PHP program you usually only use MySQL comments if you create a backup from phpMyAdmin or if you have a .sql file to create your database structure and set up data when doing an install of your program.

Comments come in different flavors in MySQL:

➤ Use a # character to comment everything from the character to the end of the line.

➤ Use -- (double-dash plus space/tab/newline) to comment everything from the dashes to the end of the line.

➤ Use /* to */ for commenting multiple lines as in PHP.

Do not nest comments. There are times when it works, but many more when it doesn't. So if you have a block of statements to comment out, don't try to do it by surrounding the block with /* */ if there are comments within the statements.

TRY IT

Available for download on Wrox.com

In this Try It, you create a database for the Case Study. Based on part of the database analysis from the previous lesson, you create the Contacts table and fill it with data. You back up the database and restore it in a second database.

> *You can download the code and resources for this Try It from the book's web page at* www.wrox.com. *You can find them in the Lesson19 folder in the download. You will find code for the* smithside.sql *file.*

Lesson Requirements

Your computer needs to be able to run as a web server with PHP and MySQL. XAMPP is a package of software that installs the web server, PHP, and MySQL for you. You can find instructions for downloading and installing XAMPP in Lesson 1.

You need a working copy of phpMyAdmin, which comes as part of XAMPP. You can download a free copy at www.phpmyadmin.net.

Hints

See the database analysis done for the Case Study in the Try It section of Lesson 18.

Make sure that you are in the right level, whether it is global, database, or table. Use the indicators on the left column or the breadcrumbs at the top of the window.

Step-by-Step

Create the Case Study database.

1. Open phpMyAdmin.

2. In the input box labeled Create New Database enter **smithside**.

3. Change the Collation drop-down from `Collation` to `utf8-general-ci`.

4. Click the Create button. Your results look similar to Figure 19-19.

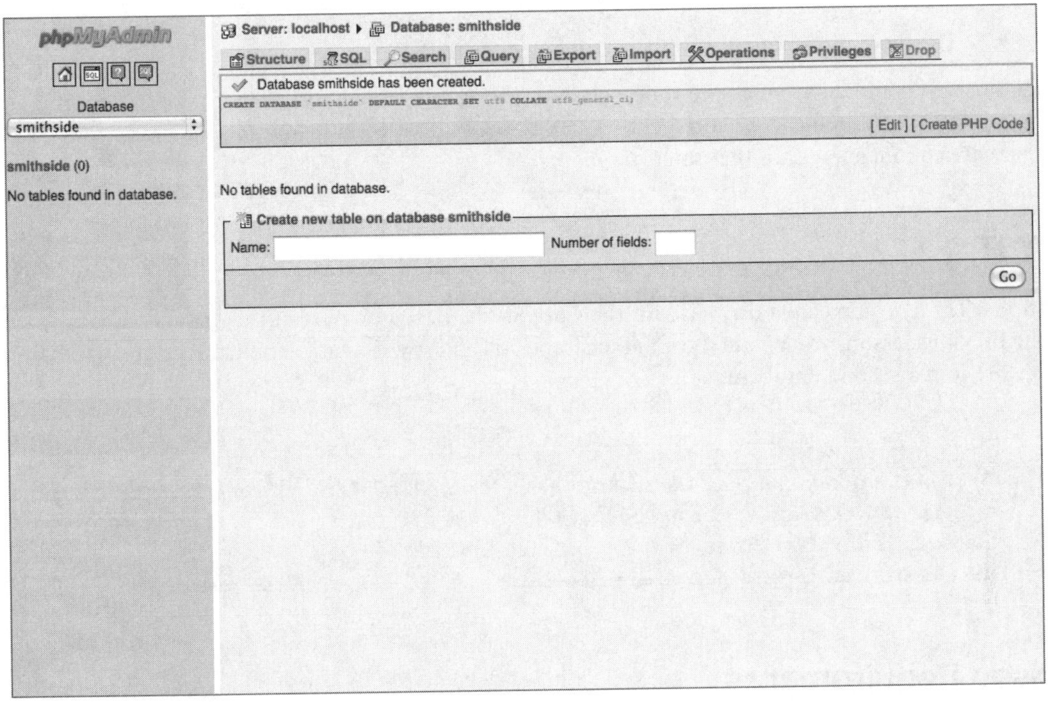

FIGURE 19-19

Create the contacts table with the fields id, first name, last name, position, email, and phone.

1. In the fieldset called Create New Table on Database smithside, type **contacts** as the name.

2. Type **6** for the Number of Fields.

3. Click Go to see a window that looks similar to Figure 19-20. Because there are several fields, each of the field definitions stretches horizontally, instead of vertically in the lesson example.

4. The first field is id. Fill in the following information, scrolling the screen to see the rest of the window as necessary. Steps 4 through 9 are shown in Figure 19-21.

   Field: **id**

   Type: **INT**

Length: **11**

Default: **None**

Attributes: **UNSIGNED**

Index: **PRIMARY**

A_I: Check this box for AUTO_INCREMENT

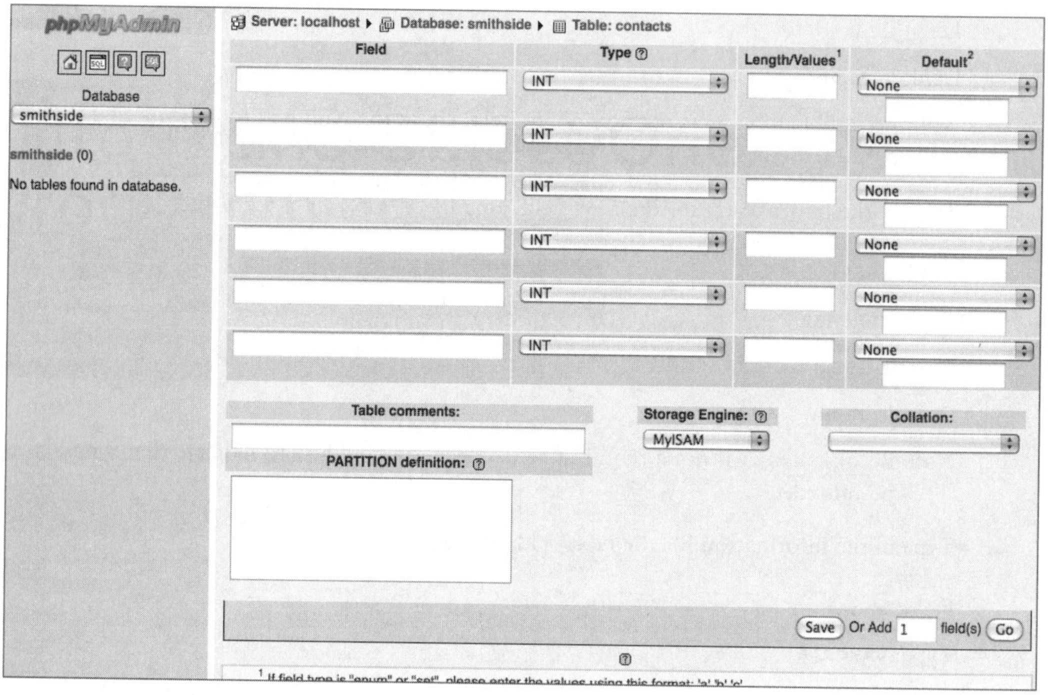

FIGURE 19-20

5. Type in the information for the next field, first name. This is a text field of up to 50 characters. VARCHAR stands for Variable Characters and lets you specify a maximum number of character positions. You learn more about types in Lesson 21.

Field: **first_name**

Type: **VARCHAR**

Length: **50**

Default: **None**

6. Type in the information for the next field, last name.

Field: **last_name**

Type: **VARCHAR**

Length: **50**

Default: **None**

7. Type in the information for the next field, position.

Field: **position**

Type: **VARCHAR**

Length: **50**

Default: **None**

Null: Because **position** is not a required field, check the Null box to indicate that a null is permitted.

8. Type in the information for the next field, email.

Field: **email**

Type: **VARCHAR**

Length: **255**

Default: **None**

Null: Because **email** is not a required field, check the Null box to indicate that a null is permitted.

9. Type in the information for the next field, phone.

Field: **phone**

Type: **VARCHAR**

Length: **20**

Default: **None**

Null: Because **phone** is not a required field, check the Null box to indicate that a null is permitted.

Field	Type [?]	Length/Values[1]	Default[2]	Collation	Attributes	Null	Index	A_I
id	INT	11	None			☐	PRIMARY	☑
first_name	VARCHAR	50	None			☐	---	☐
last_name	VARCHAR	50	None			☐	---	☐
position	VARCHAR	50	None			☑	---	☐
email	VARCHAR	255	None			☑	---	☐
phone	VARCHAR	20	None			☑	---	☐

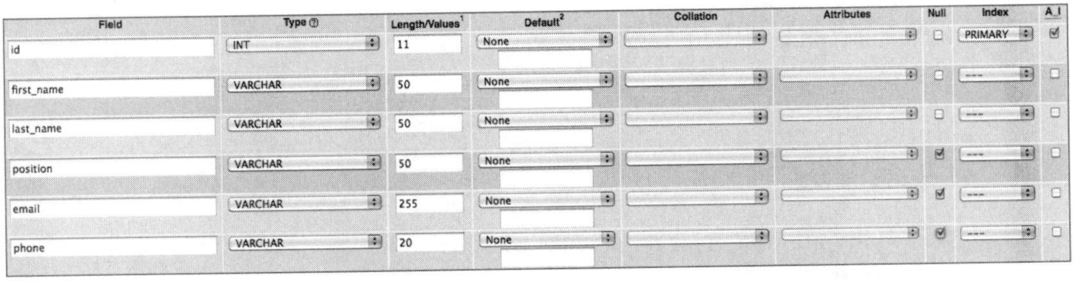

FIGURE 19-21

10. Click the Save button. Your results should look similar to Figure 19-22.

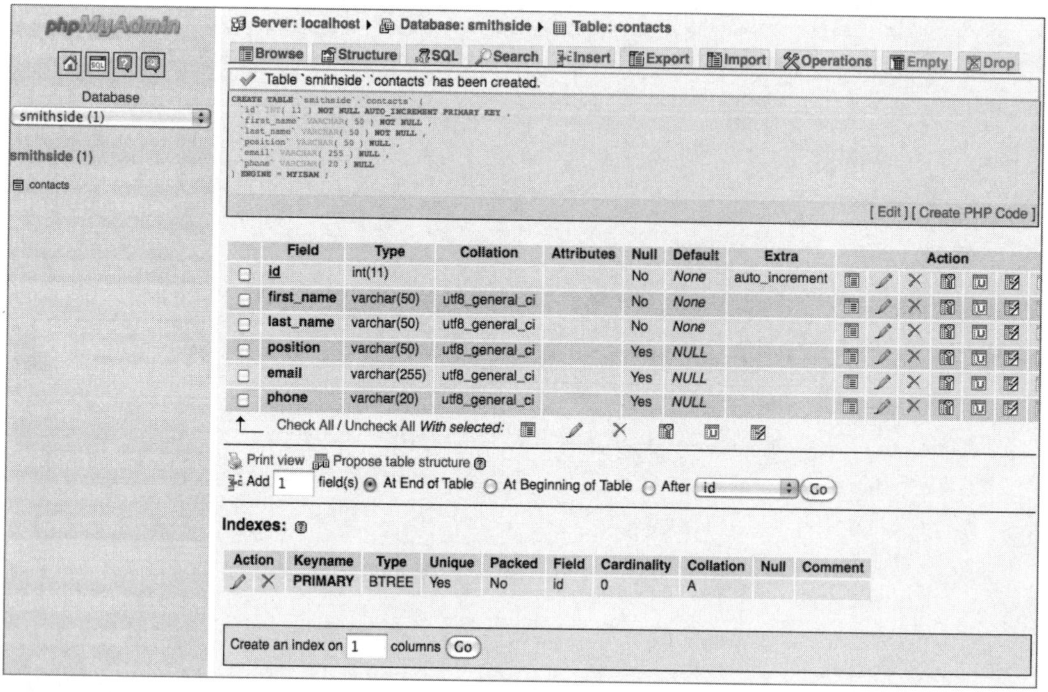

FIGURE 19-22

Create six contact records. You can use the data from the Case Study or create your own.

1. In phpMyAdmin in the contacts table, click the Insert tab.

2. At the bottom of the page, change Restart Insertion With to 10 rows.

3. Enter the contacts. Leave the ids blank so that they are automatically calculated. Do not click the Go button until you have entered all six contacts. Use the Tab key to navigate. If you press Enter, whatever you have entered so far is saved. If that happens, click the Insert tab and insert the remaining contacts. If you were in the middle of a contact, see step 4 to fix that contact. Your result should look like Figure 19-23.

   ➤ Martha Smith, position: none, martha@example.com

   ➤ George Smith, postion: none, george@example.com, 515-555-1236

   ➤ Jeff Meyers, hip hop expert for shure, jeff@example.com

   ➤ Peter Meyers, position: none, peter@example.com, 515-555-1237

   ➤ Sally Smith, position: none, sally@example.com, 515-555-1235

   ➤ Sarah Finder, Lost Soul, finder@a.com, 555-123-5555

4. Click the Browse tab to see your contact data as shown in Figure 19-24. If you need to change any of the data, click the pencil at the beginning of the row you need to change.

FIGURE 19-23

FIGURE 19-24

Back up your database and restore it in a different database.

1. Click the database smithside on the left column.

2. Click the Export tab to see the window shown in Figure 19-25.

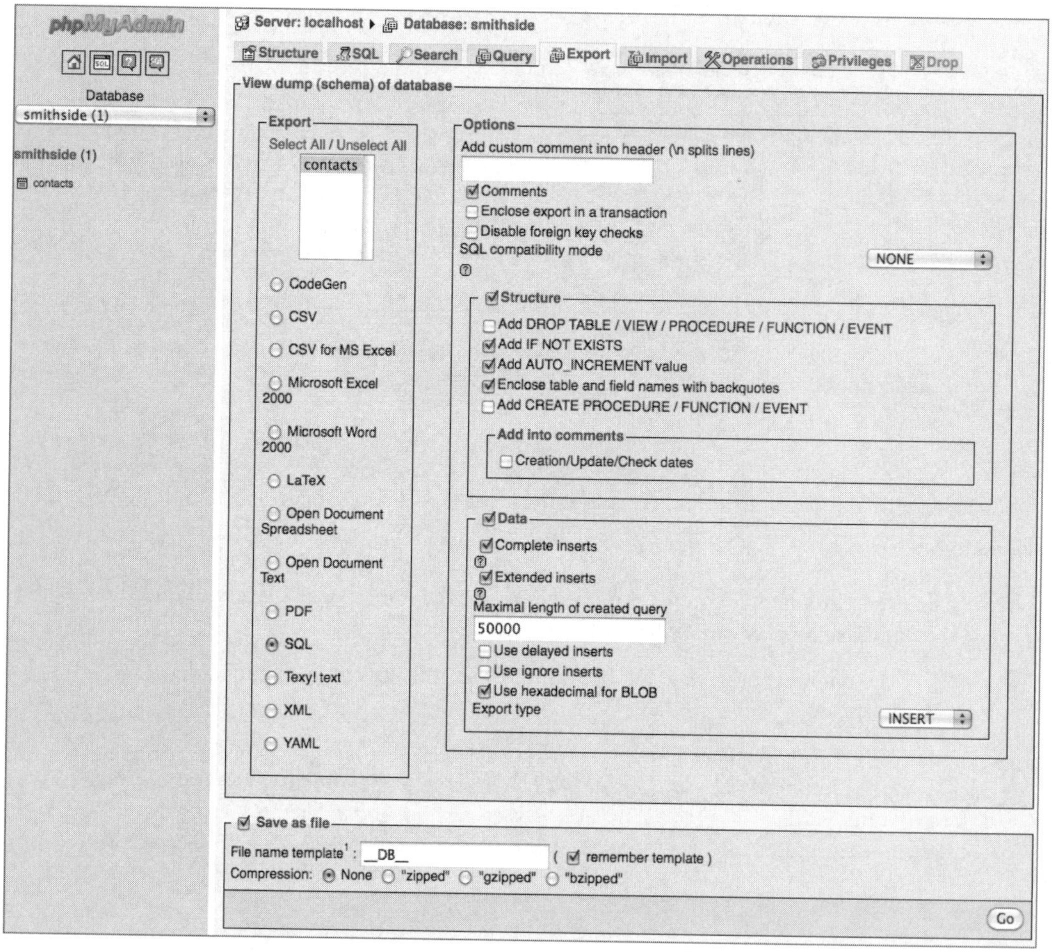

FIGURE 19-25

3. Save the `smithside.sql` file.

4. Click the house icon on the upper-left side.

5. Create a database called **ssbackup** with the `utf8_general_ci` collation. You should see Database: ssbackup appear in the breadcrumbs at the top of the window.

6. Click the Import tab to see the window shown in Figure 19-26.

7. Click the Browse tab. Find and select the `smithside.sql` file you saved.

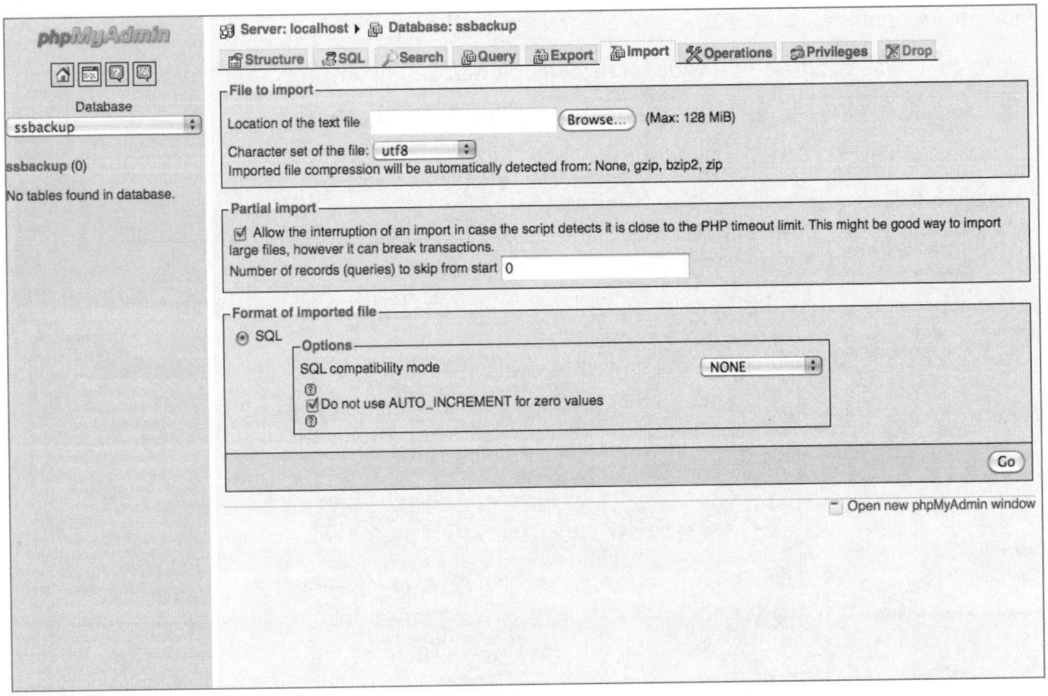

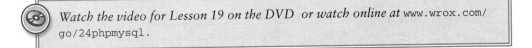

FIGURE 19-26

8. Click the Go button. You get a message saying the import was successful and the table(s) in the database display on the left column.

9. Click the contacts table in the left column to see the six contacts you added.

> Watch the video for Lesson 19 on the DVD or watch online at www.wrox.com/ go/24phpmysql.

20

Creating and Connecting to the Database

In this lesson, you learn the interfaces that PHP has to communicate with a MySQL database. The original method was with an extension to PHP called mysql. You can still find this in older code, but it has been replaced by the mysqli extension for PHP 5. Mysqli is an improved, more secure version that takes advantage of features added to newer versions of MySQL. It is recommended for new work.

PDO (PHP Data Objects) is an extension to PHP for connecting to various databases, not just MySQL. The same PHP code enables you to connect to MySQL, PostreSQL, and SQLite databases, among others. You use different drivers to switch from one database type to the other.

CONNECTING WITH MYSQL/MYSQLI

Mysql was the traditional way to communicate with MySQL. When mysqli came along in PHP 5, it added the following features:

➤ **Object-oriented interface:** Mysqli has the `mysqli` class, the `mysql_stmt` class for queries, and the `mysqli_result` class for results. Each of these has properties that give you information on the connection, the request you are making, or the data you have retrieved. They also have methods that enable you to perform actions. There is still a procedural interface similar to mysql if you prefer to use that.

➤ **Support for prepared statements:** With prepared statements you set up the request once and then send the particulars for the actual request. Reusing the same type of requests works faster than creating a new request each time. More importantly, it is more secure because it cuts down on injection attacks.

➤ **Support for multiple statements:** You can process multiple statements at a time rather than one by one.

➤ **Support for transactions:** You use transactions when you have multiple changes to a database that should be thought of as a group. An example is when you transfer money from one account to another. A transaction ties the subtraction from one account to the addition to the other so that if one action fails the other fails as well.

To connect to MySQL you need to know the hostname (which is usually localhost), username, and password. You create an instance of the class `mysqli` to establish a connection. The following code connects to MySQL running on localhost and uses the username `root` and the password `12345`. The object `$connection` can be called anything. Other common variable names are `$db`, `$dbh`, and `$mysqli`.

```php
<?php
$connection = new mysqli('localhost', 'php24sql', 'hJQV8RTe5t');
```

If there is an error with the connection, the error is put in the property `connect_error` for the object you just created. Use the `if` statement to check for errors. The following example displays the error message if there is an error. If you are in a production site you should give a message to the user without details because the details could be used to hack the system. If there is no error a success message is displayed. The `@` before the `new` suppresses the normal error handling. Without the `@`, errors with the connection are automatically displayed. Use the `@` if you want to handle the errors yourself. Remember to change the configuration information to match your setup. Your results should look similar to Figure 20-1.

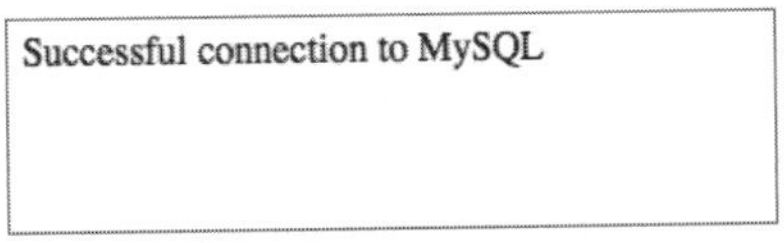

> Successful connection to MySQL

FIGURE 20-1

```php
<?php
$connection = @new mysqli('localhost', 'php24sql', 'hJQV8RTe5t');
if ($connection->connect_error) {
  die('Connect Error: ' . $connection->connect_error);
} else {
  echo 'Successful connection to MySQL';
}
```

You should have one place to go for the connection information. That way you have one place to go to if you change a username or password and you have the ability to store the information separately such as in a configuration file. One way is to use constants as the following code does:

```php
<?php
define("MYSQLUSER", "php24sql");
define("MYSQLPASS", "hJQV8RTe5t");
define("HOSTNAME", "localhost");

$connection = @new mysqli(HOSTNAME, MYSQLUSER, MYSQLPASS);
if ($connection->connect_error) {
  die('Connect Error: ' . $connection->connect_error);
} else {
  echo 'Successful connection to MySQL';
}
```

You have successfully connected to MySQL, but before you can use a database, you need to connect to the database. The database must already exist before you can connect to it. In the previous lesson,

you created a database called smithside in phpMyAdmin. Adding the database name as the fourth parameter selects that particular database.

```php
<?php
define("MYSQLUSER", "php24sql");
define("MYSQLPASS", "hJQV8RTe5t");
define("HOSTNAME", "localhost");
define("MYSQLDB", "smithside");

if ($connection = new mysqli(HOSTNAME, MYSQLUSER, MYSQLPASS, MYSQLDB)) {
  echo 'Successful connection to MySQL';
}
```

You are now at the same point as you were in the previous lesson when you opened phpMyAdmin and clicked on a database. In phpMyAdmin you could see a list of the tables. You can use your new database connection object to get a list of the tables in the database.

The mysqli class has a method called query(). You pass it a MySQL statement and it returns an object of the mysqli_result class. You then use the properties and methods of that object to see your results. The MySQL command to see a list of tables is SHOW TABLES. The MySQL command names are not case sensitive, but it is standard practice to capitalize them. Assuming that $connection is your connection object, the following code executes the SHOW TABLES command and creates $result as an object based on the mysqli_result class:

```php
$result = $connection->query("SHOW TABLES");
```

The mysqli_result class property num_rows contains the number of rows. Because $result is based on the mysqli_result class it also has num_rows as a property.

```php
$count = $result->num_rows;
```

The mysqli_result class method fetch_array() returns the results in the form of an array for each record, which in this case is each table. The first element in the array contains the table name.

```php
$row = $result->fetch_array();
echo $row[0];
```

This finds only the first table. To get a list of all the tables you use a while loop. The script continues to loop through the results until it reaches the end.

```php
while ($row = $result->fetch_array()) {
  echo $row[0]. '<br />';
}
```

The following is what the full code looks like to create a connection and list the tables in the database. Your results should look similar to Figure 20-2.

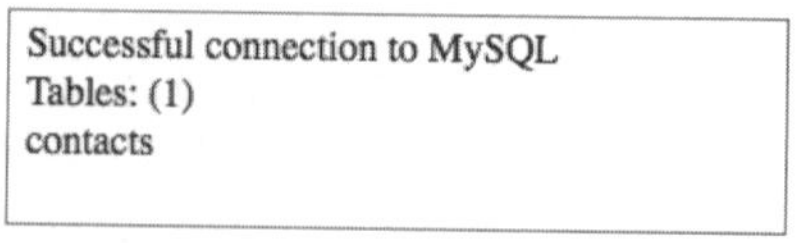

```php
<?php
define("MYSQLUSER", "php24sql");
define("MYSQLPASS", "hJQV8RTe5t");
define("HOSTNAME", "localhost");
define("MYSQLDB", "smithside");
```

Successful connection to MySQL
Tables: (1)
contacts

FIGURE 20-2

```php
$connection = @new mysqli(HOSTNAME, MYSQLUSER, MYSQLPASS, MYSQLDB);
if ($connection->connect_error) {
  die('Connect Error: ' . $connection->connect_error);
} else {
  echo 'Successful connection to MySQL <br />';
  if ($result = $connection->query("SHOW TABLES")) {
    $count =$result->num_rows;
    echo "Tables: ($count)<br />";
    while ($row = $result->fetch_array()) {
      echo $row[0]. '<br />';
    }
  }
}
```

You have been learning the object-oriented style of mysqli. There is also a procedural type of mysqli. The following is the same program using the procedural style:

```php
<?php
define("MYSQLUSER", "php24sql");
define("MYSQLPASS", "hJQV8RTe5t");
define("HOSTNAME", "localhost");
define("MYSQLDB", "smithside");

$connection = @mysqli_connect(HOSTNAME, MYSQLUSER, MYSQLPASS, MYSQLDB);
if (mysqli_connect_error()) {
  die('Connect Error: ' . mysqli_connect_error());
} else {
  echo 'Successful connection to MySQL <br />';
  if ($result = mysqli_query($connection, "SHOW TABLES")) {
    $count = mysqli_num_rows($result);
    echo "Tables: ($count)<br />";
    while ($row = mysqli_fetch_array($result)) {
      echo $row[0]. '<br />';
    }
  }
}
```

> *For a complete list of the properties and methods of the mysqli classes see the documentation at* www.php.net/manual/en/mysqli.summary.php.

Whether you use the object-oriented style or the procedural style, you use the variable that contains the connection (in this case $connection) to access the database throughout your program. Many older programs use a global variable to hold the connection. The connection itself goes in an initial program such as the following code:

```php
<?php
define("MYSQLUSER", "php24sql");
define("MYSQLPASS", "hJQV8RTe5t");
define("HOSTNAME", "localhost");
define("MYSQLDB", "smithside");
```

```php
$connection = @new mysqli(HOSTNAME, MYSQLUSER, MYSQLPASS, MYSQLDB);
if ($connection->connect_error) {
  die('Connect Error: ' . $connection->connect_error);
}
```

When the database is needed, the `$connection` variable is declared as global:

```php
<?php
global $connection;
if ($result = $connection->query("SHOW TABLES")) {
  $count = $result->num_rows;
  echo "Tables: ($count)<br />";
  while ($row =$result->fetch_array()) {
    echo $row[0]. '<br />';
  }
}
```

The other way is to create a database class that contains the connection. You can also use this class to contain other database-related functions. Start by defining the database connection information as properties. The properties are private because they should be seen only inside the class. Make them static. Static variables are associated with the class rather than a specific object.

```php
<?php
class Database
{
  private static $_mysqlUser = 'php24sql';
  private static $_mysqlPass = 'hJQV8RTe5t';
  private static $_mysqlDb = 'smithside';
  private static $_hostName = 'localhost';
```

Add a property for the connection variable, initializing it to NULL:

```php
protected static $_connection = NULL;
```

Create a method to get the connection. Make this a public static function that returns the connection property. Remember that you address static properties and functions with `self::` instead of `$this->`.

```php
public static function getConnection() {
  self::$_connection = new mysqli(self::$_hostName, self::$_mysqlUser,
    self::$_mysqlPass, self::$_mysqlDb);
  if (self::$_connection->connect_error) {
    die('Connect Error: ' . self::$_connection->connect_error);
  }
  return self::$_connection;
}
```

If you leave the method as it is, every time you create a new object you create a new database connection, which uses extra memory. The solution is to make the class a *singleton*. A singleton class is limited to a single instance. Each time you use the class, you get the same instance instead of creating a new object every time you use the database.

Check first thing to see if the connection already exists. If it doesn't, then create the object and do the error checking. Whether the connection already existed or you just created it, return the

connection. That way, you only make the connection the first time through. All the rest of the time you just return the $_connection.

```
public static function getConnection() {
    if (!self::$_connection) {
        self::$_connection = new mysqli(self::$_hostName, self::$_mysqlUser,
          self::$_mysqlPass, self::$_mysqlDb);
        if (self::$_connection->connect_error) {
            die('Connect Error: ' . self::$_connection->connect_error);
        }
    }
    return self::$_connection;
}
```

To prevent programmers from creating an object by using new Database you make the $__construct() method private:

```
private function __construct(){}
```

Outside of the class, call the getConnection method to get the $connection property. To call this static method in the Database class, use Database::getConnection as shown in the following code:

```
<?php
$connection = Database::getConnection;
if ($result = $connection->query("SHOW TABLES")) {
    $count = $result->num_rows;
    echo "Tables: ($count)<br />";
    while ($row = $result->fetch_array()) {
        echo $row[0]. '<br />';
    }
}
```

PHP closes the database connection when the script is done, but you can close it yourself if you are done with the database. The object-oriented version looks like this:

```
<?php
$connection = Database::getConnection();
$connection->close();
```

This is the procedural style for closing a database:

```
<?php
$connection = Database::getConnection();
mysqli_close($connection);
```

> *Mysqli has an object-oriented style and a procedural style. You also have the choice of sharing the connection using a global variable or using the object-oriented method. These two decisions are separate. You can use the object-oriented mysqli with the global variable or with a static singleton class.*

CONNECTING WITH PDO

Mysqli uses an extension that is created specifically to talk to the MySQL database. As such it is able to take advantage of all the features of the MySQL database. However, if you want PHP programs that are more portable — that are able to be easily adapted to other flavors of databases — then the PDO extension is the extension to use. The following is a list of PDO features.

➤ **Object-oriented interface:** PDO has the main PDO class, the PDOStatement class for prepared statements, and the PDOException class for errors.

➤ **Support for prepared statements:** With prepared statements you set up the request once and then send the particulars for the actual request. Reusing the same type of requests works faster than creating a new request each time. More importantly, it is more secure because it cuts down on injection attacks. Prepared statements in PDO are easier to use than the mysqli prepared statements.

➤ **Support for transactions:** You use transactions when you have multiple changes to a database that should be thought of as a group. An example is when you transfer money from one account to another. A transaction ties the subtraction from one account to the addition to the other so that if one action fails the other fails as well.

The concepts for using PDO are similar to using mysqli. The following code connects to MySQL running on the localhost and uses the username php24sql and the password hJQV8RTe5t. It sets up a connection to the smithside database and displays a message when it successfully connects. Your results should look similar to Figure 20-3.

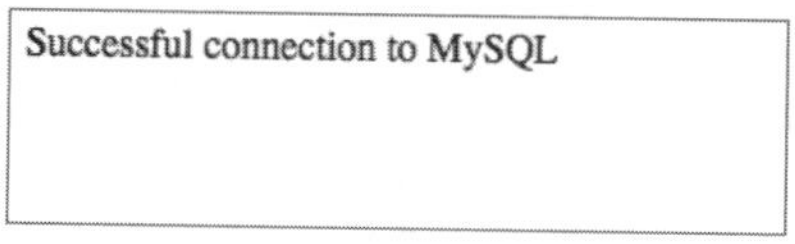

> Successful connection to MySQL

FIGURE 20-3

```php
<?php
if ($connection = new PDO('mysql:host=localhost;dbname=smithside', 'php24sql',
  'hJQV8RTe5t')) {
  echo 'Successful connection to MySQL';
}
```

As with mysqli, you can use constants to set up the connection:

```php
<?php
define("MYSQLUSER", "php24sql");
define("MYSQLPASS", "hJQV8RTe5t");
define("HOSTNAME", "localhost");
define("MYSQLDB", "smithside");

if ($connection = new PDO('mysql:host='.HOSTNAME.';dbname=' . MYSQLDB,
  MYSQLUSER, MYSQLPASS)) {
  echo 'Successful connection to MySQL';
}
```

The PDO class has a method called query(). You pass it a MySQL statement and it returns an object of the PDO class. You then use the properties and methods of that object to see your results.

The MySQL command to see a list of tables is SHOW TABLES. Assuming that $connection is your connection object, this code executes the SHOW TABLES command and creates $result as an object based on the PDO class:

```
$result = $connections->query("SHOW TABLES")
```

The PDO class method fetch(PDO::FETCH_NUM) returns the results in the format specified, which in this case is a numeric array. The format is in the form of an array for each record, which in this case is each table. The first element in the array contains the table name.

```
$row = $result->fetch(PDO::FETCH_NUM);
echo $row[0];
```

This finds only the first table. To get a list of all the tables you use a while loop. The script continues to loop through the results until it reaches the end. The following is what the full code looks like to create a connection and list the tables in the database. Your results should look similar to Figure 20-4.

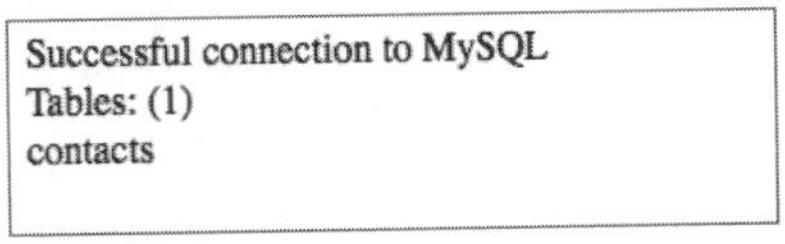

> Successful connection to MySQL
> Tables: (1)
> contacts

FIGURE 20-4

```php
<?php
define("MYSQLUSER", "php24sql");
define("MYSQLPASS", "hJQV8RTe5t");
define("MYSQLDB", "smithside");
define("HOSTNAME", "localhost");

// set up the Database connection
if ($connection = new PDO('mysql:host='.HOSTNAME.';dbname=' . MYSQLDB,
  MYSQLUSER, MYSQLPASS)) {
    echo 'Successful connection to MySQL<br />';
  if ($result = $connection->query("SHOW TABLES")) {
    echo "Tables:<br />";
    while ($row =$result->fetch(PDO::FETCH_NUM)) {
      echo $row[0]. '<br />';
    }
  }
}
```

> For a complete list of the properties and methods of the PDO classes, see the documentation at www.php.net/manual/en/book.pdo.php.

PDO can share the connection using either a global variable or the singleton class described in the mysqli section.

CREATING THE DATABASE

In the previous lesson, you created a database using phpMyAdmin. That is the normal way to create databases. Because you need more privileges to create databases than you do to use them, the creation is often a separate function from standard programs. In this example you need to use your root user or any user that has the privilege of creating databases.

To create a database, connect to MySQL and run the CREATE DATABASE command. This is the MySQL command to create a database called mydatabase:

```
CREATE DATABASE 'mydatabase';
```

After you have created the database, you need to select it for use before you can use it. Running the following code gives you a result similar to Figure 20-5:

```
<?php
define("MYSQLUSER", "root");
define("MYSQLPASS", "p##V89Te5t");
define("HOSTNAME", "localhost");

if ($connection = new mysqli(HOSTNAME, MYSQLUSER, MYSQLPASS)) {
  echo 'Successful connection to MySQL <br />';
  if ($result = $connection->query("CREATE DATABASE 'mydatabase'")) {
    $connection->select_db('mydatabase'); // use the database
    echo "Database created";
  } else {
    echo "Problem creating the database. Is the user not allowed
       to create database or does the database already exist?";  }
}
```

> Successful connection to MySQL
> Database created

FIGURE 20-5

Note that the preceding code uses an equal sign in the if statement:

```
if ($result = $connection->query("CREATE DATABASE 'mydatabase'")) {
```

The way that this statement is processed is that the statement on the right is evaluated first, which attempts to create the database. That function returns a value, which in this case is TRUE or FALSE. That value is then assigned to $result, which is then evaluated to determine if the code enclosed by the if statement should be run.

TRY IT

Available for download on Wrox.com

In this Try It, you create a database class for the Case Study. It holds a mysqli object-oriented type of connection to the database.

> You can download the code and resources for this Try It from the book's web page at www.wrox.com. You can find them in the Lesson20 folder in the download. You will find code for both before and after completing the exercises.

Lesson Requirements

Your computer needs to be able to run as a web server with PHP and MySQL. XAMPP is a package of software that installs the web server, PHP, and MySQL for you. You can find instructions for downloading and installing XAMPP in Lesson 1.

You need a text editor that can produce plain-text files. You can find instructions for downloading and installing Eclipse PDT in Lesson 1. Other text editors that you can use are Adobe's Dreamweaver in code mode, Notepad, TextWrangler, or NetBeans.

If you are following along with the Case Study, you need your files from the end of Lesson 17. Alternatively, you can download the files from the book's website at www.wrox.com.

Hints

Static properties and functions belong to the class, not to individual objects. Normally when you refer to properties or functions within a class, you use the $this->propertyname construction. The $this refers to the objects' values so when you don't have an object, you have no $this. Use self::$ instead.

Step-by-Step

In the Case Study, create a database class to connect to the smithside database.

1. Create a file called **database.php** in the includes/classes folder.

2. Create a class called **Database**:

```php
<?php
/**
 * Database class
 * For one point of database access
 */
class Database
{
// rest of the code will go here
}
```

3. Within the class, create properties for the username, password, database, and hostname. Default the properties to the appropriate values. These values won't change and they should only be seen inside the class, so make them private and static. Because they are private, start the class names with an underscore.

```php
/**
 * User name to connect to database
 * @var string $_mysqlUser
 */
private static $_mysqlUser = 'php24sql';
/**
 * Password to connect to database
 * @var string $_mysqlPass
 */
private static $_mysqlPass = 'hJQV8RTe5t';
/**
 * Database name
 * @var string $_mysqlDb
 */
private static $_mysqlDb = 'smithside';
/**
 * Hostname for the server
 * @var string $_hostName
```

```
*/
private static $_hostName = 'localhost';
```

4. You also need a property called $_connection to hold the actual connection:

```
/**
 * Database connection
 * @var Mysqli $connection
 */
private static $_connection = NULL;
```

5. Set up a public static function called getConnection(). Connect to the database using the object-oriented mysqli extension. The new object is assigned to the $_connection property. If there is an error, print the error and end the program. Return the connection. Because this is a static method, use the self::$propertyname construction to refer to the properties.

```
/**
 * Get the Database Connection
 *
 * @return Mysqli
 */
public static function getConnection() {
  self::$_connection =
    new mysqli(self::$_hostName, self::$_mysqlUser, self::$_mysqlPass,
      self::$_mysqlDb);
  if (self::$_connection->connect_error) {
      die('Connect Error: ' . self::$_connection->connect_error);

  }
  return self::$_connection;
}
```

6. You want to do the connection only once so surround the connection with an if statement that checks to be sure there is no connection before it tries to connect. The full getConnection() method looks like the following code:

```
public static function getConnection() {
  if (!self::$_connection) {
    self::$_connection = @new mysqli(self::$_hostName, self::$_mysqlUser,
      self::$_mysqlPass, self::$_mysqlDb);
    if (self::$_connection->connect_error) {
      die('Connect Error: ' . self::$_connection->connect_error);
    }
  }
  return self::$_connection;
}
```

7. You want to control this class so that it cannot be used to create an object using the new Database construct. Making the __construct() method a private method prevents that.

```
/**
 * Constructor
 */
private function __construct(){
}
```

To test your database class, temporarily display a statement on the Home page on the Case Study to show what database you are connected to.

1. In the `index.php` file, find `<div class="message">`. Enter all the following code in that div. Get the connection by making a static call to the `Database` class `getConnection()` method.

    ```php
    <?php
    $connection = Database::getConnection();
    ```

2. `SHOW DATABASE()` is the MySQL command to display the database name. Enter the following data to run the command:

    ```php
    if ($result = $connection->query("SELECT DATABASE()")) {
      $row = $result->fetch_array(MYSQLI_NUM);
      echo '<p>*** Using database ' . $row[0] . ' ***</p>';
    } ?>
    ```

3. Run the program. Your results should look similar to Figure 20-6.

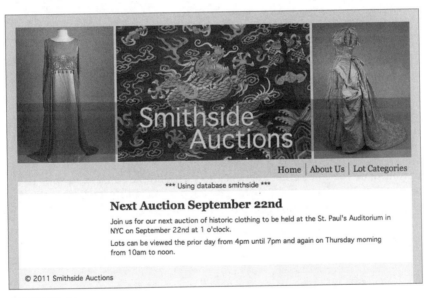

FIGURE 20-6

4. Remove the test message from `index.php` that you just added in steps 1 and 2.

 Watch the video for Lesson 20 on the DVD or watch online at www.wrox.com/ go/24phpmysql.

21

Creating Tables

In this lesson you learn how to set up detail specifications of MySQL tables. First you learn about the different data types and attributes and then you learn how to use that information to create the tables.

You learn what the different data types are and how to assign them to fields. You learn how to set up a field so that it is automatically assigned a value when a row is added, whether that is a MySQL-calculated value to be used as an arbitrary key or a constant value to be used as a default.

You also learn advanced functions in phpMyAdmin to create and change tables and how to do the same thing in PHP. Finally, you learn how to create and use a text file to perform MySQL commands.

UNDERSTANDING DATA TYPES

Just as in PHP, MySQL has different data types for the fields. The data types in MySQL are stricter than in PHP and there is not a one-to-one correlation.

Strings

There are two types of strings in MySQL. The first is text strings, which have character sets and collations. This is the type of string that you use most often. Text strings are further defined as follows:

➤ CHAR: This is the character data type. You define exactly how many characters are stored. For example, if you want a field to be exactly six characters long, you define it as CHAR(6). If you pass it data that is less than that, it pads with spaces at the end. If you pass it more, the extra characters are truncated. Whether you are truncating blanks or non-blank characters and what error reporting you have set determines what, if any, errors you see. You can go all the way up to 255 characters. Note that some character

sets require more than 1 byte to store some characters. The size limits for the text strings are based on the number of characters, not the number of bytes. Trailing spaces are removed when you retrieve the data.

➤ VARCHAR: This data type has a variable number of characters. You specify the maximum number of characters, up to 65,535. If you have a field that could contain up to 50 characters but would likely contain less, you define it as VARCHAR(50). There is a little overhead when using VARCHAR rather than CHAR because 1 or 2 bytes are used to store the length. Trailing spaces are not removed when you retrieve the data.

➤ TEXT: There are four TEXT types — TINYTEXT, TEXT, MEDIUMTEXT, and LONGTEXT. Like VARCHAR, the TEXT types contain a variable number of characters. The difference between the four types is the maximum number of characters. The type defines the maximum number of characters; you do not. See Table 21-1.

TABLE 21-1: TEXT Type Sizes

TEXT TYPE	MAXIMUM CHARACTERS
TINYTEXT	255
TEXT	64K
MEDIUMTEXT	16M
LONGTEXT	4G

The second type of string is binary strings, which have no character sets or collations. Character strings contain text, whereas binary strings contain raw data such as images and other media. The binary types are subdivided in the same way that the text strings are, but the size limits are based on the number of bytes, not the number of characters.

➤ BINARY: This is the binary data type. You define exactly how many bytes are stored. For example, if you want a field to be exactly 6 bytes long, you define it as BINARY(6). You can go all the way up to 255 bytes.

➤ VARBINARY: This data type has a variable number of bytes. You specify the maximum number of bytes, up to 65,535. If you have a field that could contain up to 50 bytes but would likely contain less, you define it as VARBINARY(50). There is a little overhead when using VARBINARY rather than CHAR because 1 or 2 bytes are used to store the length.

➤ BLOB: There are four BLOB types — TINYBLOB, BLOB, MEDIUMBLOB, and LONGBLOB. Like VARBINARY, the BLOB types contain a variable number of bytes. The difference between the four types is the maximum number of bytes. The type defines the maximum number of bytes; you do not. See Table 21-2.

TABLE 21-2: BLOB Type Sizes

BLOB TYPE	MAXIMUM BYTES
TINYBLOB	255
BLOB	64K
MEDIUMBLOB	16M
LONGBLOB	4G

Numeric

As in PHP, numbers that do not have a decimal point are integers. MySQL has different integer types that are based on the size of the integer. Additionally, if the integer is SIGNED — that is, has both negative and positive values — the range starts in the negative numbers. If the field is flagged as UNSIGNED, the values start at 0 and go twice as high, as you see in Table 21-3.

TABLE 21-3: Integer Types

INTEGER TYPE	RANGE IF SIGNED	RANGE IF UNSIGNED
TINYINT	–128 to 127	0 to 255
SMALLINT	–32,768 to 32,767	0 to 65,535
MEDIUMINT	–8,388,608 to 8,388,607	0 to 16,777,215
INT (or INTEGER)	–2,147,483,648 to 2,147,483,647	0 to 4,294,967,295
BIGINT	–9,223,372,036,854,775,808 to 9,223,372,036,854,775,807	0 to 18,446,744,073,709,551,615

You may see these types written with a length such as TINYINT(1) or TINYINT(4). This refers to the number of digits to be displayed. It does not affect the value that is stored or the space needed to store the value.

If you need decimals you use either a floating-point data type or a fixed-point data type. The floating-point types are similar to PHP floating-point types. FLOAT uses 4 bytes of storage and DOUBLE (also called DOUBLE PRECISION or REAL) takes 8. MySQL allows you to specify the total number of digits and the number of digits after the decimal point. So to specify a number between –999.9999 and 999.9999 you use FLOAT(7,4). MySQL rounds the decimal when storing it rather than truncating it if it is too long.

Just as in PHP, floating-point numbers are inexact because of how the computer stores them. You use the exact value data type of DECIMAL (also called NUMERIC) if you need to store exact numbers. Exact values take up more room than the floating-point numbers. Currency is often stored using the decimal format. As with the FLOAT data type, you can specify the total number of digits and the number of digits after the decimal point. DECIMAL(10,2) has a range of –99999999.99 to 99999999.99.

> ⊗ *The* DECIMAL *data type has been evolving in MySQL to come closer to the SQL standard. You may come across different behaviors in earlier versions of MySQL.*

Date and Time

MySQL stores dates and times in the format of YYYY-MM-DD HH:MM:SS, unlike PHP. Your MySQL server dictates where you can store invalid dates or whether all invalid dates should be converted to zeros.

> ➤ DATETIME contains the date and the time. It has a range from the year 1000 through the year 9999.

> ➤ DATE contains just the date value.

> ➤ You can use TIMESTAMP to automatically contain the initial value or automatically update when something changes on the row. It has a range from 1970 through early 2038. It stores all values as of the UTC time zone.

> ➤ TIME displays the time portion of a date or an elapsed time.

> ➤ YEAR displays the year. It can be either YEAR(2) or YEAR(4) for two- or four-digit representation of the year. It has a range from the year 1901 through 2155. Two digits between 00 and 69 are converted to 2000 through 2069 and 70 to 99 are converted to 1970 through 1999.

You can specify dates and times in several ways. Here are examples for January 8, 2013, at 8:30 a.m. Remember that the # starts a comment.

```
'2013-01-08 08:30:00' # the full information
'13-01-08 08:30:00'   # two digit year is fine
'13-1-8 8:30'         # you do not need leading zeros
'13^1+8 8/30'         # any punctuation works
'130108083000'        # no delimiters is fine
'13.01.08' # just the date, if that's all you need
'13/01/00' # you can use 00 for a missing part (not TIMESTAMP)
```

If you are updating TIME, using colons indicates a time rather than elapsed time:

```
'0830' # is an elapsed time of 8 mins, 30 secs
'08:30' # is 8:30 am
```

Other Data Types

MySQL has a data type ENUM that restricts the field to values from an enumerated list of values. Although you can use numbers as values, it is not recommended because errors can easily occur. Numbers can be misinterpreted as an index of a value instead of the value itself.

```
ENUM('small', 'medium', 'large')
```

Although you can put your business logic here, if there's any chance it might change, it would be better to put the value checking in your program where it would be easier to make changes.

MySQL has two other data types that you may come across:

➤ SET includes zero or more values from a defined list.

➤ BIT stores data at the bit level using binary values.

USING AUTO_INCREMENT

You learned in Lesson 18 that the primary key for a table should have the following characteristics:

➤ Unique

➤ Not Null

➤ Not optional

➤ Never needs to be changed

➤ Does not violate security policies

In addition, a short simple key that can be retrieved quickly helps performance. It can be difficult to find a data field that meets all of these requirements. For that reason, tables are often given artificial keys — arbitrary keys that have no meaning other than to be a primary key.

MySQL supports this policy with the AUTO_INCREMENT attribute. You assign this attribute to a field and MySQL generates a unique sequential number for each new row. You can assign AUTO_INCREMENT to either an integer or a floating-point data type, though an integer is the most common. Make sure that the data type you choose is large enough to hold the highest number you need. The following snippet of code shows the typical specifications for an artificial primary key. The name of the field is id; it is an integer data type that is unsigned, is a required field, will be automatically filled by MySQL, and is assigned as the primary key.

```
`id` INT UNSIGNED NOT NULL AUTO_INCREMENT PRIMARY KEY,
```

The table keeps track of the next number to be assigned. It starts with 1 unless you tell it differently when you create the table.

In Lesson 22, you learn how to add data to the tables. When you add the data, if you do not assign a value to id for new rows, or you assign a NULL or 0, a value is automatically assigned. MySQL

has a function, `LAST_INSERT_ID()`, that contains the last `AUTO_INCREMENT` value. PHP also has a function that can retrieve this number if you need it.

UNDERSTANDING DEFAULTS

Default values are used to automatically assign a value to a field when you create a new row and you do not assign a value to that field. If you have a required field (`NOT NULL`), you should either always assign a value through your program, assign a default, or, in appropriate cases, set it up as `AUTO_INCREMENT`.

Defaults must be constants. You cannot use MySQL functions, except that you can define a field of the `TIMESTAMP` data type to default to `CURRENT_TIMESTAMP`. The following line of code, included when you create a table, creates a field called `dept` that is up to 20 characters long, is required, and defaults to `Office` on new rows unless a different value is assigned:

```
`dept` VARCHAR(20) NOT NULL DEFAULT 'Office',
```

The following code is for a field called `startdate` that is a date, is required, and defaults to zeros on new rows unless a different value is assigned:

```
`startdate` DATE NOT NULL DEFAULT '0000-00-00'
```

A field does not need to be required to have a default. The following code is for a field called `display_number` that is an integer with a maximum range of 255 that defaults to 20:

```
`display_number` TINYINT UNSIGNED NULL DEFAULT '20'
```

Defaults are not allowed on the `TEXT` or the `BLOB` types. If you need to assign a default and the size permits it, create the field as a `VARCHAR` or `VARBINARY` data type instead.

There are implicit defaults on some data types. These implicit defaults are used if you don't assign a value or you assign the value of `NULL` and you have no explicit default. If you have `NOT NULL` specified and the implicit default has to be used, you get an error depending on the strictness of your error reporting. These are the implicit defaults:

➤ Numeric data types default to 0

➤ Date and time (except for `TIMESTAMP`) are set to the appropriate version of `0000-00-00 00:00:00`

➤ `TIMESTAMP` defaults to the current date and time

➤ Strings default to an empty string

➤ `ENUM` defaults to the first value

CREATING TABLES IN PHPMYADMIN

Now that you understand the details behind creating fields, go back to phpMyAdmin and create another table in the test database. You did this in Lesson 19, but now you should understand what you are doing. Open phpMyAdmin and select the test database or create a new database. Your window should look similar to Figure 21-1.

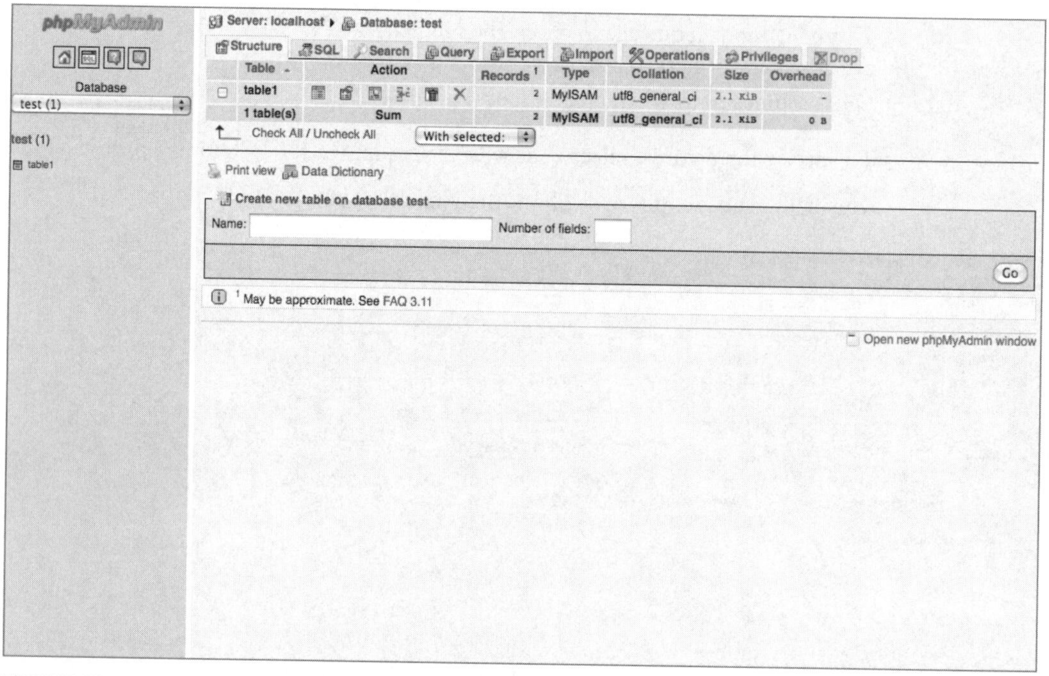

FIGURE 21-1

You create a table called `products` with the following fields: `id`, `product`, `description`, `source`, `date_created`.

Type in the new table name **products** and the number of fields as **5** and click the Go button.

Enter the following information in the five fields as shown in Figure 21-2:

➤ `id`: integer, unsigned, required, auto increment (primary key)

➤ Select UNSIGNED under the Attribute drop-down.

➤ Required is the same as NOT NULL, so do not check the Null checkbox.

➤ AUTO_INCREMENT is the A.I. checkbox. Check that box.

➤ This is the primary key, so select PRIMARY from the Index drop-down.

➤ `product:` up to 20 characters, required

➤ `description:` long description, required

➤ `source:` up to 20 characters, default to `External`

    ➤ To specify the default, select `As Defined` in the Default drop-down and then type **External**.

    ➤ This field is not required, so check the Null checkbox.

➤ `date_created:` timestamp when created

    ➤ To specify the default, select `CURRENT_TIMESTAMP` in the Default drop-down.

    ➤ This field is not required, so check the Null checkbox.

Field	Type ⓘ	Length/Values¹	Default²	Collation	Attributes	Null	Index	A_I	
id	INT		None		UNSIGNED	☐	PRIMARY	☑	
product	VARCHAR	20	None			☐	---	☐	
description	TEXT		None			☐	---	☐	
source	VARCHAR	20	As defined: External			☑	---	☐	
date_created	TIMESTAMP		CURRENT_TIMESTAMP			☑	---	☐	

Table comments: Storage Engine: ⓘ   MyISAM   Collation:

PARTITION definition: ⓘ

                                                                (Save) Or Add 1   field(s) (Go)

¹ If field type is "enum" or "set", please enter the values using this format: 'a','b','c'...
ⓘ If you ever need to put a backslash ("\") or a single quote ("'") amongst those values, precede it with a backslash (for example '\\xyz' or 'a\'b').
² For default values, please enter just a single value, without backslash escaping or quotes, using this format: a

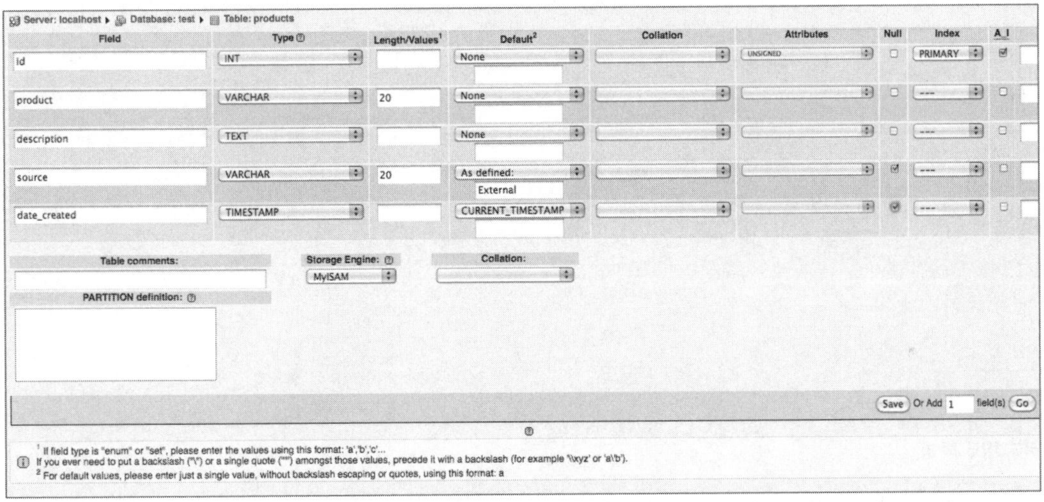

FIGURE 21-2

Below the list of fields are the attributes for the table itself. You should already be familiar with the collation from creating databases. Usually you can leave this blank. It defaults to the database collation.

The Storage Engine either defaults to MyISAM or to InnoDB. You can think of storage engines like the engines in a car. Different engines are good for different things. MySQL has several engines each with their own capabilities; the most common are MyISAM and InnoDB. MyISAM has been the default for many years. It's a very good basic engine with very good performance. InnoDB has more capabilities, but those capabilities can come with a performance hit. If you create applications with complex transactions, you should use InnoDB. For the database you are creating for this website, MyISAM is a good choice. The newest versions of MySQL are now shipping with InnoDB as the default.

Click the Save button to create the table. You see a window similar to Figure 21-3.

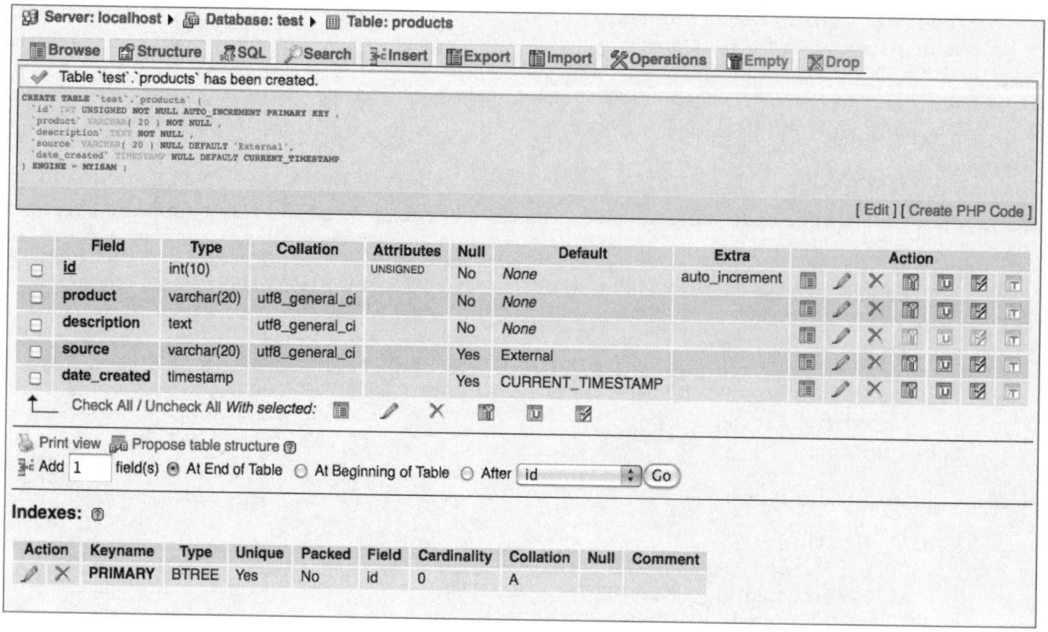

FIGURE 21-3

The MySQL command that was used to create the table is displayed at the top of the window. Copy that and paste it into a text file for the next section.

If you need to change fields after you have created them, go to the Structure tab and click the pencil icon for the field you want to change. Make your changes and click the Save button. To add fields, use the Add fields form below the list of fields as shown in Figure 21-4.

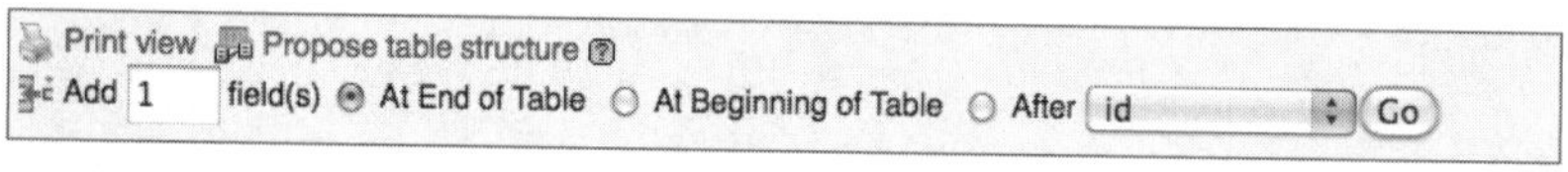

FIGURE 21-4

To add fields, select the number of fields that you want to add and whether they are to be added at the end of the table, at the beginning of the table, or after a given existing field. Click the Go button to go to the form to add fields. Enter the information for the fields and click the Save button to create the fields.

To change table attributes, go to the Operations tab, where you can change the name, the engine, the next AUTO_INCREMENT value to use, and the collation.

USING .SQL SCRIPT FILES

In the preceding section you created a table using phpMyAdmin. You copied the following code to a text file:

```
CREATE TABLE `test`.`products` (
`id` INT UNSIGNED NOT NULL AUTO_INCREMENT PRIMARY KEY ,
```

```
`product` VARCHAR( 20 ) NOT NULL ,
`description` TEXT NOT NULL ,
`source` VARCHAR( 20 ) NULL DEFAULT 'External',
`date_created` TIMESTAMP NULL DEFAULT CURRENT_TIMESTAMP
) ENGINE = MYISAM ;
```

The online MySQL manual uses 200 lines to show the syntax of the CREATE TABLE command at http://dev.mysql.com/doc/refman/5.6/en/create-table.html. This is a simplified version:

```
CREATE [TEMPORARY] TABLE [IF NOT EXISTS] tbl_name (
    col_name data_type [NOT NULL | NULL] [DEFAULT default_value]
      [AUTO_INCREMENT] [UNIQUE [KEY] | [PRIMARY] KEY]
      [COMMENT 'string'],
    col_name data_type [NOT NULL | NULL] [DEFAULT default_value]
      [AUTO_INCREMENT] [UNIQUE [KEY] | [PRIMARY] KEY]
      [COMMENT 'string']
) table_options;
```

Here are the valid data types:

```
    BIT[(length)]
  | TINYINT[(length)] [UNSIGNED] [ZEROFILL]
  | SMALLINT[(length)] [UNSIGNED] [ZEROFILL]
  | MEDIUMINT[(length)] [UNSIGNED] [ZEROFILL]
  | INT[(length)] [UNSIGNED] [ZEROFILL]
  | INTEGER[(length)] [UNSIGNED] [ZEROFILL]
  | BIGINT[(length)] [UNSIGNED] [ZEROFILL]
  | REAL[(length,decimals)] [UNSIGNED] [ZEROFILL]
  | DOUBLE[(length,decimals)] [UNSIGNED] [ZEROFILL]
  | FLOAT[(length,decimals)] [UNSIGNED] [ZEROFILL]
  | DECIMAL[(length[,decimals])] [UNSIGNED] [ZEROFILL]
  | NUMERIC[(length[,decimals])] [UNSIGNED] [ZEROFILL]
  | DATE
  | TIME
  | TIMESTAMP
  | DATETIME
  | YEAR
  | CHAR[(length)]
      [CHARACTER SET charset_name] [COLLATE collation_name]
  | VARCHAR(length)
      [CHARACTER SET charset_name] [COLLATE collation_name]
  | BINARY[(length)]
  | VARBINARY(length)
  | TINYBLOB
  | BLOB
  | MEDIUMBLOB
  | LONGBLOB
  | TINYTEXT [BINARY]
      [CHARACTER SET charset_name] [COLLATE collation_name]
  | TEXT [BINARY]
      [CHARACTER SET charset_name] [COLLATE collation_name]
  | MEDIUMTEXT [BINARY]
      [CHARACTER SET charset_name] [COLLATE collation_name]
  | LONGTEXT [BINARY]
      [CHARACTER SET charset_name] [COLLATE collation_name]
  | ENUM(value1,value2,value3,...)
      [CHARACTER SET charset_name] [COLLATE collation_name]
```

```
| SET(value1,value2,value3,...)
   [CHARACTER SET charset_name] [COLLATE collation_name]
| spatial_type
```

Here are some common table options:

```
ENGINE [=] engine_name
AUTO_INCREMENT [=] value
[DEFAULT] CHARACTER SET [=] charset_name
[DEFAULT] COLLATE [=] collation_name;
```

Words in uppercase are keywords and words in lowercase are to be replaced with the actual values. The keywords do not need to be in uppercase, though it is convention to use uppercase for them. In some cases, such as `tbl_name` and `col_name`, you can put anything as long as it conforms to the proper naming requirements. In other cases, such as `data_type` and `engine_name`, you are restricted to actual data types and engines.

Items in the square brackets (`[]`) are optional, choices are separated by the pipe symbol (`|`), and the list of fields is contained within the parentheses. This example shows two fields but you can enter as many fields as you need. Commas separate the fields and there is no comma before the final parenthesis. After the list of fields come the table attributes, which are separated by commas. The command ends with a semicolon.

You can create temporary tables by using the TEMPORARY keyword. The table is automatically deleted when the connection is closed and can be seen only by that connection.

If you try to create a table and it already exists you get an error unless you have specified IF NOT EXISTS. If the table exists and you have added IF NOT EXISTS, the new table is not created and you get no error message. Any commands that follow — for instance, to add rows — work on the already existing table. There is no way in MySQL to verify that the table has the same structure. If you want to totally replace any table that exists, use the DROP TABLE `tbl_name` command before CREATE TABLE IF NOT EXISTS `tbl_name`.

The table name can be just the table name, if it is in the default database, or you can specify the database using the dot notation:

```
CREATE TABLE `mydatabase`.`myproduct`
```

If you quote the names, remember that the quote is a back tick (`` ` ``) not a single quote (`'`) and that you quote the database and the table separately.

In the text file you created, change the name of the `products` table to **products2** and save the file with a `.sql` extension. The extension is just a convention. You could call it anything you want, but the `.sql` extension lets you and other programmers know that the file consists of SQL commands. The export file that you created in the prior lesson was the same type of `.sql` file.

Go to phpMyAdmin, select the database, and go to the Import tab. Browse for the text file you just saved. You see a window that looks similar to Figure 21-5.

Click the Go button to run the commands in the `.sql` file to create the `products2` table. Click the `products2` table that appears on the left column to see the list of fields shown in Figure 21-6.

By putting your commands in a file, you can save them, modify them, and rerun them when needed. This is a good place to put those commands that you need to create your database for your application in case you need to re-create it.

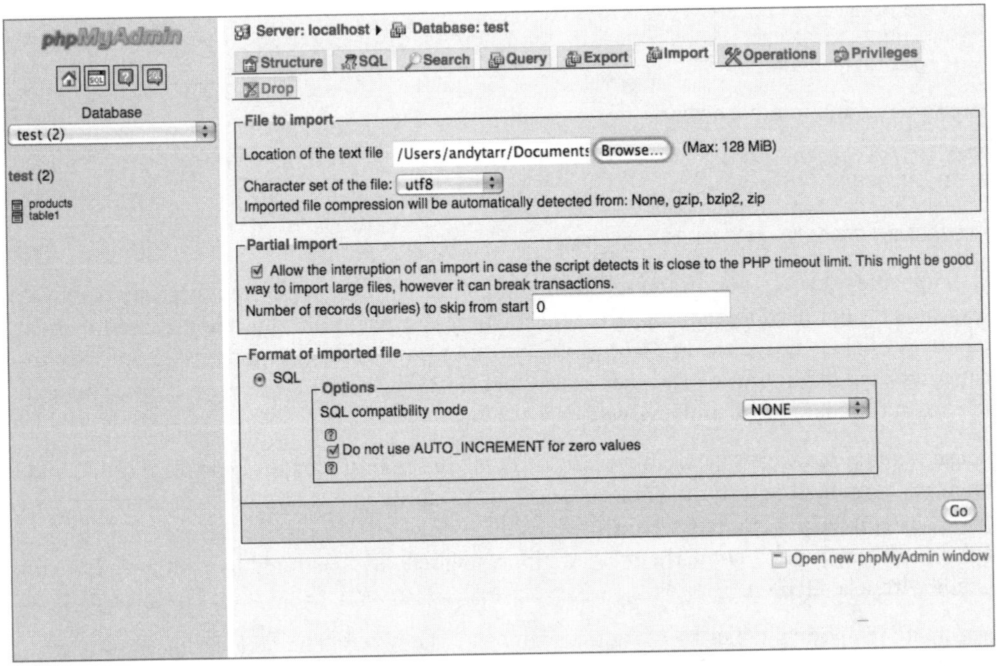

FIGURE 21-5

To change a table after it has been created, use the `ALTER TABLE` command. Many of the specifications are the same as for creating a table. For the details, see the online MySQL manual at `http://dev.mysql.com/doc/refman/5.6/en/alter-table.html`.

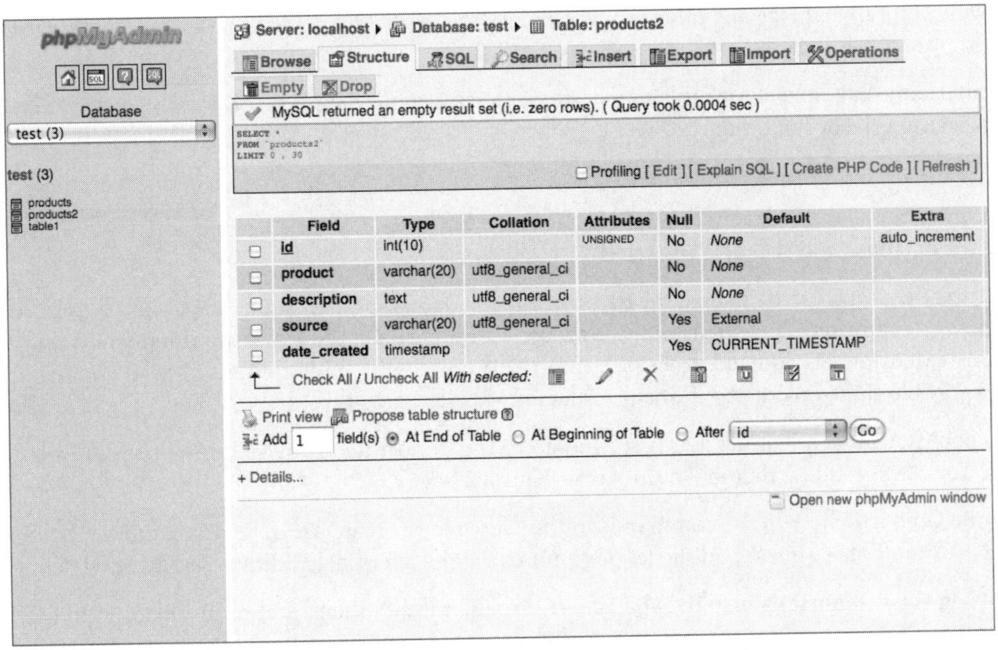

FIGURE 21-6

ADDING MYSQL TABLES TO PHP

Normally you create the tables for your application ahead of time either through a program like phpMyAdmin or by running a `.sql` file. However, there are times when you want to create them within your PHP program. If you do create tables in a PHP program, the MySQL user needs the structure privilege of CREATE. For this example, use your root user. Use the following steps:

1. Make a connection to the database.

2. Create a safe query with the command.

3. Run the query.

The following code uses the same MySQL command as in the previous section to create the table `products3`. You could just enclose the command in double quotes and assign it to the `$query` variable. It is not good practice to have extremely long lines and in practice you might need to add in PHP variables. You can use double quotes around appropriate sections of the command and put them back together with the concatenation operator (`.`). The `query()` method does only one statement at a time and does not use a semicolon at the end of the MySQL statement. Your results should look similar to Figure 21-7.

```php
<?php
define("MYSQLUSER", "root");
define("MYSQLPASS", "p##V89Te5t");
define("HOSTNAME", "localhost");
define("MYSQLDB", "test");

// Make connection to database
$connection = @new mysqli(HOSTNAME, MYSQLUSER, MYSQLPASS, MYSQLDB);
if ($connection->connect_error) {
  die('Connect Error: ' . $connection->connect_error);
} else {
  echo 'Successful connection to MySQL <br />';
  // Create the MySQL command by copying the command and
  // splitting into shorter lines and concatenating with periods
  // Drop the final semicolon on the MySQL commmand
  // but don't forget the semicolon for ending the PHP command
  $query = "CREATE TABLE `test`.`products3` ( "
    . "`id` INT UNSIGNED NOT NULL AUTO_INCREMENT PRIMARY KEY , "
    . "`product` VARCHAR( 20 ) NOT NULL , "
    . "`description` TEXT NOT NULL , "
    . "`source` VARCHAR( 20 ) NULL DEFAULT 'External', "
    . "`date_created` TIMESTAMP NULL DEFAULT CURRENT_TIMESTAMP"
    . ") ENGINE = MYISAM";
  // Run the query and display appropriate message
  if (!$result = $connection->query($query)) {
    echo "Unable to create table<br />";
  } else {
    echo "Table successfully created<br />";
  }
  // Show the tables
  if ($result = $connection->query("SHOW TABLES")) {
    $count = $result->num_rows;
    echo "Tables: ($count)<br />";
    while ($row =$result->fetch_array()) {
```

```
            echo $row[0]. '<br />';
        }
    }
}
```

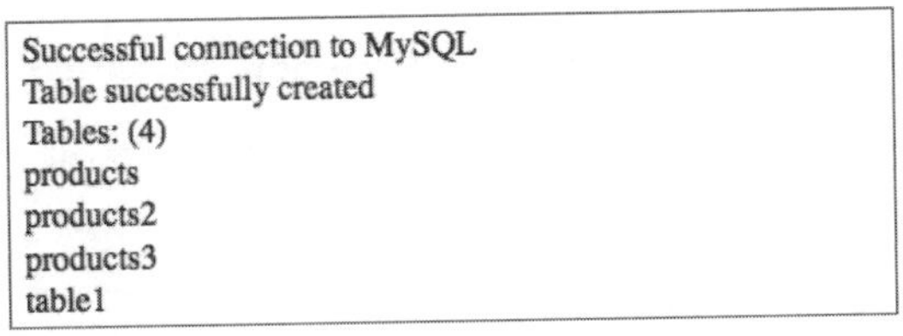

```
Successful connection to MySQL
Table successfully created
Tables: (4)
products
products2
products3
table1
```

FIGURE 21-7

TRY IT

In this Try It, you create the tables for the lots and lot categories in the Case Study using the database analysis you created in Lesson 18.

You use the classes corresponding to the tables in the Case Study, so this is a good time to start creating the classes for the lots and lot categories.

You created a class for the contacts in a Lesson 13 and then in Lesson 19 you created the table. In this Try It, you add the missing table fields to the Contact class.

> *You can download the code and resources for this Try It from the book's web page at www.wrox.com. You can find them in the Lesson21 folder in the download. You will find code for both before and after completing the exercises.*

Lesson Requirements

Your computer needs to be able to run as a web server with PHP and MySQL. XAMPP is a package of software that installs the web server, PHP, and MySQL for you. You can find instructions for downloading and installing XAMPP in Lesson 1.

You need a text editor that can produce plain-text files. You can find instructions for downloading and installing Eclipse PDT in Lesson 1. Other text editors that you can use are Adobe's Dreamweaver in code mode, Notepad, TextWrangler, or NetBeans.

If you are following along with the Case Study, you need your files from the end of Lesson 20. Alternatively, you can download the files from the book's website at www.wrox.com.

Hints

Code to create the contacts, categories, and lots tables is in the `install.sql` file in the downloadable code.

You can use the `includes/classes/contact.php` file as a basis for your new classes.

Step-by-Step

Create the `categories` and `lots` tables.

1. Based on the database analysis from Lesson 18, create the `categories` table with the following characteristics:

Table: `categories`

`cat_id`: Integer, positive number, required, primary key, auto increment

`cat_name`: Text, up to 50 characters long, required

`cat_description`: Text, up to 5 or 6 lines of text

`cat_image`: Text, up to 255 for the name of the file

You can use the graphical interface in phpMyAdmin, copy the following code into the SQL tab for the Case Study database, or copy the code to a `.sql` file and import it.

```
CREATE TABLE `smithside`.`categories` (
`cat_id` INT UNSIGNED NOT NULL AUTO_INCREMENT PRIMARY KEY,
`cat_name` VARCHAR(50) NOT NULL,
`cat_description` TEXT NULL,
`cat_image` VARCHAR(255) NULL
) ENGINE = MYISAM;
```

2. Based on the database analysis from Lesson 18, create the `lots` table with the following characteristics:

Table: `lots`

`lot_id`: Integer, positive number, required, primary key, auto increment

`lot_name`: Text, up to 50 characters long, required

`lot_description`: Text, up to 5 or 6 lines of text

`lot_image`: Text, up to 255 for the name of the file

`lot_number`: Integer, positive number

`lot_price`: Numeric, up to $100,000.00, default to 0

`cat_id`: Integer, positive number, link to `categories` table

You can use either the graphical interface in phpMyAdmin, copy the following code into the SQL tab for the Case Study database, or copy the code to a `.sql` file and import it.

```
CREATE TABLE `lots` (
  `lot_id` INT(11) UNSIGNED NOT NULL AUTO_INCREMENT PRIMARY KEY,
  `lot_name` varchar(50) NOT NULL,
  `lot_description` TEXT NULL,
  `lot_image` VARCHAR(255) NULL,
  `lot_number` INT(11) UNSIGNED NULL,
  `lot_price` DECIMAL(10,2) DEFAULT '0' NULL,
  `cat_id` INT(11) UNSIGNED NULL
) ENGINE=MyISAM
```

Create `category.php` and `lot.php` in the includes/classes folder with classes for each of the tables.

1. Create the file `includes/classes/category.php`.

2. Enter the file documentation and the `Category` class:

```php
<?php
/**
 * category.php
 *
 * Category class file
 *
 * @version    1.2 2011-02-03
 * @package    Smithside Auctions
 * @copyright  Copyright (c) 2011 Smithside Auctions
 * @license    GNU General Public License
 * @since      Since Release 1.0
 */
/**
 * Category class
 *
 * @package    Smithside Auctions
 */
class Category
{
}
```

2. Inside the class, add a property for each of the fields in the `categories` table. Make these protected properties.

```php
/**
 * Category ID
 * @var int
 */
protected $cat_id;

/**
 * Category Name
 * @var string
 */
protected $cat_name;

/**
 * Category Description
 * @var string
 */
```

```
protected $cat_description;

/**
 * Category Image path
 * @var string
 */
protected $cat_image;
```

3. Following the properties, add a __construct method to fill the properties based on an array input:

```
/**
 * Initialize the Item
 * @param array
 */
public function __construct($input = false) {
  if (is_array($input)) {
    foreach ($input as $key => $val) {
      // Note the $key instead of key.
      // This will give the value in $key instead of 'key' itself
      $this->$key = $val;
    }
  }
}
```

4. Add in methods to get the protected properties:

```
/**
 * Return Category ID
 * @return int
 */
public function getCat_id() {
  return $this->cat_id;
}

/**
 * Return Category Name
 * @return string
 */
public function getCat_name() {
  return $this->cat_name;
}

/**
 * Return Category Description
 * @return string
 */
public function getCat_description() {
  return $this->cat_description;
}

/**
 * Return Category Image path
 * @return string
 */
public function getCat_image() {
  return $this->cat_image;
}
```

5. Create a similar file for the `lots` table. This file is `includes/classes/lot.php`.

```php
<?php
/**
 * lot.php
 *
 * Lot class file
 *
 * @version    1.2 2011-02-03
 * @package    Smithside Auctions
 * @copyright  Copyright (c) 2011 Smithside Auctions
 * @license    GNU General Public License
 * @since      Since Release 1.0
 */
/**
 * Lot class
 *
 * @package    Smithside Auctions
 */
class Lot
{
    /**
     * Lot ID
     * @var int
     */
    protected $lot_id;

    /**
     * Lot Name
     * @var string
     */
    protected $lot_name;

    /**
     * Lot Description
     * @var string
     */
    protected $lot_description;

    /**
     * Lot Image path
     * @var string
     */
    protected $lot_image;

    /**
     * Lot Number
     * @var int
     */
    protected $lot_number;

    /**
     * Lot Price path
```

```
     * @var float
     */
    protected $lot_price;

    /**
     * Lot Catalog ID
     * @var int
     */
    protected $cat_id;

    /**
     * Initialize the Item
     * @param array
     */
    public function __construct($input = false) {
        if (is_array($input)) {
            foreach ($input as $key => $val) {
                // Note the $key instead of key.
                // This will give the value in $key instead of 'key' itself
                $this->$key = $val;
            }
        }
    }

    /**
     * Return Lot ID
     * @return int
     */
    public function getLot_id() {
        return $this->lot_id;
    }

    /**
     * Return Lot Name
     * @return string
     */
    public function getLot_name() {
        return $this->lot_name;
    }

    /**
     * Return Lot Description
     * @return string
     */
    public function getLot_description() {
        return $this->lot_description;
    }

    /**
     * Return Lot Image path
     * @return string
     */
    public function getLot_image() {
```

```
      return $this->lot_image;
  }

  /**
   * Return Lot Price path
   * @return string
   */
  public function getLot_price() {
    return $this->lot_price;
  }

  /**
   * Return Lot Category ID
   * @return string
   */
  public function getCat_id() {
    return $this->cat_id;
  }

}
```

Add the id field to the Contact class in includes/classes/contact.php.

1. Add id as a protected property at the beginning of the Contact class:

```
/**
 * ID
 * @var int
 */
protected $id;
```

2. Add a public getter method to access the id property. Add this at the start of the rest of the getter methods.

```
/**
 * Return ID
 * @return int
 */
public function getId() {
  return $this->id;
}
```

Watch the video for Lesson 21 on the DVD or watch online at www.wrox.com/
go/24phpmysql.

Entering Data

In this lesson you learn how to enter data into the MySQL tables you built. You learn to use both the MySQL INSERT command to add rows and to load a file of information with the LOAD DATA command.

The main way that you get — data from users on websites is through forms. In this lesson you go through the whole process from creating a form, error checking the data, adding the data to the tables, and informing the user of the success or failure of the update. You learn how to use the MySQL commands in a PHP program.

UNDERSTANDING THE INSERT COMMAND

The examples in this section are based on the table1 table that you created in Lesson 19. This is the command that creates that table:

```
CREATE TABLE IF NOT EXISTS 'table1' (
  'id' int(11) NOT NULL AUTO_INCREMENT PRIMARY KEY,
  'description' text,
  'code' int(11) NOT NULL DEFAULT '42'
) ENGINE=MyISAM
```

The MySQL INSERT command adds new rows to a table. You tell MySQL the table to use and then give it the values for all the fields in the new row. The following code creates a new row, assigning 1 as the value of the first field, abc as the value of the second field, and 15 as the value of the third field:

```
INSERT INTO 'table1' VALUES ('101','abc','15');
```

The name of the table is enclosed with back ticks, which is optional for simple names. Enclose the value in quotes, regardless of whether the value is text or numeric. The quotes can be either single or double quotes. If there is a quote as part of the value, you must either use the other type of quote to enclose it, double the quote, or escape the quote in the value. To escape

a quote, prefix it with a backslash (\). All of the following methods work when the value of the second field is a'bc:

```
INSERT INTO 'table1' VALUES ("102","a'bc","15");
INSERT INTO 'table1' VALUES ('103','a''bc','15');
INSERT INTO 'table1' VALUES ('104','a\'bc','15');
```

To add more than one row at a time, add additional parentheses groups separated by commas. This code adds three more rows:

```
INSERT INTO 'table1' VALUES ('105','def','23'), ('106', 'ghi','23'), ↵
('107', 'jkl','15');
```

If a field has the AUTO_INCREMENT attribute, MySQL automatically assigns the next number if you assign a 0, empty quotes, or the keyword NULL. Keywords are not enclosed in quotes. Assuming that the first field has the AUTO_INCREMENT attribute, the following code creates rows with the values of 108, 109, and 110. You can use multiple lines to make the code easier to read.

```
INSERT INTO 'table1' VALUES
('0','mno','15'),
('', 'pqr','23'),
(NULL, 'stu','42');
```

Use the DEFAULT keyword to indicate that the default should be used. If the default for the third field is 42, the following code inserts 42 as the value for the third field:

```
INSERT INTO 'table1' VALUES (NULL,'vwx',DEFAULT);
```

Figure 22-1 shows the rows added by the code in this section as seen in phpMyAdmin.

			101	abc	15
			102	a'bc	15
			103	a'bc	15
			104	a'bc	15
			105	def	23
			106	ghi	23
			107	jkl	15
			113	mno	15
			114	pqr	23
			115	stu	42
			116	vwx	42

FIGURE 22-1

Rather than listing a value for all of the fields, you can list the fields to be added. Any fields not listed use the default as defined in the table definition or the implied default based on the data type. If the missing field is defined as NOT NULL and there is no appropriate default, you get an error. The version of MySQL and the level of error reporting determine exactly what produces errors and whether those errors prevent the command from completing. The following code adds a row with the field description set to yza. The first field defaults with the AUTO_INCREMENT and the last field defaults to the explicit default of 42.

```
INSERT INTO 'table1' ('description') VALUES ('yza');
```

If you try to add a row that has the same primary key as an existing row, you get an error and the row is not added. To prevent the error, add the IGNORE keyword. If a duplicate is found, the new line is ignored without issuing errors or killing the command in the middle. Assuming that a row with the primary key 101 already exists and row 118 does not, the following command ignores the request to add 101 and still adds row 118:

```
INSERT IGNORE INTO 'table1' VALUES ('101','bcd','99'), ('118','efg','23');
```

If you want to do something special if you get a duplicate key, specify ON DUPLICATE KEY UPDATE. MySQL updates the existing record for any duplicates based on what you specify after the UPDATE keyword.

```
INSERT INTO 'table1' VALUES ('101','bcd','15'), ('118','efg','23') ↵
ON DUPLICATE KEY UPDATE code = '99';
```

To replace the row with the new values, you use the REPLACE statement. The REPLACE statement has the same syntax as the INSERT statement. The only difference is that if you try to add a row with the same primary key, the existing row is replaced rather than causing an error message or being ignored.

EXECUTING MYSQL COMMANDS IN PHP

You won't very often create databases or tables using PHP because then the MySQL used to make the database connection has to have extensive privileges, which is unsafe. However, you will frequently add data to MySQL tables using PHP. Entering data through a PHP program using MySQL command takes three steps:

1. Make a connection to the database.

2. Create a safe query with the command.

3. Run the query.

The following code uses the MySQL INSERT command to add rows to the table table1. You could enclose the command in double quotes and assign it to the $query variable. However, it is not good practice to have extremely long lines. Use the double quotes around appropriate sections of the command and put them back together with the concatenation operator (.). The query() method does only one statement at a time and does not use a semicolon at the end of the MySQL statement. Your results look like Figure 22-2. When you look in phpMyAdmin you see the rows in Figure 22-3.

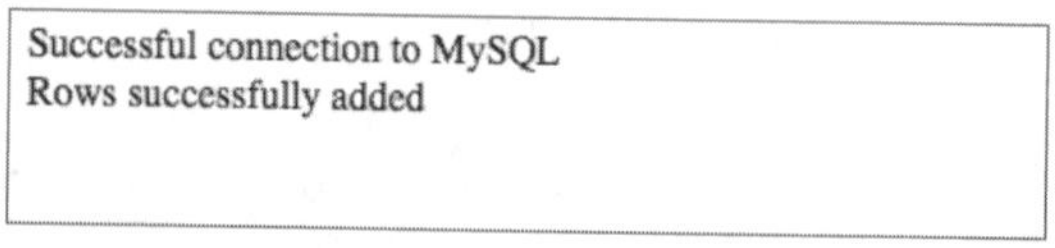

```php
<?php
define("MYSQLUSER", "php24sql");
define("MYSQLPASS", "hJQV8RTe5t");
define("HOSTNAME", "localhost");
define("MYSQLDB", "test");

// Make connection to database
$connection = @new mysqli(HOSTNAME, MYSQLUSER, MYSQLPASS, MYSQLDB);
if ($connection->connect_error) {
  die('Connect Error: ' . $connection->connect_error);
} else {
  echo 'Successful connection to MySQL <br />';
```

```
Successful connection to MySQL
Rows successfully added
```

FIGURE 22-2

```php
// Set up the query
$query = "INSERT INTO 'table1' ('description', 'code') VALUES "
 . " ('hij','15'), "
 . " ('klm','23'), "
 . " ('nop', DEFAULT)";

// Run the query and display appropriate message
if (!$result = $connection->query($query)) {
  echo "Unable to add rows<br />";
} else {
  echo "Rows successfully added<br />";
  }
}
```

☐	✎	✕	120	hij	15
☐	✎	✕	121	klm	23
☐	✎	✕	122	nop	42

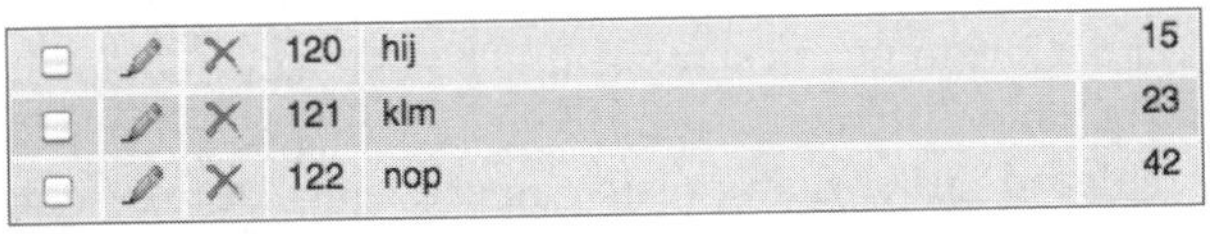

FIGURE 22-3

You can use variables to create the query statement. In the following examples I am hardcoding in the values of the variables to make the examples clearer. In real life these variables may be coming from forms, parameters or other sources. Even though you can see what the value is, assume the value could be anything. The following code is an example where the data passed to MySQL comes from variables. You add the row shown in Figure 22-4.

```php
<?php
define("MYSQLUSER", "php24sql");
define("MYSQLPASS", "hJQV8RTe5t");
define("HOSTNAME", "localhost");
define("MYSQLDB", "test");

// Make connection to database
$connection = @new mysqli(HOSTNAME, MYSQLUSER, MYSQLPASS, MYSQLDB);
if ($connection->connect_error) {
  die('Connect Error: ' . $connection->connect_error);
} else {
  echo 'Successful connection to MySQL <br />';

  $desc = "qrs";
  $code = "15";

  // Set up the query
  $query = "INSERT INTO 'table1' ('description', 'code') VALUES "
   . " ('$desc', '$code')";

  // Run the query and display appropriate message
  if (!$result = $connection->query($query)) {
    echo "Unable to add rows<br />";
  } else {
    echo "Rows successfully added<br />";
  }
}
```

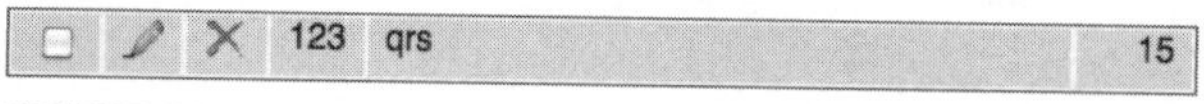

FIGURE 22-4

Earlier in this lesson you learned that you need to put quotes around the values and that you can use either single quotes or double quotes and if you have a quote within the value, you need to either enclose with the opposite type of quote or escape the quote in the value. In the preceding example you have the line `$desc = "qrs";`. If you replace that with `$desc = "qr's";` you might think you are following all the rules and that it will work. However, when you do that, as demonstrated in the following code, the rows do not update because that single quote in `$desc` is then enclosed by single quotes in `$query`, which is invalid in MySQL as shown in Figure 22-5.

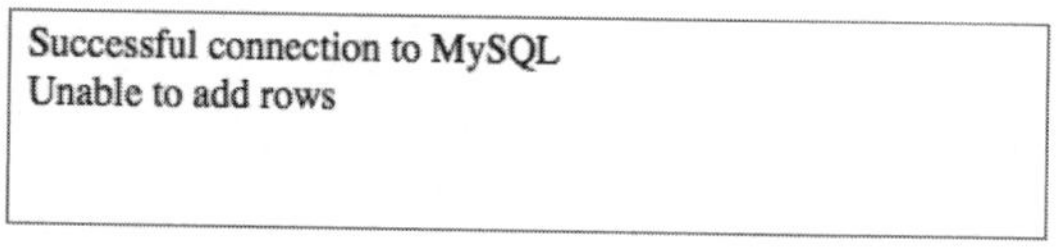

```php
<?php
define("MYSQLUSER", "php24sql");
define("MYSQLPASS", "hJQV8RTe5t");
define("HOSTNAME", "localhost");
define("MYSQLDB", "test");

// Make connection to database
$connection = @new mysqli(HOSTNAME, MYSQLUSER, MYSQLPASS, MYSQLDB);
if ($connection->connect_error) {
  die('Connect Error: ' . $connection->connect_error);
} else {
  echo 'Successful connection to MySQL <br />';

  $desc = "qr's";
  $code = "15";

  // Set up the query
  $query = "INSERT INTO 'table1' ('description', 'code') VALUES "
   . " ('$desc', '$code')";

  // Run the query and display appropriate message
  if (!$result = $connection->query($query)) {
    echo "Unable to add rows<br />";
  } else {
    echo "Rows successfully added<br />";
  }
}
```

FIGURE 22-5

You could fix this by using double quotes around `$desc` in the `$query` assignment. However, with a dynamic site you do not know whether the data contains single or double quotes (or both) so you need a solution that properly prepares the variables for insertion into the database. The answer to that is to escape any quotes in the variables by prefixing each quote character with a backslash (\). PHP has a function that does this for you. In mysqli it is the method `mysqli::real_escape_string` if you are using the object-oriented style or the function `mysqli_real_escape_string()`. This code escapes any quotes in `$desc` so that it works in the MySQL statement. The added line seen in phpMyAdmin looks similar to Figure 22-6.

```php
<?php
define("MYSQLUSER", "php24sql");
define("MYSQLPASS", "hJQV8RTe5t");
define("HOSTNAME", "localhost");
define("MYSQLDB", "test");
```

```
// Make connection to database
$connection = @new mysqli(HOSTNAME, MYSQLUSER, MYSQLPASS, MYSQLDB);
if ($connection->connect_error) {
  die('Connect Error: ' . $connection->connect_error);
} else {
  echo 'Successful connection to MySQL <br />';

  $desc = "qr's";
  $code = "15";

  $desc = $connection->real_escape_string($desc);

  // Set up the query
  $query = "INSERT INTO 'table1' ('description', 'code') VALUES "
    . " ('$desc', '$code')";
echo $query;

  // Run the query and display appropriate message
  if (!$result = $connection->query($query)) {
    echo "Unable to add rows<br />";
  } else {
    echo "Rows successfully added<br />";
  }
}
```

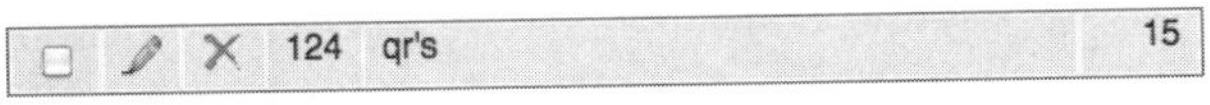

□ ✎ ✕	124	qr's	15

FIGURE 22-6

If you are using the procedural style the command looks like this instead:

```
$desc = mysqli_real_escape_string($connection, $desc);
```

There is one more wrinkle to consider — magic quotes. PHP recognized that this need to escape quotes was inconvenient and inexperienced programmers would neglect to do it. So PHP started doing it automatically. You used to be able to turn this behavior on or off in the php.ini file by turning on or off magic_quotes_gpc. Unfortunately this led to more problems and the use of magic quotes is now strongly discouraged; it will eventually be removed. However, if it happens to be on when you use the recommended mysqli::real_escape_string or mysqli_real_escape_string you get undesirable results. Before you escape your variables, you need to see if magic_quotes_gpc is on and if so, you need to strip out the escapes it added before using the recommended function. Use the get_magic_quotes_gpc() function to see if it is active:

```
<?php
define("MYSQLUSER", "php24sql");
define("MYSQLPASS", "hJQV8RTe5t");
define("HOSTNAME", "localhost");
define("MYSQLDB", "test");

// Make connection to database
$connection = @new mysqli(HOSTNAME, MYSQLUSER, MYSQLPASS, MYSQLDB);
if ($connection->connect_error) {
  die('Connect Error: ' . $connection->connect_error);
} else {
  echo 'Successful connection to MySQL <br />';
```

```
$desc = "qr's";
$code = "15";

if (get_magic_quotes_gpc()) {
  $desc = stripslashes($desc);
}
$desc = $connection->real_escape_string($desc);

// Set up the query
$query = "INSERT INTO 'table1' ('description', 'code') VALUES "
  . " ('$desc', '$code')";

// Run the query and display appropriate message
if (!$result = $connection->query($query)) {
  echo "Unable to add rows<br />";
} else {
  echo "Rows successfully added<br />";
}
}
```

Another reason for escaping the quotes is that it helps prevent SQL injection. Notice that you only escaped the $desc variable and not $code. $desc is a string field and $code is an integer. Best practices deal with different types of fields differently. If a field is an integer data type, the best check is to be sure that it is an integer.

```
<?php
define("MYSQLUSER", "php24sql");
define("MYSQLPASS", "hJQV8RTe5t");
define("HOSTNAME", "localhost");
define("MYSQLDB", "test");

// Make connection to database
$connection = @new mysqli(HOSTNAME, MYSQLUSER, MYSQLPASS, MYSQLDB);
if ($connection->connect_error) {
  die('Connect Error: ' . $connection->connect_error);
} else {
  echo 'Successful connection to MySQL <br />';

  $desc = "qr's";
  $code = "15";

  if (get_magic_quotes_gpc()) {
    $desc = stripslashes($desc);
  }
  $desc = $connection->real_escape_string($desc);
  $code = (int) $code;


  // Set up the query
  $query = "INSERT INTO 'table1' ('description', 'code') VALUES "
    . " ('$desc', '$code')";

  // Run the query and display appropriate message
  if (!$result = $connection->query($query)) {
    echo "Unable to add rows<br />";
```

```
    } else {
      echo "Rows successfully added<br />";
    }
  }
```

These examples are inserting only one row at a time. If you are inserting more than one row, the same principles apply. Add in other error-checking for the fields and you can see that there is significant preparation for each field that is used to update a database field. This is a place where creating functions for preparing variables for insertion is helpful.

PROCESSING DATA ENTRY FORMS IN PHP

In this section you take everything that you've learned about processing forms, passing tokens, preparing data, and updating the database and use it to program a form to add rows to a database table. Start by creating a basic input form with two required fields for getting the description and code as shown in Figure 22-7. Add a spot for any messages in $message to be displayed.

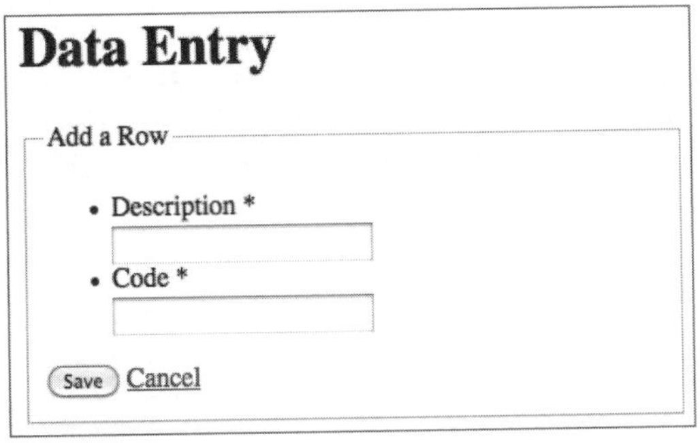

FIGURE 22-7

```
<html>
<head>
<meta http-equiv="Content-Type" content="text/html; charset=UTF-8" />
<title></title>
</head>
<body>
<h1>Data Entry</h1>

<p><?php echo $message; ?></p>

<form action="lesson22j.php" method="post" name="maint" id="maint">

  <fieldset class="maintform">
    <legend>Add a Row</legend>
    <ul>
      <li><label for="desc">Description *</label><br />
        <input type="text" name="desc" id="desc" /></li>
      <li><label for="code">Code *</label><br />
        <input type="text" name="code" id="code" /></li>
    </ul>

    <input type="submit" name="save" value="Save" />
    <a class="cancel" href="lesson22j.php">Cancel</a>
```

```
    </fieldset>
  </form>

  </body>
  </html>
```

Because you are updating a database, you want to add the security of a token. Start a session at the very beginning of the file:

```
<?php
session_start();
?>
```

Within the form fieldset, create a token and post it to the session as a hidden input:

```
<?php
// create token
$salt = 'SomeSalt';
 $token = sha1(mt_rand(1,1000000) . $salt);
 $_SESSION['token'] = $token;
 ?>
 <input type='hidden' name='token' value='<?php echo $token; ?>'/>
```

You can either create a file for the form and a different one for the processing or do everything in one file. In this example, you use one file so the next task is to add the processing of the form. After session_start(), initialize the $message variable, add a check to see if there is a form to process, and then check for a good token, as in the following code:

```
$message = '';

if (isset($_POST['save']) AND $_POST['save'] == 'Save') {
  // check the token
  $badToken = true;
  if (empty($_POST['token']) || $_POST['token'] !== $_SESSION['token']) {
    $message = 'Sorry, try it again. There was a security issue.';
    $badToken = true;
  } else {
    $badToken = false;
    unset($_SESSION['token']);
```

Next make your connection to the database and get the data from the POST array. For the description input, sanitize the data coming from the form as string data. To allow quotes without encoding them (such as ' remaining as a ' and not changing to '), add the FILTER_FLAG_NO_ENCODE_QUOTES filter. Filter the code input by forcing it to an integer. Verify that data exists in both $desc and $code. If the data passes all those requirements, prepare the data for insertion into the database and then set up the query and add it to the database. Errors or success messages are posted to $message, which is then displayed. Close out all of the if statements.

```
        define("MYSQLUSER", "php24sql");
        define("MYSQLPASS", "hJQV8RTe5t");
        define("HOSTNAME", "localhost");
        define("MYSQLDB", "test");

        // Make connection to database
        $connection = @new mysqli(HOSTNAME, MYSQLUSER, MYSQLPASS, MYSQLDB);
        if ($connection->connect_error) {
          die('Connect Error: ' . $connection->connect_error);
        } else {
```

```
        // Get the data
        $desc = filter_input(INPUT_POST,'desc',
FILTER_SANITIZE_STRING,FILTER_FLAG_NO_ENCODE_QUOTES);
        $code = (int) $_POST['code'];

        // Verify the data
        if (!$desc OR !$code) {
          $message .= 'Description and Code are required <br />';
        } else {

          // Prepare the data
          if (get_magic_quotes_gpc()) {
            $desc = stripslashes($desc);
          }
          $desc = $connection->real_escape_string($desc);
          $code = (int) $code;

          // Set up the query
          $query = "INSERT INTO 'table1' ('description', 'code') VALUES "
           . " ('$desc', '$code')";

          // Run the query and display appropriate message
          if (!$result = $connection->query($query)) {
            $message .= "Unable to add rows<br />";
          } else {
            $message .= "Row successfully added<br />";
          }
        }
      }
    }
  }
?>
```

Enter data into the form as shown in Figure 22-8. Click Save. You get a message that the row has been successfully saved, as shown in Figure 22-9.

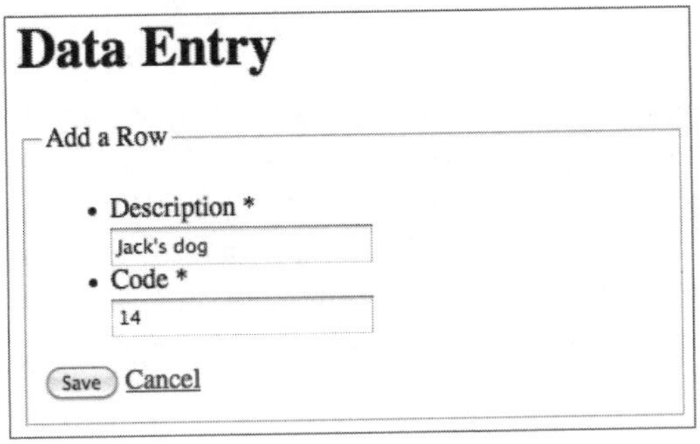

Data Entry

┌─ Add a Row ─────────────────────┐
│   │
│ • Description *   │
│   Jack's dog   │
│ • Code *   │
│   14   │
│ (Save) Cancel   │
└─────────────────────────────────┘

FIGURE 22-8

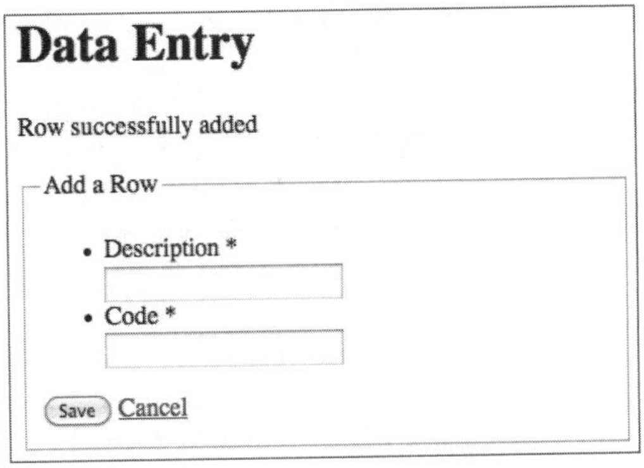

Data Entry

Row successfully added

┌─ Add a Row ─────────────────────┐
│   │
│   • Description *   │
│   │
│   • Code *   │
│   │
│ (Save) Cancel   │
└─────────────────────────────────┘

FIGURE 22-9

Go to phpMyAdmin to verify that the data was added. You should see a row similar to Figure 22-10. Note that because the id was automatically created your id might be different.

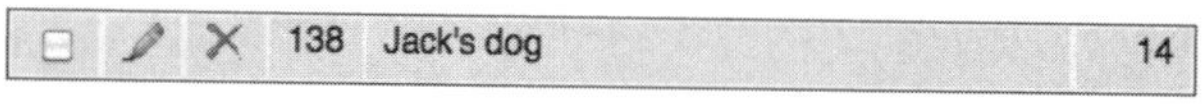

FIGURE 22-10

TRY IT

In this Try It, you add the ability to add contacts to the Case Study. You add a form to the website to get the data and then use that to add rows to the contacts table. You also create a method in the Database class for preparing data for insertion into the database.

> You can download the code and resources for this Try It from the book's web page at www.wrox.com. You can find them in the Lesson22 folder in the download. You will find code for both before and after completing the exercises.

Lesson Requirements

Your computer needs to be able to run as a web server with PHP and MySQL. XAMPP is a package of software that installs the web server, PHP, and MySQL for you. You can find instructions for downloading and installing XAMPP in Lesson 1.

You need a text editor that can produce plain-text files. You can find instructions for downloading and installing Eclipse PDT in Lesson 1. Other text editors that you can use are Adobe's Dreamweaver in code mode, Notepad, TextWrangler, or NetBeans.

If you are following along with the Case Study, you need your files from the end of the Lesson 21. Alternatively, you can download the files from the book's website at www.wrox.com. To re-create the database tables, create an empty database and then import the install.sql file in phpMyAdmin.

Hints

You learned about forms in Lesson 11, including working with header redirects and sessions.

If you have trouble with your database updates, try adding a var_dump($query) after assigning it the value. This displays the actual MySQL command that is run. Copy that and paste it into the SQL tab in phpMyAdmin to see errors.

One of the files in the downloadable code is install.sql. This file contains all the MySQL code needed to re-create your database. To use it you need an existing database. In phpMyAdmin either copy the code into the SQL table and run it, or import the file. It deletes or creates tables as needed and inserts data.

Step-by-Step

Create a form (see Figure 22-11) to enter contacts. Add processing to add the data from the form to the database and handle the messaging and page redirections.

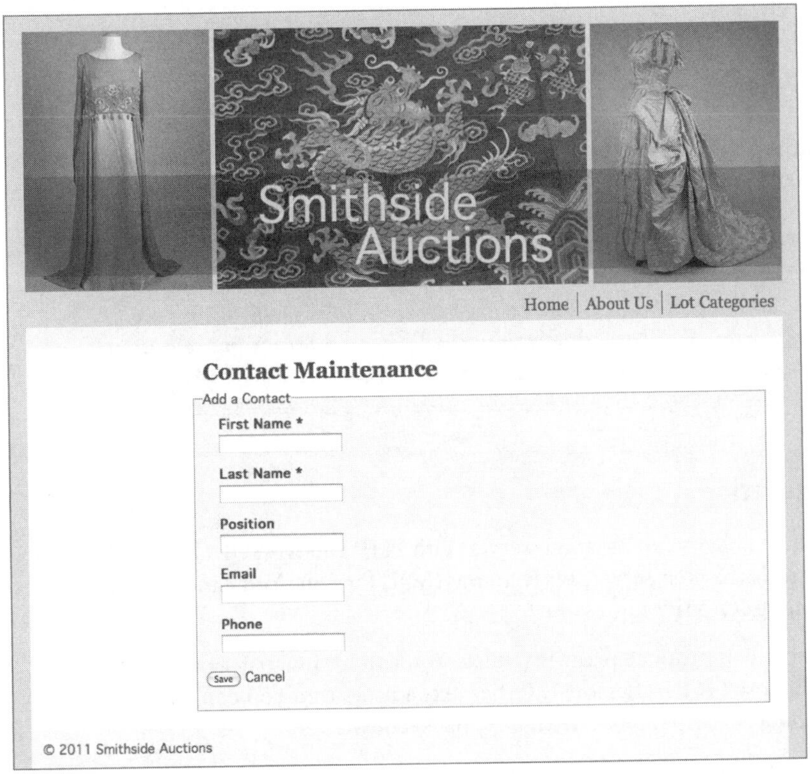

FIGURE 22-11

1. In `content/about.php` add a link in the `<h1>` to the data entry form you are creating.

   ```
   <h1>About Us<a class="button" href="index.php?content=contactmaint&id=0 ↵
   ?>">Add</a></h1>
   ```

2. Create a new file called `content/contactmaint.php`. This contains the HTML form. Use an empty `Contact` object to define the data fields. This isn't required for this window but is used when you turn it into a maintenance page. Pass a hidden input for the `id` for the row. This is blank for new contacts. Pass a hidden input for a task so you know what form you are processing. Create and pass a token to confirm this is a legitimate form.

   ```php
   <?php
   /**
    * contactmaint.php
    *
    * Maintenance for Contacts
    *
   ```

```
 * @version    1.2 2011-02-03
 * @package    Smithside Auctions
 * @copyright  Copyright (c) 2011 Smithside Auctions
 * @license    GNU General Public License
 * @since      Since Release 1.0
 */
$item = new Contact;
?>
<h1>Contact Maintenance</h1>

<form action="index.php?content=about" method="post" name="maint" id="maint">

  <fieldset class="maintform">
    <legend>Add a Contact</legend>
    <ul>
      <li><label for="first_name" class="required">First Name</label><br />
        <input type="text" name="first_name" id="first_name" class="required"
        value="<?php echo $item->getFirst_name(); ?>" /></li>
      <li><label for="last_name" class="required">Last Name</label><br />
        <input type="text" name="last_name" id="last_name" class="required"
        value="<?php echo $item->getLast_name(); ?>" /></li>
      <li><label for="position">Position</label><br />
        <input type="text" name="position" id="position" class="required"
        value="<?php echo $item->getPosition(); ?>" /></li>
      <li><label for="email" >Email</label><br />
        <input type="text" name="email" id="email"
        value="<?php echo $item->getEmail(); ?>" /></li>
      <li><label for="phone" >Phone</label><br />
        <input type="text" name="phone" id="phone"
        value="<?php echo $item->getPhone(); ?>" /></li>
    </ul>

    <?php
    // create token
    $salt = 'SomeSalt';
    $token = sha1(mt_rand(1,1000000) . $salt);
    $_SESSION['token'] = $token;
    ?>
    <input type="hidden" name="id" id="id" value="<?php echo $item->getId();
?>" />
    <input type="hidden" name="task" id="task" value="contact.maint" />
    <input type='hidden' name='token' value='<?php echo $token; ?>'/>
    <input type="submit" name="save" value="Save" />
    <a class="cancel" href="index.php?content=about">Cancel</a>
  </fieldset>
</form>
```

3. Create a constant in `includes/init.php` called `MAGIC_QUOTES_ACTIVE` that contains the result of `get_magic_quotes_gpc()`. This contains a 1 if magic quotes are on. Creating a constant once rather than running the function each time you need it is quicker.

```
define('MAGIC_QUOTES_ACTIVE', get_magic_quotes_gpc());
```

4. Create a public static method called `prep()` in `includes/classes/database.php` to prepare the data for insertion into the database. The data is passed to the function as a parameter. To refer to the connection property, use the static construction of `self::$_connection`.

```php
public static function prep($value) {
    if (MAGIC_QUOTES_ACTIVE) {
        // If magic quotes is active, remove the slashes
        $value = stripslashes($value);
    }
    // Escape special characters to avoid SQL injections
    $value = self::$_connection->real_escape_string($value);
    return $value;
}
```

5. In the `includes/init.php` file, move the `require_once 'includes/functions.php';` to just below the magic quotes constant.

6. Add processing to the `includes/init.php` file. This file works as the traffic cop to decide what task needs to be done. Up until now the implied task has been to display pages. Set up a switch to check for tasks with a `case` block where the condition is equal to `contact.maint`. Break out at the end of the `case` block.

```php
// Process based on the task. Default to display
$task = filter_input(INPUT_POST, 'task', FILTER_SANITIZE_STRING);
switch ($task) {
    case 'contact.maint' :
    break;
}
```

7. Within the `case` block you created in step 5, run a function to process the task. The `$results` return consists of an array where the first element is a redirect to different content page, if any. The second element contains a message, which is assigned the `$message` variable. If there is a redirect page, move the message to a SESSION variable and redirect. Change the code to this code:

```php
// Process based on the task. Default to display
$task = filter_input(INPUT_POST, 'task', FILTER_SANITIZE_STRING);
switch ($task) {
    case 'contact.maint' :
    // process the maint
    $results = maintContact();
    $message .= $results[1];
    // If there is redirect information
    // redirect to that page
    if ($results[0] == 'contactmaint') {
        // pass on new messages
        if ($results[1]) {
            $_SESSION['message'] = $results[1];
        }
        header("Location: index.php?content=contactmaint");
        exit;
```

```
        }
      break;
    }
```

8. Because you are using a SESSION variable you need to start the session at the very beginning of the file, just after the documentation:

```
session_start(); // starts new or resumes existing session
```

9. Add processing to check the SESSION for a message and move it to $message and then remove it from the SESSION with an unset. Put this before the task processing.

```
// Initialize message coming in
$message = '';
if (isset($_SESSION['message'])) {
  $message = htmlentities($_SESSION['message']);
  unset($_SESSION['message']);
}
```

10. Add the maintContact() function in includes/functions.php. Start by initializing the $results variable. If the Save button was clicked and equals Save, check the token. If there is a problem, put a message in the result. Otherwise, filter the data from the form and put it in an array called $item. Use that array to create a new Contact object. Run the addRecord() method of the object to add the row to the database, putting the results in $results.

```
function maintContact() {
  $results = '';
  if (isset($_POST['save']) AND $_POST['save'] == 'Save') {
    // check the token
    $badToken = true;
    if (!isset($_POST['token'])
       || !isset($_SESSION['token'])
       || empty($_POST['token'])
       || $_POST['token'] !== $_SESSION['token']) {
      $results = array('','Sorry, go back and try again. There was a ↵
security issue.');
      $badToken = true;
    } else {
      $badToken = false;
      unset($_SESSION['token']);
      // Put the sanitized variables in an associative array
      // Use the FILTER_FLAG_NO_ENCODE_QUOTES to allow names like O'Connor
      $item = array ( 'id' => (int) $_POST['id'],
                  'first_name' => filter_input(INPUT_POST,'first_name',
FILTER_SANITIZE_STRING,FILTER_FLAG_NO_ENCODE_QUOTES),
                  'last_name'  => filter_input(INPUT_POST,'last_name',
FILTER_SANITIZE_STRING,FILTER_FLAG_NO_ENCODE_QUOTES),
                  'position'   => filter_input(INPUT_POST,'position',
FILTER_SANITIZE_STRING,FILTER_FLAG_NO_ENCODE_QUOTES),
                  'email'      => filter_input(INPUT_POST,'email',
FILTER_SANITIZE_STRING),
```

```
                        'phone'        => filter_input(INPUT_POST,'phone',
        FILTER_SANITIZE_STRING)
                 );

            // Set up a Contact object based on the posts
            $contact = new Contact($item);
            $results = $contact->addRecord();
        }
    }
    return $results;
}
```

11. Add the public method `addRecord()` in `includes/classes/contact.php`. This function calls the method `_verifyInput()`. If the data is verified, get the database connection. Set up the data by creating the `INSERT` statement. Use the `Database::prep()` method to prepare the data. Create the array `$result()` where the first element is blank for normal processing, or `contactmaint` if there is an error where the user should stay on the `contactmaint` page. The second element contains a success message or an error message.

```php
public function addRecord() {

    // Verify the fields
    if ($this->_verifyInput()) {

        // Get the Database connection
        $connection = Database::getConnection();

        // Prepare the data
        $query = "INSERT INTO contacts(first_name, last_name, position, email,
phone)
            VALUES ('" . Database::prep($this->first_name) . "',
            '" . Database::prep($this->last_name) . "',
            '" . Database::prep($this->position) . "',
            '" . Database::prep($this->email) . "',
            '" . Database::prep($this->phone) . "')";
        // Run the MySQL statement
        if ($connection->query($query)) {
            $return = array('', 'Contact Record successfully added.');

            // add success message
            return $return;
        } else {
            // send fail message and return to contactmaint
            $return = array('contactmaint', 'No Contact Record Added. Unable to ↵
create record.');
            return $return;
        }
    } else {
        // send fail message and return to contactmaint
        $return = array('contactmaint', 'No Contact Record Added. Missing ↵
required information.');
        return $return;
    }

}
```

12. Add the protected function _verifyInput() in includes/classes/contact.php. This method checks that the required fields have been filled in. It returns false if there is an error.

```
protected function _verifyInput() {
  $error = false;
  if (!trim($this->first_name)) {
    $error = true;
  }
  if (!trim($this->last_name)) {
    $error = true;
  }
  if ($error) {
  return false;
  } else {
  return true;
  }
}
```

13. In index.php change the <div class="message"> section to just display the $message variable:

```
<div class="message">
  <?php echo $message; ?>
</div><!-- end message -->
```

Watch the video for Lesson 22 on the DVD or watch online at www.wrox.com/go/24phpmysql.

23

Selecting Data

In this lesson you learn how to retrieve data from the database. The SELECT command is arguably the most common MySQL command you use in PHP programs. It is also one of the most complex, with clauses that enable you to choose what table(s) you use, which columns are returned, what conditions must be met before a row is selected, what order to sort the data in, and whether and how to group and summarize the data.

You work with a single table at a time in this lesson. In the next lesson you learn how to use multiple tables. The table used to illustrate this lesson is shown in Figure 23-1 and is created from the following code:

```
CREATE TABLE IF NOT EXISTS 'table1' (
  'id' int(11) NOT NULL AUTO_INCREMENT PRIMARY KEY,
  'description' text,
  'code' int(11) NOT NULL DEFAULT '42'
) ENGINE=MyISAM;

INSERT INTO 'table1' ('id', 'description', 'code') VALUES
(101, 'abc', 99),
(102, 'a''bc', 15),
(103, 'a''bc', 15),
(104, 'a''bc', 15),
(105, 'def', 23),
(106, 'ghi', 23),
(107, 'jkl', 15),
(108, 'mno', 15),
(109, 'pqr', 23),
(110, 'stu', 42),
(111, 'vwx', 42),
(112, 'yza', 42),
(118, 'efg', 99);
```

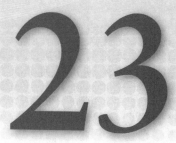

id	description	code
101	abc	99
102	a'bc	15
103	a'bc	15
104	a'bc	15
105	def	23
106	ghi	23
107	jkl	15
108	mno	15
109	pqr	23
110	stu	42
111	vwx	42
112	yza	42
118	efg	99

FIGURE 23-1

USING THE SELECT COMMAND

The easiest form of the SELECT command is to select all fields and rows from a single table:

```
SELECT * FROM 'table1';
```

The asterisk (*) indicates that all fields are to be selected and FROM 'table1' tells which table to use. By default all rows are selected.

To select only some of the fields to show, specify those fields instead of using an * as in the following code and shown in Figure 23-2:

```
SELECT 'id', 'description' FROM 'table1';
```

Whatever order you put the fields in is the order in which they are displayed as shown in the following code and Figure 23-3. This change in order is just for the display. The SELECT command does not change anything in the database itself.

```
SELECT 'description', 'id' FROM 'table1';
```

id	description
101	abc
102	a'bc
103	a'bc
104	a'bc
105	def
106	ghi
107	jkl
108	mno
109	pqr
110	stu
111	vwx
112	yza
118	efg

description	id
abc	101
a'bc	102
a'bc	103
a'bc	104
def	105
ghi	106
jkl	107
mno	108
pqr	109
stu	110
vwx	111
yza	112
efg	118

FIGURE 23-2   **FIGURE 23-3**

> *It is very tempting to always use the asterisk (*) to select your fields instead of writing out just the ones you need. You will see this done a lot, especially by programmers who don't know MySQL well. However, the * is more resource intensive and you should avoid it if it is not needed.*

The SELECT statement is made up of *clauses*. These clauses are the building blocks for creating the statement. You are already using two clauses: the *select expression* where you chose the fields and

the FROM clause. There is a list of the clauses in the MySQL documentation at http://dev.mysql
.com/doc/refman/5.6/en/select.html. The other common clauses include WHERE, ORDER BY,
and LIMIT.

> It is important that the clauses are in the right order. If you have problems with a
> SELECT command, check the manual to see that you have the different clauses in
> the right order. In general you start with the SELECT expression and then follow
> with FROM, WHERE, GROUP BY, HAVING, ORDER BY, LIMIT, PROCEDURE, and INTO.
> It's outside the scope of this book to go over all the different clauses.

The SELECT expression clause has many possibilities. You can rename using *aliases*. This code
renames the id field to myid. See Figure 23-4.

```
SELECT 'id' AS 'myid', 'description' FROM 'table1';
```

myid	description
101	abc
102	a'bc
103	a'bc
104	a'bc
105	def
106	ghi
107	jkl
108	mno
109	pqr
110	stu
111	vwx
112	yza
118	efg

FIGURE 23-4

A common select expression is COUNT(). If you use an *, the result is a count of all the
rows selected. If you use a field then the result is the count of all the rows selected
where that field is not NULL. See Figure 23-5.

COUNT(*)
13

FIGURE 23-5

```
SELECT COUNT(*) FROM 'table1';
```

Another keyword that comes in handy is the DISTINCT keyword. This
indicates that if duplicates exist, only one is used. In the following
example you count the different descriptions that are in the table. See
Figure 23-6.

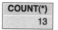

COUNT(DISTINCT `description`)
11

FIGURE 23-6

```
SELECT COUNT(DISTINCT 'description') FROM 'table1';
```

You can make complex expressions. You can use string functions on text fields. String functions are listed at `http://dev.mysql.com/doc/refman/5.6/en/string-functions.html`. Some common functions are `CONCAT()` to join fields, `CONCAT_WS` to concatenate with a separator, `TRIM()` to remove leading and trailing spaces, and `SUBSTR()` or `SUBSTRING()` to return part of the field. With numeric fields you can use numeric functions. Numeric functions are listed at `http://dev.mysql.com/doc/refman/5.6/en/numeric-functions.html`. MySQL automatically makes simple conversions but occasionally you may need to change the data type of the field. Use the cast functions that are listed at `http://dev.mysql.com/doc/refman/5.6/en/cast-functions.html`. The following code takes the description and appends it with a comma, a space, and the first letter of the description and then calls the result `item`. The result is shown in Figure 23-7.

item
abc, a
a'bc, a
a'bc, a
a'bc, a
def, d
ghi, g
jkl, j
mno, m
pqr, p
stu, s
vwx, v
yza, y
efg, e

FIGURE 23-7

```
SELECT CONCAT( 'description', ', ', SUBSTRING('description',1,1 )) AS
'item'
FROM 'table1';
```

When you use MySQL with PHP, you can choose to perform some actions in either the MySQL statement or in PHP. Which way you choose depends on how comfortable you are with each language and what the performance implications are. Some people always select all fields with the * rather than take the time to enter just the fields that they need. This has an advantage if you later want to use another field from that selection, but it means that you are taking a performance hit on the query. If your tables are small, the hit is irrelevant. However, if you have blobs of data or a large number of records, it could become significant. On the other hand, complex selections can take longer than simple selections so you could be better off doing the manipulations in PHP.

If you entered some of the commands in this lesson in phpMyAdmin, you may have noticed that they often append the LIMIT clause. The LIMIT clause is a way to limit the number of rows returned at one time. There are limits, in both MySQL and PHP, in the amount of server processing time used before an error is thrown. Using LIMIT allows you to receive your results in digestible bits. LIMIT is frequently used for pagination as well. There are two different syntaxes for LIMIT. The following code gives three ways to select the first five rows:

```
SELECT * FROM 'table1' LIMIT 5;
SELECT * FROM 'table1' LIMIT 0, 5;
SELECT * FROM 'table1' LIMIT 5 OFFSET 0;
```

And here are two ways to select the next five rows:

```
SELECT * FROM 'table1' LIMIT 5, 5;
SELECT * FROM 'table1' LIMIT 5 OFFSET 5;
```

The limiting is based on selected, ordered rows.

The ORDER BY clause enables you to return the rows in a given sequence. You specify the field or alias and whether the order should be ascending or descending. If you don't specify a direction,

ascending is assumed. The following code returns the rows in order by the description in ascending order as shown in Figure 23-8.

```
SELECT * FROM 'table1' ORDER BY 'description' ASC
```

You can string together multiple fields/directions to create more complex orders. The following code orders by the code in reverse order and then by the description (see Figure 23-9):

```
SELECT * FROM 'table1' ORDER BY 'code' DESC, 'description' ASC
```

id	description ▲	code
102	a'bc	15
103	a'bc	15
104	a'bc	15
101	abc	99
105	def	23
118	efg	99
106	ghi	23
107	jkl	15
108	mno	15
109	pqr	23
110	stu	42
111	vwx	42
112	yza	42

FIGURE 23-8

id	description	code
101	abc	99
118	efg	99
110	stu	42
111	vwx	42
112	yza	42
105	def	23
106	ghi	23
109	pqr	23
102	a'bc	15
103	a'bc	15
104	a'bc	15
107	jkl	15
108	mno	15

FIGURE 23-9

USING WHERE

The WHERE clause is the clause that you use to pick which rows to select. If there is no WHERE clause then all rows are selected. A WHERE clause can be as simple as it is in the following command in which it selects the row with the id of 105 as shown in Figure 23-10:

id	description	code
105	def	23

FIGURE 23-10

```
SELECT * FROM 'table1' WHERE 'id' = 105;
```

A WHERE clause can use most of the functions and operators that MySQL uses. For complete information, see the following pages in the online manual:

➤ **Expression Syntax:** This explains things like how to use expressions such as AND and OR (http://dev.mysql.com/doc/refman/5.6/en/expressions.html).

➤ **Comparison Functions and Operators:** This explains the different ways that you can compare values. See Table 23-1 for common operators or the manual for all the functions and operators (http://dev.mysql.com/doc/refman/5.6/en/comparison-operators .html#operator_not-between).

TABLE 23-1: MySQL Comparison Operators

OPERATOR	DESCRIPTION
=	Equal (Notes: PHP uses a double equal sign but MySQL uses a single; If a NULL is on either side, the result is NULL.)
>	Greater than
<	Less than
>=	Greater than or equal
<=	Less than or equal
!=	Not equal to
<>	Not equal to
<=>	Equal to (NULL is safe. NULL<=>NULL is true. NULL<=> other things is false.)
IS NULL	Is the value NULL
IS NOT NULL	Is the value not NULL
IS	IS TRUE, IS FALSE, IS NOT TRUE, IS NOT FALSE
LIKE	Match to a pattern character by character % wildcard matches any number of characters including zero; _ (underscore) wildcard matches any single character
NOT LIKE	Does not match to the pattern
BETWEEN... AND...	Checks to see if a value is within this range This does data type casting, but you should use CAST ( ) to explicitly convert date and time values to the same type
NOT BETWEEN... AND...	Checks to see if a value is not within this range

➤ **Literal Values Syntax:** This explains things such as when you need to use quotes and how to specify dates and times. (Hint: In general, you don't need quotes for numbers but you do for strings.) See the details at `http://dev.mysql.com/doc/refman/5.6/en/literals.html`.

➤ **Functions and Operators:** The table of contents for all the functions and operators is at `http://dev.mysql.com/doc/refman/5.6/en/functions.html`.

SELECTING DATA IN PHP

You frequently select data in a MySQL table using PHP. Selecting data through a PHP program using a MySQL command takes four steps:

1. Make a connection to the database.

2. Create a safe query with the command.

3. Run the query.

4. Read the results.

The following code makes the connection and creates a safe query. Rather than just running the query, use it as the right side of an assignment. This creates a `mysqli_result` object that you use to read the results via methods in the result object. This example takes each row, one at a time, and puts it into an associative array. It uses a `while` loop to loop through the results and prints each row as it retrieves it. See the results in Figure 23-11.

```
Successful connection to MySQL
Array ( [id] => 102 [description] => a'bc [code] => 15 )
Array ( [id] => 103 [description] => a'bc [code] => 15 )
Array ( [id] => 104 [description] => a'bc [code] => 15 )
Array ( [id] => 107 [description] => jkl [code] => 15 )
Array ( [id] => 108 [description] => mno [code] => 15 )
```

FIGURE 23-11

```php
<?php
define("MYSQLUSER", "php24sql");
define("MYSQLPASS", "hJQV8RTe5t");
define("HOSTNAME", "localhost");
define("MYSQLDB", "test");

// Make connection to database
$connection = @new mysqli(HOSTNAME, MYSQLUSER, MYSQLPASS, MYSQLDB);
if ($connection->connect_error) {
  die('Connect Error: ' . $connection->connect_error);
} else {
  echo 'Successful connection to MySQL <br />';

  // Set up the query
  $query = "SELECT * FROM 'table1' "
  . " WHERE 'code' = 15"
  . " ORDER BY 'description' ASC "
  ;

  // Run the query
  $result_obj = '';
  $result_obj = $connection->query($query);

  // Read the results
  // loop through the result object, row by row
  // reading each row into an associative array
  while($result = $result_obj->fetch_array(MYSQLI_ASSOC)) {
```

```
        // display the array
        print_r($result);
        echo '<br />';
    }
}
```

The example prints out the array, but you can do anything with it at that moment before it is over-written with the next row. This code copies the array to another array so you end up with an array of arrays, which it prints after it has finished collecting all the rows. See Figure 23-12.

```
// Read the results
// loop through the results, row by row
// reading each row into an associative array
while($result = $result_obj->fetch_array(MYSQLI_ASSOC)) {
    // collect the array
    $item[] = $result;
}
// print array when done
echo '<pre>';
print_r($item);
echo '</pre>';
```

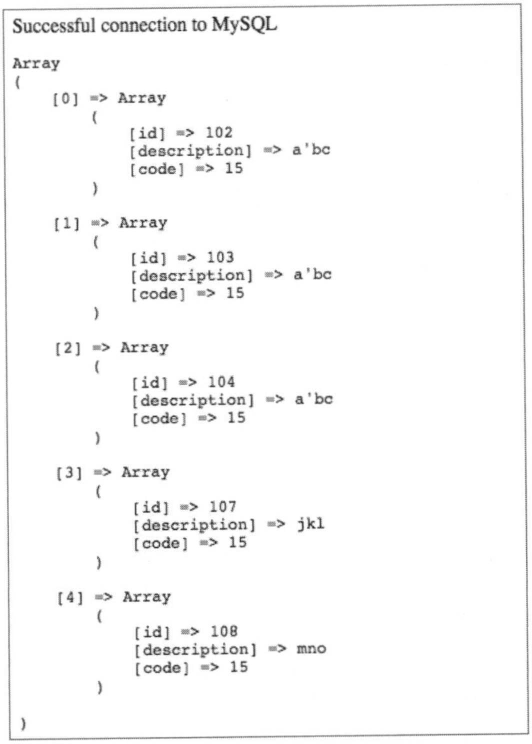

```
Successful connection to MySQL

Array
(
    [0] => Array
        (
            [id] => 102
            [description] => a'bc
            [code] => 15
        )

    [1] => Array
        (
            [id] => 103
            [description] => a'bc
            [code] => 15
        )

    [2] => Array
        (
            [id] => 104
            [description] => a'bc
            [code] => 15
        )

    [3] => Array
        (
            [id] => 107
            [description] => jkl
            [code] => 15
        )

    [4] => Array
        (
            [id] => 108
            [description] => mno
            [code] => 15
        )

)
```

FIGURE 23-12

The online PHP manual lists the different methods that you can use to read the results at www.php .net/manual/en/class.mysqli-result.php. Here are examples of some of them.

➤ `fetch_array(MYSQLI_ASSOC)`: This returns an associative array. Loop through to get all the rows. Same as `fetch_assoc()`.

➤ `fetch_array(MYSQLI_NUM)`: This returns a numeric array. Loop through to get all the rows. Same as `fetch_row()`.

➤ `fetch_array(MYSQLI_BOTH)`: This returns both an associative array and a numeric array with the same data. Loop through to get all the rows. This is the default if no type is specified.

➤ `fetch_all(MYSQLI_ASSOC)`: This returns all the rows as an associative array.

➤ `fetch_all(MYSQLI_NUM)`: This returns all the rows as a numeric array.

➤ `fetch_all(MYSQLI_BOTH)`: This returns all the rows both as an associative array and a numeric array with the same data.

➤ `fetch_object(`*`$class_name`*`)`: This returns an object of the row. Loop through to get all the rows. If you give it a class name, it uses that class to create the object. If there is no class name it will create a `stdClass` object, which is a predefined class.

These are also available as ordinary functions, which need the mysqli result variable as a parameter. You don't need it for the object method form because the object already knows that information.

➤ `mysqli_fetch_array($result, MYSQLI_ASSOC)`: This returns an associative array. Loop through to get all the rows. Same as `mysqli_fetch_assoc($result)`.

➤ `mysqli_fetch_array($result, MYSQLI_NUM)`: This returns a numeric array. Loop through to get all the rows. Same as `mysqli_fetch_row($result)`:

➤ `mysqli_fetch_array(MYSQLI_BOTH)`: This returns both an associative array and a numeric array with the same data. Loop through to get all the rows. This is the default if no type is specified.

➤ `mysqli_fetch_all($result, MYSQLI_ASSOC)`: This returns all the rows as an associative array.

➤ `mysqli_fetch_all($result, MYSQLI_NUM)`: This returns all the rows as a numeric array.

➤ `mysqli_fetch_all($result, MYSQLI_BOTH)`: This returns all the rows both as an associative array and a numeric array with the same data.

➤ `mysqli_fetch_object($result, `*`$class_name`*`)`: This returns an object of the row. Loop through to get all the rows. If you give it a class name, it uses that class to create the object. If there is no class name, it creates a `stdClass` object, which is a predefined class.

⬇ TRY IT

In this Try It, you retrieve data from the Case Study database and use it to populate the website instead of using hardcoded data. You start with the About Us page, pulling the information from the `contacts` table. Then you do the same for the Lot Categories page. Because you don't have any data in the `categories` table, you also create a maintenance page to add data to the `categories` table.

> You can download the code and resources for this Try It from the book's web page at www.wrox.com. You can find them in the Lesson23 folder in the download. You will find code for both before and after completing the exercises.

Lesson Requirements

Your computer needs to be able to run as a web server with PHP and MySQL. XAMPP is a package of software that installs the web server, PHP, and MySQL for you. You can find instructions for downloading and installing XAMPP in Lesson 1.

You need a text editor that can produce plain-text files. You can find instructions for downloading and installing Eclipse PDT in Lesson 1. Other text editors that you can use are Adobe's Dreamweaver in code mode, Notepad, TextWrangler, or NetBeans.

If you are following along with the Case Study, you need your files from the end of Lesson 22. Alternatively, you can download the files from the book's website at www.wrox.com. To re-create the database tables, create an empty database and then import the install.sql file in phpMyAdmin.

Hints

Use empty square brackets to add a value as a new element in an array.

The Lot Category maintenance page is set up the same way you set up the Contacts maintenance page in the previous lesson.

Step-by-Step

Change the About Us page to get the contact information from the database.

1. In contents/about.php the information is currently hardcoded in to the $items array. Replace those 30 lines with a static call to the Content class method getContacts():

```
// Get the contact information
$items = Contact::getContacts();
?>
```

2. When the information was hardcoded, you had total control over what it was. By pulling information from the database, you don't have the same control. There could be malicious information and there could be characters, such as ampersands, that should be encoded as HTML entities, such as &. To fix this, pass all string information through the htmlspecialchars() function:

```
<h2><?php echo htmlspecialchars($item->name()); ?></h2>
<p>Position: <?php echo htmlspecialchars($item->getPosition()); ?><br />
<?php echo htmlspecialchars($item->getEmail()); ?><br />
Phone: <?php echo htmlspecialchars($item->getPhone()); ?><br /></p>
```

3. In includes/classes/contact.php add the getContacts() public static method to retrieve the rows and fill the array. Use the fetch_object() method with the Contact class to read the rows into objects.

```
static function getContacts() {
  // clear the results
  $items = '';
  // Get the connection
  $connection = Database::getConnection();
  // Set up query
  $query = 'SELECT * FROM 'contacts' ORDER BY first_name, last_name';
  // Run the query
  $result_obj = '';
  $result_obj = $connection->query($query);
  // Loop through the results,
  // passing them to a new version of this class,
  // and making a regular array of the objects
  try {
    while($result = $result_obj->fetch_object('Contact')) {
      $items[]= $result;
    }
    // pass back the results
    return($items);
  }

  catch(Exception $e) {
    return false;
  }
}
```

Create a maintenance page so you can add lot categories into the categories table. Add the lot categories into the categories table. Change the Lot Categories page to get the information from the database.

1. In contents/categories.php add documentation at the beginning of the file:

```
<?php
/**
 * categories.php
 *
 * Content for Categories page
 *
 * @version    1.2 2011-02-03
 * @package    Smithside Auctions
 * @copyright  Copyright (c) 2011 Smithside Auctions
 * @license    GNU General Public License
 * @since      Since Release 1.0
 */
```

2. Follow that with the code to load the $items variable using the static getCategories() method from the Category class. If nothing is returned, initialize $items to an array so that later use of the variable doesn't create errors.

```
// Get the category information
$items = Category::getCategories();
```

```php
   if (empty($items)) {
     $items = array();
   }
   ?>
```

3. In the `<h1>` header, add a link to the new data entry page. Give it the class `button` for the CSS styling.

```html
<h1>Categories<a class="button"
href="index.php?content=categorymaint&cat_id=0">Add</a></h1>
```

4. Wrap the first `<li>...</li>` in a `foreach` loop to loop through the `$items` array.

```php
<?php foreach ($items as $i=>$item) : ?>
  <li class="row0">
  ...
  </li>
<?php endforeach; ?>
```

5. Change the `<li>` class to calculate the class for either `row0` or `row1` based on the `$i` key variable:

```php
<li class="row<?php echo $i % 2; ?>">
```

6. Set up the images. The table has a field for the name of the file in the images folder. There is another file with the same name in the images/thumbnail folder. You want to check to see if these files exist before trying to display them, to prevent broken links and also verify that what you display is an actual filename in a specific folder. If a file doesn't exist, display a generic image instead.

```php
<?php
  $image = 'images/'. $item->getCat_image();
  if (!is_file($image)) {
    $image = 'images/nophoto.jpg';
  }
  $image_t = 'images/thumbnails/'. $item->getCat_image();
  if (!is_file($image_t)) {
    $image_t = 'images/thumbnails/nophoto.jpg';
  }
?>
```

7. Change the image references to the new image variables:

```php
<div class="list-photo">
  <a href="<?php echo $image; ?>">
  <img alt="" src="<?php echo $image_t; ?>"/></a>
</div>
```

8. Change the `<h2>` link to assign the `content=` parameter based on the category name. Change `<h2>` text to the category name as well. Change the description to use the category description and change the `content=` parameter in the `<a>` tag link to the category name in lowercase.

```php
<div class="list-description">
  <h2>
  <a href="index.php?content=<?php echo ↵
htmlspecialchars($item->getCat_name()); ?>&amp;sidebar=catnav">
```

```
<?php echo htmlspecialchars (strtolower($item->getCat_name())); ?></a>
</h2>
<p><?php echo htmlspecialchars($item->getCat_description()); ?></p>
<a class="button display" href="index.php?content=<?php echo ↵
htmlspecialchars (strtolower($item->getCat_name())); ?>&amp;sidebar=catnav">
   Display Lots</a>
</div>
```

9. Remove the rest of the `<li>` groups.

10. In `includes/classes/category.php` add the `getCategories()` public static method to retrieve the rows and fill the array. Rather than directly creating the `Category` object, use `fetch_array(MYSQLI_ASSOC)` to retrieve the row. Use that array to create a new `Category` object that is added as an element in the `$items` array. This is a different way of creating the same `$items` array as is created in the `Contact` class using the `fetch_object()`.

```php
static public function getCategories() {
   // clear the results
   $items = '';
   // Get the connection
   $connection = Database::getConnection();
   // Set up the query
   $query = 'SELECT * FROM 'categories' ORDER BY cat_name';

   // Run the query
   $result_obj = '';
   $result_obj = $connection->query($query);
   // Loop through getting associative arrays,
   // passing them to a new version of this class,
   // and making a regular array of the objects
   try {
     while($result = $result_obj->fetch_array(MYSQLI_ASSOC)) {
       $items[]= new Category($result);
     }
     // pass back the results
       return($items);
   }

   catch(Exception $e) {
     return false;
   }

}
```

11. Add the `addRecord()` method to add rows to the `categories` table:

```php
public function addRecord() {

   // Verify the fields
   if ($this->_verifyInput()) {

     // Get the Database connection
     $connection = Database::getConnection();

     // Prepare the data
```

```
$query = "INSERT INTO categories(cat_name, cat_description, cat_image)
  VALUES ('" . Database::prep($this->cat_name) . "',
    '" . Database::prep($this->cat_description) ."',
    '" . Database::prep($this->cat_image) . "')";

// Run the MySQL statement
if ($connection->query($query)) {
  $return = array('', 'Category Record successfully added.');

    // add success message
    return $return;
} else {
    // send fail message and return to categorymaint
  $return = array('contactmaint', 'No Category Record Added.
    Unable to create record.');
  return $return;
  }
} else {
    // send fail message and return to categorymaint
  $return = array('categorymaint', 'No Category Record Added.
    Missing required information.');
  return $return;
}
```

12. Add the _verifyInput() method to verify that a category name was entered:

```
protected function _verifyInput() {
  $error = false;
  if (!trim($this->cat_name)) {
    $error = true;
  }
  if ($error) {
    return false;
  } else {
    return true;
  }
}
```

13. Create content/categorymaint.php, which is the form for data entry of the categories:

```
<?php
/**
 * categorymaint.php
 *
 * Maintenance for the Categories table
 *
 * @version  1.2 2011-02-03
 * @package  Smithside Auctions
 * @copyright Copyright (c) 2011 Smithside Auctions
 * @license  GNU General Public License
 * @since    Since Release 1.0
 */
$item = new Category;
?>
<h1>Category Maintenance</h1>
```

```
    <form action="index.php?content=categories" method="post" name="maint"
id="maint">

      <fieldset class="maintform">
        <legend>Add a Category</legend>
        <ul>
        <li><label for="cat_name" class="required">Category</label><br />
          <input type="text" name="cat_name" id="cat_name" class="required"
          value="<?php echo $item->getCat_name(); ?>" /></li>
        <li><label for="cat_description">Description</label><br />
          <textarea rows="5" cols="60" name="cat_description"
          id="cat_description"><?php echo $item->getCat_description(); ?>
          </textarea></li>
        <li><label for="cat_image" >Image</label><br />
          <input type="text" name="cat_image" id="cat_image"
          value="<?php echo $item->getCat_image(); ?>" /></li>
        </ul>

        <?php
        // create token
        $salt = 'SomeSalt';
        $token = sha1(mt_rand(1,1000000) . $salt);
        $_SESSION['token'] = $token;
        ?>
        <input type="hidden" name="cat_id" id="cat_id"
          value="<?php echo $item->getCat_id(); ?>" />
        <input type="hidden" name="task" id="task" value="category.maint" />
        <input type="hidden" name='token' value='<?php echo $token; ?>'/>
        <input type="submit" name="save" value="Save" />
        <a class="cancel" href="index.php?content=categories">Cancel</a>
      </fieldset>
    </form>
```

14. In includes/init.php add a case block in the switch statement for category.maint to process the category maintenance form:

```
case 'category.maint' :
// process the maint
$results = maintCategory();
$message .= $results[1];
// If there is redirect information
// redirect to that page
if ($results[0] == 'categorymaint') {
  // pass on new messages
  if ($results[1]) {
    $_SESSION['message'] = $results[1];
  }
  header("Location: index.php?content=categorymaint");
  exit;
}
break;
```

15. Add the function maintCategory() to includes/functions.php:

```
function maintCategory() {
  $results = '';
```

```
if (isset($_POST['save']) AND $_POST['save'] == 'Save') {
  // check the token
  $badToken = true;
  if (!isset($_POST['token'])
    || !isset($_SESSION['token'])
    || empty($_POST['token'])
    || $_POST['token'] !== $_SESSION['token']) {
    $results = array('','Sorry, go back and try again.
      There was a security issue.');
    $badToken = true;
  } else {
    $badToken = false;
    unset($_SESSION['token']);
    // Put the sanitized variables in an associative array
    // Use the FILTER_FLAG_NO_ENCODE_QUOTES
    // to allow quotes in the description
    $item  = array ('cat_id' => (int) $_POST['cat_id'],
      'cat_name' => filter_input(INPUT_POST,'cat_name',
        FILTER_SANITIZE_STRING),
      'cat_description' => filter_input(INPUT_POST,'cat_description',
        FILTER_SANITIZE_STRING,FILTER_FLAG_NO_ENCODE_QUOTES),
      'cat_image' => filter_input(INPUT_POST,'cat_image',
        FILTER_SANITIZE_STRING)
    );

    // Set up a Category object based on the posts
    $category = new Category($item);
    $results = $category->addRecord();
  }
}
return $results;
}
```

16. Go to the new entry screen and add the lot categories shown in Figure 23-13.

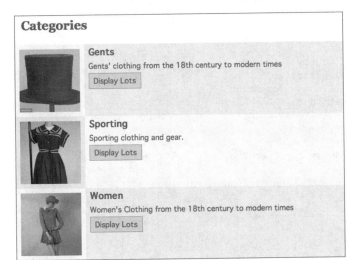

Categories

Gents
Gents' clothing from the 18th century to modern times
Display Lots

Sporting
Sporting clothing and gear.
Display Lots

Women
Women's Clothing from the 18th century to modern times
Display Lots

FIGURE 23-13

17. Change `content/catnav.php` to use the categories in the `categories` table rather than hardcoded links:

```php
<?php
/**
 * catnav.php
 *
 * Menu for the categories
 *
 * @version    1.2 2011-02-03
 * @package    Smithside Auctions
 * @copyright  Copyright (c) 2011 Smithside Auctions
 * @license    GNU General Public License
 * @since      Since Release 1.0
 */
$items = Category::getCategories();
?>
<h3 class="element-invisible">Lot Categories</h3>
<ul class="catnav">
  <?php foreach ($items as $i=>$item) : ?>
<li><a href="index.php?content=<?php echo
  htmlspecialchars(strtolower($item->getCat_name())); ?>&sidebar=catnav">
  <?php echo htmlspecialchars($item->getCat_name()); ?></a></li>
  <?php endforeach; ?>
</ul>
```

Watch the video for Lesson 23 on the DVD or watch online at www.wrox.com/go/24phpmysql.

24

Using Multiple Tables

In this lesson, you work with multiple tables. MySQL does not explicitly link tables together. Instead you design the tables so that they have fields that contain the information you need to link to another table. You then use that information in separate SELECT statements for each table or by using multiple tables in a SELECT statement.

The JOIN clause in the SELECT statement specifies what the links are between the tables. Subqueries let you create compound commands by using the result of one statement nested in another statement.

The examples in this lesson are based on three tables: the authors table that contains the author's name, the types table that contains the valid types of books, and the books table that lists the title along with a field whose value matches to the author's primary key plus a field whose value matches to the type's primary key. This is a simplified database where there is only one author per book and each book is in only one type.

> You can download the code for this example from the book's web page at
> www.wrox.com. You can find them in the Lesson24 folder in the download in
> a file labeled lesson24a.sql.

The first table is the authors table as shown in Figure 24-1.

The second table is the types table as shown in Figure 24-2.

The third table is the books table as shown in Figure 24-3.

id	first_name	last_name
1	Sally	Meyers
2	George	Smith
3	Peter	Gabriel
5	Dale	Mercer

FIGURE 24-1

type_id	type_name
1	History
2	Suspense
3	Science Fiction

FIGURE 24-2

id	title	author	type_id
1	A Long Day in Spring	3	1
2	Fifteen Hours in March	2	2
3	Green Trees Go Wild	1	3
4	And Then It Happened	1	1
5	Missing in Action	5	2
6	Fourteen Days in February	2	2

FIGURE 24-3

USING THE JOIN CLAUSE

With what you already know, you can work with multiple tables simply by using the information from one table as the basis for the WHERE clause for the other table. For instance, you know that the following command lists the author George Smith. See Figure 24-4.

first_name	last_name
George	Smith

FIGURE 24-4

```
SELECT first_name, last_name FROM authors WHERE id = '2';
```

The link between the books table and the authors table is that the author field in the books table and the id field (the primary key) of the authors table contain the same value. To list the books that George Smith wrote, you select from the books table all the rows where the author field is equal to 2, as shown in the following SELECT command and in Figure 24-5:

title
Fifteen Hours in March
Fourteen Days in February

FIGURE 24-5

```
SELECT title FROM books WHERE author = '2';
```

You can use more than one table in the SELECT statement. This command combines the books table and the types table. See the results in Figure 24-6.

```
SELECT title, type_name FROM books, types;
```

title	type_name
A Long Day in Spring	History
A Long Day in Spring	Suspense
A Long Day in Spring	Science Fiction
Fifteen Hours in March	History
Fifteen Hours in March	Suspense
Fifteen Hours in March	Science Fiction
Green Trees Go Wild	History
Green Trees Go Wild	Suspense
Green Trees Go Wild	Science Fiction
And Then It Happened	History
And Then It Happened	Suspense
And Then It Happened	Science Fiction
Missing in Action	History
Missing in Action	Suspense
Missing in Action	Science Fiction
Fourteen Days in February	History
Fourteen Days in February	Suspense
Fourteen Days in February	Science Fiction

FIGURE 24-6

These are probably not the results that you were intending. Every book is listed along with every type. The JOIN clause is used to specify how the tables should be merged. In this case you want to merge rows based on when the type_id in both tables is equal. Because the field name type_id is present in both tables, you need to specify the table when using the field. The following code displays a merged row of the title and type for each book as shown in Figure 24-7:

title	type_name
A Long Day in Spring	History
Fifteen Hours in March	Suspense
Green Trees Go Wild	Science Fiction
And Then It Happened	History
Missing in Action	Suspense
Fourteen Days in February	Suspense

FIGURE 24-7

```
SELECT title, type_name
FROM books JOIN types ON books.type_id = types.type_id
```

It is common practice to use aliases as a shortcut when you have to qualify names with the table. This is another way of writing the previous command:

```
SELECT title, type_name
FROM books AS b JOIN types AS t ON b.type_id = t.type_id
```

In the previous example, the linking fields had the same name. The names of the fields are irrelevant. The books table and the authors table both use the field name id for their primary keys. The fields, even though they have the same name, refer to different things. Qualifying the fields with the table name or alias removes the ambiguity.

The following code creates rows consisting of the author's last name, first name, and the book's title in order by author and then title. It joins the authors table, giving it an alias of a, and the books table, giving it an alias of b, based on the id in the authors table matching the author field in the books table. The author's name is concatenated into a single field. The result is shown in Figure 24-8.

full_name	title
Gabriel, Peter	A Long Day in Spring
Meyers, Sally	And Then It Happened
Meyers, Sally	Green Trees Go Wild
Smith, George	Fifteen Hours in March
Smith, George	Fourteen Days in February

FIGURE 24-8

```
SELECT CONCAT(last_name, ', ', first_name) AS full_name, title
FROM authors AS a
JOIN books AS b ON a.id = author
ORDER BY full_name, title;;
```

You can join more than two files. This example takes the previous example and adds the type of book to the list. See Figure 24-9.

```
SELECT CONCAT(last_name, ', ', first_name) AS full_name, title, type_name
FROM authors AS a
JOIN books AS b ON a.id = author
JOIN types AS t ON b.type_id = t.type_id
ORDER BY full_name, title;
```

full_name	title	type_name
Gabriel, Peter	A Long Day in Spring	History
Meyers, Sally	And Then It Happened	History
Meyers, Sally	Green Trees Go Wild	Science Fiction
Smith, George	Fifteen Hours in March	Suspense
Smith, George	Fourteen Days in February	Suspense

FIGURE 24-9

MySQL statements end with the semicolon, not the end of a line. Best practice is to move to a new line as needed for readability and to keep the lines from getting too long.

Notice that the author Dale Mercer is not on the list nor is the book *Missing in Action*. Only rows with matches in both tables are selected with the plain JOIN. There are different types of joins. The default is a plain JOIN, which is the same as INNER JOIN.

If you want all the rows of a table, regardless of whether they find a match in the other file, you use one of the OUTER JOIN keywords. To keep all rows of the first (left) table, use a LEFT OUTER JOIN. To keep all the rows of the second (right) table, use a RIGHT OUTER JOIN. These are the same as a LEFT JOIN and a RIGHT JOIN. Figure 24-10 illustrates the three types of joins.

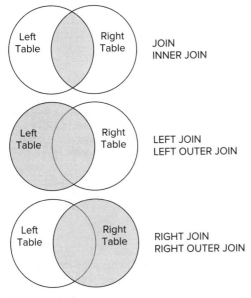

FIGURE 24-10

last_name	first_name	title
Meyers	Sally	Green Trees Go Wild
Meyers	Sally	And Then It Happened
Smith	George	Fifteen Hours in March
Smith	George	Fourteen Days in February
Gabriel	Peter	A Long Day in Spring
Mercer	Dale	*NULL*

FIGURE 24-11

In this example, Dale Mercer has no books, but using a LEFT JOIN includes him in the results. Any fields that should come from the other table are NULL. See the results in Figure 24-11.

```
SELECT last_name, first_name, title
FROM authors AS a
LEFT JOIN books AS b ON a.id = author;
```

When you use a RIGHT JOIN in the same command, all the books are listed, even if they did not match to an author in the authors table. See the results in Figure 24-12.

```
SELECT last_name, first_name, title
FROM authors AS a RIGHT JOIN books AS b ON a.id = author;
```

last_name	first_name	title
Gabriel	Peter	A Long Day in Spring
Smith	George	Fifteen Hours in March
Meyers	Sally	Green Trees Go Wild
Meyers	Sally	And Then It Happened
NULL	NULL	Missing in Action
Smith	George	Fourteen Days in February

FIGURE 24-12

When I said that all the rows from a table are included, that means all the rows that meet the other selection criteria in the other clauses such as the WHERE and LIMIT clauses. The following query asks for all authors whose last names start with an M. See the results in Figure 24-13.

last_name	first_name	title
Meyers	Sally	Green Trees Go Wild
Meyers	Sally	And Then It Happened
Mercer	Dale	NULL

FIGURE 24-13

```
SELECT last_name, first_name, title
FROM authors AS a LEFT JOIN books AS b ON a.id = author
WHERE last_name LIKE 'M%';
```

Use the JOIN clause in PHP as part of ordinary SELECT commands. The JOIN clause is also used in UPDATE and DELETE statements that you learn in later lessons.

USING SUBQUERIES

Subqueries are SELECT statements nested inside other statements. These can be a handy substitute for JOIN and can, in some cases, do things that JOIN cannot. However, if you are using large files there can be unexpected performance costs.

This code gives you a list of the author IDs in the books table as shown in Figure 24-14.

```
SELECT author FROM books;
```

author
3
2
1
1
5
2

FIGURE 24-14

The WHERE *field* IN *list* clause selects rows where the *field* is found in the *list*. You can use the SELECT statement in the preceding code to generate the list. The following example lists all the authors that have a book in the books table. See the results in Figure 24-15.

```
SELECT *
FROM authors
WHERE id IN (SELECT author FROM books);
```

id	first_name	last_name
1	Sally	Meyers
2	George	Smith
3	Peter	Gabriel

FIGURE 24-15

You need to be aware whether the subquery returns a single value, a list of single values, or a list of multiple values because it needs to match

what the outer statement expects. For instance, if you use `WHERE field = value` then `value` must be a single value, not a list. The following code returns the error "Subquery returns more than 1 row."

```
SELECT * FROM authors WHERE id = (SELECT author FROM books);
```

To fix this use either the keyword `ALL` or `ANY`. `ALL` means that all of the rows returned need to meet the criteria. In this example, using `ALL` returns an empty list of authors (but no errors), because no author wrote all the books in the `books` table. However, `ANY` means that the condition is satisfied as long as at least one of the rows satisfied the criteria. So this code also shows the result in Figure 24-15:

```
SELECT * FROM authors WHERE id = ANY (SELECT author FROM books);
```

You also get the same results writing the same statement with `JOIN` without using subqueries:

```
SELECT DISTINCT a.*
FROM authors AS a JOIN books
WHERE a.id = author;
```

id	title	author	type_id
1	A Long Day in Spring	3	1
2	Fifteen Hours in March	2	2
3	Green Trees Go Wild	1	3
4	And Then It Happened	1	1
5	Missing in Action	5	2
6	Fourteen Days in February	2	2
7	Sixteen Seconds in March	2	2

You can use the subqueries in other statements, such as the `INSERT` statement. This example uses `SELECT` queries of other tables and uses the results as the values for creating a new row. The updated `books` table looks like Figure 24-16.

FIGURE 24-16

```
INSERT INTO books (title, author, type_id)
VALUES ('Sixteen Seconds in March',
(SELECT id FROM authors WHERE first_name = 'George' AND last_name = 'Smith'),
(SELECT type_id FROM types WHERE type_name = 'Suspense'));
```

TRY IT

Available for download on Wrox.com

In this Try It, you do not use the Case Study. You create MySQL commands using `SELECT JOIN`s in phpMyAdmin and then run those commands in PHP.

> *You can download the code and resources for this Try It from the book's web page at www.wrox.com. You can find them in the Lesson24 folder in the download. You will find code for both before and after completing the exercises.*

Lesson Requirements

Your computer needs to be able to run as a web server with PHP and MySQL. XAMPP is a package of software that installs the web server, PHP, and MySQL for you. You can find instructions for downloading and installing XAMPP in Lesson 1.

You need a text editor that can produce plain-text files. You can find instructions for downloading and installing Eclipse PDT in Lesson 1. Other text editors that you can use are Adobe's Dreamweaver in code mode, Notepad, TextWrangler, or NetBeans.

Hints

Setting up complex MySQL statements first in phpMyAdmin can help you locate errors before using them in a PHP program.

If the command works in phpMyAdmin and you get errors in PHP, add a `var_dump($query);` line just after you assign the MySQL statement to `$query`. This displays the command that is processed. You can copy that and run it in the SQL tab in phpMyAdmin to find issues.

Remember that `$query` can contain only one command and no semicolons.

Step-by-Step

Create the tables to be used in this Try It. Perform the queries on the files.

1. If you followed along with the lesson, you can skip to step 4. The code for steps 1–3 is in the `Lesson24/exercise24a.sql` file and you can import it into your database in phpMyAdmin.

Create and fill the `authors` table in phpMyAdmin as shown in Figure 24-17.

```
CREATE TABLE `authors` (
  `id` int(11) NOT NULL AUTO_INCREMENT,
  `first_name` varchar(50) NOT NULL,
  `last_name` varchar(50) NOT NULL,
  PRIMARY KEY (`id`)
) ENGINE=MyISAM  DEFAULT CHARSET=utf8;
```

id	first_name	last_name
1	Sally	Meyers
2	George	Smith
3	Peter	Gabriel
4	Dale	Mercer

FIGURE 24-17

```
INSERT INTO `authors` (`id`, `first_name`, `last_name`) VALUES
(1, 'Sally', 'Meyers'),
(2, 'George', 'Smith'),
(3, 'Peter', 'Gabriel'),
(4, 'Dale', 'Mercer');
```

2. Create and fill the `types` table in phpMyAdmin as shown in Figure 24-18.

```
CREATE TABLE `types` (
  `type_id` int(11) NOT NULL AUTO_INCREMENT,
  `type_name` varchar(20) NOT NULL,
  PRIMARY KEY (`type_id`)
) ENGINE=MyISAM  DEFAULT CHARSET=utf8;
```

type_id	type_name
1	History
2	Suspense
3	Science Fiction

FIGURE 24-18

```
INSERT INTO `types` (`type_id`, `type_name`) VALUES
(1, 'History'),
(2, 'Suspense'),
(3, 'Science Fiction');
```

3. Create and fill the `books` table in phpMyAdmin as shown in Figure 24-19.

id	title	author	type_id
1	A Long Day in Spring	3	1
2	Fifteen Hours in March	2	2
3	Green Trees Go Wild	1	3
4	And Then It Happened	1	1
5	Missing in Action	5	2
6	Fourteen Days in February	2	2
7	Sixteen Seconds in March	2	2

FIGURE 24-19

```
CREATE TABLE `books` (
  `id` int(11) NOT NULL AUTO_INCREMENT,
  `title` varchar(50) NOT NULL,
  `author` int(11) DEFAULT NULL,
  `type_id` int(11) DEFAULT NULL,
  PRIMARY KEY (`id`)
) ENGINE=MyISAM  DEFAULT CHARSET=utf8;

INSERT INTO `books` (`id`, `title`, `author`, `type_id`) VALUES
(1, 'A Long Day in Spring', 3, 1),
(2, 'Fifteen Hours in March', 2, 2),
(3, 'Green Trees Go Wild', 1, 3),
(4, 'And Then It Happened', 1, 1),
(5, 'Missing in Action', 5, 2),
(6, 'Fourteen Days in February', 2, 2),
(7, 'Sixteen Seconds in March', 2, 2);
```

4. List the title of the book and the first and last name of the author in phpMyAdmin as shown in Figure 24-20.

title	first_name	last_name
Green Trees Go Wild	Sally	Meyers
And Then It Happened	Sally	Meyers
Fifteen Hours in March	George	Smith
Fourteen Days in February	George	Smith
Sixteen Seconds in March	George	Smith
A Long Day in Spring	Peter	Gabriel

FIGURE 24-20

```
SELECT title, first_name, last_name
FROM books JOIN authors AS a ON author = a.id
```

5. Take the MySQL statement in step 4, sort it by title, and display it using PHP as shown in Figure 24-21.

```
A Long Day in Spring by Peter Gabriel
And Then It Happened by Sally Meyers
Fifteen Hours in March by George Smith
Fourteen Days in February by George Smith
Green Trees Go Wild by Sally Meyers
Sixteen Seconds in March by George Smith
```

FIGURE 24-21

```php
<?php
define("MYSQLUSER", "php24sql");
define("MYSQLPASS", "hJQV8RTe5t");
define("HOSTNAME", "localhost");
define("MYSQLDB", "test");

// Make connection to database
$connection = @new mysqli(HOSTNAME, MYSQLUSER, MYSQLPASS, MYSQLDB);
if ($connection->connect_error) {
  die('Connect Error: ' . $connection->connect_error);
} else {

  // Set up the query
  $query = "SELECT title, first_name, last_name "
    . " FROM books JOIN authors AS a ON author = a.id "
    . " ORDER BY `title` ASC "
    ;

  // Run the query
  $result_obj = '';
  $result_obj = $connection->query($query);

  // Read the results
  // loop through the results, row by row
  // reading each row into an associative array
  while($result = $result_obj->fetch_array(MYSQLI_ASSOC)) {
    // collect the array
    $items[] = $result;
  }
  // print array when done
  foreach ($items as $item) {
    echo $item['title']. ' by ' . $item['first_name']. ' ' . $item['last_
name'];
    //print_r($item);
    echo '<br />';
  }
}
```

6. List the type name, title, and full name of the author for any titles that contain "Day." Put in sequence by the type in descending sequence, then the title. The results are shown in Figure 24-22.

```
SELECT type_name, title, CONCAT(last_name, ', ', first_name) AS full_name
FROM books AS b
JOIN authors AS a ON author = a.id
JOIN types AS t ON b.type_id = t.type_id
WHERE title LIKE '%Day%'
ORDER BY type_name DESC, title;
```

type_name ▾	title	full_name
Suspense	Fourteen Days in February	Smith, George
History	A Long Day in Spring	Gabriel, Peter

FIGURE 24-22

7. Take the MySQL statement in step 6 and put it into a PHP statement to display as shown in Figure 24-23.

Suspense: Fourteen Days in February by Smith, George
History: A Long Day in Spring by Gabriel, Peter

FIGURE 24-23

```php
<?php
define("MYSQLUSER", "php24sql");
define("MYSQLPASS", "hJQV8RTe5t");
define("HOSTNAME", "localhost");
define("MYSQLDB", "test");

// Make connection to database
$connection = @new mysqli(HOSTNAME, MYSQLUSER, MYSQLPASS, MYSQLDB);
if ($connection->connect_error) {
  die('Connect Error: ' . $connection->connect_error);
} else {

  // Set up the query
  $query = "SELECT type_name, title,
    CONCAT(last_name, ', ', first_name) AS full_name "
    . " FROM books AS b "
    . " JOIN authors AS a ON author = a.id "
    . " JOIN types AS t ON b.type_id = t.type_id "
    . " WHERE title LIKE '%Day%' "
    . " ORDER BY type_name DESC, title "
    ;

  // Run the query
  $result_obj = '';
  $result_obj = $connection->query($query);

  // Read the results
  // loop through the results, row by row
  // reading each row into an associative array
  while($result = $result_obj->fetch_array(MYSQLI_ASSOC)) {
```

```
        // collect the array
        $items[] = $result;
    }
    // print array when done
    foreach ($items as $item) {
        echo $item['type_name'] . ': ' . $item['title']. ' by ' . $item['full_
name'];
        echo '<br />';
    }
  }
```

 Watch the video for Lesson 24 on the DVD or watch online at www.wrox.com/ go/24phpmysql.

Changing Data

In this lesson, you learn how to change the data in your database using the UPDATE command.

There are multiple ways to process MySQL data commands. You have been using variations on similar methods. In this lesson you learn a new way with *prepared statements* where you set up the statements first and then you supply the field data separately. Prepared statements are inherently safer because they discourage SQL injections.

The examples from this lesson use the same tables used in the examples in Lesson 24.

> You can download the code for this example from the book's web page at www.wrox.com. You can find them in the Lesson25 folder in the download in a file labeled lesson25a.sql.

The first table is the authors table as shown in Figure 25-1.

The second table is the types table as shown in Figure 25-2.

The third table is the books table as shown in Figure 25-3.

id	first_name	last_name
1	Sally	Meyers
2	George	Smith
3	Peter	Gabriel
5	Dale	Mercer

FIGURE 25-1

type_id	type_name
1	History
2	Suspense
3	Science Fiction

FIGURE 25-2

id	title	author	type_id
1	A Long Day in Spring	3	1
2	Fifteen Hours in March	2	2
3	Green Trees Go Wild	1	3
4	And Then It Happened	1	1
5	Missing in Action	5	2
6	Fourteen Days in February	2	2
7	Sixteen Seconds in March	2	2

FIGURE 25-3

USING THE UPDATE COMMAND

The UPDATE command is used to change the data in your tables. To change row 1 in the authors table from Sally Meyers to Sarah Meyers, use the following code. The result is shown in Figure 25-4.

```
UPDATE authors SET first_name = 'Sarah' WHERE id = '1';
```

id	first_name	last_name
1	Sarah	Meyers
2	George	Smith
3	Peter	Gabriel
4	Dale	Mercer

FIGURE 25-4

If you leave off the WHERE clause, all rows are updated. See Figure 25-5 for the results of the following code:

```
UPDATE authors SET first_name = 'Sarah';
```

id	first_name	last_name
1	Sarah	Meyers
2	Sarah	Smith
3	Sarah	Gabriel
4	Sarah	Mercer

FIGURE 25-5

> ⊗ *If you do not specify a WHERE clause, the default is to select all rows. With the UPDATE command that means that you could accidently update all rows if you forget your WHERE clause.*

Unlike INSERT, there is no way to update multiple rows with different data, so to restore the first names you need four rows:

```
UPDATE authors SET first_name = 'Sally' WHERE id = '1';
UPDATE authors SET first_name = 'George' WHERE id = '2';
UPDATE authors SET first_name = 'Peter' WHERE id = '3';
UPDATE authors SET first_name = 'Dale' WHERE id = '4';
```

id	first_name	last_name
1	Sally	Meyers
2	George	Smith
3	Peter	Gabriel
4	Jeff	Baamer

FIGURE 25-6

You can, however, update more than one field at a time. This code gives the results shown in Figure 25-6:

```
UPDATE authors SET first_name = 'Jeff', last_name = 'Baamer' WHERE id = '4';
```

You can use clauses you learned for the SELECT statement in the UPDATE statement. The following code updates the title field in the books table by adding an asterisk (*) to the end of the title for any books written by someone with the name of Sally. See the results in Figure 25-7.

```
UPDATE books JOIN authors AS a ON author = a.id
    SET title = CONCAT(title, '*') WHERE first_name = 'Sally';
```

id	title	author	type_id
1	A Long Day in Spring	3	1
2	Fifteen Hours in March	2	2
3	Green Trees Go Wild*	1	3
4	And Then It Happened*	1	1
5	Missing in Action	5	2
6	Fourteen Days in February	2	2
7	Sixteen Seconds in March	2	2

FIGURE 25-7

You can also use subqueries, though the table you are updating cannot be in the subquery. This code appends a double asterisk (**) to any titles in `books` that have no entry in the `authors` table. See the results in Figure 25-8.

```
UPDATE books SET title = CONCAT(title, '**')
    WHERE author NOT IN (SELECT id FROM authors);
```

id	title	author	type_id
1	A Long Day in Spring	3	1
2	Fifteen Hours in March	2	2
3	Green Trees Go Wild*	1	3
4	And Then It Happened*	1	1
5	Missing in Action**	5	2
6	Fourteen Days in February	2	2
7	Sixteen Seconds in March	2	2

FIGURE 25-8

When you INSERT new rows you get an error if you try to insert a row that already exists. This INSERT fails with a Duplicate Entry error:

```
INSERT INTO authors (id, first_name, last_name) VALUES ('4', 'Jane', 'Smith');
```

If you add an ON DUPLICATE KEY UPDATE clause to the INSERT statement, you specify that you want MySQL to update the row if it already exists. See the following code and the results in Figure 25-9.

```
INSERT INTO authors (id, first_name, last_name)
VALUES ('4', 'Jane', 'Smith')
ON DUPLICATE KEY UPDATE first_name = 'Jane', last_name = 'Smith';
```

UPDATING DATA IN PHP

Updating data through a PHP program using MySQL commands takes three steps:

id	first_name	last_name
1	Sally	Meyers
2	George	Smith
3	Peter	Gabriel
4	Jane	Smith

FIGURE 25-9

1. Make a connection to the database.

2. Create a safe query with the command.

3. Run the query.

The following code uses the MySQL UPDATE command to change fields in the table `authors`. See the result in Figure 25-10.

```
<?php
define("MYSQLUSER", "php24sql");
define("MYSQLPASS", "hJQV8RTe5t");
define("HOSTNAME", "localhost");
define("MYSQLDB", "test");

// Make connection to database
```

```php
$connection = @new mysqli(HOSTNAME, MYSQLUSER, MYSQLPASS, MYSQLDB);
if ($connection->connect_error) {
  die('Connect Error: ' . $connection->connect_error);
} else {
  echo 'Successful connection to MySQL <br />';

  $first_name = "Liam";
  $last_name = "O'Reilly";
  $id = 4;

  // Prepare the data
  if (get_magic_quotes_gpc()) {
    $first_name = stripslashes($first_name);
    $last_name = stripslashes($last_name);
  }
  $first_name = $connection->real_escape_string($first_name);
  $last_name = $connection->real_escape_string($last_name);
  $id = (int) $id;

  // Set up the query
    $query = "UPDATE `authors` "
    . " SET `first_name`= '$first_name', `last_name` = '$last_name' "
    . " WHERE `id` = '$id'";

  // Run the query and display appropriate message
  if (!$result = $connection->query($query)) {
    echo "No rows updated<br />";
  } else {
    echo $result . " row(s) successfully updated<br />";
  }
}
```

Like the INSERT you learned in Lesson 22, you need to prepare the data before you post it to the database using PHP with UPDATE and REPLACE. The preparation consists of making it safe against SQL injections and to deal with quotes in string values because the wrong type of quote in the wrong place might be seen as a MySQL control character and invalidate the command.

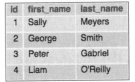

id	first_name	last_name
1	Sally	Meyers
2	George	Smith
3	Peter	Gabriel
4	Liam	O'Reilly

FIGURE 25-10

Compare these lines of code:

```php
$result_obj = $connection->query("SELECT first_name FROM authors");
$result = $connection->query("UPDATE authors SET first_name='Sally' WHERE id=4");
```

In the first line of code, the mysqli::query() method returns an object because it processes a SELECT command. In this example, I am assigning it to a variable called $result_obj as a reminder that it is an object, though it can be named anything. This object then needs to be read to get the results of the SELECT statement. You learned several ways to read the result object in Lesson 23.

In the second line of code, the mysqli::query() method returns a Boolean (TRUE or FALSE) that indicates the success of the action, in this case, the UPDATE command.

An object is returned by mysqli::query() when the command is SELECT, SHOW, DESCRIBE, or EXPLAIN. The last three commands are used to show information about the structure of the

database or internal details that can be used to optimize performance. All other commands, such as INSERT, UPDATE, REPLACE, and DELETE just return TRUE or FALSE.

You have been primarily using the object-oriented method of the mysqli connection, but the code can also be written with the procedural version as in this code and as shown in Figure 25-11:

```php
<?php
define("MYSQLUSER", "php24sql");
define("MYSQLPASS", "hJQV8RTe5t");
define("HOSTNAME", "localhost");
define("MYSQLDB", "test");

// Make connection to database
$connection = @mysqli_connect(HOSTNAME, MYSQLUSER, MYSQLPASS, MYSQLDB);
if (mysqli_connect_error()) {
  die('Connect Error: ' . mysqli_connect_error());
} else {
  echo 'Successful connection to MySQL <br />';

  $first_name = "Danny";
  $last_name = "O'Murphy";
  $id = 4;
  var_dump($connection);

  // Prepare the data
  if (get_magic_quotes_gpc()) {
    $first_name = stripslashes($first_name);
    $last_name = stripslashes($last_name);
  }
  $first_name = mysqli_real_escape_string($connection, $first_name);
  $last_name = mysqli_real_escape_string($connection, $last_name);
  $id = (int) $id;

  // Set up the query
    $query = "UPDATE `authors` "
    . " SET `first_name`= '$first_name', `last_name` = '$last_name' "
    . " WHERE `id` = '$id'";

  // Run the query and display appropriate message
  if (!$result = mysqli_query($connection, $query)) {
    echo "No rows updated<br />";
  } else {
    echo "Row(s) successfully updated<br />";
  }
}
```

id	first_name	last_name
1	Sally	Meyers
2	George	Smith
3	Peter	Gabriel
4	Danny	O'Murphy

FIGURE 25-11

USING PREPARED STATEMENTS

Prepared statements are relatively new to PHP. With prepared statements, you define a statement with placeholders and then you can rerun the statement multiple times and just give it the placeholder information. Using prepared statements has three main benefits:

➤ They are more secure. SQL injection takes advantage of input variables to pass embedded code that is unconsciously run by the processor. Prepared statements separate running code from the variable values so the embedded code has no place to run.

➤ They can have better performance. This is only true if you reuse the same prepared statement multiple times. The program does the heavy lifting when it sets up the statement and then it's cheap to send new placeholder values.

➤ They are more convenient to write. Just like templates in a word processing program, the constant data is separated out from the dynamic data, which makes the statements easier to work with. Additionally, you don't need to worry about escaping quotes because the data is separate from the command statement.

MYSQLI

The following code creates a prepared statement and then runs it to update the name of the author in row 4 and then in row 3 of the `authors` table. See the result in Figure 25-12 and Figure 25-13.

```php
<?php
define("MYSQLUSER", "php24sql");
define("MYSQLPASS", "hJQV8RTe5t");
define("HOSTNAME", "localhost");
define("MYSQLDB", "test");

// Make connection to database
$connection = @new mysqli(HOSTNAME, MYSQLUSER, MYSQLPASS, MYSQLDB);
if ($connection->connect_error) {
  die('Connect Error: ' . $connection->connect_error);
} else {
  echo 'Successful connection to MySQL <br />';

  $first_name = "Gilly";
  $last_name = "O'Donal";
  $id = 4;

  // Set up the prepared statement
  $query = "UPDATE `authors` "
    . " SET `first_name`= ?, `last_name` = ? "
    . " WHERE `id` = ?";
  // Prepare the statement
  $statement = $connection->prepare($query);
  // Bind the parameters
  $statement->bind_param('ssi',$first_name, $last_name,$id);
  // Run the query
  if (!$result = $statement->execute()) {
    echo "No rows updated<br />";
  } else {
  echo "First row successfully updated<br />";
  }

  // Assign new values to the bound variables
  $first_name = "Meg";
  $last_name = "Mitchell";
  $id = 3;

  // Rerun the statement
```

```
if (!$result = $statement->execute()) {
  echo "No rows updated<br />";
} else {
  echo "Second row successfully updated<br />";
}
// Close the statement
$statement->close();


}
```

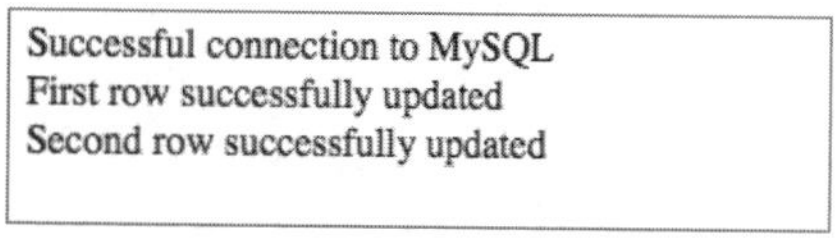

Successful connection to MySQL
First row successfully updated
Second row successfully updated

FIGURE 25-12

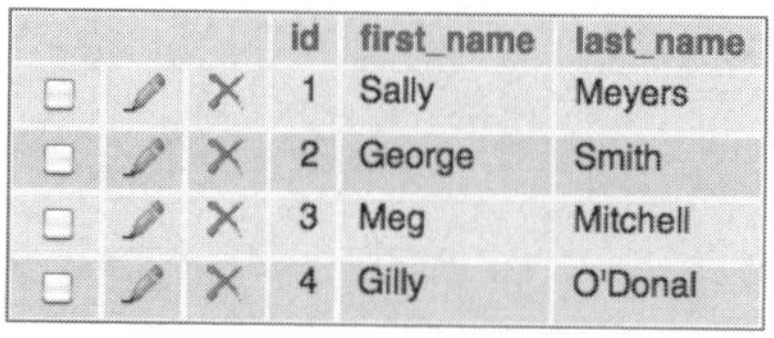

			id	first_name	last_name
☐	🖉	✕	1	Sally	Meyers
☐	🖉	✕	2	George	Smith
☐	🖉	✕	3	Meg	Mitchell
☐	🖉	✕	4	Gilly	O'Donal

FIGURE 25-13

As you see in the example, first you set up the prepared statement. To do that, replace the variables with a ? (? is the placeholder). Certain restrictions exist on what you can replace as placeholders. For the most part you can use them where you put data but not as table names or field names.

After you have set up the statement, you prepare the statement with `mysqli::prepare()`. You could do both these steps in one step, but setting up the statement in a variable first makes it easier to debug all the quotes and concatenations because you can place a `var_dump($query);` after you've created it. That displays a MySQL command that you can examine for errors.

Now that you've prepared the statement, you bind the placeholders to the statement with `mysqli::bind_param()`. This assigns the values you want to use for this processing of the prepared statement. Binding requires two pieces of information for each placeholder: the data type and the value. The placeholder parameters must be specified in the same order as they appear in the statement. In the example, the type is `'ssi'` because `$first_name` and `$last_name` are strings and `$id` is an integer. The valid codes are listed in Table 25-1.

TABLE 25-1: Parameter Data Types

CODE	DATA TYPE
i	Integer
d	Double (numeric with decimals)
s	String (Text)
b	Blob (Lots of binary characters)

After you bind the placeholder parameters, you execute the statement. Because you are binding the variables themselves, you can change the value of the variables and execute again with the different values. When you are done, close the statement. You can have only one prepared statement open at a time.

You can use prepared statements for SELECT commands as well. Here you bind the results as well as any parameters. See the results in Figure 25-14.

```php
<?php
define("MYSQLUSER", "php24sql");
define("MYSQLPASS", "hJQV8RTe5t");
define("HOSTNAME", "localhost");
define("MYSQLDB", "test");

// Make connection to database
$connection = @new mysqli(HOSTNAME, MYSQLUSER, MYSQLPASS, MYSQLDB);
if ($connection->connect_error) {
  die('Connect Error: ' . $connection->connect_error);
} else {
  echo 'Successful connection to MySQL <br />';

  $id = 4;

  // Set up the prepared statement
  $query = "SELECT `first_name`, `last_name` "
    . " FROM `authors`"
    . " WHERE `id` = ?";
  // Prepare the statement
  $statement = $connection->prepare($query);
  // Bind the parameters
  $statement->bind_param('i',$id);
  // Execute the statement
  $statement->execute();
  // Bind the results
  $statement->bind_result($first,$last);
  // Run the query
  $statement->fetch();
  echo $first . ' ' . $last . '<br />';
  // Close the statement
  $statement->close();
}
```

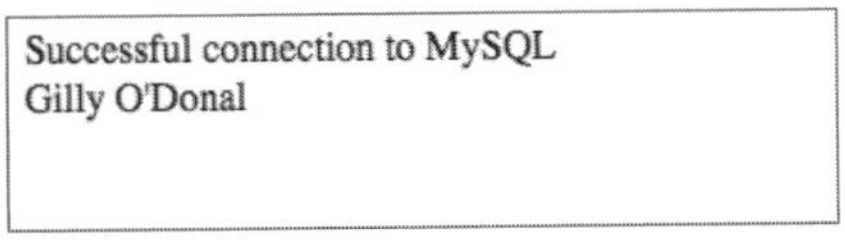

```
Successful connection to MySQL
Gilly O'Donal
```

FIGURE 25-14

PHP Data Objects (PDO)

PHP Data Objects (PDO) has its own version of prepared statements, which have some advantages over the mysqli version. You have the ability to use named parameters as well as unnamed parameters. To use named parameters, replace the question mark (?) with a name prefixed with a colon (:). The PDO_Statement::bindParm() method assigns the variable that supplies the data, as well as output data. The data type is specified with predefined PDO Constants, which are listed in Table 25-2.

TABLE 25-2: PDO Data Types

CONSTANT	DESCRIPTION
PDO::PARAM_INT	Integers
PDO::PARAM_STR	Strings
PDO::PARAM_BOOL	Boolean
PDO::PARAM_LOB	Blobs

Run the following code to see the results in Figure 25-15 and Figure 25-16:

```php
<?php
define("MYSQLUSER", "php24sql");
define("MYSQLPASS", "hJQV8RTe5t");
define("HOSTNAME", "localhost");
define("MYSQLDB", "test");

// Make connection to database
if (!$connection =
  new PDO('mysql:host='.HOSTNAME.';dbname=' . MYSQLDB, MYSQLUSER, MYSQLPASS)) {
  die('Connect Error');
} else {
  echo 'Successful connection to MySQL <br />';

  $first_name = "Paddy";
  $last_name = "O'Brian";
  $id = 4;

  // Set up the prepared statement
  $query = "UPDATE `authors` "
    . " SET `first_name`= :first_name, `last_name` = :last_name "
    . " WHERE `id` = :id";
  // Prepare the statement
  $statement = $connection->prepare($query);
  // Bind the parameters
  $statement->bindParam(':first_name', $first_name, PDO::PARAM_STR, 50);
  $statement->bindParam(':last_name', $last_name, PDO::PARAM_STR, 50);
  $statement->bindParam(':id', $id, PDO::PARAM_INT);
  // Run the query
  if (!$result = $statement->execute()) {
    echo "No rows updated<br />";
  } else {
    echo "First row successfully updated<br />";
  }
  // Change the value in the variable and rerun
  $id = 3;
  $first_name = 'Nancy';
  $last_name = 'Misson';

  // Rerun the statement
  if (!$result = $statement->execute()) {
```

```
        echo "No rows updated<br />";
    } else {
        echo "Second row successfully updated<br />";
    }
}
```

id	first_name	last_name
1	Sally	Meyers
2	George	Smith
3	Nancy	Misson
4	Paddy	O'Brian

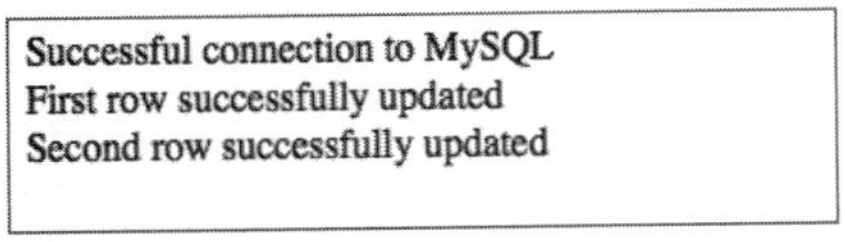

Successful connection to MySQL
First row successfully updated
Second row successfully updated

FIGURE 25-15

FIGURE 25-16

TRY IT

In this Try It, you add maintenance to the `contacts` and `categories` tables in the Case Study. You modify the add pages for the contacts and lot categories so that you can edit contacts and lot categories.

> *You can download the code and resources for this Try It from the book's web page at* www.wrox.com. *You can find them in the Lesson25 folder in the download. You will find code for both before and after completing the exercises.*

Lesson Requirements

Your computer needs to be able to run as a web server with PHP and MySQL. XAMPP is a package of software that installs the web server, PHP, and MySQL for you. You can find instructions for downloading and installing XAMPP in Lesson 1.

You need a text editor that can produce plain-text files. You can find instructions for downloading and installing Eclipse PDT in Lesson 1. Other text editors that you can use are Adobe's Dreamweaver in code mode, Notepad, TextWrangler, or NetBeans.

If you are following along with the Case Study, you need your files from the end of Lesson 23. Alternatively, you can download the files from the book's website at www.wrox.com. To re-create the database tables, create an empty database and then import the `install.sql` file in phpMyAdmin.

Hints

When adding rows, you don't need to know the primary key of the row because the primary key is automatically created. When editing rows, you need to pass that key along so that you always know what it is.

Step-by-Step

Change the contact add page so that it edits existing records.

1. In the `contents/about.php` file add an edit button to link to the maintenance page with the `id` of the current contact in the URL. This is the current `<h2>` line:

```
<h2><?php echo htmlspecialchars($item->name()); ?></h2>
```

Replace it with this new `<h2>` line:

```
<h2><?php echo htmlspecialchars($item->name()); ?>
<a class="button"
   href="index.php?content=contactmaint&id=<?php echo $item->getId(); ?>">
Edit</a></h2>
```

2. In the `contents/contactmaint.php` file check for the `id` in the URL. If it is not 0 then get the row from the table to create the `Contact` object. Do this by changing `$item = new Contact;` to the following code:

```
$id = (int) $_GET['id'];
// Is this an existing item or a new one?
if ($id) {
  // Get the existing information for an existing item
  $item = Contact::getContact($id);
} else {
  // Set up for a new item
  $item = new Contact;
}
```

3. Change the legend to show the `id` if this is an existing contact:

```
<legend><?php echo ($id) ? 'ID: '. $id : 'Add a Contact' ?></legend>
```

4. Add the `getContact()` method in the `includes/classes/contact.php` file to create a `Contact` object from a row in the `contacts` table:

```
public static function getContact($id) {
    // Get the database connection
    $connection = Database::getConnection();
    // Set up the query
    $query = 'SELECT * FROM `contacts` WHERE id="'. (int) $id.'"';
    // Run the MySQL command
    $result_obj = '';
      try {
        $result_obj = $connection->query($query);
        if (!$result_obj) {
          throw new Exception($connection->error);
        } else {
          $item = $result_obj->fetch_object('Contact');
          if (!$item) {
```

```
            throw new Exception($connection->error);
        } else {
            // pass back the results
            return($item);
        }
      }
    }
    catch(Exception $e) {
      echo $e->getMessage();
    }
  }
```

5. You need to change the processing of the `contact.maint` task. In the `includes/init.php` file, locate the `contact.maint` case. The header redirect needs the id of the row. That id is added to the `$result` array from the `editRecord()` method and passed through the `editContact()` function.

    ```
    header("Location: index.php?content=contactmaint&id=$results[2]");
    ```

6. In the `includes/functions.php` file change the `maintContact()` function to call the `editRecord()` function if the id already exists. This is the current code:

    ```
    // Set up a Contact object based on the posts
    $contact = new Contact($item);
    $results = $contact->addRecord();
    ```

    Replace it with this new code:

    ```
    // Set up a Contact object based on the posts
    $contact = new Contact($item);
    if ($contact->getId()) {
     $results = $contact->editRecord();
    } else {
     $results = $contact->addRecord();
    }
    ```

7. Back in the `includes/classes/contact.php` file add the `editRecord()` method to update the table. You need the id to create the URL to redirect to the correct page if there is an error, so add a third element to the return array.

    ```
    public function editRecord() {
        // Verify the fields
        if ($this->_verifyInput()) {

            // Get the Database connection
            $connection = Database::getConnection();

            // Set up the prepared statement
            $query = 'UPDATE `contacts`
              SET first_name=?, last_name=?, position=?, email=?, phone=?
              WHERE id=?';
            $statement = $connection->prepare($query);
            // bind the parameters
            $statement->bind_param('sssssi',
              $this->first_name, $this->last_name, $this->position,
    ```

```
        $this->email, $this->phone, $this->id);
    if ($statement) {
        $statement->execute();
        $statement->close();
        // add success message
        $return = array('', 'Contact Record successfully added.', '');
        return $return;
    } else {
        $return = array('contactmaint',
          'No Contact Record Added. Unable to create record.' ,
          (int) $this->id);
        return $return;
    }

} else {
    // send fail message and return to contactmaint
    $return = array('contactmaint',
      'No Contact Record Added. Missing required information.' ,
    (int) $this->id);
    return $return;
}

}
```

8. Go to the About Us page as shown in Figure 25-17.

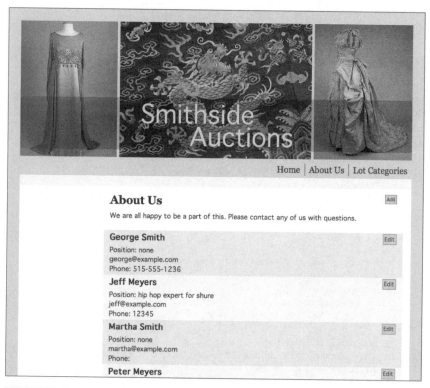

FIGURE 25-17

9. Click the Edit button on George Smith and you see a page similar to Figure 25-18. Make changes and click Save to save the changes.

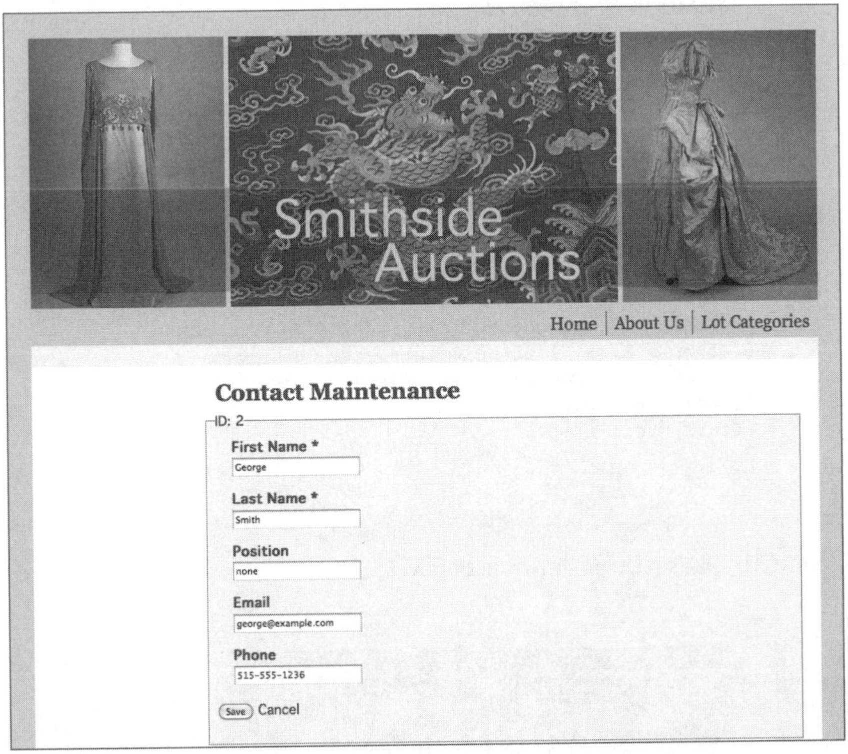

FIGURE 25-18

10. In step 7 you added a third element to the array that returns out of `editRecord()`. You need to add that element to the array that `addRecord()` returns, as shown in the following code from `includes/classes/contact.php`.

```
// Run the MySQL statement
if ($connection->query($query)) {
$return = array('', 'Contact Record successfully added.', '' );

// add success message
return $return;
} else {
// send fail message and return to contactmaint
$return = array('contactmaint', 'No Contact Record Added. Unable to ↵
create record.', '');
  return $return;
  }
} else {
  // send fail message and return to contactmaint
  $return = array('contactmaint', 'No Contact Record Added. Missing ↵
required information.', '0');
  return $return;
}
```

Change the category add page so that it edits existing records.

1. In the `contents/categories.php` file add an Edit button to link to the maintenance page with the id of the current category in the URL. Put it below the Display Lots button:

```
<a class="button edit"
  href="index.php?content=categorymaint&cat_id=<?php echo $item->getCat_id();
?>">
  Edit</a>
```

2. In the `contents/categorymaint.php` file, check for the category id in the URL. If it is not 0 then get the row from the table to create the `Category` object. Do this by changing `$item = new Category;` to the following code:

```
$id = (int) $_GET['cat_id'];
// Is this an existing item or a new one?
if ($id) {
  // Get the existing information for an existing item
  $item = Category::getCategory($id);
} else {
  // Set up for a new item
  $item = new Category;
}
```

3. Change the legend to show the id if this is an existing category:

```
<legend><?php echo ($id) ? 'ID: '. $id : 'Add a Category' ?></legend>
```

4. Add the `getCategory()` method in the `includes/classes/category.php` file to create a `Category` object from a row in the `categories` table:

```
public static function getCategory($cat_id) {
  // Get the DB connection
  $connection = Database::getConnection();
  // Prepare the query
  $query = 'SELECT * FROM `categories` WHERE cat_id="'. (int) $cat_id.'"';

  // Run the MySQL command
  $result_obj = $connection->query($query);
  try {
  while($result = $result_obj->fetch_array(MYSQLI_ASSOC)) {
     $item = new Category($result);
   }
     // pass back the results
   return($item);
  }
  catch(Exception $e) {
     return false;
  }
}
```

5. You need to change the processing of the `category.maint` task. In the `includes/init.php` file locate the `category.maint` case. The header redirect needs the id of the row. That id is added to the `$result` array from the `editRecord()` method and passed through the `editCategory()` function.

```
header("Location: index.php?content=categorymaint&cat_id=$results[2]");
```

6. In the includes/functions.php change the maintCategory() function to call the editRecord() function if the id already exists. This is the current code:

```
// Set up a Category object based on the posts
$category = new Category($item);
$results = $category->addRecord();
```

Replace it with this new code:

```
// Set up a Category object based on the posts
$category = new Category($item);
if ($category ->getGet_id()) {
 $results = $category ->editRecord();
} else {
 $results = $category ->addRecord();
}
```

7. Back in the includes/classes/category.php file, add the editRecord() method to update the table. You need the id to create the URL to redirect to the correct page if there is an error, so add a third element to the return array.

```
public function editRecord() {
   // Verify the fields
   if ($this->_verifyInput()) {

      // Get the Database connection
      $connection = Database::getConnection();

      // Set up the prepared statement
      $query = 'UPDATE `categories`
        SET cat_name=?, cat_description=?, cat_image=?
        WHERE cat_id=?';
      $statement = $connection->prepare($query);
      // bind the parameters
      $statement->bind_param('sssi',
        $this->cat_name, $this->cat_description, $this->cat_image,
        $this->cat_id);
      if ($statement) {
        $statement->execute();
        $statement->close();
        // add success message
        $return = array('', 'Category Record successfully added.', '');
        return $return;
      } else {
        $return = array('categorymaint',
          'No Category Record Added. Unable to create record.',
          (int) $this->cat_id);
        return $return;
      }

   } else {
      // send fail message and return to categorymaint
      $return = array('contactmaint',
        'No Contact Record Added. Missing required information.',
```

```
        (int) $this->cat_id);
    return $return;
  }

}
```

8. Go to the Lot Categories page as shown in Figure 25-19.

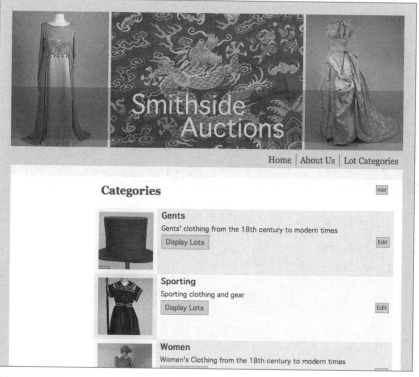

FIGURE 25-19

9. Click the Edit button on the Gents category and you see a page similar to Figure 25-20. Make changes and click Save to save the changes.

10. In step 7, you added a third element to the array that returns out of editRecord(). You need to add that element to the array that addRecord() returns as shown in the following code from includes/classes/contact.php.

```
// Run the MySQL statement
if ($connection->query($query)) {
  $return = array('', 'Category Record successfully added.','');

  // add success message
  return $return;
} else {
  // send fail message and return to categorymaint
```

```
    $return = array('contactmaint', 'No Category Record Added. Unable to ↵
create record.','');
    return $return;
    }
} else {
    // send fail message and return to categorymaint
    $return = array('categorymaint', 'No Category Record Added. Missing ↵
required information.','0');
    return $return;
}
```

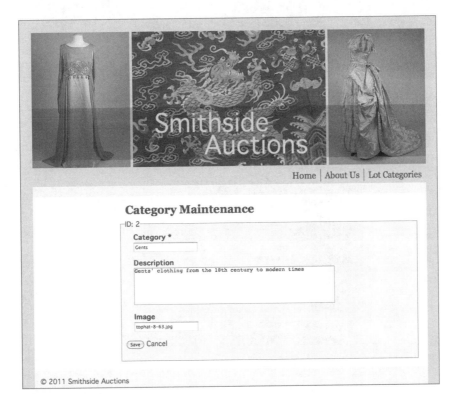

FIGURE 25-20

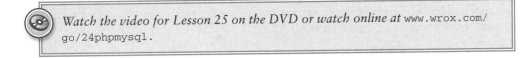

 Watch the video for Lesson 25 on the DVD or watch online at www.wrox.com/go/24phpmysql.

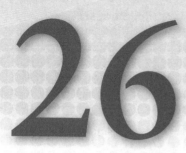

Deleting Data

In this lesson you learn how to delete rows from tables in the MySQL database. The examples from this lesson use the same tables used in the examples in Lesson 25.

You can download the code for this example from the book's web page at www.wrox.com. You can find it in the Lesson 26 folder in the download in a file labeled lesson26a.sql.

The first table is the authors table as shown in Figure 26-1.

The second table is the types table as shown in Figure 26-2.

The third table is the books table as shown in Figure 26-3.

id	first_name	last_name
1	Sally	Meyers
2	George	Smith
3	Nancy	Misson
4	Paddy	O'Brian

FIGURE 26-1

type_id	type_name
1	History
2	Suspense
3	Science Fiction

FIGURE 26-2

id	title	author	type_id
1	A Long Day in Spring	3	1
2	Fifteen Hours in March	2	2
3	Green Trees Go Wild*	1	3
4	And Then It Happened*	1	1
5	Missing in Action**	5	2
6	Fourteen Days in February	2	2
7	Sixteen Seconds in March	2	2

FIGURE 26-3

USING THE DELETE COMMAND

Later on in this lesson I ask you to restore the example tables back to this point. If you are entering the examples, then you should make a backup by exporting the files now. If you are using the downloaded file lesson26a.sql, then you can just use that file when you are asked to restore.

> *If you don't remember how to back up MySQL tables by exporting them, see "Backing Up and Restoring" in Lesson 19.*

The DELETE command is used to remove rows from your tables. To remove row 2 from the types table you use the following code. The results are shown in Figure 26-4.

type_id	type_name
1	History
3	Science Fiction

FIGURE 26-4

```
DELETE FROM types WHERE type_id = '2';
```

If you don't specify a WHERE clause, all rows are deleted from the table unless you use a LIMIT clause, in which case, the rows selected with the LIMIT clause are deleted. The following code deletes all the rows in the types table:

```
DELETE FROM types;
```

> *If you do not specify a WHERE clause, the default is to select all rows. With the DELETE command, that means that you could accidentally delete all rows if you forget your WHERE clause.*

If you want to delete all the rows in a table, best practice is to use the TRUNCATE command as shown in the following code:

```
`TRUNCATE types`
```

See what happens when you add a row back in to the types table as shown in Figure 26-5.

type_id	type_name
4	Fantasy

FIGURE 26-5

```
INSERT INTO types VALUES (NULL, 'Fantasy');
```

Notice that even though there is only one row in the table, the value automatically assigned to type_id is 4. If you are using auto_increment, deleting rows, even all the rows, does not affect it. If the next row was to be assigned 4 before you deleted all the rows, the next row you add is still assigned a 4. This is true for the MyISAM tables and, for the most part, InnoDB tables as well.

There's no way to undelete deleted rows. They are gone. You need to re-insert them if you want to restore them. If you need to synchronize the primary key with other files, you need to specify the correct value rather than letting auto_increment assign it. The following code explicitly lists the values to be used for the type_id field. As you see in Figure 26-6, these inserted rows are created with the specified values rather than being automatically generated by the next higher number.

type_id	type_name
4	Fantasy
1	History
2	Suspense
3	Science Fiction

FIGURE 26-6

```
INSERT INTO `types` (`type_id`, `type_name`) VALUES
(1, 'History'),
(2, 'Suspense'),
(3, 'Science Fiction');
```

You can use the LIMIT clause to limit how many records are deleted. You can use this if you have a lot of rows to delete that might exceed the time limit. You would run the command multiple times until all the required rows are deleted. The following example deletes one row. See the results in Figure 26-7.

			type_id	type_name
☐	✎	✕	1	History
☐	✎	✕	2	Suspense
☐	✎	✕	3	Science Fiction

FIGURE 26-7

```
DELETE FROM types LIMIT 1;
```

The ORDER BY clause determines the order in which rows are deleted. The following code deletes the first two books when the titles are in alphabetical order, as shown in Figure 26-8:

```
DELETE FROM books ORDER BY title ASC LIMIT 2;
```

id	title	author	type_id
2	Fifteen Hours in March	2	2
3	Green Trees Go Wild*	1	3
5	Missing in Action**	5	2
6	Fourteen Days in February	2	2
7	Sixteen Seconds in March	2	2

FIGURE 26-8

The WHERE clause is the same used by the SELECT statement, so it can be as complex as you need. For instance, you can use more than one condition in selecting the rows to be deleted. This example deletes any books written by author 2 that have "Days" in the title. See Figure 26-9.

```
DELETE FROM books WHERE author = '2' AND title LIKE '%Days%';
```

id	title	author	type_id
2	Fifteen Hours in March	2	2
3	Green Trees Go Wild*	1	3
5	Missing in Action**	5	2
7	Sixteen Seconds in March	2	2

FIGURE 26-9

This example uses a subquery to delete any book that has an invalid author. See Figure 26-10.

```
DELETE FROM books WHERE author NOT IN (SELECT id FROM authors);
```

id	title	author	type_id
2	Fifteen Hours in March	2	2
3	Green Trees Go Wild*	1	3
7	Sixteen Seconds in March	2	2

FIGURE 26-10

After all this deleting from the books table, only two authors in the authors table still have books in the books table. So here you use the JOIN clause to locate the orphan authors and remove them.

The LEFT JOIN selects all authors (because they are on the "left" side). Any author without any matching books has the book fields assigned as NULL values. The field author (from the books table) should always be equal to the primary key, id, in the authors table because that is what merges the rows, so if the field author is NULL, you know that no match was found. See Figure 26-11.

```
DELETE authors FROM authors LEFT JOIN books ON authors.id = author
  WHERE author IS NULL;
```

DELETING DATA IN PHP

Now that you've succeeded in deleting most of the database, restore it to the state it was in at the beginning of the lesson so you can delete it using PHP. Restore using either the lesson26a.sql file you imported at the beginning of the lesson or the file you exported at the beginning of the lesson.

id	first_name	last_name
1	Sally	Meyers
2	George	Smith

FIGURE 26-11

> *If you don't remember how to import a* .sql *file, see "Backing Up and Restoring" in Lesson 19.*

Deleting data using PHP is similar to the way you INSERT data, though you usually don't have as many fields to prepare because the only relevant fields are those you need for the selection process. Easiest of all is deleting rows when you know the primary key and that key is an integer type. The following example deletes the book with the id of 6. Figure 26-12 shows what running the PHP program looks like and Figure 26-13 shows the books table in phpMyAdmin after the deletion has taken place.

```php
<?php
define("MYSQLUSER", "php24sql");
define("MYSQLPASS", "hJQV8RTe5t");
define("HOSTNAME", "localhost");
define("MYSQLDB", "test");

// Make connection to database
$connection = @new mysqli(HOSTNAME, MYSQLUSER, MYSQLPASS, MYSQLDB);
if ($connection->connect_error) {
  die('Connect Error: ' . $connection->connect_error);
} else {
  echo 'Successful connection to MySQL <br />';

  // assign an id value for the test
  $id = 6;

  // Set up the query
  $query = 'DELETE FROM `books` WHERE id="'. (int) $id.'"';
  // Run the query and display appropriate message
  if (!$result = $connection->query($query)) {
    echo "No rows deleted<br />";
  } else {
    echo $connection->affected_rows . " row(s) successfully deleted<br />";
```

```
        }
    }
```

The `mysqli->affected_rows` is a property in the `mysqli` class that tells you the number of affected rows in the last MySQL command. In this example this is represented by the `$connection->affected_rows`.

Successful connection to MySQL
1 row(s) successfully deleted

FIGURE 26-12

id	title	author	type_id
1	A Long Day in Spring	3	1
2	Fifteen Hours in March	2	2
3	Green Trees Go Wild*	1	3
4	And Then It Happened*	1	1
5	Missing in Action**	5	2
7	Sixteen Seconds in March	2	2

FIGURE 26-13

TRY IT

Available for
download on
Wrox.com

In this Try It, you add delete capabilities to the About Us and Lot Categories pages by adding Delete buttons and a confirmation page. The Lesson26 folder on the website contains the interim files as of the end of this part.

You have been updating the About Us and Lot Categories pages piece by piece through the last several chapters to use the database instead of hardcoded data. As they say in computerese, you have created the CRUD for those tables: Create, Review, Update, and Delete. The last table, and related pages, is the `lots` table.

In this Try It, you bring the website all the way from multiple hardcoded gents, women, and sporting pages to full display and maintenance in integrated lots pages. You preselect which lots display based on the lot category they are in. You also create a drop-down input select based on the `categories` table that is used for selection of the appropriate category.

> *You can download the code and resources for this Try It from the book's web page at www.wrox.com. You can find them in the Lesson26 folder in the download. You will find code for both before and after completing the exercises.*

Lesson Requirements

Your computer needs to be able to run as a web server with PHP and MySQL. XAMPP is a package of software that installs the web server, PHP, and MySQL for you. You can find instructions for downloading and installing XAMPP in Lesson 1.

You need a text editor that can produce plain-text files. You can find instructions for downloading and installing Eclipse PDT in Lesson 1. Other text editors that you can use are Adobe's Dreamweaver in code mode, Notepad, TextWrangler, or NetBeans.

If you are following along with the Case Study, you need your files from the end of Lesson 25. Alternatively, you can download the files from the book's website at www.wrox.com.

Hints

The steps that you take to delete a row are the same basic steps you need to take to change a row: select the row and display it, process the input from the user, and then either update the table or give the user an error message.

When you display the information from the row, don't use label and input tags because you don't want the user thinking that he can change the data.

When you process the form, the only vital piece of information is the id of the row in the table. Because that is an integer, you can use (int) to force the information from the user into an integer as your safety processing.

Step-by-Step

Add delete capabilities to the About Us page.

1. In the `contents/about.php` files add a Delete button in the `<h2>` tag:

```
<h2><?php echo htmlspecialchars($item->name()); ?>
<a class="button"
href="index.php?content=contactdelete&id=<?php echo
$item->getId(); ?>">Delete</a>
   <a class="button"  href="index.php?content=contactmaint&id=<?php echo ↵
$item->
      getId(); ?>">Edit</a>
   </h2>
```

2. Create the `contents/contactdelete.php` file. This is similar to the `contactmaint.php` file except that you just display the data instead of using labels and inputs. You won't have new items on this page, so you only need to look for existing items. The submit button is a Delete button instead of a Save and the task is `contact.delete`.

```
<?php
/**
 * contactdelete.php
 *
 * Delete the Contacts
 *
 * @version    1.2 2011-02-03
 * @package    Smithside Auctions
 * @copyright  Copyright (c) 2011 Smithside Auctions
 * @license    GNU General Public License
 * @since      Since Release 1.0
 */
$id = (int) $_GET['id'];
// Get the existing information for an existing item
$item = Contact::getContact($id);
```

```
?>
<h1>Contact Delete</h1>

<form action="index.php?content=about" method="post" name="maint" id="maint">
  <fieldset class="maintform">
    <legend><?php echo 'ID: '. $id ?></legend>
    <ul>
      <li><strong>First Name:</strong>
        <?php echo htmlspecialchars($item->getFirst_name()); ?></li>
      <li><strong>Last Name:</strong>
        <?php echo htmlspecialchars($item->getLast_name()); ?></li>
      <li><strong>Position:</strong>
        <?php echo htmlspecialchars($item->getPosition()); ?></li>
      <li><strong>Email:</strong>
        <?php echo htmlspecialchars($item->getEmail()); ?></li>
      <li><strong>Phone:</strong>
        <?php echo htmlspecialchars($item->getPhone()); ?></li>
    </ul>

    <?php
    // create token
    $salt = 'SomeSalt';
    $token = sha1(mt_rand(1,1000000) . $salt);
    $_SESSION['token'] = $token;
    ?>
    <input type="hidden" name="id" id="id" value="<?php echo $item->getId();
?>" />
    <input type="hidden" name="task" id="task" value="contact.delete" />
    <input type='hidden' name='token' value='<?php echo $token; ?>'/>
    <input type="submit" name="delete" value="Delete" />
    <a class="cancel" href="index.php?content=about">Cancel</a>
  </fieldset>
</form>
```

3. In the `includes/init.php` file, add the `contact.delete` case to process the new task:

```
case 'contact.delete' :
// process the delete
$results = deleteContact();
$message .= $results[1];
// If there is redirect information
// redirect to that page
if ($results[0] == 'contactdelete') {
  // pass on new messages
  if ($results[1]) {
    $_SESSION['message'] = $results[1];
  }
  header("Location: index.php?content=contactdelete&id=$results[2]");
  exit;
}
break;
```

4. In the `includes/functions.php` file, add the `deleteContact()` function. This function checks the tokens and evokes the static `deleteRecord()` method in the `Contact` class.

Because the only piece of information you need to delete the row is the id, there is no need to create a whole object so you can use the static class method.

```
function deleteContact() {
   $results = '';
   if (isset($_POST['delete']) AND $_POST['delete'] == 'Delete') {
      // check the token
      $badToken = true;
      if (!isset($_POST['token'])
      || !isset($_SESSION['token'])
      || empty($_POST['token'])
      || $_POST['token'] !== $_SESSION['token']) {
         $results = array('',
            'Sorry, go back and try again. There was a security issue.');
         $badToken = true;
      } else {
         $badToken = false;
         unset($_SESSION['token']);

         // Delete the Contact from the table
         $results = Contact::deleteRecord((int) $_POST['id']);
      }
   }
   return $results;
}
```

5. In the `includes/classes/contact.php` file add the `deleteRecord()` method. This method deletes the row based on the id that is passed in as a parameter.

```
public static function deleteRecord($id) {
   // Get the Database connection
   $connection = Database::getConnection();
   // Set up query
   $query = 'DELETE FROM `contacts` WHERE id="'. (int) $id.'"';
   // Run the query
   if ($result = $connection->query($query)) {
      $return = array('', 'Contact Record successfully deleted.', '');
      return $return;
   } else {
      $return = array('contactdelete', 'Unable to delete Contact.', (int)
$id);
      return $return;
   }
}
```

6. Check your changes and verify that they look similar to Figure 26-14 and Figure 26-15. Test that you can delete items.

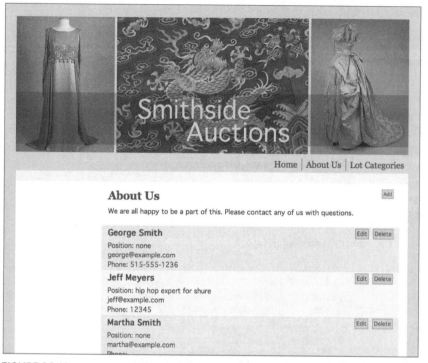

FIGURE 26-14

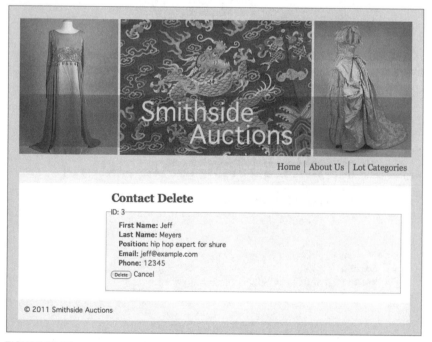

FIGURE 26-15

Now, repeat the same steps to add delete capabilities to the Lot Categories page.

1. In the `contents/categories.php` files add a Delete button just above the Edit button:

```
<a class="button edit"
   href="index.php?content=categorydelete&cat_id=<?php echo
   $item->getCat_id(); ?>">Delete</a>
```

2. Create the `contents/categorydelete.php` file. This is similar to the `categorymaint.php` file except that you just display the data instead of using labels and inputs. You won't have new items on this page, so you only need to look for existing items. The submit button is a Delete button instead of a Save and the task is `category.delete`.

```php
<?php
/**
 * categorydelete.php
 *
 * Delete for the Categories table
 *
 * @version  1.2 2011-02-03
 * @package  Smithside Auctions
 * @copyright  Copyright (c) 2011 Smithside Auctions
 * @license  GNU General Public License
 * @since    Since Release 1.0
 */
$id = (int) $_GET['cat_id'];
// Get the existing information for an existing item
$item = Category::getCategory($id);

?>
<h1>Category Delete</h1>

<form action="index.php?content=categories" method="post" name="maint"
id="maint">

  <fieldset class="maintform">
    <legend><?php echo 'ID: '. $id ?></legend>
    <ul>
    <li><strong>Category:</strong>
      <?php echo htmlspecialchars($item->getCat_name()); ?></li>
    <li><strong>Description</strong><br />
      <?php echo htmlspecialchars($item->getCat_description()); ?></li>
    <li><strong>Image:</strong>
      <?php echo htmlspecialchars($item->getCat_image()); ?></li>
    </ul>

    <?php
    // create token
    $salt = 'SomeSalt';
    $token = sha1(mt_rand(1,1000000) . $salt);
    $_SESSION['token'] = $token;
    ?>
    <input type="hidden" name="cat_id" id="cat_id"
      value="<?php echo $item->getCat_id(); ?>" />
```

```
<input type="hidden" name="task" id="task" value="category.delete" />
<input type='hidden' name='token' value='<?php echo $token; ?>'/>
<input type="submit" name="delete" value="Delete" />
<a class="cancel" href="index.php?content=categories">Cancel</a>
    </fieldset>
</form>
```

3. In the includes/init.php file, add the category.delete case to process the new task:

```
case 'category.delete' :
// process the maint
$results = deleteCategory();
$message .= $results[1];
// If there is redirect information
// redirect to that page
if ($results[0] == 'categorydelete') {
  // pass on new messages
  if ($results[1]) {
    $_SESSION['message'] = $results[1];
  }
  header("Location: index.php?content=categorydelete&cat_
id=$results[2]");
  exit;
}
break;
```

4. In the includes/functions.php file, add the deleteCategory() function. This function checks the tokens and evokes the static deleteRecord() method in the Category class. Because the only piece of information you need to delete the row is the id, there is no need to create a whole object so you can use the static class method.

```
function deleteCategory() {
  $results = '';
  if (isset($_POST['delete']) AND $_POST['delete'] == 'Delete') {
    // check the token
    $badToken = true;
    if (!isset($_POST['token'])
    || !isset($_SESSION['token'])
    || empty($_POST['token'])
    || $_POST['token'] !== $_SESSION['token']) {
      $results = array('',
        'Sorry, go back and try again. There was a security issue.');
      $badToken = true;
    } else {
      $badToken = false;
      unset($_SESSION['token']);

      // Delete the Category from the table
      $results = Category::deleteRecord((int) $_POST['cat_id']);
    }
  }
  return $results;
}
```

5. In the `includes/classes/category.php` file, add the `deleteRecord()` method. This method deletes the row based on the id that is passed in as a parameter.

```
public static function deleteRecord($id) {
  // Get the Database connection
  $connection = Database::getConnection();
  // Set up query
  $query = 'DELETE FROM `categories` WHERE cat_id="'. (int) $id.'"';
  // Run the query
  if ($result = $connection->query($query)) {
    $return = array('', 'Category Record successfully deleted.', '');
    return $return;
  } else {
    $return = array('categorydelete', 'Unable to delete Category.', (int)
$id);
    return $return;
  }
}
```

6. Check your changes and verify that they look similar to Figure 26-16 and Figure 26-17. Test that you can delete items.

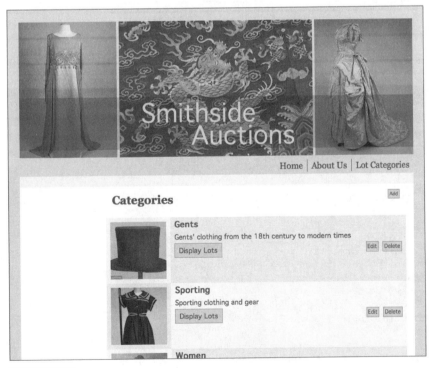

FIGURE 26-16

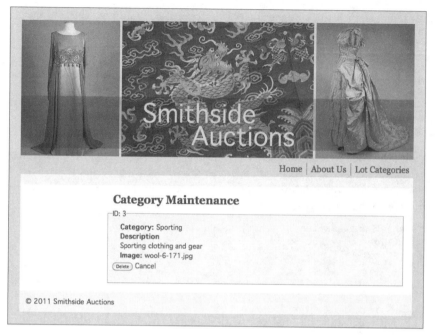

FIGURE 26-17

The rest of this Try It section turns the pages dealing with the lots from static to dynamic. First you change the multiple pages that display lots into a single page and then you add the CRUD for the tables.

Merge the `content/gents.php`, `content/sporting.php`, and `content/women.php` pages into a single `content/lots.php` page where you get the information from the database. Change the lot categories links in the `content/categories.php` file and in the `content/catnav.php` file to work with the new `content/lots.php`.

1. Copy `contents/gents.php` to a new file called `contents/lots.php` and add documentation at the beginning of the file:

```
/**
 * lots.php
 *
 * Content for Lots pages
 *
 * @version    1.2 2011-02-03
 * @package    Smithside Auctions
 * @copyright  Copyright (c) 2011 Smithside Auctions
 * @license    GNU General Public License
 * @since      Since Release 1.0
 */
```

2. The category id, that is, the value of the primary key from the categories table and the matching value in the lots table, is in the URL. Retrieve it with $_GET['cat_id']. The lots are all in this category that you use when you retrieve the lots. Category::getCategory ($cat_id_in) creates an object containing the information from the categories table for that category.

```
// Get the Category
$cat_id_in = (int) $_GET['cat_id'];
$category = Category::getCategory($cat_id_in);
```

3. Follow that with the code to load the $lots array using the static getLots() method from the Lot class. This replaces the hardcoded assignments of the existing $lots array. Pass in the category id so you can use it in the getLots() method. If nothing is returned, initialize $lots to an array so that later use of the variable doesn't create errors.

```
// Get the lot information
$lots = Lot::getLots($cat_id_in);
if (empty($lots)) {
  $lots = array();
}
?>
```

4. In the <h1> header, replace the "Gents" text with the category name and add a link to the new data entry page. Give it the class button for the CSS styling.

```
<h1>Product Category: <?php echo $category->getCat_name(); ?>
<a class="button"
   href="index.php?content=lotmaint&cat_id=<?php echo $cat_id_in; ?>&lot_
id=0">
   Add</a>
</h1>
```

5. In the <li> block change all the $lot array notations to use get methods for the object. For instance, change $lot['image'] to $lot->getLot_image(). Add an Edit button linking to the maintenance page and a Delete button to link to the delete page.

```
<div class="list-photo">
  <?php // Set up the images
  $image = 'images/'. $lot->getLot_image();

  $image_t = 'images/thumbnails/'. $lot->getLot_image();
  if (!is_file($image_t)) :
    $image_t = 'images/thumbnails/nophoto.jpg';
  endif;

  if (is_file($image)) :
  ?>
    <a href="<?php echo $image; ?>">
    <img src="<?php echo $image_t; ?>"  alt="" />
    </a>
  <?php else : ?>
    <img src="<?php echo $image_t; ?>"  alt="" />
  <?php endif; ?>
</div>
<div class="list-description">
```

```php
<h2><?php echo ucwords($lot->getLot_name()); ?></h2>
<p><?php echo htmlspecialchars($lot->getLot_description()); ?></p>
<p><strong>Lot:</strong> #<?php echo $lot->getLot_number(); ?>
  <strong>Price:</strong> $
  <?php echo number_format($lot->getLot_price(),2); ?>
  <a class="button edit"
href="index.php?content=lotdelete&cat_id=<?php echo $cat_id_in; ?>&lot_
id=<?php ↵
  echo $lot->getLot_id(); ?>">Delete
    </a>
    <a class="button edit"
href="index.php?content=lotmaint&cat_id=<?php echo $cat_id_in; ?>&lot_
id=<?php ↵
  echo $lot->getLot_id(); ?>">Edit
    </a></p></div>
```

6. In the `includes/classes/lot.php` file, add the `getLots()` public static method to retrieve the rows and fill the array. Use the parameter of `$cat_id` to select the correct lots. Rather than directly creating the `Category` object, use the `fetch_array(MYSQLI_ASSOC)` to retrieve the row. Use that array to create a new `Lot` object that is added as an element in the `$items` array.

```php
static public function getLots($cat_id) {
  // clear the results
  $items = '';
  // Get the connection
  $connection = Database::getConnection();
  // Set up the query
  $query = 'SELECT * FROM `lots`
    WHERE cat_id="'. (int) $cat_id.'" ORDER BY lot_id';

  // Run the query
  $result_obj = '';
  $result_obj = $connection->query($query);
  // Loop through getting associative arrays,
  // passing them to a new version of this class,
  // and making a regular array of the objects
  try {
    while($result = $result_obj->fetch_array(MYSQLI_ASSOC)) {
      $items[]= new Lot($result);
    }
    // pass back the results
      return($items);
  }

  catch(Exception $e) {
    return false;
  }

}
```

7. Change the links in the `content/categories.php` file to use the lots page along with the category id to the URL parameters:

```php
<h2>
  <a href="index.php?content=lots&cat_id=<?php echo (int) $item->getCat_id(); ↵
?>&amp;sidebar=catnav">
```

```
...
<a class="button display"
href="index.php?content=lots&cat_id=<?php echo (int) $item->getCat_id(); ↵
?>&amp;sidebar=catnav">Display Lots</a>
```

8. Change the link in the `content/catnav.php` file to use the lots page along with the category id in the URL parameters:

```
<li><a href="index.php?content=lots&cat_id=<?php echo
(int) $item->getCat_id(); ?>&sidebar=catnav"><?php echo
htmlspecialchars($item->getCat_name()); ?></a></li>
```

Now, create a lots maintenance page so you can add and change lots in the `lots` table.

1. Create `content/lotmaint.php`, which is the form for adding the lots. The category id is in the URL. Use `$_GET` to get the id and save it. This is used to select the right category to the new lot and for navigating back to the right lot page when saving or canceling. Because it's not displayed on the form, insert it in a hidden `<input>` so that it is available when you update the database. You also display a drop-down list of valid categories, which you create next in this Try It section. The rest of the file is similar to the maintenance files for contacts and categories.

```php
<?php
/**
 * lotmaint.php
 *
 * Maintenance for the Lots table
 *
 * @version  1.2 2011-02-03
 * @package  Smithside Auctions
 * @copyright Copyright (c) 2011 Smithside Auctions
 * @license  GNU General Public License
 * @since    Since Release 1.0
 */
// Get the Category the new lot will be in
$cat_id_in = (int) $_GET['cat_id'];
// Get the lot id. If it doesn't exist or is 0, then this is a new lot
$id = (int) $_GET['lot_id'];
// Is this an existing item or a new one?
if ($id) {
  // Get the existing information for an existing item
  $item = Lot::getLot($id);
  // set up the category dropdown
  $cat_dropdown = Category::getCat_DropDown($item->getCat_id());
} else {
  // Set up for a new item
  $item = new Lot;
  // set up the category dropdown
  $cat_dropdown = Category::getCat_DropDown($cat_id_in);
}
?>
<h1>Lot Maintenance</h1>
```

```
<form
  action="index.php?content=lots&cat_id=<?php echo $cat_id_in;
?>&sidebar=catnav"
  method="post" name="maint" id="maint">

  <fieldset class="maintform">
    <legend><?php echo ($id) ? 'Id: '. $id : 'Add a Lot' ?></legend>
    <ul>
      <li><label for="lot_name" class="required">Lot Name</label><br />
        <input type="text" name="lot_name" id="lot_name" class="required"
          value="<?php echo $item->getLot_name(); ?>" /></li>
      <li><label for="lot_description">Lot Description</label><br />
        <textarea rows="5" cols="60" name="lot_description"
         id="lot_description"><?php echo $item->getLot_description(); ?></
textarea>
      </li>
      <li><label for="lot_image" >Lot Image File</label><br />
        <input type="text" name="lot_image" id="lot_image"
        value="<?php echo $item->getLot_image(); ?>" /></li>
      <li><label for="lot_number">Lot Number</label><br />
        <input type="text" name="lot_number" id="lot_number"
          value="<?php echo $item->getLot_number(); ?>" /></li>
      <li><label for="lot_price" >Lot Price</label><br />
        <input type="text" name="lot_price" id="lot_price"
        value="<?php echo $item->getLot_price(); ?>" /></li>
      <li><?php echo $cat_dropdown; ?></li>
    </ul>

    <?php
    // create token
    $salt = 'SomeSalt';
    $token = sha1(mt_rand(1,1000000) . $salt);
    $_SESSION['token'] = $token;
    ?>
    <input type="hidden" name="cat_id_in" id="cat_id_in"
      value="<?php echo $cat_id_in; ?>" />
    <input type="hidden" name="lot_id" id="lot_id"
      value="<?php echo $item->getLot_id(); ?>" />
    <input type="hidden" name="task" id="task" value="lot.maint" />
    <input type='hidden' name='token' value='<?php echo $token; ?>'/>
    <input type="submit" name="save" value="Save" />
    <a class="cancel"
      href="index.php?content=lots&cat_id=<?php echo $cat_id_in; ↵
?>&sidebar=catnav">Cancel
    </a>
  </fieldset>
</form>
```

2. In the `includes/classes/category.php`, add the `getCat_DropDown()` method to create the `<select>` drop-down. A category id is passed in, which is used to assign which category shows as selected. If no category id is passed then the first option is set as selected. The existing `getCategories()` method is used to get a list of categories. The HTML is

collected in an array called $html. When that array is passed back, it is *imploded* with \n. Imploding takes the array and turns it into a single string variable, putting a \n between each element. The \n is a newline character, which creates a new line for each section when you view the source of the web page. Without the newline character, the entire drop-down would appear as a single line in the source code. It does not affect what shows when you view the web page.

```php
public static function getCat_DropDown($selected = '') {
  // set up first option for selection if none selected
  $option_selected = '';
  if (!$selected) {
    $option_selected = ' selected="selected"';
  }

  // Get the categories
  $items = self::getCategories();

  $html  = array();

  $html[] = '<label for="cat_id">Choose Lot Category</label><br />';
  $html[] = '<select name="cat_id" id="cat_id">';

  foreach ($items as $i=>$item) {
    // If the selected parameter equals the current category id
    // then flag as selected
    if ((int) $selected == (int) $item->getCat_id()) {
      $option_selected = ' selected="selected"';
    }
    // set up the option line
    $html[]  = '<option value="' . $item->getCat_id()
      . '"' . $option_selected . '>'
      . $item->getCat_name() . '</option>';
    // clear out the selected option flag
    $option_selected = '';
  }

  $html[] = '</select>';
  return implode("\n", $html);

}
```

3. In the includes/init.php file add a case block in the switch statement for lot.maint to process the lot maintenance form. This calls the maintLot() function.

```php
case 'lot.maint' :
// process the maint
$results = maintLot();
$message .= $results[1];
// If there is redirect information
// redirect to that page
if ($results[0] == 'lotmaint') {
  // pass on new messages
  if ($results[1]) {
```

```
        $_SESSION['message'] = $results[1];
    }
    $cat_id_in = (int) $_GET['cat_id'];
    header("Location: index.php?content=lotmaint&cat_id=$cat_id_in ↵
&lot_id=$results[2]");
    exit;
}
break;
```

4. Add the function `maintLot()` to `includes/functions.php`. Check that the token is good and then initialize an array with the information from the form. Create a `Lot` object with the data. If there is a lot id then this is an existing lot, so update the table with the `maintRecord()` method. Otherwise, create a new row with `AddRecord()`.

```php
function maintLot() {
  $results = '';
  if (isset($_POST['save']) AND $_POST['save'] == 'Save') {
    // check the token
    $badToken = true;
    if (!isset($_POST['token'])
      || !isset($_SESSION['token'])
      || empty($_POST['token'])
      || $_POST['token'] !== $_SESSION['token']) {
      $results = array('','Sorry, go back and try again.
        There was a security issue.');
      $badToken = true;
    } else {
      $badToken = false;
      unset($_SESSION['token']);
      // Put the sanitized variables in an associative array
      // Use the FILTER_FLAG_NO_ENCODE_QUOTES
      // to allow quotes in the description
      $item  = array ('lot_id' => (int) $_POST['lot_id'],
        'lot_name' => filter_input(INPUT_POST,'lot_name',
          FILTER_SANITIZE_STRING,FILTER_FLAG_NO_ENCODE_QUOTES),
        'lot_description' => filter_input(INPUT_POST,'lot_description',
          FILTER_SANITIZE_STRING,FILTER_FLAG_NO_ENCODE_QUOTES),
        'lot_image' => filter_input(INPUT_POST,'lot_image',
          FILTER_SANITIZE_STRING),
        'lot_number' => (int) $_POST['lot_number'],
        'lot_price' => filter_input(INPUT_POST,'lot_price',
          FILTER_SANITIZE_NUMBER_FLOAT,FILTER_FLAG_ALLOW_FRACTION),
        'cat_id' => (int) $_POST['cat_id']
      );

      // Set up a Lot object based on the posts
      $lot = new Lot($item);
      if ($lot->getLot_id()) {
        $results = $lot->editRecord();
      } else {
        $results = $lot->addRecord();
      }
    }
  }
```

```
        }
        return $results;
    }
```

5.   In `includes/classes/lot.php` add the `addRecord()` method to add rows to the `lots`
table. When preparing numeric data for insertion in the database, force the variables to the
proper case rather than using the `Database::prep()` method.

```php
    /**
     * Add item
     * @return array
     */
    public function addRecord() {

        // Verify the fields
        if ($this->_verifyInput()) {

            // Get the Database connection
            $connection = Database::getConnection();

            // Prepare the data
            $query = "INSERT INTO
                lots(lot_name, lot_description, lot_image, lot_number, lot_price,
    cat_id)
                    VALUES ('" . Database::prep($this->lot_name) . "',
                     '" . Database::prep($this->lot_description) ."',
                     '" . Database::prep($this->lot_image) . "',
                     '" . (int) $this->lot_number . "',
                     '" . (float) $this->lot_price . "',
                     '" . (int) $this->cat_id . "'
                  )";

            // Run the MySQL statement
            if ($connection->query($query)) {
              $return = array('', 'Lot Record successfully added.');

                // add success message
                return $return;
            } else {
                // send fail message and return to categorymaint
              $return = array('lotmaint', 'No Lot Record Added. Unable to create
    record.');
                return $return;
            }
        } else {
            // send fail message and return to categorymaint
            $return = array('lotmaint',
                'No Lot Record Added. Missing required information.');
            return $return;
        }

    }
```

6. Add the _verifyInput() method to verify that a category name was entered:

```
protected function _verifyInput() {
  $error = false;
  if (!trim($this->lot_name)) {
    $error = true;
  }
  if ($error) {
    return false;
  } else {
    return true;
  }
}
```

7. Add the editRecord() method to update records using prepared statements:

```
/**
 * Edit existing item
 * @return array
 */
public function editRecord() {

  // Verify the fields
  if ($this->_verifyInput()) {

    // Get the Database connection
    $connection = Database::getConnection();

    // Prepare the data
    // Set up the prepared statement
    $query = 'UPDATE `lots`
      SET lot_name=?, lot_description=?, lot_image=?, lot_number=?,
      lot_price=?, cat_id=?
      WHERE lot_id=?';
    $statement = $connection->prepare($query);
    // bind the parameters
    $statement->bind_param('sssidii',
      $this->lot_name, $this->lot_description, $this->lot_image,
      $this->lot_number, $this->lot_price, $this->cat_id, $this->lot_id);
    // Run the MySQL statement
    if ($statement) {
      $statement->execute();
      $statement->close();
      // add success message
      $return = array('', 'Lot Record successfully added.');
      // add success message
      return $return;
    } else {
      $return = array('lotmaint',
        'No Lot Record Added. Unable to create record.',
        '');
      return $return;
    }

  } else {
```

```
      // send fail message and return to categorymaint
      $return = array('lotmaint',
        'No Lot Record Added. Missing required information.',
        (int) $this->lot_id);
      return $return;
    }
  }
```

8. Test adding in lot rows. When you know you can successfully add lots, you can either add all the lots here or import the `insertlots.sql` file in phpMyAdmin as a shortcut.

9. Delete the `contents/gents.php`, `contents/sporting.php`, and `contents/women.php` files.

Now, add the Delete page and delete processing for the `lots` table.

1. Create `contents/lotdelete.php`. This page is similar to the `contents/lotmaint.php` file, but it displays the data from the table without allowing changes. Rather than submitting a Save button, you submit a Delete button.

```php
<?php
/**
 * lotdelete.php
 *
 * Delete for the Lots
 *
 * @version  1.2 2011-02-03
 * @package  Smithside Auctions
 * @copyright  Copyright (c) 2011 Smithside Auctions
 * @license  GNU General Public License
 * @since    Since Release 1.0
 */

// Save the category so you return to the right lots page
$cat_id_in = (int) $_GET['cat_id'];
// Get the lot id. If it doesn't exist or is 0, then this is a new lot
$id = (int) $_GET['lot_id'];
  // Get the existing information for an existing item
  $item = Lot::getLot($id);
  // get the Category name for the lot
  $cat_name = Category::getCategory($item->getCat_id())->getCat_name();
?>
<h1>Lot Delete</h1>

<form action="index.php?content=lots&cat_id=<?php echo $cat_id_in; ↵
?>&sidebar=catnav"
  method="post" name="maint" id="maint">

    <fieldset class="maintform">
      <legend><?php echo 'ID: '. $id ?></legend>
      <ul>
        <li><strong>Lot Name: </strong>
          <?php echo htmlspecialchars($item->getLot_name()); ?></li>
        <li><strong>Lot Description: </strong><br />
          <?php echo htmlspecialchars($item->getLot_description()); ?></li>
        <li><strong>Lot Image File: </strong>
```

```
            <?php echo htmlspecialchars($item->getLot_image()); ?></li>
          <li><strong>Lot Number: </strong>
            <?php echo (int) $item->getLot_number(); ?></li>
          <li><strong>Lot Price: </strong>
            <?php echo number_format($item->getLot_price(),2); ?></li>
          <li><strong>Category: </strong>
            <?php echo htmlspecialchars($cat_name); ?></li>
        </ul>

      <?php
      // create token
      $salt = 'SomeSalt';
      $token = sha1(mt_rand(1,1000000) . $salt);
      $_SESSION['token'] = $token;
      ?>
      <input type="hidden" name="cat_id_in" id="cat_id_in"
        value="<?php echo $cat_id_in; ?>" />
      <input type="hidden" name="lot_id" id="lot_id"
        value="<?php echo $item->getLot_id(); ?>" />
      <input type="hidden" name="task" id="task" value="lot.delete" />
      <input type='hidden' name='token' value='<?php echo $token; ?>'/>
      <input type="submit" name="delete" value="Delete" />
      <a class="cancel"
      href="index.php?content=lots&cat_id=<?php echo $cat_id_in; ?> ↵
&sidebar=catnav">Cancel</a>
        </fieldset>
    </form>
```

2. In the `includes/init.php` file, add the `lot.delete` case to process the delete form, which calls the `deleteLot()` function. The catalog id is also used in the URL to select the appropriate pages.

```
        case 'lot.delete' :
        // process the delete
        $results = deleteLot();
        $message .= $results[1];
        // If there is redirect information
        // redirect to that page
        if ($results[0] == 'lotdelete') {
          // pass on new messages
          if ($results[1]) {
            $_SESSION['message'] = $results[1];
          }
          $cat_id_in = (int) $_GET['cat_id'];
          header("Location:
index.php?content=lotdelete&cat_id=$cat_id_in&lot_id=$results[2]");
          exit;
        }
        break;
```

3. In the `includes/functions.php` file, add the `deleteCategory()` function, which calls the `deleteRecord()` method in the Lot class.

```
function deleteLot() {
  $results = '';
  if (isset($_POST['delete']) AND $_POST['delete'] == 'Delete') {
```

```
// check the token
$badToken = true;
if (!isset($_POST['token'])
  || !isset($_SESSION['token'])
  || empty($_POST['token'])
  || $_POST['token'] !== $_SESSION['token']) {
    $results = array('','Sorry, go back and try again.
      There was a security issue.');
    $badToken = true;
  } else {
    $badToken = false;
    unset($_SESSION['token']);

    // Delete the Lot from the table
    $results = Lot::deleteRecord((int) $_POST['lot_id']);
  }
}
return $results;
}
```

4. In the `includes/classes/lot.php` file, add the `deleteRecord()` method, which deletes the row from the `lots` table:

```
public static function deleteRecord($id) {
    // Get the Database connection
    $connection = Database::getConnection();
    // Set up query
    $query = 'DELETE FROM `lots` WHERE lot_id="'. (int) $id.'"';
    // Run the query
    if ($result = $connection->query($query)) {
      $return = array('', 'Lot Record successfully deleted.', '');
      return $return;
    } else {
      $return = array('lotdelete', 'Unable to delete Lot.', (int) $id);
      return $return;
    }
}
```

5. Check all your changes and verify that they look similar to Figure 26-18, Figure 26-19, and Figure 26-20. Test that you can delete items.

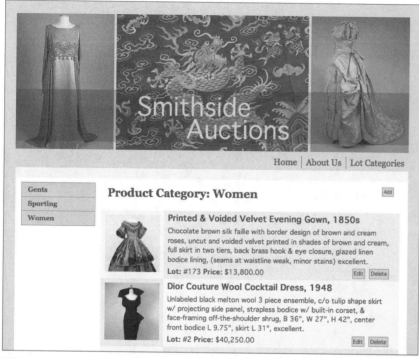

FIGURE 26-18

FIGURE 26-19

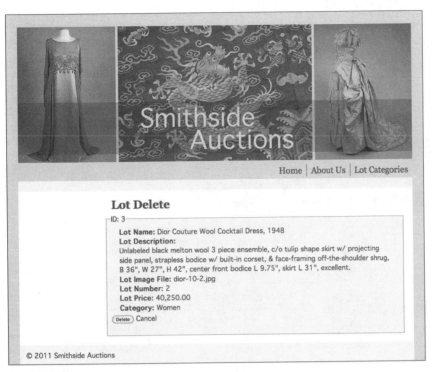

FIGURE 26-20

 Watch the video for Lesson 26 on the DVD or watch online at www.wrox.com/go/24phpmysql.

27

Preventing Database Security Issues

In this lesson, you learn the general security guidelines to use when using MySQL. Some of these guidelines are general ones that have been mentioned before in other lessons and some are particular to using a database and MySQL. They are gathered together here so that you can easily refer to them. As you are learning a new skill it can be exhilarating to just get things to work, and it's easy to ignore security issues. That can result in a painful lesson in the current climate.

Security steps must be taken to make MySQL itself more secure against attacks. These are related to your server setup and are not covered in this book. The XAMPP setup used throughout this book is for local development and is not secure for Internet access. However, the practices in this lesson are designed to make your code secure when used online.

UNDERSTANDING SECURITY ISSUES

There is no such thing as making your code completely secure against attacks. You can, however, reduce what harm can be done and make it less likely that you will be successfully hacked. Issues to be aware of are unauthorized access to your database files, unauthorized ability to change the database structure, unauthorized ability to see or change data, and SQL injection.

Unauthorized access to your database files is mostly dependent on your server setup. This is related to who has access to the MySQL files and what the permissions are on those files. MySQL is an application and as such its files are just as vulnerable to deletion and corruption as any other files on your system. If an unauthorized person can delete your whole MySQL setup, then you have a problem.

You don't want unauthorized MySQL users to have the ability to change the structure of your database. They could delete tables, for instance, if given a chance. Some hacking attacks need to exploit more than one vulnerability to be successful. When an attack succeeds in running

unplanned commands, the damage can be limited if the hackers don't have the authorization to use commands such as DROP TABLE or DROP DATABASE.

You also don't want unauthorized changing or displaying of data. If the application needs to SELECT, INSERT, UPDATE, and DELETE data, you want to make sure that that application user can do so only in a controlled manner. You need to check the data, whether it's coming from a form or a URL, to be sure that it does not contain unexpected code that also performs commands.

And that brings you to *SQL injections*. SQL injections are when additional SQL (in this case, MySQL) code is contained in seemingly innocent form fields or added to URLs. Imagine this command:

```
DELETE FROM authors WHERE id=4;
```

That command deletes a single row from the authors table. However, if you add a second condition to the WHERE clause that is always true, it deletes all the rows:

```
DELETE FROM authors WHERE id=4 OR 1=1;
```

The following innocuous-looking code deletes a single row based on a value. In this example, that value comes from $id = 4, but imagine that the value is coming from a POST or GET variable from a form. Notice how the $id is handled when assembling the command in $query. The results are shown in Figure 27-1.

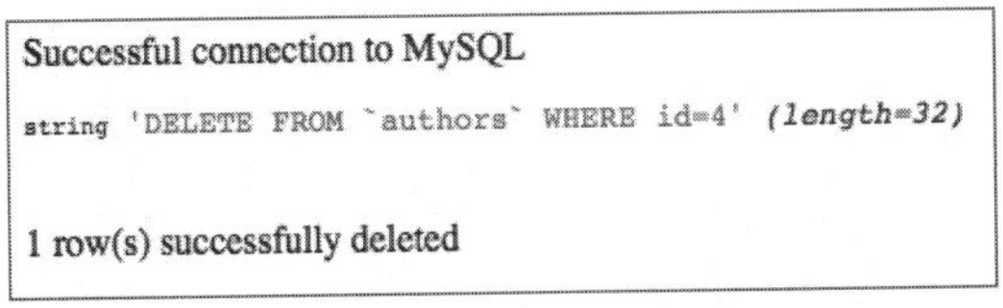

Successful connection to MySQL

string 'DELETE FROM `authors` WHERE id=4' *(length=32)*

1 row(s) successfully deleted

FIGURE 27-1

```php
<?php
define("MYSQLUSER", "php24sql");
define("MYSQLPASS", "hJQV8RTe5t");
define("HOSTNAME", "localhost");
define("MYSQLDB", "test");

// Make connection to database
$connection = @new mysqli(HOSTNAME, MYSQLUSER, MYSQLPASS, MYSQLDB);
if ($connection->connect_error) {
  die('Connect Error: ' . $connection->connect_error);
} else {
  echo 'Successful connection to MySQL <br />';

  // assign an id value for the test
  $id = 4;

  // Set up the query
  $query = 'DELETE FROM 'authors' WHERE id='. $id;
  var_dump($query); echo '<br />';
  // Run the query and display appropriate message
  if (!$result = $connection->query($query)) {
    echo "No rows deleted<br />";
  } else {
    echo $connection->affected_rows . " row(s) successfully deleted<br />";
  }
}
```

Now, assume that instead of a 4, you are passed `4 OR 1=1` from the form as a GET or POST variable. All the rows are deleted as shown in Figure 27-2.

```php
<?php
define("MYSQLUSER", "php24sql");
define("MYSQLPASS", "hJQV8RTe5t");
define("HOSTNAME", "localhost");
define("MYSQLDB", "test");

// Make connection to database
$connection = @new mysqli(HOSTNAME, MYSQLUSER, MYSQLPASS, MYSQLDB);
if ($connection->connect_error) {
  die('Connect Error: ' . $connection->connect_error);
} else {
  echo 'Successful connection to MySQL <br />';

  // assign an id value for the test
  $id = '4 OR 1=1';

  // Set up the query
  $query = 'DELETE FROM 'authors' WHERE id='. $id;
  var_dump($query); echo '<br />';
  // Run the query and display appropriate message
  if (!$result = $connection->query($query)) {
    echo "No rows deleted<br />";
  } else {
    echo $connection->affected_rows . " row(s) successfully deleted<br />";
  }
}
```

```
Successful connection to MySQL

string 'DELETE FROM `authors` WHERE id=4 OR 1=1' (length=39)

4 row(s) successfully deleted
```

FIGURE 27-2

SQL injection is a serious issue, but if you write your code using best practices and filter and prepare it properly, you prevent most SQL injections.

USING BEST PRACTICES

MySQL users and passwords are under the Privileges tab in phpMyAdmin for your local MySQL installation. The global privileges are displayed if you are at the root level. There are also specific privileges at the database and table levels. If your MySQL is online, you may not have access to the Privilege tab in phpMyAdmin. Users and passwords for MySQL may be handled by a separate program.

Following are best practices for setting up MySQL users and passwords:

➤ The only users with access to the user table in MySQL should be the root accounts.

➤ Root users must have a password. Don't make it a trivial password.

➤ All users should have a password.

➤ Only grant as many privileges as necessary. If the application is only updating data in the database and not making structural changes, then don't allow the user profile used by the application any structural privileges. Structural privileges are the ones that allow you to create, alter, and destroy tables and databases. Don't allow the user profile administration rights, which would allow the user to create other users and grant privileges. Don't confuse the MySQL user profile the application is running under with operating system users or users you might create for an application.

➤ Don't grant privileges to all hosts (%).

➤ To see what privileges a user has use the SHOW GRANTS command, the Privileges tab in phpMyAdmin, or a special program on cpanel or another hosting administration software.

➤ To remove privileges from a user, use the SHOW GRANTS command, the Privileges tab in phpMyAdmin, or a special program on cpanel or another hosting administration software.

When you are writing your application, keep these best practices in mind:

➤ Use a separate username for your application and give it only the privileges it has to have.

➤ Use the standard precautions in creating your passwords:

> ➤ No words from dictionaries.

> ➤ Don't use all numbers or all letters.

> ➤ Include some capitalization and special characters.

> ➤ Instead of using passwords, use pass phrases without spaces but with capitalization and special characters to make very strong passwords that aren't difficult to remember. "I go to the store" could look like: iGo2thest0re.

> ➤ Using the first letters of a phrase is also a good way to get seemingly random letters that are easy to remember.

➤ Don't trust data entered by users.

> ➤ This is where the SQL injections can happen.

> ➤ Embedded code can be entered in forms or URLs.

> ➤ Protect string data values with filters. See Lessons 6 and 11 for more information on filtering.

> ➤ Make sure numeric values are only numeric (preventing the OR 1=1 injection). With integers, cast to (int) in PHP or use quote marks around the numeric variables even though they aren't required.

> ➤ Escape and/or encode all data appropriately for where it is going. This helps prevent hacking by preventing suspect control characters from acting like control characters. Because you are dealing with different types of software languages (that is, MySQL on one hand and HTML on the other), different characters act as control characters

and need to be dealt with differently. Do your escaping and encoding just before using the data so you have control over how the prepared data is used:

> ➤ When passing data into a database: Use `mysqli::real_escape_string` to escape the quotes. Remember to check to see if magic quotes is already on. (See Lesson 22 for information on magic quotes.) Prepared statements do it for you, as does the PDO connection.

> ➤ When passing data to the browser for display: Use `htmlspecialchars()` to encode the special HTML characters into appropriate HTML entities. For example, < is changed to `&lt;`.

➤ If you create user logins and passwords for your application (these are separate from the MySQL users/passwords), don't store the passwords in plain text in the database. Use an encryption code such as `SHA1()` or `SHA2()` to convert the password and store that instead. MySQL has a `PASSWORD()` function, but that is for MySQL passwords and shouldn't be used for application passwords.

There are a couple tests you can try to check out your programs. Don't do the tests in place of following guidelines.

➤ Test what happens if you enter single and double quotes in web forms.

➤ Add non-numeric processing data in numeric form fields.

FILTERING DATA

You have several ways to filter and sanitize data, which you have learned through the course of this book. In Lesson 6 you learned about the `filter_var()` function. In Lesson 11 you learned how to filter `$_GET` and `$_POST` variables to make them safe. To keep your database secure, you need to use this knowledge to filter or sanitize any data going into your database.

Let's return to the example earlier in the lesson on SQL injection. The `id` in the example is an integer data type, so you can cast the variable to an integer and surround it in quotes to protect against the injection. When you change the `$query` assignment to the following code, you get the desired result in Figure 27-3. This code takes a bad input and sanitizes it to protect the database from SQL injection.

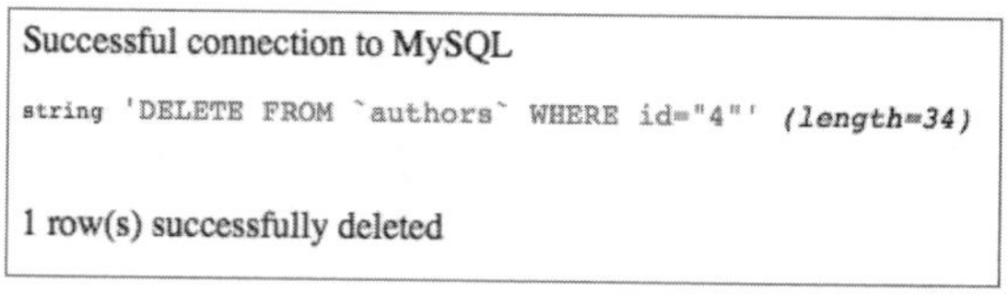

> Successful connection to MySQL
>
> string 'DELETE FROM `authors` WHERE id="4"' *(length=34)*
>
> 1 row(s) successfully deleted

FIGURE 27-3

```php
<?php
define("MYSQLUSER", "php24sql");
define("MYSQLPASS", "hJQV8RTe5t");
define("HOSTNAME", "localhost");
define("MYSQLDB", "test");

// Make connection to database
$connection = @new mysqli(HOSTNAME, MYSQLUSER, MYSQLPASS, MYSQLDB);
if ($connection->connect_error) {
  die('Connect Error: ' . $connection->connect_error);
```

```
    } else {
      echo 'Successful connection to MySQL <br />';

      // assign an id value for the test
      $id = '4 OR 1=1';
      if (get_magic_quotes_gpc()) {
        // If magic quotes is active, remove the slashes
        $id = stripslashes($id);
      }
      // Escape special characters to avoid SQL injections
      $id = $connection->real_escape_string($id);

      // Set up the query
      $query = 'DELETE FROM 'authors' WHERE id="' . (int) $id . '"';
      var_dump($query); echo '<br />';
      // Run the query and display appropriate message
      if (!$result = $connection->query($query)) {
        echo "No rows deleted<br />";
      } else {
        echo $connection->affected_rows . " row(s) successfully deleted<br />";
      }
    }
}
```

Those are a lot of quotes to keep straight. You've been seeing this in the earlier lessons, but just in case you have trouble following it, here is how it is deciphered. The final value that is passed to MySQL is a valid MySQL statement that looks like this:

```
DELETE FROM 'authors' WHERE id="4"
```

In PHP, because you are assigning this MySQL statement to a variable ($query), you have to enclose strings in either double or single quotes. You have double quotes around the 4, so you can enclose the statement in single quotes. Note that at this point you could have swapped the single and double quotes. So when the whole line is a string, the assignment looks like this:

```
$query = 'DELETE FROM 'authors' WHERE id="4"';
```

You want to replace the 4 with the variable $id. To do that, you need to break the statement into three parts (the part before the 4, the 4, and the part after the 4), make sure each part is enclosed in single quotes and concatenate them. So here you see that the crazy looking '"' is a double quote enclosed by single quotes. The assignment looks like this:

```
$query = 'DELETE FROM 'authors' WHERE id="' . '4' . '"';
```

Now you replace the '4' with the $id variable. This is a variable, not a string, so there are no quotes around it. Don't get the PHP variable itself confused with the best practice of enclosing the resulting integer value in the MySQL statement with quotes. The assignment looks like this:

```
$query = 'DELETE FROM 'authors' WHERE id="' . $id . '"';
```

Cast the $id variable to an integer so add (int) in front of the variable to get the final assignment:

```
$query = 'DELETE FROM 'authors' WHERE id="'. (int) $id . '"';
```

This is a bit of overkill for an explanation, but sometimes getting the quotes and concatenations correct can be very frustrating and it is helpful to be able to build up to the final result.

An alternative method for numeric variables is to use the `is_numeric()` function and process the request only if the variable is actually numeric. If the value is coming from a form that you are validating, you could add this test in your form validation process along with the missing fields. You will still want to put quotes around the resulting number in the MySQL statement.

For string variables, either use prepared statements, PDO, or always run variables through the `mysqli::real_escape_string()` method or `mysqli_real_escape_string()` function you learned in Lesson 22.

TRY IT

It this Try It, you test the Case Study for vulnerabilities. You've been following the best practice guidelines as you have been creating the Case Study, but sometimes the tests can point out areas where you missed something.

> *You can download the code and resources for this Try It from the book's web page at* www.wrox.com. *You can find them in the Lesson27 folder in the download. You will find code for both before and after completing the exercises.*

Lesson Requirements

Your computer needs to be able to run as a web server with PHP and MySQL. XAMPP is a package of software that installs the web server, PHP, and MySQL for you. You can find instructions for downloading and installing XAMPP in Lesson 1.

You need a text editor that can produce plain-text files. You can find instructions for downloading and installing Eclipse PDT in Lesson 1. Other text editors that you can use are Adobe's Dreamweaver in code mode, Notepad, TextWrangler, or NetBeans.

If you are following along with the Case Study, you need your files from the end of Lesson 26. Alternatively, you can download the files from the book's website at www.wrox.com.

Hints

Use the two tests listed under Best Practices:

➤ Test what happens if you enter single and double quotes in web forms.

➤ Add non-numeric processing data in numeric form fields.

Step-by-Step

Go through the following steps and correct the code if any errors are found.

1. In the website, create a new contact with the name **Mitchell "Bud" O'Reilly.**

2. Check that the double and single quotes appear as expected in the About Us page.

3. Go to the Edit page for this new contact. The first name is missing "Bud" as shown in Figure 27-4.

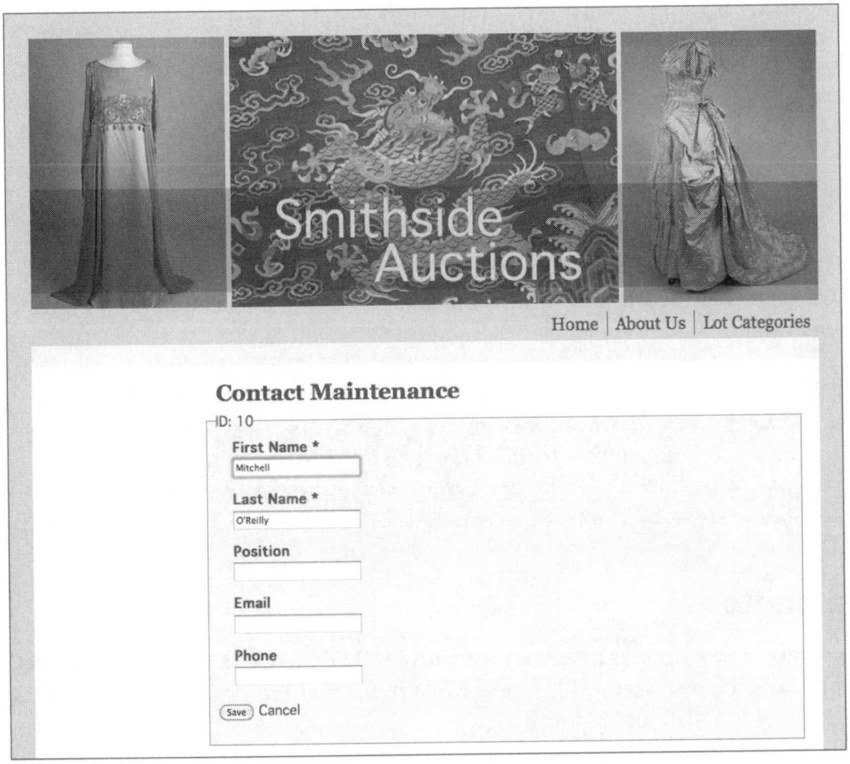

FIGURE 27-4

4. Go to `contents/contactmaint.php`. The data is contained in the value attributes for the `<input>` tags. The variable is enclosed by double quotes and is not escaped. Therefore when the browser encounters the first double quote around Bud, it thinks it is at the end of the value attribute. Enclose all the output variables with `htmlspecialchars()`. The result of refreshing the page is shown in Figure 27-5.

```
<li><label for="first_name" class="required">First Name</label><br />
   <input type="text" name="first_name" id="first_name" class="required"
   value="<?php echo htmlspecialchars($item->getFirst_name()); ?>" /></li>
<li><label for="last_name" class="required">Last Name</label><br />
   <input type="text" name="last_name" id="last_name" class="required"
   value="<?php echo htmlspecialchars($item->getLast_name()); ?>" /></li>
<li><label for="position">Position</label><br />
   <input type="text" name="position" id="position" class="required"
   value="<?php echo htmlspecialchars($item->getPosition()); ?>" /></li>
<li><label for="email" >Email</label><br />
   <input type="text" name="email" id="email"
   value="<?php echo htmlspecialchars($item->getEmail()); ?>" /></li>
<li><label for="phone" >Phone</label><br />
   <input type="text" name="phone" id="phone"
   value="<?php echo htmlspecialchars($item->getPhone()); ?>" /></li>
```

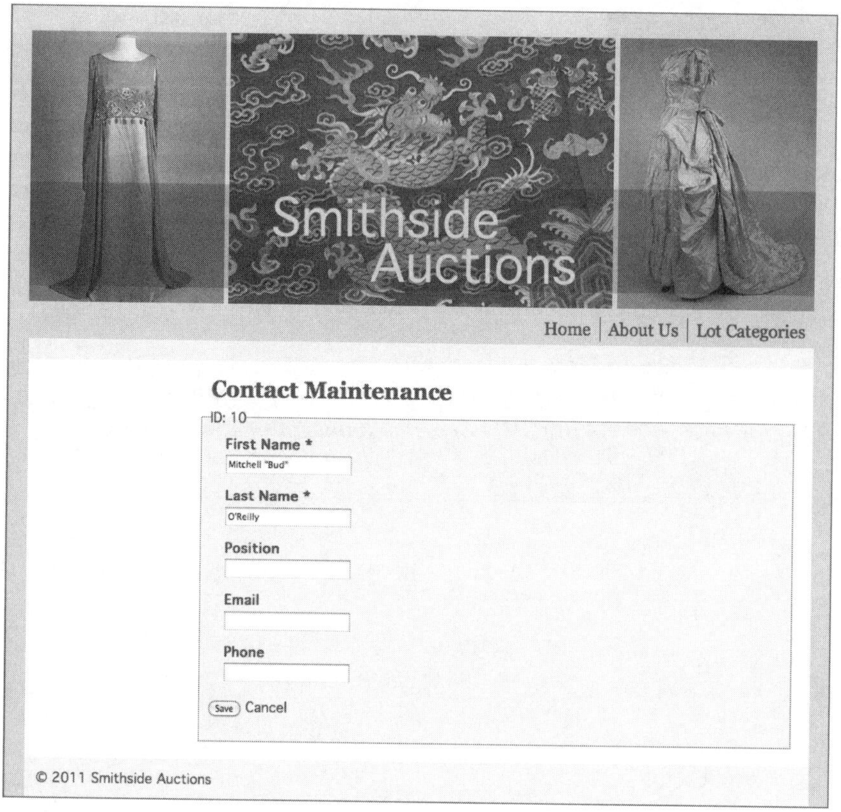

FIGURE 27-5

5. Make the same changes in `contents/categorymaint.php`:

```
<li><label for="cat_name" class="required">Category</label><br />
   <input type="text" name="cat_name" id="cat_name" class="required"
   value="<?php echo htmlspecialchars($item->getCat_name()); ?>" /></li>
<li><label for="cat_description">Description</label><br />
   <textarea rows="5" cols="60" name="cat_description"
   id="cat_description"><?php echo
htmlspecialchars($item->getCat_description()); ?></textarea></li>
   <li><label for="cat_image" >Image</label><br />
   <input type="text" name="cat_image" id="cat_image"
   value="<?php echo htmlspecialchars($item->getCat_image()); ?>" /></li>
```

6. In `contents/lotmaint.php` make the same changes to the text fields. For the lot number, cast the variable to an integer. For the price, cast the variable to a float.

```
<li><label for="lot_name" class="required">Lot Name</label><br />
   <input type="text" name="lot_name" id="lot_name" class="required"
   value="<?php echo htmlspecialchars($item->getLot_name()); ?>" /></li>
<li><label for="lot_description">Lot Description</label><br />
   <textarea rows="5" cols="60" name="lot_description"
   id="lot_description"><?php echo
htmlspecialchars($item->getLot_description()); ?></textarea></li>
<li><label for="lot_image" >Lot Image File</label><br />
```

```
    <input type="text" name="lot_image" id="lot_image"
    value="<?php echo htmlspecialchars($item->getLot_image()); ?>" /></li>
  <li><label for="lot_number">Lot Number</label><br />
    <input type="text" name="lot_number" id="lot_number"
      value="<?php echo (int) $item->getLot_number(); ?>" /></li>
  <li><label for="lot_price" >Lot Price</label><br />
    <input type="text" name="lot_price" id="lot_price"
    value="<?php echo (float) $item->getLot_price(); ?>" /></li>
  <li><?php echo $cat_dropdown; ?></li>
```

7. Add a lot, typing a non-numeric value in the lot number and price. Make sure there are no errors. Look at the row in phpMyAdmin and verify that only numbers were placed in the table.

⊛ *Watch the video for Lesson 27 on the DVD or watch online at* www.wrox.com/go/24phpmysql.

SECTION VI
Putting It All Together

- ▶ **LESSON 28:** Creating User Logins

- ▶ **LESSON 29:** Turning the Case Study into a Content Management System

- ▶ **LESSON 30:** Creating a Dynamic Menu

- ▶ **LESSON 31:** Next Steps

In this section you take what you have learned and use it to add advanced features to your site. You learn how to create user logins so that you can decide who can do what on your site. You create a table that contains content pages that you can update through your site and then have them display on your website. And, finally, you learn how to make the menuing system dynamic so that you can update it through your site rather than hardcoding in the PHP programs. This enables people who are creating text content to also create a menu item to access that content.

The examples are simple so that the concepts are easy to see.

28

Creating User Logins

In this lesson you learn how to restrict parts of your website to certain people. You learn what access control systems are and to use them to control who sees what on your site. You learn when and how to protect passwords and how to use cookies and sessions to remember who is logged in. Finally, you learn how to use that information to restrict and grant access to different parts of your site.

UNDERSTANDING ACCESS CONTROL

Access Control Lists, also known as ACLs, are the lists that are used to control who can see, add, change, or delete different elements of a system; in other words, controlling access. ACLs can be as simple as making sure someone is logged in. They can be as complex as listing what different people or groups have the ability to create, read, update, or delete specific files, tables, fields, or windows.

You can create a simple system in which you have only one type of user and all you need to know is whether she is signed on with just a table of users with usernames and passwords. When the user logs in, you check the username and password against a table to verify that the user exists and that the username and password are correct. A more complex system would have different levels of users. Some users can see but not touch. Others could see, touch, and add. Some could delete but not change.

A true ACL comes in when each of the items or groups of items (often called assets) can be addressed individually. So, for example, a user with a given access level can edit this item, but not this other type of item. You can end up with a matrix of permission levels, looking at what level is required on the asset before certain actions are allowed, looking at what level the user is, looking at whether the item or user is in a group, and what permissions might be inherited from the group.

In this lesson you keep to a simple system where the only things checked are whether the user is logged in and what his access level is. There are two hardcoded access levels: Registered and Admin.

PROTECTING PASSWORDS

Anytime you put passwords in a database, you should scramble or *hash* the password so if the database is compromised, the passwords can't be easily read. Hashing is a one-way process. You take a string of characters and pass it through a function that turns it into what looks like gibberish. This gibberish is not translated back. When someone logs in, you run the password through the same function and compare that result to the password stored in the database.

The functions used to scramble passwords are called hash functions. You used the sha1() hash function when creating tokens for validating the origin of forms. The cryptography field has developed many of these hash functions over the course of time. As problems develop with each one, newer, stronger ones are developed. Successive versions of PHP include some of the popular newer hashes as they are developed. MD5 was the hash of choice for many years but flaws have been discovered and exploited with it. SHA1 was the next favorite and is still used, though flaws have also been discovered in it. Both of these have individual functions in PHP. The following code shows a password encrypted with md5() and sha1(). See Figure 28-1 for the results.

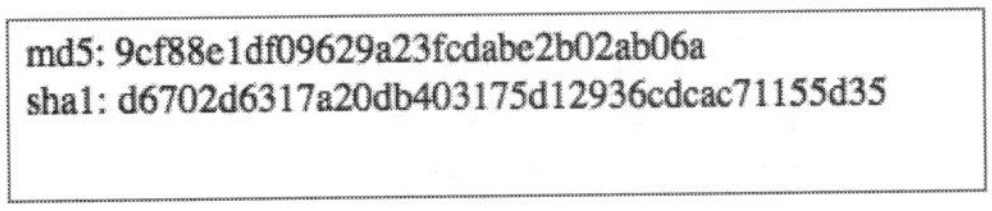

```
md5: 9cf88e1df09629a23fcdabe2b02ab06a
sha1: d6702d6317a20db403175d12936cdcac71155d35
```

FIGURE 28-1

```php
<?php
$password = 'SomePassword!';
echo 'md5: ' . md5($password) . '<br />';
echo 'sha1: ' . sha1($password) . '<br />';
```

Newer versions of PHP have the hash() function, which enables you to specify the type of hash to be used. Using a generic function with the hash engine as a parameter makes it easier for PHP to remain current. To see a list of the available hash algorithms, use the hash_algos() function as shown in Figure 28-2.

```php
<?php
echo '<pre>';
print_r(hash_algos());
echo '</pre>';
```

It is more complex to figure out what the current recommended hashes are in PHP. Currently, two of the suggested hash algorithms are sha512 and whirlpool. Note that these both create hashes that are 128 bytes long instead of the 32 and 40 of md5() and sha1(). See Figure 28-3.

```php
<?php
$password = 'SomePassword!';
echo 'md5: ' . hash('md5', $password) . '<br />';
echo 'sha1: ' . hash('sha1', $password) . '<br />';
echo 'sha512: ' . hash('sha512', $password) . '<br />';
echo 'whirlpool: ' . hash('whirlpool', $password) . '<br />';
```

In Lesson 17, you learned about salting tokens to make the hashed value more difficult to match for the hacker. The same is true for password hashes. You should always add a salt to the password. In Lesson 17 you used the same salt all the time. For passwords, it is best to use a different salt for each user. You need this salt when the user signs on. Some people store that salt in the database as well, and others use an existing field in the database that won't change, such as the id. The problem with storing the salt in the database is that if a hacker gets access to the database, he has the salt. The hash_hmac() function uses a password with a salt plus a site key that is not stored in the database. Therefore a hacker has to get access to your files and your database to be able to compromise

the passwords. The following example simulates a system using a password with a random salt that consists of the id of the user row appended to a static salt along with a site key that is a constant not stored in the database. See Figure 28-4.

```php
<?php
$password = 'SomePassword!';
$id = 42;
$salt = '!#$%jEkcy2884';
$sitekey ='d0d48339c3b82db413b3be8fbc5d7ea1c1fd3e2792605d3cbfda1HEM54!!';

echo 'sha512: ' . hash_hmac('sha512', $password . $id. $salt, $sitekey) . '<br />';
```

```
Array
(
    [0] => md2
    [1] => md4
    [2] => md5
    [3] => sha1
    [4] => sha224
    [5] => sha256
    [6] => sha384
    [7] => sha512
    [8] => ripemd128
    [9] => ripemd160
    [10] => ripemd256
    [11] => ripemd320
    [12] => whirlpool
    [13] => tiger128,3
    [14] => tiger160,3
    [15] => tiger192,3
    [16] => tiger128,4
    [17] => tiger160,4
    [18] => tiger192,4
    [19] => snefru
    [20] => snefru256
    [21] => gost
    [22] => adler32
    [23] => crc32
    [24] => crc32b
    [25] => salsa10
    [26] => salsa20
    [27] => haval128,3
    [28] => haval160,3
    [29] => haval192,3
    [30] => haval224,3
    [31] => haval256,3
    [32] => haval128,4
    [33] => haval160,4
    [34] => haval192,4
    [35] => haval224,4
    [36] => haval256,4
    [37] => haval128,5
    [38] => haval160,5
    [39] => haval192,5
    [40] => haval224,5
    [41] => haval256,5
)
```

FIGURE 28-2

```
md5: 9cf88e1df09629a23fcdabe2b02ab06a
sha1: d6702d6317a20db403175d12936cdcac71155d35
sha512: 64dd467d9f0e3b6c2fd8559009f178bad927eff588678c54453479d882400803394acae4ce73e1fc12b4cfcde1ef9ca931997b4a525926e495af57f0ffdbc895
whirlpool: 5b07fa8b6dde507cac330662d0d48339c3b82db413b3be8fbc5d7ea1c1fd3e2792605d3cbfda1a200c72d1fceb84a19c53a8848947571d0cfb4b2a038e7b69b2
```

FIGURE 28-3

```
sha512: 904e33b5a13e3c65ee197394130179ef0222c2b64f4350ed13660b8b4c0728248dc28908fc390b12e6e5cee6290c45de1cd0a5b38e96f2c8d56abca5c03f93f2
```

FIGURE 28-4

To protect the passwords you need to use a two-part login where you request both the username and the password. If you only have the password then either there's a chance that the password is unique, or you have to inform the user that the password is already taken, in which case she knows the password of another user.

As an added precaution, don't retrieve the password hash field when you query the database. Use the calculated hash in the WHERE clause of the SELECT statement but leave it out of the list of fields to retrieve. This means that you can't use an asterisk (*) and retrieve all fields.

USING COOKIES AND SESSIONS

HTTP, the protocol that runs the Web, is *stateless*. Stateless means that the system doesn't know the status of what has happened before. When the server processes requests from your website, it knows nothing more than what you've given it in that one command. It doesn't know what this user has done in the past or that he has successfully logged in.

Cookies and sessions are used to overcome this short-term memory problem. You've used cookies and sessions when working with forms. As you learned there, cookies are stored on a user's computer in plain text. Sessions, on the other hand, are stored on the server with only the id to the user session being stored in the cookie.

Security information, such as the fact that the user is logged in and what his access levels are, should be kept in a session rather than a cookie. To use a session you must always start the session before you do anything else. Start a session with session_start();. If you are using this throughout your program and you have an initialization program, put the command in there.

After you have started a session with session_start(), the session is accessed like an associative array using $_SESSION just as $_POST, $_GET, and $_COOKIE are accessed. For example, if the user data is an associative array, this code stores the user's id and access level in the session:

```
$_SESSION['user_id'] = $result['id'];
$_SESSION['access'] = $result['access'];
```

If the session is used only for logged-in users, when the user logs out, you clear the session variables, expire the cookie that points to the session, and destroy the session itself:

```php
<?php
$_SESSION = array();
if (isset($_COOKIE[session_name()])) {
  setcookie(session_name(), '', time()-360000);
}
session_destroy();
```

If you are also using the session for users who are not logged in, you unset the session variables that pertain to the logged-in user:

```php
<?php
unset($_SESSION['user_id']);
unset($_SESSION['access']);
```

PUTTING LOGINS TO WORK

Now that you have the access information in a session you can use that to allow access to specific pages or even specific pieces of information. You frequently check whether someone is logged in and what her access is, so the first thing to do is to put those checks in a function or add it as a method to a class. In these examples you use a function, though in the Case Study you use a static method in the Contact class.

Continuing with the examples you used earlier to check whether a user is logged in, create the following function:

```php
<?php
function isLoggedIn() {
  if (isset($_SESSION['user_id'])) {
    return true;
  } else {
    return false;
  }
}
```

Using this function assumes that you have called a session_start() and that you put this information in the session when the user logged in.

When you have a page that you want only a logged-in user to see, check at the beginning of the page to see if she is logged in. Display the page only if the function returns true. In this example, if the user is not logged in, she sees a message that says the page is restricted. Otherwise, if the user is logged in, she sees the private page:

```html
<html>
<title>Private Page</title>
<body>
<?php if (!isLoggedIn()) : ?>
  <p>Sorry, this page is restricted. </p>
<?php else : ?>
  <h1>Welcome</h1>
  <p>You are looking at a private page.</p>
<?php endif; ?>
</body>
</html>
```

You can use this same logic to restrict access to a part of the page as shown in the following example:

```html
<html>
<title>Private Information</title>
<body>
  <h1>Welcome</h1>
  <p>You are looking at the public part of this page.</p>

<?php if (isLoggedIn()) : ?>
  <p>And here you see private information</p>
<?php endif; ?>
```

```
    <p>And here is more public information.</p>

</body>
</html>
```

These examples only care if the user was logged in. The next level of ACL is when you have different authorizations for different people or groups. The logic is similar to checking if the user is logged in, except here you check to see that she has the appropriate access level. This function returns the actual access level if the user is logged in and false if the user is not logged in:

```
function accessLevel() {
  if (isset($_SESSION['access'])) {
    return $_SESSION['access'];
  } else {
    return false;
  }
}
```

You can then use this access level to determine what can be displayed. This page shows one link for administrators, a different link for registered users, and a third for everyone else:

```
<html>
<title>Private Information</title>
<body>
  <h1>Welcome</h1>
  <p>You are looking at the public part of this page.</p>

<?php if (accessLevel() == 'Admin') : ?>
  <a href="index.php?content=adminstuff">Admin functions</a>
<?php elseif (accessLevel() == 'Registered') : ?>
  <a href="index.php?content=registeredstuff">Registered functions</a>
<?php else : ?>
  <a href="index.php?content=publicstuff">Public functions</a>
<?php endif; ?>

</body>
</html>
```

You also can assign access levels to your assets, such as tables, fields, or rows, and then match those access levels with the access levels of the users.

TRY IT

In this Try It, you add a simple ACL system to the Case Study. You use this to restrict add, edit, and delete functions to administrators. The ACL system has two types of logged-in users: administrators and registered users.

To keep things simple, you expand the contacts to include the user information so you add username, password, and access level to the contacts table and corresponding maintenance pages and processing. In an actual system these might be two different tables.

Users need a way to sign on, so you create a login page and a logout page. Display the link to the login page to users who are not logged in and the logout link to those who are logged in.

You can download the code and resources for this Try It from the book's web page at www.wrox.com. You can find them in the Lesson28 folder in the download. You will find code for both before and after completing the exercises.

Lesson Requirements

Your computer needs to be able to run as a web server with PHP and MySQL. XAMPP is a package of software that installs the web server, PHP, and MySQL for you. You can find instructions for downloading and installing XAMPP in Lesson 1.

You need a text editor that can produce plain-text files. You can find instructions for downloading and installing Eclipse PDT in Lesson 1. Other text editors that you can use are Adobe's Dreamweaver in code mode, Notepad, TextWrangler, or NetBeans.

If you are following along with the Case Study, you need your files from the end of Lesson 27. Alternatively, you can download the files from the book's website at www.wrox.com. The password for the contacts in the database is 12345678.

Hints

There are many different ways to hash a password. The one used in this section adds three salts, each of a different kind. The first salt is a salt that is different for each user and is stored in the database. The id field is used for that. The second salt is an arbitrary list of characters hardcoded wherever hashing is needed. The third salt is a salt that is specific to the site. This is shown as a hardcoded constant. In a real program you might have that in a separate configuration file. The hashing used is sha512, which takes up 128 bytes.

Step-by-Step

Add username, password, and access level to the `contacts` table.

1. Add the following fields to the `contacts` table. You can use phpMyAdmin to add the fields to the table either with the GUI interface, in the SQL table with the following code, or by importing the `addacl.sql` file from the downloaded code.

   ```
   ALTER TABLE `contacts`
       ADD `user_name` varchar(15) NOT NULL,
       ADD `password` varchar(128) NOT NULL,
       ADD `access` varchar(10) NOT NULL;
   ```

2. Update the `content/contactmaint.php` file with the new fields. You use a drop-down for the access levels, so set that up at the very end of the first PHP block. You create this drop-down later in the Try It. You want to fill in the password only if you want to change it, so don't display the value for the password. The type should be password so that the text is not displayed when typed in. Add the attribute `autocomplete="off"`. This prevents the

password from being automatically filled in by the browser. This attribute does not validate but is needed. Add a second input for passwords to get a confirming password.

```php
// set up the access dropdown,
// setting up the selected option for existing records
  $access_dropdown = $item->getAccess_DropDown();
?>
<h1>Contact Maintenance</h1>

...

<li><label for="user_name" class="required">User Name</label><br />
  <input type="text" name="user_name" id="user_name"
  value="<?php echo htmlspecialchars($item->getUser_name()); ?>" />
</li>
<li><label for="password1" >New Password</label><br />
  <input type="password" name="password1" id="password1" autocomplete="off"  />
</li>
<li><label for="password2" >Confirm Password</label><br />
  <input type="password" name="password2" id="password2" autocomplete="off" />
</li>
<li><?php echo $access_dropdown; ?></li>
```

3. In the `includes/classes/contact.php` file, add the additional fields as properties:

```php
/**
 * User name
 * @var string
 */
protected $user_name;

/**
 * Password
 * @var string
 */
protected $password;

/**
 * Access level
 * @var string
 */
protected $access;
```

4. In the same file, add the getters for the username and the access level. Do not create one for the password.

```php
/**
 * Return User Name
 * @return string
 */
public function getUser_name() {
  return $this->user_name;
}

/**
 * Return Access
```

```
 * @return string
 */
public function getAccess() {
  return $this->access;
}
```

5. Still in the same file, create a public method that creates the HTML for a drop-down showing the options Registered and Admin:

```
public function getAccess_DropDown() {
  // set up first option for selection if none selected
  $option_selected = '';
  if (!$this->access) {
    $option_selected = ' selected="selected"';
  }

  // Get the categories
  $items = array('Registered', 'Admin');

  $html  = array();

  $html[] = '<label for="access">Choose Access</label><br />';
  $html[] = '<select name="access" id="access">';

  foreach ($items as $i=>$item) {
    // If the selected parameter equals the current category id
    // then flag as selected
    if ($this->access == $item) {
      $option_selected = ' selected="selected"';
    }
    // set up the option line
    $html[] = '<option value="' . $item . '"' . $option_selected . '>' . ↵
$item . '</option>';
    // clear out the selected option flag
    $option_selected = '';
  }

  $html[] = '</select>';
  return implode("\n", $html);

}
```

6. In the includes/init.php file, add a constant that defines a site key. This site key is used to hash the password. The value in the site key is purely arbitrary. If you later change it, none of your passwords would work.

```
define('SITE_KEY',
  'd0d48339c3b82db413b3be8fbc5d7ea1c1fd3e2792605d3cbfda1HEM54!!');
```

7. In the includes/function.php file, find the maintContact() function. Add the username and access level to the $item array. You do not add the passwords here.

```
'phone'     => filter_input(INPUT_POST,'phone', FILTER_SANITIZE_STRING),
'user_name' => filter_input(INPUT_POST,'user_name', FILTER_SANITIZE_STRING),
'access'    => filter_input(INPUT_POST,'access', FILTER_SANITIZE_STRING)
);
```

8. Back in the `includes/classes/contact.php` file, find the `_verifyInput()` function. Verify that a username exists and is at least six characters long. Run the `getContactIdByUser()` method. This method returns the id for the row with the given username. If an id is returned, it means the username is already taken. You create the method in the next step. If a password is entered, verify the length and confirm that it and the confirming password are the same. If they do not match, set an error.

```php
if (!trim($this->user_name)) {
    $error = true;
} elseif (strlen(trim($this->user_name)) < 6) {
    $error = true;
} elseif (self::getContactIdByUser(trim($this->user_name))) {
    $error = true;
}

$password1 = trim($_POST['password1']);
if ($password1) {
    if ($password1 != trim($_POST['password2'])) {
        $error = true;
    } elseif (strlen($password1) < 6) {
        $error = true;
    }
}
```

9. Create a static method that takes a username and looks up the id in the `contacts` table:

```php
public static function getContactIdByUser($user_name) {
    // Get the database connection
    $connection = Database::getConnection();
    // set up the query
    $id = '';
    $query = 'SELECT id FROM `contacts`
      WHERE user_name="'. Database::prep($user_name) .'"
      LIMIT 1';
    // Run the MySQL command
    $result_obj = '';
    // Run the MySQL command
    $result_obj = $connection->query($query);
      while($result = $result_obj->fetch_array(MYSQLI_ASSOC)) {
        $id = $result['id'];
      }
    // if user name not found, return false
    if (!$id) { // if user name not found, return with error message
      return false;
    } else {
      return $id;
    }
}
```

10. Update the `addRecord()` method by adding the processing for the new fields. Create the new row as before. This enables you to get the newly generated id with the `mysql_insert_id()` function so you can use that to help create the hash for the password. The `!hi#HUde9` is an

arbitrary salt. By hardcoding the salt here, it requires that hackers have access to your files to locate the information. You are also using the constant SITE_KEY, which you defined earlier.

Update the new row with the username, password hash, and the access level. The following code trims the password so that whitespaces are automatically used. Some people like to put deliberate whitespace at the beginning or end of the password. If you want to accommodate them, leave off the trim() around the $_POST['password1'].

```php
public function addRecord() {

    // Verify the fields
    if ($this->_verifyInput()) {
      // prepare for the encrypted password
        $password = trim($_POST['password1']);

      // Get the Database connection
      $connection = Database::getConnection();

      // Prepare the data
      $query = "INSERT INTO contacts(first_name, last_name, position, email,
phone)
      VALUES ('" . Database::prep($this->first_name) . "',
       '" . Database::prep($this->last_name) . "',
       '" . Database::prep($this->position) . "',
       '" . Database::prep($this->email) . "',
       '" . Database::prep($this->phone) . "')";
      // Run the MySQL statement
      if ($connection->query($query)) { // this inserts the row
        // update with the user name and password now that you know the id
        $query = "UPDATE contacts
        SET user_name = '" . Database::prep($this->user_name) . "',
        password = '" . hash_hmac('sha512',
          $password . '!hi#HUde9' . mysql_insert_id(),
          SITE_KEY) ."',
        access = '" . Database::prep($this->access) . "'";
        if ($connection->query($query)) { // this updates the row
          $return = array('', 'Contact Record successfully added.', '');
          // add success message
          return $return;
        } else {
        // send fail message
          $return = array('', 'User name/password not added to contact.',
'');

          return $return;
        }

    } else {
    // send fail message and return to contactmaint
    $return = array('contactmaint',
      'No Contact Record Added. Unable to create record.',
      '0');
    return $return;
    }
  } else {
    // send fail message and return to contactmaint
```

```
        $return = array('contactmaint', 'No Contact Record Added.
           Missing required information or problem with user name or password.',
 '0');
        return $return;
    }

    }
```

11. Next, update the `editRecord()` method. If a password was entered, create the hash password and update all the fields. If no password was entered, just add the username and access fields to the existing fields to be updated. The following code shows the affected part of the method:

```
// Update with a password changed
if (trim($_POST['password1'])) {
    // prepare the encrypted password
    $hash_password = hash_hmac('sha512',
      trim($_POST['password1']) . '!hi#HUde9' . $this->id,
      SITE_KEY);
    // Set up the prepared statement
    $query = 'UPDATE `contacts` SET first_name=?, last_name=?,
      position=?, email=?, phone=?,
      user_name=?, password=?, access=?
      WHERE id=?';
    $statement = $connection->prepare($query);
    // bind the parameters
    $statement->bind_param('sssssssi',$this->first_name,
      $this->last_name,
      $this->position, $this->email, $this->phone,
      $this->user_name, $hash_password, $this->access,
      $this->id);
} else {
    // update without a password changed
    // Set up the prepared statement
    $query = 'UPDATE `contacts` SET first_name=?, last_name=?,
      position=?, email=?, phone=?,
      user_name=?, access=?
      WHERE id=?';
    $statement = $connection->prepare($query);
    // bind the parameters
    $statement->bind_param('sssssssi',$this->first_name, $this->last_name,
      $this->position, $this->email, $this->phone,
      $this->user_name, $this->access,
      $this->id);
}
```

12. Change the `getContact()` method to get specific fields instead of all fields with the *. This way you don't bring in the hash password.

```
$query = 'SELECT `id`,`first_name`,`last_name`,`position`, `email`, `phone`,
  `user_name`, `access`
FROM `contacts` WHERE id="'. (int) $id.'"';
```

13. Change the `getcontacts()` method to get specific fields instead of all fields with the *.

```
$query = 'SELECT `id`,`first_name`,`last_name`,`position`, `email`, `phone`,
  `user_name`, `access`
FROM `contacts` ORDER BY first_name, last_name';
```

14. Now add usernames and passwords to the existing contacts as demonstrated in Figure 28-5. You add the Logout menu item later in this Try It.

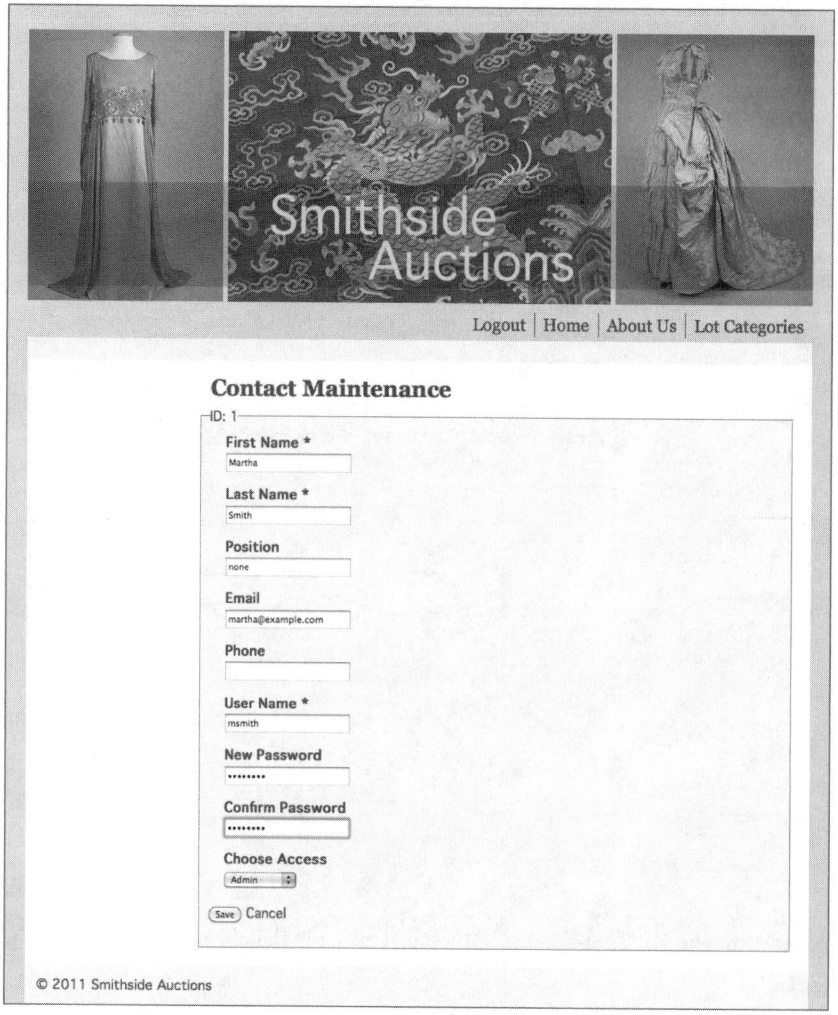

FIGURE 28-5

15. Flag `user_name` as unique in the database so that there are no duplicates in the table.

```
ALTER TABLE `contacts` ADD UNIQUE (`user_name`);
```

The next step is to create a login page so that users can log in.

1. Create a file called `content/login.php` that looks like Figure 28-6.

```php
<?php
?>
<h1>Login</h1>

<form action="index.php" method="post" name="maint" id="maint">
```

```
  <fieldset class="maintform">
    <legend>Login</legend>
    <ul>
      <li><label for="user_name" class="required">User Name</label><br />
        <input type="text" name="user_name" id="user_name" class="required"
/></li>
        <li><label for="password" class="required">Password</label><br />
          <input type="password" name="password" id="password" class="required"
/>
      </li>
      </ul>

      <?php
      // create token
      $salt = 'SomeSalt';
      $token = sha1(mt_rand(1,1000000) . $salt);
      $_SESSION['token'] = $token;
      ?>
      <input type="hidden" name="task" id="task" value="login" />
      <input type='hidden' name='token' value='<?php echo $token; ?>'/>
      <input type="submit" name="login" value="Login" />
      <a class="cancel" href="index.php">Cancel, return to Home Page</a>
  </fieldset>
</form>
```

Login

```
┌─Login────────────────────────────────────────────┐
│  User Name *                                      │
│  [                    ]                            │
│                                                   │
│  Password *                                       │
│  [                    ]                            │
│                                                   │
│  (Login) Cancel, return to Home Page              │
└───────────────────────────────────────────────────┘
```

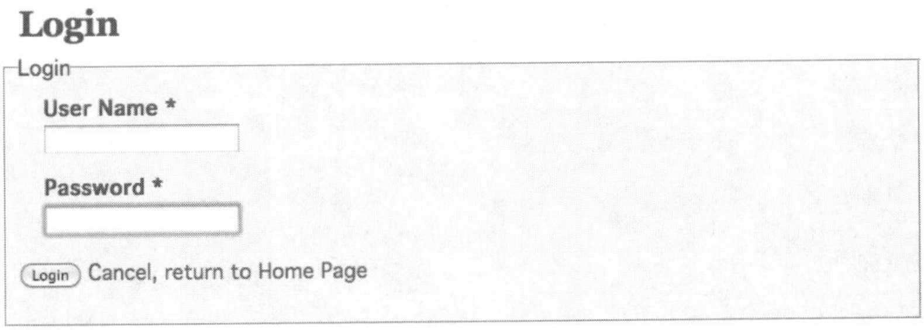

FIGURE 28-6

2. Add the `login` task to the `includes/init.php` file. This calls the `userLogin()` function.

```
case 'login' :
// process the login
$results = userLogin();
$message .= $results[1];
// If there is redirect information
// redirect to that page
// pass on new messages
  if ($results[0] == 'login') {
  // pass on new messages
  if ($results[1]) {
```

```
    $_SESSION['message'] = $results[1];
  }
  header("Location: index.php?content=login");
  exit;
}
break;
```

3. Add the `userLogin()` function to the `includes/functions.php` file. This function checks the token as usual and loads the POST variables into an array. That array is then passed to the static method `logIn()` in the `Contact` class and the results passed back to the calling function in `init.php`.

```
function userLogin() {
  $results = '';
  if (isset($_POST['login']) AND $_POST['login'] == 'Login') {
    // check the token
    $badToken = true;
    if (!isset($_POST['token'])
    || !isset($_SESSION['token'])
    || empty($_POST['token'])
    || $_POST['token'] !== $_SESSION['token']) {
      $results = array('',
        'Sorry, go back and try again. There was a security issue.');
      $badToken = true;
    } else {
      $badToken = false;
      unset($_SESSION['token']);

      $item  = array (
        'user_name' => filter_input(INPUT_POST,'user_name', FILTER_SANITIZE_
STRING),
        'password' => filter_input(INPUT_POST,'password')
        );

      // login
      $results = Contact::logIn($item);
    }
  }
  return $results;
}
```

4. Add the `logIn()` method to the `includes/classes/contact.php` file. First you check to see that the user entered both a username and a password. Use the username to get the id from the database. If there is no matching user, send the error message that, the username or password is incorrect. Never tell the user what the exact problem is because that gives hackers too much information.

Next, set up the hash for the password. Select the user based on matching both the username and hash password. In this instance you are pulling in only those fields that you need, rather

than using an * to get all fields. It is better not to pull in the hash password. Post all of those fields to SESSION variables and return a success message.

```php
public static function logIn($item) {
  if (!$item['user_name'] || !$item['password']) {
    return array('login','Sorry, invalid User Name and/or Password.');
  }
  // Get the database connection
  $connection = Database::getConnection();

  // get the id for the user
  $id = self::getContactIdByUser($item['user_name']);

  if (!$id) { // if user name not found, return with error message
    return array('login','Sorry, invalid User Name and/or Password.','');
  }

  $hash_password = hash_hmac('sha512', $item['password'] . '!hi#HUde9' . ↵
(int) $id, SITE_KEY);

  // Set up the query
  $query = 'SELECT id, first_name, last_name, user_name, access
    FROM `contacts`
    WHERE user_name="'. $item['user_name'] .'"
    AND password = "' . $hash_password . '"
    LIMIT 1';
  // Run the MySQL command
  $result_obj = '';
  // Run the MySQL command
  $result_obj = $connection->query($query);
  try {
    while ($result = $result_obj->fetch_array(MYSQLI_ASSOC)) {
      // pass back the results
      $_SESSION['user_id'] = $result['id'];
      $_SESSION['first_name'] = $result['first_name'];
      $_SESSION['last_name'] = $result['last_name'];
      $_SESSION['user_name'] = $result['user_name'];
      $_SESSION['access'] = $result['access'];
      return array('',"Welcome, {$_SESSION['first_name']}", '');
    }
    return array('login','Sorry, invalid User Name and/or Password.','');
  }
  catch(Exception $e)
  {
    return false;
  }
}
```

5. Add the Login menu item to the main menu in index.php:

```html
<li><a href="index.php?content=home">Home</a></li>
<li><a href="index.php?content=login">Login</a></li>
```

> *If you need to reset your session during your testing, an easy way is to completely close down your browser.*

The next step is to create a logout page so that users can log out.

1. Create a file called `content/logout.php`. Assuming that George is logged in, your results look like Figure 28-7.

```php
<?php
/**
 * logout.php
 *
 * Logout
 *
 * @version    1.2 2011-02-03
 * @package    Smithside Auctions
 * @copyright  Copyright (c) 2011 Smithside Auctions
 * @license    GNU General Public License
 * @since      Since Release 1.0
 */
?>
<h1>Logout</h1>

<form action="index.php" method="post" name="maint" id="maint">

  <fieldset class="maintform">
    <legend>Logout</legend>
    <p>Are you sure you want to logout, <?php echo $_SESSION['first_name'];
?>?</p>

    <?php
    // create token
    $salt = 'SomeSalt';
    $token = sha1(mt_rand(1,1000000) . $salt);
    $_SESSION['token'] = $token;
    ?>
    <input type="hidden" name="task" id="task" value="logout" />
    <input type='hidden' name='token' value='<?php echo $token; ?>'/>
    <input type="submit" name="logout" value="Logout" />
    <a class="cancel" href="index.php">Cancel, return to Home Page</a>
  </fieldset>
</form>
```

Logout

```
┌─Logout──────────────────────────────────────────────┐
│  Are you sure you want to logout, George?            │
│  (Logout) Cancel, return to Home Page                │
└──────────────────────────────────────────────────────┘
```

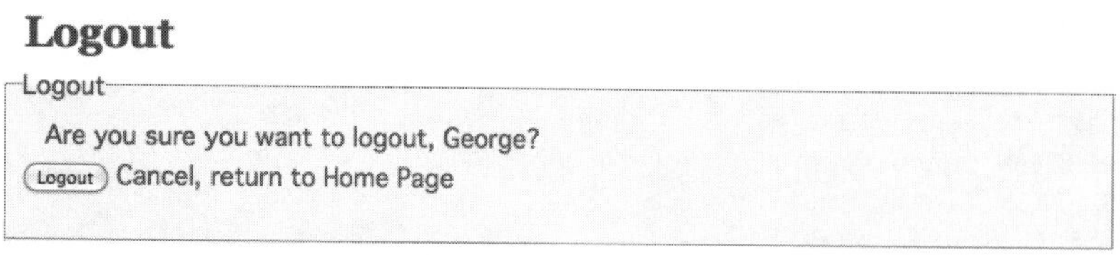

FIGURE 28-7

2. Add the `logout` task to the `includes/init.php` file. This calls the `userLogout()` function.

```php
case 'logout' :
// process the login
$results = userLogout();
$message .= $results[1];
// If there is redirect information
// redirect to that page
// pass on new messages
```

```
        if ($results[0] == 'logout') {
          // pass on new messages
          if ($results[1]) {
            $_SESSION['message'] = $results[1];
          }
          header("Location: index.php?content=logout]");
          exit;
        }
        break;
```

3. Add the `userLogout()` function to the `includes/functions.php` file. This function checks the token as usual. The static method `logOut()` in the `Contact` class is called and the results are passed back to the calling function in `init.php`.

```
    function userLogout() {
      $results = '';
      if (isset($_POST['logout']) AND $_POST['logout'] == 'Logout') {
        // check the token
        $badToken = true;
        if (!isset($_POST['token'])
        || !isset($_SESSION['token'])
        || empty($_POST['token'])
        || $_POST['token'] !== $_SESSION['token']) {
          $results = array('',
            'Sorry, go back and try again. There was a security issue.', '');
          $badToken = true;
        } else {
          // logout
          $badToken = false;
          unset($_SESSION['token']);

          Contact::logout();
          $results = array('',"You have successfully logged out",'');;
        }
      }
      return $results;
    }
```

4. Add the `logOut()` method to the `includes/classes/contact.php` file. To log the user out, you unset the `SESSION` variables.

```
    public static function logout() {
      unset($_SESSION['user_id']);
      unset($_SESSION['first_name']);
      unset($_SESSION['last_name']);
      unset($_SESSION['user_name']);
      unset($_SESSION['access']);
    }
```

5. Add the Logout menu item to the main menu in `index.php`:

```
        <li><a href="index.php?content=home">Home</a></li>
        <li><a href="index.php?content=logout">Logout</a></li>
        <li><a href="index.php?content=login">Login</a></li>
```

Finally, you add the access level checks to your program.

1. Create a static method called `isLoggedIn()` in the `Contact` class that returns true if the user is logged in. To see if a user is logged in, check to see if the `SESSION` variable `user_id` is set. In the `includes/classes/contact.php` file add this code:

```
public static function isLoggedIn() {
  if (isset($_SESSION['user_id'])) {
    return true;
  } else {
    return false;
  }
}
```

2. Create a static method called `accessLevel()` in the `Contact` class that returns the access level of the user. This is stored in the `SESSION` variable `access`.

```
public static function accessLevel() {
  if (isset($_SESSION['access'])) {
    return $_SESSION['access'];
  } else {
    return false;
  }
}
```

3. Some pages have both public and private information. Only Admin users are allowed to add, edit, or delete items. Add access level checks to those buttons in the `about.php`, `categories.php`, and `lots.php` files in the `content` folder. Here is the example for the `about.php` file:

```
// Get the contact information
$items = Contact::getContacts();
$accessLevel = Contact::accessLevel();
?>
<h1>About Us
  <?php if ($accessLevel == 'Admin') : ?>
    <a class="button" href="index.php?content=contactmaint&id=0">Add</a>
  <?php endif; ?>
</h1>

...

<h2><?php echo htmlspecialchars($item->name()); ?>
<?php if ($accessLevel == 'Admin') : ?>
  <a class="button"
    href="index.php?content=contactdelete&id=<?php echo $item->getId();
?>">Delete
</a>
  <a class="button"
    href="index.php?content=contactmaint&id=<?php echo $item->getId();
?>">Edit</a>
<?php endif; ?>
</h2>
```

4. Some pages should only be seen by Admin users. They don't have access through the program, but could still get to those pages by directly entering a URL. Check for the access level at the beginning of the content and skip the content if the user is not an Admin user.

The following files in the `content` folder should have this check: `categorydelete.php`, `categorymaint.php`, `contactdelete.php`, `contactmaint.php`, `lotdelete.php`, and `lotmaint.php`. Here is the example for the `categorydelete.php` file:

```php
$accessLevel = Contact::accessLevel();
if ($accessLevel != 'Admin') :
  echo 'Sorry, no access allowed to this page';
else :

$id = (int) $_GET['cat_id'];
// Get the existing information for an existing item
$item = Category::getCategory($id);
?>
<h1>Category Maintenance</h1>

. . .

</form>
<?php endif;
```

5. Change the menu so that Login shows for those users who are not logged in and Logout shows for those users who are logged in:

```php
require_once 'includes/init.php';
$logged_in = Contact::isLoggedIn();
?>

. . .

<li><a href="index.php?content=home">Home</a></li>
<?php if ($logged_in) : ?>
  <li><a href="index.php?content=logout">Logout</a></li>
<?php else : ?>
  <li><a href="index.php?content=login">Login</a></li>
<?php endif; ?>
```

6. Check that you can log in and out. See that the Add, Edit, and Delete buttons show only if you are logged in as an Admin user. See that the menu shows Login if you are not logged in and Logout if you are logged in.

 Watch the video for Lesson 28 on the DVD or watch online at www.wrox.com/ go/24phpmysql.

Turn the Case Study into a Content Management System

In this lesson you add the ability to create additional pages of information for the Case Study site. These could be news articles, a page listing the privacy policy, or a blog article. Instead of creating a new .php content file for each one, you create a single .php file that displays page text that you have in the database.

DESIGNING AND CREATING THE TABLE

The first step is to create the table that will contain the page data. What is the information you need in this file? There is the obvious information such as

> Title

> Text

and other information you might want to keep:

> User who created the article

> Date article was created

> User who last modified the article

> Last date the article was modified

You also need a primary key so that you can select which article you want to display. Remember that the primary key cannot change and should be unique. Therefore you do not want to use the title as the key. Use an auto-increment integer key as you have in the other file.

This example is for a freeform page, but depending on your application, you could add additional fields that you could then place in particular places on the page. For instance, if you want all the articles to start with a picture and a short introduction and be followed by a list of references, you could add fields for each of those in your table.

You might also want to put your articles into different categories the way that the lots are in the Case Study. For that, you need an article categories table and a key in the articles table that links to it. You don't use article categories for this example.

CREATING THE CLASS

After you have created the articles table, you need to create a class that describes it and contains the different actions you need to perform on the articles. This class is similar to the others that you have created, but this is a good place to list what you need in the class. In different projects that you do, you have different methods in your classes, but these are basic methods that most classes based on tables need to have.

Properties

The properties in the class match the fields in the table. They should be protected so that only this class or classes that extend this class can see them directly.

Methods

Your class needs methods to create the object and to handle the CRUD (creating, reading, updating, and deleting) of the articles.

➤ `__construct()`: This method is called when you create an object from this class. You have been using a method that takes an associative array where the indexes are equal to the properties and automatically updates the properties at instantiation. You can perform different actions in this method. In this example, you have the user who created the article and the user who last modified the article. You store the id, not the name of the user, from the contact table in the article table. If you call `Contact::getContact($this->created_by);` in this method you can assign it to a new property you create, which now contains all the information about the person who wrote the article.

➤ `getProperty_name()`: This is a getter method, where *Property_name* is the name of the property with the first letter capitalized. You need getter methods for each of the properties that are protected or private so that parts of the program outside the class are able to see what the values are.

➤ `_verifyInput()`: This method is used to verify the input used to add or update the table.

➤ `addRecord()`: This method is used to add a row to the table.

➤ `editRecord()`: This method is used to make changes to a row in the table.

➤ deleteRecord(): This method is used to remove a row from the table.

➤ getArticle(): This method is used to get the information from one row in the table, based on the id passed to the method.

➤ getArticles(): This method is used to get a list of all the rows in the table.

When you have this much code that is similar, it makes sense to reuse the same code instead of copying and pasting it into new classes. It cuts down on errors, saves you time, makes the code easier to read, and makes it easier to make changes to all the classes. For instance, instead of having four __construct() methods in four different classes, you could create a class that has a __construct() method in it and then you can extend that class.

The following class called Table has a property $id and two methods. One is the __construct() method and the other is a getter method for the $id property.

```php
<?php
class Table
{
  protected $id;

  public function __construct($input = false) {
    if (is_array($input)) {
      foreach ($input as $key => $val) {
      // Note the $key instead of key.
      // This will give the value in $key instead of 'key' itself
      $this->$key = $val;
      }
    }
  }

  public function getId() {
    return $this->id;
  }

}
```

Any class that extends the Table class automatically includes a property $id and the methods __construct() and getId(). If the child class has no property or method with the same name, it automatically uses the parent class or property version. If the child class has a property or method with the same name, then the child's property or class is used. You can still access the parent, however, by using parent as the class name. This code uses the child construct that in turn calls the parent's __construct() and then adds more code:

```php
class Article extends Table
{

  public function __construct($input = false) {
    parent::__construct($input);
    $this->author = Contact::getContact($this->created_by);
  }
}
```

You can expand this idea by moving some of the other methods that are similar across the classes into the `Table` class and then extending the `Contact`, `Category`, and `Lot` classes from the `Table` class.

CREATING THE MAINTENANCE PAGES

After you have the table and class created, you need to create the pages to maintain the table. To maintain the articles you need a page that displays a list of the articles, a page to add or change articles, and a page to delete the articles. You can use the contacts or categories pages as a model for this.

The user who creates the article, the date the article was created, the user who last modified the article, and the last date modified are already known to the system. Those fields can be automatically updated and so do not need to be on the form.

For security and validation, the title field should be run through the `htmlspecialchars()` function. This turns control characters into the HTML entities so that they display as characters rather than performing any actions. For instance, an `&` would be turned into `&amp;`.

The text field needs special consideration. If you treat it the standard way, by encoding the HTML entities, you are not able to use HTML in the text field. This is fine if you only want paragraphs, but if you want to be able to enter HTML commands you need to come up with a different solution. The `strip_tags()` function strips away HTML tags except for the ones that you specify. This lets you control what HTML you allow.

The `strip_tags()` function does not make the field entirely secure. You could still get things put into the attributes such as with JavaScript `mouseovers`. In this case, the form input is coming from within the company so it is acceptable. If this were coming from public input, you would need to program something more secure.

CREATING THE DISPLAY PAGE

To display the articles all you need to do is to create a file that looks up the article based on the id and display the fields. However, there is one additional change you need to make to the display of the text field. Figure 29-1 displays an article on the maintenance screen. Figure 29-2 displays what it looks like on the display screen.

As you can see, you have lost all the paragraphs. The text has run into a single paragraph. If you were to use `<p>` tags to surround the paragraphs you would get your paragraphs back, but there's an easier way to get them back. Control characters that signify a new line create those paragraphs. The `<textarea>` tag reads those and starts a new paragraph. Just displaying the text field does not activate those control characters. There is a function that turns those newline characters

into `<br />` tags. It is the "new line to `<br>`" function, which is written as `nl2br()`. Adding that function to the display of the text brings back the paragraphs. The results of the following code are shown in Figure 29-3.

```php
<?php echo strip_tags(nl2br($item->getText()),
    "<p><br><h2><h3><h4><strong><em><ul><ol><li><a>"); ?>
```

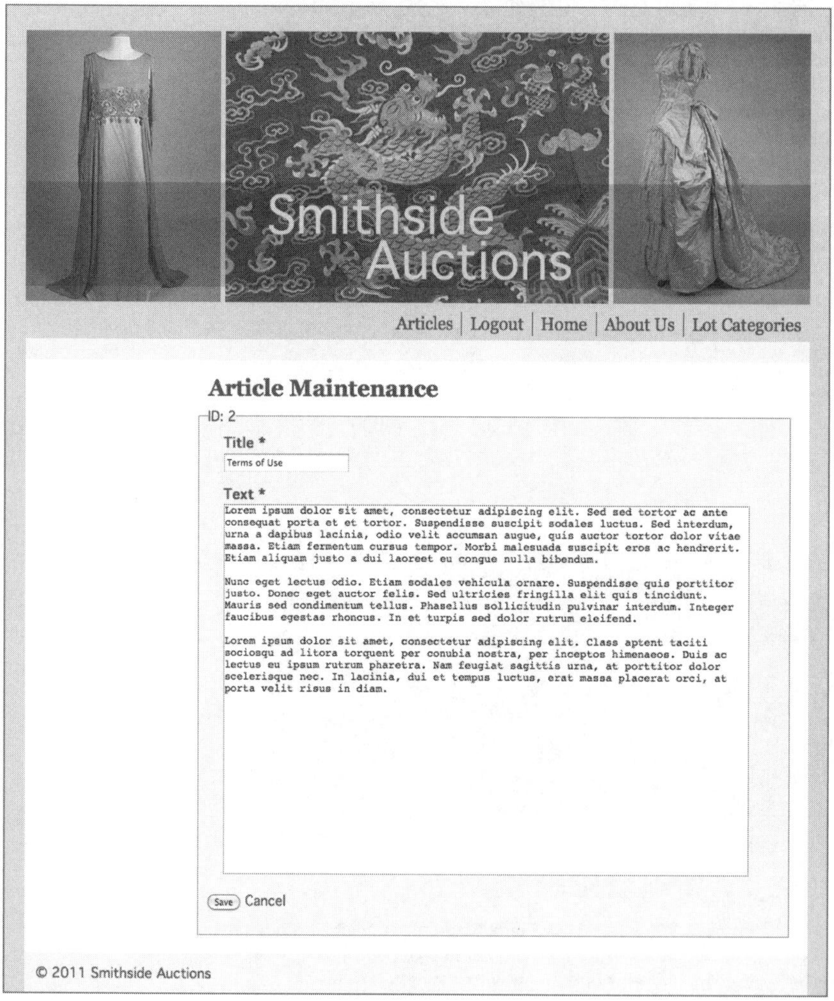

FIGURE 29-1

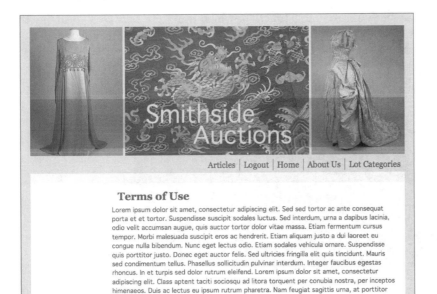

FIGURE 29-2

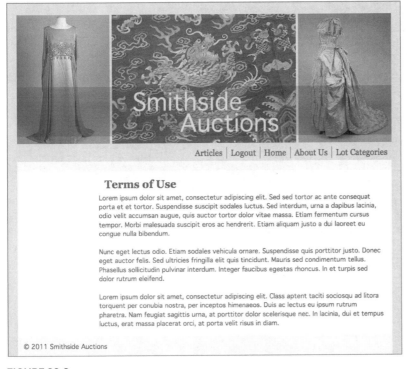

FIGURE 29-3

TRY IT

In this Try It, you add a new table to the Case Study database called `articles`. You set up maintenance pages for this new table, including all the necessary processing for adding, editing, and deleting articles. You create a new content file called `articledisplay.php` that you use to display the articles as a web page.

> *You can download the code and resources for this Try It from the book's web page at* www.wrox.com. *You can find them in the Lesson29 folder in the download. You will find code for both before and after completing the exercises.*

Lesson Requirements

Your computer needs to be able to run as a web server with PHP and MySQL. XAMPP is a package of software that installs the web server, PHP, and MySQL for you. You can find instructions for downloading and installing XAMPP in Lesson 1.

You need a text editor that can produce plain-text files. You can find instructions for downloading and installing Eclipse PDT in Lesson 1. Other text editors that you can use are Adobe's Dreamweaver in code mode, Notepad, TextWrangler, or NetBeans.

If you are following along with the Case Study, you need your files from the end of Lesson 28. Alternatively, you can download the files from the book's website at www.wrox.com.

Hints

Keep the end the `<textarea>` tag on the same line as the beginning of the text to go inside the `textarea`. If you don't, you get whitespace at the beginning of the input box.

`CURRENT_TIMESTAMP` is a MySQL constant that contains the current time. You can use that to timestamp when an article is created and when it is modified.

The user must be logged in before he has access to the maintenance screen, so the program has access to his user id in the `SESSION`. Access the `SESSION` variable to get the id to update the Article row.

Step-by-Step

Create the `articles` table.

1. Create the `articles` table with the following fields. You can use phpMyAdmin to add the fields to the table either with the GUI interface, in the SQL table with the following code, or by importing the `addarticlestable.sql` file from the downloaded code.

```
DROP TABLE IF EXISTS `articles`;
CREATE TABLE `articles` (
  `id` int(11) unsigned NOT NULL AUTO_INCREMENT,
```

```
`title` varchar(100) NOT NULL,
`text` text NOT NULL,
`created_by` int(11) NOT NULL,
`date_created` datetime NOT NULL DEFAULT '0000-00-00 00:00:00',
`modified_by` int(11) NOT NULL,
`date_modified` datetime NOT NULL DEFAULT '0000-00-00 00:00:00',
PRIMARY KEY (`id`)
) ENGINE=MyISAM;
```

2. Create the `Table` class in `includes/classes/table.php`:

```php
<?php
/**
 * table.php
 *
 * Table class file
 *
 * @version   1.2 2011-02-03
 * @package   Smithside Auctions
 * @copyright Copyright (c) 2011 Smithside Auctions
 * @license   GNU General Public License
 * @since     Since Release 1.0
 */
/**
 * Table class
 *
 * @package   Smithside Auctions
 */
class Table
{
  /**
   * id
   * @var int
   */
  protected $id;

  /**
   * Initialize the class with data from database
   * @param array
   */
  public function __construct($input = false) {
    if (is_array($input)) {
      foreach ($input as $key => $val) {
      // Note the $key instead of key.
      // This will give the value in $key instead of 'key' itself
      $this->$key = $val;
      }
    }
  }

  /**
   * Return id
   * @return int
   */
```

```
    */
    public function getId() {
    return $this->id;
    }

}
```

3. Create the `Article` class, which extends the `Table` class in `includes/classes/article.php`. You don't need the property `$id` or the method `getId()` because those are in the `Table` class. Define a `__construct()` method that calls the parent method and also creates an object of the contact who created the article. Add the `addRecord()`, `editRecord()`, and `deleteRecord()` methods, as well as the `getArticle()` and `getArticles()` methods.

```php
<?php
/**
 * article.php
 *
 * Article class file
 *
 * @version   1.2 2011-02-03
 * @package   Smithside Auctions
 * @copyright  Copyright (c) 2011 Smithside Auctions
 * @license  GNU General Public License
 * @since     Since Release 1.0
 */
/**
 * Article class
 *
 * @package  Smithside Auctions
 */
class Article extends Table
{

    /**
     * title
     * @var string
     */
    protected $title;

    /**
     * Text
     * @var String
     */
    protected $text;

    /**
     * Contact who created the article
     * @var int
     */
    protected $created_by;

    /**
```

```php
 * Date & time created
 * @var datetime
 */
protected $date_created;

/**
 * Contact who modified the article
 * @var int
 */
protected $modified_by;

/**
 * Date & time modified
 * @var datetime
 */
protected $date_modified;

/**
 * Author Information
 * @var Contact
 */
protected $author;

/**
 * Initialize the Article with data from database
 * @param array
 */
public function __construct($input = false) {
  parent::__construct($input);
  $this->author = Contact::getContact($this->created_by);
}

/**
 * Return Title
 * @return string
 */
public function getTitle() {
return $this->title;
}

/**
 * Return Text
 * @return string
 */
public function getText() {
return $this->text;
}

/**
 * Return Created by
 * @return int
 */
```

```php
public function getCreated_by() {
return $this->created_by;
}

/**
 * Return Created date/time
 * @return datetime
 */
public function getDate_created() {
return $this->date_created;
}

/**
 * Return Modified by
 * @return int
 */
public function getModifiedBy() {
return $this->modified_by;
}

/**
 * Return Modified date/time
 * @return datetime
 */
public function getModified_by() {
return $this->modified_by;
}

/**
 * Verify the Input
 * @return boolean
 */
protected function _verifyInput() {
  $error = false;
  if (!trim($this->title)) {
    $error = true;
  }
  if (!trim($this->text)) {
    $error = true;
  }

  if ($error) {
    return false;
  } else {
    return true;
  }
}

/**
 * Add a Row to the table
 * @return array (redirect content,message,id)
 */
```

```php
public function addRecord() {

  // Verify the fields
  if ($this->_verifyInput()) {
    // prepare the encrypted password

    // Get the Database connection
    $connection = Database::getConnection();

    // Prepare the data
    $query = "INSERT INTO articles(title, text, created_by,
      date_created, modified_by, date_modified)
    VALUES ('" . Database::prep($this->title) . "',
     '" . Database::prep($this->text) . "',
     '" . (int) $_SESSION['user_id'] . "',
     CURRENT_TIMESTAMP,
     '" . (int) $_SESSION['user_id'] . "',
     CURRENT_TIMESTAMP)";
    // Run the MySQL statement
    if ($connection->query($query)) {
    $return = array('', 'Article successfully added.', '');

      // add success message
      return $return;
    } else {
      // send fail message and return to contactmaint
      $return = array('articlemaint', 'No Article Added. Unable to
        create record.', '0');
      return $return;
    }
  } else {
    // send fail message and return to contactmaint
    $return = array('articlemaint', 'No Article Added. Missing
      required information.', '0');
    return $return;
  }

}

/**
 * Update a Row in the table
 * @return array (redirect content,message,id)
 */
public function editRecord() {
  // Verify the fields
  if ($this->_verifyInput()) {

    // Get the Database connection
    $connection = Database::getConnection();

    // Prepare the data
    $query = "UPDATE `articles`
```

```
            SET `title` = '" . Database::prep($this->title) . "',
                `text` = '" . Database::prep($this->text) . "',
                `modified_by` = '" . (int) $_SESSION['user_id'] . "',
                `date_modified` = CURRENT_TIMESTAMP
                WHERE id='" . (int) $this->id . "'";
            // Run the MySQL statement
            if ($connection->query($query)) {
            $return = array('', 'Article successfully updated.', '');

            // add success message
            return $return;
            } else {
            // send fail message
            $return = array('articlemaint',
                'Article not updated. Unable to update record.',
                (int) $this->id);
            return $return;
            }
        } else {
            // send fail message and return to maint
            $return = array('articlemaint',
                'Article not updated. Missing required information.',
                '0');
            return $return;
        }

    }

    /**
     * Delete a Row from the table
     * @param   int
     * @return array (redirect content,message,id)
     */
    public static function deleteRecord($id) {
        // Get the Database connection
        $connection = Database::getConnection();
        // Set up query
        $query = 'DELETE FROM `articles` WHERE id="'. (int) $id.'"';
        // Run the query
        if ($result = $connection->query($query)) {
          $return = array('', 'Article successfully deleted.', '');
          return $return;
        } else {
          $return = array('articledelete', 'Unable to delete Article.', (int)
$id);
          return $return;
        }
    }

    /**
     * Get an Article
     * @param   int
```

```php
 * @return Article
 */
public static function getArticle($id) {
  // Get the database connection
  $connection = Database::getConnection();
  // Set up the query
  $query = 'SELECT * FROM `articles` WHERE id="'. (int) $id.'"';
  // Run the MySQL command
  $result_obj = '';
    try {
      $result_obj = $connection->query($query);
      if (!$result_obj) {
        throw new Exception($connection->error);
      } else {
        $item = $result_obj->fetch_object('Article');
        if (!$item) {
          throw new Exception($connection->error);
        } else {
          // pass back the results
          return($item);
        }
      }
    }
    catch(Exception $e) {
      echo $e->getMessage();
    }
}

/**
 * Get an array of Articles
 * @return array (Article)
 */
public static function getArticles() {
  // clear the results
  $items = '';
  // Get the connection
  $connection = Database::getConnection();
  // Set up query
  $query = 'SELECT * FROM `articles` ORDER BY title';
  // Run the query
  $result_obj = '';
  $result_obj = $connection->query($query);
  // Loop through the results,
  // passing them to a new version of this class,
  // and making a regular array of the objects
  try {
    while($result = $result_obj->fetch_object('Article')) {
      $items[]= $result;
    }
    // pass back the results
    return($items);
```

```
        }

      catch(Exception $e) {
        return false;
      }
    }

  }
```

4. Add `Articles` to the menu in `index.php`. Make it so that only Admin users can get to the link. This links to a list of articles so you can add, edit, and delete them.

```
<li><a href="index.php?content=home">Home</a></li>
<?php if ($logged_in) : ?>
  <li><a href="index.php?content=logout">Logout</a></li>
  <?php if ($accessLevel == 'Admin') : ?>
    <li><a href="index.php?content=articles">Articles</a></li>
  <?php endif; ?>
<?php else : ?>
  <li><a href="index.php?content=login">Login</a></li>
<?php endif; ?>
```

5. Create `content/articles.php` to display a list of the articles as shown in Figure 29-4:

```php
<?php
/**
 * articles.php
 *
 * Content for Articles
 *
 * @version    1.2 2011-02-03
 * @package    Smithside Auctions
 * @copyright  Copyright (c) 2011 Smithside Auctions
 * @license    GNU General Public License
 * @since      Since Release 1.0
 */
$accessLevel = Contact::accessLevel();
if ($accessLevel != 'Admin') :
  echo 'Sorry, no access allowed to this page';
else :

// Get the article information
$items = Article::getArticles();
if (empty($items)) {
  $items = array();
}
?>
<h1>Articles
    <a class="button" href="index.php?content=articlemaint&id=0">Add</a>
</h1>

<ul class="ulfancy">
```

```php
<?php foreach ($items as $i=>$item) : ?>
  <li class="row<?php echo $i % 2; ?>">
    <h2><?php echo htmlspecialchars($item->getTitle()); ?>
      <a class="button"
        href="index.php?content=articledelete&id=<?php echo $item->getId();
?>">
        Delete
      </a>
      <a class="button"
        href="index.php?content=articlemaint&id=<?php echo $item->getId();
?>">
        Edit
      </a>
    </h2>
  </li>
<?php endforeach; ?>
</ul>

<?php endif; ?>
```

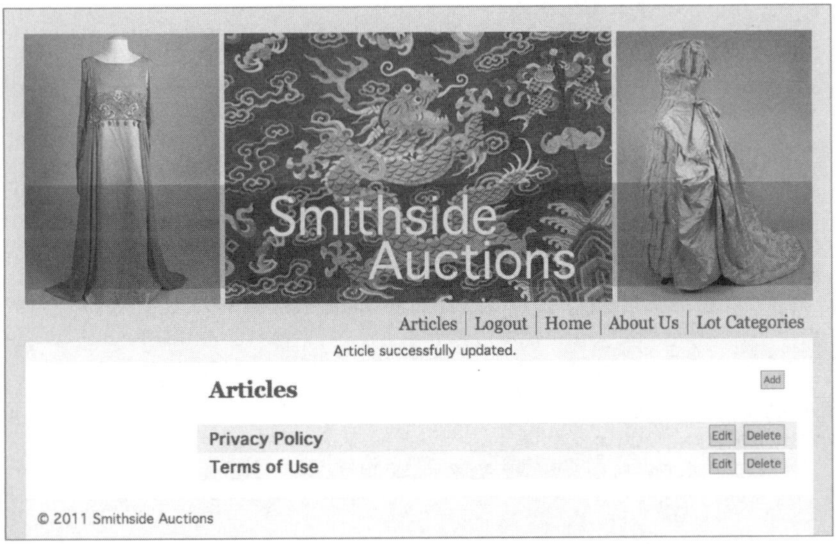

FIGURE 29-4

6. Create `content/articlemaint.php` to add and edit the articles as shown in Figure 29-5:

```php
<?php
/**
 * articlemaint.php
 *
 * Maintain the Articles table
 *
 * @version   1.2 2011-02-03
```

```php
 * @package     Smithside Auctions
 * @copyright   Copyright (c) 2011 Smithside Auctions
 * @license     GNU General Public License
 * @since       Since Release 1.0
 */
$accessLevel = Contact::accessLevel();
if ($accessLevel != 'Admin') :
  echo 'Sorry, no access allowed to this page';
else :

$id = (int) $_GET['id'];
// Is this an existing item or a new one?
if ($id) {
  // Get the existing information for an existing item
  $item = Article::getArticle($id);
} else {
  // Set up for a new item
  $item = new Article;
}
?>
<h1>Article Maintenance</h1>

<form action="index.php?content=articles" method="post" name="maint"
id="maint">

  <fieldset class="maintform">
    <legend><?php echo ($id) ? 'id: '. $id : 'Add an Article' ?></legend>
    <ul>
      <li><label for="title" class="required">Title</label><br />
        <input type="text" name="title" id="title" class="required"
        value="<?php echo htmlspecialchars($item->getTitle()); ?>" /></li>
        <li><label for="text" class="required">Text</label><br />
          <textarea rows="30" cols="80" name="text"
            id="text" class="required"><?php echo strip_tags($item-
>getText(),
            "<p><br><h2><h3><h4><strong><em><ul><ol><li><a>"); ?>
          </textarea></li>
    </ul>

    <?php
    // create token
    $salt = 'SomeSalt';
    $token = sha1(mt_rand(1,1000000) . $salt);
    $_SESSION['token'] = $token;
    ?>
    <input type="hidden" name="id" id="id" value="<?php echo $item->getId();
?>" />
    <input type="hidden" name="task" id="task" value="article.maint" />
    <input type='hidden' name='token' value='<?php echo $token; ?>'/>
    <input type="submit" name="save" value="Save" />
    <a class="cancel" href="index.php?content=articles">Cancel</a>
  </fieldset>
```

```
    </form>
    <?php endif;
```

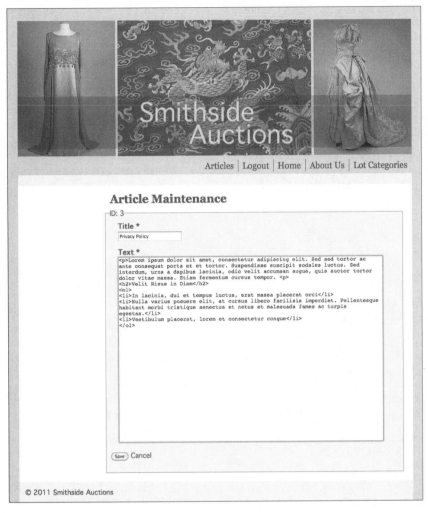

FIGURE 29-5

7. Create `content/articledelete.php` to delete articles as shown in Figure 29-6:

```php
<?php
/**
 * articledelete.php
 *
```

```php
 * Delete the Articles
 *
 * @version    1.2 2011-02-03
 * @package    Smithside Auctions
 * @copyright  Copyright (c) 2011 Smithside Auctions
 * @license    GNU General Public License
 * @since      Since Release 1.0
 */
$accessLevel = Contact::accessLevel();
if ($accessLevel != 'Admin') :
  echo 'Sorry, no access allowed to this page';
else :

$id = (int) $_GET['id'];
// Get the existing information for an existing item
$item = Article::getArticle($id);

?>
<h1>Article Delete</h1>

<form action="index.php?content=articles" method="post" name="maint"
id="maint">

  <fieldset class="maintform">
    <legend><?php echo 'Id: '. $id ?></legend>
    <ul>
      <li><strong>Title:</strong>
        <?php echo htmlspecialchars($item->getTitle()); ?></li>
      <li><strong>Text:</strong>
        <?php echo strip_tags(nl2br($item->getText()),
          "<p><br><h2><h3><h4><strong><em><ul><ol><li><a>"); ?>
    </ul>

    <?php
    // create token
    $salt = 'SomeSalt';
    $token = sha1(mt_rand(1,1000000) . $salt);
    $_SESSION['token'] = $token;
    ?>
    <input type="hidden" name="id" id="id" value="<?php echo $item->getId();
?>" />
    <input type="hidden" name="task" id="task" value="article.delete" />
    <input type='hidden' name='token' value='<?php echo $token; ?>'/>
    <input type="submit" name="delete" value="Delete" />
    <a class="cancel" href="index.php?content=articles">Cancel</a>
  </fieldset>
</form>
<?php endif;
```

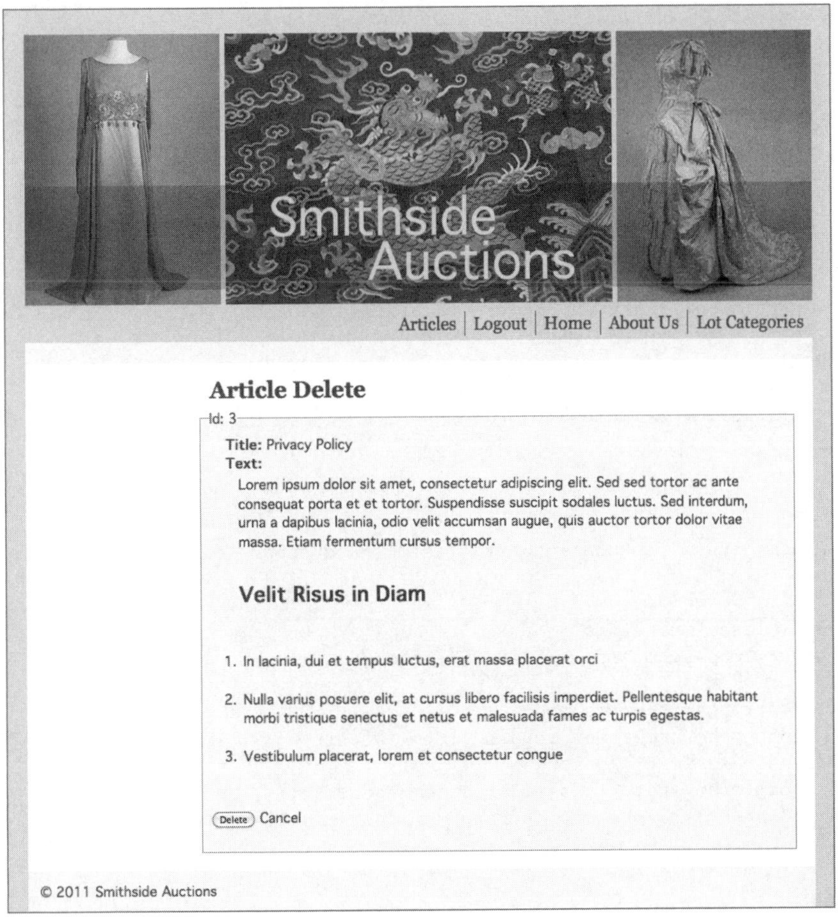

FIGURE 29-6

8. Add the `article.maint` and `article.delete` tasks to `includes/init.php`:

```
case 'article.maint' :
// process the maint
$results = maintArticle();
$message .= $results[1];
// If there is redirect information
// redirect to that page
if ($results[0] == 'articlemaint') {
  // pass on new messages
  if ($results[1]) {
    $_SESSION['message'] = $results[1];
  }
  header("Location: index.php?content=articlemaint&id=$results[2]");
  exit;
}
break;
```

```
case 'article.delete' :
// process the delete
$results = deleteArticle();
$message .= $results[1];
// If there is redirect information
// redirect to that page
if ($results[0] == 'articledelete') {
  // pass on new messages
  if ($results[1]) {
    $_SESSION['message'] = $results[1];
  }
  header("Location: index.php?content=articledelete&id=$results[2]");
  exit;
}
break;
```

9. Add the `maintArticle()` and `deleteArticle()` functions to `includes/functions.php`:

```
function maintArticle() {
  $results = '';
  if (isset($_POST['save']) AND $_POST['save'] == 'Save') {
    // check the token
    $badToken = true;
    if (!isset($_POST['token'])
    || !isset($_SESSION['token'])
    || empty($_POST['token'])
    || $_POST['token'] !== $_SESSION['token']) {
      $results = array('',
        'Sorry, go back and try again. There was a security issue.');
      $badToken = true;
    } else {
      $badToken = false;
      unset($_SESSION['token']);
      // Put the sanitized variables in an associative array
      // Use the FILTER_FLAG_NO_ENCODE_QUOTES to allow names like O'Connor
      $item  = array (
        'id' => (int) $_POST['id'],
        'title' => filter_input(INPUT_POST,'title',
          FILTER_SANITIZE_STRING,FILTER_FLAG_NO_ENCODE_QUOTES),
        'text'  => strip_tags($_POST['text'],
          "<p><br><h2><h3><h4><strong><em><ul><ol><li><a>")
      );

      // Set up a Article object based on the posts
      $article = new Article($item);
      if ($article->getId()) {
        $results = $article->editRecord();
      } else {
        $results = $article->addRecord();
      }
    }
  }
  return $results;
}
```

```
function deleteArticle() {
  $results = '';
  if (isset($_POST['delete']) AND $_POST['delete'] == 'Delete') {
    // check the token
    $badToken = true;
    if (!isset($_POST['token'])
    || !isset($_SESSION['token'])
    || empty($_POST['token'])
    || $_POST['token'] !== $_SESSION['token']) {
      $results = array('',
        'Sorry, go back and try again. There was a security issue.');
      $badToken = true;
    } else {
      $badToken = false;
      unset($_SESSION['token']);

      // Delete the Article from the table
      $results = Article::deleteRecord((int) $_POST['id']);
    }
  }
  return $results;
}
```

10. Create `content/articledisplay.php` as shown in Figure 29-7. The `id` of the article is in the URL. Use that to get the article. If an article is found, display it. Put the `title` between `<h1>` tags and the `text` in a `<div>`. Strip all the tags except the acceptable ones and change newline codes into `<br />` tags.

```php
<?php
/**
 * articledisplay.php
 *
 * Display the Article
 *
 * @version    1.2 2011-02-03
 * @package    Smithside Auctions
 * @copyright  Copyright (c) 2011 Smithside Auctions
 * @license    GNU General Public License
 * @since      Since Release 1.0
 */

$id = (int) $_GET['id'];
// Get the existing information for an existing item
$item = Article::getArticle($id);
if ($item) :
?>
<h1><?php echo htmlspecialchars($item->getTitle()); ?></h1>

<div>
 <?php echo strip_tags(nl2br($item->getText()),
    "<p><br><h2><h3><h4><strong><em><ul><ol><li><a>"); ?>
</div>
<?php endif;?>
```

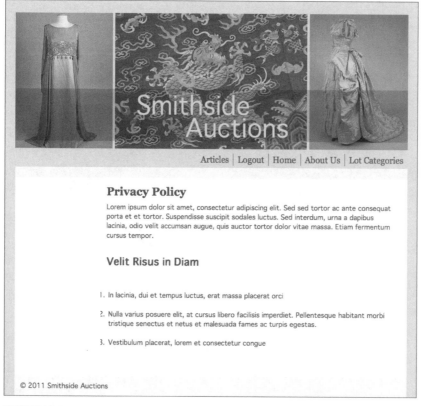

FIGURE 29-7

11. In the next lesson you add these article pages to a menu. For now, test the programs by typing in the URL manually. Assuming your article id is 1, add this to the end of your domain in the browser address bar:

```
/index.php?content=articledisplay&id=1
```

 Watch the video for Lesson 29 on the DVD or watch online at www.wrox.com/ go/24phpmysql.

30

Creating a Dynamic Menu

In this lesson, you learn how to create a menu that draws its information from the database rather than from hardcoded HTML. In the previous lesson, you created new articles through the website, but then you had to go into the index.php file to add the code to display the pages. By using a database, you are able to create menu links easily through the website as well. You create a table for the menu links, set up the maintenance for that table, and write the code to assemble and display the menu.

SETTING UP THE MENU TABLE

The first step is to create the table that will contain the menu data. Here is some information you could have in a menu table, depending on the sophistication of the menuing system. The first two items are the minimum needed for a menu:

➤ **Menu Title:** This is the text that is displayed in the menu.

➤ **Menu Link:** This is the link for the menu item.

➤ **Order By:** If you want to be able to decide in what order the links should appear, you need a field to sort the fields in a specific order.

➤ **Access Level:** If you want to be able to show only authorized links, you need a field that gives the authorization. Depending on the complexity of the ACL, this could either be the access level itself or a key to another table that contains the access level information.

➤ **Menu:** If you are creating more than one menu, you need to specify which menu the link belongs to. This should be a link to another table, which contains the information about the whole menu.

➤ **Parent:** If you are creating a menu that has multiple levels, you need to know the parent of this link.

➤ **Link Type:** If you assign different types to the rows, you can make more of the link creation automatic. If there is no link type, then all the links need to be created the same way. Take, for instance, these following three link types:

   ➤ **External:** The link is whatever the user types in.

   ➤ **Internal:** Prefix `index.php?content=` to whatever the user types in.

   ➤ **Article:** Display a drop-down with all the articles and have the user select the right article. The value on the drop-down contains the `id`. When the menu is created, prefix `index.php?content=articles&id=` to the `id`.

In this instance, the menu you create for the Case Study is very simple. All the links are in a single menu, the access levels are specified in the `menus` table, and the links are only one level deep. All the links are automatically prefixed with `index.php?` when the menu is created.

The next step is to add the maintenance for the `menus` table to the website. You do this the same way that you did for the other tables. You need a content page that displays the menu links and from there you get to the pages to add, edit, and delete the links.

ADDING THE MENU TO THE WEBSITE

After you have the links listed in a table, you need to re-create the HTML for a menu from the rows in the table. You do this with the same type of processing that you used for creating drop-downs for selecting categories. There is an additional complication here, though, which is that you aren't necessarily going to display all the menu items. Depending on the authority the user has and the access level required before viewing the menu items, different menu items are displayed for different types of users.

You can make this selection either within the MySQL SELECT statements or you can select all the rows and then filter what you need to when you create the HTML. If you have a lot of menu items, it might make sense to read only those items that you know you need. However, most menus don't have many rows so the performance hit is negligible. If you already have a method set up to get a list of the items, you can reuse that to get the information:

```
$items = self::getMenus();
```

If you have to filter the rows, now you need to get the level information for the user. The methods here look up the information from the current user and pass it back to the variable. `$logged_in` is Boolean to say if the user is currently logged in. The second one gets the actual authorized access level.

```
$logged_in = Contact::isLoggedIn();
$accessLevel = Contact::accessLevel();
```

Use an array to collect the HTML statements as you create them. Putting each line of HTML in an array element means that it is easy to implode the array with a newline control character (\n). If you do this instead of concatenating each new line, when you look at the source code, each line appears on its own line instead of being in one long row.

You initialize the array to start and add in any header information:

```
$html = array();
$html[] = '<h3 class="element-invisible">Menu</h3>';
$html[] = '<ul class="mainnav">';
```

You loop through each row and select those that pass the authorization tests. The authorizations tests can be as simple as an `if` statement using series of `and` and `or` statements. As each row passes authentication, add it as an `<a>` tag in an unordered list.

```
foreach ($items as $item) {
  if (!($item->level)
    OR ($item->level == "Public")
    OR ($item->level == "Admin" AND $accessLevel == "Admin")
    OR ($item->level == "Registered" AND ($accessLevel == "Registered" OR ↵
$accessLevel == "Admin"))
    OR ($item->level == "LoggedIn" AND $logged_in)
    OR ($item->level == "LoggedOut" AND !$logged_in)) {
      $html[] = '<li><a href="index.php?' . $item->link. '">' . $item->title. ↵
'</a></li>';
  }
}
```

When the list is complete, add any closing tags and implode it with a newline and return the variable. See the created HTML in Figure 30-1.

```
$html[] = '</ul>';
$return = implode("\n", $html);
return $return;
```

```
    <h3 class="element-invisible">Menu</h3>
<ul class="mainnav">
<li><a href="index.php?content=categories">Lot Categories</a></li>
<li><a href="index.php?content=about">About Us</a></li>
<li><a href="index.php?content=home">Home</a></li>
<li><a href="index.php?content=login">Login</a></li>
<li><a href="index.php?content=articledisplay&id=1">Terms of Use</a></li>
<li><a href="index.php?content=articledisplay&id=2">Privacy Policy</a></li>
</ul>
```

FIGURE 30-1

TRY IT

In this Try It, you create a dynamic menu that reads its links from a table in the database. The class for this table resembles those you have built for the other tables for the Case Study. You can extend the `Table` class so that you don't need to redefine what is already in that class. You need the standard processing methods to add rows, change rows, delete rows, get a list of the menu links, and retrieve a single menu link. You then create a method that creates the HTML for the menu and replaces the static links in the `index.php` file with a call to the method.

The code examples that you can download are appropriately commented, but the large docblock comments are not displayed in this Try It.

> You can download the code and resources for this Try It from the book's web page at www.wrox.com. You can find them in the Lesson30 folder in the download. You will find code for both before and after completing the exercises.

Lesson Requirements

Your computer needs to be able to run as a web server with PHP and MySQL. XAMPP is a package of software that installs the web server, PHP, and MySQL for you. You can find instructions for downloading and installing XAMPP in Lesson 1.

You need a text editor that can produce plain-text files. You can find instructions for downloading and installing Eclipse PDT in Lesson 1. Other text editors that you can use are Adobe's Dreamweaver in code mode, Notepad, TextWrangler, or NetBeans.

If you are following along with the Case Study, you need your files from the end of Lesson 29. Alternatively, you can download the files from the book's website at www.wrox.com.

Hints

The menu CRUD can be created the same way you did for the other tables in the database.

When creating a drop-down of valid level choices for menu links, you can follow the example of the drop-down of valid categories.

Step-by-Step

Create the menus table and add the standard processing for creating, updating, and deleting the data.

1.   Create the menus table with id (auto_increment, primary key), title, link, level, and orderby. You use the level field to determine who can see that link and the orderby to place the menu links in a specific order. You can use phpMyAdmin to add the fields to the table either with the GUI interface, in the SQL table with the following code, or by importing the addmenustable.sql file from the downloaded code.

    ```
    DROP TABLE IF EXISTS `menus`;
    CREATE TABLE `menus` (
      `id` int(11) NOT NULL UNSIGNED AUTO_INCREMENT,
      `title` varchar(100) NOT NULL,
      `link` varchar(255) NOT NULL,
      `level` varchar(10) NOT NULL DEFAULT 'Public',
      `orderby` int(11) NOT NULL DEFAULT '0',
      PRIMARY KEY (`id`)
    ) ENGINE=MyISAM;
    ```

2.   Create the class Menu in includes/classes/menu.php. The Menu class extends the Table class. Define the properties based on the table fields and add the getter methods. You

don't need to add the $id property because it is in the Table class. Make the properties protected.

```php
<?php
class Menu extends Table
{
    protected $title;
    protected $link;
    protected $level;
    protected $orderby;
}
```

3. In steps 3 through 10, you add the methods in the Menu class. Put these methods immediately following the list of properties. Normally you would start with a __construct() function to create the object, but you don't need one here because you already have a __construct() function coming in from the Table class. Because your properties are protected, you need to create getter functions so that you can access the properties in other parts of the program. Having your properties protected and using getter functions means that you have the option of adding processing whenever the properties are accessed. Because you want the rest of the program to use these methods, make them public. Notice that there is no getId() method in the following code because that method is coming in from the Table class.

```php
public function getTitle() {
    return $this->title;
}
public function getLink() {
    return $this->link;
}
public function getLevel() {
    return $this->level;
}
public function getOrderby() {
    return $this->orderby;
}
```

4. Add the _verifyInput() method as shown in the following code. This method performs error checking for new and changing menu fields. You only use this method within this class, so make it protected.

```php
protected function _verifyInput() {
    $error = false;
    if (!trim($this->title)) {
        $error = true;
    }
    if (!trim($this->link)) {
        $error = true;
    }

    if ($error) {
        return false;
    } else {
        return true;
```

```
      }
   }
```

5. You need to be able to add rows. The `addRecord()` method that follows adds new rows to the `menus` table. This method should be `public` because it needs to be called from outside the class. You add the code to call this class in step 16.

```php
public function addRecord() {

   // Verify the fields
   if ($this->_verifyInput()) {

      // Get the Database connection
      $connection = Database::getConnection();

      // Prepare the data
      $query = "INSERT INTO menus (title, link, level, orderby)
      VALUES ('" . Database::prep($this->title) . "',
       '" . Database::prep($this->link) . "',
       '" . Database::prep($this->level) . "',
       '" . (int) $this->orderby .  "')";
      var_dump($query);
      // Run the MySQL statement
      if ($connection->query($query)) {
      $return = array('', 'Menu item successfully added.', '');

         // add success message
         return $return;
      } else {
      // send fail message and return to contactmaint
      $return = array('menumaint',
        'No Menu Item Added. Unable to create record.',
         '');
      return $return;
      }
   } else {
      // send fail message and return to maint
      $return = array('menumaint', 'No Menu Item Added.
        Missing required information.', '');
      return $return;
   }

}
```

6. You need to be able to update rows. The `editRecord()` method that follows changes existing rows in the `menus` table. This method should be `public` because it needs to be called from outside the class. You add the code to call this class in step 16.

```php
public function editRecord() {
   // Verify the fields
   if ($this->_verifyInput()) {

      // Get the Database connection
      $connection = Database::getConnection();
```

```
        // update without a password changed
        // Set up the prepared statement
        $query = 'UPDATE `menus` SET title=?, link=?, level=?, orderby=? WHERE
id=?';
        $statement = $connection->prepare($query);
        // bind the parameters
        $statement->bind_param('sssii',$this->title, $this->link,
          $this->level, $this->orderby, $this->id);

        if ($statement) {
          $statement->execute();
          $statement->close();
          // add success message
          $return = array('', 'Menu Item successfully updated.', '');
          return $return;
        } else {
          $return = array('menumaint', 'Menu Item not changed.
            Unable to change record.', (int) $this->id);
          return $return;
        }

      } else {
        // send fail message and return to categorymaint
        $return = array('menumaint', 'Menu Item not changed.
          Missing required information.', (int) $this->id);
        return $return;
      }

    }
```

7. You need to be able to delete rows. The `deleteRecord()` method deletes rows from the menus table. This method should be `public` because it needs to be called from outside the class. This method doesn't need an object to work because it isn't using any of the properties. The only information it needs from the menus is the `id`, which is passed to it in the parameters. Therefore, make it a static function as shown in the following code. You add the code to call this class in step 17.

```
        public static function deleteRecord($id) {
          // Get the Database connection
          $connection = Database::getConnection();
          // Set up query
          $query = 'DELETE FROM `menus` WHERE id="'. (int) $id.'"';
          // Run the query
          if ($result = $connection->query($query)) {
            $return = array('', 'Menu Item successfully deleted.', '');
            return $return;
          } else {
            $return = array('menudelete', 'Unable to delete Menu item.', (int)
$id);

            return $return;
          }
        }
```

8. You need to be able to list the menu rows. The `getMenus()` method that follows reads the rows from the `menus` table in order by the `orderby` field. It creates an object from each row and puts each object in an array that is returned. This method should be `public` because it needs to be called from outside the class. It creates a bunch of objects, but doesn't need to be an object itself, so make the method `static`.

```
public static function getMenus() {
  // clear the results
  $items = '';
  // Get the connection
  $connection = Database::getConnection();
  // Set up query
  $query = 'SELECT * FROM `menus` ORDER BY `orderby` ASC';
  // Run the query
  $result_obj = '';
  $result_obj = $connection->query($query);
  // Loop through the results,
  // passing them to a new version of this class,
  // and making a regular array of the objects
  try {
    while($result = $result_obj->fetch_object('Menu')) {
      $items[]= $result;
    }
    // pass back the results
    return($items);
  }

  catch(Exception $e) {
    return false;
  }
}
```

9. You need to be able to get a single menu row from the menus table. The following method retrieves the row and creates an object from the data, which it returns. This method should be `public` because it needs to be called from outside the class. It creates an object, but doesn't need to be an object itself, so make the method `static`.

```
public static function getMenu($id) {
  // Get the database connection
  $connection = Database::getConnection();
  // Set up the query
  $query = 'SELECT * FROM `menus` WHERE id="'. (int) $id.'"';
  // Run the MySQL command
  $result_obj = '';
    try {
      $result_obj = $connection->query($query);
      if (!$result_obj) {
        throw new Exception($connection->error);
      } else {
        $item = $result_obj->fetch_object('Menu');
```

```
            if (!$item) {
                throw new Exception($connection->error);
            } else {
                // pass back the results
                return($item);
            }
        }
    }
    catch(Exception $e) {
        echo $e->getMessage();
    }
}
```

10. Finally, the last method in the Menu class is `getLevel_DropDown()`. This menu lists the level of authority required of the user before the title text appears in the menu. You use this when you add or edit menu link items. Because it needs to be called from outside the class, the method should be `public`. Unlike the previous three methods, this method works with the object so it cannot be `static`. These are the valid options to be listed:

➤ `Public`: Everyone can see the text. This is the default.

➤ `Registered`: This is the lowest level of logged-in users.

➤ `Admin`: This is the level for users who can perform admin work on the site.

➤ `LoggedIn`: This link is available for anyone who is logged in.

➤ `LoggedOut`: This link is available for anyone who is not logged in.

```
public function getLevel_DropDown() {
    // set up first option for selection if none selected
    $option_selected = '';
    if (!$this->level) {
        $option_selected = ' selected="selected"';
    }

    // Get the levels
    $items = array('Public', 'Registered', 'Admin', 'LoggedIn', 'LoggedOut');

    $html  = array();

    $html[] = '<label for="level">Choose Menu Level</label><br />';
    $html[] = '<select name="level" id="level">';

    foreach ($items as $i=>$item) {
        // If the selected parameter equals the current then flag as selected
        if ($this->level == $item) {
            $option_selected = ' selected="selected"';
        }
        // set up the option line
        $html[]  =  '<option value="' . $item . '"' . $option_selected . '>' . ↵
```

```
$item . '</option>';
      // clear out the selected option flag
      $option_selected = '';
  }

  $html[] = '</select>';
  return implode("\n", $html);

}
```

11. Create `content/menus.php` to display a list of the menus such as are shown in Figure 30-2.
This page should only be viewable by Admin-level users. Use the static `getMenus()` method
to get the menu rows to be shown. Put the results in the `$items` variable and process that
array with a `foreach` loop. Remember that the `getMenus()` method returns an array of
objects, where each object is a row from the `menus` table. Before displaying information from
the database, pass each variable through the `htmlspecialchars()` to encode the HTML
entities, which helps prevent hacks and makes valid code.

```php
<?php
$accessLevel = Contact::accessLevel();
if ($accessLevel != 'Admin') :
  echo 'Sorry, no access allowed to this page';
else :
// Get the menu information
$items = Menu::getMenus();

?>
<h1>Menu List
    <a class="button" href="index.php?content=menumaint&id=0">Add</a>
</h1>

<ul class="ulfancy">
  <?php foreach ($items as $i=>$item) : ?>
    <li class="row<?php echo $i % 2; ?>">
      <h2><?php echo htmlspecialchars($item->getTitle()); ?>
        <a class="button"
          href="index.php?content=menudelete&id=<?php echo $item->getId();
?>">
          Delete
        </a>
        <a class="button"
          href="index.php?content=menumaint&id=<?php echo $item->getId();
?>">
          Edit
        </a>
      </h2>
      <p><?php echo htmlspecialchars($item->getLink()); ?></p>
    </li>
  <?php endforeach; ?>
</ul>
<?php endif; ?>
```

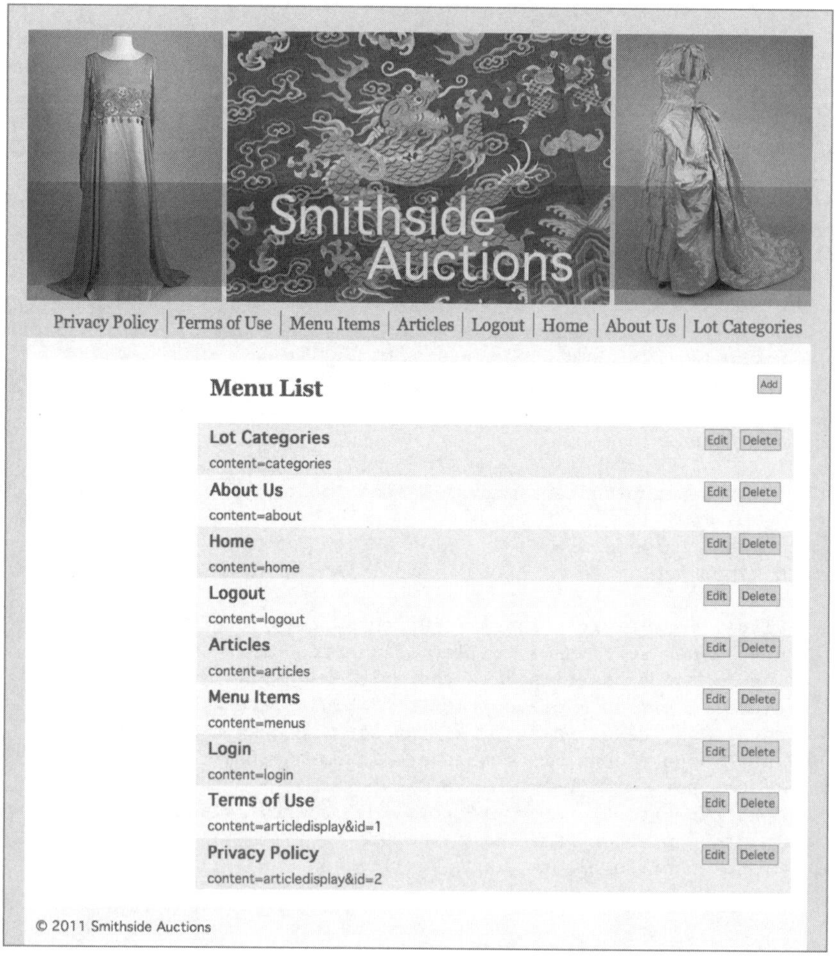

FIGURE 30-2

12. Create `content/menumaint.php` to add and edit the menu links as shown in Figure 30-3 and the following code. This page should only be viewable by Admin-level users. Pull the `id` for the menu row to be added or edited from the URL. Cast the `id` to an integer to prevent hacking. Pass that `id` to the static `getMenu()` method to get the menu row. Use the `getLevel_ DropDown()` method to create a drop-down list of valid options with the level from the existing row (or the default for a new row) selected. Create a security token to pass through the SESSION and via a POST variable. These are used when you process the form to ensure that the information is coming from a real form.

```php
<?php
$accessLevel = Contact::accessLevel();
if ($accessLevel != 'Admin') :
```

```php
    echo 'Sorry, no access allowed to this page';
  else :

$id = (int) $_GET['id'];
// Is this an existing item or a new one?
if ($id) {
  // Get the existing information for an existing item
  $item = Menu::getMenu($id);
} else {
  // Set up for a new item
  $item = new Menu;
}
  // set up the level dropdown, setting up the selected option for existing
records
  $level_dropdown = $item->getLevel_DropDown();
  ?>
<h1>Menu Maintenance</h1>

<form action="index.php?content=menus" method="post" name="maint" id="maint">

  <fieldset class="maintform">
    <legend><?php echo ($id) ? 'ID: '. $id : 'Add a Menu Item' ?></legend>
    <ul>
      <li><label for="title" class="required">Title</label><br />
        <input type="text" name="title" id="title" class="required"
        value="<?php echo htmlspecialchars($item->getTitle()); ?>" /></li>
      <li><label for="link" class="required">Link</label><br />
        <input type="text" name="link" id="link" class="required"
        value="<?php echo htmlspecialchars($item->getLink()); ?>" /></li>
      <li><label for="orderby">Order By</label><br />
        <input type="text" name="orderby" id="orderby" class="required"
        value="<?php echo (int) $item->getOrderby(); ?>" /></li>
      <li><?php echo $level_dropdown; ?></li>
    </ul>

    <?php
    // create token
    $salt = 'SomeSalt';
    $token = sha1(mt_rand(1,1000000) . $salt);
    $_SESSION['token'] = $token;
    ?>
    <input type="hidden" name="id" id="id" value="<?php echo $item->getId();
?>" />
    <input type="hidden" name="task" id="task" value="menu.maint" />
    <input type='hidden' name='token' value='<?php echo $token; ?>'/>
    <input type="submit" name="save" value="Save" />
    <a class="cancel" href="index.php?content=menus">Cancel</a>
  </fieldset>
</form>
<?php endif;;
```

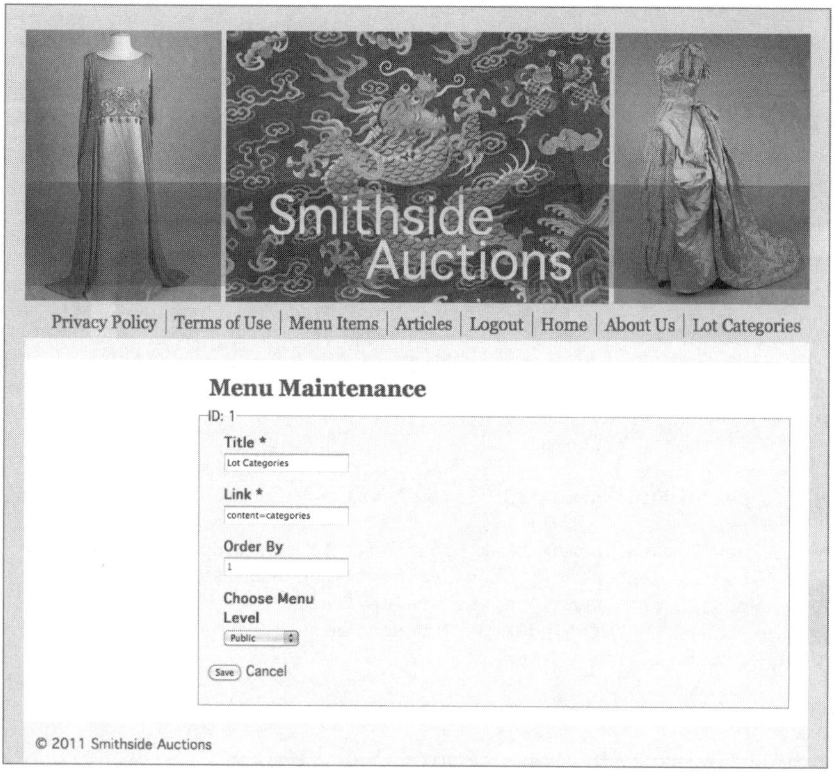

FIGURE 30-3

13. Create `content/menudelete.php` to delete menu links as shown in Figure 30-4 and the following code. This page should only be viewable by Admin-level users. Pull the `id` for the menu row to be deleted from the URL. Cast the `id` to an integer to prevent hacking. Pass that `id` to the static `getMenu()` method to get the menu row. Display the information from the row for the user to verify that this is the menu option she wants to delete.

```php
<?php
$accessLevel = Contact::accessLevel();
if ($accessLevel != 'Admin') :
  echo 'Sorry, no access allowed to this page';
else :

$id = (int) $_GET['id'];
// Get the existing information for an existing item
$item = Menu::getMenu($id);

?>
<h1>Menu Delete</h1>
```

```php
<form action="index.php?content=menus" method="post" name="maint" id="maint">

  <fieldset class="maintform">
    <legend><?php echo 'Id: '. $id ?></legend>
    <ul>
      <li><strong>Title:</strong>
        <?php echo htmlspecialchars($item->getTitle()); ?></li>
      <li><strong>Link:</strong>
        <?php echo htmlspecialchars($item->getLink()); ?></li>
    </ul>

    <?php
    // create token
    $salt = 'SomeSalt';
    $token = sha1(mt_rand(1,1000000) . $salt);
    $_SESSION['token'] = $token;
    ?>
    <input type="hidden" name="id" id="id" value="<?php echo $item->getId();
?>" />
    <input type="hidden" name="task" id="task" value="menu.delete" />
    <input type='hidden' name='token' value='<?php echo $token; ?>'/>
    <input type="submit" name="delete" value="Delete" />
    <a class="cancel" href="index.php?content=menus">Cancel</a>
  </fieldset>
</form>
<?php endif;
```

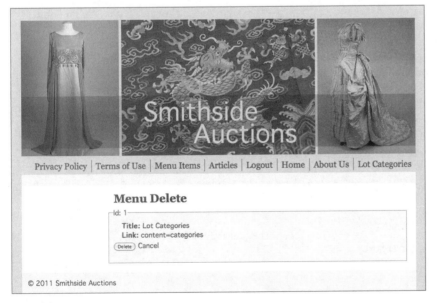

FIGURE 30-4

14. Add the `menu.maint` task to `includes/init.php`. The following code adds a `case` block to the existing `switch` statement to process this task. The task performs the function `maintMenu()` and, based on the results, either sends a success message or redirects back to the form page for corrections.

```
case 'menu.maint' :
// process the maint
$results = maintMenu();
$message .= $results[1];
// If there is redirect information
// redirect to that page
if ($results[0] == 'menumaint') {
  // pass on new messages
  if ($results[1]) {
    $_SESSION['message'] = $results[1];
  }
  header("Location: index.php?content=menumaint&id=$results[2]");
  exit;
}
break;
```

15. Add the `menu.delete` task to `includes/init.php`. The following code adds a `case` block to the existing `switch` statement to process this task. The task performs the function `deleteMenu()` and, based on the results, either sends a success message or redirects back to the form page for corrections.

```
case 'menu.delete' :
// process the delete
$results = deleteMenu();
$message .= $results[1];
// If there is redirect information
// redirect to that page
if ($results[0] == 'menudelete') {
  // pass on new messages
  if ($results[1]) {
    $_SESSION['message'] = $results[1];
  }
  header("Location: index.php?content=menudelete&id=$results[2]");
  exit;
}
break;
```

16. The following code adds the `maintMenu()` function to the `includes/functions.php` file. This function is called in the `menu.maint` task you created in step 14. It verifies that the appropriate POST values exist that the form would have submitted and verifies that the proper token exists and matches with the SESSION token. You then sanitize the information coming in through the POST variables and use them to create an array of the data. You then use that array to create an object out of the `Menu` class. If this is a new row, you call the `addRecord()` method, which verifies the data and adds a row to the database. If it is an

existing row, you call the `editRecord()` method, which verifies the data and updates the database.

```php
function maintMenu() {
  $results = '';
  if (isset($_POST['save']) AND $_POST['save'] == 'Save') {
    // check the token
    $badToken = true;
    if (!isset($_POST['token'])
    || !isset($_SESSION['token'])
    || empty($_POST['token'])
    || $_POST['token'] !== $_SESSION['token']) {
      $results = array('',
        'Sorry, go back and try again. There was a security issue.', '');
      $badToken = true;
    } else {
      $badToken = false;
      unset($_SESSION['token']);
      // Put the sanitized variables in an associative array
      // Use the FILTER_FLAG_NO_ENCODE_QUOTES to allow names like O'Connor
      $item = array (
        'id' => (int) $_POST['id'],
        'title' => filter_input(INPUT_POST,'title',
          FILTER_SANITIZE_STRING,FILTER_FLAG_NO_ENCODE_QUOTES),
        'link'  => filter_input(INPUT_POST,'link', FILTER_SANITIZE_STRING),
        'orderby'   => (int) $_POST['orderby'],
        'level'       => filter_input(INPUT_POST,'level',
          FILTER_SANITIZE_STRING),
          );

      // Set up a Menu item object based on the posts
      $menu = new Menu($item);
      if ($menu->getId()) {
        $results = $menu->editRecord();
      } else {
        $results = $menu->addRecord();
      }
    }
  }
  return $results;
}
```

17. The following code adds the `deleteMenu()` function to the `includes/functions.php` file. This function is called in the `menu.delete` task you created in step 15. It verifies that the appropriate POST values that the form would have submitted exist and verifies that the proper token exists and matches with the SESSION token. Cast the `id` from the POST variable to an integer and pass it to the static method `deleteRecord()` to delete the row from the `menus` table.

```php
function deleteMenu() {
  $results = '';
  if (isset($_POST['delete']) AND $_POST['delete'] == 'Delete') {
```

```
        // check the token
        $badToken = true;
        if (!isset($_POST['token'])
        || !isset($_SESSION['token'])
        || empty($_POST['token'])
        || $_POST['token'] !== $_SESSION['token']) {
          $results = array('',
            'Sorry, go back and try again. There was a security issue.', '');
          $badToken = true;
        } else {
          $badToken = false;
          unset($_SESSION['token']);

          // Delete the menu item from the table
          $results = Menu::deleteRecord((int) $_POST['id']);
        }
      }
    return $results;
  }
```

18. Add the menu link temporarily to the `index.php` menu. If you want, you can skip this step and just add the `index.php?content=menus` manually in the address bar for the next step because you will be removing all these links in the `index.php` file in the step after that.

```
<li><a href="index.php?content=menus">Menu Items</a></li>
```

19. Add the menu links for the main menu listed in the `index.php` file to the `menus` table using your new maintenance pages. The results are as shown in Figure 30-5. Now if someone creates an article page, she can also add it to the menu through the website.

id	title	link	level	orderby
1	Lot Categories	content=categories	Public	1
2	About Us	content=about	Public	2
3	Home	content=home	Public	3
4	Logout	content=logout	LoggedIn	4
5	Articles	content=articles	Admin	5
6	Menu Items	content=menus	Admin	6
7	Login	content=login	LoggedOut	7
8	Terms of Use	content=articledisplay&id=1	Public	8
9	Privacy Policy	content=articledisplay&id=2	Public	9

FIGURE 30-5

20. Remove the menu links from the `index.php` file and replace them with a call to the static `setMenu()` method in the `Menu` class. You create this method in the step 21.

```
<div id="navigation">
  <?php echo Menu::setMenu(); ?>
  <div class="clearfloat"></div>
</div><!-- end navigation -->
```

21. Create the static `setMenu()` method in the `Menu` class. This method calls the `getMenus()` method and then creates the HTML for an unordered list of the links read from the database, based on the authorization of the user and the access level requirements of the menu link. Because you use this method outside of the class, it needs to be `public`:

```php
public static function setMenu() {
   $items = self::getMenus();
   $logged_in = Contact::isLoggedIn();
   $accessLevel = Contact::accessLevel();

   $html = array();

   $html[] = '<h3 class="element-invisible">Menu</h3>';
   $html[] = '<ul class="mainnav">';

   foreach ($items as $item) {
     if (!($item->level)
       OR ($item->level == "Public")
       OR ($item->level == "Admin" AND $accessLevel == "Admin")
       OR ($item->level == "Registered" AND ($accessLevel == "Registered" OR ↵
$accessLevel == "Admin"))
         OR ($item->level == "LoggedIn" AND $logged_in)
         OR ($item->level == "LoggedOut" AND !$logged_in)) {
            $html[] = '<li><a href="index.php?' . $item->link. '">' . ↵
$item->title. '</a></li>';
       }
     }

   $html[] = '</ul>';
   $return = implode("\n", $html);
   return $return;
  }
```

 Watch the video for Lesson 30 on the DVD or watch online at www.wrox.com/ go/24phpmysql*.*

31

Next Steps

Over the course of this book you have taken a static website and, piece by piece, turned it into a dynamic website run from a database using PHP and MySQL. You learned the basics of programming and PHP: how to set up your computer so that it runs PHP, how to add PHP to your HTML page, and how to write PHP code. You learned what variables are, how to work with them, and how to debug your programs. You learned how to have your program make logical decisions and to loop through code, how to create functions and process forms, and how to work with objects and classes. You learned best practices and how to write secure code.

You learned how databases work and how to design one, how to use phpMyAdmin to work with MySQL, and different ways of connecting to MySQL through PHP. You learned how to create tables, enter data, select data, change data, and delete data. And finally, you learned how to combine all of these things into creating a mini content management system with a dynamic menu.

Now that you know the basics of programming in PHP and working with a MySQL database, there are different "next steps" that you can take. One is to look back at the code that you wrote for the Case Study and take it to the next level. As you worked, you probably noticed that you did a lot of copying and pasting. When you start seeing a lot of similar code, it means you have code you should be reusing instead of copying. It's time to *refactor*, which is rewriting your code to make it smaller, more secure, and more efficient. You started this process when you created the master parent Table class that you extended to create the Article and Menu classes. To finish that refactoring you redo the other classes to also extend the Table class and remove the duplicate code. You also add additional methods to the Table class by looking at what other methods, or parts of methods, are similar across the classes. You will find that there is a core of functionality you need that is the same from project to project.

Other programmers have found the need for that same "core of functionality," which has led to the development of *frameworks*. Frameworks are ordinary program files that have functions and master classes of commonly needed functionality that you can include in your program. A good next step is to become familiar with a framework. There is a learning curve to learn a specific framework, but once you do, you start each project with the base functionality of your

code in place, bug tested and, presumably, secure. CakePHP, CodeIgniter, Symfony, Yii, and Zend are examples of PHP frameworks that are available.

If you are building websites, popular open-source content management systems are available that are built on PHP and MySQL, such as Joomla!, Drupal, and WordPress, which have done the heavy lifting for you. For instance, Joomla is based on Joomla Platform, an object-oriented framework with classes you can extend. Each of these systems has its own way of doing things. If you use one of these CMSs, a good next step is to learn how to extend that CMS.

Seeing how others do things is a good way of learning, so examine how existing programs are written. However, you need to be cautious when studying or copying someone else's code. Coding styles in PHP have changed in the last decade and what was considered perfectly good code five years ago may not be how you should be coding today. Newer versions of PHP enable you to take advantage of programming best practices, including encapsulation and object-oriented programming, that older versions of PHP did not handle. In addition, the increasing availability of sophisticated hacking scripts means that you need to use programming techniques that are more secure than what used to be common practice.

In the same way, examining existing databases is a way to see how other programmers have organized their data into tables. An interesting website for seeing how databases are organized is `www.databaseanswers.org/data_models/index.htm`. This site shows examples of databases for various types of businesses and needs.

Try visiting `http://stackoverflow.com/` when you have questions that need to be answered. Use the search function to find out if an answer already exists for the question you have. I recommend that you include "php" or "mysql" as part of your search because this site covers many programming languages and database types. If you can't find your answer, you can post a specific question yourself.

Finally, to get more information on the PHP functions that you have learned and find out about additional functions you come across, use the online PHP Manual at `http://php.net/manual/en/index.php`. You learned about this manual in Lesson 3. This manual gives the syntax of the function, lists the parameters available, and what the function returns. It also contains comments from users that can be enlightening, though some of them are old and have been superseded by newer PHP versions.

For more information on MySQL, use the online MySQL Reference Manual at `http://dev.mysql.com/doc/refman/5.6/en/index.html`. There is a manual for each of the different versions, which you can easily switch to using the menu on the left of the page. If you are looking for a specific statement, go to Chapter 12, "SQL Statement Syntax," at `http://dev.mysql.com/doc/refman/5.6/en/sql-syntax.html`. Data definition statements are the statements that deal with the structure of the database, such as creating and altering tables, or listing what fields are in a particular table. Data manipulation statements are the ones that deal with the actual data such as the INSERT, UPDATE, and SELECT statements.

A

What's on the DVD?

This appendix provides you with information on the contents of the DVD that accompanies this book. For the latest and greatest information, please refer to the ReadMe file located at the root of the DVD. Here is what you will find in this appendix:

➤ System Requirements

➤ Using the DVD

➤ What's on the DVD

➤ Troubleshooting

SYSTEM REQUIREMENTS

Most reasonably up-to-date computers with a DVD drive should be able to play the screencasts that are included on the DVD.

USING THE DVD

To access the content from the DVD, follow these steps:

1. Insert the DVD into your computer's DVD-ROM drive. The license agreement appears.

> *The interface won't launch if you have autorun disabled. In that case, click Start ⇨ Run (for Windows 7, click Start ⇨ All Programs ⇨ Accessories ⇨ Run). In the dialog box that appears, type **D:\Start.exe**. (Replace D with the proper letter if your DVD drive uses a different letter. If you don't know the letter, check how your DVD drive is listed under My Computer.) Click OK.*

2. Read through the license agreement, and then click the Accept button if you want to use the DVD.

    The DVD interface appears. Simply select the lesson number for the video you want to view.

WHAT'S ON THE DVD?

Each of this book's lessons contains a Try It section that enables you to practice the concepts covered by that lesson. The Try It includes a high-level overview, requirements, and step-by-step instructions explaining how to build the example program.

This DVD contains video screencasts showing my computer screen as I work through key pieces of the Try Its from each lesson. In the audio I explain what I'm doing step-by-step so you can see how the techniques described in the lesson translate into actions.

I don't always show how to build every last piece of a Try It's program. For example, if the requirements ask you to do the same thing multiple times, I may only do the first one and let you do the rest so you don't need waste time watching me do the same thing again and again.

I recommend using the following steps when reading a lesson:

1. Read the lesson's text.

2. Read the Try It's overview, requirements, and hints.

3. Read the step-by-step instructions. If the code you write doesn't work, use the code provided to find your problem. Look for places where my solution differs from yours. In programming there's always more than one way to solve a problem, and it's good to know about several different approaches.

4. Watch the screencast to see how I handle the key issues.

You can also download all of the book's examples and solutions to the Try Its at the book's websites.

TROUBLESHOOTING

If you have difficulty installing or using any of the materials on the companion DVD, try the following solutions:

➤   **Reboot if necessary.** As with many troubleshooting situations, it may make sense to reboot your machine to reset any faults in your environment.

➤   **Turn off any anti-virus software that you may have running.** Installers sometimes mimic virus activity and can make your computer incorrectly believe that it is being infected by a virus. (Be sure to turn the anti-virus software back on later.)

➤   **Close all running programs.** The more programs you're running, the less memory is available to other programs. Installers also typically update files and programs; if you keep other programs running, installation may not work properly.

➤ **Reference the ReadMe.** Please refer to the ReadMe file located at the root of the DVD for the latest product information at the time of publication.

CUSTOMER CARE

If you have trouble with the DVD, please call the Wiley Product Technical Support phone number at (800) 762-2974. Outside the United States, call 1(317) 572-3994. You can also contact Wiley Product Technical Support at `http://support.wiley.com`. John Wiley & Sons will provide technical support only for installation and other general quality control items. For technical support on the applications themselves, consult the program's vendor or author.

To place additional orders or to request information about other Wiley products, please call (877) 762-2974.

INDEX

Symbols

: (colon)
   alternative syntax, 102
   parameters, 350
:: (colon-double), scope
   resolution operator, 195
, (comma), 285
. . . (ellipsis), parameters, 38
. (period), concatenation operator,
   48, 287
; (semicolon), 35
   errors, 59
   MySQL statements, 333
   PHP statements, 92
   $query, 337
& (ampersand)
   element variable, 113
   htmlspecialchars(), 52
   parameters, 81, 130
&& (ampersand-double), AND, 99
* (asterisk)
   COUNT(), 315
   fields, 314, 402
   numeric operator, 51
** (asterisk-double), UPDATE, 345
@ (at sign), errors, 264
\ (backslash)
   escape, 47, 60
   MySQL, 254
   variables, 299
` (backtick), MySQL, 60, 254,
   295
{} (curly brackets)
   classes, 167, 171
   errors, 59, 102
   formatting style, 34

if, 91
   properties, 174
   variables, 47
- (dash)
   classes, 170
   numeric operator, 51
-- (dash-double)
   comments, 255
   numeric operator, 51
$ (dollar sign), 170
   constants, 74
   errors, 60
   functions, 136
   properties, 168, 170
   variables, 45, 178
= (equal sign)
   assignment operator,
      46, 51
   comparison operator, 318
   conditional PHP statements,
      92
   errors, 60
   numbers, 50
   variables, 45
== (equal sign-double)
   comparison operator, 94
   errors, 60
   if, 92
=== (equal sign-triple), 92
   comparison operator, 94
! (exclamation mark), not
   operator, 100
> (greater than), comparison
   operator, 94, 318
>> (greater than-double),
   perspectives, 66
(hash mark), comments, 255

< (less than), comparison operator,
   94, 318
() (parentheses), functions, 48,
   126
% (percent sign), numeric operator,
   51
| (pipe sign)
   E_ALL, 58
   SQL tables, 285
|| (pipe sign-double), OR, 98
+ (plus sign)
   forms, 147
   numeric operator, 51
++ (plus sign-double)
   increment operator, 108
   numeric operator, 51
? (question mark)
   parameters, 81, 350
   placeholders, 349
   ternary operator, 96
" " (quotes-double), 28
   errors, 60
   variables, 47, 299, 392
' ' (quotes-single), 28,
   295–296
   arrays, 72
   classes, 218
   errors, 60
   MySQL, 253–254,
      295–296
   security best practices, 390
   variables, 47, 299, 392
/ (slash), numeric operator, 51
// (slash-double), comments, 39
[] (square brackets)
   arrays, 179, 322
   checkboxes, 142–143

errors, 59
MySQL tables, 285
name, 143
parameters, 81
~ (tilde), 58
E_NOTICE, 58
_ (underscore)
MySQL, 254
properties, 189
variables, 45
__ (underscore-double)
magic methods, 187
methods, 181
*/
block comments, 39
comments, 255
*= , assignment operator, 51
-= , assignment operator, 51
!= , comparison operator, 94, 318
>= , comparison operator, 94, 318
<> , comparison operator, 94, 318
<= , comparison operator, 94, 318
<=> , comparison operator, 318
%= , assignment operator, 51
+= , assignment operator, 51
?> , 35
comments, 41
ending tag, 57
headers, 153
/* , comments, 39, 255
/**
block comments, 39
Eclipse, 171
/- , assignment operator, 51

A

About Us, 25, 32, 185
comments, 44
databases, 233
about.html, 29
about.php, 30, 43, 183, 417
abstract, 196
abstract classes, 163, 196
Access Control Lists (ACLs), 399, 443
accessLevel(), 417

addRecord(), 325, 356, 420, 427, 448
Admin, 451
advanced techniques, 187–203
class initialization, 187–188
inheritance, 192–196
scope, 188–192
static methods and properties, 197–199
aliases, 315, 333
ALL, 336
All Privileges, 9
ALTER TABLE, 286
alternative syntax, 102–103, 112
&amp, 53, 55
AND, 99
AND/OR, 100
ANY, 336
Apache, 7, 8
files, 12
MySQL, 239
php.ini, 59
XAMPP, 5, 6
apachefriends.org, 4, 6
/ApplicationsXAMPP/
Xamppfiles/etc, 58
areatype, 149
$areatypes, 149
arguments
functions, 130
methods, 180–181
parameters, 128
returns, 131
arrays, 179, 322. See also
associative arrays
for, 111
$areatypes, 149
complex data, 71–73
fetch_array(), 265
foreach, 112, 113
functions, 132
HTML statements, 444
index, 115
multi-dimensional, 71, 73
numeric, 72
parameters, 128
print_r(), 61, 72, 179
Unix timestamps, 80
variables, 61, 207

article link, 444
artificial keys, 230
assignment operators, 46, 50, 51
associative arrays, 72
foreach, 113
$_SESSION, 402
values, 132
variables, 86–87
AUTO_INCREMENT, 252, 279, 280, 296
auto_increment, 245, 279–280
MySQL, 245, 279–280
primary key, 248
rows, 362
values, 252
__autoload(), 164, 187–188, 199, 214

B

backup, MySQL, 250–253
base class, 192
best practices
methods, 180
MySQL security, 389–391
passwords, 389–390
security, 390
workspace, 40
BETWEEN... AND..., 318
BIGINT, 277
BINARY, 276
binary strings, 243, 276
binding, 349
BIT, 279
BLOB, 276–277, 351
Boolean
PDO, 351
UPDATE, 346
variables, 73, 207

, 423
break, 114–115
breakpoints, 67, 69
built-in functions, 80–85
business rules, 230–231

C

CakePHP, 462
"Call to undefined function," 59
case, 101, 327, 378
case sensitivity, 46, 74, 167
changing data, 343–360
CHAR, 275–276
character set, 242–243
checkboxes, 142–143, 149–150
child class, 192, 195
Class, 167
classes, 195, 218
    case sensitivity, 167
    CMS, 420–422
    __construct(), 192
    defining, 167–175
    echo, 179
    extending, 163, 192
    files, 167
    initialization, 187–188
    instantiation, 162, 177–178
    methods, 162, 169–173,
        420–422
    objects, 178–182, 420
    OOP, 162–163, 167–175
    PHPDoc, 168
    properties, 162, 168–169, 420
    require_once, 177
    scope, 192
    static functions, 272
    static properties, 272
    subclasses, 192
    syntax, 167
Class Constants and Static
  Methods, 163
class functions. See methods
class variables. See properties
class="button display", 105
classes, 174
clauses, 314–315
__clone(), 192
CMS. See content management
  system
$code, 301
CodeIgniter, 462
collation, 242–243
col_name, 285
columns, 227, 244–248

comments, 255. See also PHPDoc
    Eclipse, 39, 171
    HTML, 39
    methods, 171
    MySQL, 255
    .php, 40–43
    single line, 39
    About Us, 44
    workspace, 39–40
Compare With, 17
comparison operators, 94–96,
  317–318
complex data, 71–89
    arrays, 71–73
    built-in functions, 80–85
    constants, 74
    dates, 74–80
    logical variables, 73–74
    objects, 86
concatenation operators, 48, 287
condition, 110
conditional PHP statements, 92
configuration
    workspace, 12–18
    XAMPP, 9–10
    Xdebug, 62–65
confirmation page, 220
connect_error, 264
$connection, 264, 266–267,
  268
$_connection, 273
constants, 74
$_construct(), new Database,
  268
__construct(), 163, 180–181,
  273, 420, 421
    classes, 192
    extending, 195
    inheritance, 193
    magic methods, 187
Constructors, 163
$contact, 111, 130
$contacts, 170
content, 104, 139
$content, 105, 139
content management system (CMS),
  419–441, 462
    classes, 420–422
    display page, 422–424

    maintenance pages, 422
    tables, 419–420
content/about.php, 43
content/home.php, 43
continue, 114–115
control characters, 47
Control Panel, 5, 6
$_COOKIE, 82, 83, 120, 402
cookies, 82–83, 402
Copy, 17
COUNT(), 315
$count, 127
counters, 109
CREATE, 287
CREATE DATABASE, 271
CREATE TABLE, 284
cross-site request forgeries (CSRF,
  XSRF), 217, 220
cross-site scripting (XSS), 217
CRUD, 446
CSRF. See cross-site request
  forgeries
.csv, 228
ctype_digit(), 207
CURRENT_TIMESTAMP, 280, 282,
  425
c:\xampp\php, 58

D

data
    changing
        MySQL, 343–360
        mysqli, 348–350
        PDO, 350–352
        prepared statements,
          347–348
    deleting
        MySQL, 361–386
        PHP, 364–365
    entry, 248–250, 295–311
        MySQL, PHP forms,
          302–304
    selection, 314–319
    validity, 206
Data fieldset, 252
data types, 228, 275–279
    business rules, 231
    MySQL, 228, 275–279

PDO, 350–351
placeholders, 349
databases, 227–237. *See also*
MySQL
business rules, 230–231
character set, 242–243
collation, 242–243
columns, 244–248
flat files, 228
information gathering, 228
menu, 443–460
normalization, 231–232
tables, 229, 244–248
About Us, 233
databaseanswers.org, 462
data_type, 285
DATE, 278
date(), 75–77
dates, 24–25, 74–80
date_created, 282
DATETIME, 278
date/time, 75–80, 278
$db, 264
_DB, 252
$dbh, 264
Debug As, 17
debugging, 57–70
error display, 57–59
text editors, 57
XAMPP, 65
Xdebug, 62–67
decision making, 91–106
alternative syntax, 102–103
if/else, 91–97
logical operators, 97–100
switch, 100–102
decrement operator, 108, 110
default, 101
$default, 139
Default PHP Web Server, 62
defaults
parameters, 130
values, MySQL, 280
define(), 74
DELETE, 361–364
JOIN, 335, 363–364
LIMIT, 362, 363
NULL, 364
ORDER BY, 363

rows, 362–364
WHERE, 362, 363
deleteCategory(), 371
deleteMenu(), 458
deleteRecord(), 427
includes/classes.php,
368
menu, 449, 458
rows, 421, 449
deleting data, 361–386
deprecated variables, 121–122
$desc, 299, 303
DESCRIBE, 346
description, 245
die(), 61, 220
display page, 422–424
displayApps(), 193
display_errors, 57–59, 207
DISTINCT, 315
<div>, 52
<div class="message">, 274
Doctype, 47
DOCUMENT_ROOT, 121–122
DOUBLE PRECISION, 277
do/while, 109
DROP DATABASE, 250, 388
DROP TABLE, 248, 250, 251, 388
drop-down menu, 446
Drupal, 462
Duplicate Entry error, 345
DUPLICATE KEY UPDATE,
297, 345

E

E_ALL, 58
echo, 36–37
for, 112
classes, 179
$contact, 130
errors, 59
HTML, 111
if, 60
PHP, 27–29
print_r(), 61
variables, 60
echo $i++;, 108
echo $i--;, 108

echo ++$i;, 108
echo --$i;, 108
Eclipse, 11–12
comments, 39, 171
first time use, 14–18
htdocs, 14
parameters, 171
perspectives, 18
splash screen, 15
Xdebug, 62–67
eclipse.exe, 12
editRecord(), 420, 427
includes/classes/
contact.php,
354, 358
menu, 448, 458
passwords, 410
prepared statements, 381
$result, 354
elements, 116
element variable, 113
else
comparison operators, 94–96
decision making, 91–97
errors, 214
PHP statements, 92–93
ternary operators, 96–97
elseif, 93
encapsulation
functions, 119
local variables, 161
OOP, 161
endfor, 112
engine_name, 285
ENUM, 279
$_ENV, 120
error_report, 58
errors, 59, 60, 102, 205–215, 264
data validity, 206
debugging, 57–59
Duplicate Entry, 345
fatal, 137
fields, 296
IGNORE, 297
$message, 303
MySQL, 264
PDO, 269
PHP, 209
redundancy, 231

resources, 206
testing, 205–210
try/catch, 210–211
values, 206
variables, 206
web pages, 60
escapes, 47, 60
MySQL, 254, 295–296
security best practices, 390
SQL Injections, 301
E_STRICT, 58
E_USER_ERROR, 207
E_USER_NOTICE, 207–208
E_USER_WARNING, 207
Exception, 210–211
expandType(), 134
EXPLAIN, 346
Export fieldset, 251
Expression Syntax, 317
extending classes, 163, 192
external links, 444

F

FALSE, 73, 95–96, 346–347
false, 131
fatal errors, 137
fetch(PDO::FETCH_NUM), 270
fetch_all(MYSQLI_ASSOC), 321
fetch_all(MYSQLI_BOTH), 321
fetch_all(MYSQLI_NUM), 321
fetch_array(), 265
fetch_array(MYSQLI_ASSOC),
321
fetch_array(MYSQLI_BOTH),
321
fetch_array(MYSQLI_NUM), 321
fetch_object(), 321
fields, 227, 296, 314, 402
aliases, 333
forms, SQL injections, 388
getContact(), 410
keys, 229
SESSION, 414
tables, 229
files
Apache web server, 12
classes, 167

flat, 228
plain-text, 41, 83, 86, 103
reusing code, 137
URL, 210
workspace, 12–14
file paths, 24, 212
file_exists(), 209, 212
$_FILES, 120
filters, 84–85, 391–393
FILTER_FLAG_NO_ENCODE_NO_
QUOTES, 303
filter_input, 219
FILTER_SANITIZE_EMAIL,
84
FILTER_SANITIZE_ENCODED, 84
FILTER_SANITIZE_NUMBER_
FLOAT, 84
FILTER_SANITIZE_NUMBER_INT,
84
FILTER_SANITIZE_SPECIAL_
CHARS, 84
FILTER_SANITIZE_STRING, 84
FILTER_SANITIZE_URL, 84
FILTER_VALIDATE_BOOLEAN,
85
FILTER_VALIDATE_EMAIL, 85
FILTER_VALIDATE_FLOAT, 85
FILTER_VALIDATE_INT, 85
FILTER_VALIDATE_URL, 85
filter_var(), 84–85, 219
final, 195
Firefox, 82
first normal form (INF), 231
flat files, 228
floating-point numbers, 50, 52,
207, 278
folders, 210
index.html, 222
index.php, 219
root, 222
subfolders, 221
for
id, 142
, 142
loops, 110–112
foreach
$contacts, 170
getMenus(), 452
$item, 184

<li>, 184–185
loops, 112–114
foreign keys, 229–230
<form>, 141, 142
forms, 141–159
checkboxes, 142–143
CSRF, 220
fields, SQL injections,
388
GET, 146–147
$_GET, 147
header(), 153–154
header redirection,
153–154
HTML, 141
HTTP, 147
JavaScript, 142, 219
PHP, MySQL data entry,
302–304
POST, 146–147
$_POST, 147
processing, 146–152
radio buttons, 142, 148
setting up, 141–146
formatting style, PHP, 33–34
frameworks, 461
Zend Framework,
34, 462
FROM, 315
functions, 168. *See also specific
function types*
arguments, 130
arrays, 132
built-in, 80–85
comparison functions and
operators, 317
date/time, 75–80
defining, 126–127
encapsulation, 119
false, 131
hash, 400, 405
local variables, 129
methods, 169
parameters, 127–131
properties, 168
returns, 131, 132
reusing code, 125–140
static, 272
string functions, 316

strings, 48–50
time zones, 74–75
true, 131
using, 132–136
values, 131–132
variables, 127, 136
whitespace, 126
function.php, 139

G

GET, 103
    forms, 146–147
    headers, 153
    hidden values, 220
    home, 105
    include, 104
    parameters, 154
    passwords, 81
    SQL injections,
      388–389
    Submit button, 147
    values, 220
get, 142
$_GET, 80–81, 120,
  147, 402
getArticle(), 421
getArticles(), 421
getCategory(), 357
getConnection(),
  268, 273
getContact(), 410
getCount(), 127
getdate(), 80
getLevel_DropDown(),
  451
getMenus(), 450, 452
getName(), 129
get*Property_name*(),
  420
getter methods, 190, 191
global, 120
global variables
    functions, 129
    mysqli, 268
    scope, 120–122
    static properties, 198
$GLOBALS, 120

H

<h1>, 111
hardcoding, 133, 183
    salts, 405
    user logins, 399
hash(), 400
hash functions, 400, 405
hash_algos(), 400
hash_hmac(), 400
header(), 153–154
header redirection, 153–154, 305,
  354
hidden parameters, 151
hidden values, 143, 220
home, 105
Home page, 29, 32
home.php, 43
.htaccess, 219
htdocs, 12, 14
HTML
    comments, 39
    Doctype, 47
    dynamic menu, 444
    file paths, 24
    forms, 141
    list tag, 112
    maintenance pages, 422
    menu, 454
    multi-dimensional arrays, 73
    \n, 444
    PHP, 23, 111
      while, 107
    security best practices, 391
    statements, 444
$html, 378
.html, 24, 30
<html>, 47
htmlspecialchars(), 49, 52,
  218, 391, 422
    menu, 454
HTTP, 120, 147, 153, 402
$HTTP_COOKIE_VARS, 121
$HTTP_ENV_VARS, 121
$HTTP_GET_VARS, 121
http://localhost, 7
$HTTP_POST_FILES, 121
$HTTP_POST_VARS, 121
HTTP_REFERER, 121–122

$HTTP_SERVER_VARS, 121
$HTTP_SESSION_VARS, 121
HTTP_USER_AGENT, 121–122

I

$i, 87, 108, 112
id, 142
    hidden parameters, 151
    myid, 315
$id, 388, 392, 421
id $query, 388
identifiers, 254
if
    comparison operators, 94–96
    decision making, 91–97
    echo, 60
    errors, 214
    PHP statements, 91–94
    $result, 271
    ternary operators, 96–97
IF NOT EXISTS, 252, 285
IGNORE, 297
imploding, 378
include, 66, 104, 137
    $content, 139
    index.php, 31, 32
    PHP, 27–29
    reusing code, 125
include_once, 137
includes, 174
includes/classes/contact.
  php, 289
    addRecord(), 356
    editRecord(), 354, 358
    getCategory(), 357
    logIn(), 413
    logOut(), 416
includes/classes.php, 368
includes/functions.php, 371,
  413, 416
includes/init.php, 327
increment, 110
increment operators, 108, 110
indentation, 34
index, 115, 116, 228
indexes, 228
index.html, 29, 30, 221, 222

index.php, 29, 30, 199, 423
   __construct(), 182
   content, 104
   <div class="message">, 274
   folders, 219
   include, 31, 32
   loadContent(), 139, 140
   menu link, 459
   require_once, 138, 200
index.php?content=, 444
INF, 231
infinite loops, 108
inheritance, 192–196
.ini, 228
init, 110
init.php, 413
INNER JOIN, 334
InnoDB, 282
<input>, 142, 143
<input type="button">, 142
INSERT, 252, 295–297, 336, 345
installation
   text editors, 11–12
   XAMPP, 3–10
install.sql, 288
instantiation, 162, 177–178
INT, 277
int, 366
INTEGER, 277
integers, 50, 207, 277, 351
internal links, 444
IS, 318
IS NOT NULL, 318
IS NULL, 318
is_array(), 207
is_bool(), 207
is_double(), 207
is_file(), 209, 212
is_float(), 207
is_int(), 207
isLoggedIn(), 417
is_null(), 207
is_numeric(), 206, 207, 393
is_object(), 207
isset(), 104
   checkboxes, 149–150
   variables, 209

is_string(), 207
$item, 183–184
iterations, 108

J

JavaScript, 142, 219, 422
JOIN
   DELETE, 335, 363–364
   multiple tables, 332–335
   SELECT, 331
   subqueries, 335–336
   UPDATE, 335
Joomla!, 462

K

keys, 228–230
   artificial, 230
   foreign, 229–230
   primary, 229–230, 248, 331, 352
keystroke tracking, 217

L

<label>, for, 142
LAST_INSERT_ID(), 280
LEFT JOIN, 334
   DELETE, 364
LEFT OUTER JOIN, 334
<li>, 112, 184–185
LIKE, 318
LIMIT, 316, 335, 362, 363
line length, 34
Linux, 239
list tag, 112
Listen 80, 8
Listen 8080, 8
listItem(), 196
literal values, 253–254
Literal Values Syntax, 318
LOAD DATA, 295
loadContent(), 139, 140
local variables
   encapsulation, 161
   functions, 129
   scope, 119–120

localhost, 82, 241, 264, 269
LoggedIn, 451
$logged_in, 444
LoggedOut, 451
logical operators, 97–100
logical variables, 73–74
logIn(), 413
login, 412
logins. *See* user logins
logOut(), 416
LONGBLOB, 276–277
LONGTEXT, 276
loops, 107–118
   for, 110–112
   break, 114–115
   continue, 114–115
   do/while, 109
   foreach, 112–114
   infinite, 108
   parameters, 128
   while, 107–109, 265, 270, 319
loosely typed language, 206

M

Mac OS X
   Apache, 8
   cookies, 82
   htdocs, 12
   MySQL, 239
   php.ini, 58
   wphp24, 82
   XAMPP, 6–8, 24
magic methods, 187, 199
magic_quotes_gpc, 300
maintenance pages, 422
many-to-many relationships, 230
MD5, 400
md5(), 400
MEDIUMBLOB, 276–277
MEDIUMINT, 277
MEDIUMTEXT, 276
menu
   adding to website, 444–445
   addRecord(), 448

databases, 443–460
  tables, 443–444
  `deleteRecord()`, 449, 458
  `editRecord()`, 448
  links, 443–444
    `index.php`, 459
  title, 443
  `_verifyInput()`, 447
$message, 302, 303
`method`, 142
methods, 169, 180
  arguments, 180–181
  best practices, 180
  classes, 162, 169–173, 420–422
  comments, 171
  functions, 169
  getter, 190, 191
  `mysqli`, 266
  PDO, 270
  properties, 169, 180
  `public`, 191
  `return`, 171
  scope, 169, 191
  setter, 190, 191
  `static`, 197–199
  values, 178
  variables, 169
`method="get"`, 80
`method="post"`, 81
`mktime()`, 79
Model-View-Controller (MVC), 161
mouseovers, 422
multi-dimensional arrays, 71, 73
`multiple`, 143
multiple tables, 331–341
  `JOIN`, 332–335
  MySQL, 331–341
  subqueries, 335–336
MVC. *See* Model-View-Controller
`myid, id`, 315
MyISAM, 282
MySQL, 60, 239–262
  Apache web server, 239
  `auto_increment`, 245, 279–280
  backup, 250–253
  business rules, 231
  changing data, 343–360

comments, 255
comparison operators, 318
`CURRENT_TIMESTAMP`, 425
data entry, 248–250, 295–311
  PHP forms, 302–304
Data fieldset, 252
data selection, 314–319
data types, 228, 275–279
date/time, 278
default values, 280
deleting data, 361–386
errors, 264
escapes, 254, 295–296
Export fieldset, 251
floating-point numbers, 278
identifiers, 254
indexes, 228
integers, 277
literal values, 253–254
`localhost`, 264, 269
multiple tables, 331–341
`NULL`, 280
numbers, 277–278
passwords, 9, 389–390
PDO, 269–271
PHP, 241, 263–274, 297–302
  statements, 263
phpMyAdmin, 239–253
Reference Manual, 462
restore, 250–253
security, 387–396
  best practices, 389–391
  sanitation filters, 391–393
`SELECT`, 314–317
strings, 253, 275–277
syntax, 253–255
tables, 275–294, 331–341
`UPDATE`, 344–347
`WHERE`, 317–318
XAMPP, 5, 6
`mysql`, 263–268
`mysqli`, 263–268
  changing data, 348–350
  global variables, 268
  `mysqli->affected_rows`, 365
`mysqli->affected_rows`, 365
`mysqli_fetch_all($result, MYSQLI_ASSOC)`, 321

`mysqli_fetch_all($result, MYSQLI_BOTH)`, 321
`mysqli_fetch_all($result, MYSQLI_NUM)`, 321
`mysqli_fetch_array($result, MYSQLI_ASSOC)`, 321
`mysqli_fetch_array($result, MYSQLI_BOTH)`, 321
`mysqli_fetch_array($result, MYSQLI_NUM)`, 321
`mysqli::query()`, 346
`mysqli::real_escape_string`, 299, 300, 391
`mysqli::real_escape_string()`, 393
`mysqli_real_escape_string()`, 393
`mysqli_result`, 263, 265
`mysql_real_escape_string`, 218
`mysql_stmt`, 263

N

`\n`, 378, 444
`name`, 142, 143
$name, 129, 130
`new Database`, 268
normalization, 231–232
`NOT BETWEEN... AND...`, 318
`NOT LIKE`, 318
`NOT NULL`, 280, 296
not operator, 100
notices, 58
`NULL`, 280
  `AUTO_INCREMENT`, 296
  `DELETE`, 364
  `if`, 95
  MySQL, 280
  variables, 74, 207
$number, 60
numbers, 277–278
  floating-point, 50, 52, 207, 278
  MySQL, 277–278

strings, 52, 206
variables, 50–51, 207
number_format(), 52
numeric arrays, 72
numeric operators, 51
num_rows, 265

O

objects. *See also* PHP Data
Objects
classes, 178–182, 420
complex data, 86
__construct(), 182
foreach, 112
MySQL, 254
OOP, 162–163
value, $this, 272
variables, 207
object-oriented programming
(OOP), 161–165
classes, 162–163,
167–175
mysqli, 266
one-to-many relationships,
230
one-to-one relationships, 230
OOP. *See* object-oriented
programming
operator precedence, 100
operators
assignment, 46, 50, 51
comparison, 94–96, 318
comparison functions and
operators, 317
concatenation, 48, 287
decrement, 108, 110
increment, 108, 110
logical, 97–100
not, 100
numeric, 51
precedence, 100
resolution, 195
ternary, 96–97
<option>, 143
OR, 98
ORDER BY, 316–317, 363
OUTER JOIN, 334

P

<p>, 422
parameters, 38, 350
arguments, 128
arrays, 128
defaults, 130
Eclipse, 171
functions, 127–131
GET, 154
$_GET, 81
hidden, 151
loops, 128
parent class, 195
parent class, 192, 195
Pass by Reference, 163
passwords, 9, 389–390
best practices, 389–390
editRecord(), 410
GET, 81
hash functions, 400, 405
PHP, 400–402
user logins, 400–402
Paste, 17
PDO. *See* PHP Data Objects
PDO, 269
PDOException, 269
PDO::PARAM_BOOL, 351
PDO::PARAM_INT, 351
PDO::PARAM_LOB, 351
PDO::PARAM_STR, 351
PDOStatement, 269
PDO_Statement::bindParm(),
350
Pear Coding Standards, 34
Perl, 3
perspectives, 18, 66
PHP
case sensitivity, 46
data selection, 319
deleting data, 364–365
echo, 27–29
errors, 209
formatting style, 33–34
forms, MySQL data entry,
302–304
HTML, 23, 107, 111
while, 107
include, 27–29

loosely typed language, 206
MySQL, 241, 263–274
commands, 297–302
forms, 302–304
tables, 287–288
OOP, 163–164
passwords, 400–402
scope, 119
statements, 91–94, 263
superglobal variables, 120
syntax, 33–44
Unix timestamps, 74
UPDATE, 345–347
web pages, 23–32
whitespace, 126
.php, 24, 30, 35, 40–43
<?php, 24, 28, 35, 41, 104
PHP Code, 244
PHP Data Objects (PDO), 263,
350–352
changing data, 350–352
MySQL, 269–271
PHP Debug, 66
PHP Explorer, 17
PHP Servers, 62
php24sql, 269
PHPDoc
block comments, 39–40,
174
about.php, 183
properties, 169
classes, 168
phpinfo(), 57, 58
php.ini, 58, 228
Apache web server, 59
display_errors, 57
time zones, 75
variables, 121
Xdebug, 65
phpMyAdmin, 239–253
MySQL, 239–253
statements, 337
tables, 281–283
XAMPP, 9, 239–253
PHP_SELF, 121–122
placeholders, 349
plain-text files, 41, 83,
86, 103
ports, 8

POST
    forms, 146–147
    headers, 153
    menu, 453
    SQL injections, 388–389
    values, 220
post, 142
$_POST, 81–82, 402
    forms, 147
    sanitation filters, 84–85
    superglobal variables, 120
<pre>, 73, 180
Preferences, 82
prepared statements, 343
    changing data, 347–348
    editRecord(), 381
    SELECT, 350
    var_dump($query), 349
PRIMARY, 282
primary keys, 229–230, 248, 331, 352
print_r(), 61, 72, 73, 179, 180
Privacy tab, 82
private, 168, 188, 189, 195
Privileges, 9, 389, 390
proper coding, 218–220
Properties, 17
properties, 174
    static, 197–199, 267, 272
protected, 168, 188, 189, 195
Public, 451
public, 168, 169, 188–189
    addRecord(), 448
    getMenus(), 450
    methods, 191
    setMenu(), 460

Q

query(), 265, 269, 287
$query, 337, 388, 392
query statements, 298
query strings, 147

R

radio buttons, 142, 148
REAL, 277
records, 227

redundancy, 231
Refactor, 17
refactoring, 109, 110, 461
reference, 130, 163
Reference Manual, 462
Refresh, 17
Registered, 451
register_globals, 121–122
relational database management systems, 228
relationships, 228, 229–230
REPLACE, 346
$_REQUEST, 120
REQUEST_URI, 121–122
require, 137
require_once, 137, 138, 177, 200
resolution operator, scope, 195
resources, 206
restore, 250–253
$result, 265, 270, 271, 354
return, 171
returns, 48
    arguments, 131
    functions, 131, 132
    MySQL statements, 265
    strlen(), 125
    values, 132
reusing code
    files, 137
    functions, 125–140
RIGHT JOIN, 334
RIGHT OUTER JOIN, 334
root directory, 221
root folder, 222
rows, 227
    addRecord(), 420
    auto_increment, 362
    DELETE, 362–364
    deleteRecord(), 421, 449
    editRecord(), 420, 448
    LIMIT, 335
    OUTER JOIN, 334
    primary key, 352
    type_id, 362
    WHERE, 335
"row0", 184

S

$salt, 220
salts, 220, 405
sanitation filters, 84–85, 391–393
scope, 119–123, 188–192
    global variables, 120–122
    local variables, 119–120
    methods, 169, 191
    PHP, 119
    resolution operator, 195
    variables, 194
SCRIPT_FILENAME, 121–122
SCRIPT_NAME, 121–122
search engine optimization (SEO), 154
second normal form (2NF), 232
security, 217–225
    best practices, 390
    MySQL, 387–396
        best practices, 389–391
        sanitation filters, 391–393
    proper coding, 218–220
    threats, 217–218
    XAMPP, 4
SELECT, 314–317
    dynamic menu, 444
    JOIN, 331
    MySQL, 314–317
    mysqli::query(), 346
    prepared statements, 350
    subqueries, 335–336
    UPDATE, 344
    WHERE, 402
<select>, 143
self::, 197, 267
SEO. *See* search engine optimization
$_SERVER, 120, 121–122
SERVER_NAME, 121–122
SESSION, 414, 425, 453
$_SESSION, 120, 402
sessions, 220, 221, 303, 402
session_start(), 221, 303, 402, 403
SET, 279
setcookie(), 82–83
setMenu(), 460
setter methods, 190, 191

sha1(), 220, 400
Sharing & Permissions, 13
SHOW, 346
SHOW DATABASE, 274
SHOW GRANTS, 390
SHOW TABLES, 270
SIGNED, 277
single line comments, 39
singletons, 267
SITE_KEY, 409
size, 143
Skype, 8
SMALLINT, 277
source code, 67
spaghetti code, 115
splash screen, 15
.sql, 253, 283–286
SQL injections, 217, 388–389, 390
    escapes, 301
    prepared statements, 343, 347
stackoverflow.com, 462
stateless protocol, 402
statements, 265, 287, 333, 337. See
    also prepared statements
        HTML, 444
        MySQL, 265, 287, 333, 337
        PHP, 91–94, 263
        query, 298
static, 197, 199, 450
static functions, 272
static methods, 197–199
static properties, 197–199, 267, 272
static variables, 127
stdClass, 321
strftime(), 77–79
string, 38
strings
        binary, 243, 276
        floating-point numbers, 52
        functions, 48–50
        MySQL, 253, 275–277
        numbers, 52, 206
        PDO, 351
        query, 147
        variables, 46–47, 206
string functions, 316
$stringNumber, 52
strip_tags(), 422
strlen(), 49, 59, 125

strtolower(), 50
strtotime(), 79–80
strtoupper(), 50
subclass, 192
subfolders, 221
Submit button, 141, 142, 147
subqueries, 335–336, 345
superglobal variables, 120
switch, 100–102, 115, 327, 378
Symfony, 462
syntax, 168, 253–255
        alternative, 102–103, 112
        classes, 167
        Expression Syntax, 317
        Literal Values Syntax, 318
        MySQL, 253–255
        PHP, 33–44
        properties, 168
        try/catch, 210

T

tables, 227, 275–294, 331–341. See
    also columns; fields; rows
        addRecord(), 420
        aliases, 333
        CMS, 419–420
        databases, 229, 244–248
        deleteRecord(), 421
        editRecord(), 420
        menu, 443–444
        multiple, 331–341
            JOIN, 332–335
            MySQL, 331–341
            subqueries, 335–336
        MySQL, 275–294,
            331–341
            PHP, 287–288
            .sql, 283–286
        phpMyAdmin, 281–283
        relationships, 229–230
        .sql, 283–286
        type_id, 332
tbl_name, 285
TEMPORARY, 285
ternary operators, 96–97
testing errors, 205–210
TEXT, 245, 276

text editors
        debugging, 57
        installation, 11–12
        <?php, 28
        plain-text files, 41, 86, 103
textarea, 425
<textarea>, 143, 422, 425
third normal form (3NF), 231, 232
$this, 272
$this->, 168, 188, 197
$this->someProperty, 169
$this->yourMethod(), 169
3NF. See third normal form
TIME, 278
time(), 75
time zones, 74–75
TIMESTAMP, 280
TINYBLOB, 276–277
TINYINT, 277
TINYTEXT, 276
tokens, 220, 303
transactions, 264, 269
trigger_error(), 207
trim(), 49
troubleshooting. See also
    debugging
        XAMPP, 8
TRUE, 73, 95–96, 346–347
true, 131
TRUNCATE TABLE, 248
try/catch, 210–211
2NF. See second normal form
type_id, 332, 362
type="radio", 142
type="reset", 143
typos, 59

U

ucfirst(), 49
ucwords(), 49
Universal Binary, 6
Unix, 239
        timestamps
            arrays, 80
            PHP, 74
unset($value), 113
UNSIGNED, 277

UPDATE, 344–347
    Boolean, 346
    JOIN, 335
    MySQL, 344–347
URL
    files, 210
    SQL injections, 388
user logins, 399–418
    ACLs, 399
    cookies, 402
    passwords, 400–402
    sessions, 402
userLogin(), 412, 413
userLogout(), 416
UTF-8, 243

V

Validate, 17
validation filters, 85
value, 142
values
    associative arrays,
        132
    auto_increment,
        252
    databases, 227
    defaults, MySQL, 280
    errors, 206
    fields, 296
    functions, 131–132
    GET, 220
    hidden, 143, 220
    literal, 253–254
    methods, 178
    objects, $this, 272
    placeholders, 349
    POST, 220
    returns, 132
    salt, 220
    variables, 207
var, 189
VARBINARY, 276, 280
VARCHAR, 257, 276, 280
var_dump(), 61
var_dump($query), 305,
    337, 349

variables, 45–56, 178, 188,
    299, 392
    arrays, 61
    associative arrays, 86–87
    binding, 349
    Boolean, 73
    concatenation operators, 48
    echo, 60
    errors, 206
    file paths, 212
    functions, 127
    isset(), 209
    logical, 73–74
    methods, 169
    NULL, 74
    numbers, 50–51
    php.ini, 121
    properties, 188
    query statements, 298
    reference, 130
    scope, 194
    sessions, 221
    static, 199
    strings, 46–47, 206
    values, 207
    Xdebug, 67
variable functions, 136
variables
    deprecated, 121–122
    element variable, 113
    global
        functions, 129
        mysqli, 268
        scope, 120–122
        static properties, 198
    local
        encapsulation, 161
        functions, 129
        scope, 119–120
    logical, 73–74
    static, 127
    superglobal, 120
VARS, 120
_verifyInput(), 326, 381, 420,
    447
Visibility & Final, 163
void, 38

W

web pages
    errors, 60
    PHP, 23–32
WHERE, 317–318, 344, 402
    DELETE, 362, 363
    MySQL, 317–318
    rows, 335
    SQL injections, 388
    subqueries, 335–336
$where, 139
while, 108, 109, 265, 270, 319
whitespace, 35, 126
    formatting style, 34
    textarea, 425
Windows
    htdocs, 12
    MySQL, 239
    php.ini, 58
    XAMPP, 4–6
Word, 11
WordPress, 462
workspace
    best practices, 40
    comments, 39–40
    configuration, 12–18
    Eclipse, 14–18
    files, 12–14
    PHP syntax, 35–39
wphp24, 82

X

XAMPP, 5, 6
    Apache web service, 5, 6
    configuration, 9–10
    Control Panel, 5, 6
    debugging, 65
    display_errors, 57
    installation, 3–10
    Mac OS X, 6–8, 24
    MySQL, 5, 6
    phpMyAdmin, 9,
        239–253
    security, 4
    time zones, 75

troubleshooting, 8
Universal Binary, 6
Windows, 4–6
ZIP, 4
Xdebug
    configuration,
      62–65
    debugging, 62–67
    php.ini, 65
    using, 66–67

XHTML, 218
XSRF. *See* cross-site request
    forgeries
XSS. *See* cross-site scripting

Y

YEAR, 278
Yii, 462
yourMethod(), 169

Zend Framework, 34, 462
ZIP, 4

SOFTWARE LICENSE AGREEMENT

Important - Read carefully before opening software package.

This is a legal agreement between you, the end user, and John Wiley & Sons, Inc. ("Wiley").

The enclosed Wiley software program and accompanying data (the "Software") is licensed by Wiley for use only on the terms set forth herein. Please read this license agreement. Registering the product indicates that you accept these terms. If you do not agree to these terms, return the full product (including documentation) with proof of purchase within 30 days for a full refund. In addition, if you are not satisfied with this product for any other reason, you may return the entire product (including documentation) with proof of purchase within 15 days for a full refund.

1. **License:** Wiley hereby grants you, and you accept, a non-exclusive and non-transferable license, to use the Software on the following terms and conditions only:

   (a) The Software is for your personal use only.

   (b) You may use the Software on a single terminal connected to a single computer (i.e., single CPU) and a laptop or other secondary machine for personal use.

   (c) A backup copy or copies of the Software may be made solely for your personal use. Except for such back up copy or copies, you may not copy, modify, distribute, transmit or otherwise reproduce the Software or related documentation, in whole or in part, or systematically store such material in any form or media in a retrieval system; or store such material in electronic format in electronic reading rooms; or transmit such material, directly or indirectly, for use in any service such as document delivery or list serve, or for use by any information brokerage or for systematic distribution of material, whether for a fee or free

   of charge. You agree to protect the Software and documentation from unauthorized use, reproduction, or distribution.

   (d) You agree not to remove or modify any copyright or proprietary notices, author attribution or disclaimer contained in the Software or documentation or on any screen display, and not to integrate material from therefrom with other material or otherwise create derivative works in any medium based on or including materials from the Software or documentation.

   (e) You agree not to translate, decompile, disassemble or otherwise reverse engineer the Software.

2. **Limited Warranty:**

   (a) Wiley warrants that this product is free of defects in materials and workmanship under normal use for a period of 60 days from the date of purchase as evidenced by a copy of your receipt. If during the 60-day period a defect occurs, you may return the product. Your sole and exclusive remedy in the event of a defect is expressly limited to the replacement of the defective product at no additional charge.

   (b) The limited warranty set forth above is in lieu of any and all other warranties, both express and implied, including but not limited to the implied warranties of merchantability or fitness for a particular purpose. The liability of Wiley pursuant to this limited warranty will be limited to replacement of the defective copies of the Software. Some states do not allow the exclusion of implied warranties, so the preceding exclusion may not apply to you.

   (c) Because software is inherently complex and may not be completely free of errors, you are advised to verify your work and to make backup

copies. In no event will Wiley, nor anyone else involved in creating, producing or delivering the Software, documentation or the materials contained therein, be liable to you for any direct, indirect, incidental, special, consequential or punitive damages arising out of the use or inability to use the Software, documentation or materials contained therein even if advised of the possibility of such damages, or for any claim by any other party. In no case will Wiley's liability exceed the amount paid by you for the Software. Some states do not allow the exclusion or limitation of liability for incidental or consequential damages, so the above limitation or exclusion may not apply to you.

(d) Wiley reserves the right to make changes, additions, and improvements to the Software at any time without notice to any person or organization. No guarantee is made that future versions of the Software will be compatible with any other version.

3. **Term:** Your license to use the Software and documentation will automatically terminate if you fail to comply with the terms of this Agreement. If this license is terminated you agree to destroy all copies of the Software and documentation.

4. **Ownership:** You acknowledge that all rights (including without limitation, copyrights, patents and trade secrets) in the Software and documentation (including without limitation, the structure, sequence, organization, flow, logic, source code, object code and all means and forms of operation of the Software) are the sole and exclusive property of Wiley and/or its licensors, and are protected by the United Sates copyright laws, other applicable copyright laws, and international treaty provisions.

5. **Restricted Rights:** This Software and/or user documentation are provided with restricted and limited rights.

Use, duplication, or disclosure by the Government is subject to restrictions as set forth in paragraph (b)(3)(B) of the Rights in Technical Data and Computer Software clause in DAR 7-104.9(a), FAR 52.2227-14 (June 1987) Alternate III(g)(3)(June 1987), FAR 52.227-19 (June 1987), or DFARS 52.227-701 (c) (1)(ii)(June 1988), or their successors, as applicable. Contractor/manufacturer is John Wiley & Sons, Inc., 111 River Street, Hoboken, NJ 07030.

6. **Canadian Purchase:** If you purchased this product in Canada, you agree to the following: the parties hereto confirm that it is their wish that this Agreement, as well as all other documents relating hereto, including Notices, have been and will be drawn up in the English language only.

7. **Technical Support:** Wiley will respond to all technical support inquiries within 48 hours.

8. **General:** This Agreement represents the entire agreement between us and supersedes any proposals or prior Agreements, oral or written, and any other communication between us relating to the subject matter of this Agreement. This Agreement will be construed and interpreted pursuant to the laws of the State of New York, without regard to such State's conflict of law rules. Any legal action, suit or proceeding arising out of or relating to this Agreement or the breach thereof will be instituted in a court of competent jurisdiction in New York County in the State of New York and each party hereby consents and submits to the personal jurisdiction of such court, waives any objection to venue in such court and consents to the service of process by registered or certified mail, return receipt requested, at the last known address of such party. Should you have any questions concerning this Agreement or if you desire to contact Wiley for any reason, please write to: John Wiley & Sons, Inc., Customer Sales and Service, 10475 Crosspoint Blvd, Indianapolis, IN 46256.

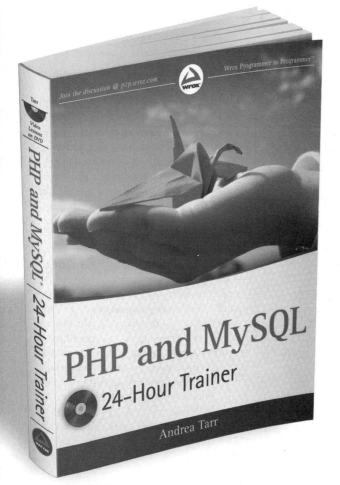